Legal Aspects of Optometry

John G. Classé, O.D., J.D.
Assistant Professor
School of Optometry/The Medical Center
University of Alabama at Birmingham
Member of the Bar, State of Alabama

Butterworths
Boston London Singapore Sydney Toronto Wellington

Every effort has been made to ensure that the drug dosage schedules within this text are accurate and conform to standards accepted at time of publication. However, as treatment recommendations vary in the light of continuing research and clinical experience, the reader is advised to verify drug dosage schedules herein with information found on product information sheets. This is especially true in cases of new or infrequently used drugs.

Library of Congress Cataloging-in-Publication Data
Classé, John G.
Legal aspects of optometry/John G. Classé
p. cm.
Bibliography: p.
Includes indexes.
ISBN 0-409-95043-2
1. Optometrists—Legal status, laws, etc.—United States.
2. Optometrists—Malpractice—United States.
3. Optometry-Practice—United States. I. Title.
KF2915.06C58 1989
344.73′041—dc19 87-27749
[347.30441] CIP

British Library Cataloguing in Publication Data
Classé, John G.
Legal aspects of optometry.
1. Opticianry—Law and legislation—United States
I. Title
347.304′41 KF2913.06
ISBN 0-409-95043-2

Butterworth Publishers
80 Montvale Avenue
Stoneham, MA 02180

10 9 8 7 6 5 4 3 2 1

Printed in the United States of America

For my mother and my father

Contents

PART EIGHT / CLINICOLEGAL ASPECTS OF SPECIALTY PRACTICE

PART NINE / THE OPTOMETRIST IN COURT

PART TWELVE / CONTRACTS

PART THIRTEEN / ECONOMICOLEGAL CONSIDERATIONS

Foreword

Ever since optometrists were first licensed in the United States—in Minnesota in 1901—and as a consequence of having had the parameters of the profession established by statutory demarcation, optometry has been inextricably intertwined with the law.

Over the years, due to an ever-expanding educational base, and with greater public acceptance of its proper place in the health-care delivery system, the optometric profession has continued to grow and evolve.

As a result of this recognition of their professional status, individual optometrists are no longer exempt from the more general legal maxims that have long been applied to other doctors. Decisions requiring professional judgments by optometrists formerly were almost always limited to those scientific or practical matters that related to patient care. Today these decisions are complicated by difficult legal considerations as well.

Optometry has always been affected by revisions in the state statutes defining the profession and by interpretative court rulings of these statutes. Now, however, each individual optometrist is directly affected by "optometricolegal" developments.

Thus, it is no longer sufficient for an optometrist to be conversant with those concerns and constraints that are unique to the practice of optometry. Today's doctor of optometry must also be aware of those legal principles that are applicable to providers of primary health care.

This book, *Legal Aspects of Optometry*, like any other massive effort, builds upon the past contributions of other knowledgeable authors who have addressed portions of this subject in their research. From Dr. Henry W. Hofstetter's *Optometry: Professional, Economic, and Legal Aspects* in 1948, through the efforts of Drs. George Elmstrom, James E. Gregg, George M. Milkie, Monroe J. Hirsch, and Ralph E. Wick, to Seymour Coblens' 1976 primer, *Optometry and the Law*, there has been valuable information presented for optometrists concerned about meeting their responsibilities to their patients.

However, *Legal Aspects of Optometry* does more than merely update the past. It breaks new ground, as it is the first comprehensive work to fully delineate an optometrist's professional and legal responsibilities. The author, John G. Classe, O.D., J.D., writes from a particularly appropriate vantage point. An Assistant Professor at the School of Optometry of the University of Alabama at Birmingham, he is an optometrist who teaches and participates in clinical practice. A member of the Alabama Bar, he is an experienced trial lawyer who has litigated medicolegal issues in the courtroom. With expertise in both optometry and law, John is one of those rare geniuses who can ably assimilate two disparate disciplines. His studied understanding of the history and precedents of legal scholarship, and his practical appreciation of the art and science of optometry are joined in this quintessential text.

The reader may wonder (as I have wondered and have been unable to deduce), is John an optometrist who has a law degree, or a lawyer with a degree in optometry? This inability to discern which of John's *schizos*, if you will, dominates, is evidence to me of his skills in synthesizing this material into an integrated whole. He dissects complicated legal philosophies and proceedings and makes them intelligible to non-lawyers. Similarly, he describes pertinent vision care precepts and procedures in terms understandable by laypersons.

Be cautioned, however; this is not light reading. It is not really meant to be—the subject matter is too significant for that. Indeed, it will be, I am sure, the leading text on its subject in optometry schools. More importantly, it will be an outstanding reference for practicing optometrists and for the attorneys representing them.

Legal Aspects of Optometry is a valuable contribution to the literature of two professions. Practitioners—both legal and optometric—and optometry students will gain wise counsel and practical guidance from this book.

Thomas E. Eichhorst, J.D., L.H.D.
Counsel, American Optometric Association

Preface

This book is an attempt to achieve what is admittedly a virtually impossible task: to write a text that is suitable both for students and for practitioners. The motivation to assume such a difficult undertaking arises from my experiences as an educator at the University of Alabama at Birmingham, and as a lecturer at optometric educational seminars. It has been my privilege to come to know students and practitioners of optometry throughout the nation, and to learn firsthand of the many vexing legal issues that complicate the contemporary practice of optometry. This experience has imbued me with a deep sense of respect for the clinical practice of this profession and with a profound admiration for the dedicated individuals who are the primary providers of eye care in our country. Indeed, there is much to admire in optometry, which today must be regarded as very much an American success story. The reason for the profession's rapid advancement during the past several decades can be found in the unique genius of the American system, and particularly in its system of laws.

For the advancement of optometry is directly related to changes in the legal status of the profession, an evolutionary process that even now continues unabated within the legislatures and courts of the United States, as optometrists seek the best means and methods to serve the vision care needs of the people. However, these advances have also engendered newfound responsibilities, and nowhere are these responsibilities more evident than in the everyday clinical practice of optometry, which has been irrevocably altered by the legal developments of the 1970s and 1980s. As a result of these changes, optometric clinicians have found themselves confronted by the same legal issues that have perplexed other providers of health care. Students of optometry have similarly found it necessary to grapple with numerous legal problems before feeling truly prepared to enter the practice of the profession. It is for these reasons that I have embarked upon this effort: to provide in one text the information sought by optometrists in clinical practice and by students looking to careers as practitioners of optometry.

The book is divided into fourteen parts, and although I realize that curriculum requirements at the various schools and colleges of optometry will differ, the text is designed to be used during the entire four years of professional education.

Parts One through Four describe the history and ethics of the profession; the legislative, judicial, and administration functions of the legal system; and the regulation of optometrists by state boards and by various third parties. These sections are designed for first-year students of optometry, so that these students will conclude the first year of training with an understanding of the fundamental ethical and legal requirements that are necessary to the practice of their chosen profession.

Parts Five and Six are intended to be used in the second professional year, as students are preparing for the clinical phase of their education. I feel strongly that legal obligations inherent in the doctor-patient relationship and principles of professional liability should be taught to optometry students before they enter the teaching clinics of the schools. Furthermore, appropriate recordkeeping and documentation, which are emphasized in the text, are habits that will benefit not only the schools but also will improve the clinical practice of these students after they have graduated.

Parts Ten through Fourteen may be used in the third or fourth year of the professional program, and discuss legal issues that relate to a student's entry into the world of private practice, including the various types of business entities; the use of contracts for associateship, partnership, or the formation of a professional corporation; income and business taxes; legal paper—loans, purchase agreements, and leases—and the economic problems of credit and collections; and the complexities of life, disability, and personal insurance protection.

Parts Seven through Nine describe liability issues in some detail and are probably best taught in the fourth year. These sections are concerned with the major sources of liability claims against optometrists; with the specific legal problems of contact lens, binocular vision, and low vision practice; and with the particular difficulties of serving as an expert witness in the legal forum.

Although the book is designed to serve as a teaching text, the depth of information included in each section clearly goes beyond that needed to introduce optometry students to these issues. I assume that optometric educators will limit discussions and reading assignments as they deem appropriate since some topics may be covered in more depth than necessary for optometry students. The reason for this detail is because *Legal Aspects of Optometry* is also intended to serve as a reference for practitioners, who are both the mainstay and the future of the profession. Optometry has entered its most revolutionary period, and the legal issues facing the profession are varied and complex. Hopefully, this text clarifies these issues and assists optometrists in meeting the demands of clinical practice.

I owe a huge debt of gratitude to an inordinate number of people for their assistance in the preparation of this manuscript, but I would be remiss if I did not begin these acknowledgments with special thanks to Tom Eichhorst. Tom, who is the counsel for the American Optometric Association (AOA), has been a constant source of expertise, advice, and encouragement, and I am deeply appreciative for his assistance. Others in the office of counsel who have given of their time are Mark Adams, Brian Andrew, and Sally Bowers. Several members of the AOA staff have been kind enough to review portions of my manuscript and offer advice, and I sincerely thank Dave Lewis, Joan Weinstock, Al Katz, Steve Miller, and Gloria Lemmex for their efforts. And I have been most grateful for the assistance of Maria Dablemont of the International Library, Archives and Museum of Optometry, and her able staff for helping me prepare the historical portions of this text.

Various individuals have been kind enough to review the manuscript and to offer useful criticism, and I am pleased to acknowledge the contributions of Drs. Norman Haffner, John Amos, James Gregg, James Scholles, Jimmy Bartlett, Jack Runninger, and Frank Watkins. And I wish to thank Dr. Larry Alexander for encouraging me to develop a format that has proven useful for the presentation of information concerning "clinicolegal aspects of practice."

A number of individuals here at the University of Alabama at Birmingham School of Optometry have worked diligently in the preparation of the manuscript, and I am indeed thankful for the hours of typing and proofing by Debbie Hicks, Affie Martin, Ann Simpson, Donna Rhodes, and Debbie Hodgson, and for the copying services provided by Ann Honeycutt. The drawings that accompany the text are due to the skills of UAB illustrator Ken Norris.

This project has taken far longer than anyone envisioned, especially my publisher, and I cannot conclude these acknowledgments without saluting the technical assistance, dedication to excellence, unremitting patience, and ultimate perseverence of Susan Gay, Margaret Quinlin, Julie Stillman, Esther Hanlon, Arlyn Powell, Kristina Smead, and Barbara Murphy, all of Butterworth Publishers, whose support has been remarkable, to say the least.

Last, I must recognize the one person who, more than any other, has contributed to the realization of this book—my wife Jeanne. From its beginnings as an idea, through the years of writing and editing the manuscript, and during the intense weeks of preparing for production, she has been a constant source of strength, understanding, and encouragement. To her I owe the greatest acknowledgment of all—and my love.

PART ONE

HISTORY

Chapter 1

Optometry—A Legal History

What's past is prologue.
—William Shakespeare, *The Tempest*

Genesis (1892–1924)
In Dubious Battle (1925–1954)
The Great Leap Forward (1955–1970)
Revolution! (1971–Present)

The development of optometry as a clinical discipline in the United States has been discussed by a number of distinguished authors.[1] For the most part, these accounts have focused on the scientific and sociological development of optometry, as it progressed from trade to profession. This rather remarkable transformation occurred because of (and at times in spite of) changes in the legal status of optometry, which became the true measure of progress; optometry's metamorphosis into a profession was complete only when recognized by the courts and legislatures. The arduous struggle waged by optometry to attain legal recognition is a rich story deserving of its own history, for the events of the past century say much about where optometry has been and foretell accurately where optometry is going.

It is a story that would not need retelling at all—indeed, there would be no optometry to recount the history of—had there not been a hardy cadre of men in the United States at the end of the nineteenth century dedicated to preserving the right of opticians to practice refraction. As historians have shown, refraction and dispensing of eyewear were nonmedical functions that were perfected over several centuries by tradesmen who became popularly known as opticians.[2] Physicians frequently disparaged the use of glasses to correct eye problems and usually restricted themselves to those remedies that were strictly medical in origin, the use of drugs and surgery.[3] As a result, the practice of the eye physician was rather restricted. Because the overwhelming majority of people needed nonmedical services, the opticians prospered; since they practiced neither medicine nor surgery, they were not in direct competition with physicianry. And since the physicians eschewed the use of refraction, they were not in direct competition with the opticians. In 1864 Frans Donders, a physician, published *On the Anomalies of Accommodation and Refraction of the Eye*; it was a primer on the practice of optometry and heralded the invasion of opticianry by physicians that was then beginning.[3]

In America, refraction and dispensing had been the exclusive domain of opticianry until about the time of Donder's book. Physicians, becoming increasingly interested in refraction, were taught the skill by American opticians and began using it in their practices.[4] At around this same time—the mid- and late-nineteenth century—modern medical practice acts began to be enacted by the several states. The laws were written in such a way as to be all-inclusive, granting to physicians a monopoly over the entire field of health care.[5] Despite the presence of these laws, by the end of the 1870s a tripartite eye care system had evolved: eye physicians, refracting opticians, and dispensing opticians.[6]

Eye physicians were known as oculists or ophthalmologists. Oculists were physicians who had been granted a license to practice medicine by a state and had thereafter decided to limit their practice to the eye; they had no formal training (such as a residency) in their area of specialty. In addition to the oculists there were a number of general practitioners who performed refraction but did not term themselves oculists; they had received no formal training either. Those who had received formal education in eye medicine and eye surgery were known as ophthalmologists. They also offered refraction in addition to their more medical functions of treating eye disease and performing eye surgery. They did no dispensing.

Refracting opticians offered not only refraction and related services but also dispensed spectacles. They treated no disease but rather referred to physicians any patients that they detected as having eye disease. Since they determined the prescription needed for spectacles (and whether spectacles were needed at all) they performed a service that required judgment, and in so doing they were in competition with eye physicians.

Dispensing opticians performed no refractions and offered no services. Theirs was a business only and depended upon the prescriptions of eye physicians for a source of income. Since they were not in competition with physicians and in fact relied on them, there was no friction between these two groups. But they were in direct competition with their colleagues, the refracting opticians, who also dispensed (whether upon their own or a physician's prescription).

It is not surprising that, by the 1890s, physicians regarded refraction and related services to be part of the practice of medicine. After all, the state medical practice acts made it so. But they were not able to enjoy the monopoly that the law implied was theirs because of the presence of the rival refracting opticians. It was of small consequence that the large majority of eye physicians (the G.P.s and oculists) had received a paucity of training in optics and refraction, whereas the refracting opticians had a system of schools and apprenticeship that ensured at least some measure of competence on the part of the practitioner. Skill was not to be the issue; rather, it was to be the "infringement upon medicine" by the nonmedically trained refracting opticians.[7]

And so eye physicians, based on this rather convoluted logic, regarded refracting opticians as their unlawful rivals and wished that they would go away. The more militant among them began to search for ways to legally disenfranchise this competition. It was a situation ripe for confrontation, and the confrontation did not take long in coming, arising in New York in 1892.

Genesis (1892–1924)

It is of historical interest that the impetus for the legal basis of optometry originated with an insult. The recipient was Charles F. Prentice,[8] a refracting optician who practiced in New York City (Fig. 1.1). Prentice did not limit his examination solely to refraction and dispensing services but employed the ophthalmoscope and other techniques to detect disease. When ocular disease was present, Prentice referred the patient to a physician for treatment. In December of 1892 Prentice referred a patient with an "ocular inflammation" to Henry D. Noyes, an ophthalmologist practicing within the city. For his efforts, Prentice received an unexpected rejoinder, a letter from Noyes that was ostensibly a thank you for the referral but was in actuality a slap at Prentice for having the audacity to charge a fee for his services. Noyes did not express himself subtly:

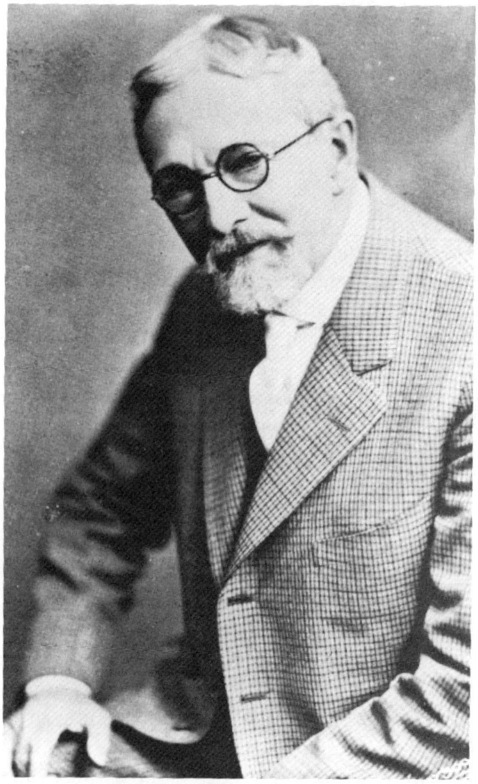

Figure 1.1. Charles F. Prentice. It was the leadership of Charles Prentice that began the effort to "legalize" the practice of optometry. The defeat of his "one board" bill by New York physicians was one of the most significant milestones in the legal history of optometry, because it resulted in the creation of autonomous state boards independent of medicine. His view that the law should be used to effect the "legalized ideal eye specialist" well-versed in both optics and medicine has withstood the test of time. (Photograph courtesy of the International Library, Archives, and Museum of Optometry)

> I consider the matter to be serious . . . because an injustice is done the public by the fact that in charging a fee you assume that you have the qualifications which entitle you to a fee for advice.[9]

Prentice, who was a feisty individual, was not inclined to defer to the opinion of Noyes or of any person with regard to the manner in which he should conduct his practice. In an impassioned reply[10] he defended his custom of charging $3.00 for his services and "but one price for glasses," deploring both the "superficially informed" optician who charged nothing for an examination while exacting an "extortionate price for the glasses" and the young medical graduate who received a "few weeks" of optical training (and a diploma), thereby enabling "the poorly instructed dupe nefariously to practice upon the public." Prentice's description of his plight was a classic depiction of a man caught in the middle.

The beneficiary of a professional education and possessing skill in a trade, Prentice was unwilling to stoop to commercialism but unacceptable to medicine. Of course, he was not the only optician performing refractions who found the situation intolerable. But he was suddenly to become the most visible.

Noyes sent Prentice's letter to a militant ophthalmologist, D.B. St. John Roosa. In a disparaging reply, Roosa voiced his opinion that Prentice was "violating the law" by charging a fee for his services and by prescribing glasses based upon his findings. Noyes concurred and advised Prentice as such. He also sent Prentice Roosa's letter, which probably more than anything spurred Prentice toward an interest in legal reform.[11] It was not until 1895, however, that significant progress was made by Prentice in mobilizing opticians to oppose the efforts of medicine, with Roosa again playing a role in galvanizing Prentice into action.[12]

Prentice initiated his effort by writing to Frederick Boger, editor of the *Optometric Journal*, warning of a declaration by Roosa that he intended to change the New York state law so as to prevent refraction by opticians. Prentice felt that opticians in New York needed to unite to combat this potential threat. Boger, who was the proponent of a national association of opticians, used the journal to propose a national convention, to be held in New York in September 1895. A series of meetings was arranged by Boger in order to form a steering committee for the convention, but the meetings in actuality were used by Prentice to lay the groundwork for a state optical society, which was founded in February 1896. The purpose of the Optical Society of the State of New York was "to elevate the optician to the highest proficiency of his calling" and to secure passage of regulatory legislation for opticianry.[13] The spectre of Roosa, however, once more haunted Prentice's plans. At the Society's first official meeting in February, legal counsel for the Society was asked to describe the reaction of Roosa to the news that a bill would be sought in the legislature:

> Dr. Roosa . . . flew into a rage and said: "I know who is as the bottom of this—that man Prentice, he is foxy, and I'm only waiting for the opportunity to put him behind prison bars; and, if any optician undertakes to join this movement, I shall see that he is punished. Besides, I shall fight you in Albany to the last ditch."
>
> When counsel had finished this recital, all of the dispensing opticians arose, their spokesman, in the absence of Mr. Meyrowitz, saying: "Well, gentlemen, we are sorry, but it will be impossible for us to be connected with this movement. We shall, therefore, have to retire, though we wish you good luck." After they departed the original eleven men and Mr. Boger remained in the room.[14]

Undeterred by the desertion of the dispensing opticians, the remaining members, eleven in number, resolved to proceed with the organization's plans. The first officers were elected and dues ($150 each) were collected.[15]

Accordingly, on January 28, 1897, "An Act to Regulate the Practice of Optometry in the State of New York"[16] was introduced in the New York State Assembly and was referred to the Committee on General Laws, where a series of hearings was held. The bill was favorably reported out by the Committee but failed by three votes to pass the full chamber. The bill was then introduced in the Senate and referred to the Public Health Committee, where it remained until too late to be acted upon during the legislative session.[17]

The demise of the bill was preordained. Besides having but eleven backers, it proposed to regulate *all* persons practicing "optometry," be they opticians or physicians. Optometry was defined as:

> The employment of subjective and objective means to determine the accommodative and refractive states of the eye and the scope of its functions in general, or the act of adapting glasses to the eye by using such skilled means as will determine their choice.[18]

The bill also proposed a panel of four persons—the State Board of Examiners in Optometry—to test and certify all those who desired to practice "optometry" in New York. This meant that the Board would control all persons who performed refractive services. That Prentice, who wrote the bill, intended this to be so was made manifestly clear:

> Through the bill it is proposed to unite opticians and medical men, who now practice optometry upon divergent lines, and to lead them upon convergent lines of practice to a point where in time their interest, both educational and otherwise, will have become so amalgamated as to have created the legalized ideal eye-specialist.[19]

The principal opposition was mounted by physicianry (oculists and ophthalmologists), but opticianry (dispensing opticians) also actively sought to defeat the bill. Yet despite this formidable opposition, an offer of compromise was extended to Prentice and his forces: If they would agree to one Board member being a physician, the bill would be acceptable. They acquiesced, and the bill was reported out of committee, only to be defeated by the full vote of the Assembly. Later, after the bill was introduced in the Senate, Prentice and his colleagues were told that it would be without opposition if they stipulated that all four members of the Board be "physicians versed in optometry." This demand was likewise agreed to, but the bill never made it to the Senate floor for a vote.[20] Why the representatives of medicine and opticianry, their "compromises" complied with, refused to allow the bill to pass is not readily understandable. With physicians entrenched in all four Board positions, and the Board empowered to regulate all refracting opticians, present and future, the bill could hardly have been regarded as a threat. Indeed, it placed in the hands of physicianry a means of preventing the licensure of opticians altogether, but the physicians failed to seize the opportunity. As Rosemary Stevens was to comment in her book, *American Medicine and the Public Interest*, "After this date no state attempted to include physicians under their optometry laws. A golden opportunity was lost, and the two camps were fixed in mutual distrust."[21]

Following the defeat of the New York bill, Prentice withdrew from active participation in legislative affairs, and it was through the efforts of A.J. Cross and E.E. Arrington that an optometry law was eventually passed in New York in 1908. By that time twelve states had enacted optometry laws, none modeled after Prentice's bill.[22]

The *bruit* engendered by the unsuccessful battle in New York spread across the nation. Commentaries proliferated in journals and newspapers and debates became common fare at society meetings and in casual conversation. The events in New York and the formation of the American Association of Opticians heightened legislative interest in those states previously unorganized, one of which was Minnesota.

It was not until June 1900 that the Minnesota State Optical Association was organized, but it was to achieve remarkable success in less than a year.[23] Soon after the association was founded, it set out to enact an optometry law. The Minnesota leaders—Alexander Sweningson, C.A. Snell, J.W. Granger, F.A. Uphan, and H.M. Hitchcock—found the same state of affairs as their predecessors in New York: a divided camp within opticianry and indivisible opposition by physicianry. Hitchcock, in assessing the argument against the law, countered with what was to become the driving force behind the Minnesota bill and all the others that were to follow: the need for professionalism.

> If we should judge by what is said by those who oppose the law and by some who favor it, we would conclude that its chief—and perhaps, only—purpose, is to give to the registered optician a monopoly of the optical business and to protect him from competition. If this is its only aim and result—if it has no wider scope or further benefit I am free to say that we have had no right to ask for it and legislators could not in justice grant it.
>
> As I understand it, the chief purpose of all of our organized effort is to encourage and promote among opticians a higher degree of professional attainment.
>
> This is our greatest need.[24]

Thus it was that, *ab initio*, legislation to regulate the practice of optometry had as its aim not only the protection of the optician's right to perform refraction but also the recognition of the optician's right to serve the public better through improved standards and stringent self-regulation. Hitchcock, a member of America's first Board of Examiners in Optometry (Fig. 1.2), understood that the law was an "experiment," but he also saw that the law was an opportunity to create a practitioner who "will become a more worthy *co-laborer* [emphasis added] with the general practitioner and the specialist in medicine and surgery."[25]

The Minnesota law was enacted on April 13, 1901; it was a political compromise. On the one hand it defined the practice of optometry, established an all optician board, and provided for licensure and for punishment of violators of the act. But on the other hand it permitted every refracting optician in practice automatically to receive a license and granted exemptions from the act's provisions both to physicians and to dispensing opticians (who were described as "persons who sell spectacles or eye-glasses without attempting to traffic upon assumed skill in adapting them to the eye").[26]

These latter two provisions became popularly known as the grandfather clause and the physician's exemption; they were politically expedient because the bill would not have been passed without them,

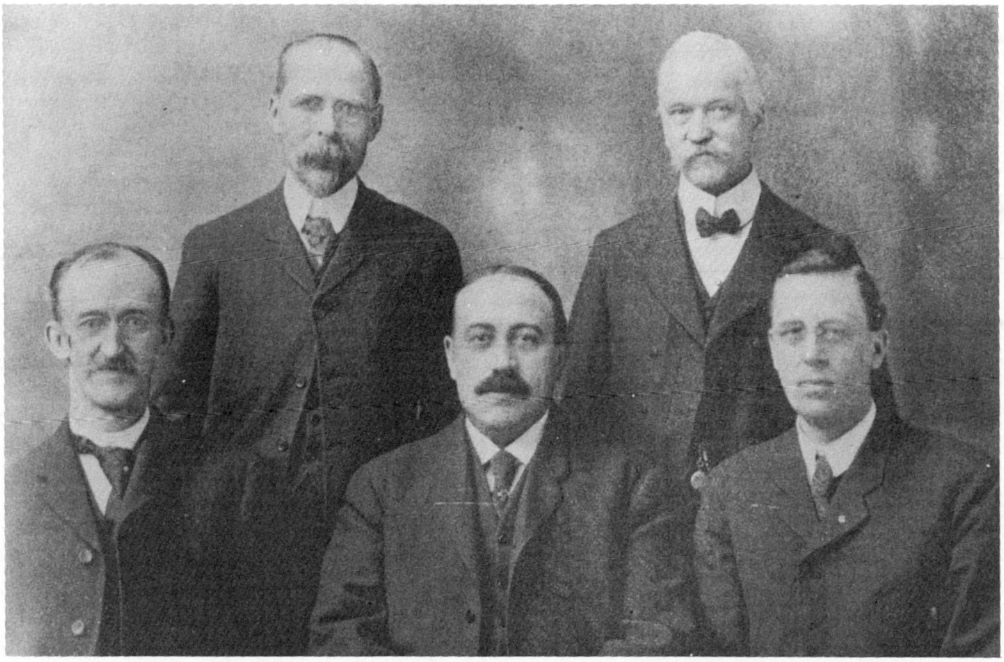

Figure 1.2. The First Optometry Board in the United States: Minnesota, 1902. From left to right: Clifton A. Snell, Hiram M. Hitchcock, Frank A. Upham, J.W. Grainger, and Alexander Sweningson. Part of the motivation for the first state optometry law apparently came from A.J. Cross, who—while on a visit to Minnesota in 1900—scoffed at the notion that the state's practitioners could enact an optometry practice act before the optometrists of New York could obtain one there. (Photograph courtesy of the International Library, Archives, and Museum of Optometry)

but they set into motion a debate that was to persist for decades.[27] The physician's exemption was particularly divisive since its effect was to permit any licensed physician to practice optometry without the necessity of ever having been tested in optometric skills. Every optometry law, however, was to be fettered with clauses containing these provisions.[28]

The legal effect of these provisions was quite significant. Many grandfathered opticians, unschooled in optics and of the opinion that refraction was merely a sideline to their occupation as jeweler or businessman, did not aspire toward the ideals of professionalism and imbued the practice of optometry with a commercial taint that never quite disappeared. Exempted physicians, unmindful of the fact that optometric skills did not evolve from physicianry, used the legally unrestricted nature of their profession to incorporate the practice of optometry into the practice of medicine, thereby creating a rivalry that has persisted for the greater part of a century.[29]

At the same time that optometrists were turning to the legislatures, physicians were turning to the courts. One testing ground was Illinois, where the state law defined the practice of medicine as being "to treat, operate on, or prescribe for any physical ailment or any physical injury to or deformity of another."[30] Lincoln Smith, a traveling optician in that state, advertised in the public press, inviting persons "afflicted with blurring, dizziness, neuralgia, headaches, spots before the eyes, inflammation, granulation, winking, trembling spells, cataracts, burning and smarting of the eyes, and various nervous brain afflictions" to call on him. His advertisements specified that he did not give medical or surgical treatment.[31] Smith would test those seeking his services, determine the appropriate lenses for their condition, have the lenses ground to his specifications and placed in frames, and then deliver the spectacles. For these actions he was prosecuted by the Illinois Board of Health for practicing medicine without a license. The litigation was a drawn-out battle spread over five years; the ultimate result was vindication for Smith and a significant setback for physicianry. The court, in holding that Smith's activities did not constitute the practice of medicine, clearly enunciated what was to become the prevailing view: that optometric services were independent of those of the medical practitioner.

> It is a well-known fact that headaches, dizziness, and other similar ailments often result from defective vision, which may be relieved by the use of spectacles; but it cannot be seriously contended that the person who sells such spectacles, or who tests the eyes and fits such glasses, practices medicine or surgery or professes to cure or treat diseases or deformities thereby.[32]

Another key confrontation occurred in 1914, in the state of Pennsylvania. By 1914 several interesting events had transpired: The national association of opticians envisioned by Boger of New York had come to pass in 1898, as thirty-one states had joined together to form the American Association of Opticians[33]; in 1904 the Association had adopted the term *optometrist* to designate those opticians who performed refraction and related services[34]; schools of optics or optometry had proliferated across the United States, totaling some sixty in number and churning out graduates at an unprecedented rate[35]; and thirty states had followed Minnesota's example and had enacted optometry practice acts, with the addition of two other states in 1914 upping the total to thirty-three.[36]

Alarmed by this evidence of growing optometric strength, a group of physicians in Pennsylvania decided to draw the line. In 1911 the state legislature enacted a statute creating a Bureau of Medical Education and Licensure, and in 1913 amended the statute to provide for its application to any "branches" of medicine, so that any practitioner of a branch of medicine thereafter would have to be licensed by the bureau. Not surprisingly, in 1914 the bureau adopted a regulation to the effect that optometry was considered to be a "minor branch" of medicine and that optometrists would thereafter be licensed and regulated by the bureau.

The prospect of regulation by a medical board was not unwelcome in Pennsylvania. In fact, a number of optometrists seemed to be in favor of such regulation; sixteen years of fruitless efforts to obtain an optometry law had created a feeling that licensure, from whatever quarter, was an advance toward professionalism. But on the very night that the state optometric association met to approve the regulation, a young Philadelphia optometrist named Albert Fitch spoke forcefully and convincingly against it.

> I said in effect, if the Medical Profession had been sincere in its friendship to Optometry, their leaders could have shown their friendship before this and at least conferred with us before having the Medical Act amended so as to include Optometry as a minor branch of Medicine. To me, I said, this procedure looked as if they had now worked out a legal means of eliminating Optometry. I also pointed out that it didn't make any difference how the optometrists voted at this meeting, for all the Medical Board needed to do was to license a few optometrists to put the law into operation and then under one pretext or another to prosecute the rest of us for practicing unlawfully. I maintained urgently that what was needed now was for us to attack the Amendment in the Courts, because I believed the Amendment to be unconstitutional insofar as it applied to Optometry.[37]

Those in attendance heeded Fitch's warning, and a campaign against medical regulation was launched. The result was a lawsuit filed against the medical board, seeking to enjoin it from enforcing the regulation pertaining to the licensure of optometrists.[38] During the trial, key testimony was given by James Cook McAllister, who established that refraction was a skill first practiced in America by opticians, and that opticians had subsequently taught it to physicians.[39] At the conclusion of the trial, the court rendered an important opinion: Optometry was not a branch of medicine and hence was not subject to the medical board's regulation.

> We cannot regard the fact that the work done by the eye specialist physician and that done by the optometrist, to a certain limited extent, lap over each other, constitutes the optometrist a practitioner in medicine. Such work on the part of the optometrist was done by him perhaps and probably long before the eye specialist among physicians had either the knowledge or the skill to do the work which is now done by both physician and optometrist.[40]

This decision, although historic, was not precedent setting. In order to constitute a precedent, the decision had to be reviewed by the Supreme Court of Pennsylvania. The case was duly appealed to the state's highest court, and in 1915 another decision favorable to optometry—this time a precedent—was rendered. Optometry was regarded as an independent calling in Pennsylvania and not subject to the dictates of medicine.[41]

This early victory was an important part of optometry's legal development, because without it optometry would not have emerged in the law as a calling separate and distinct from that of medicine.[42] Albert Fitch, in his memoirs, *My Fifty Years in Optometry*, referred to the decision of the Pennsylvania court as optometry's "Magna Carta."[43] Fitch himself was to become an optometric leader of importance as the founder and President of the Pennsylvania College of Optometry and the advocate of many progressive pieces of optometric legislation, including the first optometry drug bill and the first unrestricted optometry law[44] (Fig. 1.3). In 1923, the Pennsylvania College of Optometry also became the first school to award the Doctor of Optometry (O.D.) degree.

As the enactment of optometry laws proceeded inexorably throughout the United States, medicine was to make one last effort at subjugation. By 1919 there remained but seven jurisdictions in which optometry practice acts had not received legislative approval; one of these was Texas.

The optometrists of Texas had suffered through many bountyless legislative years by 1919. Their efforts to enact an optometry practice act had brought them nothing but frustration. Worse yet, the Attorney General of Texas had issued an opinion that, there being no optometry statute, optometrists fell under the provisions of the medical practice act.[45] Dissatisfied with this state of affairs, the Texas optometrists decided to resort to the judicial system for relief, through a test case in the courts.[46] The guinea pig was Fred R. Baker, a member of the state optometric association and a prominent Dallas optometrist.[47] On March 22, 1920, Baker performed an optometric examination on one F.F. McHenry, was arrested for "unlawfully practicing medicine" and within a week had been tried, found guilty, and sentenced to one day in jail plus a $50 fine.[48] This was according to plan because the Texas optometrists wanted a conviction that could be appealed to the Texas Court of Criminal Appeals, where, they hoped, a precedent-setting decision in favor of optometry would be rendered.

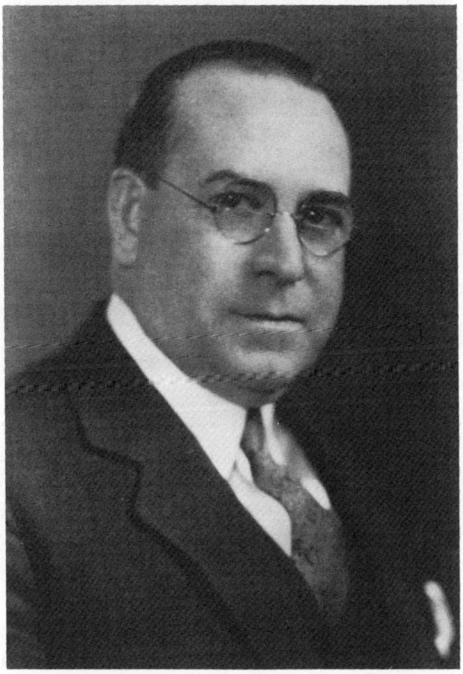

Figure 1.3. Albert Fitch. One of the great figures in the history of the profession, this Philadelphia optometrist rallied his Pennsylvania colleagues to challenge the efforts of physicians who sought to regulate optometry as a "minor branch" of medicine. The resulting case established that optometry was a profession separate from medicine and that optometrists could regulate themselves free of the dominion of physicianry. (Photograph courtesy of the Pennsylvania State College of Optometry)

The appropriate Texas law provided that any person would be regarded as practicing medicine "who shall treat or offer to treat any disease or disorder, mental or physical, or any physical deformity or injury, by any system or method or to effect cures thereof, and charge therefor, directly or indirectly, money or other compensation."[49] Physicians in Texas were understandably interested in the implications raised by the optometrists' legal challenge. They realized that if optometrists could be subjected to the law, then a means was readily at hand to ensure that all facets of eye care would be within the dominion of medicine. This led to some interesting concessions on their part: their argument before the Texas appellate court maintained that optometry was a "profession," that optometrists "diagnosed" disorders, and that they "cured" these disorders; for these reasons physicians considered optometry an aspect of medicine.[50] In countering these arguments, the optometrists of Texas proffered a rather ill-conceived defense: that optometry was a "business," that optometrists "discovered" disorders, and that they "corrected" these disorders instead of curing them. It was a defense that did not find favor with the Texas Court of Criminal Appeals. One June 1, 1921, the court found Fred R. Baker guilty—and optometry along with him—of violating the Texas Medical Practice Act:

> The power of the legislature to put the optometrists in a separate class, as it has done dentists and nurses, is without question.... Until it is done, or the optometrist...is expressly exempted from the operation of the Medical Practice Act, he, in our judgment, is required thereby to obtain from the state a license showing that he possessed the knowledge requisite to the pursuit of the practice of medicine.[51]

Baker was told to serve his one day jail sentence and to pay the $50 fine. Optometrists throughout the state were shocked.[52] In Texas an optometrist was in violation of the law for doing the very same things that an optometrist in any other state of the union was legally protected in doing. (All forty-seven other states had enacted optometry laws by this time.) Throughout the nation optometrists wondered if the adverse ruling would lead to a move to banish optometry altogether. There was considerable doubt about what to do: appeal to the U.S. Supreme Court, petition the Texas court for a rehearing, or resort to the legislature (a barren resort in the past) for an optometry practice act.[53]

The Texas optometrists decided to petition for rehearing, with Baker voicing a confidence that most of his peers did not share: "Say to my friends that we have not lost; that we have just started to fight, and the opposition is not as strong as it seems."[54] But the medical establishment was already savoring the taste of victory and warning of what was to come: "The fact that there are ophthalmologists sufficient to care for the eye requirements of the public leads to the inevitable conclusion that there is no need for such a profession as optometry."[55]

Yet it was to be a Pyrrhic victory for medicine. Public opinion slowly gathered behind the "outlawed" optometrists, newspaper editorials began to assail the court's decision, and the Texas legislature agreed to take up the question of a separate optometry law. Fund raising for the *Baker* case became a national pastime within the optometric profession.[56] It was needed; Baker was in financial straits and his wife in poor health.[57] In a bittersweet week during August 1921, Baker's wife died and Texas finally enacted an optometry practice act. Even though this signified victory for Texas optometrists in general, it was not the final solution for Baker, who still had to fight the criminal conviction that he had so cavalierly brought about.

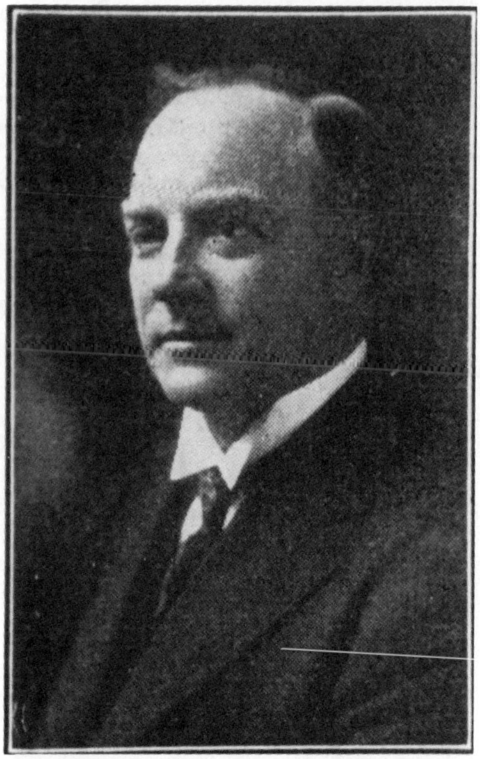

Figure 1.4. Fred R. Baker. Prosecuted for the unlawful practice of medicine, optometrist Baker's plight caught the attention of both the profession and the public and led to the passage of an optometry law in Texas. The *Baker* case dashed the hopes of medicine that a legal means had been found to "outlaw" the practice of optometry. (Photograph courtesy of the International Library, Archives, and Museum of Optometry)

A petition for rehearing was granted by the Texas Court of Criminal Appeals, and on February 22, 1922, the Texas court—in a bit of legal abracadabra—exempted Baker from punishment.[58] The State of Texas petitioned for another hearing, but the court turned them down,[59] and on April 26, 1922, a little more than two years after his arrest, Fred R. Baker—the court's decision safely recorded in the law reporters—could at last retire to enjoy his remaining years (Fig. 1.4). The case bearing his name became a significant chapter in optometry's legal history, demonstrating medicine's determination to eradicate the profession and the profession's ability to muster the legislative and political strength to defeat such efforts. The case is the most famous example to date of criminal prosecution of an optometrist for "unlawfully practicing medicine."[60]

Although the events in New York, Pennsylvania, Illinois, and Texas were resolved in optometry's favor, each of these legal confrontations had taken place in states where there were no optometry statutes. In those states where optometry laws had been enacted, the provisions and constitutionality of these statutes were tested in the courts.

One significant decision, *McNaughton v. Johnson*, rendered in 1917 by the U.S. Supreme Court (its first with respect to optometry), challenged the constitutionality of the California Optometry Practice Act, which provided for the licensure of optometrists and contained the customary exemption for physicians.[61] Kate McNaughton, a drugless "ophthalmologist,"[62] sought to enjoin the enforcement of the statute since it exempted physicians but not other eye-care practitioners, of which she was one. Her argument, based on constitutional considerations of equal application of the law, was rejected by the Supreme Court, which —in deciding the case—held that the right to practice optometry was one that the states could lawfully limit through licensure. After this decision, there could be no dispute over the power of the states to regulate optometry. The dispute turned instead to what optometry was.[63] Through the process of trial and appeal in the state courts, the question of what constitutes the practice of optometry began to find its answer.

Another California case, *Ex parte Rust* (1919),[64] held that optometry was not included in the science of osteopathy and that a person holding a license as an osteopath did not have the legal right to practice optometry. In Massachusetts (1920),[65] the optometry law withstood the legal challenge of an ophthalmologist who maintained that the law was class legislation that discriminated against him and, therefore, an interference with his rights. But in Illinois (1919),[66] the state supreme court struck down the optometry practice act as unconstitutional because it included the selection of glasses by a customer as part of the practice of optometry (which was defined as being "the employment of any means other than the use of drugs, medicine, or by surgery for the measurement of the powers of vision, and the adaptation of lenses for the aid thereof"). The Illinois statute holds the dubious distinction of being the only original optometry law that had to be passed twice; after the high court's ruling the Illinois Optometry Practice Act was changed, resubmitted to the state legislature, and re-enacted into law.[67]

By August 27, 1921, Texas had passed its optometry law, the last state to do so. Only one jurisdiction remained without a statute regulating the practice of optometry, and that was the District of Columbia.[68] When the nation's capital enacted its law on May 28, 1924, it signified the completion of the profession's genesis (Table 1.1). It had taken more than two decades for optometrists to persevere, but persevere they had, against the formidable opposition of both physicianry and opticianry (and even the federal government).[69] Of course, in hewing

Table 1.1. Historical Milestones: 1892–1924

1892	Charles Prentice of New York conceives of a means to "legalize" the practice of optometry through the enactment of a statute by the state legislature.
1896	The Optical Society of the State of New York is founded by Prentice and others; the purpose of the society is to secure the legal recognition of optometry.
1897	"An Act To Regulate the Practice of Optometry in New York" is introduced in the New York legislature and defeated by physicians and dispensing opticians opposed to the regulation of "optometry" by a single board.
1898	The American Association of Opticians is founded; in 1904 the association adopts the term *optometrist* to designate those opticians who perform refraction and related services; in 1910 the association changes its name to the American Optical Association; and in 1919 the name is again changed, this time to the American Optometric Association.
1901	Minnesota optometrists, under the leadership of H.M. Hitchcock, Alexander Sweningson, C.A. Snell, J.W. Granger, and F.A. Upham, secure the passage of the first state law regulating the practice of optometry.
1903	The Illinois Supreme Court, in the case of *People for Use of State Board of Health v. Smith*, holds that the selling of spectacles and the treatment of defective vision is not part of the practice of medicine or surgery.
1915	The Pennsylvania Supreme Court, in the case of *Martin v. Baldi*, rules that optometry is a calling separate from medicine and cannot be regulated by the state board of medicine as a "minor branch" of that profession; this precedent is achieved because of the leadership of Albert Fitch, who convinces the state optometrists to pursue legal action.
1917	The United States Supreme Court, in the case of *McNaughton v. Johnson*, holds that states may rightfully regulate the practice of optometry through licensure, thereby establishing the constitutional basis for an independent profession.
1921	The Texas Court of Criminal Appeals finds Fred Baker guilty of violating the Texas medical practice act in *Baker v. Texas*; Baker is fined and sentenced to jail for unlawfully practicing medicine, but public opinion mounts behind the "outlawed" optometrists and an optometry practice act is enacted by the Texas legislature; Baker is exempted from punishment by the court in 1922.
1923	The Pennsylvania College of Optometry awards the first Doctor of Optometry (O.D.) degree.
1924	The District of Columbia becomes the last jurisdiction to enact an optometry law, completing the genesis of "legalized" optometry.

optometry a place within the edifice of the law, certain compromises had been made. The most significant were the limited professional definition (no use of drugs and no surgery) and the exemption of physicians and opticians from regulation.

In retrospect, it would seem that these first optometry practice acts were probably the best that could be achieved at the time and that the conflict with physicianry and opticianry were as inevitable as the internecine struggle that would arise within optometry's own ranks during the forthcoming decades. But these were problems that would become the legacy of future generations of optometrists. For the moment, it was enough that optometry existed at all.[70]

In Dubious Battle (1925–1954)

The three decades that followed the legalization of optometry were to be the most trying in the profession's history (Table 1.2). Although optometrists had achieved an important first victory—legal recognition of their right to earn a living—they were soon to discover that statutory sanction was no panacea. In particular, the exemptions granted to physicians and to dispensing opticians were to prove vexing; and then there were the inevitable difficulties of self-regulation to contend with, as Boards of Examiners in Optometry sought to exercise their powers and to fulfill their duties.[71] But the greatest problem was the obvious inadequacy of the new state laws to protect the public from profiteering, illegal practices, shoddy materials, superficial examinations, and the other evils associated with a marketplace-oriented philosophy.

These failings compelled optometrists to return repeatedly to their state legislatures during the decades of the 1920s, 1930s, and 1940s, seeking modifications to the original optometry practice acts. Optometry boards, bolstered by these new laws and seeking to exercise their new powers, initiated an uncommon amount of litigation, the purpose of which was to achieve professionalization.[72] The urge for

Table 1.2. Historical Milestones: 1925–1954

1927	The Pennsylvania Supreme Court, in *Harris v. State Optometrical Examiners*, rules that the selling of spectacles by itinerant opticians can be prohibited by the state board of optometry.
1928	The New York Commissioner of Education obtains passage of a bill that allows only graduates of a school of optometry affiliated with a university to qualify for the state board examination, thereby initiating the end of the apprenticeship system of licensure.
1929	The United States Supreme Court, in *Roschen v. Ward*, rules that a New York statute requiring the presence of an optometrist where ready-made spectacles are sold is constitutional, thus determining that the commercial practice of optometry is subject to regulation by the states.
1933	The Iowa Supreme Court, in *State v. Kindy Optical Co.*, upholds the right of the state to limit the practice of optometry to individuals, thereby barring the practice of optometry by corporations within the state; this case is the first of dozens of cases brought to test the powers of state legislatures to restrict or prohibit the corporate practice of optometry.
1935	The United States Supreme Court, in *Semler v. Oregon State Board of Dental Examiners*, rules that a state board may regulate truthful advertising by professionals.
1937	A bill defining the practice of optometry as being whatever is taught in approved schools and colleges of optometry is defeated in the Pennsylvania legislature.
1941	The Association of Schools and Colleges of Optometry is formed.
1942	Arkansas becomes the first state to define optometry as a "learned profession"; the Arkansas Supreme Court, in *Melton v. Carter*, holds that the state legislature may rightfully designate optometry as a learned profession and that this designation may not be challenged by the courts.
1945	The Attorney General of Colorado becomes the first legal authority to recognize that the fitting of contact lenses is within the definition of optometry, and thus may be barred to opticians.
1947	The first patent is awarded for corneal contact lenses.
1948	*Optometry: Professional, Economic, and Legal Aspects*, by Henry W. Hofstetter, is published.
1950	The first patent for thin, interpalpebral contact lenses is awarded.
1954	The optometry school at Columbia University is closed.

this reform came both from within and without: A group of optometrists, most of whom were well educated, sought to elevate optometry above the for-profit, street-level enterprise of its beginnings to an ethical, service-oriented calling on a plane with medicine[73]; and a group of ophthalmologists, aware of this desire, dangled the carrot of recognition by medicine before these optometrists while at the same time striking at them for attempting to effect change.[74] Ophthalmology's posture is best reflected in a series of resolutions passed by the American Medical Association (AMA) at the instigation of its Section on Ophthalmology. But ophthalmology was not the only obstacle and in fact was not the greatest obstacle to reform.[75]

The path to professionalism was blocked by other forces as well, all of whom were opposed to changes in the status quo. First, there were the corporations and business enterprises that employed optometrists for the merchandising of glasses, a profitable arrangement that they did not wish to have curtailed. Second, there were the grandfathered optometrists, many of whom had acquired their skills through on-the-job training in mercantile establishments and thus regarded the effort to professionalize as a direct threat to their livelihoods and an infringement of their rights. Third, there were the exempted dispensing opticians, eager to enact regulatory legislation of their own and, eventually, to incorporate aspects of the practice of optometry into the scope of their calling.

This opposition was formidable, but a two-pronged plan was designed to overcome it: improve educational standards so as to produce professionally oriented graduates[76] and modify state optometry laws so as to banish corporate practice and unfair business tactics.[77] In setting out to effect these changes, optometry was attempting to emulate medicine, which had been dealt a severe blow by the Flexner report in 1910, only to achieve dramatic reforms by 1925.[78] Like medicine, optometry instituted significant changes in its educational system, thereby uplifting educational standards considerably, but the legal system proved a more challenging adversary, and by the mid-1950s optometrists who looked back over the preceding three decades would wonder if the small rewards had been worth the effort.[79]

A year after the last jurisdiction had enacted an optometry practice act, the physicians of Pennsylvania proposed legislation that would create a board with the responsibility to license all health care professions. The so-called one-board bill would have required all applicants for licensing to pass examinations administered by the board, which was to be composed primarily of physicians.[80] Optometry was to be one of the disciplines subject to the board's regulations; fortunately, the bill was defeated, as was an effort during the next legislative session to include optometry within a study of the healing arts to be conducted by an investigative commission authorized by the legislature at the instigation of medicine.[81] These legislative proposals in Pennsylvania illustrate the continuing interest of medicine to bring optometry under its purview. It was, perhaps, these and other legislative defeats that led ophthalmologists to turn to medical ethics as a means of exercising some control over optometry.

But medicine's opportunity to bring all of eye care under its dominion had dwindled with the passage of the optometry practice acts. Each of the state laws defined the practice of optometry and vested enforcement powers in a board, and it was these state boards that initiated the next phase of legal activity. Beginning in the mid-1920s the optometry boards began to exercise their authority over those practitioners and organizations that they deemed to be acting outside the scope of the law.[82] The confrontations frequently turned to the courts for adjudication and resulted in some notable decisions that further clarified the scope of optometric practice.[83]

In 1925 the Pennsylvania legislature amended the optometry practice act, conferring upon the state board the authority to regulate "branch offices and outside practices" of optometry.[84] A licensed optometrist who sold spectacles door-to-door was found by the board to be in violation of the statute and his license was revoked. The optometrist fought the decision, but the state supreme court eventually held against him.[85] Throughout the nation, like laws began to be adopted, and the itinerant spectacle peddler began to disappear.

In New York, a 1928 amendment to the state Education Law made it unlawful to sell ready-made spectacles (glazed goods) in a store or business unless an optometrist was present to supervise. The amendment was challenged by the S.S. Kresge Company, a multistate retail chain that commonly sold such spectacles (spherical-convex lenses used for reading) in its stores. After losing the case in the New York District Court,[86] Kresge appealed to the U.S. Supreme Court. In a decision upholding the constitutionality of the law, *Roschen v. Ward* (1929), Justice Oliver Wendell Holmes made it clear that there were limits to the commercial sale of eyeglasses and that it was the proper function of the state legislatures to set these limits:

> It is obvious that much good would be accomplished if eyes were examined in a great many cases where hitherto

> they have not been, and the balancing of the considerations of advantage and disadvantage is for the Legislature, not for the courts. We cannot say, as the complainants (Kresge) would have us say, that the supposed benefits are a cloak for establishing a monopoly and a pretense.[87]

This was the first victory for optometrists who sought to curb the growth of corporate incursions into eye care.[88]

New York also led the way in educational reform. In 1928 the state Commissioner of Education obtained passage of a bill that allowed only a graduate of a school or college of optometry affiliated with a university to qualify for the state board examination. The effect of this law was to end the apprenticeship system of licensure in optometry because each of the states soon followed New York in amending educational requirements.[89] And there was another benefit as well. Harold Kohn, the legal counsel for the American Optometric Association (AOA) at this time, was later to observe that "strengthening the educational requirements started a new trend in legislative activity. Bills were introduced and enacted into law which amended the definitions of optometry in the respective states."[90] Kohn was to become an indispensable figure in national legal strategy during these years (Fig. 1.5).

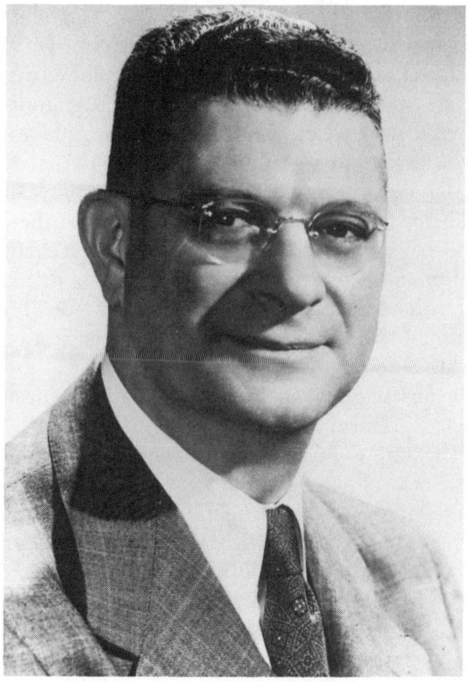

Figure 1.5. Harold Kohn. Counsel for the American Optometric Association, Mr. Kohn served in that capacity for almost 35 years, and was one of the principal proponents of the effort to "professionalize" optometry by improving educational standards, eliminating commercial practice, and developing a code of ethics. (Photograph courtesy of the International Library, Archives, and Museum of Optometry)

The culmination of these efforts occurred in the mid-1930s in political battles fought in Indiana and Pennsylvania. Indiana was the first state to embrace a comprehensive definition of the practice of optometry, enacted in 1935 after a fierce legislative struggle. The statute was constructed so as to define optometry as including "the employment of any means, for the purpose of detecting any diseased or pathological condition of the eye."[91]

This progressive development would have been taken a step further in 1937 had there not been a bit of chicanery in the Pennsylvania legislature. Albert Fitch, the president of the Pennsylvania State College of Optometry, had assisted in the introduction of a bill redefining optometry so that the scope of practice was to be whatever was taught in approved schools or colleges of optometry.[92] The proposed legislation made its way through the first two readings and seemed destined to pass when a physician-legislator made a sobbing appeal to have the bill referred to his committee, solemnly promising that it would be reported back to the full chamber the next day with a recommendation for its passage. Fitch describes what occurred next:

> It so happened that this physician told a deliberate falsehood, as he really had no authority to speak for his committee. He was simply following orders of the medical lobby, which will stoop to any dishonesty to defeat a bill which they oppose. However, in spite of the sobbing appeal, the untruthful statements and the false promise, the vote was close, ninety in favor of referring the bill and eighty-eight opposed. As the reader can well imagine, this bill never came back to the floor for a final vote.[93]

Had this bill been passed in 1937, the legal position of optometry could have been quite different during the 1940s and 1950s. The restricted nature of virtually all state definitions was to lead to further legal skirmishes during the succeeding decades. For example, it was not until 1945 that the first state law expressly mentioned contact lenses as being within the scope of optometry, and attorneys' general opinions and judicial decisions concerning contact lens practice continued to affect optometry throughout the 1960s and 1970s.[94] Tonometry was likewise subjected to attorney general and judicial review before becoming a legally accepted aspect of the practice of optometry.[95]

A second motivation for change came from medicine. A well-publicized address before the American Medical Association in 1928 by a prominent ophthalmologist held out the promise that, if optometry could divest itself of corporate practice, it would be a profession with which eye physicians could cooperate:

> The great obstacle to consultations between physicians and optometrists is *commercialism*. The practice of optometry is too much a matter of business. *It must become a profession*. If as and when, the optometrists organize a group of members who will set up professional standards and maintain them, consultation and cooperation will be welcomed by many eye physicians.[96]

Spurred on by educational improvements and the prospects of acceptance by medicine, it is little wonder that the optometrists interested in professional standards plunged into the uncertain waters of reform with such vigor. During the 1930s and 1940s there were legal skirmishes in probably every state between boards of optometry (or state attorneys general acting on their behalf) and corporations providing optometric services. An uncommon number of these disputes were eventually decided by appellate courts, with numerous precedents being established.[97] The outcome of a particular case was determined by the status of the state optometry practice act: If the law *permitted* corporations to practice optometry through licensed employees, the courts would generally uphold the law as valid; if the law expressly *prohibited* the corporate practice of optometry, the courts would likewise usually uphold the constitutionality of the statute; but if the law was *silent*, the courts were split, with the key factor being the determination as to whether optometry was a "mechanical art" or a "profession."[98] It was the latter cases that most damaged the self-image of optometrists, as decisions based on like facts ended up at complete odds with each other, one favorable, the other negative.

Looking back on these cases, it is easy to assume that this litigation was initiated prematurely. It was only through the judicial process, however, that optometrists could enforce the legislative enactments that had been won at the cost of so much labor and sacrifice. Such efforts were probably inevitable.[99]

And the remarkable interest in legal reform exhibited at the time doubtless made legislative and judicial activity impossible to suppress. The reform movement received another boost in 1935, when the U.S. Supreme Court rendered a landmark decision concerning advertising by health care professionals.[100] The court held that a state law prohibiting advertising by dentists was a proper application of the state police power, despite the fact that the advertising was "truthful." The case provided optometrists with a legislative means of prohibiting the use of advertising within their own ranks, assuming that the appropriate statutes could be enacted in each of the forty-eight states. Thus began a second front of conflict, as optometrists fought to pass new laws or to enforce existing ones. Ophthalmic advertising was frequently linked to bait-and-switch tactics that took unfair advantage of the public, and "downstairs" locations were oftentimes distinctly unprofessional in the solicitation of their clientele.[101] Optometrists waged a two-headed campaign that not only attempted to get their own house in order but also sought to end the abuse of advertising of ophthalmic goods altogether.[102]

In the litigation that ensued,[103] the courts held that statutes restricting or prohibiting advertising by optometrists or regulating or prohibiting the advertisement of prices for the sale of glasses were constitutional.[104] The effort to prohibit advertising by optometrists was eventually quite successful, and the campaign to restrict the advertising of ophthalmic materials succeeded in the majority of states.[105]

During the late 1930s and early 1940s, a series of events typified optometry's uneasy status as a quasi-profession: Courts began to hold that optometrists could be found liable for failing to refer patients to medical practitioners[106]; a national magazine advanced the argument that optometrists were not able to recognize and diagnose ocular pathology or ocular manifestations of systemic disease[107]; the American Optometric Association, eager to prevent bait and switch retailers from drafting a national standard that could regulate fair competition among providers of ophthalmic goods, participated in the development of a Code of Fair Competition for the Retail Optical Trade, with the attendant implication that optometrists were no more than retailers[108]; congressional proposals to expand social security legislation (the Wagner bill and its sequelae) did not include optometrists as providers under the law, a position strongly supported by medicine[109]; and optometrists called to duty during World War II did not receive commissions, although physicians, dentists, and other health care providers (including nurses) were routinely commissioned as officers.[110]

These experiences forced optometrists to take a closer look at themselves. In 1944 a national survey revealed that a mere 29 percent of all practitioners were located in "exclusive upstairs" (i.e., professional) offices.[111] Of such stuff is a desire for ethical reform born. The result was the most extensive effort ever undertaken to recast the ethics of a health-care profession.[112]

In 1944 the American Optometric Association adopted a new Code of Ethics, in 1946 a Supplement to the Code of Ethics, and in 1950 a stringent set of guidelines for the private practitioner, the Rules of Practice.[113] Even so, in 1952, the Office of Price Administration (an agency of the federal government) proposed regulations which held that, since optometry was a "trade," optometrists were subject to price ceilings on their services.[114] The ruling was eventually reversed, due in large part to the efforts of William P. MacCracken, Jr. (Fig. 1.6), who was to become an important and influential figure in optometric affairs in the nation's capital.[115]

Mr. McCracken was also an integral part of optometry's first significant federal legislative victory.[116] Title X of the Social Security Act stipulated that only physicians could examine persons seeking aid

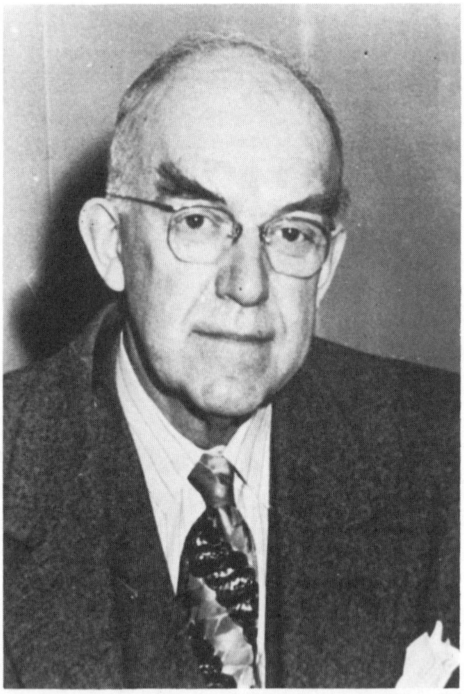

Figure 1.6. William P. MacCracken, Jr. As Washington counsel for the American Optometric Association for nearly a quarter century, Mr. MacCracken was a key man in the development of optometric legislative strength at the federal level, dealing not only with the U.S. Congress but also with federal administrative agencies, the armed forces, and agencies responsible for grants for research and education. (Photograph courtesy of the International Library, Archives, and Museum of Optometry)

to the blind under the act. In North Carolina and Oklahoma, the state welfare agencies used this provision to bar optometrists from participating in welfare programs.[117] Mr. McCracken drafted language to amend the Social Security Act so that it read, "In determining whether a person is blind, there shall be an examination by a physician skilled in diseases of the eye, or by an optometrist, whichever the individual may select." The political maneuvering necessary to marshal this and other legislation through the House and Senate constitutes some of the most colorful episodes in optometric legislative history.[118]

Another significant development during this period was the publication of the book, *Optometry: Professional, Economic, and Legal Aspects*, by optometric educator Henry W. Hofstetter[119] (Fig. 1.7). It was the first serious effort to describe the legal and ethical problems faced by practitioners of optometry.

The relationship between optometry and ophthalmology was a rocky one during these decades, as might be expected of two groups in direct economic competition. Although they did not clash in the legal forum, a war of words was waged over the years, with the principals being the American Medical Association and the American Optometric Association.[120]

The first exchange began in 1935, when the AMA (at the instigation of its Section on Ophthalmology) adopted a resolution that physicians could no longer ethically teach or consult with optometrists.[121] This resolution, although discountenanced by many physicians, remained on the AMA books until 1950, when it was rescinded "in order to disseminate information intended to prevent blindness."[122] During the post–World War II period, ophthalmologists began to promote the development of physician's assistants as ancillary personnel for private practitioners. The physician's assistants would be able to perform refraction, fit contact lenses, even apply drops under the protection of their physician-employer's license.[123] Fearing that unlicensed practitioners could invade the eye-care field, in 1954 the AOA passed a resolution calling for a study of all optometry laws to determine if exemptions should be eliminated and if encroachments by "untrained, unqualified, and unlicensed" individuals should be prevented.[124]

The resolution was seized upon by both medicine and opticianry as evidence that optometry was seeking to usurp "all" of eye care[125]; as a result, relations plummeted to an all-time low.[126]

The low water mark was soon evident, for in 1954 the AMA approved two important resolutions: the

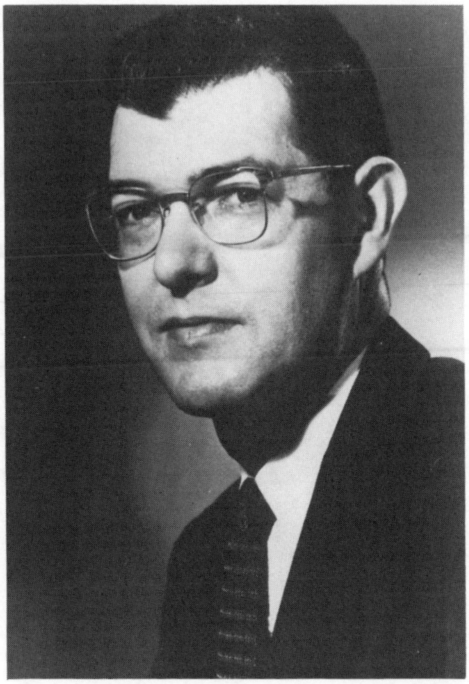

Figure 1.7. Henry W. Hofstetter. The author of the first optometric textbook to discuss legal issues affecting optometry, Dr. Hofstetter's text introduced optometrists and optometry students to principles of law and ethics and their relationship to professional practice. (Photograph courtesy of the International Library, Archives, and Museum of Optometry)

first reinstated the ban on teaching and consultation by ophthalmologists for the benefit of optometrists[127]; the second reversed more than a century of medical ethics and permitted ophthalmologists to dispense spectacles and contact lenses as long as there was "no exploitation of the public."[128] This acceptance of a dispensing role by ophthalmology required no legal approval; dispensing was within the scope of the medical practice acts, and so optometrists had no legal recourse available to them, although by adopting this stance ophthalmology had completely subsumed the field of optometry. Ophthalmologists also began introducing nuisance legislation requiring mandatory referral by optometrists.[129] Even worse, the school of optometry at Columbia University in New York was closed. There is little wonder that, as 1955 dawned, a general sense of malaise permeated optometry.[130] Few of the optometrists of the day would have suspected that the profession was poised at the start of its most progressive era.

The Great Leap Forward (1955–1970)

The fifteen years commencing with 1955 were remarkably fruitful years for optometry: It was a period of unprecedented technological advance, as the contact lens and the tonometer began to reform the nature of optometric practice; it was a period during which relations between optometry and ophthalmology warmed, chiefly because of the willingness of the AOA to go to extreme lengths in order to make peace; and it was a period of improvement in the standard of clinical practice, with some important court victories adding to the hard work of optometrists across the nation, resulting in a marked dimunition in commercialism. The optometry of 1970 was not only a far cry from that of 1955, it was prepared for revolution.

In 1955 the AOA made the first of several moves designed to improve relations with ophthalmology. With the unfortunate resolution of 1954 in mind, the association approved a new resolution that stated unequivocally the intention of optometry to live in peace with ophthalmology and disavowed any intent on the part of optometry to invade the province of medicine (medical treatment and surgery).[131] This overture was regarded with suspicion by eye physicians, but in 1961 the AOA observed this commitment by not supporting a Pennsylvania bill authorizing optometrists to utilize drugs "for diagnosis only," which died in committee. The AOA also decided against bringing an antitrust lawsuit against the AMA, and instead spent two years collecting information in order to file a complaint with the U.S. Department of Justice, alleging restraint of trade and conspiracy on the part of physicians and several medical organizations.[132]

Then, in 1964, a Chicago optometrist, Cyrus Bass, filed a lawsuit against the AMA and nine Chicago ophthalmologists, alleging that the defendants had conspired to monopolize the examination of eyes and the production, marketing, and sale of ophthalmic eyewear and that they had conspired to restrain trade and commerce in the dispensing of eyeglasses.[133] Amidst considerable publicity, Bass devised a plan whereby optometrists throughout the country would be allowed to participate in the legal fund needed to finance the lawsuit.[134] The case drew the attention of practitioners and organizations, including the International Association of Boards of Optometry (IAB), and became a source of debate within the profession. Despite the interest generated by the lawsuit, Bass—who was not an AOA member—did not receive the financial support he had envisioned.[135]

But in 1966—while the suit was still pending—the House of Delegates of the AMA voted to rescind the antioptometry resolution of 1955, declaring that:

> The full benefit of medical progress and existing opportunities for the prevention of blindness can be realized if there is no avoidable delay between the onset of abnormalities or their symptoms and the provision of medical care by qualified physicians. The improvement of educational standards of optometry is a laudable objective. Doctors of medicine may as teachers participate in the education of optometrists within the legitimate scope of optometric practice.[136]

In April 1967, the *Bass* case was settled, with the judge noting that the AMA resolution was "a great step forward in enhancing continued improvements of relationships which the Court suggests should be fostered by both the medical profession and optometrists."[137] Because of the AOA's complaint with the Justice Department, the *Bass* lawsuit, and conferences between organized optometry and medicine, the inflammatory AMA resolutions ended in 1966.

The internal battle with commercialism was also of concern in 1955; particularly important was a lawsuit involving the optometry practice act of Oklahoma.[138] A federal court had ruled that the act—which was a model law designed to eliminate commercialism in Oklahoma—was unconstitutional because it: (1) prohibited the advertisement of spectacles, frames, or other optical appliances, (2) prohibited an optician from fitting or duplicating lenses without a prescription from an optometrist or ophthalmologist, (3) exempted from regulation sellers of ready-to-wear glasses, and (4) barred operators of retail stores from furnishing space to any person purporting to do eye examinations or to render eye care.[139] In the case of *Williamson v. Lee Optical of Oklahoma* (1955), the U.S. Supreme Court reversed the federal court on all points, holding that the law was constitutional in every respect.[140] In discussing the prohibition on leasing space within retail stores, Justice William O. Douglas (Fig. 1.8) made clear the threat of commercialism:

> This regulation is on the same constitutional footing as the denial to corporations of the right to practice dentistry. It is an attempt to free the profession, to as great an extent as possible, from all taints of commercialism. It certainly might be easy for an optometrist with space in a retail store to be merely a front for the retail establishment. In any case, the opportunity for that nexus may be too great for safety, if the eye doctor is allowed inside the retail store. Moreover, it may be deemed important to effective regulation that the eye doctor be restricted to geographical locations that reduce the temptations of commercialism.[141]

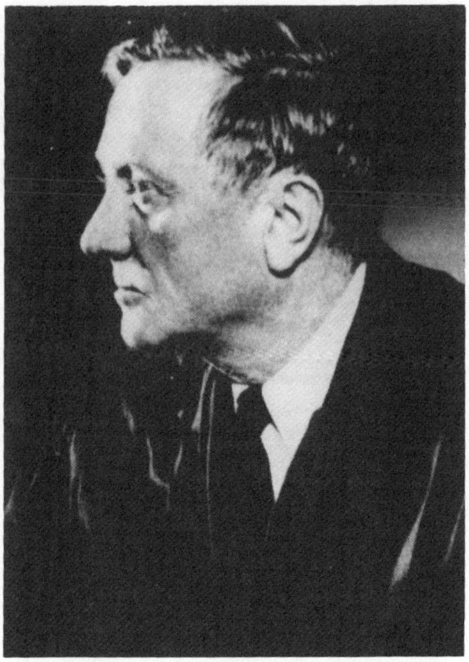

Figure 1.8. William O. Douglas. The Justice's opinion in the case of *Williamson v. Lee Optical of Oklahoma* remains the clearest enunciation of the dangers of commercial practice within optometry. (Photograph courtesy of the International Library, Archives, and Museum of Optometry)

Buoyed by this decision, optometrists lobbied for legislation based on the Oklahoma model. Unfortunately, securing passage in the state legislatures was an arduous and time-consuming activity. But after two decades of effort, laws were enacted in forty-five states, restricting various aspects of commercial practice, until social and legal changes in the 1970s reversed these gains.[142]

In 1963 another optometry case was accepted for review by the Supreme Court. This time the dispute involved advertising within the state of New Mexico by a commercial optometrist located in Texas. Optometric advertising was permitted in Texas but prohibited in New Mexico; despite the prohibition, the Texas optometrist advertised in New Mexico newspapers and radio stations. In deciding the case, *Head v. New Mexico Board of Examiners in Optometry* (1963), the Supreme Court ruled illegal the cross-border advertising of the Texas optometrist and set further limits on the advertising of ophthalmic goods and services.[143]

By 1968 the movement toward professionalism had yielded tangible results; the AOA felt that the time had come to amend the Rules of Practice, which was achieved without significant debate.[144] And Hirsch and Wick, in their book, *The Optometric Profession*, estimated the percent of optometrists eligible for admission to the Academy of Optometry (and hence practicing ethically) at 70 percent.[145] Although commercialism had not been eradicated, it had been relegated to an increasingly smaller minority, and the legal means of control was at hand. It was now a matter of hard work within the legislatures, trying to convince the lawmakers that reform was needed.

As important as the peacemaking with ophthalmology and the turn of the tide against commercialism was the technological revolution of the late 1950s and 1960s. The two major developments were the improvement of the contact lens and the invention of the Mackay-Marg tonometer. Both were due to the inspiration of optometrists.

In 1950 the first patent was taken out for a corneal contact lens made from plastic, and during this decade many practitioners contributed to the improvement of hard lens design and fitting techniques: Drs. John Neill, Irving Filderman, Gordon Butterfield, Newton Wesley, George Jessen, Alfred Rosenbloom, C.A. Boyshore, Maurice Poster, William Feinbloom, and numerous others advanced the art and science of adapting contact lenses to the eye.[146]

In 1960 Otto Wichterle discovered the cross-linked hydrophilic polymer, which was to usher in the era of the soft contact lens.[147] But the evolution of the contact lens initiated a new source of litigation as well as a new service for patients. The most troublesome predicament for optometrists was the unsupervised fitting of contact lenses by opticians.[148] Part of the problem was that many optometry practice acts did not specify the fitting of contact lenses as a part of optometry. Optometrists once again resorted to the legislatures to have the necessary amendments enacted.

In some states opticians maintained they were qualified to fit contact lenses, and optometrists were forced to turn to the courts for relief. The leading case occurred in Oregon, *State of Oregon ex rel. Reed v. Kurzurian* (1961), and held that the fitting of contact lenses was a skilled and professional task that only optometrists and ophthalmologists were authorized to perform.[149] But with the authority for fitting contact lenses came a concurrent legal responsibility to do it reasonably, and a new source of malpractice litigation arose within the profession.[150]

In 1958 Elwin Marg, O.D., Ph.D., (Fig. 1.9) of the School of Optometry, University of California (Berkeley), was on sabbatical leave in Stockholm.

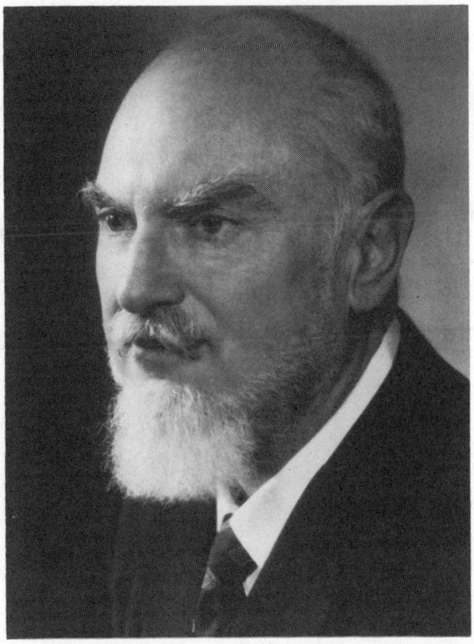

Figure 1.9. Elwin Marg. The transformation of optometry into a health care profession received an important boost with the development of a tonometer that could be used without anesthesia. The Mackay-Marg tonometer began an era of unprecedented technological achievement for the profession. (Photograph courtesy of the International Library, Archives, and Museum of Optometry)

Another Berkeley faculty member, R. Stuart Mackay, a physicist, also on sabbatical in Stockholm, discussed with Marg the theoretical basis for a new electronic tonometer, and by 1959 they had convinced the university to take out a patent for their technique.[151] Although initial ophthalmological reaction was skeptical, a joint M.D.-O.D. study undertaken at Berkeley in 1959–1960 revealed a high correlation between the pressures obtained with the Mackay-Marg and the Goldmann tonometers.[152] And the Mackay-Marg did not require anesthesia to test intraocular pressure, which made it available to optometrists for routine glaucoma assessment. The new instrument was praised in optometric literature during the 1960s and received wide acceptance throughout the profession. At schools of optometry renewed emphasis was placed on glaucoma and glaucoma detection using the new instrument and its successor, the noncontact tonometer, developed by Bernard Grolman, O.D., at American Optical Corporation, and patented in 1971[153] (Fig. 1.10). It was the start of a movement toward a more health-oriented role for optometry.

In fact, it is arguable that the contact lens and the

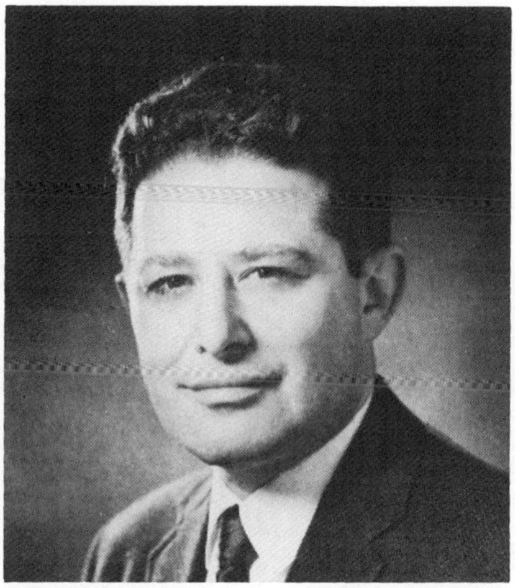

Figure 1.10. Bernard Grolman. The leader in the development of the non-contact tonometer, Dr. Grolman continued the technological advance of instrumentation created for ocular health assessment by optometrists. (Photograph courtesy of the International Library, Archives, and Museum of Optometry)

tonometer first brought optometrists into direct contact with the eye, for refractive services did not require physical interaction with the eye, nor did the treatment of anomalies of binocular vision. But the fitting and assessment of contact lenses required direct involvement with ocular tissues and the use of various ophthalmic solutions and dyes. Likewise, tonometry was a skill that demanded the touching of the ocular surface and, in some states, was performed with the use of topical anesthesia. These events thrust optometrists into an unfamiliar role but one which the profession found to its liking, and—responding to its changing perception of the scope of optometric services—optometry entered the 1970s in a mood to contribute even more within the health-care system (Table 1.3).

Technological changes also had a significant influence upon the economics of the profession. Economic surveys conducted during the decades of the 1920s, 1930s, 1940s, and 1950s had consistently demonstrated optometry to be a moderately successful calling in terms of financial remuneration, but the advent of contact lenses and the increased emphasis on health care effected a remarkable transformation in earnings. Over the course of ten years—from the late 1950s to the late 1960s—optometric income more than doubled, and during this period optometry was one of three fastest growing professions (in terms of income) in the United States. This consistent growth in earnings has continued throughout the decade of the 1970s and into the 1980s[154] (Table 1.4).

The increased emphasis toward a health oriented role came at a time when health care was itself being changed by the federal government. In 1960 the U.S. Congress approved the Kerr-Mills program (medical assistance for the aged), but by January 1965 it had been put into effect in only forty-four of fifty-four possible jurisdictions.[155] In 1965 an expanded version of the program was initiated under Title 19 of the Social Security Act, known as Medicaid.[156]

Although the federal law authorized payments for optometric services and materials, it was left to the states to determine whether or not the benefits of optometric care would be included within the services provided under the new program. Several states omitted optometric services altogether, while others permitted optometric participation but established fees at ridiculously low levels that discouraged widespread utilization of the program.[157] Medicaid marked the first occasion that optometric fees and services became the subject of legal regulation.[158]

In 1965 the Congress also enacted the Medicare program under Title 18 of the Social Security Act.[159] This law proved to be even a larger source of consternation than had Medicaid because it excluded reimbursement for ordinary refractive services when performed by an optometrist as part of a routine eye examination.[160] The only participation allowed optometrists was for "prosthetic devices," which was limited to the services and materials involved in supplying an aphakic patient with ophthalmic lenses, and originally this required referral of the patient to the optometrist after cataract surgery by the ophthalmologist. Medicare-eligible persons seeking "medical" services could be examined by physicians —who would receive at least partial reimbursement for their services—and these patients could also receive aphakic surgery and lenses from physicians, who were reimbursed for these services and materials by Medicare. In comparison, optometrists could only supply aphakic services and materials when patients were referred by a physician.[161] This law effectively denied Medicare patients freedom of choice among eye care practitioners, a defect that required 15 years to obtain even a partial remedy.[162] It was not until 1986 that optometrists were able to achieve parity with physicians, as the Medicare law was amended to permit optometrists to receive payment for services rendered to non-aphakic Medicare-eligible patients.[163] Today, any *medical* services within the scope of licensure can be rendered by optometrists

Table 1.3. Historical Milestones: 1955–1970

1955	The United States Supreme Court, in *Williamson v. Lee Optical of Oklahoma*, upholds the right of the states to pass legislation that restricts the commercial practice of optometry, even in certain "geographical locations" in proximity to for-profit stores. The first 20/40 mandatory referral bills are introduced by physicians and defeated in the state legislatures.
1958	The Mackay-Marg tonometer is conceived by Elwin Marg and Stuart Mackay of the University of California, Berkeley, faculty, and a patent is awarded.
1960	Otto Wichterle discovers the cross-linked hydrophilic polymer that ushers in the era of the soft contact lens; patents for the polymer and variations thereof abound in the decades that follow.
1961	Pennsylvania optometrists introduce a bill in the state legislature to authorize the use of ophthalmic diagnostic pharmaceutical agents but it is defeated.
1963	In the case of *Head v. New Mexico*, the United States Supreme Court recognizes the right of the states to regulate the advertising of commercial optometry across state borders.
1964	The American Optometric Association files a complaint with the U.S. Department of Justice, alleging restraint of trade and conspiracy on the part of the AMA, physicians, and several medical organizations. The antitrust case, *Bass v. The American Medical Association*, is filed; it is settled three years later without trial. The Attorney General of Oregon rules that optometrists in the state may lawfully use the tonometer for the detection of glaucoma.
1965	The Congress of the United States enacts Medicare and Medicaid.
1970	The Alabama state legislature authorizes the establishment of a school of optometry, the first to be an integral part of a medical center.

and paid for by Medicare. This legislation was rightfully hailed as the greatest legislative achievement in the profession's history.[164]

Medicaid and Medicare were sweeping social changes that reflected the politics of the times. It is ironic that, in an era devoted to the elimination of social discrimination, these programs should initiate such an array of legislation—both federal and state—that had the effect of discriminating against optometrists as vision care providers. The legislative and judicial struggle to reverse the effects of these laws continues until this day.[165]

These two pieces of legislation were landmark signs of the intrusion of the federal government into what had previously been left to the private sector of American life. Medicare, Medicaid, and third-party payment programs were to become vital to the profession during the 1970s, when it became evident that full optometric participation was an absolute necessity for economic survival. But even more, these programs had reformed the American health-care delivery system and had begun to change the attitudes of health care providers themselves. As a result, during the 1970s and 1980s increased emphasis began to be placed on vision service plans. Optometric participation in these plans, however, remains far below its potential.[166] Third-party vision service plans will be a key economic and legal factor in the profession's future.

Another indication of federal intrusion into health care was the 1965 Hart bill, which was introduced to "strengthen the antitrust laws by prohibiting the payment to or receipt by persons licensed to engage in the practice of medicine, of profit, rebates, refunds, commissions, discounts, rentals, or other valuable considerations in connection with the supplying to patients drugs, devices, or other products prescribed by such licensees."[167] The dispensing of glasses and contact lenses by ophthalmologists was specifically discussed in the ensuing hearings, with Senator Hart concluding that the dispensing of eyewear should be exempted from the bill.[168] However, this antimonopolistic attitude toward ophthalmic products was not to last.

Table 1.4. Earnings of Optometrists: 1929–1987

Year	Median Income ($)
1929	3,750
1944	5,950
1958	9,970
1968	20,926
1977	37,403
1987	57,190*

*Mean net income.

Source: American Optometric Association, Annual Economic Surveys, 1929–1987.

By 1970 optometry had changed significantly, offering expanded services, an improved image, and a new set of goals. This change was exemplified by the approval in 1970 of a new school of optometry by the Alabama legislature (the first school to be established in two decades). What was significant about the school was that it was to be an integral part of a medical center, with a sharing of the same faculty used to educate medical and dental students. It was a first for the profession, a harbinger of the revolutionary things that were to occur during the decade to come.

And so, in 1971, the revolution began.

Revolution! (1971–Present)

Seventy years after the profession of optometry had first been defined by a state statute, after Prentice and others had won legislative approval for optometry by using phrases such as "A Lens Is Not A Pill,"[169] after several resolutions had been approved by the AOA declaring that optometry was a drugless profession that would never invade the province of medicine,[170] and after years of clandestine use of drugs in at least ten states where the optometry law did not expressly prohibit their use,[171] there was revolution.

On July 16, 1971, the first diagnostic drug bill was signed into law in the state of Rhode Island. The inspiration for the bill originated with the keynote address given to members of the New England Council of Optometrists in 1968 by Alden N. Haffner, O.D., Ph.D., Director of the Optometric Center of New York[172] (See Fig. 1.11). Dr. Haffner had perceptively recognized that optometry, as a primary entry point into the health-care system, could perform its role more effectively and more efficiently if it was able to make use of the improved ophthalmic pharmaceutical agents developed for the diagnosis of conditions of the eye. Because of Dr. Haffner's speech, the optometrists of Rhode Island, led by Morton W. Silverman, O.D., David W. Ferris, O.D., and Richard I. Albert, O.D., initiated the effort that led to the passage of the first diagnostic drug bill (Fig. 1.12).

Within the space of ten years, thirty more states followed suit.[173] It was a movement that clearly galvanized the profession; optometrists began to think of themselves as an integral part of the health-care system and looked to improve the diagnostic skills that could help them better perform their responsibilities. As might be expected, the Rhode Island act was attacked as unconstitutional in the courts, but the state supreme court ruled that the ophthalmologists filing the case could not establish the injury necessary to bring such a challenge, thereby allowing the law to stand as enacted.[174]

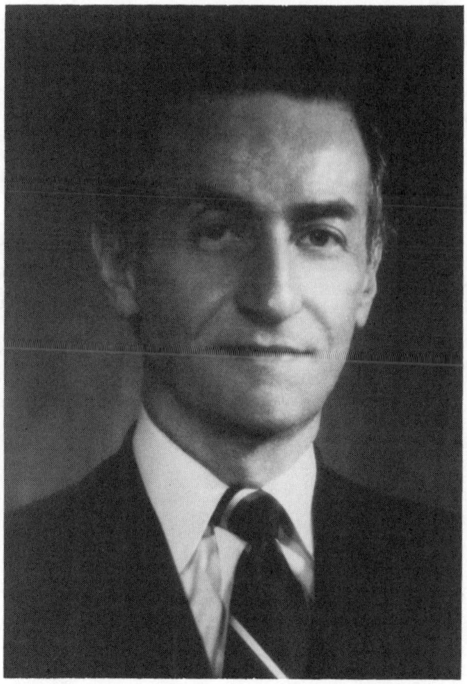

Figure 1.11. Alden N. Haffner. The inspiration for "medical" optometry began with a speech given by Dr. Haffner in 1968. Three years later the optometrists of Rhode Island succeeded in passing the first diagnostic drug bill in the United States, thereby initiating the most revolutionary era in the history of optometry. (Photograph courtesy of the State University of New York)

On March 4, 1976, the profession took another legal step destined to alter significantly the future of optometry; the legislature of West Virginia embraced the concept of primary care for optometrists by enacting (over the governor's veto) a therapeutic drug law.[175] For the first time in the nation's history, optometrists were legally recognized as able to treat eye disease. The passage of the West Virginia law was due in large part to the efforts of David (John) Janney, O.D., John Casto, O.D., and Walter S. Ramsey, O.D., (Fig. 1.13) who believed that the clinical role of optometry should involve primary care, a role that—due to the unique education, skills, and distribution of optometrists—was ideally suited to encompass the management of common eye diseases. In the years that have followed, the wisdom of their vision has been borne out.[176]

The passage of these laws irrevocably changed the direction of the profession, which once again

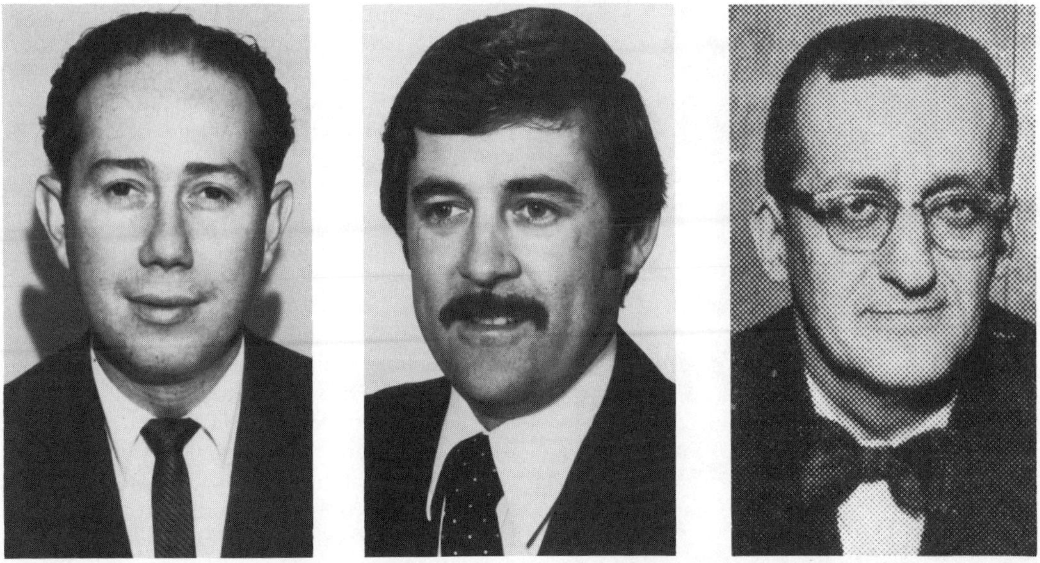

Figure 1.12. Leaders of the Rhode Island Diagnostic Drug Bill of 1971. From the left: Morton W. Silverman, David W. Ferris, and Richard I. Albert. The culmination of three years of work, the bill passed the House 31–26 and the Senate 25–16, despite the admonition of one legislator that "Practically all the people in the field of medicine are diametrically opposed to this." (Photographs courtesy of the International Library, Archives, and Museum of Optometry)

became fiercely divided on an internal issue. Although medicine charged optometry with entering into a field for which it had no preparation, the new optometry practice acts took great pains to ensure that the practitioners legally entitled to use drugs were educationally qualified to do so. The constitutionality of the West Virginia law was challenged in the courts, but the outcome of the case established that therapeusis could be the legal province of optometry, with the trial court's decision indicating the desire of the judiciary to leave the definition of professional skills to the legislatures.[177]

Contact lenses also became the subject of significant legal action. In 1976 the U.S. Food and Drug Administration classified contact lenses as a "drug," and a Colorado ophthalmologist alleged that the fitting and dispensing of this drug by optometrists was prohibited by law.[178] The physician also sought to have it declared illegal for optometrists to employ tonometers to test for glaucoma. The result was a ruling in favor of optometry on both counts, establishing a legal precedent for the use of tonometers by optometrists.[179]

During the 1970s, the battle within optometry entered its most decisive era, with judicial decisions effecting significant changes. Commercial optometrists, relegated to a decided minority, vigorously fought legislative efforts by professional optometrists that were aimed at restricting or eliminating corporate practice and advertising. And they also fought in the courts. The leading battle occurred in Alabama and ended up being decided by the U.S. Supreme Court.

The case was initiated after the Alabama law had been amended to no longer expressly permit the corporate practice of optometry.[180] The Alabama State Board of Optometry thereafter attempted to discipline several commercial practitioners, but the commercialists obtained an injunction blocking the board's actions. The case was appealed to the U.S. Supreme Court, which ruled in *Gibson v. Berryhill* (1973), that the organization of the Alabama Board was unconstitutionally composed—it consisting solely of professional practitioners—and that since the board had a pecuniary interest in its decisions which was quite opposed to that of the commercialists, it was assumed to be biased against them.[181] As a result of this decision, the method of choosing optometry board members had to be revised throughout the nation.

In 1976 events occurred that were to have an even more significant effect in blunting the decades-old struggle to divest optometry of commercialism; these events arose in the U.S. Supreme Court and the Federal Trade Commission (FTC). In a far-reaching reversal of precedent, the Supreme Court held that the professions had a legally protected right to advertise. The leading cases involved pharmacy, *Virginia*

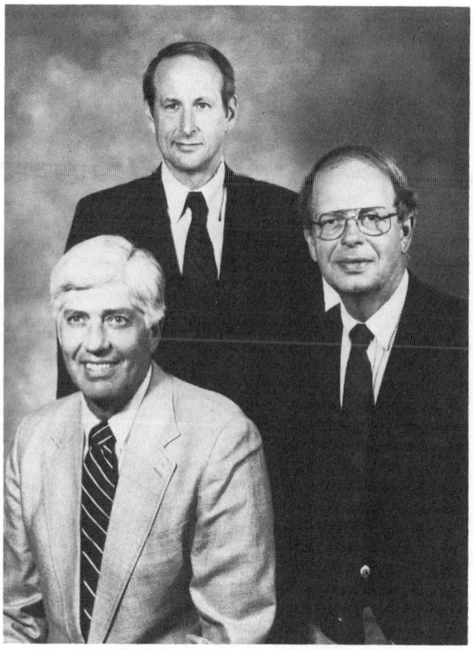

Figure 1.13. Leaders of the West Virginia Therapeutic Drug Bill of 1976. Seated, from left: David (John) Janney, John E. Casto. Standing: Walter S. Ramsey. Although the bill was vetoed by the governor, the House voted to override the veto by 59–39 (only 51 percent of the vote is necessary to override in West Virginia) and the Senate by 27–6. (Photograph courtesy of the International Library, Archives, and Museum of Optometry)

State Board of Pharmacy v. Virginia Citizens Consumer Council (1976),[182] and law, *Bates v. State Bar of Arizona* (1977),[183] but they were applicable to optometry, medicine, dentistry, and all other professions. State laws prohibiting truthful advertising by professionals became unenforceable as a result of these decisions.

This was accompanied by a trade regulation rule proposed by the FTC in 1978 that purported to preempt the laws of forty-five states—laws passed with great difficulty by optometry—laws prohibiting or restricting commercial solicitation and advertising.[184] After a series of hearings the FTC rule was put into effect, the so-called Eyeglasses I Rule.[185] The AOA sued, alleging that the preemption of state law was outside the power of the FTC and that the recent Supreme Court decisions made such a rule unnecessary.[186] In 1979 the case was decided in favor of the AOA; the only portion of the Eyeglasses I Rule left in effect was a prescription release requirement.[187] The forty-five state laws remained intact, although most of them had to be modified to meet the requirements of the Supreme Court, as expressed in the pharmacy and law cases. At the time of these events the U.S. Senate Subcommittee on Monopoly (of the Small Business Committee) announced that hearings on "the restrictive and anticompetitive practices in the pricing of eyeglasses" would be held.[188] The series of congressional hearings further fueled the debate over restrictions on price advertising of ophthalmic goods.[189]

The consumerist mood of the nation was clearly *contra* to optometry's efforts to clean its house and attain a uniform level of professionalism. But in 1979 another U.S. Supreme Court decision indicated that there would be limits to the consumerist movement. A Texas case, *Friedman v. Rogers* (1979),[190] involving the use of trade names in the practice of optometry, was heard by the Supreme Court; the case tested the constitutionality of a section of the Texas Optometry Practice Act that prohibited optometrists from practicing under a trade name (e.g., Texas State Optical). The case also tested the constitutionality of the organization of the Texas State Board of Op-

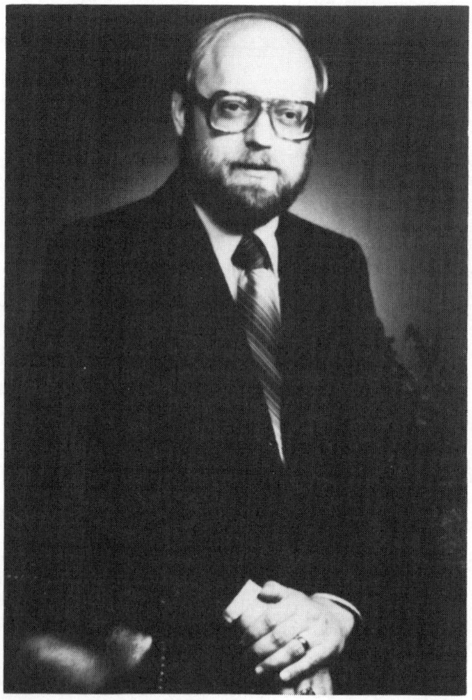

Figure 1.14. Thomas E. Eichhorst. Counsel to the AOA since 1965, Mr. Eichhorst has been an integral part of the most successful legislative era in the history of optometry, as the profession has developed a more health-oriented philosophy and has turned to primary care as the most effective means to serve the public need for eye and vision care services. (Photograph courtesy of the International Library, Archives, and Museum of Optometry)

tometry, which was split two-thirds to one-third in favor of professional practitioners. Although the law was ruled unconstitutional by the Texas high court,[191] the U.S. Supreme Court upheld it on both counts, thereby limiting the possibility of commercial incursion into an area previously uncertain.[192]

In another event of importance to professional optometry, the FTC announced in 1980 the results of its investigation into the services offered by professional and commercial practitioners.[193] While maintaining that the quality of materials between the two types of optometrists was not significantly different, the FTC was forced to concede that professional examinations were more "thorough."[194] Still ongoing is the FTC's effort to make unenforceable all state restrictions and limitations upon the commercial practice of optometry, known as Eyeglasses II.[195] In 1988 the FTC Commissioners voted to approve Eyeglasses II, a decision that will doubtless be challenged in the courts.[196]

The growing importance of third-party health-care plans, within both the public and the private sector, has also generated legislative and judicial activity by optometrists seeking to reduce what they perceive as discriminatory provisions under these laws. In particular, Medicare, Medicaid,[197] and vision services funded through public or private plans at the state level[198] have been the recipients of this activity. The 1970s and 1980s have demonstrated a clear trend, at least at the federal level, toward increased state control and more liberal utilization of optometrists as providers.[199] Within the states optometry has enjoyed a measure of success in eliminating discrimination in public reimbursement programs for vision care, but efforts directed at ending discriminatory practices among private plans

Table 1.5. Historical Milestones: 1971–Present

1971	Rhode Island enacts the first law that expressly authorizes the use of ophthalmic pharmaceutical agents for diagnostic purposes by optometrists. Bernard Grolman develops the noncontact tonometer at American Optical Corp.
1973	The United States Supreme Court, in *Gibson v. Berryhill*, holds that boards of optometry must be constituted so as to provide commercial optometrists with an opportunity for representation.
1974	The case of *Rhode Island Ophthalmological Society v. Cannon* upholds the constitutionality of the Rhode Island diagnostic drug law.
1976	The West Virginia legislature enacts the first optometry bill expressly allowing the use of drugs for therapeutic purposes; the constitutionality of the bill is challenged by state ophthalmologists and is upheld in the case of *Esposito v. Shapero*. The Colorado Court of Appeals, in *Winograd v. Johnson*, rules that a soft contact lens is not a "drug" that is prohibited to state optometrists; the court also declares that optometrists in the state may lawfully employ tonometry.
1977	In the case of *Bates v. Arizona State Bar* the United States Supreme Court ends decades of precedent and determines that professionals may utilize truthful advertising.
1978	The Federal Trade Commission issues a trade regulation rule allowing ophthalmic advertising by optometrists, ophthalmologists, and opticians; in *American Optometric Association v. Federal Trade Commission*, a federal court of appeals holds that the rule is moot except for the portion pertaining to prescriptions for glasses and contact lenses.
1979	The United States Supreme Court, in *Friedman v. Rogers*, rules that a state may lawfully restrict the use of trade names by optometrists.
1980	The Virginia Supreme Court, in *Blue Cross of Virginia v. Commonwealth of Virginia*, upholds the constitutionality of a state prepaid medical plan that requires payments to optometrists, podiatrists, and psychologists if the same services are paid for by the plan when rendered by physicians.
1981	The Congress of the United States expands optometric coverage under Medicare to enable optometrists to receive reimbursement for health-related procedures performed on aphakic patients.
1986	Medicare parity legislation, which allows optometrists to be reimbursed for health-related services performed on nonaphakic patients, is enacted by the U.S. Congress.
1988	The Federal Trade commission approves a trade regulation rule rendering unenforceable state restrictions or prohibitions on the commercial practice of optometry.

have not always achieved the desired result.[200] As private plans proliferate, this will continue to be a source of legal activity. Indeed, much of optometric litigation in the 1980s has centered around the discriminatory aspects of private and governmental plans for vision services, and a continuation of this legal activity can be expected in the future.

Optometry presently faces a legal horizon filled with opportunities, and although the transformation into a health-care profession has been primarily due to the efforts of grass roots optometrists, the American Optometric Association has clearly seized the initiative and is providing leadership in issues such as scope of practice, discrimination in third-party health-care plans, corporate incursions into health care, and governmental efforts to commercialize optometry. Clearly, one of the leading forces behind the AOA's successful legal strategies has been counsel Thomas E. Eichhorst (Fig. 1.14), who has supplied needed guidance and assistance in obtaining reforms at both the national and state levels.

As the preceding review has illustrated (see Table 1.5), optometry approaches the 1990s as a profession in transition, still plagued by the problems of the past yet able to reshape itself to meet the challenges of the future. Optometry's role within the growing complexities of the U.S. health-care system has become that of a primary care profession, although the extent of this role cannot be determined at present due to the evolutionary nature of the laws establishing the scope of optometric services. Since the past is prologue to the future, however, it seems likely that optometric involvement in health care will surpass its present level.

If nothing else, the legal developments of the past eight decades affirm the remarkable foresight exhibited by Charles Prentice, who nearly 100 years ago realized that the public would best be served by an "idealized eye specialist" who was a combination of optometrist and physician. Prentice's prediction in this regard has come true, as ophthalmology first turned to refraction, then dispensing, to be followed by optometry, which incorporated diagnosis and treatment of ocular disease into its services. Although legally distinct, the clinical division between optometrist and ophthalmologist has become increasingly ill-defined, and—as Prentice has indicated—this can be expected to continue, for it is in the public good.

Notes

1. See Arrington, E., *History of Optometry*, White Printing House, Chicago, 1929; Cox, M., *Optometry, The Profession*, Chilton, Philadelphia, 1947; Hofstetter, H., *Optometry*, C.V. Mosby Co., St. Louis, 1948; Gregg, J., *The Story of Optometry*, Ronald Press Co., New York, 1965; Hirsch, M. and Wick, R., *The Optometric Profession*, Chilton, Philadelphia, 1968; Gregg, J., *A History of the American Optometric Association*, American Optometric Assn., St. Louis, 1972.
2. An account of the evolution of the optometric service can be found in Hirsch and Wick, *The Optometric Profession*, supra note 1, pp. 45–147.
3. Donders, who was Dutch, had his work translated into English and published in England. His book described the fundamentals of clinical optometry, using optics as the basis of clinical procedures, and recognized the scientific nature of prescriptions for spectacles. It became the foundation of modern clinical optometry.
4. The entry of physicians into optometry in America is documented in the famous case of *Martin v. Baldi*, 249 Pa. 253, 94 A. 1091 (1915), in which the testimony of James Cook McAllister, a Philadelphia optician (quoted in note 39 infra), established that refraction was a skill taught by opticians to eye physicians in that state.
5. The development of medical licensure in the United States is an interesting and complex matter in its own right, having progressed through several phases of discord and disfavor before resulting in the regulatory scheme found today. In large measure, licensure was an attempt to regulate the practice of medicine by governmental action due to the inability of physicians (or government) to exercise control over the quality of medical education. Because the issuance of diplomas (some by mail) could not be regulated, minimum standards were established by the states for the practice of medicine, and through this mechanism undesirable graduates were prevented from practicing. The state definitions of medicine were written in very broad language that made it possible to subject all possible practitioners of the healing art to governmental control, and it was against this barrier that optometry was to find itself when it sought legal definition by the states. The history of U.S. medical licensure is recounted by Shryock, R.H., *Medical Licensing in America, 1650–1965*, Johns Hopkins University Press, Baltimore, 1967.
6. The competitive nature of this system was described by Charles Prentice in his book, *Legalized Optometry and Memoirs*, Casperin Fletcher Press, Seattle, 1926, pp. 11–13.

> Yet, as oculists had elected to prescribe glasses and did not generally supply them, they were compelled to send their patients to visit certain specially appointed opticians to practically execute their prescriptions for lenses that were to be mounted as spectacles or eye glasses. Of course, these collusively appointed opticians were not permitted to fit glasses to the sight, since that would have

produced an undesirable competition between the aforesaid optical merchants and the learned doctor.

Hence, opticians soon became divided among themselves, even though only a minority of them were induced by oculists to denounce their time-honored privilege to fit glasses, in order to cater exclusively to an imperious medical dictum.

Such opticians came to be eventually known as "dispensing opticians," in distinction from those who continued their vested right to fit glasses, as so-called "refracting opticians."

During this unwarranted split among opticians, the dispensing opticians and oculists prospered to a degree before unknown within the annals of specialized professionalism. Eventually dispensing opticians vied with each other to secure the oculists' prescription-business, until a system of monetary rebates was established that gave to the oculists handsome cash returns upon the prices of glasses sold by dispensing opticians to unsuspecting patients. Of course, this also offered a tempting opportunity to the general practitioner who intended to practice as an eye specialist after having absolved a three or six-months post-graduate experience at some hospital, as he could later be assured of dual income from the patient and the dependent optician, while waiting for patients to gain confidence in his ability also to treat ocular disease or to perform a delicate surgical operation.

The prescribing of spectacles among novitiate medical eye practitioners thus became the foundation upon which to build their cherished and more lucrative practice of ocular medicine and surgery.

During this period of unethical collusion some of the long established refracting opticians were not only confronted by a younger set of men, generally watchmakers or jewelers, who were being taught to examine the eyes at so-called trade schools, where attendance for various elective short periods enabled the student to secure a diploma that often carried with it a new phase of the doctorate. This pandemonium of pseudo-professionalism often caused a bewildered and uninformed public to seek eye-service from amateur oculists—who unwarrantably advocated use in eyes of harmful drops—or from the self-confessed optical incompetent, who shamelessly advertised, "Eyes Examined Free." Of course, both of these methods were reprehensible and are fortunately at present less frequently in vogue.

7. Despite the history of refraction as a nonmedical science, it had become so associated with the practice of ophthalmology in some physicians' minds that by the end of the 1800s the refracting opticians were considered to be interlopers in their own calling. An example of this can be found in Prentice's book, in which he recounts the accusation of an ophthalmologist, D.B. St. John Roosa, that Prentice had "entered into the practice of ophthalmology" by prescribing glasses. See Prentice, *Legalized Optometry and Memoirs*, supra note 6, p. 25.
8. In *Legalized Optometry and Memoirs*, supra note 6, pp. 14–15, Prentice is described as follows:

   Charles F. Prentice, M.E.—An American optician, whose father, James Prentice, of London England—also a noted optician established in New York City in 1842—had foreseen the need of a thorough technical education among future opticians and who, in the absence of a school for opticians, had his son educated in the department of mechanical engineering at the Polytechnicum, Karlsruhe, Baden, Germany. Upon the demise of his father in 1888, Charles F. Prentice succeeded him in the conduct of a lucrative general optical business, which thereafter gradually developed into a strictly professional one. Through close application and original research in optics he soon became widely known as the author of many highly technical articles in the leading ophthalmological journals in this country, a fact which gave him immediate recognition among ophthalmogists of international eminence, such as Helmholtz, Knapp, Noyes, Wood, Burnett and others.
9. Id. at 19–20.
10. Id. at 20–25.
11. Id. at 25–28. It is interesting to read the rather patronizing and dogmatic words of Roosa, which did so much to move Prentice to seek legislative reform. Is there not a parallel to the more contemporaneous efforts of certain ophthalmologists who pen similar expressions in a current-day periodical and for whom the reward has been the same as that received by Roosa, renewed legislative success by optometry?
12. Roosa displayed a vituperative attitude toward those who opposed him. In id. at 32, it is recorded that Roosa caused the passage of an unconscionable resolution by the New York County Medical Society relative to opticians:

    However, in the month of February, 1895, one of Mr. Prentice's friendly physicians informed him that Dr. Roosa, having recently discovered that he and other physicians were giving their support to a non-medical man, had appealed to the members of the New York County Medical Society to desist from such unethical practice.

    In fact, "Roosa made such strenuous objection to it that, at his insistance a resolution was passed to eject members from the Society who essayed to send patients to opticians to have glasses fitted." Moreover, Roosa had vehemently declared "he would have the medical practice act so amended as to deprive men of Prentice's cult from meddling with ophthalmology."
13. Id. at 35.
14. Id. at 38.
15. Id. at 40. The officers were: President—Charles F. Prentice, Vice President—George R. Bausch,

Treasurer—A.J. Cross, and Secretary—Frederick Boger.

16. The law in full can be found in id. at 128–133.
17. Id. at 134.
18. Id. at 131.
19. How prophetic Prentice's concept of the evolution of education in the eye care professions was to be, with both optometry and ophthalmology eventually absorbing one another's skills so as to better serve the public. See id. at 143.
20. Another compromise, proposed by a member of Prentice's committee, was to exempt all physicians from the provisions of the law. This offer was readily accepted by the physician lobby, but it made no difference in the outcome. Id. at 134.
21. Rosemary Stevens, in *American Medicine and the Public Interest*, Yale University Press, New Haven, Conn., 1977, at 103–109, describes the lost opportunity for joint regulation of both optometrists and physicians in New York, and how optometry originated from the failure of physicianry to successfully defend its contention that refraction and related services were a part of medicine.
22. The failure of the New York law in 1897 is of historical significance, as is the passage of the Minnesota law in 1901. But the first optometry law to be proposed in the United States was in Colorado in 1889. J.C. Bloom, writing in the January 15, 1941, issue of the *Optical Journal and Review* ("Early Optometry, Here and Abroad"), described his efforts to obtain an optometry law for his state and to form a state association.

    I believe I have the distinction of being the first man in the United States to have introduced in a state legislature a bill for the regulation of Optometry. In 1889 I had such a bill drawn, requiring a certain amount of both formal and practical education. I appeared before the legislature of that year and had the bill introduced, but it failed to pass. For several sessions of the legislature I worked alone and single handed. In 1892, I undertook to organize a jeweler's and optician's association. I finally succeeded and was elected its first president. Before the year was out the organization was dissolved, being made into two organizations. I held the offices of president of the jewelers, and secretary of the opticians. When we met in convention, one day was devoted to the jewelers and the other day to the opticians. I then mustered up some assistance toward an optical law, and worked from 1889 to 1913 until our bill was passed and signed.

    So far as is known, this makes Colorado first in introducing legislation (1889) and in forming an association (circa 1892).
23. Many of the details of the remarkable achievement of this group of men have been lost, but some commentaries about their motivation, problems, and their personal lives can be found in the following articles: Address Before The Minnesota State Optical Association, Sept. 4, 1901, by H.M. Hitchcock of the State Board of Examiners, *The Optical Journal*, vol. 8, no. 10, Oct. 1901, p. 929; C.A. Snell, *The Optical Journal*, vol. 13, no. 10, Apr. 28, 1904, p. 707; Secretary C.A. Snell To Retire from State Board and from Active Practice, *The Optical Journal and Review of Optometry*, vol. 31, no. 1, Dec. 26, 1912, p. 55; and Minnesota Men Hold Convention, *The Optical Journal and Review of Optometry*, vol. 31, no. 10, Feb. 27, 1913, p. 607. A historical perspective on the first law can be found in The Father of Optometry Laws, *Optometry*, Nov. 1916, pp. 218–222.
24. Address Before The Minnesota State Optical Association, Sept. 4, 1901, by H.M. Hitchcock of the State Board of Examiners, supra note 23, at 929.
25. Id. at 933
26. The text of the Minnesota law can be found in Hirsch and Wick, *The Optometric Profession*, supra note 1, at 315–317.
27. The debate over optometric legislation and the exemptions granted to physicians and grandfathered opticians was one that persisted for decades, not unlike the current debate over ophthalmic drugs that has occupied the profession over the past several years. Examples of the dispute abound in the literature. Sample articles are as follows: Cook, H.J., Optometrical Legislation, *The Optical Journal*, vol. 22, no. 7, Aug. 13, 1908, pp. 343–345; Palmer, B.S., Organization and Legislation, *The Optical Review*, vol. 1, no. 2, May 1907, pp. 27–30; Petty, J.H., The Common Abuse of the Optometric Statute, *The Optometric Weekly*, vol. 18, no. 38, Nov. 24, 1927, pp. 1371–1372; Editorial, Exemption of the Physicians, *Optical Journal and Review of Optometry*, vol. 62, no. 6, Aug. 10, 1928, pp. 17–18; Ryer, E.L., and F.E. Hotaling, The House Divided Cannot Stand, *Optical Journal and Review of Optometry*, vol. 62, no. 8, Aug. 24, 1928, pp. 23–24; Editorial, Genesis of the Medical Men's Exemption Clause in Optometry Laws, *Optical Journal and Review of Optometry*, vol. 72, no. 11, June 1, 1935, p. 22; and Editorial, National Optometry Law Proposed—Not Possible Under U.S. Constitution—Uniform State Amendments Only Substitute, *Optical Journal and Review of Optometry*, vol. 72, no. 18, Sept. 15, 1935, p. 29.
28. An annotation, Optometry As Within Statute Relating To Practice Of Medicine, can be found in 22 A.L.R. 1173. This annotation summarizes the legal struggle to have optometry recognized as a calling separate from that of medicine.
29. In legislatures across the nation, the battle was joined over the issue of legal recognition of optometry as a calling apart from medicine. With medical opposition to optometric licensure certain and strong, a counter argument had to be devised, and the optometrists of the day found it in the proposition that optometry was not a branch of medicine and thus was deserving of the right of self-regulation. Physicians, however, felt that the recognition of optometry was an infringe-

ment upon the medical practice acts. Slogans of the era proclaimed that "Physics is not physic," "A lens is not a pill," and "A lens treats light," and illustrated the separation between optometric science and medical science. (A discussion of the ophthalmological viewpoint can be found in Jackson, E., The Optometry Question and the Issues Behind It, *Journal of the American Medical Association*, vol. 57, no. 4, July 22, 1911, p. 265. It can be said, perhaps, that adopting this political stance caused the optometric practitioners of the day to make a virtue out of necessity. The position espoused by optometrists, however, that optometry deserved legal sanction as a separate profession, has become the basis for the independent position of optometry today.

30. This case was an important test of the use of medical practice acts to prosecute optometrists for quasi-medical acts that could be construed as being within the province of medicine. See *People for use of State Board of Health v. Smith*, 208 Ill. 31, 69 N.E. 810 (1904), *affirming* 108 Ill. App. 499 (1903). Smith was prosecuted for the same offense (and to the same end) in *Smith v. People*, 92 Ill. App. 22 (1900), *reversed on other grounds*, 199 Ill. 20, 63 N.E. 972 (1900).
31. He did tout himself, however, as "The famous Chicago eye expert." See *People for use of State Board of Health v. Smith*, 208 Ill. 31, 69 N.E. 810 (1904).
32. Ibid.
33. Gregg, J., *A History of the American Optometric Association*, American Optometric Assn., St. Louis, Mo., 1972, pp. 9–10.
34. Id. at 26–27. In 1910 the Association changed its name to the American Optical Association, and in 1919 to the American Optometric Association. See id. at 47 and 80.
35. Gregg, J., *The Story of Optometry*, supra note 1, at 219.
36. Id. at 365.
37. Fitch, A., *My Fifty Years In Optometry*, vol. I, Press of the Pennsylvania State College of Optometry, Philadelphia, 1955, pp. 7–8.
38. Fitch describes the decision to pursue litigation in id. at 9–15.
39. The testimony of McAllister is quoted by Fitch verbatim, id. at 15–16:

    QUESTION: What is your profession?
    ANSWER: Optician.
    QUESTION: How long have you been engaged in that profession?
    ANSWER: Forty-three years.
    QUESTION: You are of the house of McAllister that has been a optician house since some time in 1700?
    ANSWER: Yes.
    QUESTION: Do you happen to know who was the first man that measured the first pair of eyes in Pennsylvania for glasses and fitted them?
    ANSWER: My grandfather, John McAllister, Jr.
    QUESTION: Do you happen to know the first man who taught the oculists in Philadelphia how to measure eyes?
    ANSWER: My father, William Young McAllister, and James W. Queen.
    QUESTION: That is to your personal knowledge, you were in the store at that time?
    ANSWER: Yes.
    QUESTION: Who were the first oculists to your knowledge in Philadelphia?
    ANSWER: Peter Keyser, George Strawbridge, Richard Levis.
    QUESTION: After they had acquired their degree of Doctor of Medicine, to whom did they go to learn refracting?
    ANSWER:They got their knowledge of lenses and use of the test case from my father principally, and other members went to James W. Queen. Those three men came to my father.
    QUESTION: Then the profession of oculist came in as a separate profession, or as a specialty in medical work, about when to your personal knowledge?
    ANSWER: In the 70's, early 70's.
    QUESTION: And the work of what is called the optometrists was done up to that time entirely by whom?
    ANSWER: By the opticians.

    The remarkable McAllister clan is described by Kelly, C., McAllister: Five Generations of Optometrists, *Optical Journal and Review of Optometry*, vol. 112, no. 13, 1975, pp. 10–17.
40. Decision of the court of Common Pleas of the County of Philadelphia, October 10, 1914. See Fitch, supra note 37, at 16. The court's decision was technically based on the title of the bill in 1913 that amended the Bureau of Medical Education and Licensure's powers to include regulation of "branches" of medicine. The court reasoned that the title of the bill did not give reasonable or fair notice to optometrists that they would be embraced within its purposes, thereby depriving them of the opportunity to protest or testify against the bill. This was so, according to the court, because optometrists did not practice surgery or diagnose diseases, said acts being necessary to qualify optometry as constituting a "branch" of medicine.
41. *Martin v. Baldi*, 249 Pa. 253, 94 A. 1091 (1915).
42. But optometry was to find this decision judicially confining later in the century, for in the court's words optometry was restricted to a surgery-less, drug-less, diagnosis-less occupation that, for these reasons, could not be considered a "branch" of medicine or surgery. See id.
43. The importance of this case was also recognized in Hirsch and Wick, supra note 1, at 142–143. Fitch details subsequent efforts by the Medical Board of Ohio to classify optometry as a "minor branch of medicine," only to reverse this decision following the initiation of a lawsuit by the state's optometrists, who clearly were following the results in Pennsylvania

in attacking the Ohio Board's position. See Fitch, supra note 40, at 30–32.

44. Albert Fitch is unquestionably one of the great early leaders in optometry. His memoirs offer an interesting account of the formative years of the profession and stand as compelling evidence of his own leadership and farsightedness.
45. *Baker v. Texas*, 91 Tex. Cr. R. 521, 240 S.W. 924 (1921).
46. An account of the *Baker* case can be found in Gregg, J., supra note 33, at 79–80.
47. Baker's own account of what can only be termed an ordeal is contained in The *Baker* Case—Public Sentiment Reacts for Optometry—Medical Men Expect to Proceed Slowly, *Optical Journal and Review of Optometry*, vol. 48, no. 1, July 7, 1921, pp. 40–41; and From Michigan To Texas, *Optical Journal and Review of Optometry*, vol. 49, no. 23, July 8, 1922, p. 12.
48. The developments leading to the case brought against Dr. Baker are summarized in Optometry Fight In Texas, *Optical Journal and Review of Optometry*, vol. 43, no. 17, Apr. 17, 1919, p. 1090.
49. Tex. Rev. Penal Code, art. 755, §2 (1911).
50. The medical arguments that ultimately prevailed are discussed in Medical Views on the *Baker* Case, *Optical Journal and Review of Optometry*, vol. 46, no. 14, Sept. 30, 1920, pp. 939–941. The arguments in favor of *Baker* are summarized in Arguments in *Baker* Case, *Optical Journal and Review of Optometry*, vol. 46, no. 15, Oct. 7, 1920, pp. 997–999.
51. *Baker v. Texas*, supra note 45. See also 22 A.L.R. 1173.
52. Optometry Is Hamstrung in Texas, *Optical Journal and Review of Optometry*, vol. 47, no. 23, June 9, 1921, p. 45.
53. Optometrists To Appeal to the Supreme Court of the United States, *Optical Journal and Review of Optometry*, vol. 47, no. 23, June 9, 1921, p. 45.
54. Motion for Rehearing in *Baker* Case To Be Argued in October—Texas Legislature To Hold Special Session, *Optical Journal and Review of Optometry*, vol. 47, no. 25, June 23, 1921, p. 81.
55. The *Baker* Case, supra note 47, at 41 (quoting from *The Texas Medical Journal* of July 7, 1921).
56. The Baker Fund—A Testimonial, *Optical Journal and Review of Optometry*, vol. 48, no. 6, Aug. 11, 1921, p. 30.
57. The Fred Baker Testimonial, *Optical Journal and Review of Optometry*, vol. 48, no. 9, Sept. 1, 1921, p. 47.
58. The decision of the court is quoted in Court Opinion In Baker Case, *The Optical Journal and Review of Optometry*, vol. 49, no. 10, Mar. 9, 1922, p. 53.
59. The court's decision is quoted in Optometry Wins Final Decision in *Baker* Case, *The Optical Journal and Review of Optometry*, vol. 49, no. 18, May 4, 1922, p. 41.
60. Instances in which it has been alleged that optometrists have transgressed the borderline between optometry and medicine are rare. An overview of the legal issues involved in such determinations can be found in the following annotations of the *American Law Reports: Baker v. State of Texas*, 22 A.L.R. 1173; Practicing Medicine, Surgery, Dentistry, Optometry, Podiatry, or Other Healing Arts Without License as a Separate or Continuing Offense, 99 A.L.R.2d 654; What Constitutes Practice of Optometry, 88 A.L.R.2d 1290; and Validity of Governmental Regulation of Optometry, 22 A.L.R.2d 939.
61. *McNaughton v. Johnson*, 242 U.S. 344, 37 S. Ct. 178 (1917). For optometric opinion of the case, see United States Supreme Court to Pass on the Constitutionality of the California Optometry Law, *Optical Journal and Review of Optometry*, vol. 38, no. 24, Dec. 7, 1916, p. 1451; and California State Board's Annual Report—Legal Victories, Including U.S. Supreme Court Decision Upholding Optometry Law, *Optical Journal and Review of Optometry*, vol. 41, no. 26, June 20, 1918, p. 1743.
62. Ms. McNaughton was not a physician but rather "a graduated ophthalmologist, which is a school of scientific learning and practice confined to the testament of the inflammation of the eye and its membranes and in fitting glasses to the human eye," *McNaughton v. Johnson*, supra note 61, at p. 178. Thus she was a drugless practitioner just like an optometrist, even though she did not call herself such (or seek licensure from the optometry board).
63. For annotations describing the legal development of the practice of optometry, see 121 A.L.R. 1455, 141 A.L.R. 883, and 88 A.L.R. 2d 1290.
64. *Ex parte Rust*, 181 Cal. 73, 183 P. 548 (1919).
65. *Commonwealth v. Houtenbrink*, 235 Mass., 320, 126 N.E. 669 (1920).
66. *People v. Griffith*, 280 Ill. 18, 117 N.E. 195 (1917). The Illinois Supreme Court expressed its view as follows:

> What the defendant did was to try different lenses, and when the customer said she could read the letters at a distance she practically decided what glasses would suit her and contracted for them. If changing lenses until the customer was suited...is measurement of the power of vision and the adaptation of lenses, it is no more than the measurements made by any person who undertakes to fit a person where the (latter) person himself decides what answers the purpose. Such "measurements," if they are so called, have no relation to the public health, comfort, safety, or welfare, such as to require a course of previous study and an examination and payment of a license fee. No reason is given by counsel how the comfort, health, welfare, or safety of society is to be promoted by requiring a license for such acts as were done by the defendant. A statute which singles out a particular class of persons and imposes burdens upon them from which other similar classes are exempt violates their constitutional

rights, and cannot be sustained.

67. The optometry law was repassed as amended on April 19, 1919.
68. The difficulty in enacting an optometry practice act for the District of Columbia lay within the fact that the law had to be passed by the U.S. Congress.
69. In 1920 the Fess-Capper Physical Education Bill was introduced in Congress. Its purpose was to supply federal financial assistance to the physical education programs conducted by the states, through the creation of a Division of Child Hygiene in the Public Health Service, with authority over children six to eighteen years old in public or private schools. The implementation of the program was to be conducted by medical examiners and nurses, which created opposition from optometrists and other independent health care professionals.

    Optometric commentary on the bill can be found in the following articles: Modify or Defeat the Tess Bill, *Optical Journal and Review of Optometry*, vol. 46, no. 16, Oct. 14, 1920, pp. 1073–1074; Judge Rogers Prepares Able Analysis of Fess Bill and Gives His Reasons for Urging Its Defeat, *Optical Journal and Review of Optometry*, vol. 47, no. 4, Jan. 27, 1921, p. 42; Michigan Legislature Endorses Fess Bill—Strong Protest Sent to Legislators by Optometry Board's President, *Optical Journal and Review of Optometry*, vol. 47, no. 8, Feb. 24, 1921, pp. 39–40; and AOA Counsel Explains to Rotarians the Evils of the Fess Bill and the Proposed Changes, *Optical Journal and Review of Optometry*, vol. 47, no. 11, Mar. 17, 1921, p. 48.
70. A retrospective on this era and the legal heritage it brought to the profession can be found in the following article: Kohn, H., A Legal and Anecdotal History of Optometry, *Journal of the American Optometric Association*, vol. 38, no. 11, Nov. 1967, pp. 949–955.
71. The number of legal actions instituted by boards of optometry during this era is overwhelming. An appreciation for the wide range of litigation instituted by these boards can be obtained by reviewing annotations in the *American Law Reports*: One Who Fills Prescriptions Under Reciprocal Arrangement with Physician or Optometrist as Subject to Charge of Practice of Medicine or Optometry Without License, 121 A.L.R. 1455; What Constitutes Practice of "Optometry," 141 A.L.R. 883 and 88 A.L.R.2d 1290; Constitutionality of Statutes and Validity of Regulations Relating to Optometry, 98 A.L.R. 905; Validity of Governmental Regulation of Optometry 22 A.L.R.2d 939; Right of Corporation, or Individual Not Himself Licensed, To Practice Optometry Through Licensed Employee, 102 A.L.R. 343 and 128 A.L.R. 585; and Fitting of Contact Lenses as Practice of Optometry, 77 A.L.R. 3d 810.
72. During this period the literature abounded with blow-by-blow descriptions of the legal struggle to "purify" the practice of optometry from commercial taint. Examples of these reports can be found in the following articles: Corporations Knocked Out of Optometry Practice In West Virginia, *Optical Journal and Review of Optometry*, vol. 72, no. 2, Jan. 15, 1935, pp. 20–21; Corporation Cannot Practice Optometry, *Optical Journal and Review of Optometry*, vol. 72, no. 6, Mar. 15, 1935. pp. 18–20; Glorious Victory—Profession Gets Perpetual Injunction From Ohio's Court of Appeals Against Department Store Practicing Optometry Directly or Indirectly, *Optical Journal and Review of Optometry*, vol. 72, no. 14, July 15, 1935, p. 25; Short "Ad" Texts, *Optical Journal and Review of Optometry*, vol. 72, no. 18, Sept. 15, 1935, p. 28; Effect of Two Supreme Court Decisions Upon Optometry Legislation and Rules of Boards of Examiners, *Optical Journal and Review of Optometry*, vol. 72, no. 20, Oct. 15, 1935, pp. 20–21; Legality of Corporate Practice of Optometry, *Optical Journal and Review of Optometry*, vol. 74, no. 13, July 1, 1937, pp. 24–29; Massachusetts Victory, *Optical Journal and Review of Optometry*, vol. 74, no. 19, Oct. 1, 1937, p. 38; New California Optometry Rules, *Optical Journal and Review of Optometry*, vol. 74, no. 18, Sept. 15, 1937, pp. 24–25; A Court Decision of Great Importance, *Optical Journal and Review of Optometry*, vol. 81, no. 16, Aug. 15, 1944, pp. 22–23; Revocation Of Optometrist's License for Practicing for Unlicensed Employer, *Optical Journal and Review of Optometry*, vol. 81, no. 18, Sept. 15, 1944, pp. 24–26, and vol. 81, no. 19, Oct. 1, 1944, pp. 24–25; Divergent Opinion on City Ordinances Banning Eyeglass Price Advertising, *Optical Journal and Review of Optometry*, vol. 82, no. 8, Apr. 15, 1945, pp. 25–27; and New Jersey Ban on Displays Upheld—Branch Offices Limited to Two—Examination Records Held Property of Prescribing Optometrist, *Optical Journal and Review of Optometry*, vol. 87, no. 21, Nov. 1, 1950, p. 50.
73. The rationale for elevating the practice of optometry is well described by Hirsch and Wick, supra note 1, at 123–177.
74. A summary of the attitude of ophthalmology during this period can be found in Eger, M., The Degradation of a Profession, *Journal of the American Optometric Association*, vol. 53, no. 6, June 1982, pp. 453–454.
75. Although the professionalization of optometry was opposed by an array of foes, it often seemed as though optometrists were attempting to emulate the Pogo cartoon, in which Pogo exclaims, "We have met the enemy, and the enemy is us." For an example of the type of internal struggle that raged within, see Hutchinson, E.A., Optometry, Or What Have You?, *Optical Journal and Review of Optometry*, vol. 74, no. 22, Nov. 15, 1937, p. 24; and the opposing view expressed by Glazer, W.H., A New Eye Man Must Be Born, *Optical Journal and Review of Optometry*, vol. 74, no. 23, Dec. 1, 1937, p. 24.
76. For an assessment of the progress of optometric education during this formative era, see Hutchinson,

E.A., Optometric Education 1891–1951, *Optical Journal and Review of Optometry*, vol. 88, no. 2, Jan. 15, 1951, pp. 78–88; and Gregg, J.R., New Era in Optometric Education, *Journal of the American Optometric Association*, vol. 35, no. 4, Apr. 1964, pp. 291–294. See also Hirsch and Wick, supra note 1, at 157–170.

77. Part of the motivation for the intense legislative struggle was the search for identity that gripped optometrists during these turbulent decades. This struggle manifested itself in the legislative arena with the efforts of optometrists to obtain a satisfactory definition of optometry. For an interesting analysis of this still ongoing process, see Haffner, A.N., The Definition of Optometry, *Optical Journal and Review of Optometry*, vol. 103, no. 22, Nov. 15, 1966, pp. 31–39.
78. A review of the Flexner report and its dramatic aftermath can be found in Stevens, supra note 21, at 68.
79. The malaise which permeated optometry in the mid-1950s is well captured by Gregg, supra note 33, at 223–268.
80. Described in Fitch, supra note 37, at 160.
81. Id. at 239–242.
82. The legal actions instituted by boards of optometry can be found in the following *American Law Reports* annotations: 98 A.L.R. 905, 22 A.L.R.2d 939; 102 A.L.R. 343, 128 A.L.R. 585; 121 A.L.R. 1455, 141 A.L.R. 883, 88 A.L.R.2d 1290, and 77 A.L.R.3d 810.
83. The courts also exhibited a notable degree of confusion over optometry's status under the law. One example will demonstrate the courts' uncertainty over the nature of the optometric service. In *Silver v. Lansburgh and Brothers*, 111 F.2d 518 (D.C. Cir. 1940), the court attempted to justify its decision to permit the corporate practice of optometry with this rationale:

    But we prefer to rest our views upon the broader distinction arising out of the traditional relationship between physician and patient and attorney and client, a relationship which does not exist in optometry. . . . In this view we may very well concede that optometry is a profession, as the term is now colloquially used, but that fact is not enough to bring the rule into effect. There is no more reason to prohibit a corporation, organized for the purpose, from employing licensed optometrists, than there is to prohibit similar employment of accountants, architects, or engineers.

    Contrast this opinion with the views expressed in *State of Kansas ex rel. Beck v. Goldman Jewelry Co.*, 142 Kan. 881, 51 P.2d 995 (1935), in which the court—in deciding against the corporate practice of optometry—stated (quoting from *Stern v. Flynn*, 154 Misc. 609, 278 N.Y.S. 598, at 602–603):

    The relationship between an optometrist and his patient is of a personal and confidential nature, not unlike the relationship between an attorney and client, or physician and patient. The examination of an optometrist may not only indicate an eye condition, but may disclose other ailments and bodily afflictions of a more or less personal nature. True, the optometrist may not lawfully treat his patient for these ailments, but his patient is entitled to the assurance that the knowledge obtained in such examination shall be held inviolate and not become a record in the files of a business corporation. The practice of law by a corporation in this state is prohibited by statute, but quite apart from the statute, it is and was before the enactment of the statute against the public policy of this state.

    Such divided opinions required decades to resolve. Today, optometry is universally accepted as a profession and, in some jurisdictions, as a learned profession.
84. This episode, which details the end of the itinerant seller of spectacles, is found in Fitch, supra note 37, at 195.
85. *Harris v. State Board of Optometrical Examiners*, 287 Pa. 531, 135 A. 237 (Pa. 1926), the decision of which is transcribed in id. at 200–206.
86. *Roschen v. Ottinger* and *Kresge v. Ottinger*, 29 F.2d 762 (S.D. N.Y. 1928).
87. *Roschen v. Ward*, 279 U.S. 337, 49 S. Ct. 336 (1929).
88. At the time of the founding of the American Academy of Optometry (1922), according to Hirsch and Wick, supra note 1, at 153, only "a handful" of the nation's optometrists could meet the modest qualifications for membership. Thus this decision, although of little importance today, represented an important milestone for optometrists of the 1920s.
89. In every state an apprenticeship of one, two, or three years permitted a candidate for licensure to take the state board examination.
90. Interestingly, a similar educational impetus in the 1960s led to the second generation of optometry laws that were first enacted in the 1970s.
91. Ind. Code §25-24-1-4 (1982). This statute has been subjected to legal attack in recent years by the Indiana Academy of Ophthalmology and Otolaryngology, by way of a lawsuit against the State Board of Optometry, State Board of Pharmacy, and State Board of Health, questioning the use of legend drugs by optometrists under a "Joint Statement of Agreement or Understanding" between the three boards. This action was ultimately dismissed by the court, in *Indiana Academy of Ophthalmology and Otolaryngology, Inc. v. Indiana State Board of Registration and Examination in Optometry*, Superior Court, Marion County, S 480 0191, 1983. The Indiana Court of Appeals subsequently upheld the dismissal. See 481 N.E.2d 179 (Ind. 1985).
92. The idea of defining optometry on the basis of what is taught in schools of optometry has re-emerged in recent years and poses an interesting alternative to the confining and limited statutes of the past. See Chapter 9.
93. Described in Fitch, supra note 37, at 350.

94. Apparently the earliest efforts to recognize the fitting of contact lenses as part of the practice of optometry arose out of Attorneys' General opinions in the states of Colorado (1945), California (1946), and Illinois (1946). See California Opinion Upholds Drugless Contact-Lens Fitting by Optometrists–Bars Dispensers, *Optical Journal and Review of Optometry*, vol. 83, no. 5, Feb. 15, 1946, p. 44; and 1946 Illinois Atty. Gen. Rep. No. 427 at 165.

    Many court cases evolved from attempts by opticians to incorporate the fitting of contact lenses into opticianry. Where the optometry statute expressly included the fitting of contact lenses as part of the definition of optometry, the courts have uniformly held that opticians who fitted lenses were in violation of the law. See *New Jersey State Board of Optometrists v. Reiss*, 83 N.J. Super. 47, 198 A.2d 816 (1964); *Kelly ex rel. Michigan Board of Examiners v. Peterson*, 4 Mich. App. 612, 145 N.W.2d 386 (1966); and *Melton v. Ezell*, 250 S.C. 183, 156 S.E.2d 871 (1967).

    When the optometry statute did not specifically mention contact lens fitting within the definition of optometry, the courts have generally held that the fitting of contact lenses constitutes the practice of optometry. Perhaps the leading case in this regard is *People ex rel. Watson v. House of Vision*, 59 Ill. 2d 508, 322 N.E.2d 15 (1974), but see also *Delaware Optometric Corp. v. Sherwood*, 36 Del. Ch. 223, 128 A.2d 812 (1957); *State of Oregon ex rel. Reed v. Kuzirian*, 228 Or. 619, 365, P.2d 1046 (1961); *Ketring v. Sturges*, 372 S.W.2d 104 (Mo. 1963); *Louisiana State Board of Optometry Examiners v. Pearle Optical, Inc.*, 177 So.2d 164 (La. App. 1965), *annulled on other grounds*, 184 So.2d 10; and *Pennsylvania Optometric Association v. DiGiovanni*, 45 Pa. D.&C. 2d 245 (1968).

    Some courts have held that the fitting of contact lenses by opticians is not the practice of optometry where the fitting is made in accordance with a prescription written by an optometrist or physician. See *High v. Ridgeway's Opticians*, 258 N.C. 626, 129 S.E.2d 301 (1963); *State Board of Optometry v. Chester*, 251 Miss. 250, 169 So.2d 468 (1964); *Florida Association of Dispensing Opticians v. Florida State Board of Optometry*, 238 So.2d 839 (1970), *conformed to* 239 So.2d 520 (Fla. App. 1970); *State of Kansas ex rel. Londerholm v. Doolin*, 209 Kan. 244, 497 P.2d 138 (1972); and *State of Oklahoma ex rel. Clifton v. Reeser*, 543 P.2d 1379 (1975). Contra: *Fields v. District of Columbia*, 232 F.2d 300 (D.C. Cir. 1967); *State of Missouri ex rel. Danforth v. Dale Curteman, Inc.*, 480 S.W.2d 848 (1972); and *New Jersey State Board of Optometrists v. Reiss*, 83 N.J. Super. 47, 198 A.2d 816 (1964).

95. Perhaps the leading case on the use of tonometry by optometrists is *Winograd v. Johnson*, 561 P.2d 1274 (Colo. App. 1976), in which the court held that, under the state statute, optometrists were permitted to employ tonometry.

96. Lancaster, W.B., The Optometry Problem, *Journal of the American Medical Association*, vol. 91, no. 24, Dec. 15, 1928, pp. 1847–1848. Also reported in the *Optometric Weekly* of Dec. 27, 1928, with subsequent commentaries on pp. 1575–1576; and in *The Optical Journal and Review of Optometry*, vol. 62, no. 18, Dec. 21, 1928, p. 35. For another account of Lancaster's remarks and the interest they generated, see Fitch, supra note 37, at 298–306.

97. For an annotation of cases, see 102 A.L.R. 343 and 128 A.L.R. 585.

98. A description of these cases is presented by Haffner, A.N., The Definition Of Optometry, *Optical Journal and Review of Optometry*, vol. 103, no. 22, Nov. 15, 1966, pp. 31–39.

99. According to AOA Counsel Harold Kohn, who was a participant and observer during this period, these cases were an inevitable part of the struggle to improve the profession and had to be maintained, despite the roller-coaster effect they had on the times. See Kohn, H., A Legal and Anecdotal History of Optometry, supra note 70.

100. *Semler v. Oregon State Board of Dental Examiners*, 294 U.S. 608, 55 S. Ct. 570 (1935). Much of the decision, written by Chief Justice Hughes, is quoted by Hirsch and Wick, supra note 1, at 181–184.

101. For an example of how damaging the tactics of the unscrupulous could be, see Riis, R., Optometry On Trial, *Reader's Digest*, Aug., Sept., and Oct. 1937, and commentaries in the *Optical Journal and Review of Optometry* that resulted from this article (which severely injured the self-esteem of optometrists of the day): The End of the Trial, vol. 74, no. 19, Oct. 1, 1937, pp. 24–25; and Some Public Reactions, vol. 74, no. 20, Oct. 15, 1937, p. 21. The *Reader's Digest* articles are also discussed by Hirsch and Wick, supra note 1, at 251–255.

102. The campaign against advertising and the moral justification for the professionalization of optometry are well described by Hirsch and Wick, supra note 1, at 170–177.

103. The legal campaign even involved the use of city ordinances to ban price advertising. See Simpson, J., Divergent Opinion on City Ordinances Banning Eyeglass Price Advertising, *Optical Journal and Review of Optometry*, vol. 82, no. 8, Apr. 15, 1945. pp. 25–27.

104. See Annot., Validity of Governmental Regulation of Optometry, 22 A.L.R.2d 939.

105. When the Federal Trade Commission published its trade regulation rule in 1976, investigators maintained that forty-five states had laws that restricted ophthalmic advertising in some form. Thus the reform effort was certainly a successful one, albeit not completely so.

106. Apparently the first appellate case alleging optometric malpractice was *Hampton v. Brackin's Jewelry and Optical Co, Inc.*, 237 Ala. 212, 186 So. 173 (1939).

107. Riis, supra note 101.

108. This unfortunate episode is recounted by Fitch, supra note 37, at 295–296, and in Gregg, supra note 33, at 141–142.
109. The Wagner Bill is discussed by Koch, C.C., Possible Effects of Public Health Programs Upon Optometry, *American Journal of Optometry and Archives of American Academy of Optometry*, vol. 22, no. 3, Mar. 1945, pp. 135–139.
110. This problem is discussed by Gregg, supra note 33, at 184–185. A sense of outrage spurred many of the optometrists who had been forced to serve as enlisted men to agitate for change. See also Hofstetter, supra note 1, at 108–119. Although a separate corps for optometrists was approved by Congress, it died by Presidential veto, never to be revived. Commissioned rank for optometrists, however, has become a reality, and although there are still inequities between physician and optometrist benefits in the armed services, the situation is a completely different one than during World War II.
111. According the Hofstetter, supra note 1, at 129–131:

> In the earliest years of the century practically all optometrists were in "stores," and therefore in "downstairs" locations. As soon as the new supply of optometrists began coming through institutional channels instead of through apprenticeship channels there was started a trend to establish practices in "upstairs" offices. . . . Although statistics showing the trend are not available for the early years, it is apparent from the reminiscences of the older practitioners of today that the merits of the idea were quickly recognized, and that many profession-minded optometrists previously established in "downstairs" locations also made the change, so that by 1925 almost one-fourth of the optometrists were in "upstairs" offices.

112. The reforms urged by the American Academy of Optometry and the American Optometric Association were all-encompassing and by their pervasiveness managed to cast optometrists in a new light, one which gradually illuminated the path to professionalism. Examples of the passion of the day can be found throughout the literature: Andreae, J.F., AAO Calls on AOA for Drive Against Store Fronts, Display Windows, Neon Signs, and Inside Show Cases, *Optical Journal and Review of Optometry*, vol. 72, no. 23, Dec. 1, 1935, p. 28; AOA Department of Ethics and Economics, at Cincinnati Conference, Sets Up Guide Lines for Professional Advancement, *Optical Journal and Review of Optometry*, vol. 81, no. 20, Oct. 15, 1944, p. 32; Kintner, G.E., Report of the Conference of the Department of Ethics and Economics of the AOA, *Journal of the American Optometric Association*, vol. 15, no. 11, Nov. 1944, pp. 91–92; Listing of Optometrists in Telephone Directories (survey), *Optical Journal and Review of Optometry*, vol. 82, no. 22, Nov. 15, 1945, pp. 26–27; AOA Department Considers Code of Ethics and the Ethics and Economics of Industrial Optometry and Contact Lens Fitting, *Optical Journal and Review of Optometry*, vol. 83, no. 1, Jan. 1, 1946, p. 40; Ethics-Economics Meeting in Cincinnati, *Journal of the American Optometric Association*, vol. 17, no. 1, Jan. 1946, p. 165; Palmer, J.A., Ethics and Economics, Parts 1 and 2, Publications of the Professional Advancement Program of the American Optometric Association, 1943; Kintner, G.F., Ethics and Economics, *Optical Journal and Review of Optometry*, vol. 83, no. 17, Sept. 1, 1946, pp. 34–35; AOA-Recommended Standards for Outdoor Signs, Upstairs and Street Level Lettering, *Optical Journal and Review of Optometry*, vol. 85, no. 8, May 1, 1948, p. 59. There followed a Code of Ethics, a Supplement to the Code, and The Rules of Practice (see Chapter 3).
113. These guidelines were tremendously detailed, providing a comprehensive guide for the daily practice of optometry, including fees; restrictions on soliciting, advertising, displays, guarantees, and offers of free examinations; listings in public directories; names and initials used on cards; stationery; billheads; signs; patents; and numerous other matters.
114. Attorney MacCracken, who was already an influential voice in optometric political matters at the time, was able to effect a change in this policy so that optometry was reclassified as a profession. See also *Hofstetter*, supra note 1, at 102–103; *Optometric Weekly*, vol. 43, no. 26, June 26, 1952, p. 1064; and Gregg, supra note 33, for multiple references to "Mr. Mac," beginning at p. 180.
115. Mr. McCracken was more than just an influential attorney. He was also one of America's premier aviators. His life is interestingly chronicled by Michael Osborn and Joseph Riggs in "*Mr. Mac*," Southern College of Optometry, Memphis, 1970.
116. Described in "*Mr. Mac*," supra note 115, at 204–205.
117. The key legislator was the chairman of the House Ways and Means Committee, who was from North Carolina. The Congressman drafted his own amendment to the law, which specified that any state welfare program, in order to get funds, would have to provide that the applicant for aid was free to have his eyes examined by an optometrist or physician skilled in diseases of the eye. His initiative eventually prevailed in both House and Senate. See "*Mr. Mac*," supra note 115, at 204–205.
118. According to Gideon Lang, O.D., a North Carolina optometrist who was active in AOA political affairs during the 1940s, 1950s, and 1960s, a 1964 Senate hearing over the participation of optometrists in Title 16 of the Social Security Act provided this amusing confrontation between optometry and ophthalmology:

> When the bill came up before the Senate Finance Committee we were ready. Medicine had brought its top lawyers from Chicago to crush us at the hearing. We had gotten wind of the fact that they had cases to show that optometrists had

missed pathology and that patients had gone blind. Mr. Mac and Harold Kohn, the congenial General Counsel of the AOA, sent out word to optometrists all over the country to send in reports of cases of pathology that had been referred but the ophthalmologist missed the pathology or ruled it insignificant, so that the patient had to be referred to another physician. We received 39 reports in time for the hearing (later the total exceeded 2,500). Two of the 39 had been brain tumor cases. It was decided the night before at Mr. Mac's office—and over his protest—that we would play a trick. He was the most respectable and honest person anywhere, and the plan did not originate with him. We decided to bring a dolly into the hearing room and have it loaded with empty boxes, with the 39 cases in the box on top. Dave Sharman, who had opened an office for the AOA in Washington, obtained the dolly. He, John Costabile and I pushed this apparently very heavy dolly into the Senate hallway across from where 7 or 8 ophthalmologists and lawyers from the AMA were standing. Mr. Mac went to speak with them, as he knew the attorneys from his Bar Association relationships. He pointed to the dolly and told them that he was going to put "every one" of these cases into the Congressional Record, some of which were brain tumors that had been missed by ophthalmologists, and that they would be so busy defending malpractice suits that they would never get back to Washington in their lifetime. Then he walked away. The look of shock that came over the group was one I'll never forget.

Optometry had never been up against medicine this way. We had Dr. John O'Shea, the AOA President from Massachusetts, and myself among those to testify. We had agreed among ourselves to temper the amendment so we would not be on a par with physicians skilled in diseases of the eye, which was a mistake. Fortunately, the AMA lawyers called Mr. Mac back over and said they would not oppose our amendment as proposed in the Senate and the bill passed. When the House and Senate Conference Committee convened and got to our amendment, the House version was kept intact. It is still the law today.

From *History of Optometry*, by Gideon Lang, O.D., a personal memoir to be published in the *Journal of the American Optometric Association*. The author is grateful to Dr. Lang for sharing this interesting episode.

119. Hofstetter, supra note 1.
120. An interesting account of the dispute between the American Optometric Association and the American Medical Association can be found in Stevens, supra note 78, at 103–114.
121. See id. at 108–109 for a review of how ethical restrictions were used by ophthalmology against optometry.
122. A description of the 1950 AMA resolution, and the developments that led to its adoption, can be found in Gregg, supra note 33, at 223–224.
123. As a result of the use of physician's assistants by ophthalmologists, legislative efforts were mounted by optometrists to limit the ability of physician's assistants to perform refractions, an effort that eventually led to restrictions in forty-five states. *Bulletin from the Counsel of the AOA*, vol. 42, no. 15, Sept. 6, 1983.
124. The text of this unfortunate resolution can be found in Gregg, supra note 33, at 251–252.
125. The October 1954 issue of *Guildcraft* was by and large devoted to the issue of "The Stated Purposes Of Optometry As Disclosed By Official Utterances At The National Level" and contained the observation that "There is no limit expressed as to how much of the visual care field optometry wants; for frankly, it wants it all."
126. Gregg, supra note 33, at 254, understates the interprofessional difficulties that shook both optometry and ophthalmology during this period. See also Koch, C.C., Resolutions Dealing with Interprofessional Relations, *American Journal of Optometry and Archives of the American Academy of Optometry*, vol. 32, no. 8, Aug. 1955, pp. 432–434.
127. Resolution No. 77, adopted by the House of Delegates of the AMA in June, 1955, provided that "it is unethical for any doctor of medicine to teach in any school or college of optometry, or to lecture to any optometric organization, or to contribute scientific material to the optometric literature, or in any way to impart technical medical knowledge to non-medical practitioners." Commentary on this resolution can be found in Elmstrom, G., Return to the "Status Quo Ante"—Time for Self-Evaluation, *Optical Journal and Review of Optometry*, vol. 92, no. 21, Nov. 1, 1955, pp. 39–40.
128. Ophthalmologists had begun to practice dispensing years before the resolution was adopted, a change in the ethics of the profession that was not greeted with favor in all sectors. See Medical Ethics and Philosophy Involved in Dispensing of Glasses by Ophthalmologists, *American Journal of Ophthalmology*, vol. 37, no. 3, Mar. 1954, pp. 439–443. The AMA resolution can be found in *Optical Journal and Review of Optometry*, vol. 92, no. 14, July 1955, pp. 43–44.
129. The old expression that nothing is new can be applied to the current efforts of certain ophthalmologists who have propounded and even introduced mandatory referral legislation. These 20/40 referral laws were being proposed—with equal lack of success—back in the 1950s. See Nuisance Legislation?, *Optometric Weekly*, vol. 46, no. 19, May 12, 1955, p. 775. For a contemporary commentary, see Pavlichko, J.L., Taking Medicine's Pulse, *Review of Optometry*, vol. 120, no. 1, Jan. 1983, pp. 35–43.
130. The tone of the era was perfectly captured by AOA president James Wahl at the Heart of America Contact Lens Congress in 1953, when he gave an address

entitled Creeping Death. See Gregg, supra note 33, at 241–242.

131. The resolution that was passed unanimously contained these provisions:

Whereas, the purpose of both optometry and ophthalmology has been and is to give the best professional care to the public, and any misunderstanding between ophthalmology and optometry can only work to the detriment of the public and of both professions; now, therefore be it

Resolved, first, that the American Optometric Association does hereby declare that it is not the intention of the profession to eliminate exemption now granted ophthalmology;

Resolved, second, that the American Optometric Association does hereby declare that it is not the intention of optometry to enter into or engage in the practice of ophthalmology, and the American Optometric Association reiterates and reaffirms Resolution No. 3 adopted at the 41st Annual Congress on June 26, 1938, which reads as follows:

Whereas, the physiological eye care known as optometry and surgical eye care known as ophthalmology are two separate and distinct professions, each requiring the whole time, thought and attention of the practitioners of each respective art and science; now therefore, be it

Resolved, that the American Optometric Association goes on record as desiring the complete cooperation of the two professions, with emphasis on the fact that optometry has no desire to extend its practice to include any limited or other form of medical eye care.

See id. at 253 for the full text.

132. Shortly after the AOA's brief of complaint was filed with the Justice Department, Bass announced his lawsuit against the AMA, causing the Justice Department to suspend action on the AOA complaint. This doubtless was a major cause of the lack of enthusiasm on the AOA's part for the *Bass* case. See Bailey, J.H., Carel C. Koch Memorial Lecture: The Four-Eyed Man, *American Journal of Optometry and Physiological Optics*, vol. 6, no. 60, 1983, pp. 421–424.

133. *Dr. Cyrus Bass v. The American Medical Association*, Civil Action 64 C 1279, United States District Court for the Northern District of Illnois, July 24, 1964. A detailed summary of the proceedings of the case can be found in Bass's *Report to the Optometric Profession*, a copy of which can be obtained from the International Library, Archives, and Museum of Optometry, St. Louis.

134. The case began as a relatively modest item, as noted in the optometric literature (see Optometrists File Suit Against The AMA, *Optical Journal and Review of Optometry*, vol. 101, no. 16, Aug. 15, 1964), but by its conclusion had generated sufficient controversy to make it a leading subject for review. See Some Facts in the Case of Bass Versus the AMA, *Optometric Weekly*, vol. 58, no. 22, June 1, 1967, pp. 27–28; A Special Report: U.S. Court Stipulation Order Ends Bass Versus AMA Suit, *Optometric Weekly*, vol. 58, no. 22, June 1, 1967, pp. 15–18; Bass Anti-Trust Action Against American Medical Association Dismissed on Stipulation—Memorandum Opinion of Court, *Optical Journal and Review of Optometry*, vol. 104, no. 11, June 1, 1967, pp. 29–31.

135. Bass's view of how the AOA's opposition affected his case is voiced in his *Report to the Optometric Profession*, supra note 133. Decades later, the argument over the case continues within the profession. See Optometry Under Siege! Will History Repeat Itself?, *Optometric Management*, vol. 16, no. 8, Aug. 1980, p. 34.

136. Quoted in the memorandum opinion of Judge Abraham Marovitz of 28 April 1967, a copy of which can be found in *Optical Journal and Review of Optometry*, vol. 104, no. 11, June 1, 1967, p. 30.

137. The complete opinion is quoted in *Optometric Weekly*, vol. 58, No. 22, June 1, 1967, pp. 15–18.

138. *Lee Optical of Oklahoma v. Williamson*, 120 F. Supp 128 (D.C. Okla. 1954).

139. The optometrists of Oklahoma had been able to secure passage of a model law that regulated the practice of optometry within the state. The statute was immediately attacked by commercial optometrists and opticians, who argued that the law was unconstitutional and filed suit in federal court. The decision of the federal court was, surprisingly, in favor of the commercialists, although the seeds of this decision may be contained in the definitions of the various factions adopted by the court. Ophthalmologists were referred to as pure professionals, opticians as skilled artisans, and optometrists as quasiprofessionals. Id. at 131.

140. 348 U.S. 483, 75 S. Ct. 461 (1955).

141. 75 S. Ct. at 466.

142. The Federal Trade Commission Staff Report issued in 1977 as part of the Eyeglasses I trade regulation rule found that twenty-five states had legal restrictions prohibiting all forms of media advertising by optometrists. A total of thirty-five states prohibited advertising of discounts or premiums; twenty-five limited telephone directory listings; and thirty prohibited the employment of optometrists by lay persons or firms.

143. 70 N.M. 90, 370 P.2d 811, *affirmed* 374 U.S. 424, 83 S. Ct. 1759 (1963). Discussed in *Optical Journal and Review of Optometry*, vol. 100, no. 13, July 1, 1963, p. 34.

144. The Rules of Practice, when proposed in 1952, caused widespread internal dissention in the AOA. See Gregg, supra note 33, at 233–234. The profound changes wrought by the rules over the following two decades are chronicled by Dr. Gregg at 302–303, 306, 312, 317, and 322.

145. Hirsch and Wick, supra note 1, at 175.

146. A chronological list of contact lens patents can be found in Appendix II of Filderman, I.P., and P.F.

White, *Contact Lens: Practice and Patient Management*, Chilton, Philadelphia, 1969.
147. Wichterle, O., and D. Lim, Hydrophilic gels for biological use, *Nature*, vol. 185, 1960, pp. 117–118.
148. Discussed by Gregg, supra note 33, at 271–272. An example of the interest within the profession can be found in a special report, *New Jersey State Board of Optometrists v. Reiss, American Journal of Optometry and Archives of American Academy of Optometry*, vol. 41, no. 7, July 1964, pp. 438–445.
149. See *State of Oregon ex rel. Reed v. Kuzirian*, 288 Or. 619, 365 P.2d 1046 (1961). See also 88 A.L.R.2d 1284.
150. See Feld, L.G., The Optometrist and Contact Lenses: Legal Liability Without Fault!, *Optical Journal and Review of Optometry*, vol. 107, no. 9, May 1, 1970, pp. 32–35; and Lane, M.J., The Legal Risks You Run Prescribing Contacts, *Optometric Management*, vol. 13, no. 3, Mar. 1977, pp. 53–61.
151. The tonometer was described in Mackay, R.S., and E. Marg, Fast, Automatic, Electronic Tonometer Based on an Exact Theory, *Acta Ophthalmologica*, vol. 37, 1959, pp. 495–507.
152. Moses, R.A., E. Marg and R. Oechsli, Evaluation of the Basic Validity and Clinical Usefulness of the Mackay-Marg Tonometer, *Investigative Ophthalmology*, vol. 1, no. 1, Feb. 1962.
153. Grolman, B., A New Tonometer System, *American Journal of Optometry and Archives of American Academy of Optometry*, vol. 49, no. 8, Aug. 1972, pp. 646–660.
154. All figures are based on economic surveys conducted by the American Optometric Association. The 1929 and 1944 figures are quoted by Hofstetter, supra note 1, at 152–154. The 1958 survey was published as a report by the AOA. The 1968 and 1977 figures have been published in the *AOA News*. The 1987 figure may be found in the March 1, 1988 edition of the *AOA News*.
155. For background information on the evolution of Medicaid, see Newcomb, R., and J. Jolley, *Public Health and Community Optometry*, Charles C. Thomas, Springfield, Ill., 1980, pp. 262–265.
156. See 42 U.S.C. §1395 et seq.
157. There were early warnings about the impact of Medicaid and its effect on medical control of eye care, the setting of fees for optometrists, and professional standards for services and materials. See Editorial, The progress of "Medicaid"—Bigger than "Medicare"?, *Optical Journal and Review of Optometry*, vol. 103, no. 22, Nov. 15, 1966, p. 52; and Haffner, A.N., Title 19: When a Sleeper Wakes Up, *Optometric Management*, vol. 3, no. 7, July 1967, pp. 15–24.
158. The increasing federalization of Medicaid and the erosion of optometric services are discussed by Haffner, A.N., The Destruction of Medicaid, *Optometric Weekly*, vol. 67, no. 15, Nov. 4, 1976, pp. 13–16.
159. Public Law 89–97, 42 U.S.C. §1395 et seq. For the history of Medicare, see Newcomb and Jolley, *Public Health and Community Optometry*, supra note 155, at 258–262.
160. Section 1862, titled Exclusions from Coverage, provides that no payment shall be made for services:

   (7) Where such expenses are for routine physical checkups, eyeglasses or eye examinations for the purpose of prescribing, fitting, or changing eyeglasses, hearing aids, or examination therefor, or immunizations.

   Thus reimbursement for routine refractive services has never been allowed under Medicare.
161. The difficulty faced by optometrists was that patients sent to ophthalmologists for cataract surgery could be managed after surgery by the ophthalmologist, including the dispensing of ophthalmic materials, thus preventing the optometrist's participation in patient care altogether. The situation is described by AOA General Counsel Harold Kohn as follows: "As a result of our conference, we arrived at the understanding that when, after surgery, *a patient is referred to an optometrist*, and the optometrist provides the patient with the prosthetic lenses, payment can be made to him for the lenses, including payment for his services in making the refraction" (emphasis added). Kohn also delicately observed that "It was recognized that there are practical considerations involved with respect to the matter of referrals. This primarily is the relationship between the ophthalmologist and the optometrist. If the ophthalmologist retains the patient, this is a matter in which the administration [the Social Security Administration] definitely stated it cannot become involved." *Bulletin from the General Counsel*, vol. 25, no. 34, Oct. 10, 1966.
162. The necessity for amending Medicare was recognized immediately. See Editorial, A Vital Amendment to Medicare Is Recommended, *Optometric Weekly*, vol. 58, no. 2, Jan. 19, 1967, pp. 33–34. The AOA's efforts were vigorously opposed by ophthalmology and organized medicine. See Optometry Inclusion In Title 18 Opposed, *AMA News*, May 15, 1967; H.E.W. Report and Optometry and Medicare, *Eye Physician*, Feb. 1969, pp. 17–19. The right of optometrists to receive reimbursement for health-related services rendered to aphakic Medicare recipients was not achieved until 1981. The basis for the congressional decision to permit reimbursement of optometrists for eye health services rendered to aphakic patients was due, in part, to a H.E.W. report released in 1976 that recommended the expansion of Medicare to include these services. A lawsuit was filed by the Physician's Education Network to have the report rescinded, but the suit was dismissed by the district court and the dismissal was upheld in the U.S. Court of Appeals. See *Physicians Education Network, Inc. v. the Department of Health, Education, and Welfare*, 653 F.2d 621 (D.C. Cir. 1981). See *AOA News*, June 1, 1980, and May 15, 1981, for accounts of the case.
163. The details of the historic legislation are reported in

the March 1987 edition of *Optometric Management* (vol. 23, no. 3) and the March 15, 1987 edition of *Review of Optometry* (vol. 124, no. 3). See also Garland, J., Optometric Parity Legislation under Medicare, *Journal of the American Optometric Association*, vol. 58, no. 6, 1987, pp. 518–519.

164. AOA President David Ferris proclaimed the Medicare amendment to be "the greatest legislative achievement in the history of optometry." For details see The *AOA News* of Nov. 1, 1986, and Classe, J., 1986: Optometry in the Eyes of the Law, *Optometric Management*, vol. 23, no. 2, 1987, pp. 47–52.

165. Despite the judicial and legislative success achieved by optometrists, as of 1987 the Texas Medicaid program refuses to reimburse optometrists for health-related services rendered to Medicaid-eligible patients, choosing instead to reimburse physicians only for these services.

166. For a discussion of the importance of third-party vision service plans, see Newcomb and Jolley, supra note 155. Other examples of the fight mustered by optometrists to participate in vision service benefit plans include CHAMPUS and Blue Cross/Blue Shield. In 1979, after several years of disagreement, the Civilian Health and Medical Program of the Uniformed Services (CHAMPUS) "clarified" its position to include optometrists as eligible providers of health-related vision services "essential to the diagnosis and treatment of illness and injury," the same services for which physicians could receive reimbursement. And in 1981, five Pennsylvania optomerists were elected to district membership in the state Blue Cross/Blue Shield corporation, the first time optometrists had been represented on a Blue Cross/Blue Shield corporation in the United States.

167. See Drucker, S., The Challenge of the Hart Bill: Take the Profit Out of Eyeglasses, *Optical Journal and Review of Optometry*, vol. 103, no. 8, Apr. 15, 1966, p. 44.

168. See Statement by Senator Hart, *Guild Guide*, vol. 8, no. 4, Apr. 1967, pp. 13–14.

169. Described by Prentice, supra note 6, at 94–96.

170. For example, see the resolution of 1938, re-adopted in 1955, which stated bluntly that, "optometry has no desire to extend its practice to include any limited or other form of medical eye care." See note 131 supra.

171. If the use of drugs was not specifically described in the state optometry practice act, practitioners in the state could reasonably infer that drug use was not prohibited. (But the definition of optometry in the majority of states contained an express prohibition against the use of drugs.) As of 1971 there were ten states in which the law was "silent" in this regard. See Field, K.K., Optometry and Drugs—Present and Future, *Optical Journal and Review of Optometry*, vol. 108, no. 24, Dec. 15, 1971, pp. 21–22.

172. See Trumbell, N., Why Rhode Island Optometrists Saw Red, *Optometric Management*, vol. 9, no. 9, Sept. 1973, pp. 29–35.

173. The amendments to optometry practice acts that permitted the use of pharmaceutical agents are chronologically organized in Chapter 8.

174. *Rhode Island Ophthalmological Society v. Cannon*, 317 A.2d 124 (1974). The decision of the Rhode Island Supreme Court can be found in *The Citation*, vol. 29, no. 7, July 15, 1974.

175. The passage of the West Virginia law was aided by the state's unusual legislative procedure that requires only a simple majority (rather than two-thirds) of the legislators to vote to override the governor's veto. The house vote was fifty-nine to thirty-nine and the senate vote was twenty-seven to six. *Bulletin from Counsel of the AOA*, vol. 34, no. 62, Mar. 8, 1976.

176. A post facto report on the therapeutics amendment, prepared by the West Virginia Optometric Association in 1981 (five years after the passage of the bill), averred that since the bill's passage seventy-two different ophthalmic pharmaceutical agents had been employed by optometrists; a total of 47,121 patients had been treated during this period; since referral was not necessary in these cases, the treatment represented a savings of 620,000 miles in travel to these patients; and fifty-two different pathological conditions had been diagnosed and treated by the state's optometrists.

177. The West Virginia law was challenged by state ophthalmologists in *Esposito v. Shapero*, C.A. 76 1214, Cabell County Circuit Court, December 16, 1976. The trial court decision in favor of optometry was appealed to the state supreme court, but review was denied by the court on June 6, 1977, thereby permitting the lower court's determination to stand. *Bulletin from Counsel of the AOA*, vol. 37, no. 10, Sept. 7, 1978.

178. An account of the dispute can be found in *The Denver Post*, Dec. 28, 1976. The case, *Winograd v. Johnson*, 561 P.2d 1274 (Colo. App. 1976), is discussed by Coblens, S., *Optometry and the Law*, American Optometric Association, St. Louis, 1976, p. 25.

179. Classe, J., A Review of Professional Liability Cases Affecting the Practice of Optometry, *Journal of the American Optometric Association*, vol. 57, no. 1, 1986, pp. 66–71.

180. The outcome of the lawsuit in the state of Alabama was an injunction against the state board, prohibiting the board from holding hearings to investigate charges of unprofessional conduct against the commercial optometrists. See 331 F. Supp. 122. From this decision of the federal district court the Alabama State Board of Optometry appealed to the U.S. Supreme Court. An account of the case can be found in Coblens, S., The *Berryhill* Case: a Critique and a Prediction, *American Journal of Optometry and Archives of American Academy of Optometry*, vol. 51, no. 5, May 1974, pp. 347–350.

181. *Gibson v. Berryhill*, 411 U.S. 564, 93 S. Ct. 1689, (1973).

182. 425 U.S. 748, 96 S. Ct. 1817.

183. 433 U.S. 350, 97 S. Ct. 2691.
184. See *The Federal Register*, May 24, 1978.
185. Trade regulation rule on the advertising of ophthalmic goods and services, 16 C.F.R. § 456.
186. For a discussion of the rule and its effects upon the clinical practice of optometry, see Classe, J., The Effects of FTC Rulings on the Practice of Optometry, *Southern Journal of Optometry*, vol. 21, no. 5, May 1979, pp. 20–24. See also, Swallowing the FTC's Bitter Pill, *Review of Optometry*, vol. 115, no. 12, Dec. 15. 1978, p. 41.
187. *American Optometric Association v. Federal Trade Commission*, 626 F.2d 896 (D.C. Cir. 1980).
188. A review of the proceedings of the Nelson hearings can be found in the following issues of *Optometric Weekly*: vol. 68, no. 6, Feb. 10, 1977; vol. 68, no. 16, Apr. 28, 1977; and vol. 68, no. 17, May 5, 1977.
189. The impact of the Nelson hearings was analyzed by Topaz, P., Nelson Does It Again!, *Optometric Weekly*, vol. 68, no. 18, May 12, 1977, pp. 11–14.
190. 440 U.S. 1, 99 S. Ct. 887.
191. 438 F. Supp. 428 (D.C. Tex. 1977).
192. It is ironic to note, however, that in Texas, where the *Friedman* case originated, after the decision of the U.S. Supreme Court commercial optometrists were able to secure the legislative strength necessary to pass a law permitting trade name advertising by optometrists. Thus, even though a state may regulate trade name advertising by optometrists, the opposite result may be obtained if the state legislature is so inclined. For an example of enforcement of trade name restrictions on an optometrist, see *Department of Professional Regulation v. Cohen*, Case No. 0007114 (Florida Board of Optometry), Jan. 28, 1981, reported in *Bulletin From Office of Counsel of the AOA*, vol. 41, no. 23, Jan. 7, 1983.
193. *Effects of Restrictions On Advertising and Commercial Practice in the Professions: The Case Of Optometry*, released May 15, 1980. A description of the report can be found in the *AOA News* of June 1, 1980.
194. The FTC study indicated that in nonrestricted cities, nonadvertising, traditional optometrists give more thorough eye examinations and charge higher prices than advertising and chain firm optometrists. See *AOA News*, June 1, 1980. Evidence of a more compelling kind was gathered in a study performed in 1985 by Robert R. Nathan and Associates in New York City. This study determined that professional optometrists detect ocular pathology, complex refractive conditions, and anomalies of binocular vision twice as frequently as commercial optometrists (less than one-third of whom detected these conditions at all). Not surprisingly, the study also establishes that the time spent with patients is more than twice as long for professional optometrists. A summary of the study can be found in *AOA News*, June 15, 1985. The Nathan firm, in written testimony before the FTC during the Eyeglasses II hearings, also commented that the FTC studies "simply do not provide the sound empirical foundation for a regulation which would affect the vision health and care of the general public." Thus the FTC studies would seem to be flawed, a conclusion also reached by the officer who presided over the Eyeglasses II hearings. See Greenan, J., *Report of the Presiding Officer on Proposed Trade Regulation Rule: Ophthalmic Practice Rules 16 CFR 456*, Federal Trade Commission, Washington, D.C., 1986.
195. *State Restrictions on Vision Care Providers: The Effects On Consumers*, released in July, 1980.
196. The FTC decision will be challenged on a constitutional basis, with the courts being asked to decide if the U.S. Congress has granted the FTC the authority to supercede state laws prohibiting or restricting commercial practice. Interestingly, the head of the FTC—who was the only commissioner to vote against implementing Eyeglasses II—used this lack of legal authority as his reason for refusing to back the rule. See the *AOA News*, March 1, 1988.
197. Some optometrists turned to the courts in an effort to end the discrimination inherent in the reimbursement policies of Medicare and Medicaid. But the Medicare lawsuit—which challenged the constitutionality of sections of the Medicare law—was dismissed by the 5th Circuit Court of Appeals. See *Pushkin v. Califano*, 600 F.2d 486 (5th Cir. 1979). An important case involving Medicaid had a happier outcome. The 5th Circuit Court of Appeals held that the Louisiana freedom-of-choice law prohibited the state from reimbursing ophthalmologists but not optometrists for Medicaid services that were within the scope of practice of optometry. See *Sandefur v. Cherry*, 744 F.2d 1157 (5th Cir. 1984). The case, brought in 1980, has a remarkable history. See 547 F. Supp. 418 (1982), *vacated and remanded* 718 F.2d 682 (1983), and *certified* 721 F.2d 511 (1983).
198. See *Blue Cross of Virginia v. Commonwealth of Virginia*, 269 S.E.2d 827 (1980).
199. See Chapter 11. The litigation of the 1980s and perhaps the 1990s will feature continuing efforts by optometrists to eliminate discriminatory practices in health care reimbursement plans.
200. As of 1985, fourty-five states have adopted statutes prohibiting discrimination in public plans, and fourty-nine states have statutes that prohibit discrimination in private plans. The laws relating to private plans, however, have a much narrower application than do those relating to public plans. See *Bulletin from Office of Counsel of the AOA*, vol. 44, no. 7, July 31, 1985.

Chapter 2

A Short History of Liability in Optometry

The liability of an optometrist to a patient is to be tested by standards analogous to those used to test physicians and surgeons—"whether or not he did fail to exercise the amount of care, skill and diligence as (an optometrist) which is exercised generally in the community. . .in which he was practicing by (other practitioners) in the same field."
—From the decision of Chief Judge Hammond, *Tempchin v. Sampson, 277 A. 2d 67 (1971)*

Legal Basis for Liability Claims
Duty to Refer
Liability for Ophthalmic Materials
Standard of Care
Toward a Medical Standard

Legal Basis for Liability Claims

The responsibility for patient care is, ultimately, a legal responsibility, based on the nature of the duty that is owed by the practitioner to the patient. That duty is established through legislative enactment and judicial interpretation of the resulting law. All fifty states and the District of Columbia have enacted optometry practice acts that define the practice of the profession and, thereby, establish the responsibilities owed by optometrists to their patients. When optometrists have been charged with failing to observe these responsibilities, the courts have been required to analyze their conduct, using statutory requirements and existing common law as guides. From these decisions have emerged precedents that can be applied to optometrists acting under the same or similar circumstances. The brief review that follows describes the leading decisions concerning the professional liability of optometrists decided by appellate courts since the profession's legally authorized beginning in 1901.

The first reported case of optometric malpractice occurred in 1939 in Alabama and established that optometrists would be held to the standard of care expected of professionals.[1]

The services of an optometrist who worked for a jewelry store were advertised in a local paper. A woman who was experiencing difficulty in performing her work saw the advertisement and went to the store for the purpose of receiving an examination and being fitted for glasses. After receiving the glasses, she attempted to wear them but they seemed to hurt her eyes and she returned to the store several times over a period of about six months. Despite these difficulties she was advised to continue wearing the glasses. On the last visit, however, the optometrist discovered that the sight in one of her eyes was "completely gone" and referred her to a physician, who diagnosed the condition as being a detached retina secondary to glaucoma. She sued the optometrist and his employer, the jewelry store, for negligence. After the jury decided against her, she appealed the case to the Alabama Supreme Court. The court, in affirming the decision in favor of the defendant doctor, noted that the state optometry practice act did not require, or even authorize, the diagnosis and treatment of eye disease by an optometrist and that there was no evidence to establish that the glaucomatous condition of her eyes should have been detected by a skillful optometrist in the performance of his professional duties. But the court established several important guidelines to be applied in future cases: (1) expert testimony would be necessary in order to determine the standard of care expected of an optometrist; (2) under this standard an optometrist could be held responsible for the detection of disease; and (3) if disease were detected, an optometrist was required to refer the patient to the appropriate practitioner for treatment.[2]

Although liability was not proven by the evidence in this particular instance, the case established that failure to adhere to the prevailing standard of care expected of optometrists under the circumstances would result in liability for damages legally caused by such conduct. This is the rule that prevails today throughout the United States for negligence claims against optometrists.

Because optometrists not only perform professional services but also sell a product—ophthalmic materials—there is another basis for professional liability claims that has received legal recognition. Interestingly, the first reported case discussing this application of the law also arose in Alabama in 1939.

A woman visited a store with an optical department and was examined by an optometrist, who fitted her with glasses. About two months later, while wearing the glasses, she tripped down the steps of her home and severely injured herself. She sued the department store for damages, alleging that the glasses had been negligently fitted and were not suitable for the purpose for which they had been sold, but the trial court dismissed her claim. She appealed to the Alabama Supreme Court, and in discussing the basis for the woman's claim, the court observed that whenever a buyer makes known to a seller of goods—either expressly or by implication—the particular purpose for which the goods are required, and relies upon the seller's skill and judgment as to their selection and suitability, there arises an implied warranty that the goods are reasonably fit for the purpose for which they are sold. The court held that this implied warranty of fitness could be applied to the glasses sold by the optometrist and to the optometrist's employer. The decision of the trial court was reversed and the case was remanded for further disposition.[3]

The legal theory on which this case was based—warranty—is still applicable to situations where glasses are sold through a separate dispensary or optical shop. It has served as the legal foundation for product liability law, the successor to warranty law and an evolving source of liability claims against optometrists. The application of product liability law to the practice of optometry will be discussed subsequently.

Duty to Refer

The leading cause of large malpractice claims against optometrists is misdiagnosis, which is inevitably linked to allegations of failure to refer. The responsibility of optometrists to refer patients for appropriate therapy was discussed in a 1958 District of Columbia case that involved a patient with an intraocular tumor.

A patient went to an optical shop seeking to obtain a pair of glasses, but because the optometrist who worked for the optician was on vacation the patient was sent to a nearby optometrist for examination. The optometrist detected a small intraocular tumor about the size of a pea, but instead of informing the patient, the optometrist telephoned the optician who ran the optical shop, recommending that the patient be sent to a physician for consultation. The optician dispensed glasses to the patient, however, and said nothing of the pathology. This lack of disclosure ultimately resulted in total vision loss in the affected eye. The patient sued both the optician and the optometrist, and in assessing the responsibility of the optometrist in the case, the court held that although the optometrist was not required by law to make the correct diagnosis, professional standards necessitated disclosure and referral.[4]

Therefore, it is clear that the duty of an optometrist is to fully inform the patient of any pathological findings and to see that proper referral is obtained. The timeliness of the referral is also an important consideration, and the optometrist will be held responsible for damages suffered by the patient as a result of misdiagnosis that causes the patient to delay seeking necessary care.

An optometrist examined a patient who complained of "tired eyes." Opacities were detected in the lens of each eye. The patient alleged that she was told the spots were cataracts and that she would be referred to a medical practitioner in two or three years; the optometrist alleged that she was told to see an ophthalmologist immediately. The patient continued to experience difficulties with her vision, and eleven days after her visit to the optometrist she consulted a physician, who diagnosed her condition as uveitis and hospitalized her for treatment. Despite his efforts, she eventually lost sight in one eye and suffered a severe reduction in vision in the other. She sued the optometrist for malpractice, and the key issue at trial was whether or not the optometrist had made the referral. There was a notation to this effect in his records, but it was made in a color of ink that was different from the other entries. The optometrist testified that it was his custom to make notes on his records after the patient visit was concluded and that he had a number of pens at his desk which he used for this purpose. The jury, however, believed the patient's assertion that she had not been referred and awarded a judgment in her favor.[5]

Subsequent cases upholding the legal obligation to refer have involved patients with retinal detachment,[6] glaucoma,[7] and tumors.[8] Litigation has also resulted from allegations that a patient was repeatedly denied access to a medical provider despite an optometrist's referral[9] and that a patient was wrongfully denied spectacles despite an optometrist's determination that he needed them.[10]

Liability for Ophthalmic Materials

The preponderance of professional liability claims against optometrists involve ophthalmic materials. In the past, the majority of these claims were due to injuries from spectacle lenses and frames, but today the largest cause of litigation is the contact lens. Although contact lens related claims arise with more frequency, claims involving ophthalmic lenses usually allege greater injury and thus demand greater damages. The legal theory most commonly used to sustain these claims is malpractice—negligence—which requires evidence that the optometrist did not conform to the standard of care. Malpractice, however, is not the only liability issue that faces sellers of ophthalmic products.

Over the past few decades another cause of action, based on product liability law, has established that a manufacturer, designer, or seller of a product may be held strictly liable for injuries caused by a defect in the product. Ophthalmic products have been the subject of numerous product liability claims, with the majority of these cases involving glass spectacle lenses that allegedly were not in compliance with standards for impact resistance and thus unreasonably dangerous. A 1977 Missouri case illustrates how product liability theory may be applied to ophthalmic lenses.

An ophthalmologist's prescription for glass spectacle lenses for a 6-year-old hyperope specified that they were to be tempered. The lenses were heat-treated by the optical laboratory filling the prescription and dispensed to the child. Six months later, one of the lenses was struck by a rock thrown by a playmate and shattered, two slivers penetrating the youngster's eye. He suffered a traumatic cataract and corneal scarring that, after surgery, left him with a permanent vision defect. The child sued the laboratory, alleging that the lenses had been improperly heat-treated and that the laboratory had failed to perform the drop-ball test on them as required by ANSI Z-80.1 standards adopted by the federal government. Although the jury's verdict was in favor of the defendants, upon appeal this judgment was reversed, the court holding that "the object of heat treatment was to reduce the dangers from the slivers when a lens fractured. A jury could find from the evidence here that the lens, when used in a reasonably to be anticipated manner, failed to fulfill its purpose because of defects which might have been found to exist."[11]

Although the usual defendant in product liability cases is the optical shop that sells the defective lenses to the patient,[12] the optical laboratory that fabricates the lenses in a defective manner,[13] or the manufacturer of the lenses,[14] optometrists may also be found liable for the fitting and dispensing of unsafe ophthalmic lenses.[15] But applying product liability theory to the fitting and dispensing of contact lenses has thus far not been recognized by the courts.

An optical chain employing more than 100 optometrists advertised contact lenses in newspapers and on radio and television. The lenses were sold for a set price regardless of the difficulty or simplicity involved in the fitting process and despite the number of visits required to fit the patient. A young man was examined by an optometrist employed by the chain and fitted for hard contact lenses, but the result was not satisfactory to the patient, who spent a number of months being reexamined and refitted in an attempt to lessen the pain and discomfort he experienced. After sixteen months he gave up attempting to wear the lenses, but a subsequent examination revealed that he suffered from unusual corneal scars in both eyes. The patient sued the optical chain, alleging that the poor lens fit had caused the scarring and that the lenses were an unsafe product not reasonably fit for their intended use. The jury found in the patient's favor and the optical chain appealed. The Texas Supreme Court reversed, holding that an implied warranty of fitness would not be extended to the fitting and sale of contact lenses and that product liability would not be imposed since the lenses were not defective in themselves and were not a finished product offered to the general public through regular channels of trade. The court also noted that the professional judgment required of an optometrist in the fitting of the lenses made an action based on negligence a more appropriate remedy.[16]

There have been no reported cases applying product liability law to the fitting and sale of hard or soft daily wear lenses. Because injury from contact lenses is due to extrinsic factors not necessarily related to defective design, manufacture, or sale of the lenses, it seems unlikely that product liability law will be extended to encompass contact lenses. But the development of extended wear lenses has created new legal considerations that add another dimension to this issue.[17]

Standard of Care

In order to establish that an optometrist is liable for malpractice, evidence must be introduced to show that he or she did not conform to the standard of care expected of an optometrist under the circumstances. If it can be proven that the optometrist's conduct did not measure up to the standard of care and that the optometrist's actions (or failure to act) were the legal cause of the patient's injury, then liability will issue. Proof of the standard of care is established through expert testimony, and traditionally only practitioners of the same "school" have been considered to be competent to offer this testimony. Therefore, only optometrists would be allowed to testify as to the standard of care that was applicable to other optometrists.

Over the years, however, the rules of evidence have become more liberal, and physicians have been allowed to testify as to the standard of care to be applied to optometrists. A 1941 Georgia case illustrates how a medical standard may be imposed upon a defendant optometrist.

A youngster was examined by an optometrist and fitted with prescription eyeglasses. He was instructed to wear the glasses full-time, but despite efforts to wear them, he allegedly suffered from headaches and nausea. He returned to the optometrist, was re-examined, and was again told to continue wearing the glasses full-time. Because the youngster continued to experience difficulties, his mother took him to an ophthalmologist, who performed a cycloplegic examination and recommended a different prescription. Consequently, the youngster sued the optometrist for malpractice, alleging that the optometrist's eyeglasses were incorrect and that they could retard the proper development of the child's eyes. At the trial, the ophthalmologist testified that it was not possible to examine the child's eyes properly without dilation and that the optometrist's prescription had been incorrect as a result of his failure to employ cycloplegia. Even though Georgia state law did not allow the optometrist to use drops, the court, relying on the testimony of the ophthalmologist, found the optometrist liable.[18]

Because of the primary care orientation of optometry and the increased use by optometrists of medical techniques, it has become apparent that the clinical differences between optometry and ophthalmology have become less distinct. As a result, the standard of care for optometrists has begun to reflect this growing medical orientation. Likewise, the decisions of courts asked to review malpractice judgments against optometrists have reflected the perception of judges that optometry is a health-care profession and that optometrists are responsible for the detection of medical conditions that affect vision, even conditions that are rare. A 1977 Louisiana case illustrates this trend.

A woman who was a patient of a Health Maintenance Organization (HMO) sought the services of an eye-care practitioner because of decreased visual acuity in one eye. She was examined by an optometrist, who found she had 20/40 acuity in the affected eye but who attributed this finding to cataract, which was diagnosed without the use of dilation. (The use of mydriatic drugs by optometrists was not permitted under state law at the time.) About two months later, the patient was found to have a retinal detachment secondary to Von Hippel-Lindau disease, and despite two surgeries she was unable to regain normal vision. She sued the optometrist and the HMO, alleging that he was negligent in failing to diagnose the retinal detachment, but the trial court awarded a judgment in the optometrist's favor. The woman appealed, and the Louisiana Court of Appeals reversed, finding—among other things—that the optometrist had undertaken the diagnosis of a medical condition, cataract, and that consequently he should be held to a medical standard of care, which required dilation in order to confirm the diagnosis. The failure to employ dilation

—just as a physician would have done—in order to rule out the presence of a retinal detachment constituted negligence, in the court's opinion, and justified the awarding of damages to the patient.[19]

Even difficult cases in which physician experts disagree can result in liability, as is demonstrated by a 1978 Alaska case involving a military optometrist.

An optometrist examined a 4-year-old esotrope and prescribed glasses, scheduling the patient to return for a follow-up examination five weeks later. At this second visit, the optometrist found 20/30 acuities but "no good reflex" in one eye, which a dilated fundus examination revealed to have a dark vitreous hemorrhage. The optometrist did not refer the patient, however, since the blood appeared to be old or from an inactive cause. At a follow-up examination four months later, the optometrist found the acuity in the eye was limited to light perception only. The patient was referred to an ophthalmologist and subsequently examined by another ophthalmologist and a pediatrician, with the cause of the child's reduced acuity being diagnosed as a retinal detachment. But because there was uncertainty as to the cause of the detachment, the youngster was sent to San Francisco for examination by a team of physicians. Despite their efforts, ultimately the eye had to be enucleated. The optometrist was sued for negligence by the child and was held to be liable by the trial court for failure to diagnose the detachment—which was held to be due to *Toxocara canis*—and to refer the patient promptly for treatment. The trial judge specifically rejected testimony that an optometric standard of care did not require referral and based his decision on the opinion of ophthalmologists. The youngster was awarded substantial damages.[20]

Therefore, in cases alleging misdiagnosis and failure to refer, the likelihood is great that medical testimony will be allowed to determine the standard of care expected of the defendant optometrist. But misdiagnosis has always been a significant clinical and legal concern for optometrists, ever since the very beginnings of the profession when early practitioners successfully defended their right to use the ophthalmoscope. Optometrists have consistently maintained that the detection of ocular or systemic disease is a valuable service and that the responsibility for performing this service is an implicit part of an optometrist's duty to his patients. Court decisions have reflected this standard of care, one that the profession has imposed upon itself, in cases involving ocular foreign bodies,[21] cataract,[22] glaucoma,[23] tumors,[24] and systemic disease with ocular manifestations.[25]

Toward a Medical Standard

If a medical standard of care is to be applied to the conduct of optometrists, a significant body of precedent becomes available for use in optometric liability cases. Some states[26] have adopted by statute a medical standard of care for optometrists, and it may be argued that court decisions involving physicians have already begun to exert an influence upon the practice of optometry. One of the most notable of these cases was decided in the state of Washington in 1974.

A 22-year-old patient was fitted with contact lenses by two ophthalmologists. During the next nine years she was examined on numerous occasions by the doctors but her intraocular pressure was never tested. When tonometry was finally performed and her visual fields measured, she was found to be suffering from open-angle glaucoma, which had reduced her field of vision to less than ten degrees. She sued the physicians for malpractice. They defended the claim on the basis that the reasonable and ordinary standard in ophthalmology did not require routine testing for glaucoma in patients under forty, due to the low incidence of the disease in that age group (1 in 25,000). The state supreme court held that the standards of the profession were too low to adequately protect the patient and ruled against the ophthalmologists, stating that failure to test for glaucoma constituted negligence as a matter of law.[27]

The court's decision created quite a stir,[28] and because of the widespread publicity given to it in legal and medical journals, testing for open-angle glaucoma became a concern for optometrists. It also doubtless affected the frequency with which tonometry was employed by optometrists.[29]

A similar effect was achieved by a case involving the doctrine of informed consent. Although there have been no precedent-setting informed consent cases involving optometrists, a 1979 decision involving a Washington ophthalmologist again brought the issue of glaucoma testing to the attention of optometrists.[30]

A 54-year-old woman who was highly myopic and who complained of blurring and of gaps in her vision was examined by an ophthalmologist. The physician performed Schiotz tonometry and obtained readings of 23.8 mm Hg in each eye, but he said nothing of these findings to the patient and did not perform ophthalmoscopy with dilation or test the patient's visual field. The patient was examined at the ophthalmologist's clinic on a dozen occasions over a two-year period, but she was never given the additional tests. At the end of that time she was functionally blind. Eventually open-angle glaucoma was diagnosed as the cause of her loss of vision, and she brought suit against the physician, alleging that his failure to diagnose the disease was negligent and that his failure to warn her of the borderline intraocular pressure (IOP) readings and to advise her of the availability of additional tests for glaucoma constituted a lack of informed consent. At trial she was unable to prove that the conduct of the ophthalmologist did not conform to the prevailing standard of care within the profession, and a judgment was awarded in favor of the defendant doctor. She appealed to the Washington Supreme Court, and the court held that, under the doctrine of informed consent, the ophthalmologist had a duty to inform her of an abnormality (such as the IOP reading) discovered during a routine examination and to discuss with her diagnostic procedures that could be used to determine the significance of the abnormality. The court found that the ophthalmologist's conduct breached this duty and he was held liable for her injury.[31]

Similarly, cases involving physicians have made it clear that optometrists have a duty to warn patients of impaired vision and that the doctor's liability in some circumstances can be extended to include injuries suffered by third parties.[32] Other physician-litigated causes of liability may be expected to influence optometry as well.

The preceding discussion of professional liability cases involving optometrists has illustrated how the courts have imposed a standard of care for optometrists that is the same as that for physicians, dentists, and other members of the healing arts, e.g., that minimum degree of skill, care, and learning that is ordinarily exhibited by members of the profession. Concomitantly, there has been a movement, thus far limited, to impose strict liability (e.g., a judicially established standard), which is best illustrated by decisions involving ophthalmic products. The growing medical orientation of optometrists and of optometry practice acts has been recognized in the courts, as judges have begun to use a medical standard of care to assess the conduct expected of optometric clinicians. Although optometry is an independent healthcare profession, it does not exist in isolation, and legal developments that affect clinical practice within comparable professions such as medicine can be expected to exert significant influence upon the standards within optometry as well (see Table 2.1).

Table 2.1. Liability Milestones: 1939–1984

1939	The Alabama Supreme Court, in the case of *Hampton v. Brackin's Jewelry and Optical Co., Inc.*, holds that optometrists will be subject to the same rules of negligence as will be applied to professionals.
1958	In *Evers v. Buxbaum*, the federal Court of Appeals for Washington, D.C., rules that an optometrist has a duty to refer patients with ocular pathology to other health care providers for treatment.
1968	The Supreme Court of Texas, in the case of *Barbee v. Rogers*, holds that contact lenses will not be subject to the law of warranty or to product liability law when sold by an optometrist.
1970	The Seventh Circuit Court of Appeals, in *Filler v. Rayex Corp.*, rules that spectacles will be subject to warranty and product liability law.
1974	In a case involving ophthalmologists, the Supreme Court of Washington holds that failure to test for glaucoma is negligence as a matter of law; the case, *Helling v. Carey*, is the first to apply strict liability to the negligence of a health care professional.
1977	In *Fairchild v. Brian*, the Supreme Court of Louisiana holds an optometrist to the standard of care expected of a physician; the court also rules that an optometrist must be identified by academic degree when in a multidisciplinary setting.
1979	In *Gates v. Jensen*, a case involving an ophthalmologist, the Supreme Court of Washington holds that the doctrine of informed consent requires disclosure of suspicious findings revealed during an examination so that the patient can determine if further testing is necessary.
1984	The Alabama Supreme Court, in *Wills v. Klingenbeck*, rules that an optometrist's duty to refer a patient with systemic disease is not ended because the patient is concurrently under the care of a physician.

Notes

1. This is the first case to appear in a state reporter, i.e., the first appellate case, and thus is the first *reported* case involving an optometrist.
2. *Hampton v. Brackin's Jewelry and Optical Co., Inc.*, 237 Ala. 212, 186 So. 173 (1939).
3. *Gilbert v. Louis Pizitz Dry Goods Co.*, 237 Ala. 249, 186 So. 179 (1939).
4. *Evers v. Buxbaum*, 102 App. D.C. 334, 253 F.2d 356 (D.C. Cir. 1958).
5. *Tempchin v. Sampson*, 262 Md. 156, 277 A.2d 67 (1971).
6. *Whitt v. Columbus Cooperative Enterprises*, 64 Ohio St. 2d 355, 415 N.E.2d 985 (1980).
7. There have been several cases involving the failure of optometrists to detect open-angle glaucoma, but none of the appeals were based on the argument that there was no duty to test for the disease. Rather, they have been based on technical arguments that seek to avoid this issue. See *McMahon v. Glixman*, 393 N.E.2d 875 (Mass., 1979); *Collins v. American Optometric Association*, 693 F.2d 636 (7th Cir. 1982); and *Holmes v. Iwasa*, 104 Idaho 179, 657 P. 2d 476 (Idaho 1983).
8. *Wills v. Klingenbeck*, 455 So. 2d 806 (Ala. 1984).
9. *Freeman v. Lockhart*, 503 F.2d 1016 (8th Cir. 1974). This case involved a prisoner who suffered from tuberculosis, the ocular symptoms of which could be relieved by surgery, according to the prison optometrist. But the prisoner was repeatedly denied access to a surgeon, and he brought an action under the Civil Rights Act for damages.
10. *Di Febo v. Keve*, 395 F. Supp. 1350 (D.C. Del. 1975). A prisoner sued prison officials and the prison optometrist, alleging that his vision had been injured due to their negligence in failing to replace his broken spectacles. The court held that the complaint did not state a cause of action under the Civil Rights Act.
11. *Kopp v. C.C. Caldwell Optical Co.*, 547 S.W.2d 872 (Mo. App. 1977). The leading case discussing liability for ophthalmic materials is *Filler v. Rayex Corp.*, 435 F.2d 336 (7th Cir. 1970).
12. See *Newgent v. Toler*, 21 ATLA L. Rep. 113, Apr. 1978, in which an Indiana optical shop was held liable for selling lenses made of glass (rather than plastic) to a policeman who was injured when the glasses were broken in a job-related altercation.
13. For a report on such a case, see R. Marks, Product Liability: The New Malpractice Menace, *Optometric Management*, vol. 13, no. 1, Jan. 1977, pp. 26–27. The case involved a young child who was injured when she slipped and struck a wooden stake, causing the glass lens of her spectacles to shatter, resulting in some permanent loss of vision in the affected eye. The claim against the optical lab concerned the edging of the glass lens, which was alleged to have been performed in such a way as to divest it of its impact-resistance.
14. A discussion of ophthalmic product liability can be found in *American Optical Co. v. Wiedenhamer*, 404 N.E.2d 606 (Ind. App. 1980), which describes in some detail the legal standards applicable to ophthalmic lenses.
15. See *Hayes v. Hamberg*, 14 ATLA L. Rep. 372, Oct. 1971, in which a Pennsylvania optometrist was held liable for ocular injury due to ophthalmic lens breakage.
16. *Barbee v. Rogers*, 425 S.W.2d 342 (Tex. 1968).
17. As of this writing, there are several cases in litigation involving extended wear lenses in which product liability is the basis for the claim. The ultimate outcome of these cases cannot be predicted. See J. Classe, Liability in Contact Lens Practice, *Southern Journal of Optometry*, vol. 4, no. 3, July 1986, pp. 52–57; and Classe, J., and M.G. Harris, Liability and Extended Wear Contact Lenses, *Journal of the American Optometric Association*, vol. 58, no. 10, 1987, pp. 848–854.
18. *Kahn v. Shaw*, 65 Ga. App. 563, 16 S.E.2d 99 (1941).
19. *Fairchild v. Brian*, 354 So. 2d 675 (La. App. 1977). Further commentary on this case can be found in J. Classe: A Review of Professional Liability Cases Affecting the Practice of Optometry, *Journal of the American Optometric Association*, vol. 57, no. 1, Jan. 1986, pp. 66–71.
20. *Steele v. United States*, 463 F. Supp. 321 (D.C. Alas. 1978).
21. *Kime v. Aetna*, 66 Ohio App. 277, 33 N.E.2d 1008 (1940). This case was brought to determine if removal of a foreign body was within the scope of practice for Ohio optometrists.
22. *Fairchild v. Brian*, 354 So. 2d 675 (La. App. 1977); see also *Boothe v. Weiss*, 107 A.D.2d 730, 484 N.Y.S.2d 598 (1985).
23. Cases involving allegations of misdiagnosis of open-angle glaucoma include *Hampton v. Brackin's Jewelry and Optical Co., Inc.*, 237 Ala. 212, 186 So. 173 (1939); *McMahon v. Glixman*, 393 N.E.2d 875 (Mass. 1979); *Collins v. American Optometric Association*, 693 F.2d 636 (7th Cir. 1982); and *Holmes v. Iwasa*, 657 P.2d 476 (Idaho 1983).
24. *Fairchild v. Brian*, 354 So. 2d 675 (La. App. 1977); and *Wills v. Klingenbeck*, 455 So. 2d 806 (Ala. 1984).
25. *Whitt v. Columbus Cooperative Enterprises, Inc.*, 64 Ohio St. 2d 355, 415 N.E.2d 985 (1980). This case involved a patient with diabetes.
26. For example, Wyoming, Iowa, and Florida have adopted a medical standard of care as part of the optometry statute. See *Fla. Stat. Ann.* 463.0135 (1987), *Iowa Code Ann.* 154.10 (1987), and *Wyoming Stat.* 33-23-102 (1987).
27. *Helling v. Carey*, 83 Wash. 2d 514, 519 P.2d 981 (1974). For a review of the saga of this case, see also *Gates v. Jensen*, 92 Wash. 2d 246, 595 P.2d 919 (1979); *Meeks v. Marx*, 15 Wash. App. 571, 550 P.2d 1158 (1976); and *Harris v. Groth*, 99 Wash. 2d 438, 663 P.2d 113 (1983).
28. Wechsler, S., and J. Classe, *Helling v. Carey: Caveat*

Medicus (Let the Doctor Beware), *Journal of the American Optometric Association*, vol. 48, no. 12, Dec. 1977, pp. 1526–1529.

29. A study at two schools of optometry found that the routine use of tonometry was significantly higher after the *Helling* decision. See Godio, L., J. Ruskiewicz, and W. Chao: The Impact of a Court Decision on the Actual Practice of Eye Care, *American Journal of Optometry and Physiological Optics*, vol. 59, no. 3, Mar. 1982, pp. 207–210. See also Classe, J., *Helling* Revisited: How the 'Tale' Wagged the Dog, *Journal of the American Optometric Association*, vol. 58, no. 4, 1987, pp. 343–345.
30. Thal, L.S., *Gates v. Jensen*: Another Precedent for Glaucoma Testing, *Journal of the American Optometric Association*, vol. 52, no. 4, Apr. 1981, pp. 349–353.
31. *Gates v. Jensen*, 92 Wash. 2d 246, 595 P.2d 919 (1979).
32. For a review of cases involving the duty to warn of impaired vision, see Gold, A., Failure to Warn, *Journal of the American Optometric Association*, vol. 57, no. 4, Apr. 1986, pp. 317–319, and Classe, J., Optometrist's Duty to Warn of Vision Impairment, *Southern Journal of Optometry*, vol. 4, no. 1, Jan. 1986, pp. 66–69. For an example case, see *Welke v. Kuzilla*, 144 Mich. App. 245, 375 N.W.2d 403 (1985).

PART TWO

ETHICS

Chapter 3

The Ethics of Health Care

Undershaft: *Well, come! Is there anything you know or care for?*
Stephen (rising and looking at him steadily): *I know the difference between right and wrong.*
Undershaft (hugely tickled): *You don't say so! What! No capacity for business, no knowledge of law, no sympathy with art, no pretension to philosophy; only a simple knowledge of the secret that has puzzled all the philosophers, baffled all the lawyers, muddled all the men of business, and ruined most of the artists: the secret of right and wrong. Why, man, you're a genius, a master of masters, a god! And at the age of twenty-three!*
—George Bernard Shaw, *Major Barbara*

Historical Perspective

Ethics is not a legal concept; it is a moral one. It is not something that can be legislated, created by the pen of a judge, or voted into existence. It is a human attribute, just as honesty, integrity, and fairness are human attributes. It is also an attribute that is fundamental to the concept of professionalism.

Defined as "formal or professional rules of right and wrong; a system of conduct or behavior," and identified as coming from the Greek word *ethos* (moral character), ethics has interested many of the great minds of history.[1] That it has engendered such widespread and persistent discussion—not to mention differences of opinion—is inherent in the definition quoted: ethics purports to establish "professional rules of right and wrong." As George Bernard Shaw points out, any such attempt is bound to be met by widely varying opinions as to what actually constitutes right and wrong.

Nevertheless, ethics has been a concept with which all professionals have wrestled.[2] Beginning in antiquity, practitioners of the healing arts have pondered the moral basis of their calling and have propounded codes or treatises that discuss their general duties and obligations. Perhaps the most famous of these is the oath attributed to Hippocrates, written between the fifth and fourth century B.C., and the related treatises, known as the *Corpus Hippocraticum*.[3] The oath prescribed a strict and refined personal ethic, requiring a high sense of morality from those who would practice medicine. It has survived, in the Christian version, to become a valued tradition of the medical profession in contemporary times. The Hippocratic Oath, however, was not an oath taken by all physicians, and there is speculation that it may not have been taken by anyone before the end of antiquity.[4] Even into the first centuries of the Christian era, there was no common ethical code binding on the medical practitioner.[5]

Despite the high ethical ideals expressed in the Hippocratic Oath, the practice of medicine remained, on the whole, at a much lower plane for a considerable period of time.[6] This was especially true during the Middle Ages, when the conduct of surgeons—who were held in much lower esteem than physicians in terms of social and professional standing—seemed to signify a retreat toward deceitfulness and posturing.[7] The literature of this period is replete with satiric references to the moral inadequacies of physicians and surgeons.[8]

But in 1803, an English physician, Thomas Percival (Fig. 3.1), published a book entitled *Medical Ethics*. It was to become one of the leading works

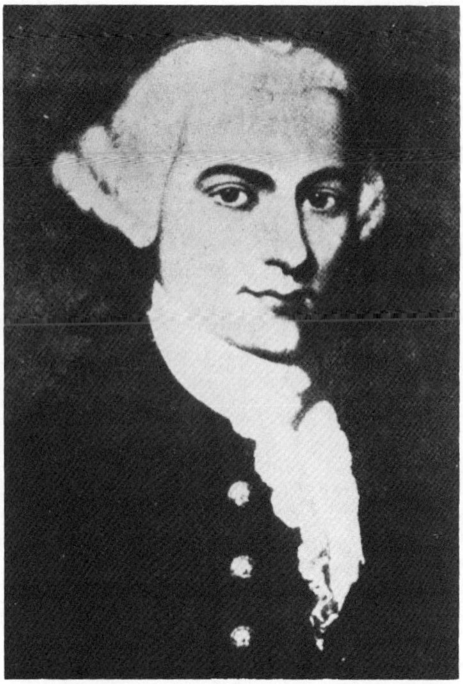

Figure 3.1. Thomas Percival. The author of *Medical Ethics* not only influenced the Code of Ethics of the American Medical Association, but also the Supplement to the Code of Ethics of the American Optometric Association, adopted by the AOA in 1946. (Photograph courtesy of the International Library, Archives, and Museum of Optometry)

of the medical Enlightenment. More importantly, when the American Medical Association (AMA) was formed in 1846 and set as one of its top priorities the formulation of a Code of Ethics, it was to Percival's book that the drafters of the AMA code turned.[9] Consequently, the 1847 Code of Ethics of the American Medical Association drew heavily on the words of Percival for inspiration.

The 1847 AMA code attempted to provide guidelines for virtually all areas of a physician's life. It was composed of three major sections, each devoted to a particular set of duties: physician to patient, physician to physician, and physician to the public. The ideals were high, and although the code itself contained no enforcement capability, over the years the alignment of state medical groups with the AMA and the ability of such state medical groups to punish local violators (principally through the suspension of licenses, expulsion from the society, or efforts that could result in the withdrawal of hospital privileges) became a potent weapon that could be used to subject the "advisory" AMA code on all physicians.[10]

The code was modified in 1903, 1912, 1949, 1957, and 1980. These modifications were used, in a general sense, to improve the image of the U.S. physician. But they were also used (just as the original code was) to reduce internal dissention and to minimize competition among physicians.[11] Another effect of the code was to assist in the preservation of the medical monopoly, which was under attack from several directions. Although physicians had won the passage of medical practice acts during the mid-1800s, these laws were uniformly weak and did not give the states the control over medical licensure that would prevent incompetent "doctors" from preying on the public.[12] But beginning in the 1870s modern laws began to be enacted that preserved for physicianry the full scope of medical care, to the exclusion of a number of emerging professions, including dentistry, chiropody (podiatry), chiropractic, osteopathy, clinical psychology, and optometry.[13] Each of these professions was at conflict with some segment of medicine; the optometry-ophthalmology conflict was merely one of a number of battles being fought between physicians and nonphysician health-care providers. The AMA Code of Ethics was but one of several devices used by physicians to prevent incursions into their monopoly.

In addition to these extrinsic influences on medicine, there was internal disagreement about many fundamental matters, including what constituted the ethical practice of medicine. This variance of opinion resulted in a code that often struggled with what should be considered ethical and what should not.[14] For example, in three rather basic areas of practice—fees, consultations, and advertising—the course advocated by the AMA was not always consistent. Over a hundred years of medical ethics is summarized in Table 3.1, which illustrates how the official stance of the AMA varied concerning these three aspects of medical practice.[15]

Fees

Physicians have displayed a decided uncertainty about how to set their fees. Percival advocated a sliding scale (so that the wealthy paid more than the poor for a physician's services), but the AMA's 1847 code established a fixed fee schedule (the same charge for the same service for all patients). By 1903 the AMA had reversed itself and had decided that Percival was right; the physician could charge more if the patient could pay more. For a number of years, the AMA codes did not mention fees at all (due to a fear of antitrust actions), but in 1957 the AMA took a rather contradictory stand: a fixed fee per service that could be escalated with the patient's ability to

Table 3.1. Selected Aspects of Medical Ethics: 1847–1957

Year	Fees	Advertising	Consultations
1847	Fixed fees (one charge for all patients per service)	Total prohibition	Consultations prohibited with any practitioner "whose practice is based upon an exclusive dogma"
1903	Sliding fees (can be changed to meet the "minimum pecuniary acknowledgement of patients")	Prohibited	Only referrals to "irregular," nonmedical practitioners considered unethical
1912	No mention of fees (due to the antitrust fervor of the time)	Prohibited	May receive referrals from "cultists"
1949	No mention of fees	Prohibited	Consultations with "cultists" prohibited; cannot send to or receive from such practitioners
1957	Fees can be "commeasurate with the service rendered and the patient's ability to pay"	"A physician... should not solicit patients"	Consultations permitted in "doubtful or difficult cases," "upon request," or "whenever the quality of medical services may be enhanced"

pay. Apparently this position was an attempt to state a policy that would be unobjectionable to everyone.[16]

Consultations

If fees were a problem, the AMA policy on consultations with nonphysicians was a paradox: There seemed to be no answer. Initially, the AMA policy prohibited all consultations with those "whose practice is based on an exclusive dogma." But this policy clearly cost physicians patients, and so in 1903 the revised code allowed physicians to accept referrals from (but not to send them to) such practitioners, who by 1912 were called cultists. The hypocrisy of this stance was apparent by 1949, however, at which time a total prohibition was reinstated. This was in turn reversed in 1957, to permit consultations under various conditions.[17] Again, as with the 1957 position on fees, the conditions were general enough to prevent dissent.

Advertising

As for advertising, the AMA initially adopted a very strict policy, but over the years it received less and less attention, being reduced in the 1957 code to a terse, "A physician...should not solicit patients." This policy, like the others, was at conflict with the social changes gripping the United States in the 1960s and 1970s and eventually had to be modified.

The advent of consumerism brought fundamental changes to the way of life enjoyed by professionals. Consumerism and professionalism frequently found themselves at odds, and in the end consumerism prevailed, particularly in the courts, where a series of cases decided by the U.S. Supreme Court altered the relationship between professionals and the public by permitting truthful advertising. As a result, codes of ethics had to be revised.[18]

The AMA revision was finally completed in 1980 and, reflecting the changing times, tacitly accepted the idea of physician advertising. The 1980 Principles of Medical Ethics were limited to seven points (Table 3.2), and the changes were rather sweeping: no advice about fees whatsoever, recognition that physicians could work in the environment they wanted, and an admission that other health care professionals could ethically participate with physicians in the delivery of health care.[19]

But the removal of anticompetitive language did not signify the end of competition with other health care disciplines. The long and often bitter fight between optometry and ophthalmology, which was itself reflected in a series of AMA resolutions, has continued to generate controversy. How medicine used ethics to wage its economic warfare with optometry is the subject of the following section.

The War of Words

Ophthalmologists formed the American Ophthalmological Society in 1864, two of the organization's charter members being Henry Noyes and D.B. St. John Roosa.[20] In 1888 the AMA approved a Section

Table 3.2. Principles of Ethics, American Medical Association: 1980

I. A physician shall be dedicated to providing competent medical service with compassion and respect for human dignity.
II. A physician shall deal honestly with patients and colleagues, and strive to expose those physicians deficient in character or competence, or who engage in fraud or deception.
III. A physician shall respect the law and also recognize a responsibility to seek changes in those requirements which are contrary to the best interests of the patient.
IV. A physician shall respect the rights of patients, of colleagues, and of other health professionals, and shall safeguard patient confidences within the constraints of the law.
V. A physician shall continue to study, apply, and advance scientific knowledge; make relevant information available to patients, colleagues, and the public; obtain consultation; and use the talents of other health professionals when indicated.
VI. A physician shall, in the provision of appropriate patient care, except in emergencies, be free to choose whom to serve, with whom to associate, and the environment in which to provide medical services.
VII. A physician shall recognize a responsibility to participate in activities contributing to an improved community.

Source: American Medical Association, 1980.

on Ophthalmology, and the American Academy of Ophthalmology had its beginnings in 1895.[21] These rather standard developments for a medical specialty were joined in 1916 by a precedent-setting event: the creation of the American Board for Ophthalmic Examinations.[22] In 1933 the board's name was changed to the American Board of Ophthalmology; it was the first medical specialty board in the United States.[23]

The impressive push by ophthalmology to become the first legitimate specialty left a wide wake because in proclaiming themselves the exclusive eye specialists, it was necessary to disenfranchise their rivals, the optometrists. The first manifestation of this came in 1899 when—at the urging of the ophthalmology section—the AMA passed a resolution that physicians should restrict their optical consultations only to other physicians.[24] A decade later (1910), the House of Delegates of the AMA commended its Bureau of Medical Legislation for working on behalf of ophthalmologists to defeat "objectionable optometric legislation."[25] In the same year, the Section on Ophthalmology passed a resolution maintaining that ophthalmologists serving on examining boards for optometry were in violation of the 1903 AMA Code of Ethics.[26]

But this was just the beginning of a long war of words. In 1934 the AMA agreed that it should try and stop optometrists from prescribing glasses in hospitals.[27] The following year the AMA declared it unethical for any AMA member to teach or consult with anyone not associated with actual medical service.[28] This unfortunate resolution was passed at the urging of the Section on Ophthalmology; the target group was obvious. And although the Section on Ophthalmology voted to rescind the resolution in 1939 and 1941,[29] it was not officially rejected until 1950, when a new resolution was passed that superceded it. The new position made it ethical for an ophthalmologist to engage in lectures, demonstrations, or other measures designed to disseminate information to nonmedical groups for the purpose of preventing blindness.[30]

In the 1940s, the ethics of ophthalmologists became a legal issue when the U.S. government filed an antitrust suit against several hundred ophthalmologists and a number of optical companies and optical wholesalers.[31] The root of the legal problem was a decades-old system of rebates from opticians to ophthalmologists. The ophthalmologist would examine a patient, write a prescription, and send the patient to an optician for the prescription to be filled. Then the optician would send the ophthalmologist part of his profit on the sale of the glasses, a transaction about which the patient knew nothing. In 1946 the suit was settled, with the defendant ophthalmologists in essence agreeing to drop the practice.[32] Despite this, the use of rebates continued within ophthalmology, a practice that responsible members of the profession found to be deplorable.[33]

During the early 1950s, ophthalmologists began to use physician's assistants as ancillary personnel for the purposes of refraction, examination, and treatment. With this in mind, in 1954 the American Optometric Association passed a resolution which held that, since visual care should be exclusively the field of optometry, a study of state optometry laws was needed for the purpose of ending exemptions and eliminating encroachments by untrained, unqualified, and unlicensed individuals.[34] This resolution was taken as an affront by ophthalmology.[35] Opticianry interpreted it as signifying optometry's intention to take over *all* of eye care.[36] Despite a clarifying resolution by the AOA in 1955, relationships between optometry and the other two professions soured.[37]

At the Section on Ophthalmology's urging, the AMA passed another resolution prohibiting optometric education by ophthalmologists.[38] The AMA also passed a resolution that ophthalmologists could dispense their own prescriptions as long as there was no "exploitation of the public," thereby ending a century of ophthalmological abstinence from dispensing and interjecting eye physicians fully into the practice of optometry.[39] Ophthalmologists escalated the paper war even further by organizing the National Medical Foundation for Eye Care, which in 1958 published a paper entitled "Optometry and the Public Interest" that was very critical of the optometric profession (and that drew a sharp rejoinder from the AOA).[40] Despite another resolution by the AOA in 1959 proclaiming the desire of the profession to get along with its medical counterpart and declaring that it was not the purpose of optometrists to "invade medicine," the official relationship of the two professions remained strained.[41]

In the midst of these exchanges came an unexpected intervention by the courts. An antitrust lawsuit was filed in 1964 by an optometrist, Dr. Cyrus Bass, against the AMA and seven ophthalmologists, alleging that the defendants had conspired to control eye care.[42] The suit did not receive sufficient financial support, and the case was eventually settled out of court, but the settlement came after the AMA had rescinded its resolution prohibiting ophthalmologists from educating optometrists, a fact of which the trial judge took note.[43] The 1966 AMA resolution permitting the education of optometrists was carefully worded to limit the knowledge to be imparted to that "within the legitimate scope of optometric practice."[44] During this period, the AOA filed a brief with the U.S. Department of Justice, alleging restraint of trade and antitrust activities by the AMA,[45] and in 1965 the Judicial Council of the AMA issued an official opinion concerning optometry that indicated clear acceptance of optometric services: "At no time have optometrists been officially declared sectarian or cult practitioners. Indeed, it may be doubted that optometry is a sectarian practice comparable to osteopathy, chiropractic, or naturopathy."[46]

Seen in retrospect, this opinion shows a grudging willingness on the part of medicine to make a truce with optometry, especially in light of medicine's subsequent actions toward osteopathy, which was a "cult" in the mid-1960s and an integral part of the medical profession by the mid-1970s. Although optometrists and ophthalmologists continued to have their differences, it was a backseat show to the battle that raged between medicine and chiropractic. Unfortunately, the lull was short-lived.

In 1971 optometry reversed its oft-extolled and legally sanctioned status as a drugless profession when a diagnostic drug bill was passed in Rhode Island.[47] Over the next few years, a number of bills permitting optometric diagnostic drug use were passed by state legislatures, to be followed in 1976 by the nation's first therapeutic drug bill, enacted in West Virginia over the governor's veto.[48] To ophthalmologists it signified the start of a new era of confrontation; to optometrists it signified a new era of opportunity.[49] The war of words resumed once more, with some ophthalmologists resorting to yellow journalism and legislative efforts designed to retard the passage of optometry drug laws.[50] Even so, there were no more pronouncements by the AMA; it was left to ophthalmological organizations to deplore the change in the status quo.[51]

The winds of consumerism affected both professions in the late 1970s, as advertising, the entrance of large corporations into the ophthalmic market, and changes in the number and distribution of ophthalmologists began to cause meaningful shifts in the traditional roles of both professions.[52] Nevertheless, at the moment, the war of words has become a classic standoff between two competing professions that find themselves in direct economic competition.[53] Looking back over the past several decades, it seems unlikely that anything productive, particularly in terms of the public interest, was realized by this discord between the two professions. If anything, the lesson to be learned from these events is the obvious vulnerability of codes of ethics to exploitation.

Yet ethical problems continue to plague both medicine and optometry, as they have for all practitioners of the healing arts over the past twenty-five centuries. Each of the health-care professions has been confronted by ethical issues, which have a unique way of returning to haunt succeeding generations, and even though the questions remain the same, answers to these issues vary, thereby demonstrating the difficulty in determining what is "right" and what is "wrong." The experiences of medicine, just reviewed, illustrate this. And the experiences of optometry can expect to be no different (see Table 3.3).

In fact, the ethical problems faced by optometry have been equal to—if not more substantial than—those of medicine. For optometry was born as a house divided, with one foundation solidly immersed in commercial enterprise and another equally set in professional practice. This ethical dichotomy has threatened to break optometry apart, but after more than seventy-five years, the profession continues to prosper and to meet its responsibilities to the public. In finding its way, optometry has had to devise its

Table 3.3. Medical Ethics and Optometry: 1846–1966

1846	American Medical Association is created and a Code of Ethics drafted.
1864	American Ophthalmological Society is formed.
1888	Section on Ophthalmology of the AMA is chartered.
1895	American Academy of Ophthalmology is founded.
1899	The AMA passes a resolution requiring physicians to restrict their consultations only to other physicians.
1910	The AMA Section on Ophthalmology declares that ophthalmologists serving on examining boards for optometry are in violation of the AMA Code of Ethics.
1916	The American Board for Ophthalmic Examinations is founded; in 1933 the name is changed to the American Board of Ophthalmology.
1935	The AMA declares it is unethical for any AMA member to teach or to consult with anyone not associated with actual medical service.
1946	The U.S. government brings an antitrust suit against 3,221 ophthalmologists and several optical companies for "rebating"; the case is settled in 1948 by consent decree with the defendants agreeing to drop the practice.
1950	The AMA passes a resolution declaring that ophthalmologists may engage in lectures, demonstrations, and other measures designed to disseminate information to nonmedical groups for the purpose of preventing blindness.
1955	The AMA adopts a resolution maintaining that it is unethical for physicians to teach in schools of optometry, to lecture to any optometric organization, to contribute scientific material to the optometric literature, or in any way to impart technical medical knowledge to nonmedical practitioners. The AMA also declares that ophthalmologists and other physicians may dispense their own prescriptions as long as there is no "exploitation of the public."
1964	Dr. Cyrus Bass files an antitrust lawsuit against the AMA; the AOA submits information on antitrust activities by medicine to the U.S. Department of Justice; the *Bass* case is settled in 1967 without trial.
1966	The AMA rescinds the resolution of 1955 stating that ophthalmologists may participate in the education of optometrists as long as the information imparted is "within the legitimate scope of optometric practice."

own codes of conduct for dealing with the ethical problems that have threatened optometrists' ability to serve the public interest. The development of these codes is discussed in the following chapter.

Notes

1. *Funk and Wagnalls, Standard College Dictionary*, Harcourt, Brace, and World, New York, 1963.
2. The following comments, taken from the Preface to *Ethics in Medicine*, by Reiser, S.J., A.J. Dyck, and W.J. Curran (eds.), The MIT Press, Cambridge, Mass., 1977, summarize the importance of ethics to practitioners of the healing arts:

   The term "medical ethics" is currently being used in a variety of ways. In one of its oldest but still current usages, medical ethics refers to a body of thinking and codes of conduct developed by the medical profession. Self-conscious reflection on standards of conduct is one of the defining characteristics of a profession. Therefore, it is not surprising that the development of medical ethics as a form of professional self-regulation has a history as long and venerable as the history of medicine itself. . . . Although the idea still persists that medical ethics is restricted to what is thought and practiced by health professionals, a critical reflection on moral issues is more lively today in fields outside medicine than at any other time in the modern period. New scientific, social, and legal developments have directed the attention of society to the values that inform medical decisions and have prompted health professionals to join with patients and experts in other disciplines to work toward resolving the moral problems of medical care.
3. Jones, W.H.S. (translator), *Hippocrates*, vol. 1, pp. 164–165, Harvard University Press, Cambridge, Mass., 1923.
4. Ludwig Edelstein, *Bulletin of the History of Medicine*, vol. 30, 1956, Johns Hopkins University Press, Baltimore, discusses the "Professional Ethics of the Greek Physician," and makes the following observation: "Scribonius Largus, perhaps the first to mention the Oath, maintains that Hippocrates began medical instruction by administering this vow. This of course is mere conjecture."
5. Ibid. Edelstein comments that, "But the Hippocratic Oath originally was a literary manifesto, a programme

laid down by one who wished to set matters right in accordance with his own convictions. It was not an oath taken by all physycians, if indeed it was ever taken at all by any one before the end of antiquity. Throughout Hellenistic times and in the first centuries of the Christian era no common agreement existed concerning an ethical code binding for the medical practitioner." Quoted in Reiser et al., supra note 2, at 40–51.

6. For an account of the development of English medicine during this period, see Kealey, E.J., *Medieval Medicus, A Social History of Anglo-Norman Medicine*, Johns Hopkins University Press, Baltimore, 1981.
7. French surgeon Henri de Mondeville decried the moral conduct of surgeons during the middle ages (thirteenth and fourteenth centuries):

   A rich man has the beginning of an inflammation. He calls in an upright surgeon, who says after examining him, "Seigneur, there is no need for any operation here, because nature will relieve herself, etc; but if the inflammation gets worse, send for me." It then happens that the patient calls in another man who is a quack, and he is told, "Seigneur, you have a great deal of inflammation, I can feel it inside, and if you are not treated at once you will certainly regret it." This surgeon then sets to work and makes an inflammation, which he afterwards cures, so that the whole proceeding redounds to his credit and profit, for he discovered an inflammation which did not exist, whilst the first surgeon is damaged both in his reputation and his pocket because he did not find out what was not there.

   Michel de Montaigne, the noted sixteenth century French philosopher, bitingly described the *mores* of the physicians of his time:

   Whoever saw one physician approve of the prescription of another, without taking something away, or adding something to it? By which they sufficiently betray their art, and make it manifest to us, that they therein more consider their own reputation, and consequently their profit, than their patient's interest.

   For a perspective of the evolution of ethics in medicine, see Reiser et al., supra note 2.
8. In the seventeenth century French farce, *Le Medecin Malgre Lui* (The Physician in Spite of Himself), Moliere satirized the "medical etiquette" and affectations of physicians of the day:

   They have made me a physician . . . and if things go on this way, I am resolved to stick to this profession all my life. I find that it is the best trade of all; for, whether we manage well or ill, we are paid just the same. Bad workmanship never recoils on us; and we cut the material we have to work with pretty much as we like. A shoemaker, in making a pair of shoes, cannot spoil a scrap of leather without having to bear the loss; but in our business we may spoil a man without its costing us a farthing. The blunders are never put down to us, for it is always the fault of the fellow who dies. The best of this profession is, that there is the greatest honesty and discretion among the dead; for you never find them complain of the physician who has killed them.
9. A copy of the tenets of ethics espoused by Percival may be found in Reiser et al., supra note 2, at 18–25. The development of the American Medical Association is recounted by Shryock, R.H., *Medical Licensing in America, 1650–1965*, Johns Hopkins University Press, Baltimore, 1967; and Starr, P., *The Social Transformation of American Medicine*, Basic Books, New York, 1983, pp. 79–144.
10. See Starr, supra note 9. The first code of medical ethics of the American Medical Association may be found in Reiser et al., supra note 2, at 26–34.
11. See Berlant, J.F., *Professions and Monopoly: A Study of Medicine in the United States and Great Britain*, University of California Press, Berkeley, 1975.
12. For a review of the efforts of U.S. medicine to effect reform, see Stevens, R., *American Medicine and the Public Interest*, Yale University Press, New Haven, 1977, pp. 55–74.
13. See Shryock, supra note 9, at 149–176.
14. See Pilcher, L.S., *An Ethical Symposium: Being a Series of Papers Concerning Medical Ethics and Etiquette from the Liberal Standpoint*, G.P. Putnam's Sons, New York, 1983, pp. 42–55.
15. For a more detailed discussion, see Berlant, supra note 11, at 86–119.
16. Berlant, supra note 11, at 109–119, comments:

    This passage apparently tries to combine uniform fees with a sliding scale, without making clear that these are separate and somewhat contradictory philosophical positions. At best this passage represents a return to Percivalean fee discrimination. Why the issue of the patient's ability to pay reentered medical ethics in America at this late date also seems to require an explanation in terms of the profession's political setting. . . .
17. The 1957 Principles of Medical Ethics stated: "A physician should seek consultation upon request; in doubtful or difficult cases; or whenever it appears that the quality of medical service may be enhanced thereby." Reiser et al., supra note 2, at 38–39.
18. After U.S. Supreme Court decisions had made it evident that advertising by professionals would be permissible, the restrictions of professional associations notwithstanding, the American Medical Association began the process of revising its Principles of Ethics. The AMA was sued by the Federal Trade Commission during this period, and the suit—which ultimately was heard by a federal appellate court—was decided after the AMA had completed its revision. The opinion of the court supported the FTC allegation that the 1957 Principles of Ethics interfered with physicians' rights to advertise and therefore were in restraint of trade. See *American Medical Association v. Federal Trade Commission*, 638 F.2d 443 (2d Cir. 1980).
19. Despite the changes in the Principles of Ethics approved by the AMA, the lawsuit with the FTC continued on to

the U.S. Supreme Court, where the decision in favor of the FTC was affirmed. See id., *mem. dec.*, 455 U.S. 676, 102 S. Ct. 1744 (1982).

20. See Stevens, supra note 12, at 101–102.
21. Ibid.
22. Id. at 111–114.
23. Ibid.
24. Id. at 108.
25. Ibid. According to Stevens, "This and the following AMA actions are reported in the *AMA Digest of Official Actions, 1858–1958*, pgs 538–540; and *Supplement to the Digest of Official Actions, 1959–1963*, pp. 215–217."
26. Ibid.
27. Ibid.
28. Ibid.
29. Ibid.
30. The resolution was phrased, in part, as follows:

    Whereas, ophthalmic subjects, such as vascular diseases, glaucoma, retinal disorders and optic nerve disease, considered as potential causes of blindness are matters of grave importance to the public; and

    Whereas, the prevention of blindness is one of the chief obligations of ophthalmologists; therefore, be it

    Resolved, That the Section on Ophthalmology of the American Medical Association declares that it is entirely within the definition of medical ethics for its members to engage in lectures, demonstrations, the preparation of pamphlets and other measures suitable for the dissemination of information designed to prevent blindness and directed to any nonmedical group.

    Journal of the American Optometric Association, vol. 25, no. 2, Feb., 1954, pp. 386–388.
31. The issue of "rebating" was a volatile one in ophthalmology for years before the federal government brought its antitrust suit against 3,221 ophthalmologists, Bausch and Lomb Optical Company and four of its subsidiaries, and the American Optical Company. The case, brought in 1946, was settled in 1948 with agreement on the part of the defendants that they would no longer continue the practice. For a historical perspective, see the following articles: Two Problems, *American Journal of Ophthalmology*, vol. 24, no. 8, Aug. 1941, pp. 951–954; Hidden Fees, *American Journal of Ophthalmology*, vol. 25, no. 8, Aug. 1942, pp. 1001–1003; Medical Ethics and Optometry-Related Matters, *Optical Journal and Review of Optometry*, vol. 81, no. 23, Dec. 1, 1944, p. 24; Acceptable Practices for Dispensing Glasses, *American Journal of Ophthalmology*, vol. 28, no. 2, Feb. 1945, pp. 211–214; Rebates and the "Agency Dispensing Policy," *American Journal of Ophthalmology*, vol. 27, no. 1, January 1946, pp. 84–86; Federal Investigation of Rebating, *American Journal of Ophthalmology*, vol. 29, no. 10, Oct. 1946, pp. 1313–1315; Optical Rebates, *American Journal of Ophthalmology*, vol. 30, no. 8, Aug. 1947, pp. 1030–1032; The Rebate Cases, *American Journal of Ophthalmology*, vol. 31, no. 9, Sept. 1948, pp. 1177–1178; Income-Tax Deductions for Kickbacks, *American Journal of Ophthalmology*, vol. 33, no. 9, Sept. 1950, pp. 1456–1458; Medical Ethics and Philosophy Involved In Dispensing of Glasses By Ophthalmologists, *American Journal of Ophthalmology*, vol. 37, no. 3, Mar. 1954, pp. 439–443. The problem did not disappear because of the lawsuit, nor did the ethical issues raised by the practice. An article, Should Eye Doctors Sell Glasses? by Irwin Ross, appeared in the December, 1966, issue of *Reader's Digest*. It spawned further debate. See Should Eye Doctors Sell Glasses?—A New Conflict, *Optometric Weekly*, Vol. 57, no. 49, Dec. 8, 1966, pp. 29–30. At this same time hearings were held in the U.S. Senate by Senator Hart to investigate this same issue. (See Chapter 1, notes 167 and 168.)
32. The "rebate" cases also caused an interesting legal dispute that ultimately was decided by the Supreme Court. The issue was whether or not the "rebates" paid by optical companies qualified as usual and customary business expenses and thus were tax deductible. Although the Tax Court and the U.S. Court of Appeals ruled they were not, the U.S. Supreme Court reversed these decisions and allowed the deductions. See *Lilly et ux v. Commissioner of Internal Revenue*, 343 U.S. 90, 72 S. Ct. 497 (1951).
33. In the March 1954 issue of the *American Journal of Ophthalmology* at 439–443, an editorial deplores the profiteering in ophthalmology from the sale of ophthalmic materials and goes on to observe:

    It is for professional men to lead in establishing a code of conduct, and not to be led away from one. We should shape tendencies rather than be controlled by them. . . . We can best distinguish ourselves from the various groups trained to fit and sell glasses who would compete with us by adhering to such a code. One might add, incidentally, that some of these groups are striving to attain a similar code of ethics in their endeavor to be regarded as professional men, and are manifesting more pride in striving to attain professional stature than are those of us who advocate relinquishing traditional professional standards.
34. The text of this resolution can be found in Gregg, J.R., *A History of the American Optometric Association*, AOA, St. Louis, 1972, pp. 251–252.
35. Id. at 354 describes the interprofessional difficulties that gripped the two professions at this time. See also Koch, C.C., Resolutions Dealing With Interprofessional Relations, *American Journal of Optometry and Archives of American Academy of Optometry*, vol. 32, no. 8, Aug. 1955, pp. 432–434.
36. The October 1954 issue of *Guildcraft* was by and large devoted to the issue of The Stated Purposes of Optometry As Disclosed By Official Utterances At The National Level, and contained the observation that,

"There is no limit expressed as to how much of the visual care field optometry wants; for frankly, it wants it all." See also, Koch, C.C., Diversionary Attack Upon Optometry, *American Journal of Optometry and Archives of American Academy of Optometry*, vol. 34, no. 5, May, 1957, pp. 276–279.

37. The debate between optometry and ophthalmology was a constant feature in the issues of the *American Journal of Optometry and Archives of American Academy of Optometry*. For examples of the arguments used, see Fry, G.A., The Division of Labor Between Optometry and Opthalmology, vol. 34, no. 3, pp. 150–156; Fry, G.A., Interprofessional Relations In The Design of Eyewear, vol. 34, no. 4, Apr. 1957, pp. 212–221; Hutchinson, E.A., Optometry, Ophthalmology, and Dispensing Opticianry, vol. 34, no. 6, June, 1957, pp. 343–346; Koch, C.C., Observations On Optometry's and Ophthalmology's Interprofessional Relations, vol. 35, no. 1, Jan. 1958, pp. 39–41; and Koch, C.C., Aspects of Interprofessional Relations, vol. 35, no. 2, Feb. 1958, pp. 83–99.

38. Resolution Number 77, adopted by the House of Delegates in June of 1955 provided that "it is unethical for any doctor of medicine to teach in any school or college of optometry, or to lecture to any optometric organization, or to contribute scientific material to the optometric literature, or in any way to impart technical medical knowledge to non-medical practitioners."

39. Ophthalmologists had begun to practice dispensing years before the resolution was adopted, a change in the "ethics" of the profession that was not greeted with favor. See Medical Ethics and Philosophy Involved in Dispensing of Glasses by Ophthalmologists, *American Journal of Ophthalmology*, vol. 32, no. 3, Mar. 1954, pp. 439–443. Surprisingly, there was little commentary in the optometric literature about the formal entry of ophthalmology into dispensing. See *Optical Journal and Review of Optometry*, vol. 92, no. 14, July, 1955, pp. 43–44.

40. See Koch, C.C., Aspects of Interprofessional Relations, *American Journal of Optometry and Archives of American Academy of Optometry*, vol. 35, no. 2, Feb. 1958, pp. 83–99; and Hirsch, M.J., Avenues of Referral Should Be Kept Open, *American Journal of Optometry and Archives of American Academy of Optometry*, vol. 36, no. 3, Mar. 1959, pp. 144–147.

41. The AOA Resolution stated: "Resolved, That the American Optometric Association goes on record as desiring the complete cooperation of the two professions with emphasis on the fact that optometry has no desire to extend its practice to include any limited or other form of medical eye care." Examples of the rumblings of discord that persisted between the two professions can be found in several articles in the *American Journal of Optometry and Archives of American Academy of Optometry*: Koch, C.C., Optometry And Interprofessional Relations, vol. 36, no. 5, May, 1959, pp. 251–265; Koch, C.C., Interprofessional Relations, vol. 37, no. 12, Dec. 1960, pp. 639–641; Tubesing, R.W., The Optometric-Medical Relationship, vol. 38, no. 5, May, 1961, pp. 275–278; Fry, G.A., Optometry and Medicine, vol. 39, no. 3, Mar. 1962, pp. 163–165; Koch, C.C., Cooperation With Medicine, vol. 41, no. 3, Mar. 1964, pp. 180–181; and Hirsch, M.J., Is Ethics More Than Time And Place?, vol. 41, no. 4, Apr. 1964, pp. 261–264.

42. *Dr. Cyrus Bass v. The American Medical Association*, Civil Action 64 C 1279, United States District Court for the Northern District of Illinois, July 24, 1964. A detailed description of the of the case can be found in the *Report to the Optometric Profession*, written by Dr. Bass, a copy of which can be obtained from the International Library, Archives, and Museum of Optometry in St. Louis.

43. An account of the case and the trial judge's opinion can be found in Bass Anti-Trust Action Against American Medical Association Dismissed on Stipulation—Memorandum Opinion Of Court, *Optical Journal and Review of Optometry*, vol. 101, no. 11, June 1, 1967, pp. 29–31.

44. See Stevens, supra note 12, at 108–109.

45. The AOA brief required two years to complete, and shortly after it was submitted to the Justice Department, the *Bass* case was filed. Because the Justice Department would not investigate matters under litigation, the AOA complaint was never pursued. Bailey, J.H., The Four Eyed Man, *American Journal of Optometry and Physiological Optics*, vol. 6, no. 6, June 1983, p. 422.

46. From Opinions and Reports of the Judicial Council, Including the Jurisdiction and Rules of the Judicial Council, American Medical Association, Chicago, 1965. (Section E 3, pp. 13–14, *Manual on Medical Ethics and Discipline.*)

47. The bill was an amendment to the state optometry practice act. It was immediately attacked by ophthalmology in the courts, but the bill withstood constitutional challenge. See *Rhode Island Ophthalmological Society v. Cannon*, 317 A.2d 124 (1974).

48. Like the first state law permitting the use of diagnostic pharmaceutical agents by optometrists, the first state law authorizing therapeutic drug use by optometrists was challenged in the courts by organized ophthalmology. Again, the courts refused to intervene or overturn the law on a constitutional basis. *Esposito v. Shapero*, C A 76 1214, Cabell County Circuit Court, West Virginia, December 16, 1976. Review denied by the West Virginia Supreme Court on June 6, 1977.

49. See Primary Care, by Louis J. Catania, in Newcomb and Jolley, *Public Health And Community Optometry*, pp. 352–368, Charles C. Thomas, Springfield, Ill., 1980.

50. See Gerber, P., Optometry Under Siege! The Gathering Storm, *Optometric Management*, vol. 16, no. 7, July 1980, pp. 23–31.

51. See Special Critical Issues Report, *Optometric Weekly*, vol. 68, no. 4, Jan. 27, 1977, pp. 15–24; and Pavlichko, J.L., Taking Medicine's Pulse, *Review of Opto-*

metry, vol. 120, no. 1, Jan. 1983, pp. 35–43.

52. The conflict between the two professions, past and present, is discussed in a series of articles in *Optometric Management* in 1980. See Optometry Under Siege! The Gathering Storm, July, p. 22; Optometry Under Siege! Will History Repeat Itself?, Aug., p. 34; Optometry Under Siege! Death Blow To Primary Care?, Sept., p. 38; Optometry Under Siege! Is Peace Possible?, Oct., p. 28; and Optometry Under Siege! In Search Of Statesmanship, Nov., p. 51.
53. The economic basis of the conflict between optometry and ophthalmology is discussed by antitrust attorney Douglas J. Colton in The O.D.-M.D. Conflict: Economic Warfare, *Optometric Management*, vol. 18, no. 7, July 1982, pp. 23–27.

Chapter 4

Optometric Ethics

I hereby solemnly swear by all I hold most sacred:

- *That I will keep the visual welfare of my patient uppermost at all times;*
- *That I will retain in confidence any information imparted to me in my professional duties;*
- *That I will seek the consultation of others and refer my patients to the care of others when such is advisable;*
- *That I enhance continuously my educational and technical proficiency to the end that my patient shall receive the benefits of all acknowledged improvements in visual care;*
- *That I will maintain my office and practice in keeping with high professional standards;*
- *That I will promote and maintain cordial and unselfish relationships with members of my own profession and of other professions for the exchange of information and to the advantage of mankind;*
- *That I will conduct myself as an exemplary citizen.*

These things I do swear, so help me God.

—The Optometric Oath, quoted by Etziony, M., *The Physician's Creed*

Historical Perspective

Preoccupation with ethics has been a consistent aspect of optometry's development both as a clinical discipline and as a profession. These concerns have been expressed throughout optometry's history and have been motivated by a desire to elevate the practice of optometry to the level of practice enjoyed by medicine and dentistry. Such a goal was not compatible with the product-oriented philosophy of the marketplace (*caveat emptor*), for the philosophy of professionalism required emphasis on services.[1] From the very beginning of the effort to legalize optometry, it was recognized that both the public good and the profession's welfare depended on the willingness of optometric practitioners to embrace ethical ideals. Charles Prentice, the father of optometry, summarized the conditions facing ethical practitioners in the early days of the profession's development:

> Again, it will be sage not to patronize optical firms who advertise the free service of hired medical eye specialists and the seductive bait of $2.00 glasses, which experience will generally prove to mean a $20.00 expenditure for glasses and services of doubtful value.
>
> Reliable optometrists do not stoop to methods of deception, but follow ethical and dignified methods in their practices. They make separate charges for services and the glasses, which, being made under their personal supervision, must be duplicates of those used in making the ocular measurements. They also refer cases that need medical attention to the physicians, for it should be remembered that among millions of persons who wear glasses, only comparatively few have diseased eyes requiring medical treatment.
>
> Optometry is still in the evolutionary stage, since only the beginning has been made with the object of ultimately placing it upon a professional plane similar to that of dentistry, and which should eventually cause it to redound to the increasing glory of ophthalmology.[2]

Thus, the necessity for a code of ethics was a problem with which the organizers of optometry had to contend, just as had the organizers of medicine some fifty years previously. And if the task faced by medicine in 1847 seemed to be formidable to the physicians of the day, the task faced by optometrists five decades later must have seemed impossible: Optometry did not exist; there were no state laws defining it, no state boards regulating it, no national association to organize it. Each of these problems was to find a solution.

The American Association of Opticians was founded in 1898 and was composed of opticians from 31 states.[3] In 1901 the first state law defining the practice of optometry was enacted in Minnesota.[4] By 1908 thirteen states had passed optometry laws and the national association had grown to 42 states.[5] Despite the fact that many optometrists were little more than businessmen running "downstairs" stores that offered refractions as a means of selling glasses, there was agitation within the national association for a code of ethics. Accordingly, in 1908 a committee chaired by Andrew J. Cross (Fig. 4.1) drafted the first optometric Code of Ethics.[6] The code was brief, broadly drawn, and reflected the realities of the time.[7] Refracting opticians were urged to:

- emphasize that optometry was a "purely technical profession" that did not infringe on the medical monopoly
- "cultivate. . .sensitivities" for the medical position, an attitude that would tend to downplay criticism of ophthalmologists and lead to a more tolerant attitude between the two groups
- refrain from using the title *doctor*

Other keys points touched on by the code pertained to advertising and to fees. Publicity was to be restricted to statements of fact, a position that attempted to discourage the shameless self-promotion of some practitioners. Fees were to be placed on a sliding scale.[8]

Predictably, these modest guidelines had little effect on the manner in which optometry was practiced.[9] Commercialism continued to be a potent force, so potent that in 1922 thirteen optometrists joined together to form the American Academy of Optometry, an organization dedicated to the promotion of ethical practice.[10] The three basic requirements for membership in the Academy were (1) the optometrist had to practice in an office, (2) he had to charge an examination fee of $3.00 or more, and (3) he could not engage in advertising.[11] Unfortunately, only a handful of optometrists could meet these criteria.[12] By the time that the last jurisdiction had enacted an optometry law (the District of Columbia in 1924), less than 25 percent of all optometrists practiced in an "upstairs," ethical environment.[13]

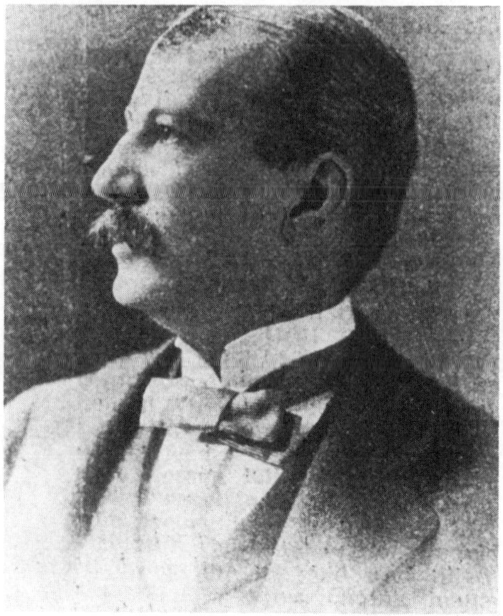

Figure 4.1. Andrew J. Cross. A leader in the New York association, "A.J." Cross was instrumental in the passage of the New York optometry law in 1908, and was chairman of the committee of the American Association of Opticians that drafted the Code of Ethics adopted by the national association in that same year. (Photograph courtesy of the International Library, Archives, and Museum of Optometry)

The depression brought hard times for everyone; optometry was no exception. Although the professional mode of practice was extolled as the ideal, economic realities exerted a contrary influence on practitioners.[14] But by 1935, external factors began to create a climate favorable to change. The United States Supreme Court, in the case of *Semler v. Oregon State Board of Dental Examiners*, held that a state had a legal right to prohibit advertising by members of a health-care profession.[15] This case raised expectations that optometric advertising could be curtailed by passing state laws prohibiting or restricting the use of advertising by optometrists. Over the next decade a remarkable amount of legislative activity ensued, and there was a flurry of litigation concerning this point. The practice of optometry by corporations was also the subject of legislative reform and legal enforcement in the courts.

Another influence on optometrists came from the American Medical Association, which in 1935 passed a resolution prohibiting ophthalmologists from consulting with optometrists.[16] The third factor in this pivotal year came from the American Optometric Association, which ended more than a quarter century of inactivity and approved a new Code of Ethics.[17] The 1935 Code was more demanding than its predecessor and proposed improvements within both clinical practice and intraprofessional relationships. To be better optometrists, practitioners were requested to[18]:

- keep the confidences of patients inviolate
- refrain from any "exaggeration" when describing a patient's condition
- stay abreast of new developments in the field
- avoid criticizing colleagues
- refrain from advertising except as permitted by the code of ethics of the optometrist's state association

The code conspicuously avoided any reference to fees, a major omission. It did offer, however, three "political" commentaries:

- It called on every optometrist to support state and national associations in their efforts to advance the profession.
- It asked optometrists to share their knowledge with one another.
- It labelled as unethical the employment of optometrists "except as the associate of a registered optometrist," a slap at both the corporate practice of optometry and the hiring of optometrists by ophthalmologists.

This Code was disseminated throughout the AOA membership amidst considerable publicity.[19] As an adjunct to the Code, a questionnaire was published so that optometrists could evaluate their level of professionalism.[20] But these efforts were not to have an opportunity to effect change. In 1937, like a bolt out of the blue, came a series of articles on optometry in a popular magazine.[21] The author chronicled, in grim detail, his futile efforts to find an honest optometrist to render a competent service. These widely read articles stung the profession[22] and initiated a determined drive for ethical reform that was given increased momentum by the discriminatory treatment of optometrists by the armed forces in World War II.[23] The leading proponent of reform was the AOA; a series of internal changes were made to strengthen emphasis on ethics and to provide practitioners with advice and help on how to become professional.[24] And in 1944, the biggest change was initiated, a new Code of Ethics that ushered in the "modern era" of ethical optometry. The Code was written by an AOA committee led by John B. O'Shea (Fig. 4.2).

The Code of Ethics of 1944 was illustrative of the professional road that optometry was determined to travel. The conspicuous intent of the Code was to improve optometric service to the public. Ethical practitioners were expected to adhere to several traditionally professional duties (Table 4.1)[26]:

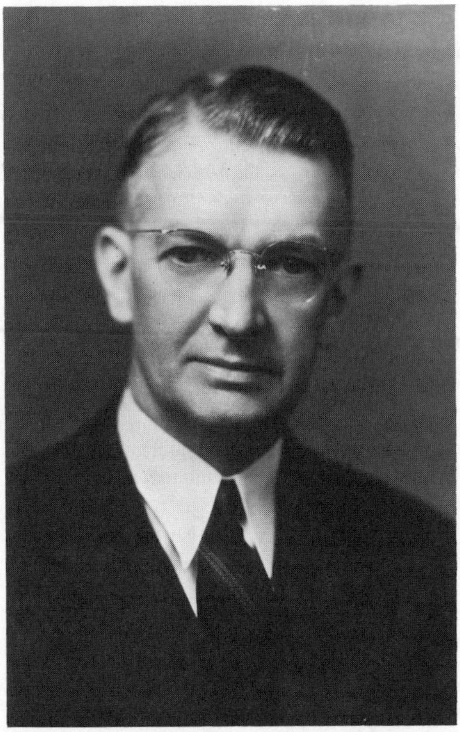

Figure 4.2. John B. O'Shea. Chairman of the committee that drafted the Code of Ethics adopted by the American Optometric Association in 1944, Dr. O'Shea later served as President of the association. (Photography courtesy of the International Library, Archives, and Museum of Optometry)

- To judge every service in terms of its benefit to the patient
- To refer the patient whenever consultation with other health-care providers (including ophthalmologists) was advisable
- To keep all patient information confidential
- To disregard the financial status of patients when rendering services
- To keep abreast of the latest advances in visual science

In addition, the optometrist was required to meet several high standards of personal conduct:

- To promote visual science "in every possible way"
- To maintain "cordial and unselfish relationships" with optometrists and other professionals (such as ophthalmologists)
- To be an exemplary citizen

Table 4.1. The 1944 Code of Ethics of the American Optometric Association

The Code of Ethics of the American Optometric Association sets forth briefly certain basic duties of its members, and it reaffirms the benevolent and humane fundamental purpose of the profession of optometry: To protect and conserve and improve human vision.

Code of Ethics

It Shall Be the Ideal, the Resolve, and the Duty of Members of the American Optometric Association:

TO KEEP the visual welfare of the patient uppermost at all times;

TO PROMOTE in every possible way, in collaboration with the Association, better care of the visual needs of mankind;

TO ENHANCE continuously their educational and technical proficiency to the end that their patients shall receive the benefits of all acknowledged improvements in visual care;

TO SEE THAT no person shall lack for visual care, regardless of his financial status;

TO ADVISE the patient whenever consultation with an optometric colleague or reference for other professional care seems advisable;

TO HOLD in professional confidence all information concerning a patient and to use such data only for the benefit of the patient;

TO CONDUCT themselves as exemplary citizens;

TO MAINTAIN their offices and their practices in keeping with professional standards;

TO PROMOTE and maintain cordial and unselfish relationships with members of their own profession and of other professions for the exchange of information to the advantage of mankind.

Source: American Optometric Association, 1944.

- To practice in an environment "in keeping with professional standards"

These duties were laudable because they set standards that were apolitical and protective of the patient. They failed, however, to set out how an optometrist was to achieve them. In particular, the Code failed to spell out the professional standards that the optometrist was expected to live up to. As a result, two very lengthy (and controversial) documents were approved by the AOA to fulfill this need: the Supplement to the Code of Ethics (1946)[27] and the Rules of Practice (1950).[28] The promulgation of these documents led to the most intensive period of ethical reform in the history of any American health-care profession.[29]

The Supplement was organized like the Percival-inspired codes of ethics adopted by the AMA; it was divided into four basic areas of conduct[30]:

- The basic responsibilities of an optometrist
- Relations between an optometrist and his patients
- Responsibilities to other optometrists and the public
- Relations between optometrists and other professionals

Taken as a whole, the Supplement provided an extremely comprehensive guide for the day-to-day practice of optometry. The Supplement discussed fees in detail and established guidelines for setting fees:

> The compensation and fees that an optometrist receives are based in general on three factors:
>
> 1. The type and character of the optometrist charging the fee
> 2. The character of the service and the skill and knowledge involved in rendering the service
> 3. The value of the service to the patient and his ability to pay
>
> The ophthalmic materials an optometrist may consume in the performance of his professional duties only interpret his services. Such materials have a value that is represented by their laboratory costs to the optometrist.
>
> It is unprofessional and unethical to accept rebates on prescription lenses or optical appliances used in the practice of optometry.[31]

This much-needed stance on fees was supplemented by a gamut of restrictions on soliciting, advertising, displays, guarantees, offers of free examinations, listings in public directories, names and initials used on cards, stationery, billheads, use of signs, profit from patents, and many other matters.[32] Additional guidelines for the conduct of practitioners were published in 1950 as The Rules of Practice, and further defined the boundaries of professional practice.[33]

The Rules of Practice put forth in fourteen clauses an even more stringent set of rules than those in the Supplement. They required the "doctor," "optometrist," or "O.D." (the only approved titles) to be subservient to the state optometry law and to the rulings of the state optometry board; not to hold himself out to be an optician or to claim any special or superior qualifications; to regulate carefully the use of diplomas, honors, official positions within the profession, signs, media, professional cards, and listings in telephone directories; to observe the Code of Ethics and other organizational guidelines published by the AOA or other professional organizations; and to keep from doing "anything inconsistent with the professional standards of the optometric and allied health professions."[34]

In addition to this mass of regulations, the Rules of Practice were given an enforcement capability: The Rules clearly stated that "Enforcement of the Provisions of the Rules of Practice shall be the duty of the various state associations."[35] Actually, there had been some sentiment to have the AOA responsible for enforcement, but in the end it was left to the states. This led to severe problems, particularly in California where the state association split into two factions, one aligned with the AOA and the other independent of the national organization.[36] Some states reported losses in membership because of reluctance to adhere to the Rules[37] and in others the Rules were not adopted.[38] But by 1968, when the Rules of Practice were revised, the revision was able to pass through the AOA voting process unamended[39]; thus, in a mere two decades a substantial change in attitude had been achieved. By 1968 Hirsch and Wick estimated that 70 percent of optometrists could qualify for membership in the American Academy of Optometry.[40] (For that matter, Academy membership was the highest it had ever been.) And by 1975, at least forty-five of the fifty states had enacted either total bans or some form of restriction upon advertising by optometrists.[41] In 1976 and 1977, however, the progress of the profession was cut short by the same entity that had given it life forty years previously, the U.S. Supreme Court.

New Rights, New Responsibilities

All of the professions are interrelated by the nexus of "professionalism," and whatever affects one profession has a way of becoming a matter of concern for the other professions as well. An example of this can be found in the U.S. Supreme Court decisions involving pharmacy, *Virginia State Board of Pharmacy v. Virginia Citizens Consumer Council (1976)*,[42] and the legal profession, *Bates v. Arizona State Bar (1977)*.[43] The holding of the high court was that consumers have a right to receive truthful, nondeceptive advertising and that professional groups could not use codes of ethics to prohibit members of the groups from publishing or disseminating such information. The effects of these two cases were felt in medicine, law, dentistry, architecture, accounting, engineering, and many other professions. They were also felt in optometry.

It was during this period that the Federal Trade Commission (FTC) proposed a trade regulation rule that would deregulate all state laws, then in effect, restricting advertising by optometrists, ophthalmologists, or opticians.[44] As an administrative agency, the FTC's powers are found in the various laws and acts which the U.S. Congress has authorized the FTC to administer. One of these laws is the Magnuson-Moss Act, which granted the FTC the right to prescribe "rules which define with specificity acts or practices which are unfair or deceptive acts or practices in or affecting commerce."[45] Maintaining that laws in forty-five states prohibited or restricted optometrists from advertising the cost and availability of eye examinations, the FTC announced that it considered this to be in restraint of commerce and formulated the "Eyeglasses I Rule" (i.e., the trade regulation rule) as an administrative remedy.[46]

The part of the rule that had the most significant effect on the ethical practice of optometry was the holding that optometrists could advertise, state laws to the contrary notwithstanding. The FTC rule in effect superseded the laws of forty-five states in an effort to return optometry to the marketplace, from which it had extricated itself with such difficulty. In 1978, after a series of hearings, the FTC put its rule into effect.[47] The AOA sued immediately, but the lawsuit was not the only response that had been made by the AOA to the crisis.[48]

Even before the *Bates* and *Virginia State Board of Pharmacy* decisions, the consumer-oriented attitude of the nation had become apparent. In order to comply with this development, the AOA found it necessary to reconsider the Supplement to the Code of Ethics and the Rules of Practice. In 1976 both were replaced by the Standards of Conduct[49] (Table 4.2).

The Standards were organized along the same lines as the Supplement; they addressed:

- the basic responsibilities of an optometrist
- relationships with the patient
- responsibilities to the public
- relationships with other optometrists
- relationships with other professionals

But the Standards of Conduct were far less comprehensive and reflected the realities of the political climate engendered by consumerism and the FTC's Eyeglasses I proceedings. The individual optometrist was left to his own judgment as to the charges for an examination but was advised to clearly separate charges for materials from professional fees.[50] As for advertising, the doctor was told to "honor the applicable provisions of valid state and federal laws

Table 4.2. Standards of Conduct

I. Basic Responsibilities of an Optometrist

Section A. **The Welfare of Humanity**

A health profession has as its prime objective the service it can render to humanity; monetary considerations should be a subordinate factor. In choosing the profession of optometry an individual assumes an obligation for personal conduct in accordance with professional ideals.

Section B. **Continuing Competence**

An optometrist should strive to keep current with every modern development in the profession, to enhance both knowledge and proficiency by the adoption of modern methods and scientific concepts of proven worth, and to contribute personally to the general knowledge and advancement of the profession. All these things should be done with that freedom of action and thought that provides first for the welfare of the public.

II. Relationships with the Patient

Section A. **Presence of a Pathological Condition**

An optometrist should give to the patient or the patient's family a timely notice of manifestations of disease or abnormality.

Section B. **Emergency Optometric Care**

A request for optometric care in an emergency should receive immediate response. Once having undertaken an emergency case, an optometrist shall neither abandon nor neglect the patient.

Section C. **Professional Fees**

Professional fees charged the patient for examination, diagnosis and treatment shall be determined by the individual optometrist.

Section D. **Charges for Materials**

Charges for materials should be clearly separated from professional fees.

III. Responsibilities to the Public

Section A. **Informing the Public**

An optometrist should honor the applicable provisions of valid State and Federal laws and rules regulating the advertising of ophthalmic materials and the disseminating of information regarding professional services.

Section B. **Patents**

It is unprofessional for an optometrist to exploit a patent for lenses, appliances, or instruments used in the practice of optometry in such a way as to deprive the public of its benefits, either through refusal to grant licenses to competent manufacturers who can assure adequate production and unimpeachable quality, or through exorbitant demands in the form of royalty; or for similar forms of monopolistic control in which the interests of the public are exploited.

Section C. **Rebates**

It is unprofessional and unethical to accept rebates on prescriptions, lenses, or optical appliances used in the practice of optometry.

IV. Relationships with Other Optometrists

Section A. **Intraprofessional Referral and Consultations**

Intraprofessional referral and consultations are encouraged when the best interest of the patient indicates additional opinion. Protocol on the relationship and responsibilities between the referring and attending optometrist that customarily is followed by health professions shall prevail.

Section B. **Official Position**

An optometrist holding an official position in any optometric organization shall avoid any semblance of using this position for self-aggrandizement.

V. Relationships with Other Professionals

Section A. **Interprofessional Referral and Consultations**

Interprofessional referral and consultations are encouraged when the best interest of the patient indicates additional opinion. Protocol of the relationship and responsibilities between the referring and attending professional that customarily is followed by health professions shall prevail.

Section B. **Public Health**

Professional responsibility demands that the optometrist actively participate in public health activities with other health professionals to the end that every step be taken to safeguard the health and welfare of the public.

Source: American Optometric Association, 1976.

and rules regulating the advertising of ophthalmic materials and the disseminating of information regarding professional services."[51] These are the guidelines that exist in optometric ethics today.

Having made these changes, the AOA was well prepared for the suit against the FTC and was in fact joined by the AMA and seventeen state attorneys general in the case, which was argued in the Court of Appeals for the District of Columbia.[52] The AOA maintained that the FTC did not have the power to preempt valid state laws and that the Supreme Court decisions concerning law and pharmacy made the FTC's ruling superfluous. The court agreed, and suspended the trade regulation rule (except for the provision unrelated to the issue of preemption requiring the "refractionist" to give a copy of the pre scription to the patient at the conclusion of the examination).[53] The outcome of the FTC's decision to implement Eyeglasses II—which seeks to end the enforceability of state laws restricting or prohibiting commercial practice by optometrists—will also depend upon a court's interpretation of the FTC's legal powers.

And so, the efforts of decades seem to be hanging in the balance. What will be the long-term effect of allowing professionals to advertise?[54] Even more importantly, what effect will these efforts by government have on professionalism? Within this latter question lies the biggest problem facing optometry today: the spectre of commercialism.

The Ethical Practitioner

Given the commercial effects of the corporate practice of optometry, the legal decisions in favor of advertising, the watering-down of codes of ethics, and the resulting decrease in authority among state boards of optometry (see Table 4.3), what will become of the professional practice of optometry?

To begin with, advertising is a problem unique to the large cities or high population areas where there is ample competition between eye-care providers. The small-town optometrist, with no or minimal competition, will not need to advertise. Hopefully, his reputation in the community will obviate the need for an advertising campaign. In larger, more metropolitan areas, it may be necessary for professional

Table 4.3. Historical Milestones: Optometric Ethics

1908	Under the leadership of Andrew J. Cross, a Code of Ethics is adopted by the American Association of Opticians (in 1919 to become the American Optometric Association).
1935	The American Optometric Association adopts a Code of Ethics, due principally to the efforts of AOA counsel Harold Kohn. The United States Supreme Court, in the case of *Semler v. Oregon State Board of Dental Examiners*, holds that states may constitutionally regulate truthful advertising by professionals.
1944	The AOA adopts a new Code of Ethics; the committee that drafted the Code is led by chairman John B. O'Shea.
1946	The AOA adopts The Supplement to the Code of Ethics.
1950	The Rules of Practice are adopted by the AOA, causing intense internal dissention among members of the association.
1955	The United States Supreme Court, in *Williamson v. Lee Optical of Oklahoma*, holds that a state may constitutionally regulate the commercial practice of optometry.
1968	The Rules of Practice are revised without difficulty.
1976	The Supplement to the Code of Ethics and The Rules of Practice are replaced by the Standards of Conduct.
1977	The United States Supreme Court, in the case of *Bates v. Arizona State Bar*, reverses four decades of precedent and holds that professionals may utilize truthful advertising.
1978	The Federal Trade Commission issues a trade regulation rule (Eyeglasses I) that preempts state laws restricting advertising of ophthalmic goods and services by optometrists, ophthalmologists, and opticians.
1980	The U.S. Court of Appeals for the District of Columbia, in the case of *American Optometric Association v. Federal Trade Commission*, refuses to enforce that portion of the FTC rule that preempts state laws restricting advertising of ophthalmic goods and services.
1988	The FTC commissioners approve a trade regulation rule (Eyeglasses II) preventing enforcement of state laws that restrict or prohibit commercial practice by optometrists.

optometrists to band together for mutual benefit and public recognition. To some extent this is already being done. But one of the chief difficulties of getting started in optometric practice—obtaining patients—has as part of its cause the historically proven reluctance of optometrists to refer patients to one another. As optometry laws evolve, bringing with them a trend toward intraprofession specialization, perhaps this will change. In any event, it is obvious that the profession as a whole must take some steps to assure the survivability of its graduates as independent private practitioners.[55]

Wherever large optical chains are able to take root in the ophthalmic market of a state, ethical practitioners are placed at a distinct disadvantage, for the ultimate emphasis of such businesses is on cost. A doctor in private practice providing quality services cannot compete with a larger, volume oriented business on the basis of price. He is placed in much the same position as the small, independent oil companies that tried to compete with the large national corporations and that were squashed in the "open market" of the early years of this century, when the open market was in effect controlled by the prices set by big business. The spectre of such an eventuality looms over all eye doctors in practice today, optometrists and ophthalmologists alike, as corporations obtain a larger share of the eye-care market.[56]

But commercialized modes of practice have already proven themselves to be no panacea.[57] They have been financial disappointments for many of the large chains funding them,[58] the optometrists employed by them,[59] and the consumers patronizing them.[60] Even so, the large corporations are pressing for increasingly larger shares of the ophthalmic market and have launched large publicity and legislative campaigns to achieve this goal. Current statistics indicate that they have been successful.[61]

Even though it is obvious that the modern-day optometrist faces an ethical crisis in the private sector, schools of optometry continue to produce approximately 1,000 new graduates a year, the great majority of whom enter into costly, ethical practices that eschew the financial stability and relative lack of risk found in the commercialized environments.[62] It is remarkable that so many young women and men are willing to dedicate themselves to less affluent beginnings in order to pursue a way of life that Corporate America (and even the U.S. government) is trying to eliminate. In very few professions is this kind of moral fiber displayed. Indeed, this willingness to incur significant personal debt and a relatively modest lifestyle while slowly building a professional practice flies in the face of the materialistic attitude of the times. But then optometry has always been a singular profession, calling for a willingness to go one's own way. The challenge that commercialism represents is the most serious threat that optometry has ever faced because it strikes at optometry's Achilles's heel: the profit that may be derived from the sale of ophthalmic materials. This issue and its implications for the future are discussed in the following chapter.

Notes

1. The basis for professional ethics is discussed by Monroe J. Hirsch and Ralph E. Wick in their fine book, *The Optometric Profession*, Chilton Book Co., Philadelphia, 1968, pp. 145–147, 170–177.
2. Prentice, C.F., *Legalized Optometry and Memoirs*, Casperin Fletcher Press, Seattle, 1926, pp. 185–186.
3. Gregg, J.R., *A History of the American Optometric Association*, American Optometric Assn., St. Louis, 1972, pp. 9–10.
4. For a historical perspective of the first optometry practice act, see Address Before the Minnesota State Optical Association, Sept. 4, 1901, by H.M. Hitchcock of the State Board of Examiners, *The Optical Journal*, vol. 8, no. 10, Oct. 1901, p. 929. The text of the law can be found in Hirsch and Wick, supra note 1, at 315–317.
5. See Gregg, supra note 3, at pp. 29–41.
6. See Code of Ethics of the American Association of Opticians, *The Optical Journal*, vol. 22, no. 8, Aug. 20, 1908, p. 379. See also Editorial, *The Optical Journal*, vol. 22, no. 11, Sept. 10, 1908.
7. The first Code of Ethics was widely viewed as inadequate, and for years following the adoption of this first ethical code, various commentaries urging a more comprehensive and useful approach could be found in the optometric literature. For examples, see A National Code of Ethics, *The Optical Journal and Review of Optometry*, vol. 50, no. 16, Oct. 19, 1922, pp. 27–28; Meyer, B., The Ethics of the Profession, *The Optical Journal and Review of Optometry*, vol. 51, no. 19, May 10, 1923, pp. 31–33; The Real Issues in Ethics, *The Optical Journal and Review of Optometry*, vol. 51, no. 22, May 31, 1923, p. 31; McFadden, F., Fundamentals in Optometric Ethics, *Optical Journal and Review of Optometry*, vol. 51, no. 22, May 31, 1923, pp. 46–47. As a result of the widespread commentary launched through the journals, the AOA appointed a committee to propose a new Code of Ethics, and in fact such a revised code was proposed but failed to be adopted in 1923. See AOA's Committee on Code of Ethics, *The Optical Journal and Review of Optometry*, vol. 52, no. 1, July 5, 1923, pp. 64–65.
8. Fees were a primary bone of contention because of the commercial element within the profession. Nearly thirty years after the adoption of this first Code of Ethics, the argument over how to set fees still raged. See Evans, E.,

Single Charge vs. Separation of Service Fee and Price of Glasses, *The Optical Journal and Review of Optometry*, vol. 72, no. 4, Feb. 15, 1935, p. 25.

9. For a review of the struggle to professionalize the practice of optometry during this era, as seen from the point of view of the membership of the AOA, see Gregg, supra note 3, at 63–136.
10. The formation of the American Academy of Optometry is described by Hirsch and Wick, supra note 1, at 152–155.
11. Ibid.
12. Ibid.
13. For a review of the development of the ethical standards within optometry, see Hofstetter, H.W., *Optometry: Professional, Economic, and Legal Aspects*, St. Louis, C.V. Mosby Co., St. Louis, 1948.
14. Ibid.
15. 294 U.S. 608, 55 S. Ct. 570 (1935). The text of this decision can also be found in Hirsch and Wick, supra note 1, at 181–184.
16. The series of resolutions passed by the American Medical Association to prevent intercourse between optometry and medicine are summarized by Rosemary Stevens in her book, *American Medicine and the Public Interest*, Yale Univ. Press, New Haven, Conn., 1977, pp. 108–109.
17. *Report of the 38th Annual Congress of the American Optometric Association National Convention*, House of Delegates, June 23–28, 1935, pp. 139–140. See also Resolution No. 1, *Journal of the American Optometric Association*, vol. 7, no. 1, Aug. 1935, p. 42.
18. See Hofstetter, supra note 13, at 120–142.
19. See AAO Calls on AOA for Drive Against Store Fronts, Display Windows, Neon Signs and Inside Show Cases, *Optical Journal and Review of Optometry*, vol. 72, no. 23, Dec. 1, 1935, p. 28.
20. Young, D., Rate Yourself, *Journal of the American Optometric Association*, vol. 7, no. 3, Oct. 1935, pp. 42–43.
21. Riis, R., Optometry on Trial, *Reader's Digest*, vol. 31, Aug. 1937, pp. 77–85; Sept. 1937, pp. 102–104; Oct. 1937, pp. 84–96.
22. See Yes, Optometry Is on Trial, *The Optical Journal and Review of Optometry*, vol. 74, no. 15, Aug. 1, 1937, pp. 22–23; "Optometry on Trial" Is a Two-Edged Sword, *Optical Journal and Review of Optometry*, vol. 74, no. 16, Aug. 15, 1937, pp. 20–21; The End of the "Trial," *Optical Journal and Review of Optometry*, vol. 74, no. 19, Oct. 1, 1937, pp. 24–25; and Some Public Reactions, *Optical Journal and Review of Optometry*, vol. 74, no. 20, Oct. 15, 1937, p. 21.
23. Sample editorials addressing the treatment of optometrists by the military can be found in The Penalty of Independence, *Optical Journal and Review of Optometry*, vol. 81, no. 16, Aug. 15, 1944; and Areas of Supremacy, *Optical Journal and Review of Optometry*, vol. 82, no. 24, Dec. 15, 1945, pp. 42–43. The consensus of opinion of the time was that commercialism had been the cause of optometry's relegation to noncommissioned status. For a personal viewpoint, see Lang, G.L., An Open Letter to the Unethical, *Optical Journal and Review of Optometry*, vol. 81, no. 22, Nov. 15, 1944, p. 26. See also Hofstetter, supra note 13, at 110–117.
24. Palmer, J.A., *Ethics and Economics*, Parts I and II, Publications of the Professional Advancement Program of the AOA, 1943; Warren, E.F., A Recent Graduate Comments on Ethics, *Optical Journal and Review of Optometry*, vol. 80, no. 23, Dec. 1, 1943, p. 25; Time to Change the System, *Optical Journal and Review of Optometry*, vol. 81, no. 2, Jan. 15, 1944, pp. 28–29; and Palmer, J.A., Report of the Department of Ethics and Economics, *Journal of the American Optometric Association*, vol. 16, no. 4, Nov. 1944, pp. 97–99.
25. Code of Ethics Adopted by the House of Delegates of the American Optometric Association, June 27, 1944, *Journal of the American Optometric Association*, vol. 16, no. 1, Aug. 1944, p. 18.
26. See Ethics and Professional Behavior, in Hirsch and Wick, supra note 1, at 170–177.
27. For a copy of the Supplement to The Code of Ethics, see Hofstetter, supra note 13, at 133–136.
28. A copy of the Rules of Practice, as adopted in 1950, can be found in Gregg, supra note 3, at 226–228.
29. The time and effort directed toward the professionalization of optometry can be said to be truly amazing. A comprehensive review of these efforts is not possible, but selective references can point out the Herculean effort undertaken throughout by practitioners: Listing of Optometrists in Telephone Directories, *Optical Journal and Review of Optometry*, vol. 82, no. 22, Nov. 15, 1945, pp. 26–27; Kintner G.F., Ethics and Economics, *Optical Journal and Review of Optometry*, vol. 83, no. 19, Sept. 1, 1946; *Principles of Ethics and Economics*, Dept. of Ethics and Economics, American Optometric Association, St. Louis, Mo., 1946; AOA Recommended Standards for Outdoor Signs, Upstairs and Street Level Lettering, *Optical Journal and Review of Optometry*, vol. 85, no. 8, May 1, 1948; and Gregg, supra note 3, at 201–246.
30. For a review of the ethics of medical practice as determined by the writings of Thomas Percival, see Chapter 2.
31. The stance of optometrists on rebating was doubtless due, in part, to the scandalous experiences of ophthalmologists who utilized this practice to derive profit from the sale of ophthalmic materials. For a discussion, see the following: Federal Investigation of Rebating, *American Journal of Ophthalmology*, vol. 29, no. 10, Oct. 1946, pp. 1313–1315; Optical Rebates, *American Journal of Ophthalmology*, vol. 30, no. 8, Aug. 1947, pp. 1030–1032; The Rebate Cases, *American Journal of Ophthalmology*, vol. 31, no. 9, Sept. 1948, pp. 1177–1178; and Income Tax Deductions for Kickbacks, *American Journal of Ophthalmology*, vol. 33, no. 9, Sept. 1950, pp. 1456–1458.
32. See Hofstetter, supra note 13, at 133–136.
33. The Rules of Practice had a stormy history. See Gregg,

supra note 3, at 223–244.
34. Id. at 227.
35. Id. at 223–244.
36. Id. at 233–234.
37. Id. at 223–244.
38. Ibid.
39. Id. at 322.
40. Hirsch and Wick, supra note 1, at 175.
41. The restrictions compiled in the Staff Report of the Federal Trade Commission can be found in the Trade Regulation Rule promulgated by the FTC in the *Federal Register* for June 2, 1978 (43 F.R. 23992-24008), 16 C.F.R. §456.
42. 425 U.S. 748, 96 S. Ct. 1817 (1976).
43. 433 U.S. 350, 97 S. Ct. 2691 (1977).
44. The FTC first proposed its trade regulation rule on January 16, 1976. See 16 C.F.R. §456. (41 F.R. 2399). The rule became effective on May 24, 1978.
45. Section 202 of the Magnuson-Moss-FTC Improvement Act, 15 U.S.C. §57a (1982).
46. This was the first trade regulation rule under the Magnuson-Moss Act published by the Federal Trade Commission, and so there were constitutional issues concerning the FTC's exercise of this power that had never been tested in a court of law. For a discussion of the rule, see Classe, J., The Effect of FTC Rulings on the Practice of Optometry, *Southern Journal of Optometry*, vol. 21, no. 5, May 1979, pp. 20–24.
47. The response of optometrists to the rule is summarized in a panel report compiled by the *Review of Optometry*, vol. 115, no. 12, Dec. 1978, pp. 41–45.
48. *American Optometric Association v. Federal Trade Commission*, Case Number 78-1461, U.S. Court of Appeals for the District of Columbia.
49. The Standards of Conduct were issued "to keep pace with the 1970's," and the AOA made it clear that they "in no way represent a change in philosophy." (From the AOA news release of March 29, 1976.) The Standards of Conduct were published in the *AOA News*, Apr. 1, 1976.
50. Ibid.
51. Ibid.
52. An account of the case can be found in the *AOA News*, June 1, 1978.
53. 626 F.2d 896 (D.C. Cir. 1980).
54. The resurrection of advertising as an issue for optometrists has once again brought forth the *angst* of professional practitioners. See Wick, R.E., The Ethical High Road, *American Journal of Optometry and Physiological Optics*, vol. 54, no. 5, May 1977, pp. 323–324. But optometry is no longer alone in the search for an answer concerning how to deal with this long-standing problem. For a medical viewpoint, see Veatch, R.M., Physician Advertising, *The New Physician*, July–Aug., 1980, pp. 35–37.
55. The average student of optometry leaves optometry school with a debt of approximately $20,000, according to a survey of graduates of the Pacific College of Optometry in 1984. A study of practice patterns of the graduates of the Illinois College of Optometry (1978–1982) revealed that 37 percent are in solo practice, 16 percent in partnership, 24 percent are in employee positions, and 7 percent are in commercial practice. A larger study, conducted by the Association of Schools and Colleges of Optometry of 72 percent of all optometry school graduates during the period 1981–1983, showed that nearly half of these graduates resorted to salaried positions rather than traditional self-employed practice and that 70 percent encountered some form of problem in entering into optometric practice. See the *AOA News*, Dec. 1, 1983.
56. The development of optical chains has become a major factor in the eye care field. According to Irving Bennett, O.D., these chains—which just a few years ago attracted a rather small portion of the patient population—enjoyed a 16 percent share of the market as of 1984 and a 22 percent share by 1988. See Special Report: State of Optometry 1988, *Optometric Management*, vol. 24, no. 4, 1988, pp. 37–43.
57. The traditional means of attracting patients to chains, advertising of low prices, convenience, and variety of products, has apparently not met with the success envisioned by the nation's two largest chains. Instead, these companies have begun touting themselves as providers of quality vision care in an effort to attract the patient population of independent, professional optometrists. See Chains Try "Quality" Care, *Review of Optometry*, vol. 121, no. 5, May 15, 1984, pp. 3–5.
58. See Pinto, D., The Drug-Optical Chains: Not Made of Gold, *Optometric Management*, vol. 16, no. 1, Jan. 1980, pp. 37–43. Contrast the reality of the chain drug store market (estimated at less than one percent) to the seeming promise of but a decade earlier. See Invasion of Optometric Dispensing, *Optometric Weekly*, vol. 67, no. 44, Oct. 28, 1976, pp. 11–13.
59. See Gerber, P., Inside Corporate Optometry—And Out Again, *Optometric Management*, vol. 15, no. 9, Sept. 1979, pp. 36–43; and Pearle's Luster Dimmed?, *Optometric Management*, vol. 15, no. 10, 1979, pp. 35–38.
60. The large commercial chains have chosen to abandon the discount market, which is a small and low-profit segment of the industry, in favor of advertising campaigns aimed toward the value market, which is made up of patients who desire quality care. This market belongs largely to independent optometrists, who are estimated to provide 52 percent of all eye examinations and to sell 43 percent of all eyewear. See Chains Try "Quality" Care, *Review of Optometry*, vol. 121, no. 5, May 15, 1984, pp. 3–5.
61. Franchising has been available nationwide since 1981 and has been reasonably successful. Serle's Pearle Vision Centers, one of the largest franchise chains, has succeeded in franchising about half of its more than 1,000 stores. The market share of franchised stores was about 16 percent in 1983 and 1984. See Bennett, I., The Ophthalmic Industry, *Optometric Management*, vol. 20, no. 5, May 1984, pp. 85–105.
62. The survey of 2,275 optometry school graduates con-

ducted by the Association of Schools and Colleges of Optometry during the period September 1981 through March 1983 revealed that 6.7 percent of those responding worked for an optical company in a commercial environment. See the *AOA News*, Dec. 1, 1983, for an account of the study's major findings.

Chapter 5

Optometry Agonistes

Frames are where the money is.
—Kurt Vonnegut, Jr., *Slaughterhouse Five*

A House Divided

One of the key concessions that was necessary in order for optometry to receive legal recognition was the so-called grandfather clause, which was a guarantee to those already in practice that they would not be deprived of their livelihoods by the optometry practice acts being enacted by the states.[1] The grandfather clause permitted all persons practicing optometry as of a stated date to receive a license, without examination, irrespective of their competence. Many of these grandfathered practitioners regarded optometry as no more than a business, or, even worse, as a sideline that merely served as an additional source of revenue. The income they enjoyed was derived from the sale of glasses. The examination was incidental to the sale and consisted of refraction almost exclusively; in many cases the examination was free and was absorbed into the charge for the glasses.[2] These practitioners were principally entrepreneurs and resented any attempts to curb either their mode of practice or their independence.

They were philosophically opposed by a small but determined group of optometrists who considered the examination to be the cornerstone of optometry and the ophthalmic goods to be an ancillary service that permitted a degree of continuity not offered by other eye-care practitioners. Besides offering refraction and ophthalmoscopy, these optometrists charged a fee for the examination that was separate and distinct from that for materials.[3] They were a decided minority, but they believed that optometry had the potential to emerge as a profession on a plane with medicine and dentistry, a sentiment often expressed by the medical leadership as well.[4] Thus, seen in a historical context, it is apparent that optometry was a house divided (not unlike the medical profession of a few decades earlier)[5] and that conflict was inevitable.

Even a cursory review of the optometric journals during the 1930s and 1940s reveals the depth of the profession's internal discord[6] and the significance of the legal forum as the ultimate arbiter of the dispute.[7] The usual protagonist was the state board of optometry (or the state acting on its behalf), seeking to prevent some activity that was in contravention to the state optometry law; the defendants were corporations or other types of business entities,[8] opticians,[9] optometrists,[10] or profit-seeking entrepreneurs.[11] The lawsuits were brought in so many jurisdictions and for so many causes that, over the course of this period (the 1930s and 1940s) nothing resembling a clear-cut opinion emerged from the decisions of the courts.[12] (In fact, these cases clearly illustrate the limitations of the judicial system when it is asked to decide ethical issues involving professionals.) By World War II there was still a large segment of optometry that opposed the movement to professionalize.

Two events tipped the balance toward the professional forces: the war and technological advances. During World War II optometrists were not accepted as commissioned officers by the armed forces,[13] and the stigma suffered by these enlisted "refractionists," accompanied by governmental discrimination,[14] initiated a call for reform that swept through optometry as never before and resulted in the most profession's intense campaign over ethics.[15] During the 1950s, two technological developments also significantly altered optometrists' view of their calling: the tonometer and the corneal contact lens. They thrust optometrists into direct contact with the eye and made ocular health an essential part of optometric care. These events provided the impetus for reform, as optometry, with the AOA as its standard bearer, grudgingly began a remarkable transformation that, within the course of two decades, brought it into full flower as a profession. This period of change produced some of the most significant legal victories in optometry's history.

Since the landmark case of *Semler v. Oregon State Board of Dental Examiners* (1935),[16] the uniform law of the land had been that states could limit advertising, even if truthful, by professionals. This law was extended to the advertising of "optical appliances" in *Williamson v. Lee Optical of Oklahoma* (1955),[17] a precedent-setting case that also curtailed the right of corporations to lease space within the corporate premises to eye-care practitioners. Another U.S. Supreme Court case, *Head v. New Mexico Board of Examiners in Optometry* (1963),[18] further limited the advertising of ophthalmic goods and services by radio and newspaper. These precedents made it clear that activities such as corporate practice and advertising could be controlled; there remained the significant problem of actually convincing state legislatures to enact the appropriate statutes. Nevertheless, by the mid-1970s, forty-five states had passed legislation intended to do just that.[19] But these victories were not without cost: Those optometrists who opposed professionalism became an ostracized minority, and the conflict with opticianry and ophthalmology escalated into more than a war of words. But the movement for professionalization also found itself up against another adversary: the consumer movement.

As has been discussed in Chapter 1, optometry was legalized in the United States in order to protect the right of a class of citizens to continue to earn a living. The refracting opticians did not contemplate that they would be accused of seeking a monopoly, since the services offered by refracting opticians were also offered by others. Even the battle over professionalism was a philosophical battle. (It must be remembered that, until the late 1950s, the average optometrist earned less than $10,000 a year and that the nonprofessional practitioners were among the highest wage earners in the profession.)[20] Thus it came as somewhat of a surprise to the optometrists who had led the movement toward professionalization to learn that they were being branded as anticompetitive and anticonsumer because of this effort.

The social revolution toward consumerism was soon reflected in the decisions of the nation's highest court. In *Gibson v. Berryhill* (1973),[21] the composition of state boards of optometry was attacked, causing far-reaching changes in the board selection process; in *Virginia State Board of Pharmacy v. Virginia Citizens Consumer Council* (1976),[22] the court recognized that certain commercial advertising should be afforded constitutional protection; and in *Bates v. State Bar of Arizona* (1977),[23] it was held that truthful commercial advertising by professionals was permissible. The effect of these cases was to eliminate the legislative restrictions prohibiting advertising and to encourage the corporate practice of optometry.

Other developments mitigated in favor of the antiprofessional forces: the Federal Trade Commission succeeded at least partially in making prescriptions for glasses an item of commerce,[24] and an economic depression made the traditional made of optometric practice (solo practitioner starting up cold) virtually unaffordable. The end result was a further depletion of the pool of professional optometrists. Large corporations seeking to profit from the sale of ophthalmic goods began an expensive and comprehensive campaign to attract optometrists and ophthalmologists into the corporate system[25] and thus initiated a new period of confrontation, with its own proliferating mass of lawsuits[26] and legislation.[27]

The current legal climate, being of relatively recent origin, promises to continue, and so it would appear that optometry, as a profession, has reached a crossroads in its development. Now the overriding issue has become the direction that the profession will take as it responds to its latest crisis.

Optometry at the Crossroads

Optometry has been a crisis-oriented profession thoughout its history and has survived because (1) it offers a service that is indispensible to the public and (2) the public welfare has demanded that it receive legal sanction and protection. Although optometry has been divided over ethical matters throughout, it has acquired a strong understanding of these problems, which perhaps will serve it well in the long run as it attempts to progress during the era of consumerism.

As explained in Chapter 1, the profession has already entered into the most revolutionary period in its history. Even so, with a multitude of new challenges awaiting it, there remains a familiar litany of problems inherited from the past. These problems, although ethical in nature, have found legal solutions (or perhaps it would be more accurate to say that legal solutions have been attempted), which in turn have generated new problems. Among the most important of these are corporate practice, advertising, fees, dispensing, and patient referral.

Corporate Practice

The initial legal battles between professional and corporate forces centered around the employment of optometrists by profit-seeking businesses. Since the primary means of profit was through the sale of ophthalmic goods, the legal issue was whether the profit motive would unduly influence the judgment of the optometrist, thus intruding on the doctor-patient relationship in a most unsatisfactory manner. The results of these cases were mixed until the landmark decision of the Supreme Court in *Williamson v. Lee Optical of Oklahoma*,[28] which held that corporations could be barred from leasing space to optometrists within their premises. In the years that followed, corporations turned to the "side-by-side" operation, whereby an optical shop leased space in a contiguous office to an optometrist, who performed the refraction for the glasses or contact lenses to be purchased at the optical shop.[29] The response to this development was the enactment of tough business codes that prohibited landlord-tenant relationships or profit sharing between optometrists and corporations in any form; these laws also frequently prohibited the sale of optometric franchises.[30] And the Supreme Court, in *Friedman v. Rogers (1977)*, upheld the right of states to prevent the practice of optometry under a trade name.[31] Despite these legal efforts, the corporate practice of optometry remains a divisive force within the profession because laws vary remarkably from state to state and big business has entered into the fray. Some professional optometrists have turned to alternative forms of delivering their services, including branch offices,[32] group practice,[33] association with physicians,[34] and the use of marketing,[35] in an effort to preserve the traditional independence of optometric practitioners. None of these efforts seem likely to reverse the trend, which is presently in favor of the commercialists.[36]

Advertising

The practice of optometry has gone full circle on the issue of advertising. Since 1935, when the famous *Semler* case was decided by the U.S. Supreme Court (and the AOA passed its first ethical prohibition), advertising has been a source of conflict among optometrists. Much litigation and legislation was instituted by the states in the 1930s, 1940s, and 1950s in an effort to rid the profession of advertising.

The greatest evil was the "bait-and-switch" tactics employed by some unscrupulous businesses, whereby cut-rate prices would be advertised but these low-priced items would be either "unavailable" or "unsuitable" for the potential purchaser, who would end up buying an expensive item instead.[37] Another reprehensible tactic was "capping and steering", which was used to lure persons seeking ophthalmic goods to a particular business.[38] Underlying these and other despicable practices was the power of advertising, which, although undeniably abused, achieved its single purpose: to attract business. Advertising is not profitable unless a volume business is sought, and it is this fundamental purpose of advertising that is at odds with the concept of professionalism.

The traditional means of "advertising," through word of mouth, contains a personal guarantee of quality; it is an implicit form of recommendation. But using electronic and printed media to advertise serves only to draw attention to the advertiser (which is itself anathema to professionalism) and contains no guarantee of quality. And if the advertising emphasizes price only, it is a virtual certainty that quality will not be a consideration.[39] Despite the efforts of professional optometrists over the decades to eradicate advertising of ophthalmic goods and services, the Supreme Court, in the precedent setting *Virginia State Board of Pharmacy* and *Bates* cases, has opened the door for all professionals to advertise. It is left to the states, and to the various professional boards, to set reasonable restrictions that conform to the court's decisions.[40] Future efforts, such as those by the FTC, may further weaken restrictions.[41]

Fees

Optometric fees have traveled a long and tortuous road over the course of the past several decades. They began as one price, a charge for ophthalmic materials, into which was subsumed the examination fee (which was often touted as free). Of course, this was primarily utilized by merchandisers of goods, be they optometrists or corporations. It was but a hearty minority of practitioners who were bold enough to charge a fee for services apart from the fee for materials.

At the root of the one charge philosophy was

economics: It was felt that an optometrist could not make a living merely performing examinations; materials had to be sold as well. Since materials were the primary source of income it seemed pointless to separate the cost of providing the examination (i.e., refraction) from the materials.

Three factors combined to erode the one-price fee structure. The first of these was taxes. Several states levied taxes on ophthalmic materials,[42] and the only way to reduce them (other than by repealing the law) was to divide fees into charges for services (which were not taxed) and for materials (which were taxed at their cost to the consumer).

Another factor was the extraordinary effort of professional optometry to reform the one charge philosophy within its membership. Entire programs were organized to educate practitioners and the literature abounds with references to the need to reform fees.[43]

A third factor was the federal government, through the Medicare and Medicaid programs and the efforts of the FTC. Since reimbursement for Medicare practitioners relied on a fee profile that was drawn from the fees being charged by practitioners in a delineated area, optometrists were forced to separate their fees in order to participate. The FTC's Eyeglasses I Rule, which required eye-care practitioners to give their patients a copy of the prescription for glasses or contact lenses at the conclusion of the examination, caused optometric fees not only to be separated into charges for services and charges for materials but also altered fee structures by causing optometrists to revise charges for services.[44] The end result of these various influences has been to modernize the current-day optometric fee structure. The trend has been toward increased emphasis on professional fees and reduced reliance on materials. This is a trend that can be expected to continue.

Dispensing

One of the major sources of conflict between medicine and optometry was optometry's involvement with ophthalmic goods as a source of profit.[45] As described in Chapter 3, however, there arose in ophthalmology an insidious system of rebating that allowed these practitioners also to derive an income from the sale of ophthalmic goods.[46] This practice was curtailed in part by the federal government through legal action and was eventually made unnecessary by the adoption of relaxed codes of ethics by the AMA in 1955, permitting ophthalmologists to own retail outlets selling ophthalmic goods and to dispense such goods directly if they so wished.[47] Although the initial reaction of optometrists to this change in medical philosophy was doubtless a feeling of satisfaction, the long-term result has been to blur distinctions between the two groups and to heighten competition.

Despite the fact that all ophthalmic providers dispense ophthalmic goods, there remains within optometry a continuing debate over the necessity of handling these goods. It has long been maintained that optometry best serves the consumer by providing both examination and materials, since this permits continuity of services and allows some guarantee of quality. That this continuity is favored by consumers would seem to be evident from results of the FTC's Eyeglasses I Rule; follow-up studies have shown that there has been no wholesale movement to abandon optometric dispensing in order to shop for ophthalmic goods from other providers.[48] Nevertheless, optometric dispensing patterns have begun to change in a fundamental fashion.

The traditional model has been one-stop service; both the examination and the dispensing were performed in one office. If the practitioner was professional, there was no advertising of fees or services. The current trend is toward "two-door" facilities that are contiguous, one being the optometrist's office and the other being an optical dispensary.[49] Ostensibly, this removes the optometrist somewhat from dealing directly with ophthalmic goods, but the dispensary sells the goods upon his prescription for a profit, and so the net effect is not changed. This trend has met with opposition within the professional segment of optometry. There is also a minority faction that advocates the abandonment of dispensing altogether.[50] This is not a feasible alternative unless the scope of practice is appreciably altered to include "medical" care.

Referral

The two instruments that differentiated optometry from opticianry were the phoropter and the ophthalmoscope. They have come to symbolize the two principal services of the profession: the determination of refractive status and the examination for disease. They also represent the responsibility that optometry has always accepted for its patients: to deliver quality vision care and to refer for medical treatment when appropriate. This second responsibility has been a feature of optometric professional liability law from the very first cases.[51] Even in those states where optometrists may employ therapeutic pharmaceutical agents, optometrists still have a clear responsibility to refer under the appropriate circumstances.

Recently there has been an effort on the part of

some members of medicine to codify the common law requirement to refer.[52] This effort has been relatively unsuccessful, and has been regarded as unnecessary regulation that would not be economically or legally practicable.[53] As the scope of practice of optometry evolves, it is likely that the responsibility of optometrists for diagnosis of disease and referral to medical specialists will increase. The clear trend in professional liability cases involving optometrists is toward expanded responsibility for disease, both ocular and systemic.

As the preceding paragraphs have shown, optometry enters its most challenging era still carrying the weighty problems of the past, problems that have not yet found resolution. Inevitably, these harbingers of the past will influence the new direction that the profession will take, as it seeks solutions to the ethical issues that have been a constant aspect of the practice of optometry. One lesson seems clear: Commercial practice offers only a continuation of these problems and cannot advance the profession in the public good.[54]

The Road Less Travelled By

The historical evolution of the role of optometrists, as seen in a legal context, is a classical illustration of "the man in the middle." The first optometry laws sought to preserve the right of refracting opticians to practice their calling while at the same time differentiating those who practiced optometry from physicians and opticians. Over the course of several decades, optometry was squeezed from both sides, as ophthalmologists turned increasingly to refraction and to dispensing ophthalmic goods and as opticians sought to incorporate the fitting of contact lenses and other optometric skills into the practice of opticianry. Each development generated its own legal actions, both judicial and legislative, and fueled the conflict between the various professions. In addition, there was the internal struggle between professional and commercial factions within optometry, which spawned a remarkable profusion of legal activity all its own.

During this period there have been significant changes in health manpower and in the delivery of vision-care services. In the past two decades, the expansion of ophthalmologists has been far greater than that of optometrists,[55] and it is projected that by 1990 the number of ophthalmologists will be in oversupply.[56] The geographical distribution of ophthalmologists will change to accommodate this influx of physicians, with ophthalmologists locating in communities previously served exclusively by optometrists. Concomitant with these changes will be an increase in the number of commercial outlets offering vision services, and it can be expected that this will significantly alter the delivery of refractive eye care.

The outlook for those in professional practice would indeed be bleak were it not for the fact that, in response to the demands of the marketplace, the profession has resorted to a more health-oriented direction. It is the culmination of the technological events of the 1950s, the federal health-care programs of the 1960s, and the revolutionary political changes of the 1970s. All of these events have combined to effect a transformation of the profession, creating a new sense of direction, one perfectly suited to optometry's heritage, mode of delivery of services, and distribution of manpower; consequently, optometry has evolved into a primary care profession within the framework of the American health care system.

Many authors have commented on the unique qualities that enable optometry to provide primary care,[57] and it is clear from a review of the professional literature that the primary care concept has been one that has been well accepted by optometrists. The challenge to optometry and optometrists is how best to fulfill the obligation to the public that this role demands. There are three major areas of endeavor in which optometry must meet this challenge: scope of services, mode of delivery of services, and education.

Scope of Services

In order to deliver primary care, the scope of services offered by optometrists will have to be enlarged to include greater involvement in the diagnosis and treatment of ocular disease. It is not inconceivable that in-office surgical procedures would be sufficiently cost-effective to also warrant inclusion within the optometric armamentarium. This would enable optometrists to serve more patients more fully, thus providing better care and reducing the cost of health care.[58] (The problem of how such changes in the scope of practice could be effected is considered in Chapter 9.) Such an increase in scope of practice would most significantly effect optometric educators, since school curricula would have to be modified substantially.

Mode of Delivery of Services

The backbone of optometry has been the sole proprietor, but economic and legal developments have combined to cause a reversal of this traditional mode of practice for optometrists. Statistics compiled by the AOA have indicated a trend toward partnership and group practice.[59] This trend has been accompanied by a move toward greater specialization within the profession.[60] If the scope of services is increased, the number of patient visits can be expected to rise for the average practitioner, which will place additional demands on the use of ancillary personnel. Therefore, a rather comprehensive change in the method of delivery of optometric services can be anticipated.

Education

Not only will optometry schools have to modify their curricula to accommodate increased optometric services, but they will have to take on an additional responsibility to educate students in the business aspects of optometry and to bring together students and practitioners for the purpose of achieving continuity of professional practices. Optometry schools have traditionally not emphasized this facet of education, and this is an oversight that must be corrected without delay.[61] Financial aid for optometry students is another education-related problem that requires remedy.[62] There is probably no aspect of optometry that requires more consideration than optometric education; it is the key to the profession's ability to meet the challenge of primary care.

As the preceding chapters have illustrated, optometry has enjoyed a full if turbulent history. It has truly been a remarkable calling that has never known a moment of complacency, and it has demanded a high degree of loyalty from its membership, which has been opposed by powerful forces as optometry evolved from a mercantile-based trade to a highly specialized profession. Indeed, optometry has required its practitioners to be willing to take the road less traveled by, and that has made all the difference.

Notes

1. The historical basis for the licensing of optometrists is described in Chapter 1. For other perspectives, see Prentice, C.F., *Legalized Optometry and Memoirs*, Casperin Fletcher Press, Seattle, 1926; Coblens, S., *Optometry and the Law*, American Optometric Association, St. Louis, 1976; and Shimberg, B., *Occupational Licensing: A Public Perspective*, Educational Testing Service, Princeton, N.J., 1982.
2. For historical views of optometrists in commercial practice and their opinions of optometric services, see the following: Evans, E., Single Charge versus Separation of Service Fee and Price of Glasses, *Optical Journal and Review of Optometry*, vol. 72, no. 4, Feb. 15, 1935, p. 26; Rukenbrod, W.H., Price Chiseling, *Optical Journal and Review of Optometry*, vol. 72, no. 6, Mar. 15, 1935, p. 21; Wilson, F.C., Radical Changes Proposed in Store and Office Environment of Optometrists—The Recent Code Regulations, *Optical Journal and Review of Optometry*, vol. 72, no. 16, Aug. 15, 1935, p. 19; Sullivan, C.H., Sink or Swim?, *Optical Journal and Review of Optometry*, vol. 7, no. 18, Sept. 15, 1937, p. 23; Hutchinson, E.A. Optometry, Or What Have You?, *Optical Journal and Review of Optometry*, vol. 74, no. 22, Nov., 1937, p. 24; Idzall, M.M., The Case for Advertising, *Optical Journal and Review of Optometry*, vol. 74, no. 21, Nov. 1, 1937, p. 24.
3. For an interesting account of the origins of this philosophy, see Defense of the Optician, in Prentice, supra note 1, pp. 43–62.
4. A well-publicized address before the American Medical Association in 1928 by a prominent ophthalmologist stated the medical attitude toward optometry: "the great obstacle to consultations between physicians and optometrists is *commercialism*. The practice of optometry is too much a matter of business. *It must become a profession*. If as and when, the optometrists organize a group of members who will set up professional standards and maintain them, consultation and cooperation will be welcomed by many eye physicians." Lancaster, W.B., The Optometry Problem, *Journal of the American Medical Association*, vol. 91, no. 24, Dec. 15, 1928, pp. 1847–1848.
5. For an understanding of the disarray that American medicine had faced a century earlier, see Stevens, R., *American Medicine and the Public Interest*, Yale Univ. Press., New Haven, Conn., 1977, pp. 55–74.
6. For a review of the literature, see Chapter 1, note 72.
7. Some of the legal actions brought by optometrists may be reviewed, in annotated form, in the American Law Reports. See One Who Fills Prescriptions Under Reciprocal Arrangement With Physician or Optometrist As Subject to Charge of Practice of Medicine or Optometry Without License, 121 A.L.R. 1455; What Constitutes Practice of "Optometry," 141 A.L.R. 883 and 88 A.L.R. 2d 1290; Fitting of Contact Lenses As Practice of Optometry, 77 A.L.R. 3d 810; Constitutionality of Statutes and Validity of Regulations Relating to Optometry, 98 A.L.R. 905; Validity of Governmental Regulation of Optometry, 22 A.L.R. 2d 939; Right of Corporation, or Individual Not Himself Licensed, To Practice Optometry Through Licensed Employee, 102 A.L.R. 343 and 128 A.L.R. 585.
8. For a representative discussion of the legal issues by a court, see *State of Kansas ex rel. Beck v. Goldman Jewelry Company*, 142 Kan. 881, 51 P.2d 995 (1935).
9. For an example, see *State v. Kindy Optical Company*, 216 Iowa 1157, 248 N.W. 332 (1933).
10. For example cases, see *Lieberman v. State Board of*

Optometry, 34 A.2d 213 (Conn. 1943), and its predecessor, *Sage-Allen Company v. Wheeler*, 119 Conn. 667, 179 A. 195 (1935).

11. Apparently, organized optometry had a running battle with a family-controlled chain of businesses that employed optometrists. This battle can be followed through a series of cases. See *Ezell v. Ritholz*, 198 S.E. 419 (S.C. 1938); *State of Iowa ex rel. Bierring v. Ritholz*, 283 N.W. 268 (1939); and *Ritholz v. Indiana State Board of Registration and Examination*, 45 F. Supp. 423 (D.C. Ind. 1937); an account of this episode can be found in A.O.A. Obtains Interlocutory Decree, Restraining Ritholzs From Bringing Harassing Lawsuits—Defendants Checked In Setting Up Imitation Association, *Optical Journal and Review of Optometry*, vol. 74, no. 20, Oct. 15, 1937, p. 30.
12. For a personal memoir of the era, see Kohn, H., A Legal and Anecdotal History of Optometry, *Journal of the American Optometric Association*, vol. 38, no. 11, 1967, pp. 949–955.
13. For a review of the status of military optometrists at the time of World War II, see Hofstetter, H.W., *Optometry: Professional, Economic, and Legal Aspects*, C.V. Mosby, St. Louis, 1948, pp. 110–117.
14. During World War II and for a period following the war, the federal government (through the office of Price Administration) set a ceiling on increases in consumer costs. Optometrists were subject to the ceiling, which had its greatest effect on practitioners who charged one price for materials and services, since the total fee was therefore subject to the ceiling. See id. at 102–103.
15. For an example of the fervor of members of the profession, particularly those who had suffered through noncommissioned rank in the military forces and who looked to commercialism as the reason for the profession's low status, see Lang, G.L., An Open Letter to the Unethical, *Optical Journal and Review of Optometry*, vol. 81, no. 22, Nov. 15, 1944, p. 26.
16. 294 U.S. 608, 55 S. Ct. 570 (1935). The text of this decision can also be found in Hirsch M. and R. Wick, *The Optometric Profession*, Chilton, Philadelphia, 1968, pp. 181–184.
17. 348 U.S. 483, 75 S. Ct. 461 (1955).
18. 374 U.S. 424, 83 S. Ct. 1759 (1963).
19. The restrictions were reported by the Federal Trade Commission in the Trade Regulation Rule on Ophthalmic Goods and Services (Eyeglasses I), 16 CFR §456, published in the *Federal Register* of June 2, 1978.
20. The National Economic Survey conducted by the AOA in 1958 received responses from 45 percent of all AOA-affiliated optometrists in the country. Based upon these responses, it was determined that the average net income of optometrists was $9,970 (*National Economic Survey*, American Optometric Association, St. Louis, 1958). A 1942 survey conducted by Sheard found that the average gross income of optometrists in "downstairs" (commercial) practices was significantly higher ($8,026) that the gross income of optometrists in "upstairs" (professional) practices ($6,662). See Hofstetter, supra note 13, at 152–153.
21. 411 U.S. 564, 93 S. Ct. 1689 (1973). For a review of the case, see Coblens, S., The Berryhill Case: A Critique and A Prediction, *American Journal of Optometry and Archives of the American Academy of Optometry*, vol. 51, no. 5, May, 1974, pp. 347–350.
22. 425 U.S. 748, 96 S. Ct. 1817 (1976).
23. 433 U.S. 350, 97 S. Ct. 2691 (1977).
24. For an account of the Eyeglasses I Rule, see Classe, J., The Effects of FTC Rulings on the Practice of Optometry, *Southern Journal of Optometry*, vol. 21, no. 5, May 1979, pp. 20–24.
25. In 1981 the major optical chains began to offer franchising, which permitted local ownership of chain optical stores. The purpose of this move, according to Irving Bennett, O.D., was "apparently in order to give optometrists that work in the stores a piece of the action." From Summary of Remarks, Opinions, and Recommendations, Delivered at Optifair '82, New York. A year later Dr. Bennett noted that 265 franchises had been sold to local owners, and two years later that the largest chain, G.D. Serle & Co., had franchised more than 40 percent of its 900-odd stores in the United States. See State of the Optical Industry, March 1, 1983, Advisory Enterprises, Inc., White Plains, New York, and The Ophthalmic Industry: 1984, *Optometric Management*, vol. 20, no. 5, 1984, pp. 85–105.
26. The biggest noncommercial market in the United States is California, and in the early 1980s G.D. Serle, the parent company of Pearle Vision Centers, began efforts designed to institute its franchising program in the state of California. These efforts resulted in a lawsuit, filed by the California Association of Dispensing Opticians (and later joined by the California Optometric Association) against Pearle Vision Centers, Inc., seeking to enjoin Pearle from instituting the franchising program. A temporary restraining order was granted by the trial court, and—following a hearing—a preliminary injunction was issued by the court, which Pearle appealed. In 1983 the California Court of Appeals upheld the injunction, making the following observation:

    The trial court's conclusion Pearle's franchise program is illegal rests upon the fundamental premise that California has a strong long-standing public policy against permitting lay persons to exercise control over the decisions made by healing art practitioners. The trial court had before it uncontested evidence of such control. From the face of the franchising agreement it is clear Pearle had the power to control many facets of the optometrist's practice of optometry. For example, with respect to real property arrangements, Pearle must approve the site of the optometrist's office. If the franchisee is purchasing an existing site from Pearle, he must also purchase all improvements. If he wishes to obtain a new site, Pearle must approve all proposed leasehold improvements, furnishings, fixtures, inventory and supplies which are obtained from anyone other than Pearle.

Pearle also exercises a variety of controls over financial aspects of a franchisee's practice. According to the circular a franchisor may "finance" franchisees, and the franchisee must pay a substantial percentage of his gross income to the franchisor as both a "franchise fee" and as an advertising contribution. Franchisees must utilize the Pearle "system" relative to operating the practice and must use the franchisor's design specifications for offices. Furthermore, the franchisee is subject to periodic audits by the franchisor. Substantial penalties can be assessed if the audit is unfavorable.

A separate and distinct specie of control lies in the franchisor's control over a variety of treatment decisions to be made by the optometrist. A franchisee is required to stock all of Pearle's approved frame lines, to carry an inventory of prescription lenses and other optical goods and supplies approved by Pearle. Pearle has the sole discretion to modify frame lines, and specifications for optical goods. Finally, the franchisee's choice of laboratory is limited to those approved by Pearle.

Reservation of this authority over an optometrist by a nonhealing arts practitioner is against public policy and clearly illegal.

See *California Assn. of Dispensing Opticians, California Board of Optometry v. Pearle Vision Center, Inc.*, 143 Cal App. 3d 419, 191 Cal. Rptr. 762 (1983) for the full decision.

27. Following the decision of the California Court of Appeals, which upheld the California statutes that formed the basis for the court's argument in favor of professional practice, bills were introduced in the California legislature to modify the California business codes so as to permit franchising and other forms of commercial practice. Although none of these bills has been enacted, the problem of commercialism in California has entered a new phase with the initiation of Eyeglasses II by the Federal Trade Commission, because the intent of the FTC's proposal is to eliminate state laws that restrict the commercial practice of optometry. See *State Restrictions on Vision Care Providers: The Effects on Consumers*, Federal Trade Commission, Washington, D.C., 1980.

28. Mr. Justice Douglas, in the opinion, expresses the reasoning of the court:

    An eyeglass frame, considered in isolation, is only a piece of merchandise. But an eyeglass frame is not used in isolation. . .it is used with lenses, and lenses, pertaining as they do to the human eye, enter the field of health. Therefore, the legislature might conclude that to regulate one effectively it would have to regulate the other. Or it might conclude that both the sellers of frames and the sellers of lenses were in a business where advertising should be limited or even abolished in the public interest. . . . The advertiser of frames may be using his ads to bring in customers who will buy lenses. If the advertisement of lenses is to be abolished or controlled, the advertising of frames must come under the same restraints; or so the legislature might think. We see no constitutional reason why a State may not treat all who deal with the human eye as members of a profession who should use no merchandising methods for obtaining customers.

    It seems to us that this regulation is on the same footing as the denial of corporations of the right to practice dentistry. . . . It is an attempt to free the profession, to as great an extent as possible, from all taints of commercialism. It certainly might be easy for an optometrist with space in a retail store to be merely a front for the retail establishment. In any case, the opportunity for that nexus may be too great for safety, if the eye doctor is allowed inside the retail store. Moreover, it may be deemed important to effective regulation that the eye doctor be restricted to geographical locations that reduce the temptations of commercialism. Geographical location may be an important consideration in a legislative program which aims to raise the treatment of the human eye to a strictly professional level. We cannot say that the regulation has no rational relation to that objective and therefore is beyond constitutional bounds.

    The full opinion of the court is reported in 348 U.S. 483, 75 S. Ct. 461 (1955).

29. See Kohn, supra note 12.
30. Ibid.
31. In ruling that the use of trade names by optometrists may be restricted, the Supreme Court decision noted that "The concerns of the Texas legislature about the deceptive and misleading use of optometrical trade names were not speculative or hypothetical, but were based upon experience in Texas with which the legislature was familiar when in 1969 it enacted the trade name statute." The intent of the statute, in the Court's eyes, was to protect the public:

    It is clear that the state's interest in protecting the public from the deceptive and misleading use of optometrical trade names is substantial and well demonstrated. We are convinced that (the trade name statute) is a constitutionally permissible state regulation in furtherance of this interest. . . . Rather than stifling commercial speech, (the trade name statute) ensures that information regarding optometrical services will be communicated more fully and accurately to consumers than it had been in the past when optometrists were allowed to convey the information through unstated and ambiguous associations with a trade name. In sum, Texas has done no more than require that commercial information about optometrical services "appear in such a form. . .as is necessary to prevent its being deceptive."

    For the full opinion, see 440 U.S. 1, 99 S. Ct. 887 (1979).

32. See Runninger, J., Are Two Offices Better Than One?,

Optometric Management, vol. 17, no. 5, May 1981, pp. 29–40.

33. See Pavlichko, J.L., Group Practice: You Can't Beat It, *Review of Optometry*, vol. 119, no. 9, Sept. 1982, pp. 23–28.
34. See Gregg, J.R., Those OD/MD Ties: How Tight the Knot?, *Optometric Management*, vol. 11, no. 8, Aug. 1975, pp. 18–23; and Runninger, J., Add An Ophthalmologist to Your Staff?, *Optometric Management*, vol. 16, no. 2, Feb. 1980, pp. 21–27.
35. See Kukula, D., Marketing in Optometry?, *Optometric Management*, vol. 15, no. 7, July, 1979, pp. 25–29; Practice Promotion: Can You Make It Pay?, *Optometric Management*, vol. 18, no. 10, Oct. 1982, pp. 27–35; and Schwartz, C.A., OD's Versus Chains: The "Yes, But" Dilemma, *Optometric Management*, vol. 21, no. 2, Feb. 1985, pp. 63–69.
36. See Private Practice: Which Way To Go?, *Optometric Management*, vol. 20, no. 10, Oct. 1984, pp. 19–35; and Bennett, I., The Independents Strike Back!, *Optometric Management*, vol. 20, no. 12, Dec. 1984, pp. 20–25.
37. For an example of how "bait and switch" tactics can lead to disciplinary action, see *Texas State Board of Examiners in Optometry v. Lane*, 306 S.W.2d 212 (Tex. Civ. App. 1957).
38. For an illustration of "capping and steering" as a cause of disciplinary action, see *Rayburn v. Minnesota State Board of Optometry*, 247 Minn. 520, 78 N.W.2d 351 (1956).
39. The power of advertising, when turned strictly to the issue of cost, does not apparently serve the advertiser in the long run. A memorandum sent to Pearle Vision Center offices by a Pearle Marketing Vice President states, "There is no question that price advertising can build short term traffic. However, it can also destroy the consumer's perception of that operation's professional abilities and hence its ability to develop a loyal customer base for the long term. Most of the retail optical offices that have gone into bankruptcy during 1980–1981 made this mistake. They became known as low price/low quality operations and went out of business as a result." Quoted by Runninger, J., Pearle Proves a Point, *Optometric Management*, vol. 18, no. 9, Sept. 1982, pp. 13.
40. The power of associations to set restrictions on advertising has clearly waned. In 1979 the Federal Trade Commission brought suit against the American Medical Association and the Connecticut and New Haven Medical Societies, arguing that the AMA's principles of ethics interefered with physician's rights to advertise and thus were in restraint of trade. In 1980 the U.S. Court of Appeals for the Second Circuit ruled in the FTC's favor, although a dissenting opinion pointed out that the AMA had modified its principles in ethics well before the suit was brought and that the FTC brought the case "to accommodate its desire to regulate the Association." The judge's opinion concludes, "Notwithstanding the mootness of the issues and the absence for years of 'a reasonable likelihood that the past wrong-doing will recur'. . . the Commission insisted on pressing for its pound of flesh. In my view the FTC is engaged in the futile business of beating a dead horse." *American Medical Assn. v. Federal Trade Commission*, 638 F.2d 443 (2nd Cir. 1980). The opinion of the court is reported in the *AOA News*, November 1, 1980.
41. The main thrust of Eyeglasses II is to pre-empt the restrictions on commercial practice which have been duly enacted by the various state legislatures. For a discussion of the rule, see FTC Unleashes Trade Rule, *Review of Optometry*, vol. 121, no. 12, Dec. 1984, p. 3. One basis for the FTC's interest is a study of contact lens practices among professional optometrists, commercial optometrists, ophthalmologists, and opticians. See FTC Study Called "Flawed," *Review of Optometry*, vol. 121, no. 1, Jan. 1984, p. 3.
42. For a review of the application of sales tax to ophthalmic materials, see Eyeglasses Or Other Optical Accessories As Subject To Sales Or Use Tax, 14 A.L.R. 4th 1370.
43. For example, an entire chapter is devoted to the subject of fees by Hofstetter, supra note 13, at 166–197.
44. See Swallowing the FTC's Bitter Pill, *Review of Optometry*, vol. 115, no. 12, Dec. 15, 1978, pp. 41–45; and Robert, L., The Great Rx Giveaway: Coping With FTC Rules, *Optometric Management*, vol. 16, no. 1, Jan. 1980, pp. 25–33.
45. See Jackson, E., The Optometry Question and the Issues Behind It, *Journal of the American Medical Association*, vol. 57, no. 4, July 22, 1911, p. 265.
46. See Federal Investigation of Rebating, *American Journal of Ophthalmology*, vol. 29, no. 10, Oct. 1946, pp. 1313–1315; Optical Rebates, *American Journal of Ophthalmology*, vol. 30, no. 8, Aug. 1947, pp. 1030–1032; The Rebate Cases, *American Journal of Ophthalmology*, vol. 31, no. 9, Sept. 1948, pp. 1177–1178; and Income Tax Deductions for Kickbacks, *American Journal of Ophthalmology*, vol. 33, no. 9, Sept. 1950, pp. 1456–1458.
47. See Fry, GA., Interprofessional Relations In The Design of Eyewear, *American Journal of Optometry and Archives of American Academy of Optometry*, vol. 34, no. 4, Apr. 1957, pp. 212–221; Fry, G.A., The Division of Labor Between Optometry and Ophthalmology, *American Journal of Optometry and Archives of American Academy of Optometry*, vol. 34, no. 3, Mar. 1957, pp. 150–156; and Hutchinson, E.A., Optometry, Ophthalmology, and Dispensing Opticianry, *American Journal of Optometry and Archives of American Academy of Optometry*, vol. 34, no. 6, June 1957, pp. 343–346.
48. Shortly after the FTC's Eyeglasses I Rule went into effect, requiring that all patients be given a copy of the prescription at the conclusion of the examination, a survey of optometrists revealed that 73 percent of the optometrists' patients obtained their ophthalmic materials from their doctors. See Swallowing the FTC's Bitter Pill, *Review of Optometry*, vol. 115, no. 12, Dec.

15, 1978, pp. 41–45.

49. See Kleinman, E.B., Competitive Dispensing: Rx for Survival in Optometry, *Optometric Management*, vol. 15, no. 5, May 1979, pp. 31–37.

50. See Gerber, P., Dispense With Dispensing?, *Optometric Management*, vol. 15, no. 5, May 1979, pp. 71–79.

51. The duty to detect disease and to refer as appropriate has always been a legal duty of optometrists. In the first appellate case discussing the liability of optometrists, the court made the following observation:

> Clearly, then, the duty resting upon the optometrist was to make examination of the plaintiff's eyes for the "purpose of ascertaining any departure from the normal. . .measuring its functional powers, and adapting mechanical means for the aid thereof." If, however, in the performance of those duties, it would be apparent to a skillful optometrist that there existed in the eye under examination a disease or malformation, we would not say that it would not be his duty to so advise his patient, so that proper medical or surgical treatment might be had.

See *Hampton v. Brackin's Jewelry and Optical Company, Inc.*, 237 Ala. 212, 186 So. 173 (1939).

52. The so-called mandatory referral laws are not really new. See Nuisance Legislation?, *Optometric Weekly*, vol. 46, no. 19, May 12, 1955, p. 775.

53. For a discussion of the economic nature of the conflict between optometry and ophthalmology, see Colton, D.J., The O.D.-M.D. Conflict: Economic Warfare, *Optometric Management*, vol. 18, no. 7, July 1982, pp. 23–27.

54. Perhaps the most convincing evidence that commercialism represents a continuation of the errors of the past can be found in the words of those who have labored in the commercial environment. There are numerous sources that could be quoted to illustrate the failings of commercialism, but the limitations of space make it necessary to select one example, the sworn statement of Mr. James Shamburger, a district manager for Pearle Vision Centers and a dispensing optician by trade, who worked for Pearle in Colorado and Texas for three years.

His allegations paint a bleak picture. For convenience, the questions and answers of the deposition are organized into extracts that are presented by selected topics.

On the Recruitment of Commercial Optometrists

QUESTION: I would like to sort of go through a chronological story of your relationship with an optometrist who would be associated with Pearle Optical. Did you recruit optometrists?

ANSWER: Yes, I did.

QUESTION: Generally what was the story or the sales pitch, so to peak, that you would tell the optometrist getting him to come to work with or for Pearle Optical?

ANSWER: I think one thing we would do would be to build the lucrativeness of the practice which you were trying to recruit him for and in many cases the figures we used were hypothetical. And naturally you tried to instill to him that there would be no loss of professionalism because the office would be owned and operated by him, that he would get his own fees, his own hours, and function as an individual entity. And from that standpoint we would try to impress upon him the size of our company and how lucrative it would be being in a location next door to us.

QUESTION: After an optometrist was signed on so to speak through the vehicle of a lease, an equipment lease, did that turn out to be the truth that he was truly independent of Pearle Optical?

ANSWER: I would have to say in reality the optometrist was never independent.

QUESTION: Was he subservient to the wishes of Pearle Optical?

ANSWER: If he wanted to continue the status of his long term lease, yes.

On the Use of the Agreement to Control the Commercial Optometrist

QUESTION: Was there any kind of termination clause in the lease whereby it could be terminated by the landlord at any time?

ANSWER: Yes, there was a thirty day cancellation clause, I should say an open termination clause, whereby giving the doctor thirty days written notice his lease could be cancelled for no apparent reason, simply at our wish to do so.

QUESTION: Was this a vehicle by which Pearle Optical exercised control over the doctors?

ANSWER: Unfortunately it was. And I might add one of the larger repercussion areas that we had was finding sound professional people to lease from us.

QUESTION: Was this a concern of the doctors: Going into this legal relationship?

ANSWER: Very definitely.

QUESTION: Either party could terminate on thirty days' notice?

ANSWER: Yes.

QUESTION: Was there any occasion to terminate the lease of any of the optometrists?

ANSWER: Yes, there was.

QUESTION: Did you or did Pearle have anything to do or say about the hours of operations or the hours that an optometrist worked at the office he leased from Pearle Vision Centers?

ANSWER: In a manipulative fashion.

QUESTION: Would you explain that for me, sir?

ANSWER: Normally in the recruiting of a doctor on the first or the second type of meeting basis naturally we tried to propose to the doctor the professionalism he could have being in a leased location next door to us, and, we did not control the hours and we did not tell him how to handle himself professionally, et cetera, et cetera, we didn't control the fees. And in actuality we did after a doctor was enticed into signing a lease and felt comfortable in a location we used certain verbal pressures at times if things weren't going the way we wanted.

QUESTION: All right. Did you suggest to the optometrists any hours?

ANSWER: Oh, yes. I probably would say the spiel that we used most of the time was that our marketing analysis marketed the best shopping hours in that area, and of course naturally you will find most O.D.'s are not that inept of business people, and so they are going to believe that in most cases.

On Review of the Commercial Optometrist's Records

QUESTION: Let's look at the referral situation then. Was there any requirement by Pearle that the doctors or optometrists to whom the space was leased refer their patients or any certain proportion of their patients to the adjoining dispensary?

ANSWER: I think there would be a common knowledge area where we had computerized cash registers geared to let us know exactly where the flow was coming from and based on the way the doctors paid their rent, we knew what their flow was. And a common knowledge area there that I can speak truthfully on would be if we were receiving less than sixty percent of what they were doing their lease probably would have been terminated.

QUESTION: All right, sir. And now, was it part of your duties to look at the records of the optometrists who leased the space from Pearle?

ANSWER: Yes, it was.

QUESTION: And how often did you do that?

ANSWER: Generally on a once a month basis.

QUESTION: For what purpose did you do that?

ANSWER: Number one: Make sure that the percentage rent check that they wrote to us did agree with their records, in other words, the volume of the examinations for the month. Number two: To do a recheck study on the percentages. As a question was asked earlier: To keep tabs on the percentage we were getting from the doctors.

QUESTION: So you would know the percentage of the prescriptions written in the optometrists' offices which were filled by the adjoining dispensary?

ANSWER: Yes.

QUESTION: Was there any case besides Dr._______in which less than sixty percent of the prescriptions written by an optometrist leasing space from Pearle was actually filled by the adjoining dispensary?

ANSWER: I would say no: in most cases the percentages ran ninety percent.

On the Control of the Commercial Optometrist's Fees

QUESTION: What about control of prices: Did Pearle Optical effectively control the price of the optometric examinations by the doctors either directly or indirectly?

ANSWER: I would say they did very effectively control the doctor's fee arrangements indirectly.

QUESTION: How was this done?

ANSWER: Naturally fees were something that was always discussed, and again in a very direct way, I know I can say that the terms used by myself normally were we would be happy if the professionals stayed within the normal boundaries of what the area calls for. And in other words, what I was saying to that doctor is if there is ninety doctors in town and ninety-five percent of them charge twenty and fifty let's stay within the ballpark. And again a preference, but I think that they pretty much were getting my message.

QUESTION: And you were discussing a range within which they need to stay?

ANSWER: Yes.

On the Profit Motive Inherent in the Corporate Ownership of Commercial Practices

QUESTION: Are the administrators and officers of Pearle and Searle in your judgment fearful of potential doctor influence or say so?

ANSWER: Yes, they are definitely afraid of any doctor having any control over any situation; the reason that some of the things happened in these big chain operations as far as bad prescriptions and a lot of other things occurring is because the upper echelon executives of the company are not optically oriented for the most part as far as I know; they don't have an optical background but they have a very good business background, but they don't know the optical business as it relates to the patients. They don't understand the problems that are incurred and they don't know how to deal with the patients in that respect; all they understand is the figures that come out of the offices as far as money is concerned and that is all they understand or want to understand.

QUESTION: Do you mean that they really do not care or are you saying that they elevate the profit motivation higher than the need for quality patient care?

ANSWER: Yes, I think they do, definitely. It is evident that they do or they would have better quality and better care; their quality and care is something to be desired, I can tell you that right now.

On the Filling of the Commercial Optometrists's Prescriptions by the Commercial Dispensary

QUESTION: Did you ever check the doctors or talk to them with respect to the number of remakes or duplications of prescriptions that they wrote that were filled by Pearle dispensaries?

ANSWER: That was a major priority, if a doctor seemed inadequate and caused the cost of goods to go up because of his inadequacies he would generally just be talked to once and generally the second time if it did not clear itself up his lease would be cancelled.

QUESTION: Was there any sort of percentage of remakes or duplications that a doctor was allowed as a standard?

ANSWER: Not in a written contract but I would say from our standpoint probably seven to nine percent would be acceptable.

QUESTION: As a rule of thumb operating—

ANSWER: As a rule of thumb if you grouped one

hundred good refractionists together I think you would find your general average to be somewhere between seven and eight percent.
QUESTION: Do you know of any doctor who was given his notice of termination of his arrangement between Pearle and the doctor because of excessive remakes?
ANSWER: I know of one doctor who was terminated and of one doctor who was moved out of a very lucrative practice to a virtually worthless practice.

On the Quality of Ophthalmic Materials

QUESTION: You mentioned earlier the number of stores in the Dallas-Fort Worth area. Of those employees in those stores that were fabricating lenses how many of them would you characterize as being top-quality from an ability standpoint, top ability?
ANSWER: One percent.
QUESTION: If you were to go out on your own and open up your own opticianry at the present time and seek employees for purposes of fabricating lenses, how many of the employees presently employed by Pearle Optical in this Dallas-Fort Worth area would you hire?
ANSWER: In the Dallas-Fort Worth area?
QUESTION: Yes.
ANSWER: There is only one of their little over one hundred employees that I would even attempt to employ.
QUESTION: So one out of one hundred persons who are presently fabricating lenses for Pearle Optical in the Dallas-Fort Worth area are truly qualified in your judgment?
ANSWER: By my standards, yes.
QUESTION: By your standards. Do you think your standards are unreasonably high?
ANSWER: No, I do not; I think that my standards probably would meet the guidelines of any individual capable of obtaining an ophthalmic license based on experience and background which should be, and, I have always been an advocate of, licensing or some type of schooling for opticianries. I think that the guidelines would follow very easily into that catagory.
QUESTION: After the doctor had issued a prescription how did you render any quality control over whether or not the prescription was in fact accurately filled by the opticians filling the prescriptions?
ANSWER: I really don't understand your question.
QUESTION: Were the lenses, the speciality lenses, ever verified by the doctor?
ANSWER: In other words, after we fabricated a pair of glasses were the patients directed to go back to the doctor for verification?
QUESTION: Yes.
ANSWER: Not to my knowledge, it wasn't a standard procedure.
QUESTION: Did you ever discuss verification procedures with the doctors?
ANSWER: No, I did not.
QUESTION: Did these doctors ever request the patient to bring their glasses back to see if in fact they had been filled accurately?
ANSWER: To my knowledge I would say no, but here again, I got very uninvolved, I almost displaced myself from how professional that doctor wanted to be and so there could have been. But to my knowledge, no.
QUESTION: Is it a standard practice, was it the rule rather than the exception for there to be no vertification by the doctor?
ANSWER: I would say in commercial optometry as a general rule the eye examination is probably extant unless the patient has a problem.
QUESTION: Can we conclude from that that the prescriptions that were filled by Pearle Optical Vision Centers were never verified by any optometrists?
ANSWER: That would be a natural assumption.
QUESTION: Getting back to the lens quality again, were there any external controls outside of the optical shop to insure that lenses were in fact correctly filled?
ANSWER: I will answer no.

On the Time Spent by Commercial Optometrists on Eye Examinations

QUESTION: And about what is the maximum length of time that the doctor can expect the patients to wait patiently in the reception area?
ANSWER: I'll say in generalities approximately twenty to twenty-five minutes.
QUESTION: And so if he had four people waiting in the reception area for examination and took longer than twenty to twenty-five minutes he would run the risks of losing that patient?
ANSWER: I will say so.
QUESTION: Would this cause then a doctor to spend no more than five or ten minutes on an examination on many occasions?
ANSWER: I would think in commercial optometry you would find as a general rule the examination time is going to be ten to twelve minutes.
QUESTION: Is this unique to Pearle Optical or is it the rule rather than the exception in all commercial optometry?
ANSWER: I would say its adherent to all commercial operations.
QUESTION: Do you think it's likely to change?
ANSWER: If the leniencies of commercialism continue and the abuse of the industry that has gone on for some odd forty or fifty years is continued, if anything. I think it will become more automated.
QUESTION: When you say abuse of the industry are you saying abuse of the optometric profession by the optical industry or just what did you mean?
ANSWER: As a general rule one hand taking care of the other. I think that commercial optometry generally takes a certain type of doctor who fits into that environment; he generally is very open to being, if I may use the term, prostituted by the optical company, per se. And so I think you are going to find a dual combination there where if society or the laws implemented into the optical industry are not changed that the advantage

will be more excessive by the large optical companies and in turn make it more lucrative for the commercial optometrists to do more eye examinations per day.

On the Doctor-Patient Relationship in Commercial Practice

QUESTION: I would like to return for a moment to the nature of the doctor-patient relationship. For the most part did the patients have continuing relationships with the doctor, was it a close relationship, would the patient remember the name of his doctor for example for six months from now?
ANSWER: From the studies I seen done in commercialism on repeat patients I would say that the loyalty to a commercial optometrists or for that matter even to the commercial optician is very low.
QUESTION: In other words, the loyalty is to the doctor next door to Pearle Optical Center regardless of who the doctor happens to be?
ANSWER: I think that the general attitude of management with the commercial operation in that the doctor himself is not an asset, his license is, because I think they know as it generally happens that the people go to that doctor because he is next door to Pearle; they could really care less if he is Dr.______or______.
QUESTION: And as a consequence they never develop a close relationship with their doctor as you normally would with your own personal physician?
ANSWER: I would say that they do not obtain relationships with them.
QUESTION: By your previous statements that the patients go to the doctor because they are next door to the Pearle Optical Center do you mean that they don't go to him because of his reputation for excellence?
ANSWER: I would say not, from my experience with Pearle, because they are a nation-wide company and they do a lot of advertising and draw a lot of traffic and generally the first question from a patient upon entering is "Hi. I need to get some new glasses. Do you all do the eye examination, too? And I can get it all done right here." And there are natural persuasions from a sales technique that there just happens to be a doctor next door there. And I believe that is where the majority of their business is coming from.
QUESTION: Are the doctors themselves aware of the patients they get because of the proximity to a Pearle Center next door rather than their own reputation?
ANSWER: I think to be associated with the setup they are, they would have to be aware of it.
QUESTION: In your judgment does the fact that they get their patients by location rather than reputation, does that lessen their incentive to perform quality work?
ANSWER: I would say yes, that it does lessen.
QUESTION: Does it lessen it to a significant degree?
ANSWER: From my experience in the business I would say yes. Commercial optometry tends to be a very mobile society and they are very seldom in a location practicing for any extreme length of time, and with that taken into consideration I would think it would have to effect their professional judgements as to how good a job they may be doing.
QUESTION: Is it fair to say then that if they develop a particularly bad relationship and do a particularly bad job on one patient they have very little fear that one incident is going to haunt them the rest of their practice career?
ANSWER: I would say that probably doesn't bother them at all because right next door they have the power of patient draw and that one patient can be forgotten easily.
QUESTION: Perhaps is that an incentive for them to spend less time with a patient than they would otherwise spend if they were in a professional private practice?
ANSWER: I'll say yes.
QUESTION: About how many patients does a Pearle Optical doctor see on a typical Saturday?
ANSWER: Probably fifteen to eighteen patients, and I have been involved in instances where commercial optometrists next door to me have done in excess of forty to fifty eye examinations on a Saturday; I think that probably the figure that I gave you earlier is not far-reached because the volume isn't there.

On the Effects of Commercialism on the Quality of Care

QUESTION: Have you observed in your years of experience as a supervisor with Pearle that the young doctors, the enthusiasm and desire for professionalism of the young doctors who first come to work for Pearle wanes as the years pass?
ANSWER: A good way to describe that would be I think they are quickly broken in spirit and professionalism to the almighty dollar.
QUESTION: Do you believe that the patients of such a doctor benefit by that deterioration of attitude?
ANSWER: Definitely not.
QUESTION: Do you believe that the quality of a doctor's product suffers as a result of that deterioration of professionalism?
ANSWER: Yes, I do.

55. For a review of manpower concerns in optometry, see Peters, H.B., Critical Optometric Manpower Issues, *Journal of Optometric Education*, vol. 4, no. 4, Spring 1979, pp. 8–12.
56. The Graduate Medical Education National Advisory Council performed a massive study of medical manpower needs in the United States, publishing its results in 1980. The study maintained that there would be 4,700 ophthalmologists more than were needed by 1990. See O.D.s And The Ophthalmology Manpower Surplus, *Optometric Management*, vol. 20, no. 9, Sept. 1984, p. 69.
57. See Catania, L.J., Primary Care, in Newcomb, R.D., and J.L. Jolley, *Public Health and Community Optometry*, Charles C. Thomas, Springfield, Ill., 1980, pp. 352–368, for an example of optometric commentary on primary care.

58. For example, in 1976 the West Virginia legislature became the first state legislature to authorize the use of therapeutic pharmaceutical agents by optometrists. Each year the West Virginia Optometric Association has reported to the legislature the experiences of West Virginia optometrists in utilizing the authority granted to them under the law. As of 1981, five years after the law's passage, the Association reported these facts: 72 different ophthalmic pharmaceutical agents had been employed by optometrists; 47,121 patients had been treated during this period; since referral was not necessary in these cases, the treatment represented a savings of 620,000 miles in travel to these patients; and 52 different pathological conditions had been diagnosed and treated by the state's optometrists.
59. In the most recently published AOA Economic Survey (1987), the percentage of solo practitioners amounted to 53.8 percent of those responding to the survey. In 1979 this percentage was 61.7 percent, and in 1968 solo practitioners constituted 73.5 percent of all respondees. See the AOA News, Mar. 1, 1988. An ASCO survey of 1979, 1980, and 1981 optometry school graduates revealed that only 54 percent entered self-employed practice opportunities. See the *AOA News*, Dec. 1, 1983. And a survey of graduates of Ferris State College of Optometry found that only 30 percent were in solo practice, with 13.8 percent in partnership or in the process of forming a partnership. See the *AOA News* of Oct. 1, 1987.
60. The AOA has studied the process whereby optometrists who specialize in certain aspects of optometry may receive certification, further emphasizing the trend. See the *AOA News* of July 15, 1983, Mar. 1, 1984, and July 15, 1984. However, no formal recognition has been granted.
61. The difficult problem of educating students in the legal, economic, and administrative aspects of practice has not been adequately addressed by optometric educators. See Classe, J., The Need For Relevant Practice Management In The Optometric Curriculum, *Journal of Optometric Education*, vol. 5, no. 2, Fall, 1979, pp. 16–18.
62. The "average" optometry school graduate departs school with his or her diploma and a $20,000 debt, according to a 1984 study of graduates of the Pacific College of Optometry.

PART THREE

THE LEGAL SYSTEM

Chapter 6

Legislative Regulation

Politics is perhaps the only profession for which no preparation is thought necessary.
—Robert Louis Stevenson, *Familiar Studies of Men and Books*

Legislative Structure
How a Bill Becomes Law

The politician has long been a source of amusement. Yet, the very foundation of the U.S. political system is the much maligned servant of the people, the elected official who conducts business at the municipal, county, state, and federal levels, producing laws that keep the government functioning and the nation running. The politician's role as lawmaker is one of vital importance to optometry because it is through legislative fiat that optometry achieved legal recognition in the first place and through continued legal sanction that the practice of optometry has continued to expand in breadth and depth.

A review of some of the legislatively approved advances for optometry demonstrates the importance of this branch of government:

- Statutory authorization for the practice of the profession
- Formulation of state boards for professional self-regulation
- Approval of and appropriations for schools of optometry
- Optometric inclusion in governmental health-care plans
- Amendment of optometry practice acts to permit use of pharmaceutical agents

These legal gains were accomplished by enacting federal and state laws intended to promote the public welfare and to improve the ability of the profession of optometry to serve the public welfare. Although federal law is preeminent over state law, health care professions—such as optometry—are defined, licensed, and regulated on a state-by-state basis,[1] which has traditionally reduced federal influence over these professions. Therefore, the state—as *parens patria*—has been the primary source of legal authority for health care and health-care programs. Only in the latter part of the twentieth century—with the advent of social welfare programs and the development of a technology and bureaucracy able to administer them—has the federal government begun to assert a leadership role in U.S. health care. As a result, health care in the United States has become the nation's second largest industry.[2]

If the shift toward increasing federal control is a phenomenon that has not yet run its course (and particularly if national health insurance ever becomes a political reality), then the pervasiveness of government can be expected to sink deeper and deeper into the health-care system.[3] Even so, the states can be expected to retain a significant amount of the health professions' regulatory mechanism, including responsibility for licensure, discipline, and internal "housekeeping" duties. In the foreseeable future, the U.S. health-care system will continue to function as a dual federal-state responsibility, with the federal government asserting leadership in those areas it wishes to preempt and the state governments grudgingly giving up those areas traditionally reserved to them. These changes in health law and administration will be accomplished through legislative reform, which bespeaks strongly of the importance of the legislative system.

The legislative process is the most prevalent and most important source of law in the United States, and—of all other sources—it is the most public and, therefore, the most accessible to optometrists. Moreover, the legislative process contains a comprehensive system of checks and balances that makes the legislative branch a most responsive branch of government in terms of giving voice to public demand without being overly susceptible to minority opinion. For these reasons, it is imperative that optometrists understand the structure of the political system, how a bill becomes law, and how the administrative agencies function.

Before proceeding, it must be mentioned that the several states have drafted constitutions and established legislatures that, although they may differ one from another, are all based on the federal Constitution, the federal Congress, and federal legislative procedure.[4] For this reason, a general model—the Congress of the United States—is used to illustrate how U.S. government is organized and how the painstaking process of creating law is undertaken. To understand the nuances of any individual state government, that state's constitution and legislative rules must be consulted.

Legislative Structure

The legislative structure of the Congress of the United States is set out in Section I, Article I of the Constitution: "All legislative powers herein granted shall be vested in a Congress of the United States, which shall consist of a Senate and House of Representatives."

These two chambers constitute the sole legislative authority of the United States government.[5] There are 100 Senators (two from each state) and 435 representatives (the number is based upon a state's population, which will be reapportioned after the 1990 census). Each state is represented by two senators and at least one representative in the U.S. Congress. Senators are elected for six-year terms whereas representatives are elected for two-year terms.

Optometrists have a special interest in the election of their federal and state legislators. Since optometry is defined and regulated on a state-by-state basis, perhaps state legislators are of more immediate interest to optometrists, but federal legislators consider many questions of importance to optometry as well (e.g., national health insurance, Medicaid and Medicare coverage, and the regulatory powers of the FTC). Each member of the U.S. House of Representatives is up for reelection every two years, as is one third of the U.S. Senate. In fact, the Congress is identified by the election of its House members: The 96th Congress is so designated because it is the 96th election of House members since the nation's founding.

Table 6.1. Key Leadership Positions: U.S. House of Representatives

Speaker of the House	The majority party's leader, who is proposed by the majority party caucus (though technically elected by the whole House), and whose chief functions are to preside over the proceedings of the House and to advise the President on the various legislative proposals before the chamber. The Speaker succeeds to the Presidency should the President and Vice-President be unable to perform their duties.
Majority Leader	Chosen by the majority party caucus, the Majority Leader is second only to the Speaker in power, and is principally responsible for the management of the House legislative agenda, working with the Speaker to effect legislative strategy.
Majority Whip	Appointed by the Speaker, the Majority Whip has the responsibility to count the votes, to persuade reluctant members of the House to side with the majority's views, and to see that legislators are present at the designated place and time for votes on key issues.
Minority Leader	Selected by the minority party caucus, the Minority Leader acts as spokesperson for the party and serves as liaison to the Majority Leader with regard to minority party legislative proposals.
Minority Whip	Appointed by the Minority Leader, this legislator serves as a floor leader for the minority party in the same fashion that the Majority Whip serves the majority party.
Caucus Chairperson	Each party caucus selects a Caucus Chairperson, who is influential in determining party positions on legislation.

Source: *Optometric Political Involvement*, American Optometric Association, Washington, D.C., 1976.

There are, of course, two principal parties within the U.S. Congress, the Democratic Party and the Republican Party. The party holding the majority of seats in either of the two houses ostensibly controls that house and has the right to elect from its membership the congressional leadership. The most important posts are described in Tables 6.1 and 6.2.

Another important aspect of legislative structure is committee organization. In the U.S. Congress, the House of Representatives has twenty-one standing committees and the Senate has eighteen. (In addition there are three joint committees with both House and Senate members.) Each of these committees has a carefully delineated area of responsibility and has been granted the power to investigate, subpoena, hold hearings, and publish reports concerning committee findings. Membership on a specific committee is conferred by the party caucus. When a Senator or Representative is elected to Congress the respective party caucus chooses the committee assignments for that individual, and these assignments usually do not change for the remainder of that individual's career (except when the Senator or Representative moves to a more powerful committee or when a vacancy has occurred through death or resignation).[6]

Table 6.2. Key Leadership Positions: U.S. Senate

President of the Senate	The Constitution provides for the Vice President of the United States to serve as President of the Senate, but this duty is not one that Vice Presidents have traditionally performed with great regularity. Although the President of the Senate presides over the activities of the chamber, only in the event of a tie does the President cast a vote.
President Pro Tempore	Elected by the members of the chamber, the President Pro Tempore presides over the Senate in the absence of the Vice President. This position usually goes to the most senior senator within the majority party.
Majority Leader	The key role insofar as the legislative agenda is concerned, the Majority Leader is elected by the majority party caucus.
Majority Whip	Elected by the majority caucus, the Majority Whip serves as floor technician for the party, much in the same fashion as the Whip in the House of Representatives.
Minority Leader	Selected by the minority party caucus, the Minority Leader is spokesman for the minority party and liaison to the Majority Leader for purposes of minority party legislative proposals.
Minority Whip	Selected by the minority party caucus, the Minority Whip serves as floor leader for the minority party.
Caucus Chairpersons	Each party caucus selects a chairperson to manage and control the respective party caucuses.

Source: *Optometric Political Involvement*, American Optometric Association, Washington, D.C., 1976.

The leadership of all committees belongs to the majority party.[7] A committee chairman is selected by the majority party caucus and usually, but not always, is the most senior majority member on a particular committee (i.e., the legislator having the most years of service on the committee). This procedure, called the seniority system, has been overruled in certain instances. The minority party caucus also selects a committee leader, again usually on the basis of seniority, who is called the Ranking Minority Member.

Each of these standing committees has subcommittees, and—like the parent committee—the subcommittee has a limited area of interest, carefully composed membership, and majority party leadership (all of which is subject to full committee approval). The subcommittees are often as important as the committees themselves.[8] Both the parent committee and its subcommittees need staff assistance to perform necessary legislative duties. These staff members conduct research, brief committee members, prepare documents and exhibits, and advise the Senators or Representatives on matters of importance. They are a vital part of the committee system and are often the ones called on to negotiate and compromise differences between various committee factions. The committees that have the most relevance for optometry are listed in Table 6.3.

Of course, despite the care with which committee jurisdiction is drawn, many issues cross committee boundary lines and become matters of interest to more than one committee. When this occurs, conferences must be arranged and compromises proposed so that differences can be alleviated through negotiation. But before a committee can consider legislation, the bill containing the proposed law must undergo a tortuous trip through the legislative process, a trip that begins in the hopper on the desk of the House or Senate clerk and ends (if successful) on the desk of the President of the United States.

Table 6.3. Committees of Importance to Optometry: U.S. Congress

Senate	Finance (particularly Health subcommittee) Labor and Human Resources Appropriations (particularly Labor, Health and Human Services, and Education subcommittee) Budget
House	Ways and Means (particularly Health subcommittee) Energy and Commerce (particularly Health and Environment subcommittee) Appropriations (particularly Labor, Health and Human Services, and Education subcommittee)

Source: *Optometric Political Involvement*, American Optometric Association, Washington, D.C., 1983.

How a Bill Becomes Law

A bill is a draft of a proposed law that is submitted to a legislative body for approval. It can be introduced in either chamber, House or Senate, by any legislator, and on introduction it is assigned a number.[9] (Legislators often prefile bills prior to the actual opening of the congressional session in order to obtain a low bill number.) See Figure 6.1 for a diagrammatic representation of the process by which a bill becomes law in a representative state (Alabama),[10] which is quite similar to the federal process described here.

After bill is filed, the presiding officer of the chamber (Speaker of the House or President of the Senate) assigns the bill to the appropriate committee. Ostensibly this means assignment to that committee that has jurisdiction over the subject matter of the bill. But jurisdiction can be a close question with many bills, and the presiding officer can use his discretion in meting out assignments (which on occasion can result in the dispatching of a bill to a committee from which it will never see the light of day).[11] The presiding officer may also refer a cross-jurisdictional bill jointly to several committees and permit them to proceed together. This is frequently the case in health-related bills. Whether a bill is the exclusive concern of one committee or of several committees, the usual course of events is for it to be referred to a subcommittee for hearings. The committee chairperson decides whether to refer it to a subcommittee and, if so, to which one.

After a bill is introduced, the legislator who has filed the bill (the author or sponsor) may wish to enlist the support of other legislators in the chamber. Those legislators who join in introducing the bill are known as co-sponsors, and their names are listed on the bill or appear in the Congressional Record as co-sponsors of a particular bill. An exceptionally popular bill may be introduced more than once.[12] Co-sponsors can be expected to support a bill and, on occasion, to exert their influence to urge others to join them in supporting the proposed legislation.[13]

A bill in committee or subcommittee is subject to the whim and fancy of the committee or subcommittee chairman, and it is within the discretion of the chairman to decide when (or if) hearings will be held on the bill. If the chairman does schedule hearings, all interested parties and organizations should be able to present their views on the merits or failings of the proposed law. Oversight hearings also may be conducted to investigate the efficacy of existing law and the bill's influence upon it. Other subjects properly discussed at oversight hearings include the role of the executive branch in executing the bill, the administration of the bill, and the necessity for ancillary legislation in the future.

These hearings have obvious importance for optometry and the health-care professions because federal interest and influence in health policy have grown dramatically during the past few decades and promise to continue in the years to come. The development of health policy, its implementation, and the responsibilities of the public and the private sectors are matters that are routinely considered at such hearings.

If the bill is referred to a subcommittee, hearings will commence at the subcommittee level. After the hearings have been concluded, the subcommittee will meet to mark up the bill (Fig. 6.2). This procedure entails a line-by-line review of the language of the bill, with revisions being proposed by subcommittee members and informal votes being cast on the individual changes, amendments, or additions being suggested. When the subcommittee completes the task of marking up the bill, it is reported out of subcommittee and referred to the full committee. The bill, in its once-revised state, again becomes the subject of a set of hearings, this time at the full committee level. Interested parties and organizations have another opportunity to argue their positions, and alterations in the bill can be proposed, put to a vote, and either accepted or rejected by the full committee at this time. Ultimately the committee will have to consider whether or not to recommend the bill, and a formal vote will be taken to determine passage of the bill out of committee. If the committee votes to report the bill favorably to the full chamber, it must write a committee report. The report usually describes the purpose and scope of the bill and the

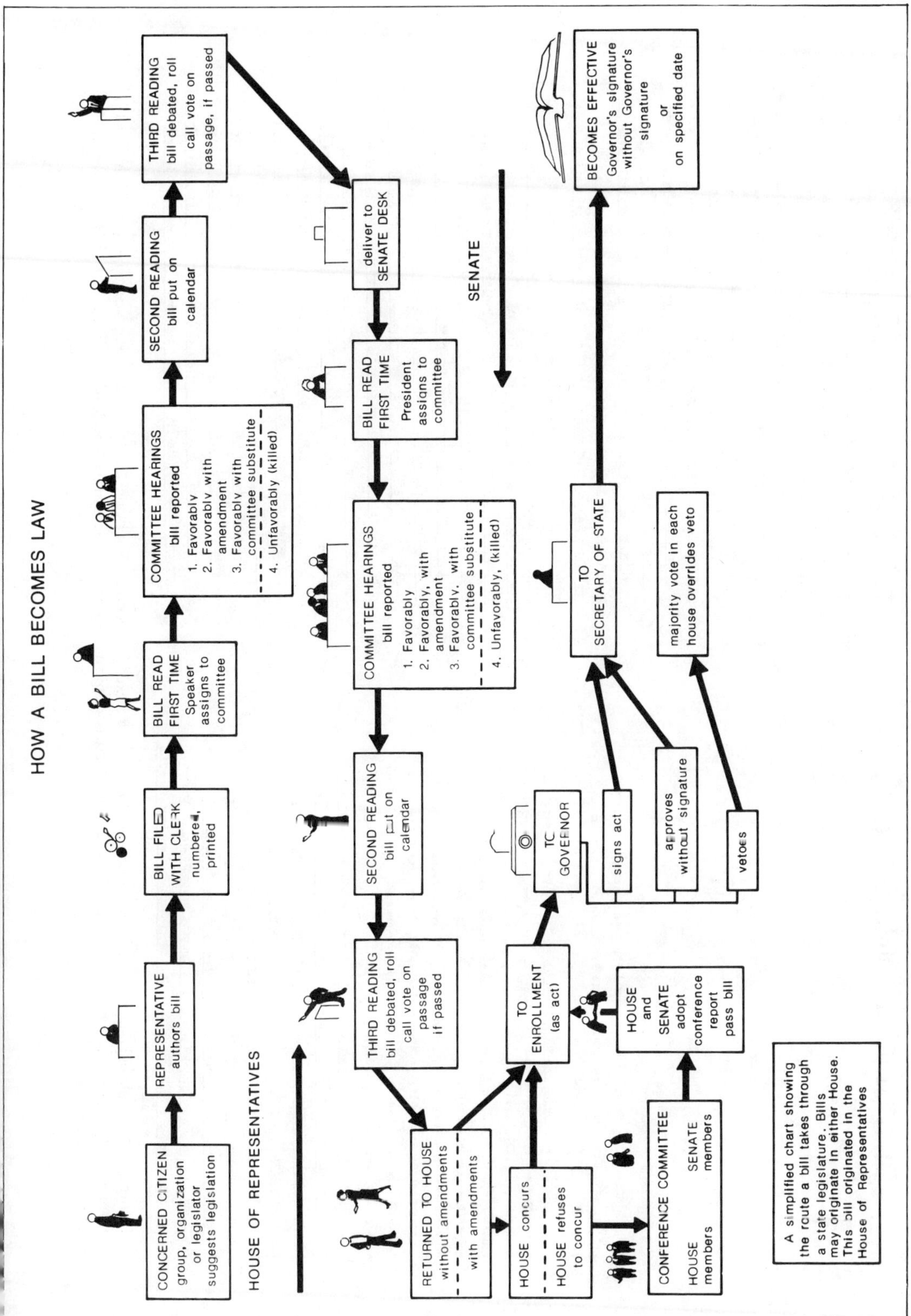

Figure 6.1. How a Bill Becomes Law

State of Rhode Island, &c.

IN GENERAL ASSEMBLY

JANUARY SESSION, A. D. 1971

AN ACT

DEFINING OPTOMETRY AND OPTOMETRISTS.

It is enacted by the General Assembly as follows:

SECTION 1. Sections 5-35-1 and 5-35-10 in chapter 5-35 of the general laws entitled, "Optometrists," is hereby amended to read as follows:

"5-35-1. Optometry and optician defined. - ~~The-practice-of optometry-is-defined-to-be-the-employment-of-any-method-or-means,-other than-the-use-of-drugs,-medicine-or-surgery,-for-the-ascertainment-of visual-defects-or-ocular-muscular-imbalances-and-the-application-of-lense and-prisms-for-the-correction-thereof.--An-optician-is-hereby-defined-to be-a-person-who-neither-practices-nor-professes-to-practice-optometry but-who-may-grind-opthalmic-lenses,-fit-spectacles-and-eyeglasses-and may-sell-spectacles-and-eyeglasses-or-lenses-or-prescription-from-either a-licensed-physician-or-licensed-optometrist.~~

Optometry is defined as the profession whose practitioners are engaged in the art and science of the evaluation of vision and the examination of vision and the examination and refraction of the human eye which includes: the employment of any objective or subjective means for the examination of the human eye or its appendages; the measurement of the powers or range of human vision or the determination of the accommodative and refractive powers of the human eye or the scope of its functions in general and the adaptation of lenses, prisms, and/or frames for the aid thereof; the prescribing, directing the use of or administering ocular exercises, visual training, vision training, or orthoptics, and the use of any optical device in connection therewith; the prescribing of contact lenses for, or the fitting or adaptation of contact lenses to the human eye; the examination or diagnosis of the human eye to ascertain the presence of abnormal conditions or functions; and the topical application of drugs to the eye, to wit, mydriatics, miotics, and the use of topical anesthetics, provided, however, that no optometrist licensed in this state shall treat by the use of these drugs or attempt or perform any surgery and shall be used only for the purpose of detecting any diseased or pathological condition of the eye, or the effects of any disease or pathological condition of the eye, further provided however, that with respect to presently licensed optometrists, only presently licensed optometrists who (i) have satisfactorily completed a course in pharmacology, as it applies to optometry, at an institution accredited by a regional or professional accreditation organization which is recognized by the national commission on accreditation, with particular emphasis on the topical application of drugs to the eye for the purpose of detecting any diseased or pathological condition of the eye; or the effects of any disease or pathological condition of the eye, approved by the board of examiners in optometry and the chief of pharmacy of the department of health, and (ii) have successfully completed an examination given by the board of examiners in optometry in conjunction with the chief of pharmacy of the department of health, shall be permitted to apply drugs topically to the eye for the purpose of detecting any diseased or pathological condition of the eye, or the effects of any disease or pathological condition of the eye. Said chief of pharmacy shall consult and advise the board of examiners in optometry with respect to that portion of the examination dealing with pharmacology.

An optician is hereby defined to be a person who neither practices nor professes to practice optometry but who may grind ophthalmic lenses, fit spectacles and eyeglasses and may sell spectacles and eyeglasses or lenses on prescription from either a licensed physician or licensed optometrist."

Figure 6.2. A sample bill illustrating how the proposed changes are marked for identification by the legislators. The language to be deleted is marked through and the proposed new language is underlined. Show here is a copy of the first two pages of the Rhode Island drug bill of 1971. (Courtesy of Thomas E. Eichhorst, Esquire)

reasons for its recommended approval. Frequently a section-by-section analysis is set forth in detail explaining precisely what each section is to accomplish.[14]

When the bill leaves the committee and is returned to the appropriate chamber, it must be placed on the chamber's calendar and assigned a calendar number. The House has five calendars and the Senate has two, each being used for specific types of legislation (summarized in Table 6.4).

Whenever a bill is placed on any of these calendars, it is numbered sequentially and voted on after all preceding bills on the calendar have been considered. (There are, however, rules in both the House and the Senate that permit the nonsequential and greatly expedited consideration of bills under certain compelling circumstances.) Both chambers have an extensive set of parliamentary rules that regulate the presentation, debate, and amendment of bills under consideration. In the House, the Rules Committee—on consent of a majority of the chamber—establishes the period of time to be allocated for debate and the procedure for offering amendments from the floor. Other than this important distinction, floor votes on proposed legislation proceed in generally the same manner in both the House and the Senate.

Table 6.4. Legislative Calendars: U.S. Congress

Calendar	Description
House	
House Consent Calendar	Reserved for bills of a non-controversial nature; requires a vote of the entire chamber to obtain passage
House Private Calendar	Reserved for bills of relief filed by individuals with claims against the U.S. government
House District of Columbia Business Calendar	Reserved for matters pertaining exclusively to the District of Columbia
House Union Calendar	Reserved for bills involving taxation or appropriation of monies
House Calendar	Reserved for any public bills that do not qualify for the House Union Calendar
Senate	
Senate Executive Calendar	Reserved for nominations to government service by the executive branch, promotions of military personnel, and approval of treaties
Senate Calendar of Business	Reserved for any legislation that does not qualify for the Senate Executive Calendar

Source: *Optometric Political Involvement*, American Optometric Association, Washington, D.C., 1976.

One important aspect of the formal voting procedure is the opportunity for any legislator to offer amendments from the floor (unless prohibited in the House by agreement with the Rules Committee). As a safeguard to prevent abuse of this privilege, the proponent of an amendment usually needs considerable support in order for approval of the amendment to be obtained.

If a bill receives a favorable vote in one chamber, it is sent to the other chamber, where it may be sent to committee, marked up, and passed back to the chamber in just the same manner as described above. It, too, must be placed on the chamber calendar and be voted on by the full chamber. (Usually the bill is introduced simultaneously in both chambers, and the two versions are known as companion bills, proposed drafts that do not differ markedly.)

If both chambers pass the bill, there are two possibilities:

1. If the two bills are identical, the chamber that passed the bill first refers its bill to the other body for approval, and then the bill is sent to the President for his signature.
2. If the bills have been amended in conflicting ways by the two chambers and do not contain identical provisions, then the chamber that passed the first version of the bill will request a conference with the other chamber in order to resolve the differing language.

When the bills differ in composition a conference committee is convened, which is a panel of House and Senate members appointed to undertake the arduous task of resolving the differences. These conferees are chosen by the Speaker of the House and the presiding officer of the Senate and are usually the senior members of the committees that reported the bill to their respective chambers. Regardless of the number of conferees appointed from either chamber, the House conferees and the Senate conferees each have one vote, and agreement is achieved only by the majority opinion of all conferees on the conference committee. Failure to obtain this consensus causes the bill to die in conference.

Even if all differences are resolved in conference committee and the revised bill is voted out of committee, a floor vote must be taken by each chamber to approve or disapprove the recommendations of the conference committee. If either chamber votes against the committee's recommendations, the bill again dies in conference. Only if both chambers agree on the conference committee's recommendations does the bill proceed to the White House for the President's signature.

Passage by the House and Senate does not automatically confer the status of law on a bill. Article I, Section 7 of the Constitution specifically provides for Presidential approval of all bills passed by the Congress: "Every bill which shall have passed the House of Representatives and the Senate, shall, before it becomes a law, be presented to the President of the United States."

The Constitution allows the President four alternatives when legislation passed by Congress reaches his desk:

1. He can sign the bill, thereby enacting it into law.
2. He can refuse to sign the bill within ten days after receiving it, but such a veto must be communicated to Congress within the ten-day limit by the President through the filling of a statement of objections and the return of the bill to the chamber from which it originated. The chamber may then vote to override the President's veto, but a two-thirds majority is required for passage. If such a majority is obtained, the bill is sent to the other chamber for another two-thirds vote. If both chambers override the veto, the bill becomes law. Otherwise, it dies and can only be revised by beginning the entire legislative process over again.
3. He can fail to sign or veto the bill, and if Congress remains in session for the ten days that the bill remains on his desk, the bill becomes law automatically.
4. He can fail to sign or veto the bill, and if Congress adjourns before ten days have elapsed (thereby preventing him from returning the bill within the allowed time period should he wish to do so), the President can pocket veto the bill by failing to act upon it at all. The pocket veto is a salutary balance granted the President as a safeguard against the numerous bills that are passed during the closing days of a legislative session.

The most famous Presidential veto affecting optometry was cast in 1946, when Harry S. Truman vetoed a bill that would have established a separate corps for optometrists in the U.S. armed forces.[15]

State constitutions authorize governors to exercise like powers in signing, vetoing, or otherwise disposing of legislation duly passed by state legislatures.[16]

Although this procedure is the manner in which the majority of federal law is enacted, there are other methods of creating federal law that are authorized by the Constitution.[17]

After enactment into law, the bill is delivered to the State Department, where it is given a serial number as either a public or a private law. Public laws (such as those affecting health care) are numbered in order of enactment: Public Law 95-626 (PL 95-626), the Health Services and Centers Amendment of 1978, was the 626th public bill signed into law during the 95th Congress. The original copy of all laws are kept by the Division of Research and Publications of the State Department; the law itself is published in the annual volume of the *United States Statutes at Large*. (See Chapter 7 for a discussion of how to find the law.)

As complex as the legislative process is, it involves only the creation of law. The administration of the law is another matter altogether and has its own complexities according to the federal (or state) agency into whose jurisdiction the statute falls. Administrative agencies exist because there have to be departments of government charged with the responsibility of seeing that duly enacted laws are discharged in accordance with the wishes of Congress. In order to perform this function, the administrative agency must interpret the law and promulgate rules designed to carry out the intent of the legislature in passing the law. In so doing, the administrative agency becomes, in effect, a quasilegislative and quasijudicial body. The procedures followed by administrative agencies, especially at the federal level, differ markedly from those followed by the legislature.[18] Since the administration of the laws of most importance to optometrists occurs at the state level, we later will discuss state administrative agencies (i.e., the state boards) separately.

Notes

1. For a contemporary review of the licensing process, see Shimberg, B., *Occupational Licensing: A Public Perspective*, Educational Testing Service, Princeton, N.J., 1982.
2. In recent years the United States has spent more money on health care than any other country in the world, both in terms of total dollars and in terms of the gross national product. The health-care industry is now the second largest industry in the country in terms of expenditures, outranked only by retail trade. See Newcomb, R.D., and J.L. Jolley, *Public Health and Community Optometry*, Charles C. Thomas, Springfield, Ill., 1980, pp. 232–236.

3. Although the general trend has been toward greater federal control, another trend—toward corporate or business control of health care—has begun to emerge in the 1980s. For-profit corporations have entered into the health-care marketplace, changing the dynamics of traditional health care economics for both institutional and ambulatory care. In optometry this trend has been manifested by the rebound of commercial interests and the growing share of the eye-care market that these interests have commanded. As improbable as it seems, through financial support to health-care institutions, business interests may one day intrude into academic environments to the point that they may direct the schools' health-care graduates into the corporate system.
4. For an overview of the workings of government, see Snider, C.F., *American State and Local Government*, 2d Ed., Appleton-Century-Crofts, New York, 1965.
5. This bicameral (two assemblies) legislative structure is repeated within forty-nine of the fifty states; only Nebraska has a unicameral legislature. Senators and representatives are elected from "districts" within the state, typically for four-year (senate) and two-year (house) terms, with both senate and house districts being based on population. Unfortunately, the criterion for "district" has been the subject of much political debate, and cries of gerrymandering have become common, so common in fact that the courts have been drawn into the argument over whether or not political districts are fairly and properly apportioned.
6. The composition of the committee to which a Senator or Representative is assigned is determined by the ratio of majority party members to minority party members for the particular congress. If the ratio of Democrats to Republicans in the House were 2:1, then the twenty-one house committees would be composed of two Democrats for every one Republican. If the Senate ratio were 3:2 in favor of the Republicans, then the eighteen Senate committees would contain three Republicans for every two Democrats. (The three joint committees retain members in the ratio of their respective chambers).
7. For example, using the ratios cited above, all committee chairpersons for the twenty-one House committees would be Democrats; the chairpersons for the eighteen Senate committees would be Republicans. Chairpersons for joint committees are alternated between the two chambers.
8. An example of such a subcommittee would be the Health and Environment Subcommittee of the Interstate and Foreign Commerce Committee, which considers matters of public health such as national health insurance.
9. There is one exception: In the U.S. Congress, all revenue bills and general appropriations bills must originate in the House.
10. For an overview of the working of the U.S. Congress, see Harris, J.P., *Congress and the Legislative Process*, 2d ed., McGraw-Hill, New York, 1972.
11. Relegating a bill to a less-than-favorably disposed committee is more often encountered in the state legislative process than in the federal congress. The author remembers vividly the efforts of Alabama optometrists to have the state optometry practice act modified, only to have the effort thwarted over several years by the mere determination of committee assignment for the bill.
12. In order to introduce the bill again, the sponsor needs twenty co-sponsors, and if they are obtained, the sponsor submits a letter of request to the Speaker. If approved, the bill is reintroduced.
13. At the state level the process of enlisting co-sponsors proceeds in much the same manner as at the federal level, with the legislatures of various states sometimes applying numerical restrictions.
14. There are two major distinctions between the federal and state legislative processes that should be noted. First, the U.S. Congress typically legislates by omnibus or all-inclusive bills. For example, all legislative changes pertaining to Medicaid or Medicare that are enacted in a given year will most likely be collected and passed in a single omnibus bill. A state legislature would enact a similar package by means of separate and distinct bills, one of which might pertain only to optometry. Second, whereas congressional committees normally hear witnesses and take action on different occasions, a state legislative committee frequently will combine these two steps into a single hearing.
15. This veto was a crushing blow for military optometrists, many of whom had suffered through World War II as enlisted members of the armed forces. The profession had mounted a herculean effort to win the bill's passage through the U.S. Congress, but Truman's veto ended all hope for a separate Optometry Corps. For a historical perspective, see Gregg, J.R., *A History of the American Optometric Association*, American Optometric Assn., St. Louis, 1972, pp. 184–185. Perhaps the most remarkable override of a veto in optometric history occurred in West Virginia in 1976, when the state legislature defeated the governor's veto of the first optometry therapeutics bill.
16. Governors can veto bills in every state except North Carolina.
17. There are three types of resolutions that can be enacted as federal law:

    1. Joint resolution—a vote of both the House and Senate on an order or resolution that has the force of statute (for example, a declaration of war); must be presented to the President for his signature or veto.
    2. Concurrent resolution—an expression of the intent of the House and Senate on an issue that does not have the effect of law (for example, a vote to censure a legislator); does not have to proceed to the President for his signature or veto.
    3. Simple Resolution—a matter affecting the operation of either chamber, House or Senate,

that is not a law and thus does not require approval from the Executive branch.

18. The following discussion will illustrate by example how the federal administrative process functions. The Federal Trade Commission (FTC) is a federal administrative agency that the U.S. Congress has charged with a number of responsibilities by statute, among them PL 93-637 (The Magnuson-Moss Warranty–Federal Trade Commission Improvement Act of 1975), Section 202 of which authorizes the Commission to: "prescribe. . . rules which define with specificity acts or practices which are unfair or deceptive acts or practices in or affecting commerce." The law further states that these rules "may include requirements prescribed for the purpose of preventing such acts or practices."

How the FTC decided to apply this rather inocuous-sounding language to optometry will serve as an example of how the administrative process works—and fails.

The first step by the FTC was taken on September 17, 1975, when—in accordance with a directive from the Commission to its Bureau of Consumer Protection—the agency initiated an investigation into the "adequacy of information disclosure by ophthalmologists, optometrists, and opticians to consumers in the eye care market." During the course of the investigation the FTC garnered information from industry representatives, consumer groups, individual consumers, state licensing boards, and other state officials. Of the Commission's findings, perhaps the most interesting are those pertaining to the distribution of the eye-care market:

> Ophthalmologists. . . in 1975. . . performed 43% of all eye examinations in the United States and dispensed 10% of all corrective lenses. . . . In 1975 optometrists performed 57% of all eye examinations and dispensed 49% of all corrective lenses. . . . In 1975, opticians supplied 41% of all corrective lenses.

These figures represent a distribution of the eye-care market that—when considering the relative numbers of ophthalmologists, optometrists and opticians—seems reasonable and in no way skewed toward any one group of providers. Nevertheless, this and other data accumulated by the Commission investigators led them to conclude that optometrists and ophthalmologists were participating in an "unfair act or practice affecting commerce," and the result was the promulgation of a Trade Regulation Rule (TRR) on January 16, 1976, which proposed:

- preemption of state or local restrictions on the advertising of ophthalmic goods or services, unless they met certain specifications
- legal sanction for optometrists and ophthalmologists to "truthfully advertise" the cost and availability of eye examinations
- a mandatory requirement that a patient's prescription for glasses or contact lenses be given to the patient at "the conclusion of the eye examination"

As required, the Commission published the proposal in the *Federal Register* and invited public commentary. This very important step in the administrative process is intended to place those who will be affected by the proposal on notice and to permit them to respond. Accordingly, the FTC was the recipient of more than 1,000 comments from consumers, officials, and organizations. (One such organization responding to the Commission was the American Optometric Association.) Thereafter the FTC scheduled public hearings in five cities across the United States, at which 175 witnesses testified. Among those testifying were consumers, state officials, representatives of opticianry, commercial interests in eye care, representatives of physicianry, and of course, representatives of optometry.

Following the public hearings the Commission offered another comment period, during which interested parties could rebut any evidence submitted at the hearings. All of this information—from the investigation, the public commentary, the hearings, and the comment period—was used by the presiding officer of the public hearings to compile a report detailing his conclusions. Not surprisingly, his report was supportive of the proposed FTC rule.

Yet another report was submitted to the Commission by its staff members within the Bureau of Consumer Protection. (Both of these reports were mandatory aspects of the administrative process.) Purporting to analyze the rulemaking record, the 307 page staff report found "the restrictions imposed on eyeglass advertising by private associations and state governments to be unfair to consumers" and recommended that the proposed Trade Regulation Rule be put into effect.

The Commission allowed a 60 day period for public commentary after the publication of the staff report. (It would be difficult to imagine, however, that any commentary *contra* to the position taken by the Commission would be given an exhaustive study at this stage of the administrative process.) Finally, on December 8, 1977, the Commission convened a special meeting, at which various proponents presented oral arguments concerning the proposed TRR. Four days later the five FTC commissioners met in a public hearing to determine the form and content of the rule and to vote on the rule's individual provisions. Although some votes were close, the commissioners adopted the TRR as proposed.

The cumbersome process begun in September 1975 reached its conclusion on June 2, 1978, some thirty-two months later, with the official publication of the new TRR in the *Federal Register*.

An administrative rule such as the TRR is accorded the force of law but cannot go into effect until thirty days after its publication in the *Federal Register*. On the day that the rule was announced the American Optometric Association requested that the FTC stay application of the rule while the AOA filed a legal challenge to the Commission's authority to promulgate such a TRR. With this act, the legislative phase of the administrative process ended and the judicial phase began.

Courts have the authority to review administrative rules under a variety of circumstances; one such circumstance would be where the rule is outside of the power of the agency publishing it. Provision is made in the law for review of a federal agency by the federal courts; for a state agency (such as a state board) review would normally proceed in the state courts. Accordingly, the AOA filed suit in the Federal Court of Appeals in Washington, D.C., against the FTC, and asked that the court stay the applicability of the rule until the legal process could determine if the rule was indeed a valid application of the Commission's powers. Both the FTC and the U.S. Court of Appeals denied the AOA's request for a stay of the rule and so the AOA applied to the U.S. Supreme Court for relief. The Supreme Court also turned down the request, (although the Chief Justice granted it initially), and on July 13, 1978, the rule officially went into effect across the United States, superseding the laws of some forty-five states and preempting the ethical codes of optometry and ophthalmology relative to advertising.

The ensuing legal battle became merely one of several being fought by the FTC against the licensed professions. The decision of an FTC judge in December of 1978 that the Code of Ethics of the AMA—which forbade advertising—was "a formidable impediment to competition in the delivery of health care service in this country" became the leading thrust of a campaign that affected dentists, anesthesiologists, nursing homes, and veterinarians (among others) in the U.S. health-care system. The ire of these various professions spilled over into the political arena, where some legislators—concerned with what they considered to be runaway authority in the writing of consumer protection trade rules—initiated a series of legislative reforms intended to curb the FTC's regulatory capability. (None of these reforms were subsequently adopted, however, by the U.S. Congress.)

On September 14, 1979, a three-judge panel of the U.S. Court of Appeals for the District of Columbia heard evidence from the FTC, the AOA, the AMA, and seventeen states; the case was heard some fifteen months after the AOA lawsuit was filed. Subsequently, the federal court suspended the FTC rule except for the requirement that patients be provided their prescriptions for glasses or contact lenses. The unanimous decision was handed down on February 6, 1980, nearly four and a half years after the FTC instituted its inquiry, and one and a half years after the TRR had gone into effect. The commission did not appeal the court's decision to the U.S. Supreme Court but let it be known that a further nonpublic inquiry into bans against commercial optometry would continue. In the 1980s the story turned to its next chapter, Eyeglasses II, and a repetition of the whole procedure.

Chapter 7

Judicial Regulation

We are under a constitution, but the constitution is what the judges say it is.
—Charles Evan Hughes, *Chief Justice, U.S. Supreme Court, 1930–1941, from a speech, May 3, 1907*

Prosperity in the United States has spawned an ever-increasing need for ules and regulations and for a forum in which to settle the inevitable disputes that arise from them. Although unique to the United States, the system that has evolved had its roots in England and the peculiar English invention known as the common law. To this common law legacy has been added an ever-expanding body of statutory law, both federal and state, which has grown to such an extent that thousands of bureaucrats are required to administer it. The result has been a "fourth branch" of government, the administrative agency, which has usurped powers traditionally belonging to the legislative and judicial branches (see Chapter 8).

The history of the United States in the twentieth century has been a story of the growing pervasiveness of government, particularly at the federal level. It has also been a period of intense social change. Part of that social change has been the slowly emerging recognition of health care as an obligation, not a privilege, of American life.[1]

This process had its beginnings in public education, which promoted the idea of equal opportunity, an idea that found favor in the business sector as well, through workman's compensation laws, whereby employers agreed to compensate workers for job-related injuries and paid the insurance premiums to finance these benefits.[2] The federal government subscribed to the same concept, organizing concomitant systems of equal access for servicemen (Veterans Administration), for federal employees (U.S. Public Health Service), and for Native Americans (Indian Health Service).[3] The courts have reinforced rights to health care, holding, for example, that emergency patients have a right to receive timely and appropriate care from hospitals with emergency room services and that patients involuntarily committed to mental health institutions have a right to treatment.[4]

In 1965 the poor and aged were granted federal assistance intended to assure equal opportunity for health care: The Medicaid and Medicare programs were founded in order to subsidize the costs of the health care received by these two populations. The next step in the evolution of the obligation to provide health care would seem to be national health insurance. This subject has been the source of a long and acrimonious debate and does not yet seem to be an idea whose day has come.[5]

Historical Perspective

The urban, industrial United States that has emerged in the twentieth century has embraced a system of English laws that evolved slowly, over the decades, in a more or less piecemeal fashion. Rarely has there been a revolutionary change in this legal structure. Rather, with each evolutionary change, a little of the old has been preserved along with a preponderance of the new. As a result, some very old concepts, such as the jury and the mortgage, are today as vital a part of the legal system as when begun in medieval times. Others have gone the way of the village blacksmith and the nickel cigar.

The famous English jurist, Blackstone, wrote his *Commentaries On The Law of England* about twenty years before the Revolutionary War.[6] In the *Commentaries*, he expressed the essence of the English common law. Unlike most of Europe, which was organized so as to make statutes (compiled into a code) the highest level of legal authority, England evolved a system of "unwritten law", as Blackstone called it. This unwritten law was not based on statute but rather on the general custom of a community, as reflected in the decisions of the common law judges. The judges were the ones who gave life to the law, by deciding cases and then publishing their opinions and the logic that fostered them. These decisions were drawn from existing principles of law, as the judges knew them, and reflected the attitudes, values, and ethical ideals of the English people. Each opinion became a precedent for succeeding generations and was modified as needed to reflect the particular needs and exigencies of the time. Therefore, in the common law reposed many of the basic rules of law that could not be found anywhere else.[7]

The common law was centered around two concepts: formal legal process[8] and the law of the land.[9] The concept of common law came to America with English settlers migrating to the New World, as did Blackstone's *Commentaries*. As a result of this inheritance, the U.S. legal system has evolved its own common law, 200 years of shared experiences that now constitute its unique law of the land. This important body of law is divided by the federal and state jurisdictions that have created a unique dual court system. And presiding over all courts, both federal and state, is the U.S. Supreme Court.

The Judicial System

The federal Constitution of 1787 created a judicial branch of government to be co-equal in powers with the legislative and executive branches. But the United States Supreme Court, although the highest court in the nation, was not given the right to review cases or controversies coming before it as to the constitutionality of the issues raised by the dispute.[10] It was Chief Justice John Marshall, in the seminal case of *Marbury v. Madison* (1803), who enunciated this important function of the court and changed forever the course of U.S. history.[11] Marshall, in this decision, stressed the preeminence of the Constitution over the laws passed by Congress:

> If then, the courts are to regard the constitution, and the constitution is superior to any ordinary act of the legislature, the constitution, and not such ordinary act, must govern the case to which they both apply.... Thus, the particular phraseology of the Constitution of the United States confirms and strengthens the principle, supposed to be essential to all written constitutions, that a law repugnant to the constitution is void, and that courts, as well as other departments, are bound by that instrument.[12]

Ever since this remarkable decision, the U.S. Supreme Court has considered constitutionality one of its responsibilities. In so doing, the judiciary has managed to achieve an important balance with the legislative and executive branches of government: Although the Congress may pass a bill, and the President may sign it into law, it is left to the Supreme Court to decide if the law is constitutional and thereby enforceable. Therefore, if a case or controversy involves a constitutional issue, the U.S. Supreme Court will have the final word.

But to reach this exalted tribunal of nine judges, a tedious appeals process must be followed, through either the federal or the state system. In fact, the cry, "I'll take it to the Supreme Court!" is a hollow one, for studies have shown that the Supreme Court annually reviews about 1 percent of the appellate decisions rendered by Courts of Appeals across the nation.[13] Appellate petitions for review—through direct appeal or the discretionary writ of certiorari—can be presented through either the federal courts or the state courts, depending on the nature of the case or controversy. A brief explanation of these two court systems will demonstrate the two alternative routes to final adjudication.

The Federal System

Through the agency of the Judiciary Act of 1789, the U.S. Congress exercised the power granted it by the U.S. Constitution to award jurisdiction to the federal courts in certain kinds of cases.[14] The most important of these are cases involving federal statutes (which are compiled in the *U.S. Code*) and cases involving disputes between citizens of two different states (diversity cases). The federal courts are the arbiters of other categories of cases as well, but they have far less relevance for optometry.[15]

The federal court system is a national multitiered system that divides the United States into thirteen circuits (including eleven numbered circuits, a circuit for the District of Columbia, and a circuit known as the Federal Circuit, which hears appeals from U.S. District Courts under certain circumstances). A number of states are in a circuit (Table 7.1 and Fig. 7.1). Each state is divided into districts, and a federal judge presides over each of these districts (Fig. 7.2). The district judge is a *trial* judge, before whom cases—both civil and criminal—are litigated. The judge's decision can be appealed, however, to the court of appeals for the entire circuit. Since there are thirteen federal circuits, there are thirteen federal Courts of Appeals within the country. A circuit appellate court is actually a panel of judges (rather than a single judge), and it can overrule or uphold or modify the decision of a district judge. If a constitutional issue is involved, appeal from the decision of a federal Court of Appeals may be made to the U.S. Supreme Court (see Fig. 7.3). But the mere fact that a party petitions for review does not ensure that the case will be heard. Under the rule of four, at least four of the justices of the Supreme Court must be willing to review a case before it can be heard.[16] The court is very judicious in its selections.

Table 7.1. Federal Circuits: U.S. Courts of Appeals

Circuit	Jurisdiction
U.S. Court of Appeals	District of Columbia
First	Maine, Massachusetts, New Hampshire, Rhode Island, Puerto Rico
Second	Connecticut, New York, Vermont
Third	Delaware, New Jersey, Pennsylvania, Virgin Islands
Fourth	Maryland, North Carolina, South Carolina, Virginia, West Virginia
Fifth	Louisiana, Mississippi, Texas, Canal Zone
Sixth	Kentucky, Michigan, Ohio, Tennessee
Seventh	Illinois, Indiana, Wisconsin
Eighth	Arkansas, Iowa, Minnesota, Missouri, Nebraska, North Dakota, South Dakota
Ninth	Arizona, California, Idaho, Montana, Nevada, Oregon, Washington, Alaska, Hawaii, Guam, Northern Mariana Islands
Tenth	Colorado, Kansas, New Mexico, Oklahoma, Utah, Wyoming
Eleventh	Alabama, Florida, Georgia
Federal	All federal judicial districts

Source: 28 U.S.C.A. §41.

The State System

Each state has original jurisdiction over cases and controversies involving its citizens.[17] Legal disputes

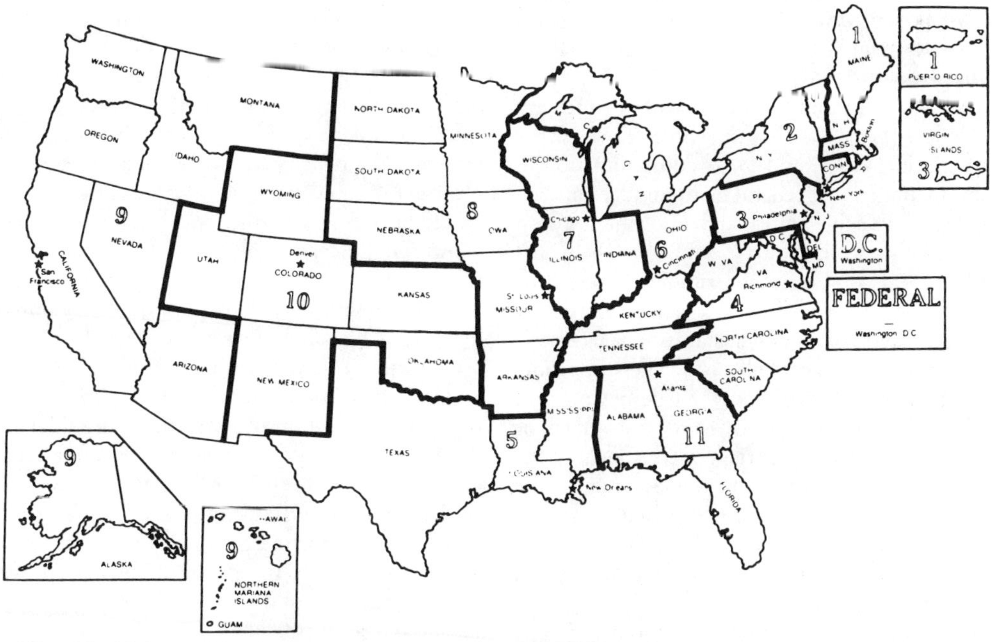

Figure 7.1. The Thirteen Federal Judicial Circuits, 1987 (see 28 U.S.C.A. §41). (Diagram courtesy of West Publishing Company)

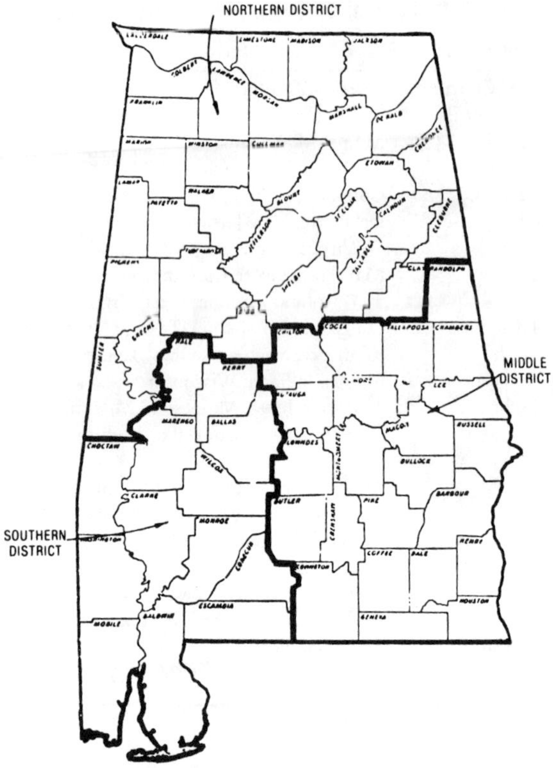

Figure 7.2. Federal Court Districts, State of Alabama.

not capable of being filed in or removed to the federal courts will be settled within the state system, which is organized very similarly to its federal counterpart.[18] Each state is divided into judicial areas that are usually composed of one or more counties, within which are several judges (Fig. 7.4). They may preside over either civil or criminal cases, and in so doing, function in the same manner as the federal district judges, i.e., as trial judges.[19] In some states, appeal of the decision or ruling of a state trial court would be to the Court of Civil Appeals or Court of Criminal Appeals for the state, depending on whether a civil or a criminal dispute was involved.[20] Other states only have one court of appeals that hears all cases. These appellate courts are panels of judges (like the federal Courts of Appeals) and have the authority to reverse, affirm, or modify the decisions of the trial court. Appeal of the decision of this tribunal is to the highest court of the state (Fig. 7.3). The opinions of the states' highest courts are final unless there is a federal issue involved that would be of sufficient interest to the U.S. Supreme Court to merit its review.

Even though dissatisfaction with the decision of a state's highest court may prompt a petition for review to the U.S. Supreme Court, the situation is the same as in the federal system, e.g., very few cases are actually selected for a hearing by the nation's top court. Therefore, the decisions of the states' highest courts settle disputes of state law the overwhelming percentage of the time, a fact that has considerable importance for optometry.

Like all professions, optometry is defined and regulated according to state law and so the decisions of state appellate courts are of considerable importance to the profession's future development. State decisions are cited most frequently within this text, but it must be realized that the applicability of these decisions is limited to the confines of the state border. A decision of a state's highest court establishes the law within that state only, just as a decision of a federal Circuit Court of Appeals establishes the law within that circuit only. These precedents may be cited by lawyers within other states or circuits as examples of law that should be adopted, but the courts of the other jurisdictions are not bound by them. The Supreme Court of the United States is the only court that can formulate a uniform law of the land.

The dual federal-state system contains a certain amount of overlapping jurisdiction, and on occasion disputes arise as to which court (federal or state) is appropriate.[21] Both courts can handle either civil or criminal cases.

A *civil* case involves injury to person or property. An automobile accident, for example, in which a person is hurt and the automobile damaged, is typical. The injured party would sue the malefactor for damages (hospital bills, doctor's bills, medications, pain and suffering), and, if the injured party prevails, would receive an award of money. Thus, money is the penalty for civil liability. The idea is to place the injured party in as good a position as he would have been in if the injury had never occurred.

A *criminal* case involves an offense to the public, through the perpetration of a crime (such as burglary, robbery, or murder). It is punishable by imprisonment or a fine or both (or, in these days, perhaps even death). The theory is to punish the one who has violated the rules of society. A felony is a crime that is punishable by imprisonment for more than a year. A misdemeanor is a crime that is punishable by imprisonment for less than a year.

There is an important difference in the burden of proof required for these two classifications of cases. In a criminal case, the prosecution must prove the accused guilty beyond a reasonable doubt, which is a substantial and difficult undertaking. But in a civil case, the plaintiff (the one who brought the lawsuit) need only prove he is entitled to compensation by a

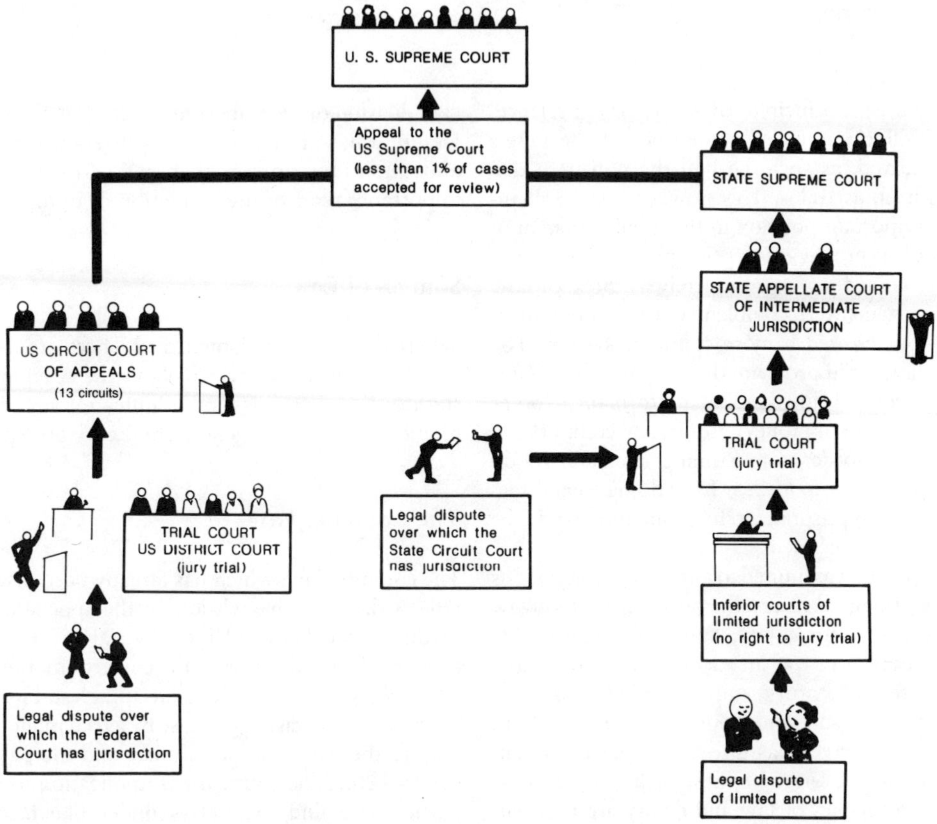

Figure 7.3. Appellate Procedure, U.S. Courts. This simplified schematic diagram shows how a legal dispute, beginning either in the state or the federal court system, may be appealed to the U.S. Supreme Court.

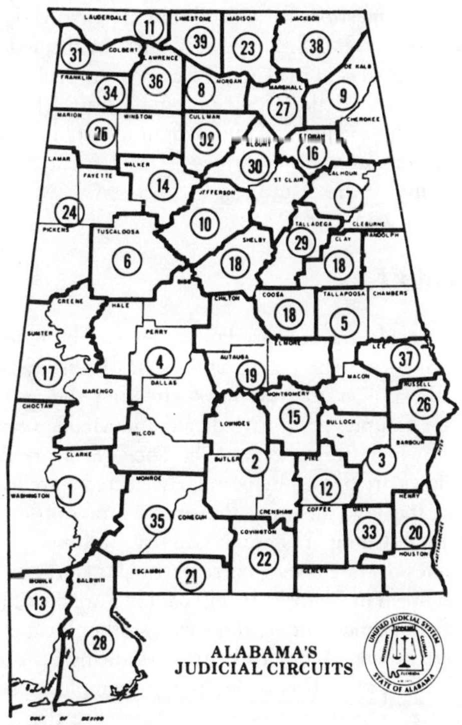

Figure 7.4. Judicial Circuits of the State of Alabama.

preponderance of the evidence, which means that he must be more believable than the defendant. This is a far less stringent burden than in a criminal case.

To sum up, judges exercise enormous power in the judicial system, through the interpretation of laws and the formulation of rulings on the constitutionality of statutes. State judges have the most authority with regard to optometry, but they are popularly elected in most states,[22] which makes their careers less long-lived than those of their federal brethren, who are appointed for life. The justices of the United States Supreme Court, whose decisions so greatly influence all our lives, are also lifetime appointees.

Equity

The English common law discussed in the preceding section was not without rival systems, particularly the interesting system known as equity.[23] The chancellor's office, the chancery, was responsible for issuing writs to the common law courts. Through a long and complex process following the Norman conquest of England, chancery itself became a court, but it did not follow the common law rules, which were rules of law. Rather, it employed principles that were in line with principles of equity or conscience. The chancellor was called the keeper of the king's conscience, and, as such, he had the power to dispense with unjust rules. This power gave the chancellor an important position in the English system of justice, and eventually rules, principles, and doctrines of equity evolved just as completely as those of law. The two systems were complementary—and contradictory—but created a more complete system. The common law could proclaim duties and rights; but it could not compel any kind of performance (other than the payment of money). Equity, by comparison, could issue an order commanding a person to do some specific act or to forbear from doing something. If disobeyed, imprisonment for contempt could be meted out as punishment.

Equity power was limited to authority over persons rather than things. As a result, courts of common law ignored doctrines of equity, and equity courts dismissed cases if there was an adequate remedy at law. In the nineteenth century, equity and law merged in England. As a result, one court administered both systems. This merger has also taken place, but incompletely, in the United States, such that, in most states, the principles of law and equity are both enforceable in one proceeding. In some states separate courts resolve equitable and legal disputes, and separate actions are still necessary.[24]

The significance of equity to optometry is found in the court's extraordinary powers; the *injunction* and the *declaratory judgment* are two of the most important remedies a chancellor can employ, and both are frequently prayed for in litigation involving optometry. For instance, an optician who is functioning outside the scope of opticianry, as defined by the pertinent state statutes, can be enjoined from performing the illegal act (e.g., using diagnostic pharmaceutical agents). Failure to adhere to the court's injuction (by continuing to use the diagnostic drugs) would constitute a contempt of court, punishable by fine or incarceration. Another equitable remedy is the declaratory judgment, by which the chancellor fixes the rights and responsibilities of the parties under a given law. The validity of a state department of revenue regulation taxing optometrists for the sale of ophthalmic materials (glasses and contact lenses)[25] but not taxing ophthalmologists for the same materials dispensed in their practices would be a valid subject for a declaratory judgment.[26] The enforceability of such a regulation could be suspended should the judge find it discriminatory.

Chancellors of Equity are members of the state court system, and in those states that have merged law and equity they will be denoted judges for the civil division of the state court instead of chancellors. Despite this subtrefuge, they will retain the unique and important powers that makes them such an important factor in the regulation of optometry.

Sources of Law

Where does the law come from? There are five generally recognized sources of law: the common law, statutory law, rulings of administrative agencies, opinions of attorneys general, and advisory opinions.

The Common Law

The common law, which has already been discussed, reflects the collective wisdom of the appellate judges of the United States. Although trial judges are the arbiters of legal disputes in the courtroom, the appellate judges make the decisions that establish legal precedents. A decision in a case by a trial judge applies only to the particular set of facts and the particular parties before the court. It has application to all like parties who find themselves under like facts only when upheld by an appellate court. And it is final only when the highest appellate court approves it. (The decisions of the highest state appellate court can, if a question of federal law is involved, be appealed to the U.S. Supreme Court. In the federal system appeal is to the Circuit Court of Appeals, and, on occasion, to the U.S. Supreme Court). Judges, through the medium of the common law, interpret the meaning of various statues, as well as the constitutionality of these statutes.

Statutory Law

Duly enacted statutes are laws; they can be federal, state, or local. The U.S. Congress has been invested with the power to pass laws affecting the several states. Examples are the Medicaid and Medicare programs, which are aspects of the Social Security Act. State laws are passed by popularly elected state legislators; the laws defining the practice of optometry and establishing a state board of optometry are examples of state laws. (These particular statutes will be discussed in Chapter 10.) Local laws are passed by counties, municipalities, and various other local units of government. A city ordinance requiring an optometrist to pay a license fee is an example of such a statute. Taken as a whole, statutes are the most immediate legal influence on a practitioner.

Rulings of Administrative Agencies

Authorized rulings by administrative agencies such as the FTC, the Food and Drug Administration (FDA), or the Internal Revenue Service (IRS) have the force of law. The FTC's Eyeglasses 1 Rule is an example of an administrative agency's use of the power ostensibly delegated to it by Congress, through the passage of various statutes authorizing the administrative agency to perform certain duties. More will be said about this subject in Chapter 8.

Opinions of Attorneys General

These opinions are not laws per se. They are advisory only and are not binding in the same sense as are statutes passed by legislatures or decisions of appellate judges.[27] Rather, they are the attorneys' general responses to particular legal questions posed to them.[28] The courts (which have the authority to interpret the law) may not agree with an attorney general if the matter is brought to litigation. In many states, attorneys general have been asked to interpret the state optometry law; whether *pro* or *con*, the decision is not binding on a court or on the average practitioner of optometry but is useful to a state agency such as a state board of optometry.[29]

Advisory Opinions

Advisory opinions are like the opinions of attorneys general because they are advisory only and are not binding on the courts. Such opinions are not permissible in the majority of states,[30] but where they are allowed they are legal questions posed to the state supreme court asking how the court would rule in a given legal situation. For example, an advisory opinion could be asked of a state supreme court as to whether or not an optometrist is eligible, under the state optometry law, to be the employee of a corporation. But even if the court issued such an opinion, it would not be bound by it should a case involving the same set of facts come before it for adjudication.

These, then, are the various ways laws are created. But how is the law recorded, and how is it found?

How to Find the Law

Entire books are devoted to helping novice legal scholars locate the burgeoning number of decisions, statutes, and opinions that make up the *corpus juris* of our nation's legal system.[31] Fortunately, legal references are compiled according to the source of the laws being sought. There is such a profusion of legal references that it is rather easy to become discouraged at the prospects of locating a particular law. Accordingly, the following discussion centers around the five sources described in the preceding section: (1) common law, (2) statutory law, (3) administrative rulings, (4) opinions of attorneys general, and (5) advisory opinions.

Common Law

In order to locate the law as determined by a particular case, certain fundamental questions must be asked: (1) If it is a state case, has it been appealed? Only if it is heard by a state appellate court is the decision formally recorded in the case reporting system; (2) Is the case in the state or the federal court? The answer to this question dictates which reporter system is to be consulted; and (3) What is the citation for the case? Appellate cases are recorded in a particular format for convenience and continuity. For example, the case of *Helling v. Carey*, which held that ophthalmologists in Washington State had a legal duty to test persons below the age of 40 for glaucoma, was reported in 83 Wash. 2d 514, which means that the decision of the Washington Supreme Court is to be found in volume 83 of the second series of the Washington Reporter at page 514 (see Table 7.2). But this is not the only reporter system in which *Helling* can be found. There is also a National Reporter System (Table 7.3) consisting of seven regional reporters, and the state of Washington is included in the Pacific Reporter. This citation is recorded as 519 P. 2d 981, which indicates that Volume 519, page 981, of the second series of the Pacific Reporter also contains the Washington high court's opinion of the case.

The National Reporter System, published by West Publishing Company, is probably the easiest source to consult once the national citation is known.[32] This system includes the decisions of the highest courts in each state (just as published in the state reporter). It also includes the decisions of intermediate appellate courts and those of the federal courts (a separate series of four different reporters).[33] These federal sources are infrequently needed, since optometry cases rarely find their way into the federal courts. An exception is *Gibson v. Berryhill*, one of the few optometry cases to be accepted for review by the U.S. Supreme Court. The *Gibson* case, which protested the composition of the Alabama State Board of

Table 7.2. State Reporter System

Reporter	Citation
Alabama Reports	Ala
Alabama Appellate Reports	Ala App
Alaska Reports	Alask
Arizona Reports	Ariz
Arkansas Reports	Ark
California Appellate Reports	Cal App
California Reports	Cal
Colorado Reports	Colo
Connecticut Reports	Conn
Delaware Reports	By name of reporter
Delaware Chancery Reports	Del Ch
Florida Reports	Fla
Georgia Reports	Ga
Hawaii Reports	Haw
Idaho Reports	Idaho
Illinois Reports	Ill
Illinois Appellate Reports	Ill App
Indiana Reports	Ind
Indiana Appellate Reports	Ind App
Iowa Reports	Iowa
Kansas Reports	Kan
Kentucky Reports	Ky
Louisiana Reports	La
Maine Reports	Me
Maryland Reports	Md
Massachusetts Reports	Mass
Michigan Reports	Mich
Minnesota Reports	Minn
Mississippi Reports	Miss
Missouri Reports	Mo
Missouri Appeal Reports	Mo App
Montana Reports	Mont
Nebraska Reports	Neb
Nevada Reports	Nev
New Hampshire Reports	NH
New Jersey Equity Reports	NJ Eq
New Jersey Reports	NJ
New Jersey Superior Court Reports	NJ Super
New Mexico Reports	NM
New York Appellate Division Reports	NY App Div
New York Miscellaneous Reports	NY Misc
New York Reports	NY
North Carolina Reports	NC
North Dakota Reports	ND
Ohio Appellate Reports	Ohio App
Ohio State Reports	Ohio St
Oklahoma Reports	Okla
Oklahoma Criminal Reports	Okla Cr
Oregon Reports	Or
Pennsylvania District and County Reports	Pa D&C
Pennsylvania Reports	Pa
Pennsylvania Superior Court Reports	Pa Sup
Rhode Island Reports	RI

Table 7.2. *Continued*

Reporter	Citation
South Carolina Reports	SC
South Dakota Reports	SD
Tennessee Reports	Tenn
Tennessee Appeals Reports	Tenn App
Texas Reports	Tex
United States Reports	US
United States Court of Appeals, District of Columbia	DC App
Utah Reports	Utah
Vermont Reports	Vt
Virginia Reports	Va
Washington Reports	Wash
West Virginia Reports	W Va
Wisconsin Reports	Wis
Wyoming Reports	Wyo

Source: Coblens, S., *Optometry and the Law*, American Optometric Association, St. Louis, 1976.

Optometry, was reported by the Supreme Court in 411 U.S. 564 and in West's own separate system, The Supreme Court Reporter, at 93 S. Ct. 1689. Both sources report the same decision, but, as with the state and national reporter systems, this duplicate recording system is intended to ensure ease of access to the law.

One other state source deserves mention. The *American Law Reports, Annotated* (A.L.R.), which is now in its fourth series, contains an annotation of numerous points of law and rules on the subject of the annotation, discusses the application of the rules, and provides definitions of cogent words and phrases.[34] The A.L.R. contains a number of annotations that pertain to optometry, and it cites and summarizes many of the leading cases involving the profession. It is a quick, fairly straightforward source to consult for a rapid understanding of any point that is the subject of annotation. For example, the Second Series of A.L.R. contains a historical annotation entitled "Liability of Optometrist or Optician for Malpractice"; the citation for this annotation is 68 A.L.R.2d 426, which refers the researcher to volume 68, page 426, of A.L.R.'s second series. There is an Index for each series that can be consulted to determine if a particular topic is the subject of annotation.[35] A.L.R., however, is not a primary source of law and should be used as an encyclopedia to obtain an overview of a particular topic.

Statutes

Statutory law can be researched on a federal, state, or local basis.[36]

Table 7.3. National Reporter System

Name of Reporter	Citation	Courts Covered	
Supreme Court Reporter	S Ct	U.S. Supreme Court	
United States Reporter	US	U.S. Supreme Court	
Federal Reporter	F	U.S. Circuit Courts of Appeal U.S. District Courts	
Federal Reporter, second series	F 2d	U.S. Courts of Appeals U.S. Court of Customs and Patent Appeals U.S. Emergency Court of Appeals	
Federal Supplement	F Supp	U.S. District Courts U.S. Court of Claims	
Atlantic Reporter Atlantic Reporter, second series	A A 2d	Connecticut Delaware Maine Maryland New Hampshire	New Jersey Pennsylvania Rhode Island Vermont District of Columbia
New York Supplement New York Supplement, second series	NY Supp NYS 2d	New York Court of Appeals Appellate Division of the Supreme Court Miscellaneous Courts	
Northeastern Reporter Northeastern Reporter, second series	NE NE 2d	Illinois Indiana New York Massachusetts Ohio	
Northwestern Reporter Northwestern Reporter, second series	NW NW 2d	Iowa Michigan Minnesota Nebraska	North Dakota South Dakota Wisconsin
Pacific Reporter Pacific Reporter, second series	P P 2d	Alaska Arizona California Colorado Hawaii Idaho Kansas Montana	Nevada New Mexico Oklahoma Oregon Utah Washington Wyoming
Southeastern Reporter Southeastern Reporter, second series	SE SE 2d	Georgia North Carolina South Carolina Virginia West Virginia	
Southern Reporter Southern Reporter, second series	So So 2d	Alabama Florida Louisiana Mississippi	
Southwestern Reporter Southwestern Reporter, second series	SW SW 2d	Arkansas Kentucky Missouri Tennessee Texas	

Source: Coblens, S., *Optometry and the Law*, American Optometric Association, St. Louis, 1976.

Table 7.4. State Statutes Defining Optometry: 1985

Alabama	Ala. Code §34-22-1
Alaska	Alaska Stat. §08.72.300(2)
Arizona	Ariz. Rev. Stat. Ann. §32-1701(6)
Arkansas	Ark. Stat. Ann. §72-801
California	Cal. Bus. & Prof. Code §3041(A) (West)
Colorado	Colo. Rev. Stat. §12-40-102(1)
Connecticut	Conn. Gen. Stat. §20-127
Delaware	Del. Code Ann. tit. 24, §2102
District of Columbia	D.C. Code Ann. §2-501
Florida	Fla. Stat. Ann. §463.002 (West)
Georgia	Ga. Code Ann. §84-1101
Hawaii	Haw. Rev. Stat. §459-1
Idaho	Idaho Code §54-1501
Illinois	Ill. Ann. Stat. ch. 91, §105.3 (Smith-Hurd)
Indiana	Ind. Stat. Ann. §25-24-1-4 (Burns)
Iowa	Iowa Code Ann. §154.1
Kansas	Kan. Stat. Ann. §65-1501
Kentucky	Ky. Rev. Stat. Ann. §320.210(2)
Louisiana	La. Rev. Stat. Ann. §37:1041(3) (West)
Maine	Me. Rev. Stat. Ann. tit. 32, §2411(1)
Maryland	Md. Ann. Code art. 43, §368(e)
Massachusetts	Mass Gen. Laws Ann. ch. 112, §66 (West)
Michigan	Mich. Comp. Laws Ann. §14.15 (17401)
Minnesota	Minn. Stat. Ann. and §§148.56, 148.571
Mississippi	Miss. Code Ann. §§73-19-1 and 73-19-103(2)
Missouri	Mo. Rev. Stat. §336.010
Montana	Mont. Code Ann. §37-10-101
Nebraska	Neb. Rev. Stat. §71-1,133
Nevada	Nev. Rev. Stat. §636.025
New Hampshire	N.H. Rev. Stat. Ann. §327-1
New Jersey	N.J. Rev. Stat. Ann. §45:12-1 (West)
New Mexico	N.M. Stat. Ann. §61-2-2
New York	N.Y. Educ. Law. (McKinney) §7101
North Carolina	N.C. Gen. Stat. §90-114
North Dakota	N.D. Cent. Code §43-13-01(1)
Ohio	Ohio Rev. Code Ann. §4725.01(A)
Oklahoma	Okla. Stat. tit. 59, §§581 and 353.1(7)
Oregon	Or. Rev. Stat. §683.010(2)
Pennsylvania	Pa. Stat. Ann. tit. 63 §244.2 (Purdon's)
Rhode Island	R.I. Gen. Laws §5-35-1
South Carolina	S.C. Rev. Code §40-37-10
South Dakota	S.D. Codified Laws Ann. §36-7-1
Tennessee	Tenn. Code Ann. §63-802(1)
Texas	Tex. Rev. Civ. Stat. Ann. arts. 4552-1.02(1) and 4505-1.(5) (Vernon)
Utah	Utah Code Ann. §58-16-11
Vermont	Vt. Stat. Ann. tit. 26, §§1703(1) and 1723
Virginia	Va. Code §54-368
Washington	Wash. Rev. Code Ann. §18-53.010
West Virginia	W. Va. Code §30-8-2
Wisconsin	Wis. Stat. Ann. §449.01
Wyoming	Wyo. Stat. §33-23-101

Source: American Optometric Association, 1985.

Laws enacted by Congress can be found in the *United States Code* (U.S.C.), which has an official edition and two annotated editions offered by private publishing houses, the *U.S. Code Annotated* and the *Federal Code Annotated*. Both are kept reasonably up to date. *The United States Law Week* also publishes the full text of important federal laws and cases, and has a rather good subject index as well. A recently enacted law can be found in *Statutes at Large*, before the law is placed in the U.S.C.

State statutes are compiled into state codes, just as the federal statutes are compiled into a federal code. These state codes may be called codes or statutes, but their format is generally the same from state to state. For example, each state code contains statutory law defining the practice of optometry (Table 7.4). Unfortunately, there is no one reference source that offers a comprehensive index to the statutes of all the states.

Local laws, such as municipal charters, codes, and ordinances rarely affect optometry. But zoning and housing laws play an obvious role in daily life, and these laws—in the form of city ordinances or resolutions—may be found collected by title or subject into a municipal code. Frequently, a telephone call and a visit to the office of the city clerk are required before the desired law can be found.

Administrative Regulations and Decisions

An overwhelming number of documents of legal effect and significance pour out of the many federal and state administrative agencies that are the offspring of "big government" and ambitious social programs.[37] Since 1935 all federal proclamations, orders, notices, regulations, and other documents have been published in *The Federal Register* (Fed. Reg.), a daily newspaper-like compilation of these governmental offerings. *The Federal Register* has a daily table of contents, a monthly index, and a codification guide that is keyed to the *Code of Federal Regulations* (C.F.R.). The first C.F.R. was published in 1938 and was an attempt to collect all administrative regulations in force; because of difficulties in updating it a second edition was published in 1949, and revisions and supplements of this second edition continue to date. The FTC's Eyeglasses I Rule, an administrative regulation with significant effects on optometry, ophthalmology, and opticianry, can be found in 16 C.F.R. §456.

Although state administrative agencies are less visible than their federal counterparts, they too have profound effects on optometry, especially the particular state entity known as the Board of Optometry. Unfortunately, problems with publication, public access to records, and control of documents have been met with little concern. Therefore, information is difficult to obtain, although most state boards will have a publication delineating the board's officers, its duties, and its powers. For a survey approach to state administrative agencies, *The Book of the States*, published by the Council of State Governments, is a very helpful beginning point.

Many federal agencies issue their own texts of rules and regulations, and some of these can be purchased through the Government Printing Office. The Internal Revenue Service's *Looseleaf Regulations System* (a five part series), is an example, and vividly illustrates the almost inhuman propensity of government to issue regulation after regulation. Federal administrative agencies also exercise judicial power in determining cases and questions involving their regulations, usually after conducting formal hearings, and thereafter publish formal opinions to justify or explain their decisions. This is in fact the procedure that the Federal Trade Commission followed to justify its Trade Regulation Ruling on Advertising of Ophthalmic Goods and Services in 1978.

Opinions of Attorneys General

These opinions are usually written in response to specific inquiries that ask the attorney general to construe statutes, interpret case law, and render legal counsel.[38] Federal opinions can be found in the *Opinions of the Attorneys General of the United States* and, at the state level, in a similarly titled series published by the individual states. Attorneys general are frequently asked to interpret optometry laws, which usually requires a determination of the scope of services that an optometrist can perform.

Advisory Opinions

On occasion, a court will agree to advise a petitioning party as to what the court would rule under a certain set of facts, statutes, or circumstances. These opinions are recorded in the same manner and under the same reporting systems as are the common law decisions discussed previously.

With this knowledge of the structure of the judicial system, the sources of law, and how the law in its various forms can be located, we will turn to a brief discussion of the regulation of optometry by the federal administrative agencies.

Notes

1. For an overview of public health policy and optometry, see Newcomb, R.D., and J.L. Jolley, *Public Health and Community Optometry*, Charles C. Thomas, Springfield, Ill., 1980, pp. 103–121.
2. Lawrence M. Friedman, *A History of American Law*, Simon and Schuster, New York, 1973, pp. 587–588, describes the purpose of workman's compensation laws in the following manner:

   > Workman's compensation was a compromise system. Each side gave a little, got a little. The worker got compensation. If he was injured on the job, he collected for it, whether the employer was negligent or not. . . . On the other hand, what the employer had to pay to an injured workman was fixed by statute. . . . Statutes . . . set a definite price for "permanent partial disability"—so many weeks' compensation for a finger, a toe, an eye, a foot, an arm. The employee could get no less; but he could also get no more.
3. The role of optometry in federal aspects of health care and health care policy is summarized in Newcomb and Jolley, supra note 1, at 281–314.
4. Another important right to health care concerns abortion. The U.S. Supreme Court, in the case of *Roe v. Wade*, 410 U.S. 113, 93 S. Ct. 705 (1973), held that certain restrictions on abortion were unconstitutional. Other examples include the right to receive voluntary sterilization and the right to privacy. Thus there has been a growing recognition in federal law of legal rights to various aspects of health care. The emerging issue of the right to health care per se is discussed briefly in Chapter 7, note 1.
5. For information on various proposals for national health insurance, see the following: Rogers, P., Before National Health Insurance—Some Points To Consider, in Conference Proceedings—The National Leadership Conference in America's Health Policy, *National Journal*, 1976; Falk, I.S., National Health Insurance for the United States, *Public Health Reporter*, vol. 92,

no. 5, Sept.-Oct., 1977, pp. 399–406; U.S. Department of Health, Education, and Welfare, Social Security Administration, *National Health Insurance Proposals*, HEW Publication No. (SSA) 76-11920, Washington, D.C., 1976. National health insurance, as a political force, has lost the momentum it held in the 1970s and no longer is viable politically.

6. Blackstone, Sir William, *Commentaries On The Laws Of England* (4 vols., 1765–1769).
7. Interestingly, the common law was not based on the legal tribulations of the common people but rather on the experiences of the English nobility. Observes Friedman, supra note 2, at 20–21:

   > Common law was, essentially, the law of the royal central courts. It was this law, basically, that the great English jurists, up to and including Blackstone, described. But the royal central courts, by and large, handled the legal problems of a tiny group of people. . . here one will find a colorful set of litigants, all drawn from the very top of English society—lords and ladies, landed gentry, high-ranking clergymen, wealthy merchants. Common law was an aristocratic law, for and of the gentry and nobility. The masses were hardly touched by this system and only indirectly under its rule.

   The one exception to the common law rule in the United States is Louisiana, which is based upon the Continental civil law system.
8. Under the English system of courts that began in the 1200s, in order for an injured party to be heard by the court a *writ* had to be filed, charging the defendant with a specific offense for which relief could be granted. These *writs* were quite formal, as was the procedure necessary for the defendant to answer and for the determination of whether or not a remedy was available under the law. For a discussion of how the procedural law influenced the development of claims based in tort (including those alleging malpractice), see Chapter 18.
9. According to Friedman, supra note 2:

   > Common law was judge-made law—molded, refined, examined, and changed in the crucible of actual decision, and handed down from generation to generation in the form of reported cases. . . . In practice, the judges relied upon their own past actions, which they modified under the pressure of changing times and changing patterns of litigation. In other words, common law adhered to precedent as a general rule.

   Thus, an essential cornerstone of the common law was *precedent*, which permitted cases involving similar facts to be decided in a similar manner, even though the cases were brought in different places or at different times. See id. at page 17.
10. Article III of the Constitution describes the powers of the Supreme Court:

    > *Section 1.* The judicial power of the United States, shall be vested in one supreme Court, and in such inferior Courts as the Congress may from time to time ordain and establish. The Judges, both of the supreme and inferior Courts, shall hold their offices during good Behaviour, and shall, at stated Times, receive for their Services a Compensation, which shall not be diminished during their Continuance in Office.
    >
    > *Section 2.* The judicial Power shall extend to all Cases, in Law and Equity, arising under this Constitution, the Laws of the United States, and Treaties made, or which shall be made, under their Authority;—to all Cases affecting Ambassadors, other public Ministers and Consuls;—to all Cases of admiralty and maritime Jurisdiction;—to Controversies to which the United States shall be a Party;—to Controversies between two or more States;—between a State and Citizens of another State;—between Citizens of different States;—between Citizens of the same State claiming Lands under the Grants of different States, and between a State, or the Citizens thereof, and foreign States, Citizens or Subjects.
    >
    > In all Cases affecting Ambassadors, other public Ministers and Consuls, and those in which a State shall be a Party, the supreme Court shall have original Jurisdiction. In all the other Cases before mentioned, the supreme Court shall have appellate Jurisdiction, both as to Law and Fact, with such Exceptions, and under such Regulations as the Congress shall make.
11. *Marbury v. Madison*, 5 U.S. (1 Cranch) 137 (1803). A review of the case can be found in Van Alstyne, A Critical Guide to *Marbury v. Madison*, 1969 *Duke Law Journal* 1.
12. After this decision the Supreme Court did not hold an act of Congress unconstitutional until more than fifty years had passed, in the case of *Dred Scott v. Sandford*, 60 U.S. (19 How.) 393 (1857).
13. See Griswold, Rationing Justice—The Supreme Court's Caseload and What the Court Does Not Do, 60 *Cornell Law Review* 335 (1975). For an interesting view of the inner workings of the Supreme Court, including the factors that influence the decisions of the court, see Woodward, B., and S. Armstrong, *The Brethren*, Simon and Schuster, New York, 1979.
14. For a scholarly discussion of the federal court system, see Wright, C.A., *The Federal Courts*, 2d ed., West Publishing Co., St. Paul, Minn., 1970.
15. Examples of how the federal court system can involve optometric disputes include cases arguing: the constitutionality of state statutes restricting the commercial practice of optometry, *Williamson v. Lee Optical of Oklahoma*, 120 F. Supp. 128 (D.C. Okla. 1954); the constitutionality of the makeup of state boards of optometry, *Gibson v. Berryhill*, 331 F. Supp. 122 (D.C. Ala. 1971); the use of trade names by optometrists, *Friedman v. Rogers*, 438 F. Supp. 428 (D.C. Tex. 1977); and the validity of the FTC's Eyeglasses I Rule, *American Optometric Association v. Federal Trade Commission*, 626 F.2d 896 (D.C. Cir. 1980).

16. See Wright, C.A., supra note 14, at 493–495.
17. To understand the state court system, see Pound, R., *Organization of Courts*, Little, Brown, Boston, 1940; Mayers, L., *The American Legal System*, Harper, New York, 1955; Council of State Governments, *State Court Systems*, The Council of State Governments, Chicago, 1956; and Abraham, H.J., *The Judicial Process*, Oxford University Press, New York, 1962.
18. Although the structure of courts will vary from state to state, in general these courts will fall into five classes:
    1. tribunals of petty jurisdiction (such as some municipal courts)
    2. courts of intermediate grade (such as small claims courts and some municipal or county courts)
    3. courts of general trial jurisdiction (usually referred to as county, district, or circuit courts)
    4. appellate courts (which stand in some states between the trial court and the state's highest tribunal)
    5. the state supreme court, which is principally intended to correct the errors of lower tribunals and to unify the interpretation of the law within the state (and which may not be denoted by the title *supreme* in some state systems).
19. In general, these courts are authorized to try civil cases without regard to the amount involved and to try criminal cases regardless of the seriousness of the charge. Although cases in these courts may be tried without juries, it is in these courts that the greatest use of juries is made.
20. The purpose of these courts is to reduce the volume of appeals to the state's highest court. In some classes of cases, the decision of the appellate court will be final, but in important matters appeal may be made to the state's highest tribunal for ultimate determination.
21. For example, if a case is brought in state court between citizens of different states and the amount in dispute exceeds $10,000, on proper motion the case may be removed to the federal court for adjudication (known as a *diversity* case).
22. The method used to select judges varies considerably among the several states, and even within a given state the method employed to select members of different tribunals may vary. Approximately three fourths of the states select most of their judges through popular election, which, arguably, is not the best means of ensuring that the most capable candidate is chosen.
23. For historical background on the evolution of courts of equity in England and the United States, see Friedman, supra note 2, at 21–23, 47–48, 130–131, and 346–347.
24. A development that must also be mentioned is the adoption by several states of the unified state court system, which is patterned after the English system, and which organizes all state courts into branches or divisions of a single, unified plan, thereby permitting specialization by judges but retaining the flexibility necessary to respond to heavy case loads or other problems.
25. For example, in *State Tax Commissioner v. Hopkins*, 234 Ala. 556, 176 So. 210 (1937), Alabama optometrists argued that the services rendered by optometric practitioners should not be subject to the sales tax and that the tax should be levied only upon the materials being dispensed to patients. The lawsuit was in the form of a declaratory judgment seeking relief from the tax.
26. Almost fifty years after the case referred to above, Alabama optometrists brought a case alleging that the tax on ophthalmic materials—which was levied against optometrists but not against ophthalmologists—was discriminatory. The trial court agreed and imposed the tax on both optometrists and ophthalmologists for the value of ophthalmic materials obtained from an ophthalmic supplier. The case was appealed to the Alabama Supreme Court and, in *Alabama Board of Optometry v. Eagerton*, 393 So. 2d 1373 (1981), the court held that optometrists could be exempt from the tax if optometry was recognized by the legislature as a learned profession. (See Chapter 9, note 37, for a further discussion of this case.)
27. A statute that is duly enacted by a state legislature has the force of law unless a state appellate court of competent jurisdiction holds otherwise. (The usual basis for holding that a law is void is unconstitutionality.) An opinion issued by an attorney general may be cited in such a dispute or reviewed by the court in making its decision, but the court is not bound by the attorney general's opinion.
28. The attorney general must be requested to make a ruling as to a specific legal point. For example, in the state of Texas the medical practice act was modified in 1981 to permit optometrists to use diagnostic pharmaceutical agents on the proper delegation of authority by a physician. Shortly after the law was enacted, the state attorney general was asked to render an opinion as to whether or not this provision of the medical practice act was unconstitutional. His ruling was that "the scheme of the statute raises serious questions about the constitutionality of delegating such public powers to private individuals who are neither members of the executive branch of government, nor answerable to the public." Opinion No. MW-499, July 30, 1982. However, a successor attorney general has ruled that, in his opinion, the statute is constitutional. See Opinion JM-454 re: "Clarification of MW-499 (1982) use of topical pharmaceutical agents by optometrists," which states, "On reexamination, we conclude that (the law). . .is not a licensing provision. Instead, it is comparable to other provisions of law whereby physicians may authorize non-physicians to administer certain drugs."
29. An example will illustrate how rulings do not necessarily affect the practitioner of optometry. In the state of Alabama, the legislature modified the optometry practice act in 1975, and the attorney general was subsequently asked to interpret the law as to whether or not, as modified, it permitted the use of diagnostic

pharmaceutical agents. The attorney general's opinion, issued in 1976, was that the law did not permit the use of these agents. Despite this ruling optometrists in the state, believing that the law did in fact permit the use of diagnostic drugs, used them in clinical practice, as did students and faculty at the school of optometry.

The attorney general was asked to reconsider his opinion several months after he had rendered his decision, which resulted in a second opinion that said that the law *did* permit the use of diagnostic agents by optometrists. A third opinion, issued the next year, reversed the attorney general's stance once more. This state of affairs persisted until 1982, when a different attorney general, when asked his opinion of the law (unchanged since 1975), issued a ruling that optometrists could use diagnostic pharmaceutical agents in clinical practice. The use of these drugs by state optometrists has been constant throughout this period. There has been no legal challenge of the statute in the courts. The state board of optometry, by following the opinion of the attorney general, avoids the possibility that individual members of the board could be held responsible if the opinion is not upheld in a legal proceeding before the state's highest court. Thus the opinion is of value to administrative agencies that enforce the law.

30. Apparently, advisory opinions are available in eleven states (Alabama, Colorado, Delaware, Florida, Maine, Massachusetts, Michigan, New Hampshire, North Carolina, Rhode Island, and South Dakota). See Snider, C.F., *American State and Local Government*, 2d ed., Appleton-Century-Crofts, New York, 1965, pp. 305–306.
31. For an excellent reference, see Roalfe, W.R., ed., *How To Find The Law*, 6th ed., West Publish Co., St. Paul, Minn., 1965.
32. Id. at 63–72.
33. Id. at 72–74.
34. Id. at 74–88.
35. There are numerous annotations that pertain to optometry that would be of interest to a researcher. The ALR Quick Index should be consulted for specific topics. Several of these annotations are listed in this text. See the Appendix.
36. See Roalfe, supra note 31, at 89–146.
37. Id. at 147–171.
38. Id. at 171.

Chapter 8

Administrative Regulation

The powers not delegated to the United States by the Constitution, nor prohibited by it to the States, are reserved to the States respectively, or to the people.
—Tenth Amendment, *Constitution of the United States*

Federal Administrative Regulation

The federal constitution does not expressly confer on the U.S. government the responsibility for the regulation of health care.[1] Therefore, under the Tenth Amendment, it is a duty that seemingly would fall to the states, but such has not been the case. Only in the area of licensure have the states been able to retain preeminence. (The unique subject of licensure will be addressed in Chapter 11.) As a result, federal statutes lawfully enacted by the U.S. Congress have exerted significant influence on health care programs, services, and expenditures.[2] The power of the federal government to regulate commerce, provide funds for education and assistance to the needy, assure the quality of food and drugs, and establish programs for the military are but a few of the reasons that the federal government has come to direct health care with increasing regularity over the past few decades.[3] With the enactment of each new law, there has been a necessity for some entity to supervise the administration of the program; this task has fallen on the federal administrative agencies.

In the preceding two chapters, we have reviewed the steps that the Congress (or a state legislature) must go through in order to enact a law. We have seen how judges, federal or state, interpret the meaning of laws and determine their constitutionality. An equally important aspect of the passage of laws is their administration; it is the responsibility of an administrative agency to ensure that a duly enacted law is carried out in the manner that the legislature intended.[4]

The agency is not a law-making body in itself since its function is but to carry out the law within the guidelines of the specific statute and the comments that constitute the congressional record of the law's enactment. But most laws are constructed of rather broad language that requires interpretation or clarification or are written in such a manner as to leave much power in the hands of those who have responsibility for the administration of the program.[5] Not infrequently critics of various federal administrative agencies complain that the agencies have gone beyond the powers delegated to them by Congress and that they have over-complicated the basic issues by generating needlessly complex rulings and regulations. Despite these criticisms, the federal administrative agencies remain an integral part of the federal rulesmaking hierarchy.

One power that is prohibited to the federal government is the licensure of health-care practitioners, a power that is relegated exclusively to the states.[6] Thus, the administrative agency that has the most direct effect on the practice of optometry—the state board—has to be considered separately from the federal agencies and will be discussed in Chapter 10.

The regulatory powers of the various agencies reflect the extensive influence that the federal government has wielded in so many areas of health affairs. After decades of growing federal dominance over the states, however, there has been a trend toward greater authority for the states in administering health-care programs, particularly those funded by federal money.[7] Concomitant with this trend has been another, a liberalization of federal laws so as to afford increased recognition of optometrists as providers or participants in health-care programs.[8] This state of affairs has been brought about in part by political developments and in part through the efforts of organized optometry. It is a trend that is expected to continue.

There is an exhaustive list of federal laws and agencies that affect the profession (see Table 8.1), and so this discussion will be limited to those agencies and programs that exert the most influence on the day-to-day practice of optometry. Among those agencies that must be discussed are the Food and Drug Administration (Department of Health and Human Services), the Social Security Administration (Department of Health and Human Services), the Drug Enforcement Agency (Department of Justice), and the Federal Trade Commission (FTC). The health-related programs regulated by these and other agencies influence virtually every aspect of optometry, including fees for services, standards for ophthalmic products, education and manpower, professional standards, and modes of practice. The following discussion is organized according to the various departments of the federal government that contain agencies regulating some aspect of the practice of optometry. Individual programs within these agencies are briefly described; appropriate sources must be consulted in order to learn the details of any particular federal program.[9]

Department of Defense

The leading Department of Defense program that involves optometric services is the Civilian Health and Medical Program of the Uniformed Services (CHAMPUS).[10] It was established to provide financial assistance for certain types of health care from civilian sources for military retirees, dependents of active duty members of the military, and children of retirees or deceased members. Since 1969, optometrists have been able to provide any covered service that is within the scope of licensure, in most instances without the need for prior referral from a physician. In 1984 CHAMPUS coverage was extended to include

Table 8.1. Federal Agencies and Programs Affecting Optometry

Agency	Program
Department of Defense	Armed Forces Entrance/Vision Consultation Requirement Armed Forces Health Professions Scholarship Program CHAMPUS
Department of Education	Education of Handicapped Act Elementary & Secondary Education Act and Block Grant Follow Through Rehabilitation Act Vocational Education
Department of Health and Human Services	Food and Drug Administration Impact-Resistant Lenses Medical Devices Classification Hydrophilic ("Soft") Contact Lenses Investigational Studies Custom Devices Headstart Health Maintenance Organizations Indian Health Medicaid EPSDT Medicare Migrant Health Centers National Institutes of Health National Institute of Occupational Safety & Health Older Americans Act Primary Care Centers (Hospital Affiliated) Professional Standards Review Organizations Public Health Service Commissioned Corps Social Security Supplemental Security Income
Department of Justice	Drug Enforcement Administration (DEA)
Department of Labor	ERISA Occupational Titles Outlook; Health Careers
Department of Transportation	Federal Aviation Administration Highway Safety Urban Mass Transportation Act
Federal Trade Commission	Price Advertising/Commercial Practice Prescription Release Requirements
Office of Personnel Management	Federal Employees Health Benefits Act (FEHBA)

Table 8.1. *Continued*

Agency	Program
	Standards for Federal Optometrists Workers Compensation (Federal Employees)
Veterans Administration	VA Optometrists VA Optometry Residency Program VA Services by Private Optometrists

Source: *Optometry in Federal Programs*, American Optometric Association, Washington, D.C., 1982.

annual eye examinations for dependents of active duty military personnel.[11] The cost of spectacles, contact lenses, or other optical devices, however, are excluded from coverage unless the materials have to be prescribed for the amelioration of certain specified conditions.[12]

Until 1975, visual or perceptual training was covered under CHAMPUS if it was for the treatment of such physical handicaps as strabismus or amblyopia, but these benefits have been limited to the CHAMPUS program for the handicapped since that date.[13] Generally, diagnosis of handicaps under this program must be made by a physician, although subsequent benefits for the visually handicapped can be furnished by a competent professional such as an optometrist. There are exceptions for children under seven years of age who suffer only from a visual handicap.[14]

Although CHAMPUS is unquestionably oriented towards medical benefits, the program has become more liberal in its policy toward optometry, and political efforts continue to reinstate visual or perceptual training as a covered benefit.

Department of Education

Federally assisted vocational rehabilitation programs were initiated in 1920 and currently are administered through the Department of Education and the provisions of the current law, the Rehabilitation Act of 1973.[15] Title I of this law is concerned with vocational rehabilitation services, and establishes a joint federal-state program under which the states must provide any goods or services necessary to render a handicapped individual employable, which includes eyeglasses and visual services, diagnostic services, and reader services for individuals who are determined to be blind. Optometrists are specified as providers under the act.[16]

Each state must provide for both preliminary and thorough diagnostic studies and for an individualized rehabilitation program; optometrists are eligible for evaluation of visual impairment, but the degree of optometric involvement in vocational rehabilitation often depends on the relationship between local optometrists and the vocational rehabilitation counselors in the state.

Title VII of the law pertains to comprehensive services for independent living, a program designed to extend vocational rehabilitation services to older blind persons and to the severely handicapped. Eyeglasses and other visual aids are included within the provided benefits.[17]

Optometrists who seek to assist in the rehabilitation process must be familiar with the provisions of state law and should be certain that the vocational rehabilitation counselors in their area are familiar with the ability of optometrists to provide low vision services.

Department of Health and Human Services

The Department of Health and Human Services (DHHS) has the greatest responsibility within the federal government for the regulation of health care. The two leading agencies within DHHS that affect the practice of optometry are the Food and Drug Administration (FDA) and the Social Security Administration (SSA). But there are numerous other responsibilities of this department that have significance for optometry, including the Headstart program,[18] health maintenance organizations,[19] financial assistance to optometric students and schools under laws intended to assist health professions education,[20] Indian health,[21] and the National Institutes of Health.[22] This discussion will be limited to the regulatory powers of the FDA and the SSA, but the impact of these other important programs should not be overlooked.

The Food and Drug Administration

The FDA exerts a regulatory influence over three aspects of optometric practice: the classification and approval of medical devices and drugs, the establishment of impact-resistance standards for ophthalmic lenses, and the institution of investigational studies.

Classification of Medical Devices

The basic law that granted the FDA authority to control medical devices was a 1938 Food, Drug, and

Cosmetic Act that was enacted to assure consumers that medical devices were not adulterated or misbranded. In 1976 additional regulatory legislation was passed that extended FDA authority to oversee the safety and effectiveness of medical devices.[23] As defined, a medical device is an instrument, apparatus, implant, or other related bodily article intended to be used in the diagnosis, treatment, or prevention of disease, or intended to affect structures or functions of the body, that does not achieve any of its principal intended purposes through chemical action or the process of metabolism. Thus all devices, regardless of how potentially hazardous they are, will be subject to control.[24] The classification of medical devices and drugs is based on the type of regulation needed to assure the safety and effectiveness of the device or drug (see Table 8.2).

Under this legislation, all soft contact lenses have been transferred from drugs to Class III.[25] PMMA (polymethylmethacrylate) hard contact lenses have been placed in Class II, and gas permeable hard contact lenses have been put in Class III.[26] Ophthalmic lenses for spectacles have been placed in Class II, with impact-resistance the only performance standard recognized (discussed below). Despite efforts to change the FDA classification, all soft lenses remain in Class III and must undergo a rigorous premarket review program prior to being granted FDA approval and being sold in the ophthalmic market.[27]

Table 8.2. U.S. Food and Drug Administration Classification of Ophthalmic Medical Devices: 1976

Classification	Device
Class I—**General Controls**	
General controls are sufficient to provide reasonable assurance of the safety and effectiveness of the device.	None
Class II—**Performance Standards**	
General controls are insufficient and performance standards are necessary. The only performance standard for dress ophthalmic lenses is impact resistance.	PMMA (polymethyl-methacrylate) contact lenses Dress ophthalmic lenses for spectacles
Class III—**Premarket Approval**	
General controls and performance standards are insufficient. The device supports or sustains human life or is of substantial importance in preventing impairment of human health. The device presents a potentially unreasonable risk of illness or injury, and premarket approval is warranted.	All gas permeable contact lenses All soft contact lenses

Source: U.S. Food and Drug Administration, 1976.

Impact-Resistance Standards for Lenses

In 1972 the FDA published regulations that required all eyeglasses and sunglasses to be made of impact-resistant material "except in those cases where the physician or optometrist finds that such lenses will not fulfill the visual requirement of the particular patient, directs in writing the use of other lenses, and gives written notification thereof to the patient."[28] The standards were put into effect during a transition period that ended in 1976, and today all prescription ophthalmic lenses must be capable of withstanding the FDA test for impact resistance, which is known as the drop-ball test.[29] In 1979 the regulations were again amended to permit methods equal or superior to the drop-ball test to be used by the lens manufacturer.[30] No state may adopt or continue to enforce any regulation with respect to ophthalmic lens standards that is different from or more stringent than the FDA requirements without first obtaining the permission of the Commissioner of the agency.[31]

Investigational Studies

The premarket approval needed for soft contact lenses requires that clinical trials be conducted by investigators approved by the FDA, who serve as members of an institutional review committee composed for that purpose.[32] Optometrists may serve as clinical investigators for these studies, which are required for all soft lenses except those that qualify as custom devices.[33]

In terms of legal consequences, the most important application of the FDA's regulatory authority is the promulgation of standards for ophthalmic lenses. These standards have been the subject of much discussion and have been applied in product liability lawsuits (discussed in detail in Chapter 27).

The Social Security Administration

This enormous administrative agency has responsibility for some of the largest government-funded health-care benefit plans in the world. The two programs that have the most significance for optometry are Medicare and Medicaid, but there are a number of other programs coordinated by the SSA that also have applicability for optometrists, including Maternal and Child Health Services,[34] Professional Standards Review Organizations,[35] Federal Old-Age, Survivors and Disability Insurance,[36] and Supplemental Security Income for the Aged, Blind, and Disabled.[37]

The passage of Medicare and Medicaid in 1965 signified a social change of some magnitude in the United States, which had lingered behind most western nations in instituting government-sponsored health care. Both programs offered limited vision benefits, but Medicare restricted optometric services in a fashion that optometrists considered to be discriminatory.[38] It required fifteen years of effort to eliminate some of the discriminatory aspects of the program,[39] and it was not until 1986 that optometrists achieved parity with ophthalmologists under the law.[40]

Medicare

Medicare was enacted in 1965 as Title XVIII of the Social Security Act and was intended to provide certain basic health services for the aged and disabled, including those who were blind.[41] Medicare benefits are divided into two parts:

- Part A provides a basic hospital insurance plan for all persons that are covered by the Social Security retirement program; it is financed through mandatory contributions.
- Part B is a supplemental medical insurance plan covering physicians' services and certain other benefits and is available on a voluntary basis to persons aged 65 or older, without regard to Social Security status, who wish to participate; it is financed through payments by participants and through government appropriations.

Since Part A only concerns hospital and post-hospital benefits, it does not provide payment for optometric services.

Part B provides for physicians' services, limited coverage for services by other providers (including optometrists), additional home health services, outpatient hospital services, and prosthetic devices.

Routine (refractive) vision care is specifically excluded since Medicare benefits are not applicable "where such expenses are for routine physical checkups, eyeglasses or eye examinations for the purpose of prescribing, fitting, or changing eyeglasses, procedures performed (during the course of any examination) to determine the refractive state of the eyes, hearing aids, or examination therefor, or immunization."[42] Thus routine eye examinations are not provided under Medicare. But Part B does allow eye-care benefits related to the diagnosis and treatment of medical conditions. The specific services provided are:

- Eye examinations performed by an optometrist or physician, except that part of the examination related to refraction, if the examination is conducted in relation to a specific patient complaint
- Surgical and related services carried out in connection with the removal of the lens
- Services related to the provision of both temporary and permanent prosthetic lenses, including both the fitting and the dispensing of the lenses themselves

Originally, doctors of optometry could be reimbursed only as suppliers of prosthetic lenses prescribed by ophthalmologists. A study of vision-care benefits conducted in 1968 recommended that no optometrist's services be reimbursible under Medicare unless the program was willing to expand its coverage to include refractive services and eyeglasses.[43] Despite the passage of new legislation in 1972[44] and a favorable report by the Health Resources Administration in 1976,[45] optometric participation remained extremely limited. A lawsuit was initiated, challenging the discriminatory aspects of this policy, but a federal appellate court ruled in 1979 that only the U.S. Congress could determine the reimbursement policies of the program.[46] In 1980, optometric providers were allowed reimbursement for "services related to the condition of aphakia," thereby permitting them to receive compensation under Medicare for both examination and dispensing services. Finally, in 1986, optometrists achieved their most significant federal political victory with the passage of parity legislation.[47] As of 1987, doctors of optometry may provide non-refractive professional services (examinations and follow-up care) for all patients covered by Medicare. Therefore, optometrists may receive reimbursement for medical services that are within the scope of licensure, thereby ending the discriminatory aspects of Medicare.

Medicaid

Medicaid was enacted as Title XIX of the Social Security Act in 1965[48] and was established to aid the states in furnishing health-care services to families on welfare (covered by the Aid to Dependent Children or Supplemental Security Income programs and defined as *categorically eligible*), or to those who otherwise had low incomes (defined as *medically needy*). The objective of Medicaid was to unify the health-assistance programs offered to the poor by the individual states so as to permit basic services to be provided by all. Financial support from the federal government for the program, which is administered by localities (cities or counties) under state guidelines, ranges from 50 to 83 percent, varying in accordance with a formula which allows greater federal contributions to those states with the lowest per capita income.[49]

Medicaid was not a program that found immediate favor with the states; participation was voluntary and there were significant requirements under the federal guidelines. Persons deemed categorically eligible had to be covered by the state program; those termed medically needy could be covered at the state's option.[50] Likewise, benefits were divided into mandatory and optional services. The mandatory services initially required by Medicaid did not include vision care but did provide for periodic screening and diagnosis of eligible persons under 21 years of age, which led to the Early and Periodic Screening, Diagnosis, and Treatment program (EPSDT) and to optometric participation (discussed infra). States were allowed to provide optional services if they so wished, and these included "medical care, or any other type of remedial care, furnished by licensed practitioners within the scope of their practice as defined by state law"[51] (which included optometric services) and "eyeglasses prescribed by a physician skilled in diseases of the eye or by an optometrist, whichever the individual may select."[52] Optometric participation in Medicaid depends on the individual state's decision to include vision services within the scope of optional services offered by the state program. As might be expected, a less-than uniform result has been achieved across the nation.[53] The only optometric services that are mandatory are those required under the EPSDT program.

Early and Periodic Screening, Diagnosis, and Treatment

Federal regulations specify that each state Medicaid agency must provide for *vision testing* and *developmental assessment* among its EPSDT screening services, and require each state to provide treatment for any defects in vision, including eyeglasses, vision therapy, or other necessary care.[54] Thus an optometrist who signs up as an EPSDT provider may offer screening, diagnostic, and treatment services within the scope of his license to Medicaid-eligible persons under the age of 21.[55] Optometrists may also participate in Medicaid for the purpose of determining an individual's eligibility for benefits on account of blindness or visual disability.[56]

Although Medicaid did not generate the outpouring of unhappiness among optometrists that Medicare did, there was frequent commentary about the fee structure of Medicaid, which was criticized as being unfairly low.[57] Even so, optometric utilization by Medicaid programs has been shown to be cost effective and of service to the public.[58] The effect that Medicaid and Medicare have had on optometric fees, freedom-of-choice legislation, and patient populations is discussed elsewhere.[59]

Department of Justice

Current federal regulations that pertain to the distribution and dispensing of central nervous system drugs with a significant potential for abuse are contained in the Comprehensive Drug Abuse Prevention and Control Act of 1970, commonly known as the Controlled Substances Act.[60] Responsibility for the enforcement of this act falls on the Drug Enforcement Administration (DEA), which is an agency of the Department of Justice.

The Controlled Substances Act was designed to regulate the manufacture, distribution, and dispensing of controlled substances by creating a closed system for the legitimate handlers of these drugs.[61] The drugs that come under the jurisdiction of the Act are divided into five schedules, ranging from Schedule I (drugs that have no accepted medical use) to Schedule V (which includes some drugs that can be dispensed without prescription). The distinctions among the five schedules are summarized in Table 8.3.

The DEA requires registration of a physician (defined as any practitioner who is authorized to administer, dispense, or prescribe controlled substances) who wishes to employ any drug that its regulated by the Controlled Substances Act. Optometrists have been defined as physicians for purposes of registration under the act and have been duly registered by the DEA.[62]

In order to register, the optometrist must submit a form to the DEA. The form is processed and, if approved, the optometrist receives a DEA registration number. The registration number must be written on all prescription orders for controlled substances, and there are other requirements that must be complied with as well.[63] Optometrists in several states

Table 8.3. Schedules of Comprehensive Drug Abuse Prevention and Control Act: 1970

Schedule	Description	Example
Schedule I	Drugs that have no accepted medical use in the United States and have high abuse potential	Heroin, marijuana, psilocybin, LSD
Schedule II	Drugs that have a high abuse potential with severe psychic or physical dependence, but have accepted medical use within strict limitations Prescriptions must be written by typewriter, in ink, or with indelible pencil, and must be signed personally by the prescribing practitioner. Prescriptions in this schedule are not refillable.	Opium, codeine, merperidine (Demerol[R]), morphine, amphetamines, phenobarbital, cocaine, oxycodone (Percodan[R])
Schedule III	Drugs with an abuse potential less than those in schedules I and II, and that have accepted medical use. Abuse may lead to low-to-moderate physical dependence or to high psychological dependence. Prescriptions may be oral or written and may be refilled up to five times in six months of issuance if authorized by the prescribing practitioner.	Nonnarcotic drugs, chlorhexadol, nalorphine, paregoric
Schedule IV	Drugs with a lower abuse potential than those in schedule III, and that have medical acceptance. Abuse may lead to limited physical dependence or psychological dependence. Prescriptions may be refilled up to five times in six months of issuance if authorized by the prescribing practitioner, and may be either oral or written.	Chloral hydrate, chlor-diazepoxide (Librium[R]), diazepam (Valium[R]), meprobamate (Equanil[R]), propoxyphene (Darvon[R])
Schedule V	Drugs with a decreased abuse potential relative to schedule IV and containing limited quantities of certain drugs used generally for antitussive and antidiarrheal purposes. Certain drugs in this schedule may be dispensed without prescription if certain specified conditions are met. Prescriptions may be refilled as authorized by the prescribing practitioner.	Robitussin-AC[R], Terpine Hydrate with Codeine[R]

Source: Bartlett, J.D., and J.W. Wood, Optometry and the Drug Enforcement Administration, *Journal of the American Optometric Association*, vol. 52, no. 6, June 1981, p. 495.

have obtained DEA registration, but it should be mentioned that individual state laws must permit the use of controlled substances by optometrists in order for registration to be approved.[64] In those states where permitted, optometrists have used such drugs for diagnosis, analgesia, and other purposes related to treatment. Optometric utilization of controlled substances has been relatively infrequent, but this may change as optometry laws evolve.

Department of Transportation

There are two agencies of the Department of Transportation that have applicability to doctors of optometry, the Federal Aviation Administration (FAA) and the Federal Highway Administration (FHA).

Federal Aviation Administration

Vision requirements for airman certification candidates, air traffic controllers, and others involved in aviation are set by the FAA (Table 8.4).[65] Optometrists are eligible to conduct eye evaluations for these individuals, within the FAA guidelines.[66] But individuals who are being referred for treatment or diagnosis of ocular disease should usually be examined by ophthalmologists.[67] Optometrists should be careful to submit the appropriate form when performing evaluations of airman certification candidates.

Federal Highway Administration

The Highway Safety Act of 1966 established state guidelines for licensing drivers (Table 8.5),[68] and subsequent FHA regulations recognized optometrists for the purpose of examining and certifying commercial drivers, who must undergo physical examination (including eye exams) every two years.[69] Since 1971 commercial drivers have been permitted to wear contact lenses while driving, as long as they have a spare set of lenses with them.[70]

State visual requirements to obtain a license to operate a motor vehicle are a separate matter, and so is the release of information by an optometrist concerning a driver's visual acuity or visual fields. These problems will be discussed in Chapters 16 and 20.

Table 8.4. Vision Standards for Pilots

	Uncorrected Visual Acuity in Each Eye	Corrected Visual Acuity in Each Eye*	Uncorrected or Corrected Near Acuity	Color Vision	Visual Fields	Phorias	Ocular Pathology
First class	20/20	No worse than 20/100 uncorrected, and correctable to 20/20	20/40 (J_3)	Normal	Normal	Not in excess of 1^{Δ} of hyperphoria, 6^{Δ} of exophoria, or 6^{Δ} of esophoria†	No acute or chronic pathological condition of either eye that might interfere with its proper function, might progress to that degree, or might be aggravated by flying
Second class	20/20	No worse than 20/100 uncorrected, and correctable to 20/20	20/40 (J_3)	Able to distinguish aviation signal red, aviation signal green, and white	Normal	Not in excess of 1^{Δ} of hyperphoria, 6^{Δ} of exophoria, or 6^{Δ} of esophoria†	No serious pathology
Third class	20/50	Correctable to 20/30	20/60 (J_6)	Able to distinguish aviation signal red, aviation signal green, and white	None	None	No serious pathology

*Correction may be either by spectacles or contact lenses.
† If phorias exceed these limits, further examination is required to determine if there is bifoveal fixation and an adequate vergence-phoria relationship.

Source: 16 C.F.R. §67.13 et seq.

Federal Trade Commission

The most-discussed administrative agency affecting optometry has been the FTC, which initiated a staff study "into the inadequacy of information disclosure in the retail ophthalmic market" in 1975 and, three years later, published a trade regulation rule that made it an unfair act for a state or local government or any person to prohibit the price advertising of ophthalmic goods and services or for a "refractionist" (optometrist or ophthalmologist) not to give a patient a copy of his prescription for glasses or contact lenses.[71] The rule purported to preempt state statutes restricting the price or availability of ophthalmic goods and services.

This trade regulation rule was challenged in the

Table 8.5. Vision Standards for Interstate Commercial Drivers

Monocular Visual Acuity	Binocular Visual Acuity	Visual Field	Color Vision	Contact Lenses
20/40 (Snellen) distance visual acuity with or without corrective lenses	20/40 (Snellen) distance visual acuity with or without corrective lenses	At least 70 degrees in the horizontal meridian of each eye	Able to recognize the colors of traffic signals and devices showing standard red, green, and amber	Permissible if there is good tolerance to the lenses and the driver has adapted to their use

Source: 49 C.F.R. §391.41(b)(10)

federal courts by the AOA on the day it was published, and the result of this lawsuit was a decision in 1980 that remanded the rule to the FTC for further consideration and suspended the majority of its provisions.[72] The only significant portion of the rule that was left in effect was the prescription requirement[73] (see Chapter 17 for a detailed discussion). Failure to conform to the provisions of the rule is punishable by a fine of up to $10,000 per offense, but there have been no efforts by the FTC to date to enforce the rule.[74]

The effect that the FTC rule—known as Eyeglasses I—has had on the retail ophthalmic market has been uncertain, since there were no prerule studies to determine its potential ramifications.[75] The rule, however, has not created a wholesale abandonment of optometric dispensers by patients, as had been predicted by some; three years after the rule went into effect, estimates were that only 20 percent of optometric patients sought to purchase their ophthalmic materials elsewhere.[76] One effect of the rule seems to have been the escalation of optometric fees for services.[77]

In 1980 the FTC instituted a new study, known as Eyeglasses II,[78] of restrictions upon commercial practice, duplication of lenses by opticians, over-the-counter sale of ready-to-wear reading glasses, and contact lens fittings by opticians. That same year, the FTC released a report comparing the effects of state optometric advertising restrictions on the cost of eye examinations and ophthalmic materials.[79] In 1983 the FTC released another study, which investigated the relative differences between contact lens fittings by optometrists, ophthalmologists, and opticians.[80] Finally, in 1984, the FTC voted to go ahead with a rulemaking proceeding on Eyeglasses II, and after holding hearings in 1986 and 1987, the FTC commissioners voted to implement the rule in 1988.[81] This trade regulation rule challenges "form of practice" restrictions (e.g., employment by corporations, practice location, branch offices, and use of trade names) but not "scope of practice" restrictions (e.g., fitting of contact lenses by opticians and duplication of lenses by opticians).[82] Since the FTC rule is in conflict with state statutes that restrict or prohibit commercial practice, the rule will become the subject of litigation, as the courts are left to determine the extent of the authority granted to the FTC by Congress.

As influential as the federal administrative agencies are, they do not direct one of the most important aspects of professional life—licensure—or mete out discipline for transgressions. These functions are the exclusive domain of the most significant of administrative agencies, the state board. The organization, powers, and duties of the state boards of optometry are described in Chapters 9, 10, and 11.

Notes

1. The growing federal role in health care must be seen as a reflection of social values that are worldwide, not just nationwide. In 1946 the World Health Organization adopted a constitution that addressed the right of citizens to good health, maintaining that: "The enjoyment of the highest attainable standard of health is one of the fundamental rights of every human being, without distinction of race, religion, political belief, economic or social condition." See World Health Organization: Basic Documents, 26th ed., World Health Organization, Geneva, 1976, p. 1. Probably the greatest foe of federal intrusion into health care, the American Medical Association, has begun to appreciate the growing recognition of health as a right of life in the United States, passing a resolution in 1969 that stated, "It is the basic right of every citizen to have available to him adequate health care." Quoted by Chapman, C.B., and J.M. Talmadge, in The Evolution of the Right to Health Concept in the United States, from *Ethics in Medicine*, Reiser, S.J., A.J. Dyck, and W.J. Curran, eds., MIT Press, Cambridge, Mass., 1977, pp. 553–572. This philosophical change has been reflected at the federal level by the passage of significant programs such as Medicare and Medicaid. The growing acceptance of the right of people to health care has met with far from universal acceptance. See Sade, R.M., Medical Care as a Right: A Refutation, *New England Journal of Medicine*, vol. 285, 1971, pp. 1288–1292.
2. For a review of the federal role in health care and its impact on optometry, see Newcomb, R.D., and J.L. Jolley, *Public Health and Community Optometry*, Charles C. Thomas, Springfield, Ill., 1980, pp. 281–314.
3. The evolution of federal concern with the public health and the profusion of laws designed to deal with public health problems are discussed by Friedman, L.M., *A History of American Law*, Simon and Schuster, New York, 1973, pp. 397–405.
4. One illustrative example of an administrative agency's efforts can be found in the Federal Trade Commission's trade regulation rules that purport to eliminate restrictions in the health-care field, 16 C.F.R. §456. The FTC has promulgated these rules under the color of authority granted to the agency by the U.S. Congress (Magnuson-Moss Act, P.L. 93-637). Whether or not Congress intended for the FTC to exercise the degree of power that it has is another issue.
5. For example, the Federal Trade Commission has used the power granted to it by the Congress to make state laws unenforceable. Whether or not the law actually confers this power upon the FTC will doubtless be determined by the courts, which will be called on to

decide the limits of the broad language used to describe the agency's responsibilities and authority.

6. For an interesting analysis of the development of licensure for health care professionals, see Stevens, R., *American Medicine and the Public Interest*, Yale University Press, New Haven, Conn., 1972, pp. 34–74.
7. See *Optometry in Federal Programs*, American Optometric Association, Washington, D.C., 1982, at Preface, in which it is stated, "The following pages reflect two contemporary themes regarding federal programs: greater authority for the states and increased recognition for optometry."
8. For example, after years of effort, in 1981 the U.S. Congress recognized the right of optometrists to receive reimbursement under Medicare for health-related services rendered to Medicare-eligible patients. The basis for the congressional decision to expand optometric involvement in Medicare was, in part, a report released in 1976 by the Department of Health, Education, and Welfare that stated:

    Based primarily on considerations of patient needs, qualifications of optometry to provide services effective in patient management, increased access of Medicare beneficiaries to vision/eye care services, and reasonable cost/administrative dimensions, the Department recommends that those covered services related to aphakia, and within the scope of optometric practice be reimbursable under Part B of Medicare when provided by optometrists.

    From *Report To The Congress Regarding Reimbursement Under Part B Of Medicare For Certain Services Provided By Optometrists*, U.S. Department of Health, Education, and Welfare, Washington, D.C., July 1976.
9. For example see *Optometry in Federal Programs*, American Optometric Association, Washington, D.C., 1982, and supplement. (Available through the AOA office in St. Louis.)
10. 10 U.S.C. §§1079–1088 (1982). See also 32 C.F.R. §§199.1 et seq., 42 Fed. Reg. 17972, Apr. 4, 1977.

    CHAMPUS provides financial assistance for certain health care from civilian sources for retirees, dependents of active duty members, children of retirees and children of deceased members, or retirees of the uniformed services (Military, Coast Guard, and commissioned corps of the U.S. Public Health Service and the National Oceanic and Atmospheric Administration). Typically, benefits are similar to those available to federal civilian employees. The program was created to address the reality that military medical facilities cannot meet all of the health care needs of military dependents. *Optometry in Federal Programs*, AOA, 1982. See also the *AOA News*, Feb. 1, 1979, for a description of optometric participation in CHAMPUS at the time.
11. The decision to expand benefits under CHAMPUS to include annual eye examinations for dependents was reported in the *AOA News*, October 15, 1984. The plan, which went into effect October 1, 1984, was a response to the recognized need of military dependents to receive eye care from civilian providers.
12. Although CHAMPUS generally forbids the prescribing of eyeglasses, spectacles, contact lenses, or other optical devices, there are a number of specified eye conditions and circumstances under Basic Program regulations (32 C.F.R. §199.10(e)(6)) where an optometrist may examine for and prescribe optical devices:
    (1) Eyeglasses or contact lenses that perform the function of the human lens, lost as the result of intraocular surgery or ocular injury
    (2) "Pinhole" glasses prescribed for use after surgery for detached retina
    (3) Lenses prescribed as treatment in lieu of surgery for the following conditions
        (a) contact lenses used for treatment of infantile glaucoma
        (b) corneal or scleral lenses prescribed in connection with treatment of keratoconus
        (c) scleral lenses prescribed to retain moisture in cases where normal tearing is not present or is inadequate
        (d) corneal or scleral lenses prescribed to reduce a corneal irregularity other than astigmatism

    See *Optometry in Federal Programs*, AOA, St. Louis, 1982.
13. *Program for the Handicapped* benefits consist of financial assistance for active duty uniformed services personnel whose spouses or children may be moderately or severely mentally retarded or seriously physically handicapped and in need of specialized institutional care, training, or rehabilitation and the required services are not available from public institutions or agencies. Thus, other programs (such as Education of the Handicapped or Crippled Children's Services) must be used before this program may apply.

    Diagnosis of the handicap must be made by a physician, although subsequent benefits may be furnished by a competent professional such as an optometrist. Under 1978 guidelines, however, if the patient is under age seven and the only problem is a visual one, the diagnosis may be made by an optometrist.

    Coverage for the partially sighted (the term visual impairment is used) is described in detail as follows (32 C.F.R. §§199.11(e)(2)(i)(a)–199.11(e)(2)(i)(f); 32 C.F.R. §199.11(e)(2)(ii)): A vision impairment will be considered serious in persons seven years of age and older if any of the following conditions occur:
    - the remaining vision in the better eye after best correction is 20/200 or less
    - the contraction of visual fields is to 10 degrees or less from the point of fixation
    - the widest diameter subtends an angle no greater than 20 degrees
    - the visual efficiency of the better eye after best correction is 20 percent or less
    - other conditions impairing visual function such as complete homonymous hemianopsia, or total bilaterial ophthalmoplegia have reached the point where the individual requires assistance to

support the essentials of daily living

See *Optometry in Federal Programs*, AOA, St. Louis, 1982.

14. A visual impairment in children under six years of age will be considered serious (even if correctable with lenses) in those cases where the visual impairment is manifested by 20/60 vision or less.

    Services covered include:

    (1) optometric professional services
    (2) certain special optical devices necessary to ameliorate the handicapping condition, limited to the following (32 C.F.R. §199.11(2)(vii)):
        (a) contact lenses necessary to correct a visual handicap that qualifies
        (b) subnormal vision corrective devices such as telescopic and isoiconic lenses
        (c) optical aids such as handheld optical devices for reading
    (3) vision therapy needed to alleviate, overcome, or adjust to a serious physical handicap, provided it is included as a part of the approved management plan

    See *Optometry in Federal Programs*, AOA, St. Louis, 1982.

15. 29 U.S.C. §§701 et seq. See also 34 C.F.R. et seq.; 34 C.F.R. §365; 34 C.F.R. §366; and 34 C.F.R. §395.1(c).

    Federally assisted vocational rehabilitation programs began in 1920. P.L. 90-391, the Vocational Rehabilitation Amendments of 1968, broadened the scope of services to include "eyeglasses and visual services as prescribed by a physician skilled in the diseases of the eye or by an optometrist." The accompanying House Report No. 90-1346 took "cognizance of the fact that optometrists can and do contribute a valuable service to the visually impaired" and urged state utilization of optometrists' services. Senate Report No. 90-139 defined visual services as including "visual training and services essential to the examination, prescription, and provision of contact lenses, telescopic lenses, and other special visual aids." The Vocational Rehabilitation Act was repealed and replaced by P.L. 93-112, the Rehabilitation Act of 1973. (29 U.S.C. §701 et seq.) See *Optometry in Federal Programs*, AOA, St. Louis, 1982.

16. This is a federal-state program under which each state plan must cover "any goods or services necessary to render a handicapped individual employable, including, but not limited to...eyeglasses and visual services as prescribed by a physician skilled in the diseases of the eye or by an optometrist, whichever the individual may select." Also covered are diagnostic services as well as reader services for individuals determined to be blind by an optometrist. Regulations (34 C.F.R. §361.1) define visual services as "visual training, and the examination and services necessary for the prescription and provision of eyeglasses, contact lenses, microscopic lenses, telescopic lenses, and other special visual aids as prescribed by a physician skilled in diseases of the eye, or by an optometrist, whichever the individual may select." See *Optometry in Federal Programs*, AOA, St. Louis, 1982.

17. Vocational rehabilitation services are available to persons "whose disabilities are so severe that they do not presently have the potential for employment but may benefit from vocational rehabilitation services which will enable them to live and function independently" (29 U.S.C. §§796(a)–796(d)). Federal grants are available to assist states, with each state drafting a plan for "providing comprehensive services for independent living to severely handicapped individuals."

    Grants are authorized to the states to provide independent living services to older blind individuals (29 U.S.C. §796(f)). Such services are to be designed by each state to "assist an older blind individual to adjust to his blindness by becoming more able to care for his individual needs," e.g.:

    (1) Services to help correct blindness such as (A) outreach services, (B) visual screening, (C) surgical or therapeutic treatment to prevent, correct, or modify disabling eye conditions, and, (D) hospitalization related to such services
    (2) The provision of eyeglasses and other visual aids

    Eligibility extends to individuals age 55 or older whose "severe visual impairment makes gainful employment extremely difficult to obtain but for whom independent living goals are feasible." See *Optometry in Federal Programs*, AOA, St. Louis, 1982.

18. 42 U.S.C. §2928. See also 45 C.F.R. §§1301–1305.8.

    This program aims to provide such comprehensive health, nutritional, educational, social, and other services as will aid low-income (primarily) preschool children in attaining their full potential. DHHS—subject to review by the states—approves and funds individual Headstart agencies in communities. One of the roles of a Headstart project is to meet certain health goals: to improve a child's present function by finding and remedying present defects; and to ensure a child's future health by providing preventive services, improving the health of all members of the child's family, and improving the health of the community in which the child lives. Among the priorities for care are conditions that may be progressive if untreated (such as strabismus) or that interfere with classroom function and require corrective treatment (such as partial sight).

    Headstart arranges for needed health services, using community resources (such as private practitioners, group practices, health centers, local health departments) and government programs (e.g., Medicaid and Crippled Children's Services) whenever possible. Optometric participation depends on the services and providers included by each individual Headstart agency. See *Optometry in Federal Programs*, AOA, St. Louis, 1982.

19. 42 U.S.C. §§300(e) et seq. See also 42 C.F.R. §§110.101 et seq.

    A qualified HMO provides a system for delivering a

broad scope of specified comprehensive, preventive health care services to its members for a fixed, negotiated fee. A federally qualified HMO may deliver services either directly or by contracting through its own staff, medical group, or individual practice association. A medical group is defined (42 U.S.C. §300(e)−1(4)) as a partnership, association, corporation or other entity which is composed of medical doctors, osteopaths, and "such other licensed health professionals" (including dentists, optometrists and podiatrists) as are necessary for the provision of health services for which the group is responsible; a majority of the members must be medical doctors or osteopaths, and the members must be in a true group setting. An individual practice association is defined (42 U.S.C. §300e−1(5)) as a partnership, corporation, association, or other entity that has arranged for the delivery of health services by health professionals (as defined above), a majority of whom are medical doctors or osteopaths.

The law mandates such services as physician services, periodic health evaluations for adults, and "preventive health services (including. . . children's eye. . . examinations conducted to determine the need for vision. . . correction)" (42 U.S.C. §300(e)−1). Any other vision care may be provided as a supplemental service (42 U.S.C. §300(e)−1). See *Optometry in Federal Programs*, AOA, St. Louis, 1982.

20. The nature and availability of federal assistance to students and schools of optometry has undergone significant change over the past few years. See *Optometry in Federal Programs*, AOA, St. Louis, 1982, for a comprehensive discussion.
21. 25 U.S.C. §450; and 25 U.S.C. §1651.

The Health Service Administration of the Public Health Service (PHS), Department of Health and Human Services (DHHS), is a basic arm of the U.S. government concerned with the delivery of quality health care. The Indian Health Service (IHS), as a major health component of PHS, is the main instrument through which the government discharges its responsibilities to native Americans.

A comprehensive range of optometric services is provided by the PHS Commissioned Corps officers, civil service personnel employed by DHHS, and private contracting individuals.

While a detailed description of the structure of vision-care delivery systems is beyond the scope of this text, it can be noted that the delivery of vision care to native Americans is accomplished through federally employed optometrists as well as civilian optometrists who contract with the IHS for vision-care services. The AOA's Washington Office has a descriptive manual entitled "Indian Vision Care," which will benefit any interested individual who is in need of a guide to contracting for vision care services relative to the Indian Health Service. See *Optometry in Federal Programs*, AOA, St. Louis, 1982.

22. NIH institutes support 60 percent of biomedical research in this country. Optometrists are participating in several of the institutes' programs. See *Optometry in Federal Programs*, AOA, St. Louis, 1982.
23. 21 U.S.C. §§351–360(k). See also 21 C.F.R. §§800–895. For a discussion of the law's enactment, see the *AOA News*, June 1, 1976.
24. Except where specifically permitted by the Commissioner of Food and Drugs upon application by a state, no state may establish or continue in effect with respect to a medical device any requirement that is different from, or in addition to, any federal requirement applicable to the device, and that relates to the safety or effectiveness of the device or to any other matter included in federal requirements that are applicable to the device.
25. At the time the U.S. Congress was considering the Medical Devices Act, a lawsuit was filed in Colorado by an ophthalmologist, alleging that soft contact lenses were "drugs" and that they could not be fitted by optometrists because the state law prohibited the use of "drugs" by optometrists. The case, which ultimately was appealed (and thereby established a precedent), was resolved in favor of optometry, with the court ruling that contact lenses were not "drugs" within the meaning of the statutory proscription. See *Winograd v. Johnson*, 561 P.2d 1274 (Colo. App. 1976). The classification of soft contact lenses as Class III by the FDA has made the question raised by the *Winograd* case moot. For a discussion of the FDA classification, see Smith, L.S., FDA Regulations Regarding Soft Contact Lenses, *International Contact Lens Clinic*, vol. 7, no. 2, Mar./Apr. 1980, pp. 45–55.
26. The Class II category includes *only* contact lenses made of PMMA. Gas permeable lens materials still remain in Class III and thus are subject to the tedious (and expensive) ritual of premarket testing.
27. In 1982 the FDA proposed a rule that would reclassify gas permeable daily wear hard contact lens materials from Class III to Class I, thus obviating the need for expensive premarket trials. In 1984, however, the FDA withdrew the proposed rule, a move that was viewed in some quarters as a victory for large contact lens manufacturers, who could afford the timely and expensive premarket approval procedures of Class III. Another result of the continuation of Class III restrictions has been the developing inability of the FDA to deal with the glut of contact lens new device applications in a timely manner. For commentary on the problem, see Guerrein, R.L., Editorial, *Review of Optometry*, vol. 121, no. 11, p. 15, and the accompanying article, Paperwork Jam Hinders FDA, at p. 3.
28. 21 C.F.R. §3.84. For optometric commentary, see Editorial, The New FDA Regulation on Impact-Resistant Lenses, *Optometric Journal and Review of Optometry*, vol. 108, no. 12, June 15, 1971; Editorial, Impact-Resistant Lenses—An Important Step for the Consumer, *Optical Journal and Review of Optometry*, vol. 109, no. 1, Jan. 1, 1972; and Editorial, The FDA Regulation on Impact-Resistant Lenses, *Optical Journal*

and Review of Optometry, vol. 109, no. 7, Apr. 1, 1972.

29. 21 C.F.R. §801.410. See also 41 F.R. 6896, Feb. 13, 1976.
30. 21 C.F.R. §801.410. See also 44 F.R. 20678, Apr. 6, 1979.
31. Although the FDA requirements are the applicable law, an interesting situation has resulted in California, where the state has enacted a statute that requires fabricators of ophthalmic lens prescriptions to meet the American National Standards Institute (ANSI) Z-80-1972 standards, which are more stringent than those approved by the FDA. Although California applied for an exemption from the FDA rule, it was denied by the agency. However, the FDA seemingly is without resources to enforce its ruling. An FDA Bureau of Devices representative is quoted as commenting, "There's really nothing the FDA can do about it. We can write them a letter, but that's about all." See the *AOA News*, March 15, 1981. A challenge to the law would have to come from a state optical laboratory, but to this date apparently none has been forthcoming and so the law remains in effect.
32. 21 C.F.R. §§813 et seq. and 21 C.F.R. §56.107.
33. 21 U.S.C. §360j(b). Federal performance standards and premarket approval requirements do not apply to: "any device which, in order to comply with the order of an individual physician or dentist (or any other specially qualified person designated under regulations...), necessarily deviates from an otherwise applicable performance standard or requirement"; if the device is not generally available in finished form for purchase or for dispensing; if the device is made in a specific form for an individual patient; and if the device is not generally available to or generally used by other health professionals. To date, the FDA has not expanded this custom device exemption to include optometrists, although the AOA has so recommended. See *Optometry in Federal Programs*, AOA, St. Louis, 1982.
34. Title V of the Social Security Act, 42 U.S.C. §§701 et seq. See also 45 C.F.R. §96.
35. Title XI of the Social Security Act, 42 U.S.C. §§1320(c) et seq.
36. Title II of the Social Security Act, 42 U.S.C. §§401 et seq. See also 20 C.F.R. §§404 et seq. Enacted in 1935, this is the familiar system of monthly cash payments to the aging, their survivors, and the disabled.

    A person who is age 55 or over and is blind and therefore is substantially limited in work, or a person who is unable to engage in any substantial gainful activity by reason of any medically determinable physical impairment which is relatively permanent, may be eligible. DHHS is to determine the "medical and other evidence" required to establish the disability (42 U.S.C. §423(d)(5)). Blindness is defined as "central visual acuity of 20/200 or less in the better eye with the use of a correcting lens." An eye "accompanied by a limitation in the field of vision such that the widest diameter of the visual field subtends an angle no greater than 20 degrees shall be considered for purposes of this paragraph as having a central visual acuity of 20/200 or less," 42 U.S.C. §416(i)(1)). There was no statutory freedom of choice between eye physician or optometrist under Title II for the determination of blindness as found under Titles X, XVI, and XIX.

    On August 20, 1968, regulations were adopted (20 C.F.R. §404.1524(c)) to permit the use of an optometrist's measurement of visual acuity and visual fields as medical evidence in cases involving visual impairments. Under revised regulations published on Aug. 20, 1980, "Acceptable medical sources are...(4) Licensed optometrists for the measurement of visual acuity and visual fields (we may need a report from a physician to determine other aspects of eye diseases)" (20 C.F.R. §404.1513).

    Appendix 1 of the 1980 regulations (Appendix 1 of Subpart P of 20 C.F.R. §404) also describes the various impairments, including blindness and other visual impairments, that may qualify a person for eligibility. They include such conditions as loss of central or peripheral vision, impaired bilateral muscle function, loss of visual efficiency, aphakia, or statutory blindness, and impairment of central visual acuity or absence of accommodative reflex in children under age 18. The criteria for making determinations of disability under Title II are also used under Title XVI (Supplemental Security Income). See *Optometry in Federal Programs*, AOA, St. Louis, 1982.
37. Title XVI of the Social Security Act, 42 U.S.C. §§1202, 1382(c)–1382(i)). See 20 C.F.R. §416.903 (c); 20 C.F.R. §§416.913(a)(4), 416.913(f), 416.981; and 20 C.F.R. Appendix 1 of Subpart P of §404.
38. The difficulty faced by optometrists was that patients sent to ophthalmologists for cataract surgery could be managed after surgery by the ophthalmologist, including the dispensing of ophthalmic materials, thus preventing the optometrist's participation in patient care altogether. The situation was described by AOA General Counsel Harold Kohn as follows: "As a result of our conference, we arrived at the understanding that when, after surgery, *a patient is referred to an optometrist*, and the optometrist provides the patient with the prosthetic lenses, payment can be made to him for the lenses, including payment for his services in making the refraction" (emphasis added). Kohn also delicately observed that, "It was recognized that there are practical considerations involved with respect to the matter of referrals. This primarily is the relationship between the ophthalmologist and the optometrist. If the ophthalmologist retains the patient, this is a matter in which the administration (Social Security Administration) definitely stated it cannot become involved." *Bulletin from the General Counsel*, vol. 25, no. 34, Oct. 10, 1966.
39. The necessity for amending Medicare was recognized immediately. See Editorial, A Vital Amendment To Medicare Is Recommended, *Optometric Weekly*,

vol. 58, no. 2, Jan. 19, 1967, pp. 33–34. The AOA's efforts were vigorously opposed by ophthalmology and organized medicine. See Optometry Inclusion in Title 18 Opposed, *AMA News*, May 15, 1967; and HEW Report and Optometry and Medicare, *Eye Physician*, Feb. 1969, pp. 17–19. The right of optometrists to receive reimbursement for health-related services rendered to eligible Medicare recipients was not achieved until 1981. The basis for the congressional decision to permit reimbursement of optometrists for eye health services rendered to aphakic patients was due, in part, to a HEW report released in 1976 that recommended the expansion of Medicare to include these services. A lawsuit was filed by the Physician's Education Newwork to have the report rescinded, but the suit was dismissed by the district court and the dismissal was upheld in the U.S. Court of Appeals. See the *AOA News* of June 1, 1980, and May 15, 1981.

40. In 1986 a bill was passed in the U.S. Congress to allow optometrists to be reimbursed for services rendered to nonaphakic Medicare recipients. Under the prior law, physicians were eligible for reimbursement for vision services provided to nonaphakic patients (except for routine examinations and refractive services). Thus patients were effectively denied economic freedom of choice in their selection of eye-care provider because reimbursement could be obtained if a physician was consulted but not if an optometrist was chosen. See the *AOA News*, June 1, 1983. An account of the argument in favor of optometric reimbursement can be found in the *AOA News*, Feb. 1, 1984.
41. 42 U.S.C. §§1395(x), 1395(y), and 1395(ll). See also 42 C.F.R. §405.232c. For background information on Medicare, see Newcomb and Jolley, supra note 2, at 258–262.
42. See 42 U.S.C. §1862(7).
43. This study, popularly known as the Cohen Report, was released in 1968 as the Independent Practitioners Study. The section on optometry was written by four M.D.s, two of them ophthalmologists, and concluded that no eye examination services by optometrists should be reimbursable unless Medicare wished to expand its coverage to include refractive services and eyeglasses.
44. In 1972, P.L. 92-603 included a clause that was designed to reimburse optometrists for examining aphakic patients. It defined doctors of optometry as physicians for the purpose of attesting to the need for prosthetic lenses. The accompanying committee report language (H.R. No. 92-231, May 26, 1971; S. No. 92-1230, Sept. 26, 1972; H. Conf. Rep. No. 92-1605, Oct. 14, 1972) effectively negated this expectation, interpreting the statutory language as only intending to recognize the optometrists' prescription of aphakic lenses as valid. See *Optometry in Federal Programs*, AOA, St. Louis, 1982.
45. In 1975, P.L. 94-182 mandated a new DHEW study of optometry, which was to be done by the Health Resources Administration using a balanced panel of experts. The study, entitled, Report to Congress: Reimbursement Under Part B of Medicare for Certain Services Provided by Optometrists, was released in June 1976. While recommending that the only change that should be made at that time was reimbursement of covered services related to aphakia, the report spoke highly of the qualifications of optometrists in providing a broad range of services beyond refraction and the provision of eyeglasses. See *Optometry in Federal Programs*, AOA, St. Louis, 1982.
46. A federal appellate court decision (*Pushkin v. Califano*, 600 F.2d 486 (1979)) effectively stated that the Congress may make "reimbursement distinctions between the diagnostic services provided by a medical doctor and those provided by an optometrist." Its impact was to confirm that any remediation of Medicare's discriminatory reimbursement policies must come from the Congress rather than from the courts or administrative regulations.
47. In 1980 the Congress broadened reimbursement of optometric aphakic services as a part of P.L. 96-499. The language expanded the definition of doctor of optometry as physician to "services related to the condition of aphakia," thus permitting reimbursement for professional as well as dispensing services (42 U.S.C. §1395x(r)(4); 42 U.S.C. §1395x(s)(8)). (See House Rep. No. 96-1167, July 21, 1980, and House Conf. Rep. No. 96-1479, Nov. 26, 1980.) In 1986 the Congress again modified the Medicare law to permit optometrists to receive reimbursement for services within the scope of licensure that were rendered to Medicare eligible patients, whether phakic or aphakic. Amendment to SSA Section 1861(r) of 42 U.S.C. §1395(r). See Garland, N., Optometry Parity Legislation Under Medicare, *Journal of the American Optometric Association*, vol. 58, no. 6, June 1987, pp. 518–519.
48. 42 U.S.C. §§1396 et seq., and 42 U.S.C. §1315. See also 42 C.F.R. §§430–456.
49. See Newcomb and Jolley, supra note 2, at 262–265.
50. 42 U.S.C. §§1396a(a)(10)(A) holds that the following services are among those that a state Medicaid plan must provide under SAA Section 1905(a) (42 U.S.C. §§1396d(a)(1)–1396d(a)(5), and 1396d(a)(17)):
    - Skilled nursing facility services (for persons 21 years or older), or "such early and periodic screening and diagnosis of individuals who are eligible under the plan and are under the age of 21 to ascertain their physical or mental defects, and such health care, treatment, and other measures to correct or ameliorate defects and chronic conditions discovered thereby, as may be provided in regulations of the Secretary," and family planning services and supplies
    - Physician services (defined as doctor of medicine or osteopathy)

    A state may also provide, among others, the following optional services from the list contained in 42 U.S.C. §§1396d(6) and 1396d(12):
    - Medical care, or any other type of remedial care, furnished by licensed practitioners within the scope of their practice as defined by state law

(this is where optometric services are covered)
- Eyeglasses prescribed by a physician skilled in diseases of the eye or by an optometrist, whichever the individual may select

See *Optometry in Federal Programs*, AOA, St. Louis, 1982.

51. Ibid.
52. Ibid.
53. A survey conducted by the American Optometric Association in 1982 of Medicaid use of optometric skills revealed that forty states covered adult optometric services, at least twenty-six states provided reimbursement for vision therapy under the EPSDT program, and that the vast majority of eye examinations conducted under the Medicaid program (estimated at 75 percent) are provided by doctors of optometry. *Bulletin from the Federal Health Programs Implementation Committee of the State Legislative Affairs Advisory Committee*, vol. 41, no. 6, Sept. 7, 1982.
54. 42 C.F.R. §441.56.
55. DHHS's Medical Services Administration *Medical Assistance Manual* (Sections 5-70-20) contains several statements that mention optometry's role in EPSDT:
    - Treatment means...optometrist's services,... eyeglasses...rehabilitative services, and any other type of medical care and services recognized under state law, to prevent, correct or ameliorate disease or abnormalities detected by screening and diagnostic procedures
    - Although screening should be performed under the supervision of a physician, dentist, optometrist, audiologist or other health care specialist, or with consultation from such persons.... Nurses, trained health aids, laboratory technicians and trained volunteers can conduct the screening activity
    - Other participants to provide screening services may be found among...optometric schools
    - Vision Testing. Administer a vision screening test appropriate to the child's age. Consultation by ophthalmologists and optometrists can be of help in determining the type of tests to be used and the criteria for determining when a child should be referred for diagnostic examination

    See *Optometry in Federal Programs*, AOA, St. Louis, 1982.
56. In determining blindness under the state's definition, a physician skilled in the diseases of the eye or an optometrist, whichever the individual selects, must examine the applicant, unless both of his or her eyes are missing (42 U.S.C. §1396a(a)(12); see also 42 C.F.R. §435.531). Under this regulation "a physician skilled in the diseases of the eye (for example, an ophthalmologist or an eye, ear, nose, and throat specialist) must review the report and determine on behalf of the (state Medicaid) agency...whether and when reexaminations are necessary for periodic redeterminations for eligibility." See *Optometry in Federal Programs*, AOA, St. Louis, 1982.
57. One interesting development concerning reimbursement of optometrists under Medicaid occurred in the state of Louisiana, where optometrists challenged the provisions of the state medical assistance plan (Medicaid), which allowed reimbursement to ophthalmologists for eye care services that were within the scope of optometry but denied reimbursement to optometrists for these same services. The lawsuit, *Sandefur v. Cherry*, 744 F.2d 1157 (5th Cir. 1984) was brought in the federal courts and had a tortuous history (see Chapter 11) but ultimately resulted in a ruling by the Fifth Circuit Court of Appeals that the Louisiana law be amended "so as to provide that optometrists who perform eye care services that are within the scope of optometric practice will receive Medicaid reimbursement to the same extent, and according to the same standards, as physicians who perform those same eye care services." The case is reviewed in the *AOA News*, Jan. 1, 1985.
58. See Rosenthal, J., J.R. Posner, and W.C. Folsom, Optometric Prescribing Patterns: A Quality Comparison of Medicaid and Non-Medicaid Practitioners, *Medical Care*, vol. 13, no. 6, June 1975, pp. 499–510.
59. It must be mentioned that, as of 1982, freedom of choice for Medicaid recipients seems to be on its way out. In several states application has been made to the Health Care Financing Administration to grant waivers so that Medicaid patients can be funneled to prepaid plans or "case managers" (physicians or HMOs), an effort that is designed to reduce Medicaid costs. As a result, Medicaid recipients will lose the right to choose the doctor they want. Reported in *Medical World News*, Sept. 1, 1982.
60. For a brief history of drug regulation in the United States and the emerging place of optometry in the regulatory scheme, see Bartlett, J.D., and J.W. Wood, Optometry and the Drug Enforcement Administration, *Journal of the American Optometric Association*, vol. 52, no. 6, June, 1981, pp. 495–498.
61. See *Physician's Manual: An Informational Outline of the Controlled Substances Act of 1970*, Washington, D.C., U.S. Department of Justice, Apr. 1978.
62. For example, in Alabama the state optometry practice act was modified in 1975, with optometrists maintaining that the amendment permitted the use of diagnostic pharmaceutical agents, despite a negative attorney general's opinion on this point. When a different attorney general held that the law permitted the use of these drugs by optometrists, the state board of optometry ruled that all licensed optometrists were eligible to use them. One state optometrist thereafter applied to the DEA for a registration number, and although a dispute ensued between the optometrist, the state board of optometry, and the DEA over the issuance of the number (which permitted the optometrist to employ cocaine for diagnostic purposes), the registration number ultimately was issued to the practitioner. *In the Matter of Thomas Jefferson R. Hicks, O.D.*, U.S. Department of Justice, Drug Enforcement Administration, Docket 82–4, 1982.
63. See Bartlett and Wood, Optometry and the Drug

Enforcement Administration, supra note 60, at 496–497.

64. Ibid.
65. 14 C.F.R. §§67.13, 67.15, 67.17. See also DeHaan, W.V., *The Optometrist's and Ophthalmologist's Guide to Pilot's Vision*, American Trend Publishing Co., Boulder, Colo., 1982.
66. As early as 1961, it has been the policy of the Federal Aviation Administration (FAA) not to refer patients of optometrists to ophthalmologists for evaluation except where there is suspected eye disease. In fact, the Office of the Federal Air Surgeon has, on several occasions, gone on record to announce that candidates for airman medical certification may have eye evaluations performed by an "eye specialist". The FAA has gone on record in 1963, 1965, and 1966 as defining "eye specialist" to mean either an optometrist or an ophthalmologist. See *Optometry in Federal Programs*, AOA, St. Louis, 1982.
67. The FAA recognizes only two forms for the eye evaluation of airman certification candidates: FAA Form 8500-7 and FAA Form 8500-14. Form 8500-7 is to be used for evaluating all airman candidates' eyes when there is no presence of suspected eye disease or previous surgical condition. When FAA patients are suspected of having eye disease or are being treated for an eye disease or previous surgical condition, FAA Form 8500-14 is used and must be signed by an ophthalmologist.
68. 23 U.S.C. §§401–404.
69. 49 C.F.R. §§386–398. P.L. 89-564, the Highway Safety Act of 1966, established guidelines for the states regarding driver licensing.

    Initial Federal Highway Administration regulations (1967 and 1968) permitted an optometrist's examination and certification to be made for "visual acuity, field of vision, and ability to distinguish colors" as part of the "physical examination" of commercial drivers (49 C.F.R. §391.43). Specific visual requirements may be found at 49 C.F.R. §391.41(b)(10). See *Optometry in Federal Programs*, AOA, St. Louis, 1982.
70. In April 1970 and 1971, the FHA added requirements that commercial drivers must undergo a physical examination (and thus an eye exam), every two years (49 C.F.R. §391.45) and that such drivers who must wear corrective lenses in order to meet minimum standards of visual acuity must wear spectacles (and not contact lenses) while they are driving. The contact lens ban (49 C.F.R. §392.9(a)) was rescinded in 1971, due to the recommendation of the AOA and others, and was replaced with language stating that "if the driver wears contact lenses while driving he must have a spare lens or set of lenses on his person while he drives."
71. 15 U.S.C. §57a. The pertinent regulation for Eyeglasses I is 16 C.F.R. §456 (43 F.R. 23992, June 2, 1978).
72. *American Optometric Association v. Federal Trade Commission*, 626 F.2d 896 (D.C. Cir. 1980).
73. Remaining in effect is 16 C.F.R. §456.7, Separation of Examination and Dispensing:

    In connection with the performance of eye examinations, it is an unfair act or practice for a refractionist to:

    (a) Fail to give to the buyer a copy of the buyer's prescription immediately after the eye examination is completed. Provided: A refractionist may refuse to give the buyer a copy of a buyer's prescription until the buyer has paid for the eye examination but only if that refractionist would have required immediate payment from that buyer had the examination revealed that no ophthalmic goods were required;

    (b) Condition the availability of an eye examination to any person on a requirement that that person agree to purchase any ophthalmic goods from the refractionist;

    (c) Charge the buyer any fee in addition to the refractionist's examination fee as a condition to releasing the prescription to the buyer. Provided: A refractionist may charge an additional fee for verifying ophthalmic goods dispensed by another seller when the additional fee is imposed at the time the verification is performed; or

    (d) Place on the prescription, or require the buyer to sign, or deliver to the buyer a form or notice waiving or disclaiming the liability or responsibility of the refractionist for the accuracy of the eye examination or the accuracy of the ophthalmic goods or services dispensed by another seller.
74. There are no reported cases to date of any refractionist being prosecuted for failure to adhere to the rule.
75. See Unclear Victory, *Review of Optometry*, vol. 119, no. 7, July 1982, p. 3.
76. Ibid.
77. See Swallowing the FTC's Bitter Pill, *Review of Optometry*, vol. 115, no. 12, Dec. 15, 1978, pp. 41–45.
78. The proposal for Eyeglasses II can be found at 16 C.F.R. §456 (45 F.R. 79823, Dec. 2, 1980). For a summary of the major provisions of the rule, see Gerber, P., Eyeglasses II: FTC's Latest Probe, *Optometric Management*, vol. 15, no. 10, Oct. 1979, pp. 31–37.
79. *Effects of Restrictions on Advertising and Commercial Practice in the Professions: The Case of Optometry*, FTC, Washington, D.C., May 15, 1980. For a review of the report's major findings, see the *AOA News*, June 1, 1980.
80. *A Comparative Analysis of Cosmetic Contact Lens Fitting by Ophthalmologists, Optometrists, and Opticians*, FTC, Washington, D.C., Dec. 15, 1983.
81. 16 C.F.R. §456. The details of the proposed rule are described in the *AOA News*, Jan. 15, 1985.
82. An analysis of the effects of the proposed rule can be found in Cohn, S., Eyeglasses II: Commercial Optometry Set Free, *Optometric Management*, vol. 21, no. 3, Mar. 1985, pp. 31–35.

PART FOUR

PROFESSIONAL REGULATION

Chapter 9

The Optometry Practice Acts

The bill was originally so formed as to logically regulate the practice of optometry by whomsoever practiced, so that interested physicians, as well as opticians, would in the future be obliged to prove their competency, to adopt glasses to the eyes, before the Regents of the State.
—Charles F. Prentice, *Legalized Optometry and Memoirs*

Legalized Optometry

Had the bill to regulate the practice of optometry proposed by Charles Prentice been enacted into law by the New York State Assembly in 1896, the history of optometry would have been far different than that described in Chapter 1, for Prentice proposed to regulate all persons who practiced optometry, irrespective of their training (either as opticians or physicians). It is even conceivable that the "idealized eye specialist" envisioned by Prentice would exist today, rather than the three separate eye-care professions that have evolved independently. But the New York bill failed to pass, and with its defeat ended the one board concept, never again to be revived.[1]

But the idea of legalizing optometry was able to germinate, eventually reaching full flower five years later (1901) in Minnesota, where the legislature passed a statute that was to be emulated by every state in the nation. The Minnesota[2] optometry practice act contained five basic provisions that have been the cornerstone of legal regulation of the profession:

- A definition of the practice of optometry
- The creation of a board authorized to carry out the provisions of the optometry law
- Requirements for licensure by the board
- Enumerated causes for disciplinary action to be instituted by the board against licensees, and procedures to be followed when instituting discipline
- Exemptions from the law

One of these provisions, the definition, has been of such importance that it is discussed separately in Chapter 10. The four other provisions, which relate to boards of optometry and their powers, will be discussed in Chapter 11. Statutory regulation of optometry by third-party reimbursement programs, and the discriminatory problems that have plagued the administration of these laws, will be described in Chapter 12.

Versions of the Minnesota law spread throughout the country, with the last jurisdiction (the District of Columbia) passing its law in 1924 (see Table 9.1).

Of course, the optometry practice acts were not the first attempts to regulate a health care profession by statute. They were in essence imitations of the legislative acts that had been passed during the 1800s to regulate medicine, laws enacted in part due to the poor quality of medical education that existed at the time. There was an abundance of proprietary schools that ground out inadequately trained "physicians" or that awarded diplomas to "graduates" through the mails, and many other "doctors" were little more than apprentices who had decided to strike out on their own.[3]

Responsible members of the medical profession felt that minimally acceptable standards had to be established, but with so many schools and no accre-

Table 9.1. Optometry Practice Acts: 1901–1924

Order	State	Date Enacted
1	Minnesota	April 13, 1901
2	North Dakota	March 4, 1903
3	California	March 20, 1903
4	Oregon	February 21, 1905
5	New Mexico	March 16, 1905*
6	Tennessee	February 12, 1907
7	Montana	March 7, 1907
8	Indiana	March 9, 1907
9(tie)	Arizona	March 14, 1907*
10(tie)	Utah	March 14, 1907
11	Idaho	March 18, 1907
12	Nebraska	March 27, 1907
13	New York	May 21, 1908
14	Vermont	January 9, 1909
15	West Virginia	March 3, 1909
16	North Carolina	March 6, 1909
17	Washington	March 11, 1909
18	Kansas	March 12, 1909
19	Maine	March 18, 1909
20	Delaware	March 22, 1909
21	Iowa	March 27, 1909
22	Rhode Island	April 16, 1909
23	Michigan	May 6, 1909
24	Florida	May 21, 1909
25	Oklahoma	February 15, 1911
26	New Hampshire	April 15, 1911
27	Massachusetts	June 1, 1912
28	South Dakota	March 12, 1913
29	Nevada	March 17, 1913
30	Colorado	May 2, 1913
31	Connecticut	June 4, 1913
32	Maryland	April 13, 1914
33	New Jersey	April 17, 1914
34	Arkansas	March 5, 1915
35	Illinois	June 29, 1915†
36	Wisconsin	July 30, 1915
37	Virginia	March 11, 1916
38	Georgia	August 7, 1916
39	South Carolina	February 13, 1917
40	Wyoming	February 16, 1917
41	Pennsylvania	March 30, 1917
42	Hawaii	April 30, 1917*
43	Alaska	May 2, 1917*
44	Louisiana	July 10, 1918
45	Ohio	April 10, 1919
46	Alabama	September 8, 1919
47	Mississippi	March 6, 1920
48	Kentucky	March 20, 1920
49	Missouri	April 7, 1921
50	Texas	August 27, 1921
51	District of Columbia	May 28, 1924

*Territorial enactment.

†This law was declared unconstitutional and was repassed as amended on April 19, 1919.

Source: American Optometric Association.

diting mechanism, the only practical route available was through the states and the power of state governments to regulate the health and welfare of its citizens. And so medical practice acts were written and state medical boards were created for the principal purpose of conducting examinations that would weed out (and keep out) the incompetents and charlatans.[4] This medical prototype was followed by optometry several decades later.

Unfortunately, the laws regulating the practice of medicine were written in such a way that the efforts of optometrists (and other health-care practitioners) to legalize their callings were regarded by physicians as being "infringements" on the medical monopoly. As a result, the optometry practice acts paid a political price for their enactment, the effects of which are still felt today.[5]

But the struggle to obtain passage of these laws was not the end of the legal battle over the practice of optometry. Indeed, it was just the beginning.

Challenge in the Courts

In Part II, we discussed the U.S. legal system and noted that, even though the legislatures are empowered to enact the nation's laws, it is the judiciary that must determine the constitutionality of these laws. This right of constitutional review has great significance for optometry, which enjoys a legal status that is predicated on statutory recognition. The constitutional basis for judicial review of laws such as the optometry practice acts lies within the *police power* granted to state governments; one application of this power is the authority to safeguard the public health and welfare. The initial cases involving the optometry laws tested the right of states to authorize the practice of optometry and to license optometrists.

California passed a law permitting the practice of optometry, which was defined as the right to measure the powers or range of vision other than by the use of drugs. Those practicing optometry had to be licensed by the state. A practitioner who called herself an "ophthalmologist"—but did not use drugs to test the eyes—attacked the statute, maintaining that it denied her equal protection under the law by making it unlawful to provide drugless eye care without first obtaining a license to practice optometry. Thus, she argued, the law was an improper application of the police power. After the California Supreme Court upheld the constitutionality of the law, the case was appealed to the U.S. Supreme Court, where a precedent-setting decision in favor of the law was rendered.[6]

Other cases were brought by physicians,[7] osteopaths,[8] chiropractors,[9] itinerant spectacle peddlers,[10] opticians,[11] and optometrists,[12] testing the constitutionality of various provisions of state laws. One particular aspect of these laws that drew constitutional scrutiny was the exemption granted to physicians and opticians.

An individual who had failed the Wisconsin optometry licensing examination on three occasions was charged with practicing without a license and responded with a defense that the law was unconstitutional. The Wisconsin Supreme Court, in reviewing this claim, took note of the exemptions granted to physicians and opticians, commenting that, "The propriety of the exemptions is so manifest that discussion of the reasons therefor would be but to attempt to demonstrate the obvious." The law was upheld as a valid exercise of the state police power and enforceable.[13]

The exemption of optometrists from provisions of state medical practice acts[14] and basic science acts[15] was likewise held to be a proper application of the police power.

With the unquestioned right of the states to regulate optometry established, cases were brought to determine what constituted the practice of optometry.[16] Although each state law defined those acts with specificity, legal issues were raised as to their validity and meaning. In particular, the relationship between the retail sale of glasses and the practice of optometry required clarification.

In Illinois, optometry was defined as being "the employment of any means other than the use of drugs, medicine, or surgery for the measurement of the power of vision and the adaptation of lenses for the aid thereof." A store sold ready-made glasses. The glasses were selected by customers after trying them on and determining which pair best suited their needs. No professional advice or assistance was given to purchasers. The store, through its employees, was charged with violating the statute. In declaring the law unconstitutional, the Illinois high court ruled that the sale of ready-made glasses had "no relation to the public health, comfort, safety, or welfare, such as to require a course of previous study and an examination and payment of a license fee." The court's ruling not only exonerated the defendant store, it necessitated the passage of a new optometry law by the state legislature.[17]

Although some states made it unlawful for any business to sell glasses at retail unless an optometrist or physician was in personal attendance,[18] and these laws did exercise some control over the commercialism of eye care, by and large retail sales of ready-made glasses have not been subject to regulation under optometry practice acts.

But the biggest difficulty for the courts arose out of efforts to determine the nature of optometric services, as set forth in the optometry practice acts. There were two principal causes for this judicial consternation: the variation from state to state in the wording and provisions of the optometry laws and the dichotomy between professional and commercial practitioners that existed in virtually every state. The difficulties experienced by the courts are best illustrated by the decisions of appellate judges asked to rule on the issues of corporate practice of optometry and advertising by optometrists.[19]

The employment of optometrists by corporations was a problem inherited by the optometry laws at the time of their enactment. Storefront locations were not uncommon because the profitability of these businesses made them a lucrative alternative to professional practice.[20] The difficulty that they posed for the courts went to the very heart of the practice of optometry: Was it a business or a profession? In deciding this question, the courts had to decide if optometry, as defined by state law, could be practiced by a corporation or could rightfully be limited by statute to individuals.

The Kansas optometry practice act specified that it was unlawful for any person to practice optometry who was not registered with the state board. A corporation engaged in the retail jewelry business leased space to an optometrist, who was required to be present during certain specified hours, to maintain and keep equipment, to make examinations on the basis of stipulated fees, and to sell glasses, frames and supplies, the purchase of these frames and lenses to be made from the corporation. For these duties the optometrist was to receive $2.75 per examination and 10 percent of the gross sales of ophthalmic materials. The lease arrangement provided for termination of the contract upon the giving of ten days notice by either party. An action in *quo warranto* was brought against the corporation to determine if it was in violation of the statute. In deciding the case in the affirmative, the Kansas Supreme Court observed,

"There is a material difference between the practice of optometry as defined in the statute and simply the sale of optical goods. . .the legislature, having in mind the protection of eyesight. . .by the enactment of the statutes with reference to optometry, recognized that it is a profession and accordingly regulated it, and. . .the practice of the profession is limited to individuals."[21]

Thus in those states where the law restricted the practice of optometry to individuals, the courts held that such a restriction was enforceable.[22] But in a number of states litigation was instituted where the law was silent (i.e., where no prohibition against the employment of optometrists by corporations was expressed in the law), and in those states the courts were divided, with opinions varying widely as to the nature of the practice of optometry.[23]

In deciding that the optometry practice act for the District of Columbia permitted the practice of optometry by a corporation, the federal appellate court commented, "But we prefer to rest our view upon the broader distinction arising out of the traditional relationship between physician and patient and attorney and client, a relationship which does not exist in the practice of optometry. . .we may very well concede that optometry is a profession, as that term is now colloquially used, but that fact is not enough."[24]

In a New York case discussing the same issue, the practice of optometry by a corporation, the New York Superior Court observed, "The relationship between an optometrist and his patient is of a personal and confidential nature, not unlike the relationship between an attorney and client, or physician and patient. The examination of an optometrist may not only indicate an eye condition, but may disclose other ailments and bodily afflictions of a more or less personal nature. True, the optometrist may not lawfully treat his patient for these ailments, but the patient is entitled to the assurance that the knowledge obtained in such examination will be held inviolate and not become a record in the files of a business corporation."[25]

The right of the states to regulate corporate practice was eventually settled by the U.S. Supreme Court, which upheld the constitutionality of an Oklahoma statute that prohibited retail stores from leasing space to optometrists.[26] Even though this decision afforded the states a means of regulating the practice of optometry by corporations, not all states were able to enact laws as rigorous as those of Oklahoma, and so corporate practice was never fully eradicated.[27]

Advertising was another difficult problem faced by the courts in deciding what constituted the practice of optometry. Statutes prohibiting fraudulent or misleading advertising of skills or method of practice,[28] prices to be charged for examinations or glasses,[29] credit terms,[30] "free" examinations for spectacles,[31] or the display of signs, licenses, or merchandise[32] were upheld in various states,[33] and the U.S. Supreme Court, in a precedent-setting decision of some importance, ruled that any advertising of materials or services, even if truthful, could be lawfully restricted,[34] concluding that, "We can see no constitutional reason why a state may not treat all who deal with the human eye as members of a profession who should use no merchandising methods for obtaining customers." Two decades later, however, the nation's highest court recognized the right of professionals to advertise truthful information.[35]

Taken as a whole, the trend of these cases was clearly toward recognition of optometry as a profession,[36] an interpretation made easier for the courts by the reform of state practice acts to include the designation of optometry as such. Even so, the practice of optometry was not on a legal plane with that of medicine because it was not considered to be a *learned* profession, a designation that the courts traditionally reserved for medicine, the law, and theology.[37] The elevation of optometry to parity with these other learned professions could be achieved, however, by state legislatures,[38] through the substitution of the appropriate language in the optometry practice act.

The Arkansas legislature amended the optometry law to redefine optometry as a learned profession. The constitutionality of this declaration, as a valid exercise of the police power, was challenged by a corporation that employed optometrists. The corporation alleged that the amendment denied them equal protection under the law by virtue of giving the state optometrists this recognition. In upholding the constitutionality of the amendment, the state Supreme court stated that, "if the General Assembly, by express language, should classify optometry as a learned profession, such determination, being an expression of public policy, would not be in excess of legislative powers."[39]

As the preceding cases illustrate, the legal progression of optometry from a mercantile business to a learned profession has been reflected in the decisions of the courts, with the ultimate result being a reformation of the original optometry practice acts.[40] These initial laws were the product of the argument that optometry, having grown from different roots than medicine, deserved to be accorded legal recognition as a profession separate and independent from that of medicine. In voicing this argument, optometrists stressed the nonmedical nature of optometric services.[41] But technological and sociological changes following World War II forced optometrists to reassess their thinking and caused the profession to resort to legislative and judicial measures in order to enable optometric practitioners to fulfill their new role as providers of primary eye care.

Legislative Reform

The original optometry laws did not envision the advent of the contact lens, improved techniques for tonometry, or advancements in ophthalmic pharmaceutical agents. In order to ensure that these new developments within eye care could be utilized by optometrists, the first significant alterations in the definition of optometry since the original practice acts had to be made. The initial changes concerned the fitting of contact lenses.[42]

In those states in which contact lenses were expressly identified in the optometry law, the fitting of contact lenses was included within the practice of optometry. But in states where the law was silent, the outcome was less certain and resulted in a plethora of legal disputes. The courts were asked to decide if measurement of the cornea for the purpose of fitting contact lenses constituted the practice of optometry,[43] if supervision was necessary for opticians fitting contact lenses pursuant to a doctor's prescription,[44] the effect of professional follow-up examinations,[45] and whether a soft lens was a "drug" and thus an aspect of the practice of medicine.[46] These cases were met by a determined effort at legislative reform on the part of opticians, and in a number of states the fitting of contact lenses became part of the practice of opticianry[47] (see Table 9.2).

Another technological advance, tonometry with-

Table 9.2. State Listing of the Status of the Fitting of Contact Lenses by Opticians as of 1985

	1	2	3	4	5	Comments	Citation
Alabama*				×			Ala. Code §34-22-4
Alaska†			×			Opticians required to work in conjunction with and under O.D./M.D. supervision—opticians must receive a written CL prescription and person is required to return to the prescribing doctor.	Alaska Stat. §08.71.240
Arizona*				×		Opticians are required to tell person to return to the examining doctor.	Ariz. Rev. Stat. Ann. §32-1671(3)
Arkansas*	×						Ark. Stat. Ann. §72-2112
California*					×	Opticians must direct person to return to prescribing doctor for evaluation.	Cal. Bus. & Prof. Code §§2560-2564.5 (Deering)
Colorado	×						Colo. Rev. Stat. §12-40-102
Connecticut*					×		Conn. Gen. Stat. §20-145
Delaware		×					Del. Code Ann. tit. 24 §2117
District of Columbia	×					Court held that opticians may not adopt lenses to persons' eyes. Actual fitting of contact lenses equals practice of optometry.	*Fields v. District of Columbia*, 232 A.2d 300, 244 A.2d 643, *app. den.* 404 F.2d 1323 (1967)
Florida*				×		Court held opticians could prepare the prescriptions if they were fully supplied by O.D./M.D.	*Florida Assn. of Dispensing Opticians v. Bd. of Optometry*, 227 So.2d 736, *aff'd in part, quashed in part* 238 So.2d 839, *vacated in part* 239 So.2d 520 (1970)
Georgia*				×		May fill a specific written prescription from O.D./M.D.	Ga. Code Ann. §84-3502

Table 9.2 *Continued*

	1	2	3	4	5	Comments	Citation
						and must return patient to the prescribing doctor for evaluation and approval.	
Hawaii*				×			Hawaii Rev. Stat. §458-13(5)
Idaho				×			Idaho Code §54-1501(4) & (5)
Illinois	×						Ill. Ann. Stat. ch. 111 §3803(3) (Smith-Hurd)
Indiana	×					Attorney General Opinion No. 69 (1946) interprets this statute to mean that fitting of contact lenses constitutes practice of optometry.	Ind. Stat. Ann. §25-24-1-4 (Burns)
Iowa*				×		Attorney General Opinion 567-3-1 of 3/6/67	Iowa Code Ann. §153A (West)
Kansas				×		Opticians may fit if they receive a complete prescription and work under direct physical supervision of O.D./M.D.	Kan. Stat. Ann. §65-1508; *Burch v. State Bd. of Ex. in Optomety Kan.*, decided 6/14/83
Kentucky			×				Ky. Rev. Stat. Ann. §326.060 (Baldwin)
Louisiana	×						La. Rev. Stat. Ann. §37:1065 (West)
Maine	×						Me. Rev. Stat. Ann. tit. 32, §2411
Maryland					×		*Bd. of Examiners in Optometry v. Spitz*, 479A.2d 363 (1984)
Massachusetts*				×		*Atty. Gen. v. Kenco Optics*, 340 NE2d 868 (1976)	Mass. Gen. Laws Ann. ch. 112, §73C (Michie/Law Coop.)
Michigan	×					Attorney General Opinion 3563 of 1/13/61	Mich. Comp. Laws Ann. §14.15 (17401) (Callaghan)
Minnesota	×						Minn. Stat. Ann. §148.56
Mississippi				×		Optician must direct person to return to prescribing doctor for evaluation.	*State Board of Optometry v. Chester*, 169 So.2d 468, 251 Miss. 250 (1964)
Missouri	×						*State ex. rel. Danforth v. Dale Curteman, Inc.*, 480 S.W. 2d 848 (1972)
Montana	×						Mont. Code Ann. §§37-10-101 and 37-10-102
Nebraska				×			Neb. Rev. Stat. §71-1, 134
Nevada*				×		Optician is required to direct person to return to the prescribing doctor.	Nev. Rev. Stat. §637.020
New Hampshire	×						N.H. Rev. Stat. Ann. §327:12
New Jersey*	×						N.J. Rev. Stat. Ann. §52-17B-41.1
New Mexico		×					N.M. Stat. Ann. §§61-2-2 and 61-2-15
New York*			×				N.Y. Educ. Law §7121 (McKinney)
North Carolina*	×					Optician must tell person, both	N.C. Gen. Stat. §90-236.1

Table 9.3 *Continued*

	1	2	3	4	5	Comments	Citation
						orally and in writing, to return to prescribing doctor for insertion, instruction on care and insertion, and to determine accuracy.	
North Dakota	×						N.D. Cent. Code §43-17-02(10)
Ohio				×		Optician must be registered for fitting contact lenses.	Ohio Rev. Code Ann. §4725.40 (Page)
Oklahoma*				×		Court held use of keratometer by optician to fit contact lenses is permissible.	*State ex rel. Clifton v. Reeser*, 543 P.2d 1379 (1975)
Oregon	×						*State v. Kuzirian*, 288 Or. 619, 365 P.2d 1046 (1961)
Pennsylvania	×						*Neill v. Wall and Ochs*, 68 Pa. D.&C. 2d 429 (1973)
Rhode Island*	×						R.I. Gen Laws §5-35-1
South Carolina*				×		Opticians must have a written prescription, and, if they are not directly supervised by an O.D./M.D., they must tell patient to return to the prescribing doctor.	S.C. Code §40-38-150 (Law Co-op)
South Dakota	×						S.D. Codified Laws Ann. §36-7-1
Tennessee*			×			Opticians must be directly supervised by O.D./M.D.	Tenn. Code Ann. §63-14-102
Texas	×						Tex. Rev. Civ. Stat. Ann. art. 4552-1.02 (Vernon)
Utah	×						Attorney General Opinion 59-089 of 10/7/59
Vermont*			×				Vt. Stat. Ann. tit. 26, §2651(3)
Virginia*			×			Both a written prescription and direct supervision by O.D./M.D. are required.	Va. Code §54-398.27
Washington*				×			Wash. Rev. Code Ann. §18.34.060
West Virginia				×		Attorney General Opinion ruled that an optician must have a contact lens prescription from an O.D./M.D. before doing any work.	Atty. Gen. Op. of 6/8/79
Wisconsin	×					Attorney General ruled fitting of a contact lens may only be performed by a licensed O.D./M.D.	36 OAG 314 (1947)—*aff'd.* in 1971
Wyoming				×			Wyo. Stat. §33-23-101
Total	22	2	6	18	3		

Key: 1 = Opticians totally prohibited from engaging in fitting of contact lenses (CL)
2 = Opticians may do CL work on O.D./M.D. premises
3 = Opticians may do CL work under O.D./M.D. supervision
4 = Opticians may do CL work if they receive a complete CL prescription from an O.D./M.D.
5 = Opticians may fit CL
* = State has enacted law requiring opticians to be registered or certified
† = Denotes sunset of law licensing opticians

Source: American Optometric Association, 1985.

out anesthesia, was added without dispute to the armamentarium of optometrists in most states because all optometry practice acts granted optometrists the right to examine eyes for *departures from the normal, abnormal conditions*, or similar phrases that conveyed the intention of the legislatures to permit optometric practitioners to examine for disease. The use of tonometry by optometrists, when challenged in the courts, was found to be within the practice of optometry.

Colorado ophthalmologists brought an action for declarative and injunctive relief against state optometrists, alleging that it was unlawful for optometrists to hold themselves out as being able to diagnose glaucoma. The Colorado appellate court, in affirming the right of optometrists to use tonometry to test for glaucoma, noted that optometrists have "a right and duty to refer or direct a patient to a physician whenever. . . a patient exhibits signs or symptoms of a disease requiring treatment by an ophthalmologist or other physician."[48]

But the most revolutionary change in optometry was the effort to amend optometry practice acts to permit the use of ophthalmic pharmaceutical agents, beginning with the initial law enacted in Rhode Island in 1971.[49] This law was the first to authorize the use of diagnostic agents by optometrists, and initiated a legislative effort that has not yet run its course. This revolutionary statute was immediately challenged as being unconstitutional.[50]

The Rhode Island statute and its sequelae were manifestations of the increased emphasis on health care within optometry. This altered view of the role of optometrists was taken a step further in 1976 with the amendment of the West Virginia optometry practice act, which authorized the use of pharmaceutical agents for therapeutic purposes by optometrists.[51] The constitutionality of this law was also subjected to immediate judicial scrutiny.[52] Both legal challenges were defeated and the laws were upheld (see Chapter 10).

The effect of these legislative reforms has been to give the profession a new direction, one that is more oriented toward ocular and systemic health. Optometry is at present undergoing a transitional period, during which further reforms may be required so that optometric practitioners may better serve the public as providers of primary care. In seeking these reforms, optometrists will return to their state legislatures, offering amendments to the optometry practice acts. In particular, they will be seeking to amend the statutory definitions of optometry, and it is to this singularly important aspect of the law that we now turn.

Notes

1. For a discussion of the history of the New York optometry bill and its significance for medicine, see Stevens, R., *American Medicine and the Public Interest*, Yale University Press, New Haven, Conn., 1977, pp. 103–109.
2. The full text of the Minnesota law is quoted by Hirsch, M.J., and R.E. Wick, *The Optometric Profession*, Chilton, Philadelphia, 1968, pp. 315–317.
3. For an account of the predicament of medicine during the late 1700s and early 1800s, see Starr, P., *The Social Transformation of American Medicine*, Basic Books, New York, 1983, pp. 30–78.
4. For the motivation for the changes in state law that resulted in the "modern" medical practice acts, see id. at 79–144.
5. The development of professional licensure and the evolution of optometry licensing laws is recounted by Coblens, S., *Optometry and the Law*, American Optometric Association, St. Louis, Mo., 1976, pp. 15–25.
6. This decision by the U.S. Supreme Court, *McNaughton v. Johnson*, 242 U.S. 344, 37 S. Ct. 178 (1917), affirmed the right of the states to regulate the practice of optometry through licensure.
7. An ophthalmologist challenged the Massachusetts optometry law on the basis that it was class legislation that discriminated against him and thus was an interference with his rights, but this argument was rejected by the court. See *Commonwealth v. Houtenbrink*, 235 Mass. 320, 126 N.E. 669 (1920).
8. In California, it was held that the practice of optometry was not within the science of osteopathy and that a person holding a license as an osteopath did not have the legal right to practice optometry. See *Ex parte Rust*, 181 Cal. 73, 183 P. 548 (1919).
9. A chiropractor argued that the exemption of optometrists from the Texas medical practice act amounted to class legislation and was discriminatory since chiropractors did not have a similar exemption under the act. This argument was rejected in *Robertus v. State*, 119 Tex. Crim. Rep. 370, 45 S.W.2d 595 (1931). A similar result was obtained in *Allison v. State*, 76 S.W.2d 527 (1934).
10. The right of optometry statutes to regulate and forbid the selling of spectacles from door to door was upheld in *Saunders v. Swann*, 155 Tenn. 310, 292 S.W. 458 (1927), and in *Harris v. State Board of Optometrical Examiners*, 287 Pa. 531, 135 A. 237 (1926).
11. The provisions of the Iowa law, which required licensure in order to practice optometry, were challenged by an optical shop as being in violation of the state and federal constitutions. The validity of the law was upheld in *State v. Kindy Optical Co.*, 216 Iowa 1157, 248 N.W. 332 (1933).
12. The right of the Connecticut Board of Optometry to revoke the licenses of optometrists for immoral, dishonorable, or unprofessional conduct was upheld as not being an unconstitutional delegation of legislative

powers in *Sage-Allen v. Wheeler*, 119 Conn. 667, 179 A. 195 (1935).
13. *Price v. State*, 168 Wis. 603, 171 N.W. 77 (1919).
14. *People v. Witte*, 315 Ill. 282, 146 N.E. 178 (1924). See also *Robertus v. State*, 119 Tex. Crim. Rep. 370, 45 S.W.2d 595 (1931).
15. *State v. Broden*, 181 Minn. 341, 232 N.W. 517 (1930).
16. Annotations discussing "What Constitutes Practice of 'Optometry'" can be found in 121 A.L.R. 1455, 141 A.L.R. 883, and 88 A.L.R.2d 1290.
17. *People v. Griffith*, 280 Ill. 18, 117 N.E. 195 (1917).
18. The U.S. Supreme Court, in *Roschen v. Ward*, 279 U.S. 337, 49 S. Ct. 336 (1929), upheld the right of the states to make it unlawful to sell at retail eyeglasses for the correction of vision unless a licensed optometrist (or physician) was present. See also *Kresge v. Ottinger*, 29 F.2d 762 (2nd Cir. 1928), which was affirmed in *Roschen v. Ward*, and *Commonwealth v. S.S. Kresge Co.*, 267 Mass. 145, 166 N.E. 558 (1929), decided on similar grounds.
19. The issue of the practice of optometry by corporations has been vigorously contested in the courts, and several annotations of the American Law Reports can be consulted for background information. See "Right of Corporation, or Individual Not Himself Licensed, to Practice Optometry Through Licensed Employees," 102 A.L.R. 343 and 128 A.L.R. 585. See also 121 A.L.R. 1455, 141 A.L.R. 883, and 88 A.L.R.2d 1290.
20. For a description of the plight of optometry in the first half of the 20th century, see Hirsch and Wick, supra note 2, at 139–147 and 170–177.
21. *State of Kansas ex rel. Beck v. Goldman Jewelry Co*, 142 Kan. 881, 51 P.2d 995 (1935).
22. For cases upholding the right of states to prohibit the practice of optometry by corporations, see the following cases: *State v. Kindy Optical Co.*, 216 Iowa 1157, 248 N.W. 332 (1933); *State of Kansas ex rel. Beck v. Goldman Jewelry Co.*, 51 P.2d 995 (Kan. 1935); *Eisensmith v. Buhl Optical Co.*, 178 S.E. 695 (W. Va. 1934); *Stern v. Flynn*, 278 N.Y.S. 598 (N.Y. 1935); *Fink Jewelry Co., v. State*, 50 P.2d 945 (Ariz. 1935); *McMurdo v. Getter*, 10 N.E.2d 139 (Mass. 1937); *State of Ohio ex rel. Bricker v. Buhl Optical Co.*, 2 N.E.2d 601 (Oh. 1936); *Neill v. Gimbel Brothers*, 199 A. 178 (Pa. 1938); *Teseshi v. Mathis*, 183 A. 146 (N.J. 1936); *Rowe v. Standard Drug Co.*, 9 N.E.2d 609 (Oh. 1937); *Ezell v. Ritholz*, 198 S.E. 419 (S.C. 1938); and *Kay Jewelry Co. v. Board of Registration*, 27 N.E.2d 1 (Mass. 1940). A keen analysis of this issue can be found in Gekoski, A.C., Legality of Corporate Practice of Optometry, *Temple Law Quarterly*, Jan., 1937.
23. Cases maintaining that a corporation may practice optometry include the following: *Jaeckle v. Bamburger & Co.*, 181 A. 181 (N.J. 1935); *Sage-Allen Co. v. Wheeler*, supra note 12; *Georgia Board of Examiners v. Frieman's Jewelers*, 189 S.E. 238 (Ga. 1936); *Dvorine v. Castleberg Jewelry Corp.*, 185 A. 562 (Md. 1936); *State v. Gus Blass Co.*, 105 S.W.2d 853 (Ark. 1937); *State of Missouri ex rel. McKittrick v. Gate City Optical Co.*, 97 S.W.2d 89 (Mo. 1936); *Golding v. Shubach Optical Co.*, 70 P.2d 871 (Ut. 1937); *State of Wisconsin ex rel. Harris v. Kindy Optical Co.*, 282 N.W. 283 (Wis. 1940); *Dickson v. Flynn*, 6 N.E.2d 102 (N.Y. 1937); *Williams v. Mack*, 278 N.W. 585 (Minn. 1938); and *State by Erwin v. Goodman*, 288 N.W. 157 (Minn. 1939).
24. *Silver v. Landsburgh & Brother*, 111 F.2d 518 (D.C. Cir. 1940).
25. *Matter of Pace*, 156 N.Y.S. 641, 154 Misc. 609 (N.Y. 1915)
26. *Williamson v. Lee Optical of Oklahoma*, 348 U.S. 483, 75 S. Ct. 461 (1955).
27. For a discussion of legal efforts to eradicate commercialism, see Kohn, H., A Legal and Anecdotal History of Optometry, *Journal of the American Optometric Association*, vol. 38, no. 11, Nov. 1967, pp. 949–955.
28. *Ritholz v. Indiana State Board of Registration & Examination*, 45 F. Supp. 423 (D.C. Ind. 1937); and *Melton v. Carter*, 204 Ark. 595, 164 S.W.2d 453 (1942).
29. *Siefert v. Buhl Optical Co.*, 276 Mich. 692, 268 N.W. 784 (1936); and *Ritholz v. Commonwealth*, 184 Va. 339, 35 S.E.2d 210 (1945).
30. *Ritholz v. Johnson*, 246 Wis. 442, 17 N.W.2d 590 (1945).
31. *Finlay Straus, Inc. v. University of the State of New York*, 270 A.D. 1060, 62 N.Y.S.2d 892 (1946).
32. *Abelson's, Inc. v. New Jersey State Board of Optometrists*, 5 N.J. 412, 75 A.2d 867 (1950).
33. For an annotation of cases, see "Validity of Governmental Regulation of Optometry," 22 A.L.R.2d 939.
34. *Semler v. Oregon State Board of Dental Examiners*, 294 U.S. 608, 55 S. Ct. 570 (1935).
35. *Bates v. State Bar of Arizona*, 433 U.S. 350, 97 S. Ct. 2691 (1977).
36. The evolution of optometry from business to profession is described by Hirsch and Wick, *The Optometric Profession*, supra note 2, at 148–177. The decisions of the courts were reflections of the professional advances made by optometry during the 1940s, 1950s, and 1960s.
37. The learned professions have traditionally been medicine, law, and the ministry, callings that not only involve a unique body of knowledge but also require undivided loyalty to those they serve. The courts have not been willing to extend this distinction to other professions unless there is clear and compelling reason to do so. By way of example, in Alabama the state optometrists sought a declaratory judgment that optometry was a learned profession, presenting witnesses and information to substantiate their claim that this distinction was due. The state supreme court, in refusing to accord optometry this recognition, stated that, "Although the contemporary scientific, educational, and clinical developments in that profession are noteworthy, nevertheless we do not denote any legislative intent to change that body's policy so as to denote the practice of optometry as the practice of a learned profession." Chief Justice Torbert, in a dissenting opinion, described the fallacy of the majority's decision:

When this court held...that dentistry is a learned profession...we departed from the traditional listing of learned professions, i.e., doctors, lawyers, and ministers of the gospel, and embarked on a course of action requiring us to distinguish the "learned" professions from all other professions. I cannot agree that optometrists are not entitled to this honor, since we are now committed to making such a distinction.

Appellants presented evidence at trial concerning the training that optometrists are required to undergo before being certified by the State Board of Optometry. The similarity to that of dentists in terms of length, course material, and practical experience is striking. Additionally, appellants introduced lengthy testimony of the great strides that have been made in the field. An optometrist is no longer a mere technician who measures the severity of a vision defect and matches to it the proper strength of eyeglasses, but he now is engaged in all aspects of testing and treating a multitude of sight problems. Although he can neither prescribe drugs nor perform surgery, he can and often does diagnose illnesses of the eyes, for treatment of which he refers the patient to an ophthalmologist. The optometrist also uses a number of mechanical devices, as well as exercises and unique eyeglass prescriptions, to correct all sorts of eye problems which he has discovered and/or diagnosed.

The materials and cosmetic attractiveness of the eyeglasses sold by optometrists are only a small part of the total cost. The major cost involved stems from the expertise he demonstrates in determining the correct prescription for the problem of the particular patient. Anyone who has ever purchased "dime store" eyeglasses knows the differential both as to price and effectiveness between them and a pair of eyeglasses prescribed and fitted by a certified optometrist. The parallel between optometry and dentistry, as well as many other branches of medicine, is obvious in this regard....

The majority makes much of the fact that optometrists are prohibited from prescribing drugs or performing surgery. Suffice it to say that a determination of "learned" as regards a profession is not based on what members of a profession cannot do, but on what they can do. While the inability to prescribe drugs or perform surgery may mean that optometrists are not medical doctors, it does not prevent them from being members of a learned profession. Neither lawyers nor ministers prescribe drugs or perform surgery, yet both the law and the ministry are considered to be learned professions....

Quoted from *Alabama Board of Optometry v. Eagerton*, 393 So. 2d 1373 (Ala. 1981).

38. Those states that have *legislatively* recognized optometry as a learned profession are Arkansas, Georgia, and Idaho. For an excellent discussion of the legal ramifications of such recognition, see *Pearle Optical of Monroeville, Inc. v. Georgia State Board of Examiners in Optometry*, 219 Ga. 364, 133 S.E.2d 374 (1963). Judicial recognition was extended in the state of New Jersey in *Abelson's Inc. v. New Jersey State Board of Optometrists*, 5 N.J. 412, 75 A.2d 867 (1950).
39. *Melton v. Carter*, 204 Ark. 595, 164 S.W.2d (1942). This was apparently the first statute to recognize optometry as a learned profession.
40. The original optometry practice acts were the laws enacted between 1901 and 1924, the laws that first recognized the legal right of optometrists to pursue their calling. See Chapter 1.
41. Precedent for the argument that optometry was not a part of medicine was established in *Martin v. Baldi*, 249 Pa. 253, 94 A. 1091 (1915).
42. A discussion of "Fitting of Contact Lenses as Practice of Optometry" can be found in 77 A.L.R.3d 817.
43. A most interesting case is *House of Vision, Inc. v. Watson*, 59 Ill. 2d 508, 322 N.E.2d 15 (1974), *cert. denied*, 422 U.S. 1008, 95 S. Ct. 2631 (1974), in which it was held that the fitting of contact lenses was within the meaning of the statute requiring the licensing of persons engaged in the practice of optometry, and that the defendant—a large optical company—should have been enjoined from permitting its employees who were not licensed as optometrists from fitting customers with contact lenses. See also *Delaware Optometric Corp. v. Sherwood*, 36 Del. Ch. 223, 128 A.2d 812 (1957), in which it was assumed that fitting contact lenses was an act of optometry; *Pennsylvania Optometric Association v. Di Giovanni*, 45 Pa. D.&C.2d 245 (1968), in which the fitting of contact lenses by an optician was enjoined as within the practice of optometry; and *State of Oregon ex rel. Reed v. Kuzirian*, 228 Or. 619, 365 P.2d 1046 (1961), which was decided on similar grounds.
44. *New Jersey State Board of Optometrists v. Reiss*, 83 N.J. Super. 47, 198 A.2d 816 (1964). An account of this case and the legal issues it presented can be found in the July 1964 issue of the *American Journal of Optometry and Archives of American Academy of Optometry*, pp. 438–445.
45. Some cases have recognized that the fitting of contact lenses, when made in accordance with the prescription of an optometrist or physician, does not constitute the practice of optometry when the patient is required to return to the optometrist or physician for follow-up. See *Florida Association of Dispensing Opticians v. Florida State Board of Optometry*, 238 So. 2d 839, *conformed to* 239 So. 2d 520 (1970); *State of Kansas ex rel. Londerholm v. Doolin*, 209 Kan. 244, 497 P.2d 138 (1972); *State Board of Optometry v. Chester*, 251 Miss. 250, 169 So. 2d 468 (1964); *High v. Ridgeway's Opticians*, 258 N.C. 626, 129 S.E.2d 301 (1963); and *State of Oklahoma ex rel. Clifton v. Reeser*, 543 P.2d 1379 (Okla. 1975). In a number of cases the courts recognized that the fitting of contact lenses constitutes the practice of optometry, and that a follow-up examination does not obviate the application of the

law. See *House of Vision, Inc. v. Watson*; 59 Ill. 508, 322 N.E.2d 15 (1974), *cert. denied*, 422 U.S. 1008, 95 S. Ct. 2631 (1974); *Fields v. District of Columbia*, 232 A.2d 300 (D.C. App. 1967), *adhered to* 244 A.2d 643 (D.C. App. 1968), *app. denied*, 131 App. D.C. 346, 404 F.2d 1323 (1967); *State of Missouri ex rel. Danforth v. Dale Curteman, Inc.*, 480 S.W.2d 848 (Mo. 1972); and *New Jersey State Board of Optometrists v. Reiss*, 83 N.J. Super. 47, 198 A.2d 816 (1964).

46. *Winograd v. Johnson*, 561 P.2d 1274 (Colo. App. 1976).
47. As of 1985, twenty-nine states and the District of Columbia did not permit the independent fitting of contact lenses by opticians, eighteen allowed fittings only if the optician had a complete prescription from an optometrist or physician, and three granted opticians this right. *Bulletin from the Office of Counsel of the AOA*, vol. 44, no. 7, July 31, 1985.
48. *Winograd v. Johnson*, supra note 46.
49. The history of the Rhode Island law is recounted in Chapter 1; the law was enacted on July 16, 1971.
50. *Rhode Island Ophthalmological Society v. Cannon*, 317 A.2d 124 (1974).
51. The history of the West Virginia law is recounted in Chapter 1; the law was enacted on March 4, 1976.
52. *Esposito v. Shapero*, Civil Action No. 76-1214 (W. Va. Circuit Court, Cabell County, Dec. 13, 1976), *cert. denied* W. Va. Supreme Court, June 7, 1977.

Chapter 10

Defining Optometry

Optometry: *Measurement of the powers of vision and correction of visual defects by optical means.*
—Funk and Wagnalls, *Standard College Dictionary*

Defining a Profession
A Creature of Statute
Apples and Oranges
Upsetting the Applecart
Future Directions

Defining a Profession

The dictionary is a logical source to consult for a definition. The definition of a *profession*, however, entails far more than the simplistic wording to be found in a dictionary because a profession is a legal entity, recognized by government and given certain rights and privileges by government. It is the governmental definition that is important, be it within a statute or in a judicial interpretation of a statute. Because the licensure of a profession is a state matter, inevitably there must be a multiplicity of definitions to contend with,[1] and although these definitions may contain basic similarities, they are free to include differences as well. This chapter will be an attempt to deal with both the similarities and the differences of the various statutes defining optometry.

Government recognition brings restriction, and the most fundamental restriction for a profession—any profession—is the definition, the function of which is to limit the duly qualified members of the profession to a well-delineated set of services. For example, by legal definition, a physician is limited to the practice of medicine, a lawyer is limited to the practice of law, and an optometrist is limited to the practice of optometry. Unfortunately, optometry is defined much more narrowly than these other professions, and this fact has been the cause of much legal activity during the past three decades.

The legal definition of a profession is found within the statute recognizing the profession. But the definition is only one small part of the statute. Other key provisions typically authorize the regulation of the profession through a state board and provide for the licensing of properly qualified individuals by the board. Lastly, there are provisions incorporated into the statute that describe the circumstances under which an individual can be disciplined (including the loss of the right to practice the profession). All of these regulations are enforced by the state board, which serves as an administrative agency. In order to carry out this function the state board serves both in a legislative capacity (by publishing rules to enable it to carry out the intent of the statute) and in a judicial capacity (by conducting hearings or investigations of alleged violations). The state board, licensing, and professional discipline will be discussed in Chapter 11.

Once a statute becomes law, there are various mechanisms for review: The attorney general can be asked to interpret the meaning of the statute, the appellate courts may be petitioned to render an advisory opinion, or—through the process of an actual lawsuit—the courts may decide a legal controversy involving the statute. Any or all of these factors can serve to *interpret* the original law duly enacted by the legislature. In addition to these influences on statutory law, the legislature has the capability to modify the existing statute at any time, as it deems proper and necessary. As a result, the definition of optometry has become fluid and variable, evolving over time into something quite different than the dictionary definition quoted at the beginning of this chapter.

A Creature of Statute

In Chapter 6 the legislative process by which a bill becomes law was discussed. Optometry is practiced in all fifty states, the District of Columbia, Guam, the Virgin Islands, and the Commonwealth of Puerto Rico, because each of these governments has recognized optometry as an essential aspect of the health and welfare of its citizenry and has passed a bill designed to define it, to regulate it, and to license qualified practitioners. Therefore, optometry can be accurately described as a creature of statute. The legalization of optometry began on April 13, 1901, when Minnesota become the first state to enact an optometry practice act.[2] The definition of optometry, as written in the 1901 statute, is:[3]

> *Section 1.* The practice of optometry is defined as follows; namely: The employment of subjective and objective mechanical means to determine the accommodative and refractive states of the eye and the scope of its functions in general.

This is not a very broad definition. In fact, it is an exceptionally narrow one focusing on *mechanical means* as the only technique by which to ascertain the accommodative and refractive abilities of the patient's visual system. Political circumstances had much to do with the wording and content of the early definitions of the profession.[4] (The problems peculiar to the initial statutes recognizing the practice of optometry are detailed in Chapter 1.) All of these original statutes conspicuously omit any reference to drugs or treatment other than for accommodative and refractive difficulties. And they all contain the physician's exemption, the intent of which was to except physicians from the provisions of the optometry practice acts.[5] The 1901 Minnesota law was the first to grant this exemption:

> *Section 16.* Nothing in this Act shall be construed to apply to physicians and surgeons authorized to practice under the law of the State of Minnesota, nor to persons who sell spectacles or eye-glasses without attempting to traffic upon assumed skill in adopting them to the eye.

These first statutes traded the assurance of governmental recognition for a narrowly defined scope of services that was not in competition with the medical eye-care practitioners of the time.[6] Cases in Pennsylvania[7] and California[8] resulted in important judicial opinions in which the courts theorized that since optometrists practiced refraction and related optical services before physicians did, and did not treat eye disease or perform surgery (the traditional physician's functions), optometry deserved recognition as a separate discipline. The trade-off of a noncompetitive legal definition for the protection of state recognition was so successful that by 1924 all fifty states and the District of Columbia had passed optometry laws.[9] But this first breath of independence for the Lilliputian optometry from the Brobdignagian physicianry was not without cost: A look at the standard definition of the practice of medicine will reveal the significant difference between the legal stature of optometry and that of medicine.

Apples and Oranges

A standard common-sense homily dictates that you can't compare apples with oranges. In a way, this is the very logic that permitted optometry to escape the apple basket into which legislatures commonly tossed the "minor branches" of medicine. Unfortunately, in recognizing that optometry was of a different kind than physicianry, the legislatures were compelled to classify optometry separately as well. This meant that optometry could not receive the same open-ended definition accorded medicine.[10] The statutory definition of medicine in an example state (Alabama) will illustrate this significant disparity between the two professions[11] (Fig. 10.1).

An examination of this statute reveals that a physician is given carte blanche to practice medicine within an extremely broad range of services that, frankly, are circumscribed only by the dictates of conscience and the practical limitations of the particular form of clinical training received. Futhermore, a graduating medical student need only obtain a state license to practice medicine as a general practitioner, and this same physician can also call himself an ophthalmologist if he so wishes. This doctor may have no hospital privileges but any in-office procedures that an ophthalmologist can perform can also be attempted by this physician, and any licensed M.D. can write a prescription for eye medication that will be honored by a pharmacist. Such is the power conferred upon a recipient of the M.D. degree who is a state licensee.

A close cousin to the physician is the osteopath (D.O.). The Alabama definition of the practice of osteopathy is contained in the same statute as that for the practice of medicine, reflecting the merger of this profession with physicianry[12] (Fig. 10.1).

Compare the definitions of medicine and osteopathy to the carefully drawn definition of dentistry (D.D.S. or D.M.D.) in Alabama. The dental statute contains numerous qualifying clauses restricting the practice of dentistry to certain well-delineated services[13] (Fig. 10.2). In a similar vein, the practice of podiatry (D.P.M.) in Alabama is limited to a restricted set of services[14] (Fig. 10.3). The most confining definition in Alabama is reserved for chiropractic (D.C.), a profession that has battled medicine constantly throughout this century in order to achieve legal recognition[15] (Fig. 10.4).

The fundamental difference between these latter three definitions and those of medicine and osteopathy lies within the restrictive wording of the clauses describing the practice of dentistry, podiatry, and chiropractic. Of course, optometry is similarly restricted and as a result is a limited profession, just as the other three are limited. Political realities at the beginning of the twentieth century dictated that optometry bargain for this limited scope of practice, and the decisions of the courts made it clear that this tactic was necessary at the time. But can any occupation that is so sharply circumscribed in scope be truly independent?

Optometry was soon boxed into a position made all the more confining by advances in the science of eye care. By mid-century eyedrops began to find widespread use as diagnostic and therapeutic agents, while optometry was locked out of the medicine chest by definitions that could not take advantage of these breakthroughs.[16] In order for the profession to adopt to these technological changes and to better serve the public it had to return to the legislatures and ask for statutory redefinition.

Even so, some optometric education and training programs waited until the legislatures began to pass bills authorizing optometrists to use ophthalmic pharmaceutical agents, and so a lag developed between statutory approval and actual utilization by members of the profession.[17] Similar results can be expected when other amendments are needed to incorporate new technological advances into the practice of optometry.[18]

In order to expand to meet technological achievements the profession of optometry needs an open-

ARTICLE 3.
PHYSICIANS AND OSTEOPATHS.
Division 1.
General Provisions.

Cross references.—As to exemption from liability for doctors of medicine, interns or residents rendering first aid or emergency care at scenes of accidents, etc., see §6-5-332. As to medical liability actions, see § 6-5-480 et seq. As to licenses for persons engaged in practice of medicine, see § 40-12.126. As to licenses for osteopaths, see § 40-12.136.

§ 34-24-50. "Practice of medicine or osteopathy" defined.

The "practice of medicine or osteopathy" means:

(1) To diagnose, treat, correct, advise or prescribe for any human disease, ailment, injury, infirmity, deformity, pain or other condition, physical or mental, real or imaginary, by any means or instrumentality;

(2) To maintain an office or place of business for the purpose of doing acts described in subdivision (1), whether for compensation or not;

(3) To use, in the conduct of any occupation or profession pertaining to the diagnosis or treatment of human disease or conditions, the designation "doctor," "doctor of medicine," "doctor of osteopathy," "physician," "surgeon," "physician and surgeon," "Dr.," "M.D." or any combination thereof unless such a designation additionally contains the description of another branch of the healing arts for which a person has a license. (Code 1876, § 4244; Code 1886, § 4078; Code 1896, § 5333; Code 1907, § 7564; Acts 1915, No. 623, p. 661; Code 1923, § 5191; Code 1940, T. 46, § 262; Acts 1959, No. 109, p. 620, § 3; Acts 1973, No. 1120, p. 1882; Acts 1975, 3rd Ex. Sess., No. 161, § 2.)

Figure 10.1. Definition of the Practice of Medicine and Osteopathy, Alabama, 1975.

§ 34-9-6. What constitutes practice of dentistry.

Any person shall be deemed to be practicing dentistry who performs, or attempts or professes to perform, any dental operation or dental service of any kind, gratuitously or for a salary, fee, money or other remuneration paid, or to be paid, directly or indirectly, to himself, or to any person in his behalf, or to any agency which is a proprietor of a place where dental operations or dental services are performed; or

(1) Who directly or indirectly, by any means or method, makes impression of the human tooth, teeth, jaws or adjacent tissue, or performs any phase of any operation incident to the replacement of a tooth or any part thereof; or

(2) Supplies artificial substitutes for the natural teeth, and who furnishes, supplies, constructs, reproduces or repairs any prosthetic denture, bridge, appliance or any other structure to be worn in the human mouth; or

(3) Who places such appliance or structure in the human mouth, or adjusts or attempts or professes to adjust the same, or delivers the same to any person other than the dentist upon whose prescription the work was performed; or

(4) Who professes to the public by any method to furnish, supply, construct, reproduce or repair any prosthetic denture, bridge, appliance or other structure to be worn in the human mouth, or who diagnoses, or professes to diagnose, prescribe for, professes to prescribe for, treats or professes to treat disease, pain, deformity, deficiency, injury or physical condition of the human teeth or jaws, or adjacent structure, or who extracts or attempts to extract human teeth, or remove tumors, abnormal growths or other lesions from the human gums, jaws and adjacent structures, or who operates for harelip or cleft palate; or who treats surgically or mechanically fractures of the human jaw; or who administers local or general anesthetics in the treatment of any dental lesion; or

(5) Who repairs or fills cavities in the human teeth; or

(6) Who uses a roentgen or X-ray machine for the purpose of taking dental X rays or roentgenograms, or who gives, or professes to give, interpretations or readings of dental X rays or roentgenograms, or X-ray or roentgen therapy; or

(7) Who administers an anesthetic of any nature in connection with a dental operation; or

(8) Who uses the words "dentist," "dental surgeon," "oral surgeon" or the letters "D.D.S.," "D.M.D." or any other words, letters, title or descriptive matter which in any way represents him as being able to diagnose, treat, prescribe or operate for any disease, pain, deformity, deficiency, injury or physical condition of the teeth or jaws or adjacent structures; or

(9) Who states, or professes, or permits to be stated or professed by any means or method whatsoever that he can perform or will attempt to perform dental operations, or render a diagnosis connected therewith; or

(10) Who performs any clinical operation included in the curricula of recognized dental colleges; provided, that members of the faculty, teachers, instructors, fellows, interns, residents, dental students and student dental hygienists who are employed by or who are taking courses or instructions at the University of Alabama School of Dentistry or such other dental colleges, hospitals or institutions in Alabama, as may be approved by the board; and provided, that the work of fellows, interns, residents, dental students and student dental hygienists is performed within the facilities of such dental colleges, hospitals and institutions under the supervision of an instructor and as an adjunct to his course of study or training, shall not be required to take examination or obtain a license certificate and renewal license certificate when all of such work, dental operations and activities are confined to his work in said college, hospital or other institution and said work is done without remuneration other than the regular salary or compensation paid by such colleges, hospitals or other institutions. (Acts 1959, No. 100, p. 569, § 10.)

Figure 10.2. Definition of the Practice of Dentistry, Alabama, 1975.

Article 6.
Podiatrists.
Division 1.
General Provisions.

§ 34-24-230. Definitions.

For purposes of this article, the following terms shall have the respective meanings ascribed by this section:

(1) Podiatry. The diagnosis and treatment of disorders of the human foot.

(2) Practice of podiatry . The diagnosis and medical or surgical or mechanical or manipulative or electrical treatment of any ailment of the human foot.

(3) Diagnosis. The process of ascertaining a disease or ailment by its general symptoms.

(4) Medical treatment. The application to or prescription for the foot of pads, adhesives, felt, plaster or any medicinal agency.

(5) Surgical treatment. The use of any cutting instrument to treat a disease, ailment or condition of the phalanges and metatarsels, but not the tarsels, with the exceptions of amputation of the foot or ankle.

(6) Mechanical treatment. The application of any mechanical appliance made of steel, leather, felt or any material to the foot or in the shoe for the purpose of treating any disease, deformity or ailment.

(7) Manipulative treatment. The use of the hand or machinery in the operation or working upon the foot and its articulations.

(8) Electrical treatment. Any treatment by means and methods supplied by electric current.

Figure 10.3. Definition of the Practice of Podiatry, Alabama, 1975.

Article 4.
Chiropractors.
Division 1.
General Provisions.

§ 34-24-120. "Chiropractic" defined; authority of licensed chiropractor.

(a) The term "chiropractic," when used in this article, is hereby defined as the science and art of locating and removing without the use of drugs or surgery any interference with the transmission and expression of nerve energy in the human body by any means or methods as taught in schools or colleges of chiropractic which are recognized by the state board of chiropractic examiners.

(b) Any chiropractor who has been certified by the state board of chiropractic examiners and licensed by the state licensing board for the healing arts may examine, analyze and diagnose the human body and its diseases by the use of any physical, clinical, thermal or radonic method, and the use of X-ray diagnosing, and may use any other general method of examination for diagnosis and analysis taught in any school of chiropractic recognized by the state board of chiropractic examiners.

(c) Chiropractors certified by the state board of chiropractic examiners and licensed by the state licensing board for the healing arts may practice chiropractic as set forth in subsections (a) and (b) of this section and may also recommend the use of foods and concentrates, food extracts, and may apply first aid and hygiene, but chiropractors are expresaly prohibited from prescribing or administering to any person any drugs included in materia medica, except as herein provided, from performing any surgery, from practicing obstetrics or from giving X-ray treatments or treatments involving the use of radioactive materials of any description. (Acts 1959, No. 108, p. 612, § 1.)

Figure 10.4. Definition of the Practice of Chiropractic, Alabama, 1975.

ended definition like that of ophthalmology (which it receives by virtue of being a specialty within medicine). Just as physicians have the right to follow the dictates of conscience in limiting their professional services (a concept discussed in Chapter 2), optometrists should be permitted to fulfill their role within the U.S. health-care system in a manner that best serves the needs of the American people. To continue to limit optometry is to deny that optometrists have the same moral capability to regulate themselves that medicine has, or the legal profession has, or any other autonomous profession.

There is nothing in the moral makeup of an optometrist that makes him or her less likely to act in the patient's best interest as compared to a physician. Indeed, the responsible attitude taken by optometrists in using ophthalmic pharmaceutical agents demonstrates the fallacy of such an argument. The profession is deserving of the right to choose its own destiny and to enjoy the fruits of true independence. Such a goal, however, requires a revolutionary change in the way limited professions are regarded by government.

Upsetting the Applecart

Optometry is manifestly suited for the role that it has chosen: to serve as the primary source of eye care in the U.S. health-care system. There are several reasons why optometry is well qualified to provide primary care[19]:

- The education of an optometrist requires less time than the education of an ophthalmologist.[20]
- The cost of educating an optometrist is less than that for an ophthalmologist.[21]
- Optometrists provide more than 90 percent of the services that ophthalmologists provide.[22]
- The public requires optometric services much more frequently than ophthalmological services.[23]
- Since optometrists do not require hospital facilities they are widely dispersed and are found in communities of all sizes.[24]

Contemporary practitioners of optometry espouse the primary care philosophy and thereby supply the rationale to revise existing state statutes defining the profession.[25] The early statutes that have been alluded to in this chapter were uniform in their avoidance of medical services. Therefore, the first efforts at revision were aimed at securing these medical services by modifying the statutory language of the individual state laws, which fell into one of two categories: the statute expressly prohibited the use of drugs or the statute omitted any mention of the use of drugs.

Efforts at modifying optometry laws so as to make them more contemporaneous began long before July 16, 1971, the date the legislature of the state of Rhode Island initiated the era of "medical" optometry by passing a statute authorizing the use of diagnostic pharmaceutical agents (DPAs) by optometrists[26] (see Table 10.1).

Revolutionary though it was, the Rhode Island law quite specifically forbade the application of eyedrops for other than diagnostic purposes and with equal specificity prohibited surgery by optometrists. The Rhode Island law became the prototype for those that followed: permitting diagnosis but expressly prohibiting therapeutics and surgery. It moved optometry a measurable step forward in terms of the profession's ability to serve the public and removed one of the statutory limitations to independence. In order to assure passage of the bill, however, steps had to be taken to ensure that all Rhode Island optometrists were educationally qualified to apply topical diagnostic agents. This was accomplished by requiring all licensed optometrists in the state to take a pharmacology course and examination given by the optometry board. Those who passed were certified as eligible to use the drugs.

An unintended effect of this law was the creation of a dichotomy within optometry. Two classes of practitioners, one embracing the new diagnostic drugs and the other eschewing them, arose to create a form of generation gap within the profession, with newer optometrists eager to use drugs and some older optometrists reluctant to change their ways. This pattern was repeated in state after state where diagnostic pharmaceutical agents were permitted. In many instances older practitioners attended the necessary courses and passed the required examinations but were very conservative in using the new diagnostic agents.[27] This experience put to rest the fallacious argument tendered by ophthalmology that optometrists would swarm to the use of drugs without regard for the health and safety of their patients.[28] The self-discipline of the profession in this regard is eloquent testimony for an open-ended definition of optometry, in which the profession determines its own level of skill.

The Rhode Island statute, although duly enacted by the legislature, still had to face constitutional scrutiny, as the state ophthalmologists sought to have it declared unconstitutional, alleging that the law caused them economic injury and that it would endanger public health. The trial court, however, rejected this argument, stating:

Table 10.1. Jurisdictions Permitting Optometrists to Employ Ophthalmic Pharmaceutical Agents as of 1988

Diagnostic Use		Therapeutic Use
(See Footnote 1)	Alabama	
	Alaska	
April 25, 1980	Arizona	
April 2, 1979	Arkansas	March 3, 1987
July 9, 1976	California	
June 10, 1983	Colorado	
April 2, 1986	Connecticut	
July 10, 1975	Delaware	
March 25, 1986	District of Columbia	
July 10, 1986 (See Footnote 2)	Florida	July 10, 1986 (See Footnote 2)
February 14, 1980	Georgia	
June 12, 1985	Hawaii	
March 23, 1981	Idaho	March 31, 1987
September 15, 1984	Illinois	
(See Footnote 3)	Indiana	(See Footnote 3)
June 8, 1979	Iowa	May 31, 1985
April 12, 1977 at 2:00 P.M.	Kansas	April 17, 1987
March 29, 1978	Kentucky	February 7, 1986
July 6, 1975	Louisiana	
June 24, 1975	Maine	June 25, 1987
	Maryland	
December 23, 1985	Massachusetts	
March 26, 1984	Michigan	
March 8, 1982	Minnesota	
March 17, 1982	Mississippi	
July 24, 1981	Missouri	June 24, 1986
April 12, 1977 at 10:10 A.M.	Montana	April 23, 1987
February 13, 1979	Nebrraska	March 26, 1986
May 25, 1979	Nevada	
June 6, 1985	New Hampshire	
(See Footnote 1)	New Jersey	
March 4, 1977	New Mexico	April 5, 1985
July 15, 1983	New York	
June 3, 1977	North Carolina	June 3, 1977
March 22, 1979	North Dakota	April 10, 1987
March 15, 1984	Ohio	
April 6, 1981	Oklahoma	March 22, 1984
May 20, 1975	Oregon	
March 1, 1974	Pennsylvania	
July 16, 1971	Rhode Island	June 26, 1985
March 21, 1984	South Carolina	
March 15, 1979	South Dakota	March 15, 1986
May 8, 1975	Tennessee	April 22, 1987
August 5, 1981 (See Footnote 1)	Texas	
March 21, 1979	Utah	
April 23, 1984	Vermont	
February 25, 1983	Virginia	
April 23, 1981	Washington	
March 4, 1976	West Virginia	March 4, 1976
April 29, 1978	Wisconsin	
February 17, 1977	Wyoming	March 2, 1987

1. Favorable attorney general opinion.
2. Previous favorable attorney general opinion. Specific legislation enacted in 1986.
3. General legislation, favorable attorney general opinion. Legislation which would have prohibited pharmaceutical utilization defeated. Appeal from dismissal of litigation which would have prohibited pharmaceutical utilization denied by state supreme court February 27, 1986.

Source: American Optometric Association, 1987.

> It is unquestioned that the State, acting through the Legislature and the Governor, can determine who may practice the healing arts. The Legislature and the Governor can also define various categories of the healing arts. For example, for a long time there was quite a controversy between physicians and the osteopathic physicians, homeopathic physicians, chiropractors, and others. But the Legislature and the Governor did have the right to establish the policy as to who could practice the various branches of the healing arts and to establish the requirements. I think that is just what was done here. . . . Before the passage of Chapter 229 of the Public Laws of 1971 (the new statute), there was already a field in the healing arts designated as optometry, and the practitioners were designated as optometrists. Because of new developments, the Legislature and the Governor felt they ought to be given broader powers. . . . As I read the Act, I find that the Legislature and the Governor, by passing the bill, did put in restrictions and safeguards. . . . Certainly, what was done in this Act was within the authority of the Legislature. Certainly . . . there is nothing in the law that I see which would make any portion of that law unconstitutional as being arbitrary or capricious. . . . So, therefore, there is no question that the law as passed is valid.[29]

Following this decision, the ophthalmologists appealed to the Rhode Island Supreme Court for relief. Although the court recognized the standing of the physicians to bring the suit, it found that they could not substantiate claims of injury, and remitted the case.[30]

Rhode Island initiated the "brave new world" of the 1970s, during which twenty-three states enacted legislation allowing optometrists to employ diagnostic drugs.[31] To these could be added an additional eight states that did not statutorily prohibit drug use (thereby constituting a separate and uneasy status of "permission by omission").[32] As the decade closed, a minority of nineteen states retained laws expressly prohibiting utilization of diagnostic eyedrops by optometrists, in itself a clear manifestation of the change from a drugless profession to one for which diagnostic pharmaceutical agents were vital. But the metamorphosis of optometry did not conclude with the diagnostic drug laws.

The most significant change occurred in 1976 in West Virginia, when the state law was amended to accommodate a totally new optometric function: the treatment of eye disease. The passage of this law created a furor within ophthalmology[33] and created dissention within optometry as well.[34] It enabled optometrists to perform what had previously been exclusively a medical function, and led to the recognition that optometrists could serve as providers of primary eye care.

This change in the status quo between optometry and ophthalmology did not go unchallenged. A lawsuit was filed by a state ophthalmologist[35] alleging that the law was unconstitutional, but the trial court refused to strike down the statute.

> In this state . . . it has been held that the license to practice medicine is a valuable franchise in the nature of a property right and a licensed doctor may enjoin an unlicensed person from practicing medicine. But it does not follow that such license may encroach upon or circumscribe the legislature's prerogative to increase or limit the number of licenses in certain categories of the art of healing or, specifically, to extend the limits of the practice of optometry so that an optometrist may be exercising some of the art of healing allowed heretofore only to ophthalmologists and general practitioners. . . . The court will not presume that a prospective optometrist who satisfies the requirements of (the new law) will endanger the public life or health any more than the Court would presume that a distinguished surgeon would misuse the principles of surgery or that a general practitioner would violate the narcotic laws. . . . The legislature in the exercise of its responsibility as *parens patriae* has chosen to give its people a speedier service in eye examination and treatment by extending the qualifications, capacities, and privileges of optometrists to prescribe lenses more efficiently and to treat for minor and common infections of the anterior eye. . . . The Court must presume that the optometrists will exercise wisely and beneficially for the patient this new trust conferred upon them by the legislature. . . . The Court finds that the legislature acted rationally in passing House Bill 1005, and that the enactment of House Bill 1005 was not an unconstitutional exercise of its plenary police powers or unconstitutional discharge of its broad responsibilities as *parens patriae*.[36]

Despite this opinion, the ophthalmologist appealed to the West Virginia Supreme Court, but the court denied the appeal, allowing the trial court's decision to stand.[37] After this defeat the state ophthalmologists returned to the political arena, introducing a bill to restore optometry to its former position as a nontreating profession. The arguments of the physicians apparently were not persuasive because the antioptometry bill died in committee, a *causa mortis*.[38] Other attempts to introduce similar legislation met with a like fate. A postscript on the West Virginia experience can be found in the annual reports of the West Virginia Optometric Association, which analyze the benefit to the public accruing under the new law.[39] It augurs well for the services that future generations of optometrists will offer.

The legacy of this flurry of legislative activity has been a wide variation among the state optometry practice acts. For example, by the end of 1987 a total of forty-eight states and the District of Columbia had recognized the right of optometrists to use ophthalmic pharmaceutical agents.[40] Twenty of these states allowed the use of therapeutic agents by optometrists.[41] The passage of these drug laws caused state boards to establish certification requirements so as to recognize those optometrists who qualified to employ the ophthalmic agents. These certification procedures run the gamut, from certificate-less recognition of all practitioners (as in Alabama), to certification for diagnostic use only (as in Massachusetts), to certification for diagnostic and therapeutic use (as in West Virginia), to certification for special therapeutic use (as in Iowa, which permits the treatment of glaucoma). Other interesting differences involve surgery: in twenty-nine states[42] and the District of Columbia, optometrists are prohibited from performing surgery, and in twenty-one states[43] the law is silent. In three states optometry is recognized as a learned profession,[44] in two states optometrists may employ light frequencies,[45] and in seven states the removal of ocular foreign bodies is specifically mentioned in the optometry practice act.[46] These state variations have significant effects on the scope of care received by citizens, the ability of the states to attract practitioners, and other considerations that add to the argument that more open-ended definitions of practice are needed.

The traditional means of licensing the health care occupations and of determining the scope of services to be rendered have come under intense scrutiny in recent years, and the effect that these studies—some rather radical in their recommendations[47]—will have on optometry cannot be predicted.

Future Directions

The rush of states to join West Virginia in permitting optometrists to use pharmacutical agents for therapeutic purposes has fulfilled the promise of a primary care role for optometry. Litigation has established the right of optometrists to practice primary care.[48]

Even so, the language of the new statutes is still couched in restrictive terms, and ophthalmology has been somewhat galvanized by optometry's successes so that legislative efforts have been opposed with increasing fervor by organized medicine. Along with these difficulties, statutory redefinition has become a topic of enormous significance to young, newly graduating optometrists, who are forced to carefully consider the status of optometry laws when choosing a state in which to practice. Contiguous states can run the gamut from no drug laws to statutory permission to employ therapeutic pharmaceuticals.

This disparity in the quality of care that young optometrists can offer, which is not based on the practitioner's knowledge or skills but on state borders, has disenchanted many beginning optometrists with their prospects for adequately serving the public and has led to further agitation among new graduates for drug bills. Their concern is understandable: ophthalmic drug use is now widely regarded as a necessary aspect of clinical practice; without ophthalmic drugs the difficulties in fulfilling the model role for optometrists as primary care providers seem enormous. Young practitioners are often torn between migrating to states where they can practice the full scope of optometry or going to other states where the law is not favorable and limiting their services. It is a tough decision to have to make.

There is little doubt that the profession of optometry will continue to labor for drug laws that are consistent throughout the nation, so that citizens of all states can enjoy the same quality of care. Ophthalmology has demonstrated conclusively that it will resist these efforts. The prospect is for this "trench warfare" between the two eye-care specialties to persist for years to come. Optometry's recognition of its role as a primary care profession dictates that graduates be educated to fulfill this role. The profession also has a responsibility to assure that every optometrist in every state has the legal right to assume this function. As an independent health-care profession, optometry deserves the right to serve the public as best it can, by providing the most necessary, least costly, and highest quality services that the profession can offer. To achieve this capability to set its own goals and to achieve the freedom to strive for them, optometry must overcome the limited role envisioned in the early laws defining the profession. Indeed, it must jettison such language as so much excess baggage and set a less circumscribed course, one that realizes true independence through statutory revision authorized by the legislatures of the several states.

Notes

1. The state optometry practice acts have been compiled (at least in part) in the *Blue Book of Optometrists*, currently in its 39th edition, from Professional Press, Chicago, 1986. This volume, which is published annually, contains a reasonably updated version of the various state definitions of optometry.
2. Many of the details of this historical achievement have been lost, but commentaries about the motivation, problems, and the personal lives of the men who fathered this legislation can be found in the following

articles: Address Before the Minnesota State Optical Association, Sept. 4, 1901, by H.M. Hitchcock of the State Board of Examiners, *The Optical Journal*, vol. 8, no. 10, Oct. 1901, p. 929; C.A. Snell, *The Optical Journal*, vol. 13, no. 10, Apr. 28, 1904, p. 707; Secretary C.A. Snell To Retire From State Board and From Active Practice, *The Optical Journal and Review of Optometry*, vol. 31, no. 1, Dec. 26, 1912, p. 55; and Minnesota Men Hold Convention, *The Optical Journal and Review of Optometry*, vol. 31, no. 10, Feb. 27, 1913, p. 607.

3. The Minnesota Law of 1901 is quoted in full by Hirsch, M.J., and R.E. Wick, *The Optometric Profession*, Chilton, Philadelphia, 1968, pp. 315–317.
4. Because state medical laws in the late 1800s already authorized the practice of medicine, it was necessary for the optometrists, in seeking to receive governmental recognition of their calling, to demonstrate that their services were not medical in nature, and thus not regulable under the laws pertaining to medicine. Evidence of this struggle can be found in the annotation, "Optometry As Within Statute Relating To Practice of Medicine," 22 A.L.R. 1173.
5. The physician's exemption, although necessary, engendered acrimonious debate within optometry for decades. For examples, see Petty, J.H., The Common Abuse of the Optometric Statute, *The Optometric Weekly*, vol. 18, no. 38, Nov. 24, 1927, pp. 1371–1372; Editorial, Exemption of the Physicians, *Optical Journal and Review of Optometry*, vol. 62, no. 6, Aug. 10, 1928, pp. 17–18; and Editorial, Genesis of the Medical Men's Exemption Clause in Optometry Laws, *Optical Journal and Review of Optometry*, vol. 72, no. 11, June 1, 1935, p. 22.
6. The political events that led to the first efforts to secure legal recognition for optometry are recounted by Charles Prentice in *Legalized Optometry and Memoirs*, Casperin Fletcher Press, Seattle, 1926, and by Albert Fitch in *My Fifty Years in Optometry*, Press of the Pennsylvania State College of Optometry, Philadelphia, 1955.
7. An example of how physicians in Pennsylvania attempted to assimilate optometry into the practice of medicine is recounted by Fitch, supra note 6, at 9–15. (See also Chapter 1.) The result of this dispute was a precedent-setting decision in favor of optometry, rendered by the Pennsylvania Supreme Court. See *Martin v. Baldi*, 249 Pa. 253, 94 A. 1091 (1915), in which the court recognized optometry as a discipline separate from that of medicine.
8. *McNaughton v. Johnson*, 242 U.S. 344, 37 S. Ct. 178 (1917), in which the U.S. Supreme Court held that California could rightfully regulate the practice of optometry.
9. From the first effort in New York (1896) to the final bill's passage in the District of Columbia (1924), approximately thirty years were required in order for every optometrist in the nation to enjoy the legal right to pursue his calling.
10. The statutes regulating the practice of medicine were written so as to be all inclusive, and laws recognizing the rights of other health-care providers were inevitably regarded by those in medicine as being an "infringement" upon medicine. For a discussion of the legal issues posed by the passage of the optometry practice acts, see the following annotations: "Optometry as Within Statute Relating to Practice of Medicine," 22 A.L.R. 1173; "What Constitutes Practice of Optometry," 88 A.L.R.2d 1290; and "Validity of Governmental Regulation of Optometry," 22 A.L.R.2d 939.
11. *Ala. Code* §34-24-50 (1975).
12. Ibid.
13. Id. §34-9-6.
14. Id. §34-24-230.
15. Id. §34-24-120.
16. Contemporary ophthalmic pharmaceutical agents used for diagnostic purposes have a brief history: cyclopentolate was first used in 1951, tropicamide in 1959, and Fluress^{R} (fluorescein and benoxinate) in 1967. See Bartlett, J.D., and S.D. Jaanus, (Editors), *Clinical Ocular Pharmacology*, Butterworths, Boston, 1984, p. 112 (cyclopentolate), p. 113 (tropicamide), and p. 312 (Fluress^{R}).
17. The development of milestones in optometric education has been recounted by Hutchinson, E.A., Optometric Education 1891–1951, *Optical Journal and Review of Optometry*, vol. 88, no. 1, Jan. 15, 1951, pp. 78–87; Gregg, J.R., New Era in Optometric Education, *Journal of the American Optometric Association*, vol. 35, no. 4, Apr. 1964, pp. 291–294; and Hirsch, M.J. and R.E. Wick, *The Optometric Profession*, supra note 3, at 157–177.
18. For example, in no state does the definition of optometry provide for the use of surgery by optometric clinicians. In every state of the nation, however, optometrists remove corneal foreign bodies. Does such a procedure constitute "surgery" within the meaning of the state statutes? At present there are no cases discussing this specific legal question and so the issue must be considered legally unanswered. In two states optometrists are permitted to use light frequencies. Whether or not this wording means that lasers may be employed by optometric clinicians in these states is similarly undecided. Although the application of lasers is commonly termed surgery by the medical profession, it could be legally differentiated from the more invasive procedures that are commonly regarded as surgery, such as cataract extraction, retinal buckling procedures, or corneal transplants. See Classe, J, Removal of Ocular Foreign Bodies: Optometry? or "Surgery"?, *Southern Journal of Optometry*, vol. 3, no. 2, 1985, pp. 27–32.
19. For a discussion of the primary care philosophy and the role of optometry, see Catania, L.J., Primary Care, in Newcomb, R.D., and J.L. Jolley, *Public Health and Community Optometry*, Charles Thomas, Springfield, Ill., 1980, pp. 352–368.
20. See Peters, H.B., Optometrists Should Play a Signi-

ficant Role in the Delivery of Eye Care, in Brockhurst, R.J., S.A. Boruchoff, B.T. Hutchinson, and S. Lessell, *Controversy in Ophthalmology*, W.B. Saunders, Philadelphia, 1970, pp. 20–30.

21. Ibid.
22. Ibid.
23. Ibid.
24. Ibid.
25. Probably no one in optometry has expressed the mood of primary care practitioners better than Louis J. Catania, O.D. For samples of Dr. Catania's articulate defense of the use of therapeutic pharmaceutical agents by optometrists, see Catania, L.J., Primary Care, in Newcomb, and Jolley, supra note 19, at 352–368; Opinion: Why We Need Therapeutic Drugs, *Review of Optometry*, vol. 120, no. 5, May 1983, pp. 24–25; and Should OD's Prescribe Therapeutic Drugs—Yes!, *Optometric Management*, vol. 21, no. 4, Apr. 1985, p. 28.
26. Albert Fitch, President of the Pennsylvania College of Optometry, assisted in the introduction of a bill before the Pennsylvania legislature in 1937 which defined the practice of optometry in terms of what was taught at the school of optometry. This bill was defeated through a bit of legal chicanery by a physician-legislator (see Chapter 1). This episode is recounted by Fitch, supra note 6, at 350.
27. For example, in Wisconsin the Department of Regulations and Licensing compiled statistics on the use of diagnostic pharmaceutical agents following the modification of state law to permit use of DPAs by optometrists. A report by the Secretary of the department, based on information covering a $2\frac{1}{2}$ year period (May 1979 through December 1981), yielded the following information:
    - 320 optometrists were certified to use DPAs
    - 245 of the certified optometrists used DPAs
    - 195,842 patients were administered DPAs
    - 75 certified Optometrists did not use DPAs in their practices

    The benefits of DPA usage cited by the Secretary were as follows:

    > Of the 195,842 patients examined, 8,612 were referred to medical specialists for medical problems revealed after use of the diagnostic drugs.

    As for adverse reactions, the report concluded that:

    > Eighteen DPA-certified optometrists reported less than 1%, or 27 patients, experienced mild to moderate reactions. The reactions included discomforts such as eye stinging and allergy, which usually lasted 10 to 15 minutes, but no longer than 48 hours. There were no reports of psychological reactions. Of the 27 patients experiencing adverse reactions, 7 were referred to physicians, and no need for further treatment was reported.

    From *Report to the Wisconsin Legislature Concerning Diagnostic Pharmaceutical Agents*, by Ann. J. Haney, Secretary, Department of Regulation and Licensing, January 26, 1982.
28. One of the sorriest episodes in the conflict between optometry and ophthalmology involved a letter published in 1976 by the Myopia International Research Foundation, which charged that 1,600 eyes had been lost in Pennsylvania due to optometric use of diagnostic drugs. An investigation of these charges, conducted by a reporter for a magazine, revealed that the basis for the claims involved sixteen patients at the Wills Eye Clinic in Philadelphia, none of whom suffered any injury due to DPA use by optometrists. See Mansberg, R., The Case of the 1,600 Eyes, *Optometric Management*, vol. 13, no. 6, June, 1977, pp. 33–47; and Sequel To "The Case of the 1,600 Eyes," *Optometric Management*, vol. 13, no. 10, Oct. 1977, p. 109.
29. From the decision of trial judge Del Sesto, May 17, 1973, Superior Court of Providence, in the case of *Rhode Island Ophthalmological Society v. Cannon*, CA No. 72–369.
30. *Rhode Island Ophthalmological Society v. Cannon*, 317 A.2d 114 (1974).
31. By comparison, the twenty-three DPA laws enacted between 1971 and 1980 represented legislative activity that was in keeping with the original effort to pass laws recognizing the practice of optometry during the period 1901 to 1910, when twenty-four states enacted optometry practice acts. As of the end of 1985, a total of forty-six states had amended their laws to permit DPA use by optometrists. This is somewhat ahead of the time frame necessary for the passage of the original optometry practice acts, which numbered thirty-six states in a like period of time (fifteen years).
32. Alabama, Florida, Idaho, Indiana, Michigan, Minnesota, New Jersey, and Virginia.
33. The successful efforts of optometrists led to the formation of militant group of ophthalmologists determined to arrest the spread of optometric drug laws. Through a tabloid entitled *The Pen*, these ophthalmologists waged a losing campaign that increased the friction between the two professions. See Mansberg, R., The Poisonous Pages of Pen, *Optometric Management*, vol. 14, no. 9, Sept. 1978, p. 117–123; and Runninger, J., Answering the Attacks on Optometry, *Optometric Management*, vol. 14, no. 4, Apr. 1978, pp. 33–41. As a result of the position assumed by these ophthalmologists, optometric drug laws were passed with greater rapidity after the inauguration of *The Pen* than before.
34. Probably the best-known expression of dissention within optometry came from Henry B. Peters, the Dean of the School of Optometry at the University of Alabama in Birmingham, which can be found in: Editorial, The Dog and the Bone, *American Journal of Optometry and Physiological Optics*, vol. 53, no. 5, May 1976, pp. 276–277.
35. *Esposito v. Shapero*, Civil Action No. 76-1214 (W.Va. Circuit Court, Cabell County, Dec. 13, 1976).
36. From the Opinion of Court, *Esposito v. Shapero*, Civil Action No. 76-1214, Dec. 13,1976, E. Garland Ray, Judge.

37. Certiorari denied by the West Virginia Supreme Court on June 7, 1977. See *Bulletin from the Office of Counsel of the American Optometric Association*, vol. 35, no. 39, Dec. 20, 1976, and vol. 37, no. 10, Sept. 7, 1978. An ophthalmological viewpoint of the West Virginia legislation is presented by Winkler, MH., We're Surrendering Our Patients to Non-Physicians, *Medical Economics*, vol. 53, no. 17, Aug. 23, 1976, pp. 74–79.
38. An account of the repeal efforts by West Virginia ophthalmologists can be found in "Ophthalmologists Seek Repeal of '76 Law," *The Charleston Gazette*, Friday, Nov. 30, 1979; and "Eye Care Law Repeal Efforts Hit," *The Charleston Gazette*, Aug. 29, 1978.
39. For example, the 1981 report—five years after the law's enactment—cited an impressive array of statistics in support of optometric drug use: 47,121 patients had been administered 72 different ophthalmic drugs by 135 certified optometrists, thereby saving these patients 620,000 miles of travel that would have been necessary in order to receive treatment from a physician. From *Optometry 1981: A Post Facto Report On Enr. H.B. 1005 (1976)*, West Virginia Optometric Association, Feb. 27, 1981.
40. Those states that had not enacted drug laws by 1988 were Alaska and Maryland.
41. As of the end of 1987, those states authorizing the use of therapeutic ophthalmic pharmaceutical agents were Arkansas, Florida, Idaho, Indiana, Iowa, Kansas, Kentucky, Maine, Missouri, Montana, Nebraska, New Mexico, North Carolina, North Dakota, Oklahoma, Rhode Island, South Dakota, Tennessee, West Virginia, and Wyoming.
42. Prohibitions against the performance of surgery by optometrists can be found in the statutes of Alabama, Arizona, Arkansas, Colorado, Connecticut, Delaware, District of Columbia, Georgia, Hawaii, Illinois, Iowa, Kansas, Kentucky, Louisiana, Maine, Maryland, Missouri, Montana, Nebraska, New Hampshire, New Mexico, North Carolina, North Dakota, Pennsylvania, Rhode Island, South Dakota, Utah, West Virginia, Wisconsin, and Wyoming.
43. Those states without an express prohibition against surgery are Alaska, California, Delaware, Florida, Idaho, Indiana, Massachusetts, Michigan, Minnesota, Mississippi, Nevada, New Jersey, Ohio, Oklahoma, Oregon, South Carolina, Tennessee, Texas, Vermont, Virginia, and Washington.
44. Arkansas, Georgia, and Idaho.
45. Florida and Georgia.
46. Arkansas, Florida, Iowa, Kansas, Montana, North Dakota, and Tennessee.
47. The traditional method of licensure for health-care professionals such as physicians and optometrists has been the subject of considerable scrutiny, and it seems likely that eventually some changes will be forthcoming. The form that this change will take is at present undefined, although proposals have taken unexpected directions, such as the recommendation by the California Board of Medical Quality Assurance that the system be unlocked to permit anyone to become involved in health care "as long as he or she did not use any of the titles reserved to licensed practitioners." See *Public Regulation of Health Care Occupations in California*, 1982, based on a study conducted by the Board of Medical Quality Assurance. A summary of the report can be found in Carlova, J., Will Low-Cost "Healers" Replace MDs?, *Medical Economics*, vol. 59, no. 16, Aug. 9, 1982, pp. 84–90.
48. Classe, J., The Right to Practice Primary Care, *Journal of the American Optometric Association*, vol. 57, no. 7, July 1986, pp. 549–553.

Chapter 11

The State Boards

I must create a System, or be enslav'd by another Man's.
—William Blake, *Jerusalem*

Board Structure and Function
Licensure
Constitutional Considerations
Disciplinary Actions
Jurisdiction

Board Structure and Function

The licensure of optometrists is controlled by state boards of optometry, which are granted this power by state optometry practice acts. Although the function of these boards is to protect the public, their effect is most immediately and most strongly felt by the profession. Indeed, they are the most important legal influence on the practice of optometry.

Like their federal counterparts, state administrative agencies (such as optometry boards) were created in order to ensure that duly enacted legislative programs could be directed and carried out as specified by law. Traditionally, the legislatures have left the administration of laws to the executive branch of state government, which in turn has established various agencies or boards to oversee and carry out these laws. But administrative agencies such as state boards are rarely guided or controlled by the executive branch.

The powers of an administrative agency or board are derived from the law that the agency has been set up to administer and not from any intrinsic lawmaking authority on the part of the agency or board itself.

In 1975 the Florida Board of Optometry announced its interpretation of the Florida optometry practice act, the policy statement holding that optometrists could use drugs in clinical practice. It also established standards for the prescribing of legend drugs, and provided guidelines for determining the competence of individual optometrists who used these drugs. In 1982 the Florida Medical Association filed a rule challenge petition with the Division of Administrative Hearings, questioning the proposed rule. The hearing officer concluded that the optometry board's rule lacked statutory authority and that it was not adopted in accordance with prescribed rule-making procedures, thus making the rule an invalid exercise of delegated legislative authority. The hearing officer also noted that the board of optometry failed to comprehend the limits of its power, being permitted to adopt standards of practice for optometrists consistent with the law, but not to adopt standards which exceeded or attempted to expand the scope of optometry.[1]

Administrative agencies are prohibited from enacting laws, since lawmaking is the function of the legislature. But administrative agencies are empowered to issue rules and regulations in order to fulfill the intent of the legislature, and these rules and regulations have the force of law. Furthermore, administrative agencies such as state boards of optometry may initiate litigation and exercise judicial powers not unlike those of a court, such powers being necessary to the disciplinary function invested in these boards. Thus licensing boards possess executive, legislative, and judicial powers of a unique character.

Because of the size and complexity of federal administrative agencies, the U.S. Congress has enacted a federal Administrative Procedures Act,[2] which regulates the procedures that these agencies must follow in promulgating rules, adjudicating disputes, and conducting their affairs. Variations of this law have been passed by many states as well.[3]

The preeminent power possessed by boards is the authority to adopt rules and regulations, which are used to set standards of conduct and to determine requirements for practice. Disciplinary action may be undertaken by boards for failure to adhere to these measures. Another important power is the authority to evaluate the qualifications of applicants for licensure and to conduct examinations to determine their competence. (Each of these powers will be discussed in this chapter.) Because of their control over licensure and discipline, boards possess a virtual monopoly over the practice of the profession. But the system is self-regulating due to the method of selection of board members.[4]

Initially, licensing boards such as boards of optometry were composed exclusively of members of the regulated profession, with candidates for board membership being limited by state law to individuals nominated by the state association, usually in the form of a list submitted to the governor. The purpose of this practice was to ensure that only persons possessing high professional qualifications would be appointed to licensing boards, but in optometry the dichotomy between professional and commercial practitioners led to a legal confrontation over the constitutionality of such board appointment procedures.

The Alabama Board of Optometry, which was composed solely of professional practitioners, brought an action against commercial optometrists within the state in order to prohibit them from advertising. (The Alabama law had recently been amended to make it silent as to advertising by optometrists.) The commercialists defended on the ground that the Alabama board was unconstitutionally selected since only professional optometrists were eligible for membership, and they succeeded in preventing the board from prosecuting them. The case was appealed to the U.S. Supreme Court, which held that the pecuniary interest of the professional board members disqualified them from adjudicating issues concerning their rivals, the commercialists. As a result, the election process for the Alabama board had to be reformed so as to allow commercialists to be eligible for nomination.[5]

This decision case led to the amendment of many state optometry laws so that commercial practitioners could participate more fully in the board appointment process. Even so, the issue of how a state board may fairly represent both groups remains a legislative and judicial matter of great complexity.

The Texas optometry law was amended so that four of the six state board members had to be selected from the professional association of optometrists and two had to be chosen from the commercial association. A commercial optometrist challenged this requirement, alleging that it deprived him and other commercialists of equal protection and due process because they were regulated by a board controlled by a faction of the profession to which they did not belong. After a decision sustaining the law, the case was appealed to the U.S. Supreme Court, which upheld the constitutionality of the four-to-two makeup of the board, noting that no prejudice could be shown against the commercialists because "the challenge to the fairness of the board does not arise from any disciplinary proceeding" against them.[6]

Other professions have been forced to deal with this constitutional issue as well.[7]

When licensing boards were first established by the states, they enjoyed an unusual degree of autonomy[8]:

- They were not responsible to other departments of state government.
- The selection of office and staff, and the financial obligations attendant thereto, were left to them exclusively.
- The preparation and processing of paperwork was performed without outside supervision.
- Such duties as the conduct of examinations, hearings, and disciplinary actions were undertaken independently, without the participation of other agencies.

Funding was also independently provided, since it was derived from licensing fees and expenditures and did not have to be justified to the legislature. Autonomous boards were the rule during the first half of this century, but centralization has begun to change the character of licensing boards. Recent studies have shown that about two thirds of the states now have central agencies overseeing some aspect of licensure.[9]

The extent to which centralization affects the autonomy of state boards varies from state to state. One review of state board structure divides it into five models, ranging from fully autonomous boards with no central agency (Model A) to central agencies with complete licensure authority that relegate boards to an advisory capacity only (Model E) (see Fig. 11.1).[10] These models, as they apply to the health-care professions, are listed on a state-to-state basis in Table 11.1.[11] Optometry boards have had to surrender some degree of independence in accordance with these changes.

Another significant development has been the adoption of *sunset laws* by state governments.[12] These laws establish termination dates for specified agencies and programs, including licensing boards.

Models Describing the Organization of Occupational Licensing in the States

Model A Boards are autonomous. They hire their own staffs; make decisions about office location, purchasing, and procedures. Each board receives and investigates complaints and disciplines licensees. Each board is responsible for the preparation, conduct, and grading of examinations. Each board sets qualifications for licensing and standards for practice. Boards collect fees and maintain financial records. Board staff prepares and mails licenses and applications for renewal and answers inquiries from licensees and the public.

Model B Boards are autonomous, but less so than in Model A. They set policy and determine standards regarding licensing and professional practice. They prepare or approve exams and decide who is qualified for licensing and professional practice. They prepare or approve exams and decide who is qualified for licensure. They handle complaints and discipline licensees. The board has responsibility for hiring and supervising its staff. A central agency may be responsible for such housekeeping matters as providing space, answering routine inquiries, collecting fees, and issuing licenses and renewals.

Model C Boards are autonomous and have decision-making authority in many areas. However, the central agency has greater authority over certain functions than in Model B. Its powers go beyond housekeeping. For example, board budgets, personnel, and records may be subject to some degree of control by the agency. Complaints and investigations and adjudicatory hearings may be handled by a central staff, even when boards continue to make final decisions with respect to disciplinary actions.

Model D Boards are not fully autonomous; that is, they do not have final decision-making authority on all substantive matters as do boards in the preceding models. While the central agency provides a wide range of services, in practice, boards may be delegated responsibility for such functions as preparing exams, setting pass/fail points, recommending professional standards, and recommending disciplinary sanctions. A crucial distinction, however, between Model D and the preceding models is that certain board actions are subject to review by the central agency.

Model E The regulatory system is run by an agency director, commission, or council, with or without the assistance of a board. When boards do exist, they are strictly advisory. The agency director, commission, or council has final decision-making authority on all substantive matters. Boards may be delegated such functions as preparing exams, setting pass/fail points, recommending professional standards, and recommending disciplinary actions. A crucial distinction between this model and Model D is that, when boards exist, they serve only in an advisory capacity.

Figure 11.1 State Board Models in the United States, 1982. (Source: Roederer, Doug, and Benjamin Shimberg. *Occupational Licensing: Centralizing State Licensure Functions*, Lexington. KY: The Council of State Governments, 1980, p. 4.)

Table 11.1. Organizational Models for Occupational Licensing

State	A	B	C	D	E	Notes/Exceptions
	Model Type*					
Alabama	×					
Alaska			×			
Arizona†		×				A = 10 boards, including accountancy, medicine, and industry B = 11 boards, including podiatry and psychology E = 3 boards
Arkansas	×					
California			×			
Colorado			×			C = 22 boards E = 3 boards
Connecticut				×		Health boards are under Department of Health Services.
Delaware			×			Boards handle investigations, complaints, and some major boards hire their own staffs.
Florida				×		
Georgia		×				Boards do not hire staff.
Hawaii			×			
Idaho†			×			A = 11 boards, including medicine, dentistry, state bar, and accountancy C = 14 boards, including barbering, ophthalmology, and architecture
Illinois					×	
Indiana	×					
Iowa†	×					A = 20 boards, including medicine, accountancy, and other business boards B = 12 health-related boards, including dentistry and psychology
Kansas	×					
Kentucky	×					B = 6 boards, including psychology and social work A = all other boards, including accountancy, dentistry, and medicine
Louisiana	×					
Maine		×				The central agency provides staff support and optional investigatory services at board request.
Maryland			×			The central agency can approve regulations of nonhealth-related boards.
Massachusetts		×				Central agency provides investigatory staff to boards.
Michigan			×			
Minnesota		×				
Mississippi	×					
Missouri			×			
Montana			×			
Nebraska†		×				B = all health boards except nursing
Nevada	×					
New Hampshire	×					
New Jersey			×			C = most professional and occupational boards
New Mexico	×					E = other boards, except that board budgets are subject to review by the legislative finance committee which then includes the board's budget in the appropriations bill
New York					×	
North Carolina	×					
North Dakota	×					A = including most professional licensing boards, i.e., health-related, accountancy, and engineering boards
Ohio	×					
Oklahoma		×				
Oregon†			×			A = health-related boards C = 11 business-related boards, including accountancy and engineering Approximately 12 other boards fit models D or E.
Pennsylvania			×			The central agency has the power of review with the right to "persuade" but not the right to vote.

Table 11.1. *Continued*

State	Model Type* A	B	C	D	E	Notes/Exceptions
Rhode Island			×			Health boards are under Department of Health.
South Carolina	×					
South Dakota	×					
Tennessee			×			19 boards are under Department of Health, while 15 boards are under Department of Insurance.
Texas	×					
Utah				×		
Vermont			×			B = boards of medicine, nursing, and real estate C = all other boards Hearings and investigations are handled by individual boards.
Virginia†			×			B = 7 health-related boards C = all other boards
Washington				×		
West Virginia	×					
Wisconsin			×			
Wyoming	×					
Totals	19	7	18	4	2	

*For a description of model types, see Figure 11.1.

†In these six states, respondents indicated that more than one model could apply. For purposes of analysis, the model which described the greatest number of boards in each state was designated as the predominant model.

From Roederer, D., and B. Shimberg, *Occupational Licensing: Centralizing State Licensure Functions*, Lexington, KY, The Council of State Governments, 1980, pp. 6–7.

Prior to the deadline, legislative hearings are conducted to determine if there is a need for the board to continue, if the board's activities are duplicated by other government agencies, and if the board is operating effectively and efficiently. If the board can justify its continued existence, it is permitted to continue functioning for a stated period of time; otherwise, "the sun sets" for the board. As of 1980, a total of thirty-four states had passed sunset laws.[13] The sunset hearings offer an opportunity for an exchange of dialogue between board members and legislators and for favorable information to be placed in the legislative record. But boards can be captured by the legislature on these occasions just as readily.

The Texas medical practice act was before the legislature for sunset review. If the statute was not automatically renewed within a certain period of time, the medical practice act would elapse. A debate over the scope of practice of optometry prevented the legislature from renewing the medical law within the requisite period of time and the statute was terminated. Before it could be re-passed by the legislature an amendment permitting the use of drugs for diagnostic purposes by optometrists was attached to it and made a part of the statute. This provision was duly enacted by the state legislature along with the elapsed medical practice act. Consequently, optometrists were allowed the use of the specified pharmaceutical agents.[14]

The future of sunset legislation is far from certain at the present date, as repeal efforts have been initiated in some states.

There has been a growing body of criticism directed at the role of licensing boards,[15] and even the basic premise of these boards—that they ensure that only competent practitioners will be permitted to practice—has itself been questioned.[16] The principal activity that has been granted to them, licensure, has been singled out as being particularly in need of reform.[17] Indeed, several proposals, some of them radical,[18] have been entertained as alternatives to the current licensing system. We will discuss the current status of licensure, as it relates to optometry, in the next section.

Licensure

Licensure can be described as "the process by which an agency of government grants permission to an individual to engage in a given occupation upon finding that the applicant has attained the minimal degree of competency necessary to ensure that the public health, safety, and welfare will be reasonably well protected."[19] Optometry is a licensed occupation, and the minimum requirements that are usually cited in the law include: a specified number of years of formal education, graduation from an accredited school of optometry, a minimum age, evidence of good moral character, and U.S. citizenship. Applicants satisfying these requirements are permitted to take a licensing examination, and if they pass, they are granted a license to practice optometry, which is a partial monopoly that entitles the licensee to perform certain acts and to employ a given title. *Licensure* is the most restrictive form of governmental regulation, differing substantially from registration and certification.[20]

Registration[21] is a form of governmental title control that prohibits individuals from employing a title rather than from engaging in a regulated occupation. The designations that are controlled are *certified* and *registered*; the state establishes standards that must be met in order for individuals to use these titles. Examples of registration would be certified public accountants and registered opticians. Although these individuals do not enjoy a monopoly in their occupation, they do receive the grant of the title from the state, which sets them apart from others in their calling.[22]

Certification is title control conducted by professions or trades in order to recognize individuals who have attained a superior level of competence or are highly qualified to perform a specialized area of practice. Since it is a nongovernmental form of title control, certification is a voluntary form of regulation that is not based on state law. Rather, a certification agency is established by a group to formulate standards and to recognize individuals satisfying these standards. An example of such a group is the American Academy of Optometry, which grants certificates to those optometrists who successfuly fulfill all requirements to be called diplomates.[23]

Licensure of optometrists embraces three components:

1. A grant of the right to perform certain acts and to use a given title, conferred upon those qualified individuals who satisfy the minimum requirements established by the state for the practice of optometry
2. Satisfaction by the individual of such requirements as are necessary to continue the eligiblity of the individual to practice optometry within the state
3. Withdrawal of the right to practice optometry or other disciplinary action initiated by the state for the failure of the individual to adhere to certain express requirements relating to personal and professional conduct

Grant of the License

A license to practice optometry is considered to be a valuable right under the law, and so legal safeguards have arisen to ensure the proper procurement, maintenance, and forfeiture of this economically valuable commodity. The requirements to obtain a license must be reasonable, and must be related to the stated mission of the board, i.e., the protection of the public against unqualified individuals who seek to practice optometry. There are two aspects to the awarding of licenses: the determination of those individuals who are qualified and the examination of these qualified applicants. A third, special consideration involves the award of licenses by reciprocity.

In order to determine if an applicant is qualified, the board must establish certain criteria that are the minimum standards to be applied in all cases. The most common of these criteria concern age, citizenship, moral character, pre-optometry education, and optometric training.

Age

Most state laws specify a minimum age for applicants, the usual age cited being 21. Since preoptometric and optometric education requires six to eight years of collegiate training after high school, this age limit is not a factor in determining the qualifications of individuals.

Citizenship

Many optometry laws maintain that applicants must be U.S. citizens, a requirement that has been held by the U.S. Supreme Court to have no relationship to an individual's ability to serve as a licensed professional[24] or as a government employee.[25] Aliens have been recognized by the nation's highest court as "persons" and thus entitled to protection against discrimination under the Fourteenth Amendment.[26] Therefore, even though these requirements remain part of some optometry laws, it is unlikely that they are enforceable.

Moral Character

All optometry practice acts include good moral character as a prerequisite for licensure and list certain offenses related to personal conduct as grounds for discipline, but the guidelines are frequently couched in vague language that is difficult to interpret. The most commonly accepted evidence of bad character is conviction of a crime,[27] which has been upheld by the courts as a reasonable basis for denial of a license to practice a licensed occupation. Since convicted persons are usually prevented from obtaining a license, moral character most often becomes an issue when licensed individuals commit acts that reflect unfavorably on their moral character and thereby threaten their right to continue as licensees.

Education

The most stringent qualification for licensure pertains to the education of the applicant; minimum high school, college, and optometry school requirements can be found in all state laws. Every state specifies that the applicant's optometric education be from an accredited school, which has significance for foreign-trained graduates. Another aspect of this issue concerns the certification of licensed individuals who have met certain special educational requirements, such as optometrists who have satisfactorily completed a specified amount of training in the use of pharmaceutical agents, thereby enabling these practitioners to employ them in the practice of optometry. In all states these certification requirements are optional rather than mandatory.

Training

In a small minority of states, some training is required (in addition to the educational requirements) in order to qualify the applicant for licensure. Internship for a stated period is provided for in three state laws (Alabama, Delaware, and Rhode Island). Residencies, however, are not required for the licensure of optometrists in any state.[28]

If the applicant satisfies the qualifications enumerated by the state optometry law, he is eligible to take the examination, which can consist of a written test, a practical test, or both. In lieu of a written test, forty-three states (as of 1987) have substituted the examination given by the National Board of Examiners in Optometry (NBEO), which is administered to second, third, and fourth year optometry students as a test of minimum competency necessary for the practice of the profession.[29] In those states where the NBEO is not accepted, the optometry practice act lists the subjects on which applicants will be tested and describes the specific procedures that individuals must follow in order to apply. Depending on the degree of centralization present, the examination may be conducted exclusively by the state board of optometry or under the aegis of a central agency. Grading policy also varies from state to state.

Many commentaries have been published on the failings of state board examinations,[30] and yet they remain a staple of the licensing machinery. Practical examinations have been singled out as exercises in subjectivity,[31] but even so they probably are a necessary aspect of testing in those states that have more liberal laws (such as those states that permit the use of drugs for therapeutic purposes). For the most part, licensing examinations are intended to test recent optometry school graduates and are rarely administered to established optometrists seeking to relocate in another state. For these practitioners, *reciprocity* offers an opportunity to obtain licensure without the necessity of examination. However, this opportunity is more often illusory than real.

Most states do not give credence to licenses issued by other states.[32] They require all individuals seeking licensure to meet current educational and training requirements and to pass the current licensing examination, a policy that discourages the relocation of established practitioners. Some states recognize the licenses of other states and have established reciprocity agreements (see Table 11.2). No exami-

Table 11.2. Reciprocity Agreements, Optometry Statutes: 1985

State	Practice Requirement (Prior to Applying for License)	Supplemental Examination Requirements
Arkansas	3 years	
Florida		
Georgia		
Indiana		Written examination on Indiana law
Iowa	3 years	
Maryland		
Missouri		Practical examination and written examination on Missouri law

Licenses are awarded by reciprocity in the above states if the applicant's state of origin will also award licenses by reciprocity to applicants from the above states.

nation is necessary; a licensee from one state will automatically be granted a license from the reciprocating state. But the determining factor is not the qualification of the licensee but rather how the licensee's state of origin treats license holders of the reciprocating state.[33]

A similar policy is known as *endorsement* and exists in a larger number of states (see Table 11.3). These states unilaterally accept licensees of another state if it can be shown that the standards of the other state are comparable to their own. In effect, the determining factor becomes the qualifications of the individual applicant rather than his state's reciprocity policy. Unfortunately, in some states a reciprocity requirement is tacked onto the comparable standards criterion, creating a complex and difficult burden for any licensee to meet[34] (see Table 11.4). The result of these restrictions has been to retard the mobility of optometrists. In several states there is no provision for licensure other than through the state examination mechanism (see Table 11.5).

Table 11.3. Endorsement Agreements, Optometry Statutes: 1985

State	Practice Requirement (Prior to Applying for License)	Supplemental Examination Requirements
Alaska	3 years	Oral and practical examinations
California		
Louisiana		
Michigan		Interview
New Jersey		
New Mexico	7 years	Practical examination
New York	5 years	
North Carolina	Practice of optometry 3 out of the 5 years prior to application	Practical examination
Oregon	3 years	
Pennsylvania	4 years	Written examination administered by the NBEO
Texas		State continuing education requirement must be equal to that of Texas
Vermont	2 years	Oral and practical examinations

Licenses are awarded by endorsement in the above states if the applicant's state of origin has standards that are comparable to the above states's standards.

Table 11.4. Endorsement Agreements Requiring Reciprocity, Optometry Statutes: 1985

State	Practice Requirement (Prior to Applying for License)	Supplemental Examination Requirements
Alabama	1 year	
Arizona	Practice of optometry 4 out of the 5 years prior to the application	Oral and practical examinations
Connecticut		
District of Columbia		
Illinois		
Kansas		
Kentucky	5 years	Oral and practical examinations
Maine	3 years	Practical examination
Massachusetts	3 years	
Minnesota	3 years	Practical examination
Mississippi		
Montana	5 years	
Nebraska	1 year	Practical examination
Nevada		
New Hampshire	3 years	
North Dakota		Practical examination
Ohio		
Oklahoma		
Rhode Island		
South Dakota		
Utah		
Virginia	1 year	
Wisconsin	5 years	Written examination

Licenses are awarded by endorsement in the above states if the applicant's state of origin has standards that are comparable to the above states' standards *and* if the applicant's state of origin will also award licenses by reciprocity to applicants from the above states.

Maintenance of the License

Once an optometrist has been granted a license, he must thereafter satisfy the requirements specified in the state law to maintain the license or suffer its forfeiture. The first licensing laws required only that practitioners pay a set fee each year by a certain deadline in order for renewal to be effected. Gradually questions began to emerge concerning the need for periodic reassessment of professional licensees, and

Table 11.5. States Not Recognizing Licensure by Reciprocity or Endorsement: 1985

Colorado	Tennessee
Delaware	Washington
Hawaii	West Virginia
Idaho	Wyoming
South Carolina	

To receive a license in these states, the applicant must satisfy the statutory requirements for examination.

alternative methods of achieving this goal, such as written examinations,[35] simulations,[36] peer reviews and audits,[37] and self-assessment[38] were proposed. But the idea that received the greatest support was mandatory continuing education.

A report issued by the U.S. Department of Health, Education, and Welfare in 1971 questioning the effectiveness of voluntary education programs intended to update professionals suggested that "professional associations and states should include specific requirements to ensure continued competence."[39] This proposal to include mandatory continuing education as a condition of continued licensure was adopted by the health-care professions with great enthusiasm, with optometry leading the way.[40] As of 1985, forty-six states had enacted mandatory continuing education requirements for optometrists, the most for any profession (see Table 11.6). The implementation of these requirements was left to the state boards, which have been granted the authority to approve programs, award credits, and in some states to set the minimum number of hours necessary for license renewal. Mandatory continuing education has been of significant benefit to optometry, which is presently undergoing a revolutionary change in its philosophy and scope of services, and these legal developments have doubtless contributed to the popularity of continuing education within the profession.

Disciplinary Actions Against the Licensee

If an optometrist pays the annual license fee and obtains the necessary hours of continuing education credit, then the license will be renewed each year until retirement or death, unless the optometrist commits an act for which he can be subjected to disciplinary proceedings by the board. The offenses for which discipline may be meted out are listed in the state optometry law and generally fall into four categories:

1. Violations related to moral character (conviction of a crime, addiction to drugs, habitual drunkenness, gross immorality, and insanity being the most common examples)
2. Proscriptions on advertising (although these requirements have been limited by recent Supreme Court decisions)
3. Prohibitions related to the commercial practice of optometry (e.g., unauthorized practice of optometry by a corporation, franchising, fee splitting, use of a trade name, and unlawful lessor-lessee arrangements)
4. Certain offenses related to improper optometric practice (failing to comply with requirements for branch offices, prescriptions, minimum examination procedures, ownership of records, or willful violations of the optometry law such as unauthorized practice, aiding in the unlawful practice of optometry by an unlicensed person, or participating in illegal rebates).

Because of the importance of these proceedings to licensees, disciplinary actions will be discussed in a subsequent section of this chapter.

The procedures to be followed by state boards when instituting disciplinary actions have been the subject of much scrutiny by the courts.[41] Since a license is a valuable right, the licensee is entitled to due process of law before it can be taken from him, a constitutional guarantee that he cannot be arbitrarily or capriciously subjected to discipline or be penalized without an opportunity to be heard.[42] As a result, the process that a board must follow when initiating disciplinary action against a licensee is spelled out with great specificity in state optometry practice acts. The legal requirements necessary to ensure that due process is observed will be discussed subsequently.[43]

The penalties that may be imposed on violators of the law include formal reprimand, suspension from practice, and revocation of the license. A *reprimand* is a form of offical censure but does not affect the right of the licensee to use his license. A *suspension* is a temporary prohibition of the right to employ the license, with reinstatement being automatic after the passage of a specified period. A *revocation* is a forfeiture of the license for an undetermined period, which may be permanent or may be subject to reinstatement at an uncertain future date. These penalties are not the only remedies that may be sought. Injunctions (and other extraordinary remedies), which are orders by courts to perform or cease from performing certain acts, may be sought by optometry boards, as may consent decrees, which are agreements by licensees that they will perform or refrain from performing certain acts. The disciplinary measures that

Table 11.6. Selected Occupations Requiring Continuing Education: 1985
Status of Mandatory Continuing Education in Selected Professionals

	Architects	CPAs	Dentists	Engineers	Lawyers	Nurses	Nursing Home Administrators	Optometrists	Psychologists	Pharmacists	Physical Therapists	Physicians	Salespersons and Brokers	Social Workers	LPNs	Veterinarians
Alabama		X					X	X		X				X		X
Alaska		X				S	X	X				X				
Arizona		X			S		X	X				X	X			X
Arkansas		X					X	X	•	X		•				X
California		X	X		S	X	X		X	X		X	X		X	
Colorado		X			X		X		X			X		X		X
Connecticut		X					X	X								
Delaware						S	X	X						X		
District of Columbia		X														
Florida		X			S	X	X	X		X			X		X	X
Georgia		X			S		X	X					X			
Hawaii		X					X	X				X				
Idaho					X		X	X		X						
Illinois								X				X				X
Indiana		X						X		X						
Iowa	X	X	X	X	XS	X	X	X	X	X	X	X	X		X	X
Kansas		X	X			X	X	X		X	X	X	X	X	X	X
Kentucky			X			X	X	X		X		•	S	X	X	X
Louisiana		X				S	X	X								
Maine		X					X	X		X		X	X	X		
Maryland		X					X	X	X			X	X	X		X
Massachusetts		X	•			X	X	X				X		X	X	
Michigan		X				•	X	X	•	X		X			X	
Minnesota	•	X	X	•	X	X	X	X	•	X		X	X			
Mississippi							X	X								•
Missouri							X	X								
Montana		X					X	X		X						X
Nebraska		X				XS	X	X		•		•			X	X
Nevada		X				X	X	X	X	X		•	X		X	•
New Hampshire						S	S	X				X				X
New Jersey			S				X	X		X						
New Mexico		X	X		S	X	X	X	X	X	X	X			X	X
New York							X						X			
North Carolina		X		•			X	X								X
North Dakota		X	X		X	•	X	X							•	X
Ohio		X					X	X		X		X				X
Oklahoma							X	X		X						

Table 11.6. *Continued*

	Architects	CPAs	Dentists	Engineers	Lawyers	Nurses	Nursing Home Administrators	Optometrists	Psychologists	Pharmacists	Physical Therapists	Physicians	Salespersons and Brokers	Social Workers	LPNs	Veterinarians
Oregon		X	X			S	X	X	•	X			X			X
Pennsylvania		X					X					S				X
Rhode Island		X						X				X				
South Carolina		X			XS			X								
South Dakota		X	X			X	X	X		X			X	X	X	X
Tennessee		X						X								
Texas		•					X	X								
Utah						S		X	•			X		X		
Vermont	•	X					X									
Virginia								X								
Washington		X			X		X	X	X	X		X				X
West Virginia							X		X							
Wisconsin					X		X					X	X			
Wyoming		X			X		X	X								

X = required by statute or regulation; • = enabling legislation passed; S = required under certain circumstances.
Note: Information obtained from national professional associations
From Louis E. Phillips, Furman University, revised June 1980.
Source: Shimberg B., *Occupational Licensing: A Public Perspective*, Educational Testing Service, Princeton, N.J., 1982, p. 128.

may be brought by boards against licensees, and the constitutional safeguards that influence them, will be described later in this chapter.

There yet remains one other aspect of licensure that must be reviewed: exemptions. The legal development of optometry has been discussed previously (see Chapters 1 and 9), and the political considerations that influenced the form and content of the original optometry practice acts have been described. These events led to the incorporation of two important exemptions within all optometry licensing laws: those granted to physicians and those granted to dispensing opticians.

Because medical practice acts regulated physicians and because the one-board concept for the practice of optometry was rejected by medicine, the optometry laws were uniformly written so as to exempt physicians from their provisions. Consequently, optometry boards have no jurisdiction over ophthalmologists, even when they practice optometry. Physician's assistants, however, are regulated in many states.[44]

The fitting of spectacles and the filling of prescriptions for spectacles or contact lenses are activities that are exempted from optometry laws, such transactions being little more than a sale of goods, but the prescribing of spectacles or contact lenses by unlicensed persons is the unauthorized and illegal practice of optometry, punishable under state optometry practice acts. An exemption is also granted to various individuals who merely determine the need for vision services.

Enforcement of the optometry statutes is the responsibility of the board of optometry, which exercises powers otherwise relegated to the judicial branch of government when attempting to uphold the law or to discipline violators. These activities often raise constitutional issues that must be settled in the courts. In the next section we will briefly review some of the more important constitutional rights that must be observed by licensing boards.

Constitutional Considerations

The purpose of government is to provide for the health, safety, and welfare of its citizenry, a role that is carried out by the states through the passage and enforcement of laws intended to achieve that end. This authority granted to the states is referred to as the *police power* and is the basis for the enactment of laws regulating the practice of optometry, medicine, dentistry, or any other of the health-care occupations.[45] Licenses to practice these occupations are regarded as valuable rights that may be terminated only in a constitutionally acceptable manner, this policy being based on the due process clause of the Fourteenth Amendment of the U.S. Constitution, which holds in part: "No state shall . . . deprive any person of life, liberty, or property without due process of law."

This clause and other federal and state constitutional provisions create legal standards that must be met by the boards when licensure or disciplinary measures are instituted. Regulation of the practice of optometry must itself satisfy the constitutional requirement that no person be deprived of property or equal protection under the law.

New Hampshire enacted an optometry practice act and set forth rules for the qualification and licensure of optometrists within the state. The law was challenged by a jewelry store (which offered optometric services) as being in contravention to the Fourteenth Amendment by allowing deprivation of property without due process and denying unlicensed persons equal protection under the law. In upholding the constitutionality of the law, the New Hampshire Supreme Court observed that, while the legislature to some degree suppressed competition by restricting the right to practice optometry only to those persons who demonstrated the competency to do so, it could not be said that unlicensed persons were unlawfully deprived of property since the purpose of the law was to protect the public health.[46]

The denial or revocation of a license due to lack of good character has been upheld as reasonable[47]: One common ground for discipline is gross immorality;[48] another constitutionally acceptable ground is conviction of a crime.[49] These offenses (and others) will be discussed subsequently.

Optometry statutes must be written with sufficient clarity to put a reasonable person on notice as to the offences for which he or she may be punished. Statutes that are vague are constitutionally unenforceable because they do not establish a definite standard, and legal disputes have centered around the vagueness of such offenses as moral turpitude,[50] advertising special ability,[51] and unprofessional conduct.[52]

An important aspect of the police power is the right of administrative agencies such as state boards to institute disciplinary proceedings (rather than restricting this right exclusively to the courts). It has been argued that the often broadly stated grounds on which discipline can be imposed constitute a constructive delegation of legislative power to boards since the boards must decide which delegations of misconduct justify the initiation of disciplinary sanctions. In deciding this issue the courts have held that the power to enforce laws may rightly be delegated to administrative agencies but that their discretion must be limited.[53]

The right to institute disciplinary proceedings raises important issues relating to procedural due process. While state board procedures may be less formal and rigorous than those followed by the courts, certain constitutional requirements must nevertheless be met. Among the most important of these are: reasonable notice of the disciplinary hearing[54] and a reasonable opportunity to present a defense.[55]

Reasonable notice requires that the accused be informed of the wrong that is alleged and the particular instances of its perpetration.[56] Adequate notice of the time and date of the hearing must also be provided.[57]

After the passage of the optometry practice act in Georgia, provisions necessary for licensure under the law were duly supervised by the Georgia State Board of Examiners in Optometry. A practitioner who satisfied all the requirements of the law applied for a certificate of registration but the board refused to issue it to him. He brought an action to compel them to award the certificate, alleging that he had been denied due process of law because he had been given no notice or hearing concerning the board's decision. In requiring the board to issue the certificate, the Supreme Court of Georgia noted, "The fundamental idea in due process of law is that of notice and hearing. It means that the citizen must be afforded notice and a hearing before he is condemned. There must be a hearing first, and judgment can be rendered only after trial."[58]

The proceeding does not have to be conducted with the same formality as a trial[59] and does not require strict adherence to the rules of evidence.[60] In many states, codes of administrative procedure have been adopted and they will dictate the manner in which the hearing is to be conducted, unless a different procedure is required in the optometry practice act.[61] In most states, the procedure the board must follow throughout the investigation and hearing is described in considerable detail. Also, the board must be fair and impartial when conducting a hearing.

An optometrist was brought before the New Mexico Board of Examiners in Optometry for allegedly making sexual advances to female patients. The Board revoked the optometrist's license and he appealed, contending that a board member should have been disqualified from the hearing because he had made comments prior to the disciplinary proceeding that the optometrist would lose his license. The state supreme court reversed the revocation and remanded the case to the board for a new hearing, holding that the failure to disqualify the board member for bias violated the optometrist's right to procedural due process. The court stated that no individual can be deprived of personal or property rights except after a hearing before a fair and impartial tribunal, and that whenever government agencies make decisions that directly affect the legal rights of individuals, it is imperative that those agencies use the procedures that have traditionally been associated with judicial process.[62]

Optometry laws not only grant to boards the right to impose discipline against licensees, they authorize licensees to obtain review of these decisions in the courts. Judicial review may be a *de novo* proceeding—a new trial—in a state court of original jurisdiction, or it may be a review by the court of the board's decision. In reviewing the case, the court will apply the substantial evidence test: The board's action should be supported by substantial evidence preserved in the written record of the hearing.

The rationale applied by the courts is that the board is better able to determine issues of fact, due to the expertise of board members, and can better weigh the credibility of witnesses, because it may observe their demeanor.

A Pennsylvania optometrist appealed a 90-day license suspension issued by the State Board of Optometrical Examiners, claiming that the board erred in finding the testimony of three of his patients more credible than his own, but the appellate court held that it was within the power of the board to base its ruling upon the credibility of witnesses observed by the board during the taking of testimony and upheld the suspension.[63]

Once a court has rendered judgment, the licensee may obtain appeal to an appellate court of competent jurisdiction. Appellate courts will reverse the rulings of lower courts as to the adequacy of evidence in support of a board's decision only when they are clearly erroneous.

An optometrist was found to be guilty of gross immorality by the California Board of Optometry, his conduct being such that it constituted "unprofessional conduct" for which the board revoked his license. The optometrist appealed the board's decision to the superior court, which concluded upon review of the record of the hearing that the accusation did not state a course of action and that cumulative nonprobative hearsay testimony was admitted, the effect of which was to prejudice the case. The court set aside the revocation.[64]

Certain unusual remedies may also be used to obtain judicial review of a board decision. Among these are the extraordinary writs of certiorari[65] and mandamus,[66] the declaratory judgment,[67] and the equitable remedy of injunction.[68]

An optometrist and his family owned a chain of optical houses located throughout the United States. A number of legal actions were brought against the owners of these businesses and against the businesses themselves, both by individuals and the U.S. government, with many of the allegations involving fraudulent practices. Consequently, the optometrist and his family filed a series of lawsuits across the nation, naming the American Optometric Association, which they believed to be the cause of their legal troubles, as the defendant. To prevent the continued perpetration of groundless lawsuits, the AOA filed for injunctive relief, asking the courts to prevent further cases from being filed. This relief, in the form of an order to the optometrist and his family, was ultimately granted by the courts.[69]

There is provision under all of the optometry practice acts for boards to revoke or suspend an optometrist's license or to issue a reprimand, and as long as the board does not abuse its discretion in determining the discipline to be imposed, it will be upheld by the appellate court.[70]

A Kansas optometrist established a corporation for the purpose of starting an optical dispensary adjacent to his optometry office. Although others were represented as owning the dispensary, the optometrist controlled business, finances, and advertising. He also arranged for patients to be sent to his office from the dispensary. The State Board of Optometry revoked his license for violations of the state optometry law involving commercialism and advertising. He appealed, alleging that the judgment against him was arbitrary, capricious, and unreasonable, but the state supreme court found that the order revoking his license was supported by substantial competent evidence and upheld the revocation.[71]

Boards are vested with the authority to reinstate licenses where it is determined that such action is warranted.

Disciplinary Actions

The types of acts for which optometry boards may initiate disciplinary proceedings vary widely from state to state, but there are common offenses that are found in virtually all laws. We will review these offenses, as applied to specific cases, in the following section. There are two basic categories that may be used when organizing such a discussion: general offenses and specific offenses.

General Offenses

Violations such as unprofessional conduct, unprofessional and dishonorable conduct, manifest incapacity, or gross immorality are general offenses that do not describe specific activities for which the optometrist will be subject to discipline. These violations have been attacked in the courts as constructive delegations of legislative authority and on the ground that they are constitutionally vague.[72] Unprofessional conduct, however, continues to find applicability as a punishable offense.

A group of optometrists had an arrangement with an optical shop whereby the store acted as a "steerer" by directing persons to them for examination, to be returned to the store for the dispensing of glasses. The optometrists would not subsequently check the glasses to determine if they were appropriate for the patient's needs but would receive a portion of the income derived from their sale. The Minnesota State Board of Optometry sought to discipline the optometrists for "unprofessional conduct," and the optometrists defended upon the basis that the law was vague and a delegation of legislative power to the board. In upholding the right of the board to proceed against them, the state supreme court noted that unprofessional conduct is "conduct that violates those standards of professional behavior that through professional experience have become established, by the consensus of the expert opinion of the members, as reasonably necessary for the protection of the public interest. In establishing the necessity for and the existence of such standards, every member of the profession should be regarded as an expert."[73]

Similarly, gross immorality may be considered sufficiently certain to serve as the basis for disciplinary action against an optometrist.

An optometrist advertised two-for-one specials for glasses and sunglasses and reduced prices for certain frames and lenses. A woman interested in the advertised glasses was examined by the optometrist, who afterwards demanded the payment of a $5 examination fee without showing the woman any of the advertised products. Upon her refusal to pay he threatened to call a detective, then deliberately pulled off her glasses, knocked them against the edge of a table, threw them on the floor, and stepped on them, damaging them to the extent that they were useless. He refused the woman's pleas to repair the glasses or assist her, even though he knew her unaided vision to be 20/400, and put her on the street. The Texas State Board of Examiners in Optometry thereafter suspended his license, basing its decision in part on the allegation that his acts constituted "gross immorality" under the state optometry laws. The optometrist appealed the board's decision, and the court of civil appeals, in upholding the suspension, noted that gross immorality "has been defined as a course of conduct so reprehensible and revolting as to shock the sensibilities of reasonable men.... [It] does not necessarily mean great and excessive but rather such a 'willfully flagrant and shameful quality' as renders a person unfit to hold his license." The court held that the optometrist's conduct was sufficient to satisfy the definition and that the disciplinary action was proper.[74]

The majority of disciplinary actions are brought for specific offenses such as those described below.

Specific Offenses

All optometry practice acts enumerate the specific types of conduct for which an optometrist may suffer suspension or revocation of his license. The most common of these offenses, as interpreted by the courts, are certain acts of untruthful advertising, improper practice by unlicensed corporations or businesses, commission of a crime, narcotics violations or habitual drunkenness, insanity, sexual misconduct, aiding nonlicensed persons to practice optometry, and offenses including moral turpitude.

Optometry boards have a long history of opposition to advertising. But with the advent of precedent-setting decisions by the U.S. Supreme Court recognizing the right of professionals to advertise, state prohibitions on advertising and their defenders, the boards, have themselves become the subjects of litigation.[75] Despite the new liberality accorded to professionals, boards may continue to initiate actions to prevent unfair or deceptive advertising of ophthalmic goods or services.[76] And, in states where the use of trade names by optometrists is prohibited, boards may rightfully enforce this prohibition.

The Texas Optometry Act prohibited the practice of optometry under an assumed name, trade name, or corporate name. A multi-outlet chain offering optometric services brought an action to prevent enforcement of the law, alleging that it was unconstitutional in that it abridged the business' right to free speech under the First Amendment. A federal court found the law to be an unconstitutional restriction upon the "free flow of commercial information," but this decision was appealed to the U.S. Supreme Court, which reversed and upheld the prohibition, declaring that,

> The use of a trade name in connection with optometrical practice conveys no information about the price and nature of the services offered by an optometrist until it acquires meaning over a period of time by associations formed in the minds of the public between the name and some standard of price or quality. Because these ill-defined associations of trade names with price and quality information can be manipulated by the users of trade names, there is a significant possibility that trade names will be used to mislead the public.[77]

Another often-enforced provision of state laws were prohibitions against the practice of optometry by unlicensed corporations or businesses.[78] These cases have been brought to prevent businesses from practicing optometry through licensed employees,[79] enforce prohibitions against lessor-lessee arrangements in commercial establishments,[80] prevent illegal side-by-side operations,[81] and uphold various provisions of state business codes that pertain to the unauthorized practice of optometry.[82] A relatively recent aspect of this latter responsibility concerns the right of states to bar optometric franchises.

The California Business and Professions Code prohibited certain acts related to employment of professionals, practice of a profession, advertising, use of an assumed name, sharing of profits between licensed and unlicensed persons, and unlawful competition. The law forbade optometric franchises and other types of landlord-tenant or profit-sharing arrangements between optical manufacturers and optometrists. A national corporation offered franchises to practitioners within the state, and legal proceedings were instituted against the company, requesting injunctive relief against the sale of these franchises. The injunction was granted.[83]

Optometrists who have been convicted of the commission of a crime may properly be the subject of license revocation or suspension hearings.[84]

An optometrist who was the employee of a retail optical outlet in Missouri was arrested and charged with Medicaid fraud. One of the allegations was that he had permitted his employer, who was not an optometrist, to perform eye examinations and to fill out Medicaid claims, which he then falsely signed as the examiner. The optometrist was permitted to plead guilty to the lesser charge of violating the state optometry law and to make financial restitution to the state. He was also placed on a year's probation and ordered to surrender his optometry license for that period of time as a condition of probation. Subsequently, the optometrist was also indicted on charges of obtaining money by false pretenses.[85]

Habitual drunkenness or narcotic addiction may also be a proper cause of disciplinary action against a practitioner.[86] Insanity is likewise a condition for which a board may initiate action seeking the suspension or revocation of the individual's license.

Sexual misconduct on the part of an optometrist may be justification for disciplinary action by the board, usually under the claim of unprofessional conduct or conduct likely to deceive the public.[87]

A woman brought her 14-year-old daughter to be examined by an optometrist and the girl was taken to an examination room while her mother waited outside. The optometrist, pretending that there was some clinical purpose to be served in so doing, required the girl to expose herself to the waist while he examined her upper body with a light. A charge of immoral conduct was brought by the State Board of Optometric Examiners of the State of Colorado, and after a hearing the optometrist's license was revoked. He appealed, alleging among other causes of error that the revocation was a penalty "so grossly excessive and unconscionable as to make it repugnant to every sense of justice." In upholding the board's decision to revoke the license, the state supreme court noted that the board had been granted discretion in awarding discipline under the law and concluded that "we cannot say as a matter of law that there was an abuse of discretion on its (the board's) part in revoking the license under the uncontradicted evidence disclosed by the record before us."[88]

If optometrists aid or permit the practice of optometry by unlicensed persons, they can be subjected to disciplinary measures intended not only to prevent future occurrences of the illegal act but also to punish the licensee who has assisted or allowed its perpetration.[89]

A New York optometrist who permitted an ophthalmic dispenser to fit contact lenses under his supervision was found to be in violation of the New York Education law, which limited the fitting of contact lenses to licensed optometrists only. As a result the Commissioner of Education suspended his license for six months, with an 18-month period of probation to follow. The Commissioner's penalty was appealed by the optometrist, but the appellate court held that the penalty was not so disproportionate to the offense as to require modification and upheld the suspension.[90]

There are certain violations that have become known as offenses involving moral turpitude,[91] and disciplinary proceedings against licensees on these grounds have been upheld by the courts.[92] Consequently, optometrists in states where offenses involving moral turpitude are listed as causes for disciplinary action may be prosecuted for violations that are regarded as belonging in this category.

Other offenses, such as acts outside the scope of practice,[93] failure to adhere to minimum examination requirements,[94] negligence,[95] improper branch offices,[96] and inadequate continuing education credit,[97] have also served as the basis for disciplinary proceedings.

Although a licensee may believe that a licensing board has proceeded unfairly against him, the institution of a claim of malicious prosecution will—except in extremely limited circumstances—not be recognized by the courts as stating a valid cause of action.

An optometrist had his license suspended for six months by the Indiana State Board of Registration and Examination in Optometry and appealed the decision. The state court reversed the board, holding that the statute upon which the suspension was based was unconstitutional. The optometrist thereafter brought a malicious prosecution claim against the board, but the claim was held not to state a cause of action because the board's decision against the optometrist was found to be conclusive of probable cause, even though it was subsequently reversed on appeal. In its decision the court described the basis for a successful claim of malicous prosecution:

> One who initiates or procures the initiation of civil proceedings against another before an administrative board which has power to take action adversely affecting the legally protected interests of the other, is subject to liability for any special harm caused thereby, if (a) the proceedings are initiated (i) without probable cause to believe that the charge or claim on which the proceedings are based is well founded, and (ii) primarily for a purpose other than that of securing appropriate action by the board, and (b) the proceedings have terminated in favor of the person against whom they are brought.[98]

Despite this lengthy litany of offenses, disciplinary proceedings against optometrists that result in license revocation are extremely rare, which is in keeping with the relative infrequency of license revocations within professions as a whole.[99] Procedural safeguards doubtless play a role in limiting the harshness of sanctions imposed by licensing boards. Procedural matters are also of importance in determining the jurisdiction of optometry boards.

Jurisdiction

A disciplinary action is initiated through the service of a complaint upon the licensee who is the defendant in the proceeding. If the licensee is thereby accorded adequate notice as to the charges against him and the nature, time, and place of the hearing, the process will pass through a period of discovery and then proceed to the hearing itself.

The boards of several states are empowered to issue subpoenas to compel the attendance of witnesses or to assure the presence of documents. The conduct of the prehearing period and the actual hearing itself will depend upon the specific provisions of the optometry practice act. But the licensee will be granted an opportunity to be heard, be represented by counsel, confront and offer witnesses, and question or use documents in his defense. Based on its findings of fact and supported by substantial evidence, the board will render a decision and pronounce such disciplinary measures as it feels, in the exercise of its discretion, are reasonable. Appeal may be had by the licensee from this decision.[100]

Optometry licensing boards are granted jurisdiction over licensed practitioners and those individuals, businesses, or entities that are unlicensed but in violation of the law.[101] Certain individuals will be expressly exempted from the provisions of the optometry practice act, and the board will not be able to exercise jurisdiction over them.[102] But activities by unlicensed individuals or businesses that constitute the practice of optometry are within the jurisdiction of the board and can be prosecuted.[103] Most optometry practice acts provide for injunctive relief (to prohibit further occurrences of the illegal act) and for criminal proceedings against the violator; the penalty for a finding of guilty being conviction of a misdemeanor or a felony.[104] The most common types of offenses involve acts such as refraction,[105] use of a keratometer,[106] unsupervised fitting of contact lenses,[107] employment of an optometrist,[108] or the issuance of prescriptions for glasses. Although injunctive relief is frequently awarded by the courts, criminal convictions are relatively rare. Thus there is some question as to the effectiveness of imposing criminal penalties against unlicensed practitioners, which has led some states to institute civil penalties as an alternative.[109]

Disputes over jurisdiction are rare between licensing boards but can occur. Where licensees are potentially subject to discipline by two boards, the board that has issued the license is virtually always the one that proceeds against the licensee, the other board recognizing this right to proceed as a matter of comity.[110] If a licensee is subjected to notice and a hearing, and the board makes a determination as to the controversy, then a second board may be barred from proceeding against the licensee on the basis of *res judicata*.[111]

Due to the evolving nature of optometry laws, some conflict has been generated between optometry boards and medical and pharmacy boards.[112] The nature of these disputes and their outcome depends in great part on the provision of the state practice acts and the structural hierarchy accorded to the boards within the healing arts. Therefore, the degree of comity between boards may vary significantly from state to state.

One thing seems certain: The one-board concept envisioned by Prentice does not appear to be the ultimate result of the licensing process that controls the practice of optometry. Even though alternatives to the traditional method of licensure have been proposed, there is little probability that the current licensing structure will soon change. The state boards, with all their inherent complexities and problems, will continue to be a vital and important aspect of the practice of optometry in the decades to come.

Notes

1. *Florida Society of Ophthalmology v. Florida Optometric Association*, 489 So. 2d 1118 (1986), *reversing* 465 So. 2d 1319 (1985). Reported in *Bulletin from the Office of Counsel of the AOA*, vol. 43, no. 46, Dec. 28, 1984.
2. The Federal Administrative Procedure Act, 5 U.S.C. §§551–559, 701–706, 1305, 3105, 3344, 5362, and 7521 (1976).
3. See 14 *Uniform Laws Annotated* at 357 (Master Edition 1980), which lists twenty-nine such jurisdictions: Arkansas, Connecticut, District of Columbia, Georgia, Hawaii, Idaho, Illinois, Iowa, Louisiana, Maine, Maryland, Michigan, Mississippi, Missouri, Montana, Nebraska, Nevada, New Hampshire, New York, North Carolina, Oklahoma, Rhode Island, South Dakota, Tennessee, Vermont, Washington, West Virginia, Wisconsin, and Wyoming. Davis, K., *Administrative Law Treatise*, vol. 1, §1:10, 2d ed., 1978, pp. 36–37, also lists Arizona, Florida, Indiana, Massachusetts, New Mexico, and Oregon as such states and notes that other states have comprehensive legislation not based on the Model Act.
4. Shimberg, B., *Occupational Licensing: A Public Perspective*, Educational Testing Service. Princeton, N.J., 1982, pp. 22–30.
5. *Gibson v. Berryhill*, 411 U.S. 564, 93 S. Ct. 1689 (1973).
6. *Friedman v. Rogers*, 440 U.S. 1, 99 S. Ct. 887 (1979).
7. *Rogers v. Medical Association of Georgia*, 244 Ga. 151, 259 S.E.2d 85 (1979).
8. Shimberg, supra note 4, at 19–34.
9. Roederer, D., and B. Shimberg, *Occupational Licensing: Centralizing State Licensure Functions*, Council of State Governments, Lexington, Ky., 1980.
10. Ibid.
11. Another analysis of state board organization, as applied to optometry, can be found in Coblens, S.L., *Optometry and the Law*, American Optometric Association, St. Louis, 1976, pp. 15–25.
12. For a review of the success of sunset laws, see Nice, D.C., Sunset Laws and Legislative Vetoes in the States, *State Government*, vol. 58, no. 1, Spring 1985, pp. 30–35.
13. Shimberg, supra note 4, at 22.
14. The Texas law was an anomaly in that it was an amendment to the medical practice act rather than to the optometry practice act and required Texas optometrists who wished to employ ophthalmic phar-

maceutical agents for diagnostic purposes to obtain standing delegation orders from a physician in order to use the drugs. The Texas Attorney General, in Opinion No. MW-499 of July 30, 1982, held that the statute was unconstitutional, but a successor Attorney General "clarified" this ruling by upholding the statute. See Opinion No. JM-454 of March 20, 1986.

15. Shimberg, supra note 4, at 5–14.
16. Ibid.
17. Ibid. In contrast to the consumer-oriented views offered by Shimberg, practitioners of optometry seem to believe that state boards do a good job with licensure, but feel that enforcement of optometry laws is poor. See Board's Policing Ability Seen Ebbing, *Review of Optometry*, vol. 120, no. 9, Sept. 1983, p. 10.
18. The traditional method of licensure for health-care professionals is currently undergoing study and it seems likely that some changes will be forthcoming in the future. The form that changes would take is at present uncertain, although proposals have entered into previously unexplored ground, such as the recommendation by the California Board of Medical Quality Assurance that the system of licensure be unlocked to permit anyone to become involved in health care, "as long as he or she did not use any of the titles reserved to licensed practitioners." A summary of these recommendations can be found in an article by John Carlova, Will Low-Cost "Healers" Replace MDs?, *Medical Economics*, vol. 59, no. 16, Aug. 9, 1982, pp. 84–90.
19. U.S. Department of Health, Education, and Welfare, Public Health Service, *Credentialing Health Manpower*, DHEW Pub. No. (05) 77-50057, Washington, D.C., July 1977.
20. For a discussion of licensure, see Shimberg, supra note 4, at 15–18.
21. Not to be confused with the requirement to register, which is a legal obligation to register with a designated government agency and which usually involves only the payment of a fee without examination or a demonstration that the individual has met any predetermined standards. See Shimberg, supra note 4, at 18.
22. See id. at 16.
23. It should be mentioned that the American Optometric Association has undertaken a study of the process of certification within optometry, creating a Commission of Optometric Specialties to make recommendations and to coordinate the certification process, if approved by the association. See the *AOA News*, Sept. 1, 1985. As of 1987, the AOA has not adopted any commission recommendations.
24. The U.S. Supreme Court has held in several cases that legal resident aliens may not be prevented from engaging in occupations and professions. Perhaps the leading case is *In re Griffiths*, 413 U.S. 717, 93 S. Ct. 2851 (1973), in which the court ruled that admission to the Connecticut Bar could not hinge upon U.S. citizenship.
25. *Sugarman v. Douglas*, 413 U.S. 634, 93 S. Ct. 2842 (1973).
26. *Graham v. Richardson*, 403 U.S. 365, 91 S. Ct. 1848 (1971).
27. See Shimberg, supra note 4, at 51–54. The usual offenses listed in state optometry practice acts are gross negligence, conviction of a felony or a misdemeanor which involves moral turpitude, gross immorality, habitual drunkeness or narcotic addiction, or willful violation of the optometry law. For a review of the status of persons convicted of crime, see Grant, W., et al., The Collateral Consequences of a Criminal Conviction, *Vanderbilt Law Review*, vol. 23, no. 5, 1970, pp. 1002, 1010.
28. The role of residencies in optometric education is still evolving, with sixty-five accredited positions available (as of mid-1985) at schools and colleges of optometry or within the Veteran's Administration system. These positions represent forty-four different programs, which had their beginning in 1977. Despite the growth of residencies and their potential impact on the educational process, it seems certain that they will have no effect on entry-level licensure.
29. A 1987 survey of state boards conducted by the National Board of Examiners in Optometry (NBEO) reveals the following:

NBEO required: no state writtens given	19 states
NBEO required/accepted: state writtens given to failing candidates	2 states
NBEO required/accepted: state writtens given for specific state requirements	22 states
NBEO useful: state writtens required	2 states
NBEO not accepted: state writtens required	5 states

The state board use of NBEO results is listed on a state-by-state basis in the *Candidate's Guide of the National Board of Examiners in Optometry, Inc.*, Washington, D.C., published yearly. The information listed above can be found in the 1988 edition of the guide.

30. For some sample commentaries, see Holen, A.S., The Effects of Professional Licensing Arrangements on Interstate Mobility and Resource Allocations, *Journal of Political Economy*, vol. 73, no. 5, 1965; Derbyshire, R., *Medical Licensure and Discipline in the United States*, Johns Hopkins Press, Baltimore, 1969; Bateman, R.H., Regulating Professions and Occupations, *Report of the New Jersey Professional and Occupational Licensing Study Commission*, Trenton N.J., Jan. 7, 1971; Shimberg, B., B. Esser, and D. Kruger, *Occupational Licensing: Practices and Policies*, Public Affairs Press, Washington, D.C., 1972; Gellhorn, W., The Abuse of Occupational Licensing, *University of Chicago Law Review*, vol. 44, no. 6, 1976; Shimberg, B., *Improving Occupational Regulation*, Educational Testing Service, Princeton, N.J.,

1976; and Stross, J.K., and W.R. Harlan, The Impact of Mandatory Education, *Journal of the American Medical Association*, vol. 239, no. 25, 1978, p. 2663–2666.

31. See Shimberg, supra note 4, at 54–64. Other sources of information include the following: U.S. Department of Health, Education, and Welfare, *Report On Licensure And Related Health Personnel Credentialing*, DHEW publication 72-11, Washington, D.C., 1971; Shimberg, supra note 30; U.S. Department of Health, Education, and Welfare, Public Health Service, *Credentialing Health Manpower*, supra note 19; and Hogan, D.B., A Study in the Philosophy and Practice of Professional Regulation (vol. I of a four-volume series, *The Regulation of Psychotherapists*), Ballinger Publishing Co., Cambridge, Mass., 1979.
32. Shimberg, supra note 4, describes the restrictions upon interstate mobility caused by licensing examinations on pages 66–68. Interestingly, whereas physicians have a relatively unrestricted right to changes states (as do nurses), dentists and lawyers face numerous restrictions that apparently impede interstate migration.
33. Id. at 64–66.
34. Ibid.
35. Id. at 122–123.
36. Id. at 124–125.
37. Id. at 125–126.
38. Id. at 132–133.
39. U.S. Department of Health, Education and Welfare, *Report On Licensure And Related Health Personnel Credentialing*, supra note 31.
40. Shimberg, supra note 4, at 126–132.
41. For example, see *Disciplinary Digest*, a collection of court decisions about disciplinary actions by state boards of medical examiners, published by the law division of the American Medical Association, Chicago, 1967. In optometry, the cases and decisions of state boards of optometry are compiled in the periodic issues of the *Bulletins from the Office of Counsel of the AOA*. The history of board litigation in optometry has been recounted in Chapter 1.
42. The phrase *due process of law* originated in England and was inserted into the Fourteenth Amendment of the Constitution by the post-civil war U.S. Congress.
43. Due process continues to have interesting applications in the health-care professions. In *Wood v. Graddick*, a 1981 state circuit court case in Montgomery, Alabama, the amendment was used to strike down a state licensing law that set limits on the practice of podiatry. The Alabama statute prohibited podiatrists from working on the tarsals of the human foot, reserving this portion of the human anatomy to the medical profession. The court found no reason why podiatrists could be considered competent enough to operate on the metatarsala and phalanges but not the tarsals. The court observed that the law kept many podiatrists out of Alabama and—comparing podiatric education favorably to medical training—stated:

    It appears that podiatrists are better qualified than osteopaths and M.D.s, by education, training, and experience, to treat the tarsals, and are at least as well qualified as orthopedists, who comprise only five percent of the medical doctor population.

    The court applied the Fourteenth Amendment, which requires that citizens be afforded equal protection of the law, and holds that distinctions in law or regulations that establish two classes of citizens and treat them differently must be rationally related to a legitimate state purpose or they will be in violation of the amendment. Finding no rational relationship between the prohibited surgery and the protection of the public, the court struck down the relevant provisions of the Alabama podiatry practice act (the only state law that contained this restriction). See State Court Stomps on Licensing Provision, *Supplement to Commission Reports*, National Commission for Health Certifying Agencies, vol. 3, no. 3, Summer 1982, p. 12.
44. According to a 1985 survey of state laws published by the American Optometric Association, forty-five states have enacted legislation to regulate physician's assistants. In thirty-eight of these states amendments pertaining to optometric services have been passed: seven states have enacted the Duffy-type amendment, in twenty-five states there is a general optometric exception, in five states physical presence is required, and in one state there is a medical/osteopathic exception. See *Bulletin from the Office of Counsel of the AOA*, vol. 44, no. 7, July 31, 1985.
45. The police power is regarded as a prerogative of state—not federal—government. It is an inherent power of states to enact laws for the protection of the health, safety, and welfare of its citizens, and these laws will be regarded as constitutional as long as they bear a reasonable relation to the end sought. This power is not without limitation, however. The due process clause of the Fourteenth Amendment is one such safeguard, intended to shield the basic rights of citizens against abuse by the state. For a discussion of the important balance between the police power and the Fourteenth Amendment, see *Barsky v. The Board of Regents of the University of the State of New York*, 347 U.S. 442, 74 S. Ct. 650 (1954).
46. *New Hampshire Board of Registration in Optometry v. Scott Jewelry Co.*, 90 N.H. 368, 9 A.2d 513 (1939).
47. *Hewitt v. State Medical Examiners*, 148 Cal. 590, 84 P. 39 (1906); see also *Lawrence v. Biry, Board of Registration in Medicine*, 238 Mass. 424, 132 N.E. 174 (1921).
48. *Meffert v. State Board of Medical Registration and Education*, 66 Kan. 710, 72 P. 247 (1903), *affirmed* 195 U.S. 625, 25 S. Ct. 790 (1903).
49. *Hawker v. People of New York*, 170 U.S. 189, 18 S. Ct. 573 (1893); see also *Barsky*, supra note 45.
50. *White v. Andrews*, 70 Colo. 50, 197 P. 564 (1921).
51. *State Medical Board of Arkansas Medical Society v. McCrary*, 95 Ark. 511, 130 S.W. 544 (1910).
52. *Foreman v. State Board of Health*, 157 Ky. 123, 162 S.W. 796 (1914); and *State Board of Medical Ex-*

aminers v. Macy, 92 Wash. 614, 159 P. 801 (1916).

53. *Matthews v. Murphy*, 23 Ky. 750, 63 S.W. 785 (1901); *In re Hyning*, 257 Mich. 146, 241 N.W. 207 (1932); *Schireson v. Walsh*, 354 Ill. 40, 187 N.E. 921 (1933); and *Colorado State Board of Medical Examiners v. Weiler*, 402 P.2d 606 (Colo. 1965).
54. *State of Missouri ex rel. Hurwitz v. North, Board of Health of the State of Missouri*, 271 U.S. 40, 46 S. Ct. 384 (1925).
55. *State of Florida ex rel. Weathers v. Davis*, 143 Fla. 250, 196 So. 487 (1940); *State v. Hanson*, 201 Iowa 579, 207 N.W. 769 (1926); and *Schireson v. State Board of Medical Examiners of New Jersey*, 129 N.J.L. 203, 28 A.2d 879 (1942), *reversed* 130 N.J.L. 570, 33 A.2d 911 (1943).
56. *Munk v. Frink*, 75 Neb. 172, 106 N.W. 425 (1905).
57. *State of Missouri ex rel. Kerr, State Board of Health v. Landwehr*, 32 S.W.2d 83 (Mo. 1930); *Colorado State Board of Medical Examiners v. Palmer*, 400 P.2d 914 (Colo. 1965).
58. *Mott v. Georgia State Board of Examiners in Optometry*, 148 Ga. 55, 95 S.E. 867 (1918).
59. Numerous cases have dealt with various aspects of disciplinary hearings.

    Manner of service: *Colorado State Board of Medical Examiners v. Palmer*, 400 P.2d 914 (Colo. 1965); *State v. Hanson*, 201 Iowa 579, 207 N.W. 769 (1926).

    The complaint: *Munk v. Frink*, 75 Neb. 172, 106 N.W. 425 (1905); *Freeman v. State Board*, 54 Okla. 531, 154 P. 56 (1916); *Davis v. Calderwood, Board of Registration in Medicine*, 251 Mass. 283, 146 N.E. 708 (1925); *Anderson v. Board of Medical Examiners*, 117 Cal. App. 113, 3 P.2d 344 (1931); *Tapley v. Abbott, State Board of Medical Examiners*, 111 Cal. App. 397, 295 P. 911 (1931); *Mississippi State Board of Health v. Johnson*, 197 Miss. 417, 19 So. 2d 445 (1944); *Schyman v. Department of Registration and Education*, 9 Ill. App. 2d 504, 133 N.E.2d 551 (1956); *State of Montana ex rel. Yuhas v. Board of Medical Examiners*, 135 Mont. 381, 339 P.2d 981 (1959); and *Shapiro v. Board of Regents of the University of the State of New York*, 16 N.Y.2d 783, 262 N.Y.S.2d 503 (1965).

    Amendment of the complaint: *Tapley v. Abbott, State Board of Medical Examiners*, 111 Cal. App. 397, 295 P. 911 (1931); and *In re Buck's License*, 200 Or. 488, 258 P.2d 124 (1953).

    Discovery: *State of Missouri ex rel. Farber v. Shot*, 304 Mo. 523, 263 S.W. 804 (1924); *Moormeister v. Golding, Director of Registration Department*, 84 Utah 324, 27 P.2d 447 (1933); and *Smith v. Department of Registration and Education of the State of Illinois*, 412 Ill. 322, 106 N.E.2d 722 (1952).

    Findings: *Adam v. Connecticut Medical Examining Board*, 137 Conn. 535, 70 A.2d 350 (1951); and *State Board of Medical Examiners v. Gandry*, 149 S.E.2d 644 (S.C. 1966).

    Venue: *In re Shortridge*, 53 N.D. 614, 207 N.W. 442 (1926); *State of Florida ex rel. Landis v. Simmons*, 104 Fla. 487, 140 So. 187 (1932); *De Gaetini v. Driskell, State Board of Medical Examiners*, 139 Fla. 49, 190 So. 461 (1939); *Wall v. American Optometric Association*, 379 F. Supp. 175 (D.C. Ga. 1974), *affirmed* 419 U.S. 888, 95 S. Ct. 166 (1974).

    Statute of limitations: *State v. Schaeffer*, 129 Wis. 459, 109 N.W. 522 (1906); *Medical Examining Board v. Stewart, 46 Wash. 79, 89 P. 475 (1907); In re Buck's License*, 200 Or. 488, 258 P.2d 124 (1953); and *Frank v. Board of Regents of the University of the State of New York*, 24 A.D.2d 909, 264 N.Y.S.2d 413 (1965).

    Burden of proof: *Schyman v. Department of Registration and Education*, 9 Ill. App. 2d 504, 133 N.E.2d 551 (1956), *cert. denied* 352 U.S. 1001, 77 S.Ct. 557; *In re Reno*, 57 Nev. 314, 64 P.2d 1036 (1937); and *Newman v. Board of Regents of the State of New York*, 270 A.D. 964, 61 N.Y.S.2d 841 (1946).

    Regularity of proceedings: *State of Missouri ex rel. Johnson v. Clark, State Board of Health*, 288 Mo. 659, 232 S.W. 1031 (1921); *Ramsey v. Shelton*, 329 Ill. 432, 160 N.E. 769 (1928); *Moormeister v. Department of Registration of the State of Utah*, 76 Utah 146, 288 P. 900 (1930); *Brown v. Hassig*, 136 Kan. 384, 15 P.2d 401 (1932); and *Werted v. Board of Regents of the University of the State of New York*, 18 A.D.2d 1032, 238 N.Y.S.2d 356 (1963).

    Bias: *Gibson v. Berryhill*, 411 U.S. 564, 93 S. Ct. 1689 (1973); and *Friedman v. Rogers*, 440 U.S. 1, 99 S. Ct. 887 (1979).
60. Representative evidentiary rulings include the following:

    Standards of admissibility: *Meffert v. State Board of Medical Registration and Education*, 66 Kan. 710, 72 P. 247, *affirmed* 195 U.S. 625, 25 S. Ct. 790 (1903); and *Tobinsky v. Board of Medical Examiners of the State of California*, 49 Cal. App. 2d 591, 121 P.2d 861 (1942).

    Quality of evidence: *Stevens v. Hill*, 74 Vt. 164, 52 A. 437 (1902); *Thrasher v. Board of Medical Examiners of the State of California*, 44 Cal. App. 26, 185 P. 1006 (1919); *Stammer v. Board of Regents of the University of the State of New York*, 287 N.Y. 359, 39 N.E.2d 913 (1942); and *Sunseri v. Board of Medical Examiners*, 224 Cal. App. 2d 309, 36 Cal. 553 (1964).

    Documentary evidence: *Tobinsky v. Board of Medical Examiners of the State of California*, 49 Cal. App. 2d 591, 121 P.2d 861 (1942); *and Davis v. Board of Medical Examiners*, 108 Cal. App. 2d 346, 239 P.2d 78 (1951).

    Witnesses: *Epstein v. Board of Regents of the University of the State of New York*, 295 N.Y. 154, 65 N.E.2d 756 (1946); *Murphy v. Board of Medical Examiners of California*, 75 Cal. App. 2d 161, 170 P.2d 510 (1946); and *Paley v. Connecticut*, 142 Conn. 522, 115 A.2d 338 (1955).

Board opinion: *Macomber v. State Board of Health*, 28 R.I. 3, 65 A. 263 (1906); *McKay v. State Board of Medical Examiners*, 103 Colo. 305, 86 P.2d 232 (1938); *Jaffe v. State Department of Health*, 135 Conn. 339, 64 A.2d 330 (1949); *Smith v. Department of Registration and Education of the State of Illinois*, 412 Ill. 322, 106 N.E.2d 722 (1952); *Board of Medical Examiners of the State of Oregon v. Mintz*, 233 Or. 441, 378 P.2d 945 (1963); and *Hake v. Arkansas State Medical Board*, 237 Ark. 506, 374 S.W.2d 173 (1964).

61. When medical boards first began to conduct hearings for the purpose of imposing discipline upon physicians, the procedures used were less formal than those employed today. The reason for this increased formality has been the adoption, by statute, of procedures to be followed in virtually every aspect of board actions. The same trend is evident in optometry board laws. Thus, the procedure to be followed can be found in the state optometry practice act. The state code of administrative procedure will control board proceedings when the optometry law is silent (see note 3 supra), but usually the optometry practice act will be found to contain the procedures to be followed by the board.
62. *Christmas v. Voyer*, 92 N.M. 722, 595 P.2d 410 (1979).
63. *Hartman v. Commonwealth*, 454 A.2d 1150 (Pa. 1983).
64. *Samalin v. Board of Optometry*, Case No. EAC-20446, Cal. Superior Ct., Los Angeles County, June 21, 1976, reported in *Bulletin from the Office of Counsel of the AOA*, vol. 37, no. 10, Sept. 7, 1978.
65. The writ of certiorari is one of review or inquiry, and the proceeding is one that requests an appellate court to review the action of an inferior tribunal or that serves as an auxiliary process to enable the appellate court to obtain further information in a pending cause. For application within optometry, see *House of Vision, Inc. v. Watson*, 59 Ill. 2d 508, 322 N.E.2d 15 (1974), *cert. denied*, 422 U.S. 1008, 95 S. Ct. 2631 (1974).
66. Mandamus is a writ that is issued by a court of superior jurisdiction to a private or municipal corporation, or any of its officers, or to an executive, administrative, or judicial officer, or to an inferior court, commanding the performance of a specific act or directing the restoration of rights or privileges to the complainant. For optometry cases involving mandamus, see *New Jersey Optometric Association v. Hillman-Kohan Eyeglasses, Inc.*, 388 A.2d 1299 (1978); and *Mott v. Georgia State Board of Examiners in Optometry*, 148 Ga. 55, 95 S.E. 867 (1918).
67. A declaratory judgment is one that simply declares the rights of the parties or expresses an opinion of the court on a question of law without an order being issued for something to be done. For an example, see *Montgomery Ward v. Board of Examiners in Optometry*, Case No. 54433 (Okla. 1983), reported in *Bulletin from Office of Counsel of the AOA*, vol. 43, no. 46, Dec. 28, 1984.
68. An injunction is writ issued by a court of equity to a defendant requiring the defendant to do or to refrain from doing a particular thing. For examples, see *Wall v. Youmans*, 233 Ga. 191, 154 S.E.2d 191 (1967); and *California Association of Dispensing Opticians, California Board of Optometry v. Pearle Vision Center, Inc.*, 143 Cal. App. 3d 419, 191 Cal. Rptr. 762 (1983).
69. See AOA Obtains Interlocutory Decree, Restraining Ritholzs From Bringing Harassing Lawsuits—Defendants Checked In Setting Up Imitation Association, *Optical Journal and Review of Optometry*, vol. 74, no. 20, Oct. 15, 1937, p. 30. Several cases can be consulted for further information: *Ezell v. Ritholz*, 188 S.C. 39, 198 S.E. 419 (1938); *Ritholz v. Indiana State Board of Registration and Examination*, 45 F. Supp. 423 (D.C. Ind. 1937); *State of Iowa ex rel. Bierring v. Ritholz*, 283 N.W. 268 (Iowa 1939); *Ritholz v. Arkansas State Board of Optometry*, 177 S.W.2d 410 (Ark. 1944); *Ritholz v. Commonwealth*, 184 Va. 339, 35 S.E.2d 210 (1945); and *Ritholz v. Johnson*, 246 Wis. 442, 17 N.W.2d 590 (1945).
70. For sample cases see the following:

Reprimand: *Administrative Hearing re: Yarborough and Wells*, North Carolina State Board of Optometry Hearing, Aug. 31, 1983 (reprimand and $2,500 costs of board hearing), reported in *Bulletin from Office of Counsel of the AOA*, vol. 43, no. 46, Dec. 28, 1984; and "Prescribing Optometrist Is Censured" reported in *The Arizona Republic*, Dec. 28, 1983 (reprimand and probation).

Suspension: *In the Matter of Marrell W. Brooks, O.D.*, North Carolina State Board of Examiners, October 1983 (suspension), reported in *Bulletin from Office of Counsel of the AOA*, vol. 43, no. 46, Dec. 28, 1984; *Department of Professional Regulation v. Cohen*, Florida Board of Optometry, Case No. 0007114, Jan. 28, 1981 (suspension and probation), reported in the *Bulletin from Office of Counsel of the AOA*, vol. 41, no. 23, Jan. 7, 1983; and *Falcone v. New York State Education Dept.*, 50 N.Y.2d 854, 407 N.E.2d 1335 (1980).

Revocation: "Convicted Optometrist Loses License," reported in the *St. Louis Globe-Democrat*, June 15, 1978, and in *Bulletin from Office of Counsel of the AOA*, vol. 37, no. 10, Sept. 7, 1978; *Cardemon v. State Board of Optometric Examiners*, 165 Colo. 520, 441 P.2d 25 (1968); *Serian v. State of West Virginia*, 297 S.E.2d 889 (W. Va. 1982); and *Edmunds v. Board of Examiners in Optometry*, 9 Alas. 482 (1939).

71. *Copeland v. Kansas State Board of Examiners in Optometry*, 518 P.2d 377 (Kan. 1974). For a different result, see *Mordhorst v. Egert*, 223 N.W.2d 501 (S.D. 1974).
72. Perhaps the leading case involving optometry is *Abelson's Inc. v. New Jersey State Board of Opto-*

metrists, 5 N.J. 412, 75 A.2d 867 (1950), in which the court held that a provision of the state optometry law—which allowed the board of optometry to refuse, revoke, or suspend a license for any conduct that the board considered to be of a character likely to deceive or defraud the public—was invalid as a delegation of power that was essentially legislative rather than administrative. For other cases, see *McCrory v. Wood, State Board of Optometry*, 171 So.2d 241 (Ala. 1965) (unethical conduct); *Haffner v. Indiana State Board of Registration in Optometry*, 333 N.E.2d 312 (Ind. App. 1975) (gross incompetence); *Wozniak v. State Board of Examiners in Optometry*, 23 Mich. App. 646, 179 N.W.2d 210 (1970) (gross incompetence); *Pushkin v. Lombard*, 279 So.2d 79 (Fla. App. 1973) (unprofessional conduct); *Walker v. State Board of Optometry*, 322 So.2d 612 (Fla. 1975) (unprofessional conduct); and *Falcone v. New York State Education Dept.*, 50 N.Y.2d 854, 407 N.E.2d 1335 (1980) (unprofessional conduct).

73. *Rayburn v. Minnesota State Board of Optometry*, 247 Minn. 520, 78 N.W.2d 351 (1956). For a discussion of incompetency as the basis for discipline, see *Kansas State Board v. Foote*, 200 Kan. 447, 436 P.2d 828 (1968).
74. *Texas State Board of Examiners in Optometry v. Lane*, 306 S.W.2d 212 (Tex. Civ. App. 1957).
75. For example, see *California Citizens Action Group v. Department of Consumer Affairs*, 407 F. Supp. 1075 (D.C. Cal. 1976), reported in *Bulletin from Office of Counsel of the AOA*, vol. 37, no. 10, Sept. 7, 1978; *Consumer Association of Kentucky v. Kentucky Board of Optometric Examiners*, CA No. 76-26 (US Dist. Court, East. Dist. of Ky., Nov. 1, 1977), reported in *Bulletin from Office of Counsel of the AOA*, vol. 37, no. 10, Sept. 7, 1978; and *Louisiana Consumer's League v. Louisiana State Board of Optometric Examiners*, CA No. 76.2921 (US Dist. Court, East. Dist. of La., Jan. 16, 1977), reported in *Bulletin from Office of Counsel of the AOA*, vol. 37, no. 10, Sept. 7, 1878.
76. *California Association of Dispensing Opticians, California State Board of Optometry v. Pearle Vision Center, Inc.*, 143 Cal. App. 3d 419, 191 Cal. Rptr. 762 (1983).
77. *Friedman v. Rogers*, 440 U.S. 1, 99 S. Ct. 887 (1979).
78. A notable series of cases were brought by boards of optometry during the 1930s, 1940s, and 1950s attempting to divest the profession of the taint of commercialism. Many of these cases have been summarized in the annotations of the *American Law Reports*. See "Right of Corporation, or Individual Not Himself Licensed, to Practice Optometry Through Licensed Employee," 102 A.L.R. 343 and 128 A.L.R. 585.
79. For an example case, see *State of Kansas ex rel. Beck v. Goldman Jewelry Co.*, 142 Kan. 881, 51 P.2d 995 (1935).
80. For an example case, see *Williamson v. Lee Optical of Oklahoma*, 120 F. Supp. 128 (1954), *reversed* 348 U.S. 483, 75 S. Ct. 461 (1955); see also *State of Arizona ex rel. Board of Optometry v. Sears, Roebuck, & Co.*, 102 Ariz. 175, 427 P.2d 126 (1967).
81. For an example case, see *State of Iowa ex rel. Bierring v. Ritholz*, 283 N.W. 268 (Iowa 1939).
82. *Terminal-Hudson Electronics, Inc. v. Department of Consumer Affairs*, 407 F. Supp. 1075 (D.C. Cal. 1976) *vacated and remanded* 426 U.S. 916, 96 S. Ct. 2619 (1976).
83. *California Association of Dispensing Opticians, California Board of Optometry, v. Pearle Vision Center, Inc.*, 143 Cal. App. 3d 419, 191 Cal. Rptr. 762 (1983).
84. For an example case involving optometry, see *Reidinger v. Optometry Examining Board*, 81 Wis.2d 292, 260 N.W.2d 270 (1977). The usual provision allows revocation of the license if the practitioner is convicted of a felony. For cases discussing various aspects of board proceedings on this basis, see *Seitz v. Ohio State Medical Board*, 24 Ohio App. 154, 157 N.E. 304 (1926); *Donnell v. Board of Registration in Medicine*, 128 Me. 523, 149 A. 153 (1930); *Page v. State Board of Medical Examiners of Florida*, 141 Fla. 294, 193 So. 82 (1940); *Mingo County Medical Society, Inc. v. Simon*, 124 W. Va. 493, 20 S.E.2d 807 (1942); *Schireson v. State Board of Medical Examiners of New Jersey*, 129 N.J.L. 203, 28 A.2d 879 (1942), *reversed* N.J.L. 570, 33 A.2d 911 (1943); and *In re Raab, State Medical Board of Ohio v. Raab*, 156 Ohio 158, 101 N.E.2d 294 (1951).
85. See "Convicted Optometrist Loses License," *St. Louis Globe-Democrat*, June 15, 1978, reported in *Bulletin from Office of Counsel of the AOA*, vol. 37, no. 10, Sept. 7, 1978.
86. Representative cases include the following: *Tompkins v. Board of Regents of the University of the State of New York*, 299 N.Y. 469, 87 N.E.2d 517 (1949); *Palmer v. Spaulding, Commissioner of Education*, 299 N.Y. 368, 87 N.E.2d 201 (1949); *Glenn v. Colorado State Board of Medical Examiners*, 131 Colo. 586, 284 P.2d 230 (1955); *Texas State Board of Medical Examiners v. McClellan*, 307 S.W.2d 317 (1957); *Strode v. Board of Medical Examiners of California*, 195 Cal. App. 2d 291, 15 Cal. Rptr. 879 (1961); *Board of Medical Registration and Education of Indiana v. Armington*, 242 Ind. 436, 178 N.E.2d 741 (1961); and *Bernanke v. Board of Regents of the University of the State of New York*, 24 A.D.2d 910, 264 N.Y.S.2d 399 (1965).
87. For a sample case involving an optometrist, see *Reid v. New Mexico Board of Examiners in Optometry*, 92 N.M. 414, 589 P.2d 198 (1979); also see *Samalin v. Board of Optometry*, No. EAC-20446 (Cal Super. Ct., Los Angeles Co., June 21, 1976), reported in *Bulletin from Office of Counsel of the AOA*, vol. 37, no. 10, Sept. 7, 1978.
88. *Cardemon v. State Board of Optometric Examiners*, 165 Colo. 520, 441 P.2d 25 (1968).

89. For cases involving the use of unlicensed persons in violation of the optometry statute, see *Beaver v. Louisiana State Board of Optometry Examiners*, 206 So. 2d 118 (La. App. 1968); and *Serian v. State of West Virginia*, 297 S.E.2d 889 (W. Va. 1982).
90. *Falcone v. New York State Education Dept.*, 50 N.Y.2d 854, 407 N.E.2d 1335 (1980).
91. Moral turpitude may be defined as conduct contrary to justice, honesty, modesty, or good morals. *Black's Law Dictionary*, 4th ed., West, St. Paul, Minn., 1968.
92. Numerous cases have been brought alleging moral turpitude as the basis for disciplinary action, including the following: *Kemp v. Board of Supervisors*, 45 App. D.C. 173 (1917) (advertising of abortion by physician); *State Medical Board v. Rogers*, 109 Ark. 266, 79 S.W.2d 83 (1935) (possession of counterfeit money by physician); *Speer v. State*, 109 S.W.2d 1150 (Tex. Civ. App. 1937) (physician convicted of smuggling narcotics); *DuVall v. Board of Medical Examiners of Arizona*, 49 Ariz. 329, 66 P.2d 1026 (1937) (conviction of physician for sale of narcotics); *Brainard v. Board of Medical Examiners of the State of California*, 68 Cal. App. 2d 591, 157 P.2d 7 (1945) (physician did not maintain adequate records of narcotics dispensed to patients); *Furnish v. Board of Medical Examiners*, 149 Cal. App. 2d 326, 308 P.2d 924 (1957) (physician guilty of income tax evasion); and *Bernstein v. Board of Medical Examiners*, 204 Cal. App. 2d 378, 22 Cal. Rptr. 419 (1962) (psychiatrist convicted of statutory rape of teenage patient).
93. For example, an Arizona optometrist was censured for prescribing pharmaceutical agents for therapeutic purposes, the state board of optometry finding that this conduct was outside the scope of practice permissible under the optometry practice act. See "Prescribing Optometrist Is Censured," *The Arizona Republic*, Dec. 28, 1983.
94. In Louisiana, a federal judge established the minimum standards for an initial optometric examination. See *Louisiana Consumer's League v. Louisiana State Board of Optometric Examiners*, Civil Case No. 76.2921, East. Dist. La., Jan. 16, 1977, reported in *Bulletin from Office of Counsel of the AOA*, vol. 37, no. 10, Sept. 7, 1978; and *LeBow v. Optometry Examining Board*, 52 Wis. 2d 569, 191 N.W.2d 47 (1971), in which the optometrist was disciplined for failing to perform a "minimum examination."
95. Gross negligence was cited as a basis for discipline in *Wozniak v. State Board of Examiners in Optometry*, 23 Mich. App. 646, 179 N.W.2d 208 (1970); and in *Blanchard v. Michigan State Board of Examiners in Optometry*, 198 N.W. 2d 804 (Mich. 1972).
96. The right of a state board of optometry to regulate branch offices is upheld in *Abelson's, Inc. v. New Jersey State Board of Optometrists*, 5 N.J. 412, 75 A.2d 867 (1950).
97. *Brown v. State Board of Examiners in Optometry*, 263 N.W.2d 490 (S.D. 1978).
98. See *Cassidy v. Indiana State Board of Registration and Examination in Optometry*, 244 Ind. 137, 191 N.E.2d 492 (1963), and the resultant malicious prosecution case, *Cassidy v. Cain*, 251 N.E.2d 852 (Ind. App. 1969).
99. See Shimberg, supra note 4, at 101–121.
100. For a discussion of the right of appeal, see *Porter v. Michigan State Board of Examiners in Optometry*, 41 Mich. App. 150, 199 N.W.2d 666 (1972).
101. For a review of the legal basis for jurisdiction, see the following annotations: "Constitutionality of Statutes and Validity of Regulations Relating to Optometry," 98 A.L.R. 905; and "Validity of Governmental Regulation of Optometry," 22 A.L.R.2d 939. See also *Williamson v. Lee Optical of Oklahoma*, 348 U.S. 483, 75 S. Ct. 461 (1955).
102. For a discussion of the exemption granted to physicians, see Coblens, S.L., *Optometry and the Law*, supra note 11, at 1–38; and Chapter 1.
103. See "Practicing Medicine, Surgery, Dentistry, Optometry, Podiatry, or Other Healing Arts Without License as a Separate or Continuing Offense," 99 A.L.R.2d 654; "One Who Fills Prescriptions Under Reciprocal Arrangement with Physician or Optometrist as Subject to Charge of Practice of Medicine or Optometry Without License," 121 A.L.R. 1455; "What Constitutes Practice of 'Optometry,'" 121 A.L.R. 1455, 141 A.L.R. 883, and 88 A.L.R.2d 1290; "Fitting of Contact Lenses as Practice of Optometry," 77 A.L.R.3d 817; and "Right of Corporation, or Individual Not Himself Licensed, To Practice Optometry Through Licensed Employee," 102 A.L.R. 343 and 128 A.L.R. 585.
104. Even where the statute is penal in nature, injunctive relief may be sought. See *Kelly ex rel. Michigan Board of Examiners v. Peterson*, 4 Mich. App. 612, 145 N.W.2d 386 (1966).
105. The definition of optometry has been interpreted to include the use of self–eye-testing devices and other subjective means of determining the patient's corrective lenses. See "What Constitutes Practice of Optometry," 141 A.L.R. 883, citing *People v. Griffith*, 280 Ill. 18, 117 N.E. 195 (1917); *State v. Etzenhouser*, 223 Mo. App. 577, 16 S.W.2d 656 (1929); and *Price v. State*, 168 Wis. 603, 171 N.W. 77 (1919).
106. See *State of Oregon ex rel. Reed v. Kuzirian*, 228 Or. 619, 365 P.2d 1046 (1961); *Ketring v. Sturges*, 372 S.W.2d 104 (Mo. 1963); *Pennsylvania Optometric Association v. Di Giovanni*, 45 Pa. D.&C.2d 245 (1968); *and State of Oklahoma ex rel. Clifton v. Reeser*, 543 P.2d 1379 (Okla. 1975). Contra: *Commonwealth v. Stemet*, 21 Pa. D.&C.2d 295 (1959); *High v. Ridgeway's Opticians*, 258 N.C. 626, 129 S.E.2d 301 (1963); and *Florida Association of Dispensing Opticians v. Florida State Board of Optometry*, 238 So.2d 839 (Fla. 1970), *conformed to* 239 So.2d 520 (Fla. App. 1970).
107. *New Jersey State Board of Optometrists v. Reiss*, 83 N.J. Super. 47, 198 A.2d 816 (1964); *Fields v. District of Columbia*, 232 A.2d 300 (D.C. App. 1967),

adhered to 244 A.2d 643 (D.C. App. 1968); *State of Missouri ex rel. Danforth v. Dale Curteman, Inc.*, 480 S.W.2d 848 (Mo. 1972); and *House of Vision, Inc. v. Watson* 59 Ill. 2d 508, 322 N.E.2d 15, *cert. denied* 422 U.S.1008, 95 S. Ct. 2631 (1974).

108. See "Right of Corporation, or Individual Not Himself Licensed, to Practice Optometry Through Licensed Employee," 102 A.L.R. 343 and 128 A.L.R. 585.

109. For example, in Texas the optometry practice act has been amended to permit civil actions by any injured party, the action to include injunctive relief, damages, court costs and reasonable attorney's fees. Section 5.11 (d) of the Texas Optometry Act (*Texas Rev. Civ. Stat. Ann.* arts. 4552-1.01 et seq. [Vernon 1965]).

110. Comity is a matter of courtesy, a willingness to grant a privilege, not necessarily as a matter of right but out of deference and good will. For a discussion of the conflict between boards and licensing laws, see Shimberg, supra note 4, at 84–100.

111. Res judicata is a rule that a final judgment or decree on the merits of a civil case rendered by a court of competent jurisdiction is conclusive of the rights of the parties (or their privies) in all later suits as to the points and matters determined by the prior suit. To be applicable, there must be identity as to the thing sued for as well as identity of the cause of action, of persons and parties to the action, and of quality in the persons for or against whom the claim is made. The rule stands for the proposition that a matter once judicially decided is finally decided. *Black's Law Dictionary*, 4th ed., West, St. Paul, Minn., 1968.

112. For example, in Florida the board of optometry issued a ruling that optometrists could use ophthalmic drugs for therapeutic purposes, but this rule was challenged by the state medical association, and the board of pharmacy refused to honor the prescriptions for therapeutic drugs written by state optometrists. Although the optometry board did not prevail in the lawsuit that followed, the Florida optometrists succeeded in passing an amendment to the state optometry practice act that expressly permitted the use of these drugs. The bill, although vetoed by the governor, was upheld as valid by a Florida appeals court on the ground that the governor's veto was cast after the bill had automatically become law. See the *AOA News*, April 1, 1985. As in any good soap opera, the fortunes of the Florida optometrists were once again reversed, as the state supreme court upheld the veto! See *Florida Society of Ophthalmology v. Florida Optometric Association*, 489 So. 2d 1118 (Fla. 1986), *reversing* 465 So. 2d 1319 (Fla. App. 1985).

Chapter 12

Third-Party Regulation

The price of optometric freedom is eternal vigilance.
—AOA Counsel Harold Kohn, *comment made at the close of every annual report to the AOA House of Delegates*

Regulation or Discrimination?
Assuring Nondiscrimination
Freedom of Choice
Obtaining Like Reimbursement
Taxation of Ophthalmic Goods

Regulation or Discrimination?

Harold Kohn, who served for more than three decades as general counsel of the American Optometric Association, was intimately acquainted with the struggle waged by optometrists to remain independent,[1] fought primarily in the legislatures of Washington, D.C. and of the various state capitals, as optometrists sought to obtain fair treatment at the hands of federal and state government. As we have seen, optometry is a creature of statute, and the many laws, regulations, and rulings emanating from the legislative and administrative branches of government have exerted a profound influence upon the socioeconomic well-being of the profession.

But the regulation of optometry by federal and state government is not limited to administrative agencies and legislatures. A less conspicuous but increasingly important form of regulation is imposed through vision service plans, which are either public or private in nature. Health insurance that includes vision services is a relatively recent development, but the clear trend is toward increased use of these plans, the potential of which has just begun to be realized.[2] The establishment and administration of vision care benefits have brought a new set of legal issues before optometry.[3] Unfortunately, these issues have included discrimination against the profession by both government and the private sector.

The California Vision Service Plan (VSP) was the first private prepaid insurance plan for vision care in the United States; begun in the 1950s, it remains the nation's largest.[4] Successor plans have proliferated throughout the nation as vision services have begun to receive wider acceptance as a benefit of employment.[5] But two major legal problems have emerged with regard to these plans: how to determine those eligible to be providers under the program (can a plan be limited to physicians only? optometrists only? to certain named doctors in a community only?) and how to establish fair reimbursement policies for these providers (can physicians be reimbursed on a different scale than optometrists? can certain services be limited to physicians only?). The regulation of vision service plans is, for the most part, a matter of state law. Only those state laws that pertain to private industry apply, however, since public funds are not involved in the financing of these plans. Thus private vision service plans enjoy a degree of independence that publicly funded plans do not.

The enactment of Medicare and Medicaid in 1965 brought the federal government into the administration of vision service plans for the first time: Through Medicare, aphakic services and materials were eligible for reimbursement, and through Medicaid, vision screening and other eyecare services for the needy were reimbursable. The eligibility of optometrists to serve as providers under these programs became a legislative and judicial issue that sparked widespread debate, and the reimbursement policies established for optometric practitioners likewise generated a flood of legal activity.[6] Although many of these issues have been resolved, legal problems continue to plague these and other federal programs.

Like the federal government, the states allow reimbursement for specified vision services provided to eligible recipients, such as under vocational rehabilitation programs for the visually handicapped. The determination of those eligible for reimbursement under these plans, and the reimbursement schedules to be applied, have served as the basis for legislative and judicial activity on the part of optometrists.[7] As a result of these activities, most states now include optometric practitioners as providers of vision services and establish equal reimbursement policies for optometrists and physicians.

The problems posed by vision service plans can be divided into three categories:

1. Assuring that optometrists are eligible to participate in covered services which are within the scope of optometric licensure (remedied through the passage of nondiscrimination legislation)
2. Establishing that patients will be permitted to choose the practitioner of their choice (whether O.D. or M.D.) for covered services (achieved through the enactment of freedom-of-choice legislation)
3. Determining that all providers (optometrists or physicians) will receive like reimbursement for the same services (obtained through the inclusion of "like reimbursement" language within the provisions of the plan).

Although vision service plans have been the cause of the majority of legal actions initiated to abolish discrimination, an unrelated government activity has likewise served as the impetus for legal efforts at reform: the taxation of ophthalmic goods. Optometrists have fought a series of legal battles over the right of state government to tax optometric services and ophthalmic goods, a struggle that has had significance for the consumer as well as for the profession. It is an issue that remains viable today.

This chapter discusses the various discriminatory problems related to vision service plans before concluding with a brief description of the legal considerations involved in the taxation of ophthalmic goods. Since in the majority of cases these problems are matters of state law, general fact situations must be used, from which general conclusions will be drawn. State statutes will have to be consulted in order to determine the applicable law in any individual case.

Assuring Nondiscrimination

Nondiscrimination legislation is intended to assure that doctors of optometry receive the same treatment under the law as physicians or other health care providers eligible to render like services. The programs to which these laws apply may be public or private in character and may involve the delivery of vision services for such matters as health insurance, certification for public assistance, assessment of visual disability, testimony in legal disputes, and similar legal issues that are within the scope of optometric practice. In some instances discrimination has been arrested through the intervention of the courts.

Public Plans

The most fundamental discrimination is the exclusion of optometrists from a vision service program, where the program offers services that are within the scope of optometric licensure. Perhaps the foremost example of this type of discrimination was the original Medicare bill, which excluded optometrists from coverage except for the dispensing of aphakic lenses. Since routine services such as refraction were excluded from Medicare, optometrists could not receive reimbursement for this service, even for aphakic patients. Physicians were not reimbursed for refractive services either, but could receive compensation under Medicare for eye health examinations. Thus began a long legislative battle to accord optometrists legal recognition as physicians under Medicare. After years of defeat in the federal congress, optometrists challenged the fairness of the Medicare law in the courts.

A group of optometrists filed suit in federal court challenging the constitutionality of the Medicare provisions that defined reimburseable services so as to exclude optometric participation. They also alleged that the distinctions in the law between optometrists and physicians were arbitrary and denied optometrists equal protection under the law. The suit was dismissed, but the optometrists appealed. In upholding the dismissal, the Fifth Circuit Court of Appeals noted that there were other courts and means of litigating the issue that had been designated by congress for challenges to the Medicare program. The court held that it had no jurisdiction over the issue.[8]

This decision forced optometry to look once again to a legislative remedy, a recourse that became more feasible when the Department of Health, Education, and Welfare issued a study that suggested fuller utilization of optometrists within Medicare.[9] This report was challenged by a group of physicians, who maintained that the report was biased and improperly compiled.

The suit was filed in federal court, seeking recission of the HEW report favoring increased utilization of optometrists by Medicare. The case was dismissed, but upon appeal it was reviewed by the District of Columbia Circuit Court of Appeals, which agreed with the lower court's analysis that the suit —which came three years after the report was issued—was not timely. The suit was dismissed.[10]

Consequently, optometrists were included under Medicare as physicians eligible for reimbursement for eye health examinations. The fee schedules established under Medicare for optometrists were based upon profiles that considered only optometric practitioners in determining the reimbursement to be paid for examinations.[11] These fees have not been subjected to legal scrutiny.

Medicaid has a similar history of legal controversy, with the dispute at first centering around participation in the program, an issue that continues to generate litigation.

Louisiana optometrists brought suit, alleging that the state medical assistance plan (Medicaid) was unconstitutional and violated the Louisiana freedom-of-choice statute. The case was heard in federal district court, which held that, because optometrists did not make *definitive* diagnoses of the existence or nonexistence of eye pathology or disease, there was no wrongful discrimination because only ophthalmologists were qualified under Louisiana law to make definitive diagnoses (and to be reimbursed under the medical assistance plan for such diagnoses). The case was appealed, and after a tortuous course through the appellate process, the Fifth Circuit Court of Appeals held that the plan was in violation of the Louisiana statute that prohibited state officials from limiting or restricting the freedom of patients to choose between an optometrist or a physician for eye care services. The court ordered the plan amended "so as to provide that optometrists who perform eye care services that are within the scope of optometric practice will receive Medicaid reimbursement to the same extent, and according to the same standards, as physicians who perform those same eye care services. The defendants must put optometrists on a precisely equal footing with ophthalmologists and other physicians with regard to reimbursement for services that optometrists are qualified to perform under Louisiana law."[12]

Medicaid was intended to encourage individual states to establish unified health assistance programs for the poor, and although minimum federal requirements had to be met by each state, a considerable degree of variability could exist from state to state. An important provision of Medicaid was that only vision screening services were mandatory, which allowed the states to determine which, if any, vision services would be offered as an optional benefit to those eligible as medically needy. In some states, only pathological eye disorders were covered under the program, a provision that was held to violate federal law.

Vermont's Department of Social Welfare prohibited the payment of Medicaid funds for glasses or for services required to correct refractive error and only allowed reimbursement for glasses if the claimant's vision problem arose from an eye disease or from surgery performed to treat an eye disease. A class action was brought challenging these regulations, and a federal court ruled that the Vermont program was being conducted contrary to federal law, holding that, by denying benefits to persons suffering from refractive error, the state was reducing the scope of a required service solely on the basis of diagnosis, type of illness, or condition, which was in contravention of Medicaid regulations.[13]

A Pennsylvania medical assistance program funded under Medicaid that provided eyeglasses only to individuals with pathological eye disorders was found to be in violation of federal law. Subsequently, the state department of public welfare decided to eliminate the program entirely but failed to give individual participants adequate notice of the termination. A suit was brought to have the program continued until the notice requirements could be complied with. In upholding the suit, the Third Circuit Court of Appeals held that the fact that the program was nominally optional did not mean that a state could terminate it without restraint.[14]

Medicaid fee schedules are determined on a state-by-state basis and have long been criticized by optometrists as being deplorably low. Legal efforts to have the courts—rather than state government—set Medicaid fees have been unsuccessful.[15]

Public vision service plans funded by the states, such as those that require certification or examination to determine eligibility for state financial assistance, are discussed in the following section on freedom-of-choice.

Private Plans

Vision service plans that are organized and funded through private sources have also been the subject of legislative and judicial scrutiny. These plans establish a panel of doctors that contracts to provide specified vision services to certain beneficiaries at a predetermined cost. Physicians have formulated panels that purposefully excluded optometrists from membership, but such plans will not necessarily be approved by the state.

A nonprofit health service plan offering a comprehensive general ophthalmological service that consisted of an examination and treatment (including medication or lenses) filed an application with the state to have the plan approved. The Pennsylvania Optometric Association objected to the plan's requirement that participating doctor membership be limited to physicians, but the plan justified the exclusion on the basis that the vision services were principally medical in nature and that optometrists were not trained or qualified to provide such services. Under state law, however, optometrists were included under the definition of health service doctor. The application was found to violate Pennsylvania law, with the state concluding, "Eligibility to register with a professional health service plan turns upon the nature of the proposed services, procedures, and materials and the qualifications of a health service doctor to provide them competently, regardless of the doctor's category of licensure."[16]

The determining factor in the legal regulation of private plans is whether or not the state law requires freedom of choice. But these statutes only apply to competing professions. The courts have held that panel membership within a profession does not have to be unrestricted and thus open to all eligible licensees.

An optometrist who sought membership on the California Vision Service Plan (VSP) filed suit seeking to compel the state optometry board to force VSP to strike from its membership criteria all advertising restrictions of the kind allowed under state law. In deciding the case, the Court of Appeals held that a nonprofit corporation such as VSP was not required to grant membership to every licensed optometrist without restriction, and that VSP did not act improperly in establishing such restrictions.[17]

Another concern is the ability of federal law—principally the Employee and Retirement Income Security Act (ERISA)—to supersede state statutes that guarantee nondiscrimination and freedom of choice. The full application of ERISA has not yet been determined.[18]

Freedom of Choice

Whereas nondiscrimination legislation was intended to provide equal treatment under the law for optometrists, freedom-of-choice legislation was intended to permit persons seeking vision services under public or private programs to select the provider of their choice rather than be limited exclusively to physicians. Freedom-of-choice laws have been enacted, in some form, in the majority of states. These laws are either public in nature (preventing discrimination by the state and its agencies) or private (prohibiting discrimination in private insurance plans). A summary of states in which freedom-of-choice legislation has been enacted can be found in Tables 12.1 and 12.2.

The language and application of these statutes varies widely from state to state. Some examples of these laws can be used to illustrate their diversity.

> *Private Plans.* No person entitled to benefits under this Act shall be denied his or her freedom of choice of any practitioner licensed under Arkansas Statutes Section 72-602 or Arkansas Statutes Section 72-801 by any insurer or agent or employee of such insurer or by any Department, Agency, or employee of this State.[19]
>
> *Public Plans.* Any state or municipal board, commission, department, institution, agency or bureau including public schools expending public money for any purpose involving eye care which is within the scope of the practice of optometry shall not deny the recipients or beneficiaries the freedom to choose an optometrist. . . .[20]
>
> *Medical foundations.* If any medical or healing arts practitioners join together to offer, through a medical foundation, medical and healing arts care and provide ophthalmologic care, such care shall include optometric care.[21]
>
> *Health Maintenance Organizations.* If a health maintenance organization offers eye care which is within the scope of the practice of optometry it shall make optometric care available to its subscribers.[22]

Freedom-of-choice laws involving optometric services have been challenged as unconstitutional and

Table 12.1. Freedom of Choice: Private Acts, 1985

State	Statute
Alabama	Ala. Code §27-19-39
Alaska	Alaska Stat. §21.87-330(8)
Arizona	Ariz. Rev. Ann. §§20-1376, 20-1406, 20-841
Arkansas	Ark. Stat. Ann. §3212.2
California	Cal. Ins. Code §§10176, 10177.6 (Deering)
Colorado	Colo. Rev. Stat. §§10-8-103, 10-16-107, 12-40-117
Connecticut	Conn. Gen. Stat. §20-138d
Delaware	Del. Code Ann. tit. 24, §2101C
District of Columbia	D.C. Code Ann. §35-530
Florida	Fla. Stat. Ann. §627.419
Georgia	Ga. Code Ann. §56-2447
Hawaii	Hawaii Rev. Stat. §431-450
Idaho	Idaho Code §41-2103(9)
Illinois	Illinois Ann. Stat. ch. 32, §§667.1, 609.10
Indiana	Indiana Stat. Ann. §§27-8-11, 27-8-6-1 (Burns)
Iowa	Iowa Code Ann. §§514.B1, 514.7, 509.3
Kansas	Kan. Stat. Ann. §§40-2, 100, 50-112
Kentucky	Ky. Rev. Stat. Ann. §§304.17-305, 304.18-095, 304.32-157 (Baldwin)
Louisiana	La. Rev. Stat. Ann. §22:664
Maine	Me. Rev. Stat. Ann. tit. 24A, §2841
Maryland	Md. Ann. Code art. 48A, §§355(b)(2), 470A; 477F
Massachusetts	Mass. Gen. Laws Ann. ch. 175, §§108,110
Michigan	Mich. Comp. Laws Ann. §21.12213
Minnesota	Minn. Stat. Ann. §§62A.03(10), 62A.15(3), 62C.14(3)
Mississippi	Miss. Code Ann. §83-41-203
Missouri	Mo. Rev. Stat. §§375.947, 375.936(11)(b)
Montana	Mont. Code Ann. §33-22-111(1)
Nebraska	Neb. Rev. Stat. §44-513
Nevada	Nev. Rev. Stat. §686A.100
New Hampshire	N.H. Rev. Stat. Ann. §§415:5(A)(8), 415.18
New Jersey	N.J. Rev. Stat. Ann. §§17B:27-51, 17:48A-29
New Mexico	N.M. Stat. Ann. §61-2-16
New York	N.Y. Ins. Law §§250(1), 221(5) (Consol.)
North Carolina	N.C. Gen. Stat. §§57-1, 58-260
North Dakota	N.D. Cent. Code §43-13-31
Ohio	Ohio Rev. Code Ann. §3923.23 (Baldwin)
Oklahoma	Okla. Stat. tit. 36, §6051
Oregon	Or. Rev. Stat. §§743.117, 750.065
Pennsylvania	Pa. Stat. Ann. tit. 40, §1502 (Purdon)
Rhode Island	R.I. Gen. Laws §40.1-3-15
South Carolina	
South Dakota	S.D. Codified Laws Ann. §58-17-54
Tennessee	Tenn. Code Ann. §§56-7-108, 56-7-109
Texas	Tex. Ins. Code Ann. §§3.70-2, 21.52 (Vernon)
Utah	Utah Code Ann. §§31-20-3, 31-33-2.5
Vermont	
Virginia	Va. Code §§38.1-824, 38.1-347.1, 38.1-347.2
Washington	Wash. Rev. Code Ann. §§48.21.140, 48.20.410
West Virginia	W. Va. Code §33-6-30
Wisconsin	Wis. Stat. Ann. §§628.36, 632.87
Wyoming	Wyo. Stat. §26-22-101

Source: American Optometric Association, 1985.

have been upheld as being within the police power of the state.

A Virginia statute required prepaid medical plans to pay for services provided by podiatrists, optometrists, psychologists, and others if the same services were paid for when provided by medical doctors. Blue Cross/Blue Shield did not comply with the statute, and when ordered by the state to do so, filed a suit challenging the constitutionality of the law. The case was ultimately decided by the state supreme court, which, in upholding the law, made the following comment:

> Here the subject of legislative attention is directly related to protection of the public health, a necessary, legitimate public purpose; the purpose is not, as defendants contend, to further the economic interests of non-physician licensed practitioners. To support this public objective, the General Assembly has authorized establishment of plans to provide prepaid medical services at reasonable costs for the general public. The focus is on services for medical care and the availability of such services. As a means to increase the accessibility of such services to the public, the legislature by the 1973 amendment has required defendants to recognize and pay for the services rendered by optometrists, opticians, and psychologists, but only if the services are those which these providers are licensed to render in Virginia. Thus, as the Commission decided, the legislature has increased the availability of mental and eye care services to the public by permitting them to choose between the services of psychiatrists and psychologists, and ophthalmologists and opticians and optometrists. The method employed by this state reasonably accomplishes its purpose and is rationally related to such objective.[23]

Table 12.2. Freedom of Choice: Public Acts, 1985

State	Statute
Alabama	
Alaska	Alaska Stat. §23.30-265
Arizona	Ariz. Rev. Stat. Ann. §§46-276, 46-301-303
Arkansas	Ark. Stat. Ann. §§83-128.4, 83-128.5
California	Cal. Welf. & Inst. Code §14053 (Deering), Cal. Bus. & Prof. Code §690 (Deering)
Colorado	
Connecticut	Conn. Gen. Stat. §20-138B
Delaware	Del. Code Ann. tit. 24, §2118; tit. 19, §2323
District of Columbia	
Florida	Fla. Stat. Ann. §463.014
Georgia	Ga. Code Ann. §89-956
Hawaii	
Idaho	Idaho Code §56-214A
Illinois	Ill. Ann. Stat. ch. 127, §535.1
Indiana	
Iowa	
Kansas	Kan. Stat. Ann. §§44-5085, 72-5376
Kentucky	Ky. Rev. Stat. Ann. §§205.560, 320.380 (Baldwin)
Louisiana	La. Rev. Stat. Ann. §§37:1066, 49:185
Maine	Me. Rev. Stat. Ann. tit. 32, §2444
Maryland	Md. Health Occ. Code Ann. §10-401(b)
Massachusetts	Mass. Gen. Laws Ann. ch. 151D, §3A
Michigan	Mich. Comp. Laws Ann. §16-601
Minnesota	
Mississippi	Miss. Code Ann. §43-13-117
Missouri	Mo. Rev. Stat. §336.210
Montana	Mont. Code Ann. §37-10-104
Nebraska	Neb. Rev. Stat. §71-1,136.04
Nevada	Nev. Rev. Stat. §636.385
New Hampshire	
New Jersey	N.J. Rev. Stat. Ann. §45:12-27
New Mexico	
New York	
North Carolina	N.C. Gen. Stat. §90-127.1
North Dakota	N.D. Cent. Code §43-13-30
Ohio	Ohio Rev. Code Ann. §4725.16
Oklahoma	Okla. Stat. tit. 56, §199
Oregon	Or. Rev. Stat. §683.435
Pennsylvania	Pa. Stat. Ann. tit. 63, §244.10
Rhode Island	R.I. Gen. Laws §40.1-3-15
South Carolina	S.C. Rev. Code §40-37-160
South Dakota	
Tennessee	Tenn. Code Ann. §14-20-313
Texas	
Utah	Utah Code Ann. §31-27-24
Vermont	
Virginia	
Washington	Wash. Rev. Code Ann. §§18.53.160, 165, 170, 175, 180, 185, 190
West Virginia	
Wisconsin	Wis. Stat. Ann. §499.01 (3)
Wyoming	Wyo. Stat. §56-214A

Source: American Optometric Association, 1985.

Unfortunately, the courts can be confused by the complexities of these statutes,[24] but freedom-of-choice laws have recently re-established the applicability of antitrust law to health insurance plans,[25] a development that has interesting and far-reaching significance for optometry.

Obtaining Like Reimbursement

Even though statutes may specify the eligibility of optometrists to participate in public or private vision service programs, there yet remains the problem of fair reimbursement, a matter that arises when optometrists and physicians are both included as providers of covered services. If the method of reimbursement differs between optometrists and physicians, there is the prospect for discrimination.

To prevent this form of discrimination, optometrists have sought legislation to assure that the amount or method of reimbursement for services provided will be the same regardless of the discipline of the provider. These statutes have required like reimbursement for services within the scope of practice of optometrists and have superceded the so-called equal fees for equal services legislation enacted in several states. The equal services laws were often attacked by physicians on the basis that procedures performed by doctors of optometry were different from the procedures performed by doctors of medicine, and hence the services were not equal. Use of the term services within the scope of practice clarifies the intent of these laws, which is to provide reimbursement for a covered service regardless of the nature of the provider, as long as the service is within the provider's scope of licensure. As a result, vision service plans can list the services for which they will provide reimbursement, and the determination of which licensee may provide those services rests with the state licensing laws.

Although the legal conflict over fair reimbursement, nondiscrimination in vision service plans, and freedom-of-choice for patients has been partially resolved in the legislatures and courts, optometrists continue to encounter situations in which discrimination is alleged. Some problem areas are:

Membership in Health Maintenance Organizations (HMOs) and Preferred Provider Organizations (PPOs)—In some HMOs and PPOs membership is restricted to physician providers only

Testimony as to visual disability—Under worker's compensation laws, injured workers are compensated for their injury in accordance with the degree of impairment; in some situations optometrist testimony as to ocular disability is not accepted

Certification for driver's licenses—The certification of visial efficiency for driver's licenses is not accepted in some states unless performed by a physician

Optometric participation in medical foundations—In many states medical foundations that offer health-care programs including vision care may bar optometrists from membership

Government-sponsored benefits programs limited to physicians—In a few states the participants in government-sponsored public assistance programs do not have freedom of choice when seeking vision care

Another source of conflict has involved the taxation of ophthalmic goods.

Taxation of Ophthalmic Goods

In a number of states sales or use taxes have been imposed upon the dispensing of eyeglasses, contact lenses, and other optical accessories.[26] Although the nature of the sales or use tax is determined by the terms of the statute under which it is imposed, there are features of these laws that are common to all. One such feature concerns the taxation of services.

For a vocation to be taxable under a retailer's occupation tax, it must be one that sells tangible personal property rather than one that renders services, and the recognition of optometry as a service-oriented profession has been obtained in all states. Thus the services of optometrists are not subject to sales or use taxes.[27]

In states where sales taxes are levied on the sale of eyewear and optical accessories, however, it has been held that the portion of an optometrist's fee that represents the cost of materials will be subject to the tax. In reaching this conclusion the courts have held that the portion of the fee attributable to services and materials is severable,[28] lump sum charges for professional services rendered that include ophthalmic goods could not avoid the tax,[29] and the dispensing of glasses was not an inconsequential element of the personal services rendered by optometrists and hence an exception to the tax statutes.[30]

One constitutional question that has been raised by the imposition of these taxes concerns their application to optometrists but not to ophthalmologists. When a sales tax is levied on the sale of ophthalmic materials to the patients of optometrists but the patients of ophthalmologists are not charged the tax for the same transaction, constitutional allegations of unequal protection under the law will be upheld.

The State of Alabama imposed a sales tax upon the sale of glasses or contact lenses by optometrists and opticians. Ophthalmologists were not required to charge the tax. Suit was brought against the state, alleging that the law was unconstitutional since it denied the patients of optometrists the same protection under the law granted to the patients of ophthalmologists—exclusion from the sales tax—and caused the majority of the tax to be paid by patients in rural areas. It was also argued that optometry was a learned profession and that the dispensing of eyewear was not a sale but rather the furnishing of a product incidental to the rendering of professional services. The state supreme court ruled that the law was being applied unfairly, but upheld its validity, requiring that it be imposed on the patients of both optometrists and ophthalmologists.[31]

Another constitutional issue that remains unresolved is the right of states to exempt the taxation of the sale of drugs, dentures, orthopedic shoes, and like prosthetic devices and yet impose a tax on the sale of eyeglasses and contact lenses. The recognition of optometry as a learned profession by the courts and thereby exempt from such taxation is another matter to be adjudicated.[32] As optometry continues its evolution toward primary care, the likelihood that these issues will be resolved in a manner favorable to the profession increases substantially.

As the preceding discussion has demonstrated, there are factors outside government (but that inevitably interact with government) exerting an important influence upon the practice of optometry. Of particular importance are vision service plans, both public and private, that affect the scope of services to be rendered, the accessibility of certain patient populations to optometrists, the remuneration to be enjoyed by optometric practitioners, and many other issues that, if not fairly regulated, could have adverse effects on the profession and those persons who rely upon its services. The spectre of discrimination has been shown to be real by the courts and the legislatures, and optometrists must continue to be vigilant in order to reduce restraints that serve the interests of defined groups rather than the populace as a whole.

Notes

1. For a reminiscence of the major legal issues faced by optometry during the years that Kohn was AOA counsel, see Kohn, H., A Legal and Anecdotal History of Optometry, *Journal of the American Optometric Association*, vol. 38, no. 11, Nov. 1967, pp. 949–955.
2. See Jolley, J.L., Third Party Payment Programs, in Newcomb, R.D., and J.L. Jolley, Editors, *Public Health and Community Optometry*, Charles C. Thomas, Springfield, Ill., 1980, pp. 253–280.
3. The optometric literature reflects the growing impact of third-party vision-care plans. See Myhre, A.G., Learning to Love Third Party Care, *Optometric Management*, vol. 14, no. 11, Nov. 1978, p. 29; Mansberg, R., Medicare Discrimination Must Stop!, *Optometric Management*, vol. 14, no. 3, Mar. 1978, p. 119; Medicaid Discrimination Can Be Stopped!, vol. 14, no. 12, Dec. 1978, p. 23; Medicare: Help Needed, *Optometric Management*, vol. 15, no. 8, Aug, 1979, p. 141; Atwood, R.E., Third Party Vision Care Today, Tomorrow, *Journal of the American Optometric Association*, vol. 51, no. 2, Feb. 1980, p. 105; Soroka, M., Optometric and Ophthalmological Eye Care Under the Medicare Program, *Journal of the American Optometric Association*, vol. 51, no. 5, May 1980, p. 462; Myhre, A.G., Coordination of Benefits: Insuring the Insurers, *Optometric Management*, vol. 16, no. 6, June 1980, p. 41; Maybury, M., and M. Morgenthalen, The Prospect of Third Party Health Care, *Optometric Management*, vol. 17, no. 7, July 1981, p. 41; Bennett, I., Your Bigger Share Under Medicare, *Optometric Management*, vol. 17, no. 8, Aug. 1981, p. 35; Gackenbach, J.G., Vision Care Benefit Plans: Understanding the Complexity of Current and Emerging Third Party Programs, *Journal of the American Optometric Association*, vol. 54, no. 4, Apr. 1983, p. 363; Soroka, M., and Rosenthal, J., Vision Care Policy, Ophthalmological Practices, and the Medicare Program, *Journal of the American Optometric Association*, vol. 54, no. 6, June 1983, p. 565; Jolley, J.L., Review of Federal Law and Regulations: Reimbursement Under Medicare, *Journal of the American Optometric Association*, vol. 54, no. 8, Aug. 1982, p. 743; Cohn, S., Alphabet Soup: A PPO that Fills the Holes, *Optometric Management*, vol. 21, no. 12, Dec. 1985, pp. 24–30; Kloos, S., Alphabet Soup: A Rewarding Career, *Optometric Management*, vol. 21, no. 12, Dec. 1985, pp. 20–24; Bennett, I., Alphabet Soup: Is It Good for Optometry?, *Optometric Management*, vol. 21, no. 12, Dec. 1985, pp. 16–20; and Kloos, S. and B. Hrozenchik, HMO's: How Can You Adapt, *Optometric Management*, vol. 22, no. 9, Sept. 1986, pp. 32–41.
4. Newcomb and Jolley, supra note 2 at 273. In 1984 revenues exceeded $117 million, with 869, 000 subscribers. See Professional News, *Optometric Management*, vol. 21, no. 8, Aug. 1985.
5. Newcomb and Jolley, supra note 2, at 267–280.
6. From the outset, optometrists considered the Medicare program to be discriminatory. See Editorial, A Vital Amendment to Medicare Is Recommended, *Optometric Weekly*, vol. 58, no. 2, Jan. 19, 1967, pp. 33–34; Optometry Inclusion in Title 18 Opposed, *AMA News*, May 15, 1967; HEW Report and Optometry and Medicare, *Eye Physician*, Feb. 1969, pp. 17–19; and Davis, K., Equal Treatment and Unequal Benefits: The Medicare Program, *Milbank Memorial Fund Quarterly*, vol. 53, no. 4, Fall 1975, p. 452. Medicaid was similarly considered to be flawed. See Editorial, The Progress of Medicaid—Bigger Than Medicare?, *Optical Journal and Review of Optometry*, vol. 103, no. 22, Nov. 15, 1966, p. 52; Brownfield, A., Medicaid: The Anatomy of the Failure of the Government Program, *Private Practice*, vol. 5, 1973, pp. 11–19; and Haffner, A.N., The Destruction of Medicaid, *Optometric Weekly*, vol. 67, no. 15, Nov. 4, 1976, pp. 13–16.
7. An interesting discussion of the legal issues attendant to reimbursement statutes enacted by state legislatures can be found in *Ketcham v. King County Medical Service Corp.*, 81 Wash. 2d 565, 502 P.2d 1197 (1972), in which a deeply divided court held a statute requiring reimbursement to optometrists under a state medical service program to be an unconstitutional exercise of the police power, impeding the freedom to contract.
8. *Pushkin v. Califano*, 600 F.2d 486 (5th Cir. 1979).
9. *Report to Congress: Reimbursement Under Part B of Medicare for Certain Services Provided by Optometrists*, Department of Health, Education and Welfare, Washington, D.C., July 1976.
10. *Physicians' Education Network, Inc. v. The Department of Health, Education, and Welfare*, 653 F.2d 621 (D.C. Cir. 1981).
11. Under Medicare, the optometrist who provides services to an eligible patient will receive as reimbursement an amount that can be no more than 75 percent of the prevailing fee for the services in a particular region. This 75th percentile amount is established by profiles of the fees charged in a given area by optometrists, and so ophthalmologists set their own fee reimbursement independent of optometrists through this same type of mechanism. For a discussion of the Medicare reimbursement system, see Jolley, J.L., Review of Federal Law and Regulations: Reimbursement Under Medicare, *Journal of the American Optometric Association*, vol. 54, no. 8, Aug. 1983, pp. 743–750.
12. *Sandefur v. Cherry*, 744 F.2d 1157 (5th Cir. 1984).
13. *Simpson v. Wilson*, 480 F. Supp 97 (D.C. Vt. 1979).
14. *Eder v. Beal*, 609 F.2d 695 (3rd Cir. 1979).
15. *New York State Optometric Association v. Blum*, 360 Medicare and Medicaid Guide (CCH) paragraph 32,

069. The New York association brought suit, contesting the validity of the Medicaid fee schedules and seeking to compel the state to increase the fee schedule for optometrists. The court dismissed the complaint for failure to raise a justiciable claim, pointing out that the judiciary had traditionally refused to grant relief involving a determination of what fees were reasonable in the marketplace and what was the proper allocation of public funds. The court also commented that "the highly developed infrastructure of the Medicaid Assistance Program clearly evidences the legislature's intention to rest the responsibility for administration and determination of policy within the plan itself." Quoted in *Bulletin from Office of Counsel of the AOA*, vol. 41, no. 23, Jan. 7, 1983.

16. *In the Matter of the Application of Medical Eye Care Foundation of Pennsylvania for a Certification of Authority*, Departments of Health and Insurance, Apr. 7, 1977. See *Bulletin from Office of Counsel of the AOA*, vol. 37, no. 10, Sept. 7, 1978.
17. *Jacobs v. State Board of Optometry*, 147 Cal. Rptr. 225, 81 Cal. App. 3d 1022 (1978).
18. The leading commentary on the application of ERISA (29 U.S.C. §1001 et seq.) may be found in *Metropolitan Life Insurance Co. v. Massachusetts*, __ U.S. __, 105 S. Ct. 2380 (1985).
19. Ark. Stat. Ann. §66-3212.
20. 63 *Pa. Cons. Stat.* §239.1.
21. *Conn. Gen. Stat. Annot.* §20-138d.
22. 40 *Pa. Cons. Stat.* §1502.
23. *Blue Cross of Virginia v. Commonwealth of Virginia*, 269 S.E.2d 827 (1980).
24. A strikingly convoluted argument that contains virtually no legal justification can be found in *Sandefur v. Cherry*, 547 F. Supp. 418 (D.C. La. 1982)—eventually overturned in 744 F.2d 1157 (5th Cir. 1984)—in which the court uses a lengthy and complex rationalization in support of discrimination that can only be called amazing.
25. A class action suit, *Blue Shield of Virginia v. McCready*, was brought in Virginia on behalf of all Blue Shield subscribers who were denied reimbursement for psychologist's services, alleging conspiracy and antitrust violations. The Fourth Circuit Court of Appeals held that the subscribers had standing to bring such a suit (649 F.2d 228 (1981)), and the U.S. Supreme Court affirmed, 457 U.S. 465, 102 S. Ct. 2540 (1982).
26. An annotation on the application of use or sales taxes to ophthalmic goods can be found in "Furnishing Glasses or Optical Accessories as Sale Within Sales Tax Law," 157 A.L.R. 578, and "Eyeglasses or Other Optical Accessories as Subject to Sales or Use Tax," 14 A.L.R. 4th 1370.
27. The general question as to what constitutes a sale at retail within the tax statutes is discussed in 68 Am. Jur. 2d, Sales and Use Taxes, §1.
28. *State Tax Commissioner v. Hopkins*, 234 Ala. 556, 176 So. 210 (1937).
29. *Kamp v. Johnson*, 15 Cal. 2d 187, 99 P.2d 274 (1940).
30. *Rice v. Evatt*, 144 Ohio St. 483, 59 N.E.2d 927 (1945).
31. *Alabama Board of Optometry v. Eagerton*, 393 So.2d 1373 (1981).
32. For a discussion of optometry as a learned profession, see *Pearle Optical of Monroeville, Inc. v. Georgia State Board of Examiners in Optometry*, 219 Ga. 364, 133 S.E.2d 374 (1963).

PART FIVE

DOCTOR AND PATIENT

Chapter 13

The Doctor-Patient Relationship

God and the Doctor we alike adore
But only when in danger, not before;
The danger o'er, both are alike requited,
God is forgotten, and the Doctor slighted.
—John Owen, *Epigrams*

Doctor and Patient

Optometry is a clinical science and is based upon the relationship between practitioner and patient, a relationship of some impermanence, as Owen points out. There are ethical considerations inherent in the relationship that the practitioner must observe (see Chapter 4) including: keeping the patient's confidences inviolate, giving timely notice of disease, rendering care regardless of the patient's financial status, responding to requests for emergency care, and referring patients to other health care providers when appropriate. But the primary focus of this chapter is upon the legal considerations that flow from the relationship of doctor and patient, including the contractual basis of the relationship, the right to refuse treatment, obligations to the patient for substitute or alternative care, professional liability issues, and the optometrist's role as fiduciary. We will discuss in some detail the best means to employ in order to document the doctor's agreement to provide services and will conclude the chapter by considering how the doctor-patient relationship may be terminated.

We begin with a description of the legal issues that form the basis for the clinical relationship of doctor and patient.

Contractual Basis for the Relationship

The relationship of doctor and patient is a legal relationship and is generally considered to be contractual in nature, even though the contract at times may be implied from the conduct of the parties rather than based upon a written agreement that specifies definite terms.[1] A contract for a doctor's services may be described as "a deliberate agreement between competent parties, upon a legal consideration, to do or abstain from doing, some act."[2] In the practice of optometry the relationship usually begins with the request of the patient for treatment and the agreement on the part of the doctor to undertake the patient's care. For a valid contract to exist, however, there must be mutuality of understanding between the parties as to the terms of the agreement. Failure to obtain this understanding is the reason that disagreements occasionally arise between doctor and patient, most frequently due to disputes over financial matters such as fees. For this reason, formalizing the contractual relationship through the use of printed materials is advisable.[3]

The contractual relationship may be created under circumstances that are far less explicit than those to be encountered in an optometrist's office. In these instances the contract may be held to be implied. An implied contract has been defined as "one not created by the explicit agreement of the parties but inferred by the law as a matter of reason and justice from their acts or conduct, the circumstances surrounding their transaction making it a reasonable, or even a necessary, assumption that a contract existed between them by tacit understanding."[4] Not every patient encounter will occur in the office, after the patient has filled out the necessary forms and clearly entered into a contract for services. Optometrists may find themselves confronted with ocular emergencies—due to trauma, chemical splashes, foreign bodies, or other injuries—outside the office and under the most informal of circumstances. The conduct of the doctor on these occasions will determine whether or not the doctor-patient relationship exists. It should be noted that services rendered gratuitously and without expectation of payment are still sufficient to create the legal relationship of doctor and patient.[5] The actions of either or both parties may be held in retrospect to constitute an implied contract, thereby creating the doctor-patient relationship (and all its attendant liabilities).[6]

Despite the consensual nature of the relationship, the patient does not consent to *treatment* merely by entering into a contract for services with the doctor, for the patient has the right to accept or reject the proposed services based upon an informed consent of the treatment involved. (Discussed in Chapter 22.) Thus the doctor is required to disclose pertinent results of the examination to the patient in order to obtain this consent. The courts, however, do not assume a guarantee or warranty from a doctor that he or she will cure the patient merely because the doctor has entered into a contractual relationship with the patient,[7] and it has long been held that a poor result following treatment does not of itself create legal liability for the doctor.[8] Even so, if an optometrist does guarantee results ("With these contact lenses you will see 20/20") or create a warranty ("The lenses of these glasses are shatterproof"), and the guaranteed results are not obtained or the warranty is breached, the optometrist may be held liable for having made these declarations to the patient and then not having achieved the specified results (see Chapter 27). The optometrist is also expected to adhere to certain standards in the care of the patient.

Liability for Care

Once an optometrist has commenced actual treatment, he is under a legal duty to conform to the standard of care expected of like practitioners acting under the same or similar circumstances. This duty is a fundamental aspect of the doctor-patient relationship and requires the doctor to meet reasonable standards of conduct in the management of the patient's condition.

For this reason, actions such as diagnosing a condition or prescribing for the patient over the telephone—particularly if the individual or the individual's history are not known in detail—are fraught with peril. For example, a patient with post-examination headache may be suffering angle closure secondary to mydriasis; a complaint of this nature is best not assessed over the telephone since such conduct would fall below reasonable standards of care. It is advisable to take the time to investigate a patient's complaint at the office, where the proper instrumentation and equipment may be employed. Failure to do so may constitute negligence.[9]

If a patient calls seeking a doctor's care and the doctor does not wish to give advice or treat the patient over the telephone, the doctor should advise the patient accordingly so that the patient may seek advice elsewhere.[10] An analogous situation concerns requests for advice at social gatherings. The doctor may wish to demur answering social inquiries, but casual questions, asked of a doctor outside of a situation in which a professional relationship would ordinarily be expected to exist, do not usually create such a relationship.[11] Therefore, opinions offered in response to questions posed at a social gathering, if given out of politeness and not in any professional capacity, would in all probability not subject the doctor to liability.[12]

The issue of professional liability is complex but must be understood by contemporary practitioners of optometry. It is discussed in detail in Chapters 18 through 22.

Limitations in the Relationship

An optometrist in private practice ordinarily has the right to refuse to see a patient, and this refusal is legally permissible even if the situation constitutes an emergency and no other doctor is available[13] (emergency care is discussed in Chapter 14). Similarly, patients have the right to refuse treatment recommended by the optometrist, even important diagnostic tests such as tonometry and dilation for ophthalmoscopy. An adult of sound mind cannot be compelled to undergo treatment because the contractual relationship between doctor and patient is consensual as to both parties. But a wise clinician will document patient refusals, either by writing a comment in the patient record or by securing the patient's signature on a form that is retained in the record.

Under some circumstances the doctor-patient relationship will be held to exist even though the contractual arrangement is made with a person other than the patient. A common example of such a relationship is when a doctor renders services for a minor. The contractual obligation should be established with the parent, who assumes the responsibility for payment. If the parents are divorced or separated, the mother typically assumes primary responsibility for the doctor's compensation, if she is the parent who arranges for the doctor's services. In most instances the father remains liable for the child's necessary expenses, even in the absence of a court order for child support,[14] and so a mother may be permitted to proceed against the father for the recovery of these expenses. To prevent financial misunderstandings when rendering services for minors, the doctor should ascertain at the beginning of the relationship which parent is to be held responsible for payment. A printed form may routinely be employed for this purpose (the use of forms is discussed later in this chapter).

Emergency care is regarded differently, and the parent remains financially liable for the minor's expenses as long as the parent is still contributing to the minor's support.[15] But if a doctor bills a child's parents for nonemergency services or materials, obtained by the child without their knowledge or consent, the parents may be able to disavow financial responsibility.

A practitioner may institute reasonable limitations upon the clinical care offered to patients. For example, an optometrist who does not wish to perform a certain clinical technique, such as dilation, may refer the patient to another practitioner for this purpose, even though the patient would prefer that the optometrist perform the test. Similarly, an optometrist may choose not to manage a particular ocular disease, even though legally permitted to do so, and may refer the patient to another doctor for management despite the patient's willingness to have the optometrist institute therapy. In the same vein, the doctor—and not the patient—has the right to determine the times and frequency of appointments.

Substitutes, Referrals, and Consultations

Like other health-care professionals, optometrists have the right to enjoy a reasonable amount of time away from their practices, and although medical practitioners must provide competent substitutes during their absence and must provide adequate notice of the substitution to affected patients, this degree of coverage is not required in most optometric practices.[16] Nevertheless, it is advisable for an optometrist to have a competent doctor available to consult with patients if the optometrist expects to be absent from the practice for an extended period of time. If a covering doctor examines a patient under such an arrangement, once the doctor has satisfied this obligation he is not legally bound to continue to treat the patient.[17] And if the covering doctor is negligent in the treatment rendered the patient, the absent optometrist is generally held to have no legal responsibility as long as due care was employed in the selection of the covering doctor.[18] Thus, as long as the optometrist has taken reasonable steps to ensure that the affected patients will be left in the care of a qualified practitioner, there will be no liability.

A problem that is common in optometric practice involves an optometrist's responsibility for the referral of a patient to a physician, optometrist, or other health-care provider for treatment. If the optometrist has used due care in the selection of the practitioner to whom the patient is being referred, the optometrist will not be liable even though the practitioner is actually negligent.[19] The optometrist, however, must have no responsibility for the patient's care while the patient is being treated by the other practitioner in order for the arrangement to be a true referral.[20] An example situation is the referral of a patient to an ophthalmologist for cataract surgery. Once the optometrist has made the referral, if the ophthalmologist negligently performs the surgery and the patient sues for damages, the optometrist will have no liability as long as the ophthalmologist was chosen with due care. Likewise, if the ophthalmologist refers the patient to the optometrist for treatment, and the optometrist is negligent, the ophthalmologist would not be responsible for the patient's injury as long as the optometrist was chosen with due care and competent to perform the necessary services.[21]

By comparison, a consultation is considered to be a joint undertaking, and so the optometrist may be jointly responsible for the negligence of the consultant. In a true consultation the patient receives diagnosis or treatment by another provider that is offered in conjunction with the care being rendered by the optometrist, and if there is negligence by either party then both parties may be held responsible for the patient's injury.[22] For example, in some cases an optometrist may undertake the treatment of an ocular disease in consultation with a physician—such as through the use of standing orders—and if the optometrist is negligent, both the physician and the optometrist may be held liable for the injury. Consequently, optometrists should choose consultants with great care.

Role as Fiduciary

Another ramification of the doctor-patient relationship is that the optometrist must assume the role of fiduciary, which can be defined as "Where there is special confidence reposed in the one who in equity and good conscience is bound to act in good faith and with due regard to the interests of the one who has reposed his confidence in him."[23] It is this legal obligation as fiduciary that places upon the optometrist an affirmative duty to disclose pertinent examination findings to the patient (discussed in Chapter 22) and creates liability for the withholding of information (see Chapter 20). Thus an optometrist has a duty to communicate pertinent information to the patient.

There are legal and ethical considerations that affect an optometrist's right to reveal patient information to third parties. The Code of Ethics of the American Optometric Association states that an optometrist has an ethical obligation to keep the personal or business matters of patients inviolate (see Chapter 4). The courts have held that health-care practitioners have a duty not to disclose information of a confidential nature revealed by their patients during the course of an examination (discussed in Chapter 16). Therefore, the disclosure of patient information to third parties requires the patient's consent in order to avoid breach of the duty to respect confidentiality.

Under some circumstances an optometrist may be required to release patient information. One common situation is when there is litigation, and the optometrist's records are needed as evidence or the optometrist is called upon to testify as to the examination findings. Unlike physicians in many states, optometrists may be compelled to testify (described in Chapter 16) and their records subjected to review. Another aspect of the release of patient information involves the prescription for glasses or contact lenses. Due to the Federal Trade Commission's Eyeglasses I rule, optometrists are required to offer a copy of the prescription to the patient at the conclusion of the examination (discussed in Chapter 17). Other information may have to be released to patients according to the requirements of federal or state law.

The Contractual Relationship

Since the basis of the doctor-patient relationship is contractual, it is important that, whenever possible, a written contract be entered into. This is today a *sine qua non* of private practice. The agreement need not be lengthy or complex, but there are fundamental matters that all contracts should include. A variety of forms may be chosen by private practitioners, both ready-made and custom printed. The matter of what form is to be used and the depth of the information it contains is not to be taken lightly. A doctor will be bound (or limited) by the form's provisions, and a patient's understanding of the doctor-patient relationship will be aided (or deterred) by its language and degree of comprehensiveness. Such forms are important and can be used for a variety of services: general examinations, contact lenses, visual training, and any procedure that requires informed consent due to its experimental nature.

Perhaps the most important forms are those used to establish the express contractual relation discussed in the preceding section. For most optometrists, the form that is necessary to settle this relationship is a Patient Information/Financial Policy Form.

Patient information is needed for obtaining baseline data, providing accurate billing, scheduling future appointments, and collecting monies due. The more complete the information, the better these goals can be met (for a sample form, see Fig. 13.1).

The Patient Information section is intended to collect personal data from the patient, and may be as general or comprehensive as the doctor wishes. The more detailed the information, the more likely the form will be useful should billing or collections efforts be necessary.[24]

The most important part of this type of form, however, is the Statement of Financial Policy. Such a statement demands that the practitioner in fact have a financial policy that will be applied to everyone. Putting it on the form and requiring the patient's signature beneath it formalizes the policy and creates an express contract. The policy used in the sample agreement (50 percent downpayment and 50 percent on delivery) is a customary means of charging for materials. Note that the examination fee (i.e., fee for services) is to be paid at the time of the exam and the mode of payment must be specified by the patient before the examination is undertaken; this prevents misunderstanding afterwards. Typically, this form is only used at the first visit. Each year that the patient returns for another examination, the form is completed and signed again.

There is another important item on the Statement of Financial Policy and that is the description of the payment terms. The purpose of this clause is to inform the patient that there is a certain period of time in which payment—in full—is expected to be received and if it is not paid the balance due may be turned

UNIVERSITY OPTOMETRIC GROUP

UNIVERSITY OF ALABAMA AT BIRMINGHAM

BIRMINGHAM, ALABAMA 35294

PATIENT'S NAME ______ BIRTHDATE: ___ / ___ / ___ AGE ___

HOME ADDRESS ______ CITY ______ STATE ______ ZIP ______

IF PATIENT IS A CHILD, SHOW PARENT'S NAME ______ HOME PHONE # ______

Show the following information on the **RESPONSIBLE** party:

MARITAL STATUS: (CIRCLE ONE) S M D W SOC. SEC. # ___ / ___ / ___ EMPLOYED BY: ______

ADDRESS ______ BUSINESS PHONE ______

SPOUSE'S NAME ______ EMPLOYED BY ______ BUSINESS PHONE # ______

IN CASE OF EMERGENCY, NOTIFY: ______ PHONE # ______

PERSON RESPONSIBLE FOR THIS ACCOUNT ______

REFERRED TO OUR OFFICE BY ______

STATEMENT OF FINANCIAL POLICY

As a service to you, this office offers several means of payment for the services and materials that you may require. It is customary to PAY THE EXAMINATION FEE at the time of the examination. You must be prepared to also pay for any required materials and/or follow-up care in the following manner:

1. Spectacles, hard/soft contact lenses — 50% when ordered, balance at dispensing.
2. Vision training, office visits, etc.: Payable on each visit.

To insure that we understand how you wish your account to be handled, please check the payment plan you prefer and sign in the space indicated. If you have any questions, please ask the receptionist before you make your choice:

CASH OR PERSONAL CHECK: ______ (check one)

MASTERCHARGE: ______ (show your card number)

VISA: ______ (show your card number)

The doctor, at his discretion, may place an UNPAID account with an attorney for collection. In the event your account is referred to an attorney for collection of unpaid charges, the patient (or person responsible for the account) agrees to pay an attorney's fee, court cost and any other reasonable costs of collection.

SIGNATURE: ______

DATE: ______ RECEPTIONIST: ______

PS-4865

Figure 13.1. Sample Patient Information/Financial Policy Form. (Courtesy University Optometric Group)

over to an attorney for collection. This clause does not obligate the doctor to resort to collections efforts, but it fulfills an important legal responsibility should the doctor be forced to do so by putting the patient on notice that in the event of failure to pay—and if a lawyer must be employed to collect an overdue and unpaid account—the patient will not only have to pay the bill but also the attorney's fee, court costs, and "any other reasonable costs of collection."[25] Every financial policy should contain a similar statement, unless barred by state law (collections are discussed separately in Chapter 51).

In addition to the Patient Information/Financial Policy Form, there are other documents that can be utilized, depending upon the services offered by the practitioner. One common example may be found in contact lens practice: For these patients, a contact lens fitting agreement and a prepaid service agreement can be indispensable (see Chapter 30 for examples). Similarly, vision training agreements can be used by a private practitioner to ensure that there is no misunderstanding as to the scope of the therapy or its costs (see Chapter 31).

The most widely employed type of form in an optometric office—the patient record—is discussed in the following chapter.

Termination of the Doctor-Patient Relationship

The doctor-patient relationship can be terminated in a variety of ways, but the most common is the completion of treatment, which renders continuation of the relationship unnecessary. Of course, the patient is free to discharge the doctor and to end the contractual relation at any time,[26] although in some instances the doctor may have a duty to warn the patient of the need for further care and to provide the successor doctor with information sufficient to permit continuation of treatment without undue delay.[27]

Similarly, written proof that the patient, not the doctor, terminated the relationship is important because these patients are the ones who—justifiably or not—are most likely to pursue legal action against the doctor. The doctor is also free to withdraw from a case for any reason satisfactory to himself, including failure of the patient to pay for services or materials or to follow proper instructions,[28] but there is the spectre of abandonment under such circumstances.

Abandonment has been defined as "the unilateral severance by the doctor of the professional relationship between himself and a patient without reasonable notice, at a time when there is still the necessity of continuing medical attention."[29] If a doctor wishes to withdraw from a case in which further care is required, it is advisable to notify the patient in writing and to retain a copy of the letter in the patient's record[30] (see Fig. 13.2). Under these circumstances, the doctor may also be obligated to provide records and information sufficient to ensure proper continuing care. For example, an optometrist who is the only eye-care provider in a community could conceivably—regardless of the provocation—have to continue seeing a patient requiring follow-up care, despite a desire to end the relationship.

Refusal to attend to a patient's needs, even though the doctor has not stated an intention to do so, may also be considered abandonment, even if the lack of attention is due to the doctor's preoccupation with other patients.[31] This type of abandonment may be found if the doctor fails to see the patient at intervals necessary for the proper treatment of the patient's condition, for frequency of attendance is usually considered by the courts to be as much a part of careful treatment as any other aspect of care. The patient has the right to expect a doctor to stay adequately informed about the patient's condition, which cannot be done if the doctor abandons the case without notice or does not see the patient frequently enough

Dear Mr./Ms. ________________,

This letter is to inform you that I find it necessary to withdraw from the performance of further professional duties in your case because ____.
Since you are still in need of treatment, I suggest that you place yourself under the care of another practitioner without delay. If you are unable to obtain the necessary services, I will continue to provide care for a reasonable period, not to exceed ______. When you determine who your provider will be, with your consent I will make availiable to this practitioner the case history and other information concerning the diagnosis and treatment that you have received from me.

Sincerely,

________________ O.D.

Figure 13.2. Sample Letter Withdrawing from the Care of a Patient Who Requires Further Treatment.

to be aware of what is happening.[32] Furthermore, the failure by a doctor to see a patient when necessary may also constitute negligence in terms of the standard for care—for both diagnosis and treatment—since the courts have held that a doctor who was properly attentive might well have known what was wrong with the patient and have treated it properly.[33] Doctors who withdraw from cases in which patients still require treatment—on the ground that the patient has not paid a past due bill—do not have a good defense to an abandonment claim.[34] Such a financial question is considered to be irrelevant to the question of the patient's care.

Although abandonment can occur either by express withdrawal by the doctor or by failure to continue to treat the patient, it should be noted that, even if abandonment occurs, the patient still must show that the delay or failure of treatment resulted in some damages. If the patient was able to contact another doctor before any harm was done, damages cannot be recovered, even if the abandonment was both legally and ethically unjustified. Consequently, abandonment claims are not a significant cause of liability. In fact, a large study of medical malpractice claims has found that the number of claims filed on the basis of abandonment is very small, constituting less than 1 percent of all the claims compiled during the study.[35] In optometry, this type of claim is even more unlikely.

If an optometrist desires to close a practice, it is best to notify active patients so that they can arrange for uninterrupted care from another provider. The best means is by a letter, sent at least three months in advance of the date the office will be closed. The closing date should be specified in any correspondence. Other practitioners may be recommended, and the optometrist should offer to transfer records or examination data upon the receipt of written authorization from the patient. If records are forwarded to another doctor, it is advisable to retain copies or to notify the doctor that access to the records may be required in the future. Records of a closed practice should be retained for a period of time sufficient to satisfy relevant statutes of limitation (discussed in Chapter 16).

The death of an optometrist creates similar obligations.

Notes

1. For discussions of the contractual and consensual nature of the doctor-patient relationship, see Morris, R.C., and Moritz, A.R., *Doctor and Patient and the Law*, 5th Edition, C.V. Mosby Co., St. Louis, 1971, pp. 135–146; and Holder, A.R., *Medical Malpractice Law*, Wiley & Sons, New York, 1975, pp. 1–39.
2. *Smith v. Thornhill*, 25 S.W.2d 597 (Tex. 1930).
3. For a practitioner's view of the importance of data collection when entering into the doctor-patient relationship, see Elmstrom, G.A., *Advanced Management for Optometrists*, Professional Press, Chicago, 1974, pp. 403–419.
4. *Landon v. Kansas City Gas Co.*, 10 F.2d 263 (8th Cir. 1926).
5. Treatment, once initiated, is usually sufficient by itself to impose the contractual relationship. See *Stohlman v. Davis*, 220 N.W. 247 (Neb. 1928); *Childers v. Frye*, 201 N.C. 42, 158 S.E. 744 (1931); and *Gross v. Partlow*, 68 P.2d 1034 (Wash. 1937).
6. For a review of cases creating liability under circumstances in which the doctor-patient relationship was implied, see *O'Neill v. Montefiore Hospital*, 11 A.D.2d 132, 202 N.Y.S.2d 436 (1960) (telephone call to doctor); *Smart v. Kansas City*, 208 Mo. 162, 105 S.W. 709 (1907) (casual comment by a medical school professor); *Lundberg v. Bay View Hospital*, 175 Ohio St. 133, 191 N.E.2d 821 (1963) (pathologist diagnosing biopsy of patient he had never met); and *Capuano v. Jacobs*, 33 A.D.2d 743, 305 N.Y.S.2d 837 (1969) (radiologist held responsible for X-ray finding despite no contact with the patient.)
7. Breach of warranty for medical services is discussed by Lane B.J., and H. Hirsh, The Broken Promise: Physician's Breach of Warranty, *Case and Comment*, Sept.–Oct. 1984, pp. 3–14.
8. See *Custodio v. Bauer*, 251 Cal. App. 2d 303, 59 Cal. Rptr. 463, 470 (1967) for a recent enunciation of this principle.
9. For an example case, see Bettman, J.W., A Review of 112 Claims in Ophthalmology, in Medicolegal Aspect of Ophthalmology, Bettman, J.W. (ed.), *International Ophthalmology Clinics*, vol. 20, 1980, pp. 131–142.
10. An implied contract can result from a telephone call. See *O'Neill v. Montefiore Hospital*, 11 A.D.2d 132, 202 N.Y.S.2d 436 (1960).
11. *Ranier v. Grossman*, 107 Cal. Rptr. 469, 31 Cal. App. 3d 539 (1973).
12. As expressed by Angela Holder, supra note 1, at 6:

    A casual question asked of a physician outside a situation in which a professional relationship would ordinarily be thought to exist, however, does not usually constitute such a relationship. A physician who is backed into a corner at a cocktail party and asked his opinion of various aches and pains by a fellow guest and who replies in an off-hand manner out of simple politeness may undoubtedly be subject to extreme social irritation at the time, but in all probability would not be liable for malpractice as the result of his comments.
13. *Hurley v. Eddingfield*, 59 N.E. 1058 (Ind. 1901).
14. *Yarborough v. Yarborough*, 290 U.S. 202, 54 S. Ct. 181 (1933); *Hachat v. Hachat*, 71 N.E.2d 927 (Ind.

1947); and *Porter v. Powell*, 79 Iowa 151, 44 N.W. 295 (1890).

15. Emergency care rendered to minors without parental consent is allowable, and parents may not recover damages on this basis. See *Luka v. Lowrie*, 136 N.W. 1106 (Mich. 1912). And in an emergency the parents remain financially responsible.
16. *Browning v. Hoffman*, 111 S.E. 492 (W.Va. 1922).
17. For an example case, see *Podvin v. Eickhorst*, 373 Mich. 175, 128 N.W.2d 523 (1964).
18. *Stacy v. Williams*, 253 Ky. 353, 69 S.W.2d 697 (1934).
19. See Law and Medicine, Duty to Refer Patient to Medical Specialist, *Journal of the American Medical Association*, vol. 204, no. 8, May 20, 1968, p. 281; and Liability of Referring Physician, vol. 204, no. 3, Apr. 15, 1968, p. 273; for medical precedents. If an optometrist refers a patient to a duly qualified specialist who enjoys a good reputation for the services he is to render, and the optometrist's involvement with the case terminates with the referral, any negligence committed by the specialist will not be imputed to the optometrist. For example cases involving physicians, see *Wallace v. Yudelson*, 224 Ill. App. 320, (1927); and *Harwick v. Harris*, 166 So. 2d 912 (Fla. 1964).
20. As explained by Angela Holder, supra note 1, at 48–49:

    When the referring physician continues to participate actively in the care of the patient, however, he may be jointly liable with the specialist. If his assistance is entirely directed by the specialist, as in a situation in which he assists in surgery planned and carried out by the specialist, or if the specialist assumes all decision-making responsibility, however, the referring physician probably would not be liable even if he continued to visit the patient in the hospital or involved himself in other cooperative ventures to that extent. The controlling factor, therefore, in any question of joint liability in a referral situation is the extent of participation by the referring physician in diagnosis and treatment.

21. The liability of optometrists and ophthalmologists for post-operative care conducted by an optometrist has not been legally tested and thus there are no precedents to be cited concerning this evolving aspect of co-management by the two professions. In the state of North Carolina, however, the state board of medicine instituted an action to censure an ophthalmologist for this practice, maintaining that to allow optometrists to be responsible for the post-operative follow-up of cataract patients constituted the unauthorized practice of medicine. This allegation was reviewed by the state attorney general, who ruled that the post-operative care of these patients fell within the practice of optometry and was not unlawful. A copy of the opinion may be found in *Bulletin from the Office of Counsel of the AOA*, vol. 45, no. 33, Oct. 23, 1986.
22. For an example case involving physicians, see *Arshanasky v. Royal Concourse Co.*, 28 A.D.2d 986, 283 N.Y.S.2d 646 (1967).
23. *Black's Law Dictionary*, 4th Edition, West, St. Paul, Minn., 1968.
24. One item that is omitted from this form is the school attended by any children. This bit of information can be very useful in trying to locate parents who have "skipped" without paying their bill, for the school records will be forwarded to the new school, which in turn will have a record of the parent's new address. See Kuhn, B.L., How to Set Up a Collections Policy that Works, *Optometric Management*, vol. 22, no. 12, Dec. 1986, pp. 43–45.
25. If the patient is put on notice before the contract is entered into—through the inclusion of a clause such as the one described—the patient agrees to pay the extra costs, if the doctor is forced to go to court, including the cost of the doctor's attorney. This agreement by the patient allows the doctor to collect the entire amount owed, rather than just a percentage of it.
26. *Miles v. Harris*, 194 S.W. 839 (Tex. 1917).
27. *Engel v. Clarke*, 346 S.W.2d 12 (Ky. 1961).
28. For a review of abandonment, see the following issues of the *Journal of the American Medical Association*: vol. 225, no. 9, Aug. 27, 1973, p. 1157; vol. 225, no. 10, Sept. 3, 1973, p. 1285; vol. 225, no. 11, Sept. 10, 1973, p. 1429; and vol. 225, no. 12, Sept. 17, 1973, p. 1511.
29. *Stohlman v. Davis*, 220 N.W. 247 (Neb. 1928).
30. *Lee v. Dewbre*, 362 S.W.2d 900 (Tex. 1962).
31. *Thomas v. Corso*, 265 Md. 84, 288 A.2d 379 (1972); and *Sinclair v. Brunson*, 212 Mich. 387, 180 N.W. 358 (1920).
32. Frequency of attention is particularly important when the patient is receiving prescription drugs. See *Boyd v. Andrae*, 44 S.W.2d 891 (Mo. 1932).
33. *Tadlock v. Lloyd*, 65 Colo. 40, 173 P. 200 (1918).
34. *Ricks v. Budge*, 64 P.2d 208 (Utah 1937).
35. In a study of malpractice claims performed by St. Paul Fire and Marine Insurance Company, the claim of abandonment accounted for only 0.8 percent of claims compiled over a five year period. For a discussion, see Curran, W.J., Malpractice Claims: New Data and New Trends, *New England Journal of Medicine*, vol. 300, no. 1, Jan. 1979 p. 26.

Chapter 14

Emergency Care

No person licensed under this chapter, who in good faith renders emergency care at the scene of the emergency, shall be liable for any civil damages as a result of acts or omissions by such person in rendering the emergency care.
—California "Good Samaritan" statute, *Cal. Codes, Bus. & Profs., §2144 (West 1961)*

Recognizing Ocular Urgencies and Emergencies

The responsibility for emergency eye care has not traditionally been an optometric function, but various factors have combined to increase the participation of optometrists in the management of these cases, including the widespread geographical distribution of optometrists, the use of specialized ophthalmic instrumentation by optometric practitioners, and the emphasis by the profession on primary care services. Consequently, optometrists have found themselves more likely to be called upon to render urgent care to patients who suffer acute or debilitating ocular problems. Practitioners who provide these services should understand the legal ramifications of their conduct, for there is significant opportunity for liability in the management of these patients.

There are four aspects of this issue that merit consideration:

1. What are ocular urgencies and emergencies?
2. What is an optometrist's legal responsibility if a patient seeks treatment for an ocular urgency or emergency?
3. What constitutes the standard of care for optometrists in the management of ocular urgencies and emergencies?
4. What is the appropriate documentation to be employed in the management of ocular urgencies and emergencies?

Duke-Elder observed that there are few true ocular emergencies and relatively few situations that require urgent attention, a comment[1] that reflects the general medical philsophy that time is almost always available to make a careful and thorough assessment before initiating therapy.[2] Although there are various ways of classifying ocular urgencies and emergencies (see Table 14.1) only two conditions—chemical burns of the cornea and central retinal artery occlusion—may be categorized as true emergencies[3], and in the great majority of cases the optometrist's care will probably be limited to first aid.

Chemical Burns

Burns caused by alkali or acid require intervention within minutes in order to minimize injury, particularly burns caused by alkaline materials, which penetrate the cornea more rapidly. Acid burns typically cause their damage within the first few hours, whereas alkali burns may continue their effect for days and may result in perforation if left in contact with the eye. Alkali burns caused by lye, fresh lime, or ammonia are the most commonly observed.[4]

Except for chemicals that react violently with water, the treatment of chemical burns must be the

Table 14.1. Ocular Urgencies and Emergencies

Situation	Condition
True Emergencies *Therapy should be instituted within minutes*	Chemical burns of the cornea Central retinal artery occlusion
Urgent Situations *Therapy should be instituted within one to several hours*	Endophthalmitis Penetrating injuries of the globe Acute angle-closure glaucoma Pupillary block glaucoma (lens or vitreous incarcerated in pupil); lens in anterior chamber Orbital cellulitis Cavernous sinus thrombosis Corneal ulcer Gonococcal ulcer Corneal foreign body Corneal abrasion Acute iritis and formation of synechias Giant cell arteritis with acute ischemia of optic nerve Acute retinal tear with hemorrhage Acute retinal detachment Descemetocele Hyphema Acute vitreous hemorrhage Lid laceration
Semi-urgent Situations *Therapy should be instituted within days whenever possible, or sometimes within weeks*	Optic neuritis Ocular tumors Exophthalmos, acute Previously undiagnosed chronic open-angle glaucoma Old retinal detachment Strabismic or other remediable amblyopias in young children Blow-out fracture of the orbit

Source: Deutsch, T.A., and D.B. Feller, *Management of Ocular Injuries*, 2d ed., Saunders, Philadelphia, 1985.

immediate and copious irrigation of the eye with water.[5] If possible, particulate chemical matter should be removed from contact with the eye, and the eyelids should be everted and the fornices of the conjunctival sac swept with cotton applicators.[6] If the irritating chemical is unknown, pH paper may be used by touching it to the involved tissue, thus determining whether the chemical is acidic or basic. After initial lavage, it may be necessary to use a topical anesthetic to reduce discomfort and to facilitate the examination. Irrigation should be continued for a minimum of one liter for each eye, and pH paper can again be employed to make certain that the pH is back within the normal range.[7] After lavage, it may be appropriate to assess the intraocular pressure (with alkali burns) and to use a cycloplegic to minimize the opportunity for adhesions between the iris and the lens.[8] Further care—or referral—will depend on the skill of the practitioner and the clinical options that are available under state law.[9] Severe chemical burns will require referral to a specialist.

Central Retinal Artery Occlusion

Occlusion of the central retinal artery most often occurs due to emboli from the carotid artery (in older patients) or the cardiac valves (in younger patients) and from thrombosis related to arteriosclerosis.[10] Treatment is directed toward efforts to dislodge the embolus, and the length of time the occlusion is permitted to persist is a critical factor in the ultimate outcome: relief within one hour may restore all vision whereas after three to four hours only peripheral vision may be spared. After this period of time, or if the macula has become a cherry red spot in an edematous retina, the visual loss is likely to be permanent.[11]

The most immediate treatment is intermittent massage of the eye, with moderate pressure applied to the globe for five seconds, then suddenly released for five seconds, then repeated.[12] Paracentesis of the anterior chamber, retrobulbar injections, and anticoagulation therapy may also be useful, and so prompt referral may be necessary.[13] Afterwards, these patients will require a careful evaluation of the cardiovascular system to determine the underlying cause of the attack.

These two conditions are the only clinical situations requiring intervention within minutes. All other conditions will be regarded as urgencies, in which the optometrist has more freedom to evaluate the patient and to determine whether or not to undertake management of the condition.

The decision to manage an ocular urgency or emergency has legal ramifications that necessitate a review of the legal basis of the doctor-patient relationship and of the duty of practitioners to undertake the treatment of these patients.

Optometrist's Duty to Treat Ocular Urgencies and Emergencies

The doctor-patient relationship is generally regarded as contractual in nature, and the contract may be implied from the actions of the parties rather than expressed in formal terms. The commencement of actual treatment is usually sufficient by itself to create the contractual relationship and to impose a duty upon the doctor to conform to certain recognized standards of conduct.

An optometrist in private practice has the right to refuse to examine a patient, for the contractual basis of the doctor-patient relationship requires the consent of both parties in order for a legally binding agreement to exist. This right to refuse treatment extends to emergency cases, even if the situation is one in which no other doctor or care is available. Numerous cases have held that physicians (and hospitals) may rightfully refuse to initiate treatment in emergency situations.[14]

In conflict with this legal right to refuse treatment is the ethical obligation of an optometrist to render emergency care. The Standards of Conduct of the American Optometric Association[15] maintain that "A request for optometric care in an emergency should receive immediate response. Once having undertaken an emergency case, an optometrist shall neither abandon nor neglect the patient."

The clear import of these words is to encourage optometrists to respond to requests for emergency eye care. Therefore, optometrists may rightfully consider it to be their obligation to volunteer, especially in communities devoid of other eye care providers or lacking specialized health care facilities. But what is the legal status of such a volunteer?

Under the common law it has long been held that a person who volunteers to assist an individual who is unable to aid, protect, or care for himself has a legal obligation to exercise reasonable care while rendering the services.[16] If the volunteer is negligent, then he or she can be held liable for any injury that is the proximate result of the negligence. This specter of liability under common law in emergency situations has proven to be a deterrent to physicians and other health-care providers, who more often than not avoided scenes of accidents and disasters out of fear that they would be exposing themselves to unnecessary legal risks. As a result of these concerns, the state legislatures began to enact Good Samaritan statutes, starting with California in 1959.[17]

Many of these laws provided immunity for physicians only, while some included other health-care providers and various types of emergency-care personnel. None specifically listed optometrists, but in a few states any persons stopping to render care were covered under the statute, a category that would obviously include optometrists.[18]

An optometrist who feels an ethical or moral obligation to assist an accident victim can do so but should understand that there is no legal duty to volunteer. Once having volunteered, the optometrist is required to use reasonable care under the circumstances and to exercise that degree of skill and learning that would ordinarily be exercised by other optometrists (or, perhaps, physicians) acting under the same or similar emergency situation.[19]

A like standard of care will be applied to an optometrist who renders in-office treatment of an ocular urgency. Since no Good Samaritan statute in any state confers immunity for this kind of service, it is the common law theory of the volunteer that prevails.

Even though the treatment given by the optometrist may not be within the scope of the state optometry practice act, it should be within the limits of the standard of care applicable to the situation (and this standard may be set by physicians in some circumstances). As long as the optometrist has complied with the standard of care, there can be no liability for negligence. In meeting this standard, the optometrist will be expected to use reasonable care, and an optometrist who is not familiar with the appropriate treatment of an ocular urgency should not undertake to treat the condition but should instead arrange immediate referral to a competent practitioner. If *any* treatment is instituted (other than referral), the common law duty applicable to volunteers will be applied, and so it is important to document any care rendered.

Although in some circumstances it may be possible to assert that an optometrist offering first aid treatment of an ocular urgency has acted outside the scope of practice and thus is subject to disciplinary action on the part of the state board of optometry, if the optometrist has met the standard of care and has acted to facilitate medical care (through referral), the likelihood of disciplinary action would be remote at best.[20] Only when a medical condition outside the scope of practice is treated under the guise of emergency care does the possibility of disciplinary action become genuine.

In summary, optometrists who treat ocular urgencies should do so only when they feel the condition is one that they are capable of managing. Otherwise, referral to another practitioner is advisable.

Documentation of Treatment

The management of ocular urgencies begins with the patient's first contact with the doctor, which is usually accomplished by telephone. It is important for optometrists to train office assistants responsible for scheduling appointments (or for otherwise communicating with inquiring patients), so that they will be familiar with the proper methods to employ in the assessment of telephone complaints, thereby ensuring that an urgency will not be overlooked or the patient subjected to an injurious delay.

The patient of an ophthalmologist telephoned for an appointment, complaining that she had recently noticed specks and flashes of light in her field of vision. The receptionist told her that the doctor was "booked up" and made a routine appointment for six weeks later. When the ophthalmologist finally examined the patient, he discovered the retina was totally detached, with periretinal proliferation, and although surgical repair of the injury was attempted, it was unsuccessful. The patient sued the physician for failure to examine her on a timely basis.[21]

Optometric assistants should be prepared to respond to patient requests for urgent care and should be able to recognize complaints and symptoms that require immediate assessment (Table 14.2). Patients should be questioned carefully, and appointments should be scheduled on a timely basis. Part of the daily schedule may in fact be set aside for the examination of patients who call or walk in with urgent complaints.

Table 14.2. Telephone Assessment of Ocular Urgencies

The person communicating with the patient should record the following information:

Baseline data: Be calm and encouraging
- Name
- Age
- Phone number

Description of symptoms: Permit the patient to describe symptoms first (usually specific if it is an urgency)
- Is there pain? (acute, chronic, sharp, dull, constant, intermittent, local, or general)
- Is there a curtain or veil that seems to block vision?
- Is there burning, stinging, or difficulty in opening the eye (especially if there has been a chemical splash)?
- Is vision reduced (noticed with or without glasses) or is there a marked difference in vision between the two eyes?
- Is there sensitivity to light?
- Are there halos around lights?
- Is there the feeling that something is in the eye?
- Are there flashes of light, spots, floaters, or other noticeable changes of vision?
- Is the field of vision reduced?

Appearance of the eye: Patient may need to look in a mirror or have someone else describe the eye
- Is there swelling or discoloration of the orbit?
- Is the eye red, bloodshot, have blood in it?
- Is there any discharge (watery or thick)? Is there excessive tearing?
- Is the cornea hazy or cloudy?
- Are the pupils equal?
- Is the eye turned in or out or unable to move in some direction?

Onset of symptoms
- How long has the patient noticed the symptoms?
- Are the symptoms getting worse?
- Is there a previous history of these symptoms?
- Have there been any eye problems before?

If there is a report of a blow or other trauma to the eye
- Is there any pain? (describe)
- Was something splashed in the eye? (have the patient bring the chemical to the office if possible, and instruct to flush eye immediately)
- What struck the eye? (bring glasses if worn at the time of the blow)
- Is there any bleeding or discharge from a wound?
- Is there double vision?
- Is there decreased vision?
- Is there any loss of the field of vision?
- Are there streaks of light? A curtain or veil? Spots or floaters?

Any emergency visit should be adequately documented in the patient record. Of particular importance is information that describes the status of patients when they are first seen. The presenting complaint or symptoms and the visual acuity must be recorded. It is particularly important to record a visual acuity, even if it is "light perception only" or "finger counting at five feet" or other descriptive language rather than Snellen notation.

Pertinent examination findings should be noted and may be greatly enhanced through the use of drawings or photography.

Another significant piece of information that must be recorded is the dispostion of the case. If therapy is prescribed, it should be described in the record. If the patient is to return for further evaluation or follow-up, the date of the recall appointment should be noted. If a referral is made, the details should be documented. When specialized care is needed, it is best to recommend a specific practitioner to the patient and to arrange the appointment while the patient is in the office (the clinicolegal management of recalls and referrals is discussed in Chapter 16).

The problem-oriented record is an excellent way to document the management of an emergency or urgency since progress notes employing the SOAP format (Subjective complaint, Objective findings, Assessment, and Plan) provide a logical and efficient description of the injury and how it was handled. The problem-oriented record will be described in Chapter 16.

Notes

1. Duke-Elder, S., and P.A. MacFaul, *System of Ophthalmology*, vol. XIV, *Injuries*, St. Louis, C.V. Mosby, 1972.
2. For a review of the management of various emergencies and urgencies, see Deutsch, T.A., and D.B. Feller, *Management of Ocular Injuries*, 2d ed., W.B. Saunders, Philadelphia, 1985; and Freeman, H.M. (ed.), *Ocular Trauma*, Appleton-Century-Crofts, New York, 1979.
3. Deutsch, T.A., and D.B. Feller, note 2 supra, p. 2.
4. Escapini, H., Trauma to the Cornea, in King, J.H., Jr, and J.W. McTigue, (eds.), *The Cornea: World Congress*, London, Butterworth, 1965, pp. 300–315; and Brown, S.I., M.P. Tragakis, and D.B. Pearce, Treatment of the Alkali-Burned Cornea, *American Journal of Ophthalmology*, vol. 74, 1972, p. 316.
5. Deutsch, T.A., and D.B. Feller, note 2 supra, pp. 93–99.
6. Ibid.
7. Ibid.
8. Ibid.
9. Since the scope of optometry is defined by state law, the degree of care an individual optometrist can offer will vary from state to state. Ideally, a clinician should do all that is necessary and appropriate to preserve vision, but after initial first aid (lavage, removal of any particulate debris, and cycloplegia), in most instances the optometrist will refer the patient to the appropriate specialist (assuming that the injury is severe enough to warrant specialized care). Further steps, such as the use of topical antibiotics and steroids and the treatment of elevated intraocular pressure (if necessary), must be left to physicians if these procedures are outside the practice of optometry. See Classe, J., Liability for Ocular Urgencies and Emergencies, *Southern Journal of Optometry*, vol. 4, no. 4, 1986, pp. 51–58.
10. Liversedge, L.A., and V.H. Smith, Neuromedical and Ophthalmic Aspects of Central Retinal Artery Occlusion, *Transactions of the Ophthalmolgical Societies of the UK*, vol. 85, 1962, pp. 571–588; and Karjalainen, K., Occlusion of the Central Retinal Artery and Retinal Branch Arterioles, *Acta Ophthalmologica*, vol. 109 (Supp.), 1971, pp. 1–96.
11. Watson, P.G., The Treatment of Acute Retinal Arterial Occlusion, in Cant, J.S. (ed.), *William MacKenzie Centenary Symposium on the Ocular Circulation in Health and Disease*, C.V. Mosby, St. Louis, 1969, p. 234.
12. Ibid.
13. Ibid.
14. *Hurley v. Eddingfield*, 59 N.E. 1058 (Ind. 1901); *Rice v. Rinaldo*, 119 N.E.2d 657 (Ohio 1951); and *Agnew v. Parks*, 343 P.2d 118 (Cal. 1959). See also Right to Refuse Necessary Treatment, *Journal of the American Medical Association*, vol. 221, no. 3, July 17, 1972, pp. 335–336.
15. Published in 1976 by the American Optometric Association in lieu of the Supplement to the Code of Ethics and the Rules of Practice.
16. *Alabama Great Southern Railway Co v. Hunt*, 204 Ala. 504, 86 So. 100 (1920); *Triestram v. Way*, 286 Mich. 13, 281 N.W. 420 (1938); *Seele v. Purcell*, 45 N.M. 176, 113 P.2d 320 (1941); *Phillips v. Delta Motor Lines, Inc.*, 235 Miss. 1, 108 So.2d 409 (1959); and *Cook v. Thomas*, 25 Wis.2d 467, 131 N.W.2d 299 (1964).
17. The history of these statutes is recounted by Morris, R.C., and A. R. Moritz, *Doctor and Patient and the Law*, 5th ed., C.V. Mosby, St. Louis, 1971. See also, Who Should Provide Emergency Care?, *Journal of the American Medical Association*, vol. 210, no. 4, Oct. 27, 1969, pp. 775–776.
18. For example, the Georgia statute covers any person who renders emergency care and has been applied to a homeowner who attempted to help a workman who fell from a ladder while working on the homeowner's house. See *Wallace v. Hall*, 145 Ga. App. 610, 244 S.E.2d 129 (1978). But in Alaska a similar statute (providing immunity to any person rendering aid) was held not to apply to a state trooper because he was, in the court's opinion, under a preexisting duty to assist persons and was thus not a true volunteer. See *Lee v. State*, 490 P.2d 1206 (Alas. 1971). And in New Mexico, the statute—which applied to lay persons as well as physicians—did not provide immunity for the transportation by automobile of a victim from the scene of an accident to a motel, this act not constituting emergency

care in the opinion of the court since no medical aid was rendered by the motorist. See *Dahl v. Turner*, 80 N.M. 564, 458 P.2d 816 (1969). For a general review of these statutes, see Good Samaritan Laws, *Southern Texas Law Journal*, vol. 21, 1982, pp. 327–354.

19. If an optometrist attempts to undertake medical treatment at the scene of an accident—such as attempting cardiopulmonary resuscitation—in a state where the Good Samaritan statute affords no legal protection for such actions, the optometrist must realize that the standard of care will be a medical one, inasmuch as the procedures undertaken to assist the stricken individual are medical. Any time an optometrist performs services that are outside the scope of optometry, he or she may be held to a medical standard rather than one established solely by optometrists.
20. Even though an optometrist performs an act outside the scope of practice, such an act may nonetheless be in keeping with ethical obligations to assist patients in an emergency. If the optometrist's actions are limited to first aid or immediate treatment, are within the standard of care, and serve to prevent loss of vision or further injury, it is difficult to understand the purpose to be served by the imposition of discipline in such a case. The ethical necessity to assist a patient in an emergency should override the technical violation of the optometry statute under these circumstances. For a discussion of medical and legal principles, see Bettman, J.W., How to Reduce Medicolegal Involvement in Cases of Trauma, *Ophthalmology*, vol. 87, no. 5, 1980, pp. 432–434.
21. Bettman, J.W., A Retrospective Look at Twenty-two Medicolegal Claims: How They Might Have Been Avoided, *Survey of Ophthalmology*, vol. 28, no. 1, 1983, pp. 55–60.

Chapter 15

Evaluation of Ocular Disability

Appellee testified that while working in appellant's mine at a cutting machine a piece of coal struck and injured his right eye; that theretofore his vision in both eyes had been good but thereafter the vision of his right eye was greatly impaired and had continued so... Dr. Steel, an optometrist, who examined appellee stated that the vision of his right eye was 20/200... about 10 percent vision. Dr. Steel also testified concerning the scar on the eye and gave as his opinion that the loss of vision was due to the scar or to the injury causing it. It will therefore be seen that if Dr. Steel was a competent witness there is unquestionably sufficient evidence to sustain the award of the board.... Upon being asked concerning his qualifications Dr. Steel testified that... the school from which he graduated trained him in diagnostic work and examination of the eyes and he was skilled at diagnosis.... Furthermore, when asked concerning matters of evidence about which the oculist had testified he displayed general knowledge concerning the subject. In view of the evidence of training and experience of Dr. Steel... we are constrained to hold that his evidence was competent.... Since the finding of the board that appellee is industrially blind in his right eye as a result of the accident is sustained by competent evidence it is conclusive and binding upon the court.

—From the opinion of Commissioner Creal, *Black Starr Coal Corp. v. Reeder, 128 S.W.2d 905 (1939)*

Legal Blindness

In the assessment of disablity an optometrist may be called upon to determine if a patient is legally blind. There are numerous reasons for which such an assessment may be necessary but among the most common are social security benefits, veteran's benefits, worker's compensation benefits, eligibility for vocational rehabilitation, deductions under the Internal Revenue Code, or other insurance benefits.

In order to make the diagnosis of legal blindness, optometrists must be familiar with the applicable definition for the benefits or eligibility being claimed. Therefore, an optometrist should always be certain that the purpose for the determination of legal blindness has been stated so that the interpretation of examination results can be properly made.

If the patient is seeking to qualify for federal benefits, then the applicable federal definition must be consulted. The most common definition used for federal purposes is that of the Social Security Administration.[1]

Under the Social Security law, blindness for purposes of the statute exists if there is:

- central visual acuity of 20/200 or less in the better eye with the use of a correcting lens
- contraction of the peripheral visual fields in the better eye:
  - (a) to 10° or less from the point of fixation or
  - (b) so the widest diameter subtends an angle no greater than 20° or
  - (c) to 20 percent or less visual field efficiency

Figure 15.1 illustrates how visual field efficiency can be calculated.

The Internal Revenue Service uses the Social Security definition in order to determine if a taxpayer is blind and thus eligible to claim the extra exemption when reporting personal income taxes on Form 1040.[2]

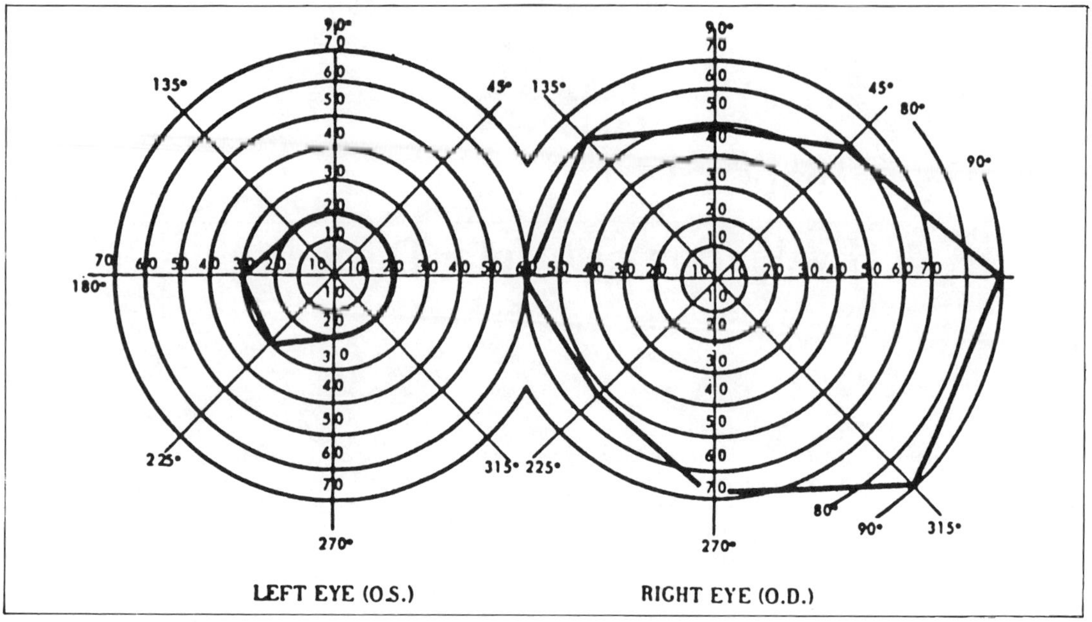

Figure 15.1. Visual Field Efficiency, Social Security Law, 1985. Diagram of right eye illustrates extent of normal visual field as tested on standard perimeter at 330 mm with a 3 mm white disc under 7 foot-candles illumination. The sum of the eight principal meridians of this field total 500 degrees. The percent of visual field efficiency is obtained by adding the number of degrees of the eight principal meridians of the contracted field and dividing by 500. Diagram of left eye illustrates visual field contracted to 30 degrees in the temporal and down and out meridians and to 20 degrees in the remaining six meridians. The percent of visual field efficiency of this field is: $6 \times 20 + 2 \times 30 = 180 \div 500 = 0.36$ or 36 percent remaining visual field efficiency, or 64 percent loss. (Source: 20 C.F.R. §416.981.)

If the program for which the patient is seeking eligibility for benefits is a state program, the state definition of blindness must be consulted. This definition may be different from the one used by the Social Security Administration.[3]

The legally blind population includes not only persons who are totally blind but those who have a severe vision impairment in both eyes. There are no actual figures available on this population for the nation as a whole or for each state. However, estimates (as of 1978) are that about 498,000 persons in the United State are legally blind.[4]

A person may not be legally blind but may yet have suffered a permanent vision impairment. Optometrists may be required to evaluate the permanent impairment of a patient's visual system for various reasons and to express this impairment in terms of diminished ability of the whole person. It is to this subject that we now turn.

Assessment of Visual Impairment

Optometrists must employ uniform criteria when evaluating the permanent impairment of the visual system. A standard set of guidelines has been developed by the Committee on Rating of Mental and Physical Impairment of the American Medical Association and has been used by the medical profession for decades.[5] These guidelines provide a ready means for determining the permanent vision impairment of an individual and how it affects the individual's ability to perform the activities of daily life. The impairment is expressed as a percentage of impairment of the visual system and as a percentage of impairment of the whole person.

The assessment of visual impairment requires that deviations from the normal be considered to the extent that they are reflected in corrected visual acuity for distance and near, visual fields, and ocular motility with the absence of diplopia.[6]

Although other aspects of vision such as anomalies of accommodation, light adaptation difficulties, epiphora, loss of stereopsis or color vision, macular pathology resulting in distortions of vision such as metamorphopsia, and disturbances of lid function such as ectropion and intropion may not be reflected in the loss of visual function related to visual acuity, visual field, or ocular motility, they should be con-

Table 15.1. Visual Acuity Notations with Corresponding Percentages of Loss of Central Vision

For Distance			
	Snellen Notations		
English	Metric 6	Metric 4	% Loss
20/15	6/5	4/3	0
20/20	6/6	4/4	0
20/25	6/7.5	4/5	5
20/30	6/10	4/6	10
20/40	6/12	4/8	15
20/50	6/15	4/10	25
20/60	6/20	4/12	35
20/70	6/22	4/14	40
20/80	6/24	4/16	45
20/100	6/30	4/20	50
20/125	6/38	4/25	60
20/150	6/50	4/30	70
20/200	6/60	4/40	80
20/300	6/90	4/60	85
20/400	6/120	4/80	90
20/800	6/240	4/160	95

For Near				
Near Snellen		Revised Jaeger	American	
Inches	Centimeters	Standard	Point-type	% Loss
14/14	35/35	1	3	0
14/18	35/45	2	4	0
14/21	35/53	3	5	5
14/24	35/60	4	6	7
14/28	35/70	5	7	10
14/35	35/88	6	8	50
14/40	35/100	7	9	55
14/45	35/113	8	10	60
14/60	35/150	9	11	80
14/70	35/175	10	12	85
14/80	35/200	11	13	87
14/88	35/220	12	14	90
14/112	35/280	13	21	95
14/140	35/350	14	23	98

Source: *Guides to the Evaluation of Permanent Impairment, 2d Ed.*, American Medical Association, 1984.

sidered by the examining optometrist and combined with these functional impairments in order to make a complete assessment.[7] If there are other ocular impairments, such as abnormal pupillary responses and opacities or disturbances of the cornea or other ocular media, they may be considered to constitute an additional 5 to 10 percent impairment of the involved eye. Permanent deformities of the orbit or cosmetic defects that do not affect vision function must be considered as individual factors that can cause up to 10 percent impairment of the whole person.[8]

In order to assess the visual impairment of patients, an optometrist needs a relatively modest amount of equipment:

- Visual acuity charts for distance and near (Snellen or Jaeger test charts are preferable)
- A standard perimeter with a radius of 330 mm
- Equipment for refraction

The assessment of visual acuity, visual field, and ocular motility should be conducted in accordance with the guidelines established by the AMA.

Visual Acuity

The standard test distance should be 20 feet (6 meters) for distance acuity and 14 inches (35 centimeters) for near acuity. The patient's vision should be recorded both with and without correction, and each eye's acuity considered separately as a percentage of loss of central vision (see Table 15.1).

In order to determine the impairment when both eyes are affected, the mean of the two percentages must be determined. Thus a 10 and 50 percent loss equals a binocular loss of 30 percent.

If the patient is a monocular aphake, this condition is considered to be an additional handicap and is assigned a value corresponding to a 50 percent decrease in the remaining visual acuity (see Table 15.2). For example, if a patient is 14/60 for near and 20/200 for distance, there is an 80 percent loss of central vision. But if the patient is also a monocular aphake with those same acuities, the percentage of impairment becomes 90 percent.

Visual Field

The patient should be tested with a three-millimeter (mm) white target at a distance of 330 mm under illumination that is not less than seven foot-candles. (If the Goldmann 30 cm bowl perimeter is used, the III/4e target in the kinetic mode should be employed.) The target is brought from the periphery until it is detected by the patient. The examiner should obtain two peripheral fields which agree within 15 degrees in each meridian. The results should be plotted on a standard visual field chart. The minimum expected values for each of the eight-principal meridians are summarized in Table 15.3. A different procedure may be required for an aphakic patient.[9]

The loss of visual field for each eye may be determined by adding the number of degrees found in the eight principal meridians for the 3W/330 isopter—

Table 15.2. Determination of Loss of Central Vision

Snellen Rating for Distance in Feet	Approximate Snellen Rating for Near in Inches													
	14/14	14/18	14/21	14/24	14/28	14/35	14/40	14/45	14/60	14/70	14/80	14/88	14/112	14/140
20/15	0*	0	3	4	5	25	27	30	40	43	44	45	48	49
	50†	50	52	52	53	63	64	65	70	72	72	73	74	75
20/20	0	0	3	4	5	25	27	30	40	43	44	46	48	49
	50	50	52	52	53	63	64	65	70	72	72	73	74	75
20/25	3	3	5	6	8	28	30	33	43	45	46	48	50	52
	52	52	53	53	54	64	65	67	72	73	73	74	75	76
20/30	5	5	8	9	10	30	32	35	45	48	49	50	53	54
	53	53	54	54	55	65	66	68	73	74	74	75	76	77
20/40	8	8	10	11	13	33	35	38	48	50	51	53	55	57
	54	54	55	56	57	67	68	69	74	75	76	77	78	79
20/50	13	13	15	16	18	38	40	43	53	55	56	58	60	62
	57	57	58	58	59	69	70	72	77	78	78	79	80	81
20/60	16	16	18	20	22	41	44	46	56	59	60	61	64	65
	58	58	59	60	61	70	72	73	78	79	80	81	82	83
20/80	20	20	23	24	25	45	47	50	60	63	64	65	68	69
	60	60	62	62	63	73	74	75	80	82	82	83	84	85
20/100	25	25	28	29	30	50	52	55	65	68	69	70	73	74
	63	63	64	64	65	75	76	78	83	84	84	85	87	87
20/125	30	30	33	34	35	55	57	60	70	73	74	75	78	79
	65	65	67	67	68	78	79	80	85	87	87	88	89	90
20/150	34	34	37	38	39	59	61	64	74	77	78	79	82	83
	67	67	68	69	70	80	81	82	87	88	89	90	91	92
20/200	40	40	43	44	45	65	67	70	80	83	84	85	88	89
	70	70	72	72	73	83	84	85	90	91	92	93	94	95
20/300	43	43	45	46	48	68	70	73	83	85	86	88	90	92
	72	72	73	73	74	84	85	87	91	93	93	94	95	96
20/400	45	45	48	49	50	70	72	75	85	88	89	90	93	94
	73	73	74	74	75	85	86	88	93	94	94	95	97	97
20/800	48	48	50	51	53	73	75	78	88	90	91	93	95	97
	74	74	75	76	77	87	88	89	94	95	96	97	98	99

*Upper figure = % loss of central vision without allowance for monocular aphakia.
†Lower figure = % loss of central vision with allowance for monocular aphakia.
Source: *Guides to the Evaluation of Permanent Impairment, 2d Ed.*, American Medical Association, 1984.

normally 500 degrees—and dividing by five. Special calculations are required for quadrantic or hemifield loss,[10] for scotomas,[11] and for enlarged blind spots.[12] The total degrees lost are then converted into the percentage of visual field lost (see Table 15.4).

For example, if the patient has a concentric contraction to 30 degrees, the extent of loss in each of the eight principal meridians is:

MERIDIAN	LOSS	DEGREE
1	Temporally	55
2	Down temporally	55
3	Down	35
4	Down nasally	20
5	Nasally	30
6	Up nasally	25
7	Up	15
8	Up temporally	25
	Total loss	260

A total loss of 260 degrees corresponds to a loss of 52 percent of the visual field.

Table 15.3. Minimal Normal Extent of Visual Field from Point of Fixation

Direction of Vision	Degrees of Field
Temporally	85
Down temporally	85
Direct down	65
Down nasally	50
Nasally	60
Up nasally	55
Direct up	45
Up temporally	55
Total	500

Source: *Guides to the Evaluation of Permanent Impairment, 2d Ed.*, American Medical Association, 1984.

Ocular Motility

The extent of diplopia must be determined for the various directions of gaze by using the perimeter at 330 mm—or a tangent screen at 1,000 mm—by testing each of the 45 degree meridians with a test light.[13]

To determine the loss of ocular motility for each eye the examiner must plot the results of the separation of two images on a visual field chart and add the percentage loss of motility caused by diplopia for each of the positions of gaze by consulting the chart illustrated in Figure 15.2

For example, if diplopia is found to affect the pa-

Table 15.4. Determination of Loss of Visual Field

Total Degrees		% of	Total Degrees		% of	Total Degrees		% of
Lost	Retained	Loss	Lost	Retained	Loss	Lost	Retained	Loss
0	500*	0	170	330	34	340	160	68
5	495	1	175	325	35	345	155	69
10	490	2	180	320	36	350	150	70
15	485	3	185	315	37	355	145	71
20	480	4	190	310	38	360	140	72
25	475	5	195	305	39	365	135	73
30	470	6	200	300	40	370	130	74
35	465	7	205	295	41	375	125	75
40	460	8	210	290	42	380	120	76
45	455	9	215	285	43	385	115	77
50	450	10	220	280	44	390	110	78
55	445	11	225	275	45	395	105	79
60	440	12	230	270	46	400	100	80
65	435	13	235	265	47	405	95	81
70	430	14	240	260	48	410	90	82
75	425	15	245	255	49	415	85	83
80	420	16	250	250	50	420	80	84
85	415	17	255	245	51	425	75	85
90	410	18	260	240	52	430	70	86
95	405	19	265	235	53	435	65	87
100	400	20	270	230	54	440	60	88
105	395	21	275	225	55	445	55	89
110	390	22	280	220	56	450	50	90
115	385	23	285	215	57	455	45	91
120	380	24	290	210	58	460	40	92
125	375	25	295	205	59	465	35	93
130	370	26	300	200	60	470	30	94
135	365	27	305	195	61	475	25	95
140	360	28	310	190	62	480	20	96
145	355	29	315	185	63	485	15	97
150	350	30	320	180	64	490	10	98
155	345	31	325	175	65	495	5	99
160	340	32	330	170	66	500	0	100
165	335	33	335	165	67			

*Or more.

Source: *Guides to the Evaluation of Permanent Impairment, 2d Ed.*, American Medical Association, 1984.

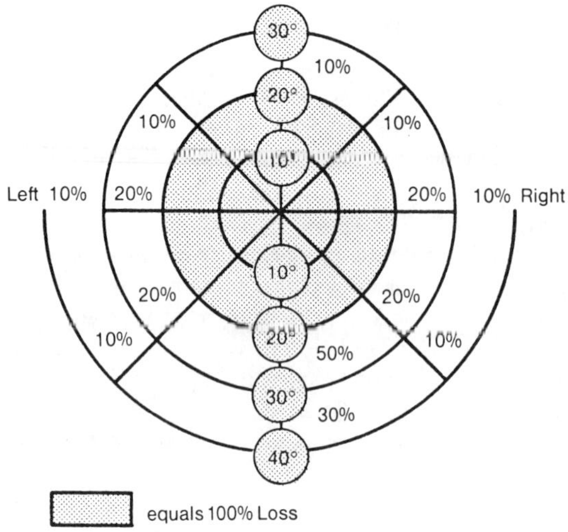

Figure 15.2. Determination of Percentage Loss of Ocular Motility in One Eye with Diplopia Fields. (Source: *Guides to the Evaluation of Permanent Impairment*, 2nd ed., American Medical Association, 1984.)

tient's side vision when looking from 20 to 30 degrees (a 20 percent loss of motility) and when looking from 30 to 40 degrees (a 10 percent loss of motility), the patient has a total loss of ocular motility of 30 degrees.

Impairment of the Visual System and the Whole Person

To assess the impairment of the visual system represented by the loss of one or more of visual acuity, visual field, and ocular motility, the examiner must consult a special chart (see Appendix).

For example, if the impairment of the right eye (the worse eye) is 20 percent, and the impairment of the left eye (the better eye) is 10 percent, the impairment to the visual system is 13 percent (see Appendix).

To assess the impairment of the visual system when all three functions have been affected, each of them must be calculated separately for each eye as percentages, and then a combined values chart (see Appendix) is consulted to (1) combine the loss of visual acuity with the loss of visual field and (2) combine the loss of ocular motility with the value for loss of visual acuity and visual field by using the chart a second time. In making this determination only the eye with the greatest loss of motility is used.

For example, if the patient's right eye has a 56 percent loss of acuity and a 32 percent loss of visual field, there is a combined value of 70 percent loss. If there is also a 25 percent loss of ocular motility, the eye has a 78 percent loss. (See Appendix for chart.)

The last step is to determine the percentage of impairment of the whole person. This assessment may be made by consulting Table 15.5.

For example, a 25 percent impairment of the visual system equals a 24 percent impairment of the whole person. Total loss of vision in both eyes represents an 85 percent impairment of the whole person.

It is necessary for doctors of optometry to be familiar with the evaluation of disability since optometrists will be called on by the courts to offer testimony

Table 15.5. Impairment of the Visual System As It Relates to Impairment of the Whole Person

% Impairment of		% Impairment of		% Impairment of		% Impairment of		% Impairment of		% Impairment of	
Visual System	Whole Person	Visual System	Whole Person	Visual System	Whole Person	Visual System	Whole Person	Visual System	Whole Person	Visual System	Whole Person
0	0	15	14	30	28	45	42	60	57	75	71
1	1	16	15	31	29	46	43	61	58	76	72
2	2	17	16	32	30	47	44	62	59	77	73
3	3	18	17	33	31	48	45	63	59	78	74
4	4	19	18	34	32	49	46	64	60	79	75
5	5	20	19	35	33	50	47	65	61	80	76
6	6	21	20	36	34	51	48	66	62	81	76
7	7	22	21	37	35	52	49	67	63	82	77
8	8	23	22	38	36	53	50	68	64	83	78
9	8	24	23	39	37	54	51	69	65	84	79
10	9	25	24	40	38	55	52	70	66	85	80
11	10	26	25	41	39	56	53	71	67	86	81
12	11	27	25	42	40	57	54	72	68	87	82
13	12	28	26	43	41	58	55	73	69	88	83
14	13	29	27	44	42	59	56	74	70	89	84
										90–100	85

Source: *Guides to the Evaluation of Permanent Impairment, 2d Ed.*, American Medical Association, 1984.

to this effect (described in Chapter 35). Optometrists should never overlook the possibility of visual rehabilitation or low vision evaluation in a patient with ocular disability (see Chapter 32).

Notes

1. 20 C.F.R. §416.981.
2. The personal exemption for blindness has been changed by the Tax Reform Act of 1986. See IRS publication 920, *Explanation of the Tax Reform Act of 1986 for Individuals.*
3. For example, in Alabama a blind person is defined as follows:

   (a) As used in this Code or any statute of this state heretofore or hereafter enacted, unless the context requires a different meaning, the term "blind person" means a natural person who has no vision or whose vision with correcting glasses is so defective as to prevent the performance of ordinary activities for which eyesight is essential, or who has central visual acuity of 20/200 or less in the better eye with correcting glasses, or whose central visual acuity is more than 20/200 in the better eye with correcting glasses but whose peripheral field has contracted to such an extent that the widest diameter of the visual field subtends an angular distance no greater than 20 degrees.

   Alabama Code §1-1-3.
4. National Society to Prevent Blindness, *Vision Problems in the United States*, National Society to Prevent Blindness, N.Y., 1980.
5. American Medical Association, *Guides to the Evaluation of Permanent Impairment*, 2d ed., American Medical Association, Chicago, 1984, pp. 141–151.
6. Ibid.
7. Ibid.
8. Ibid.
9. Ibid. For an aphakic patient who is uncorrected (not adapted to a contact lens or an intraocular implant or whose eye is fitted with aphakic spectacles) a 6-mm white target should be used at 330 mm. If a Goldmann bowl perimeter is employed, the target should be IV/4e in the kinetic mode. If the patient wears contact lenses or is a pseudophake, testing should proceed as for phakic patients.
10. To determine the loss of a quadrant or half field, it is necessary to add the total of the loss in each meridian to half the sum of the two boundary meridians. For example, assume the temporal field is lost. The visual fields are:

Up temporally	55 degrees
Temporally	85 degrees
Down temporally	85 degrees
Average up and down	55 degrees

   The total loss is 280 degrees, which is a 56 percent visual loss. From *Guides to the Evaluation of Permanent Impairment*, supra note 5, at 146.
11. Approximate values for scotomas are calculated by subtracting the width of the scotoma from the peripheral visual field at the same meridians. See ibid.
12. To determine the loss of the visual field due to enlargement of the blind spot, multiply the enlargement times eight (for each of the eight measured meridans) and divide the total degrees by five to obtain the permanent loss. For example, if the blind spot is enlarged by five degrees, the loss is 5 × 8 or 40 degrees, and when divided by five amounts an to 8 percent loss. See Ibid.
13. Ibid.

Chapter 16

Recordkeeping and Documentation

Oh that my words were now written!
—Job, Chapter 19, Verse 23, *Holy Bible*

An essential aspect of the doctor-patient relationship is the patient record. The primary reason for maintaining records is to facilitate management of the patient's case and to provide a current, comprehensive account of the care and treatment undertaken by the attending doctor. It is also the cornerstone of a doctor's defense if the doctor is forced to go to court to defend the diagnosis or treatment of a particular patient. As Louisell and Williams note in their leading treatise for plaintiff's attorneys on the subject of malpractice litigation: "The significance of patient records in malpractice cases cannot be overemphasized."[1]

All optometrists should carefully organize, maintain, and preserve their patient records and should be aware of the significant legal ramifications of recordkeeping. In this chapter we will discuss the many facets of recordkeeping in the hope that no practitioner faced with a legal dispute will have to give voice to the despair expressed by Job (above).

Form and Content

The form, organization, and content of an optometrist's patient records are best determined by professional standards and not by specific legal requirements. Therefore, the statutory and regulatory law of the individual states does not mandate a specific type of organization or content for the records of private practitioners.[2] But both legal considerations and professional standards of practice for optometrists require that entries in the patient record contain a certain minimum of information, which is intended to provide proper substantiation of the care rendered to the patient. In maintaining records it is essential to document why the patient was seen, when, what was diagnosed, and what was done in terms of treatment. The problem-oriented record is an excellent way to organize this information.[3]

The problem-oriented record system is solution oriented and enables the practitioner to manage patients in a logical and efficient manner by helping to define problems, plan for their resolution, and properly monitor their progress. When used appropriately, the problem-oriented record system also provides the documentation that is essential for clinicolegal purposes while requiring a minimum of time for recording and interpretation.

There are four steps to the problem-oriented system of recordkeeping: formulating an adequate data base, compiling a complete problem list, formulating an initial plan, and using progress notes.

Data Base

The data base begins with the collection of information sufficient to allow the practitioner to perform an adequate examination. The amount of information necessary to constitute an adequate data base will

UNIVERSITY OF ALABAMA IN BIRMINGHAM
SCHOOL OF OPTOMETRY

CLINICIAN Classe
INSTRUCTOR

Name Jo. G. SMITH Age 52 Sex W/F Data Sheet Confirmed

PATIENT HISTORY:

CC: Has trouble reading at near. No other subjective complaints.

PVH: Current Rx 10 yrs old; obtained at last exam (Dr. Springer, Anniston). Rx is satisfactory for distance. Takes Rx off for reading.

PH: Last physical 1 year ago; health is "excellent". No recent illnesses or hospitalizations. Neg hx of diabetes, hypertension, arthritis, cardiac, thyroid disease.

FPH: Father deceased (pneumonia); mother living. Neg family hx of diabetes, hypertension, heart disease, cancer.

OH: Denies hx of trauma, disease, or surgery; denies glaucoma, cataracts, squint, diplopia, ambyopia, color defects.

FOH: No family history of blindness, glaucoma, cataracts, squint, ambyopia, or surgery.

Med: Taking no medications at present; no hx of taking meds for prolonged periods.

Hyp: Denies sensitivities to drugs.

Avo: Homemaker; reads, sews; no active sports.

Old Rx

W	Sph	Cyl	Axis	Prism	Add	Seg Type	Seg Ht	CT	B.C.	±Cyl	Tint
O.D.	-0.75	-0.25	085								
O.S.	-0.75	-0.25	068								

LEE 10 yrs ago
Dr. Springer

Frame Paris/blk Eye 44 DBL 22 Temple Lib. Lens P.D. Seg dec

Other Rx's; Comments

EXAMINATION:

V_s	6m	40cm
OD	20/40	20/20-
OS	20/40	20/20-
OU	20/30-	20/20-

V	6m	40cm
OD	20/20-	20/30-
OS	20/20-	20/30-
OU	20/20	20/30-

B.P. 121/84 RAS Pupils PERRLA MG neg.
IPD 61/57 NPC TN Lids unremarkable
Stereo 6m 40cm 40 sec/arc Test Titmus
Color OD OS Test
Acc. Amp/Fac OD OS
Ductions Versions no restrictions
Cover Test: Dist. 3 XP Thru W
Near (40 cm) 6 X'P Thru W

K O.D. @ @
O.S. @ @

R O.D. -0.50 -0.50 X 075 V 20/20-
O.S. -0.75 -0.50 X 065 V 20/20-

M_1 O.D. -0.75 -0.25 X 080 V 20/20
O.S. -0.75 -0.25 X 066 V 20/20

M_2 O.D. V
O.S.

TIB
TNA O.D. +1.75 V 20/20
O.S. +1.75 V 20/20

Method MPBU Range 10 to 23" PRA NRA

BINOCULAR STATUS

FAR (Thru W)
Phoria /
NFV x / 8 / 6 PFV x / 10 / 4 (PB)
FD /
Suppression:

NEAR (40 cm. Thru W and TNA
Phoria /
NFV x / 20 / 15 PFV x / 20 / 15 (PB)
FD /
Suppression:

FORM OPT 100

ADDITIONAL TESTS, COMMENTS

No facial asymmetry
Demonstrated M_1 and TNA in trial frame; patient prefers M_1/TNA over W.

DATE 17 July 1987

Figure 16.1. Sample Data Base. (Courtesy UAB School of Optometry)

BIOMICROSCOPY Angle OD 1:½ (T) 1:1 (N) OS 1:½ (T) 1:½ (N) Method: SL

OD: Conjunctiva, cornea, media, iris unremarkable. 1^+ posterior yellowing of lens. Neg. staining w/fluorescein. Anterior adnexa unremarkable.

OS: as noted for OD.

T OD 14 mm Hg ANESTH. Fluress ___%

OS 15 mm Hg APPREHENSION (L) M H

(TAP) NCT MM TIME: 2:00 ~~a.m.~~ p.m.

OPHTHALMOSCOPY (Dilation c̄ 1 gt Myd 1% and Neo 2½%)

BIO X
DO X
MIO ___

OD: disc oval, no pallor, C/D=.2/.2, 1 D deep, margins distinct, NRR intact
A/V= 2:3, no crossing changes
macular reflex present
GRA unremarkable by BIO

OS: as noted for OD except for 4 DD size nevus at 12:00 and 3 DD from disk

VISUAL FIELDS full central fields OD/OS Method TS Stimulus 2W Dist. 1000
Performed at 7 fc; good responses

ADDITIONAL TESTS/SKETCHES ATTACHED: ___

Dx / IMPRESSIONS:

Diag Code (COIT)*		Diagnoses
	1.	CMA OD and OS
	2.	Presbyopia
	3.	Choroidal nevus OS
	4.	
	5.	
	6.	

*See Clinic Manual for listing

Comments: Warned the patient of the risks of driving while pupils dilated. Supplied mydriatic glasses.

Tx / Px

1. Prescribe M_1 for full-time wear
2. Prescribe +1.75 add
3. Monitor at next exam
4.
5.
6.

RTC: 1 yr

Comments: Photodocument nevus OS

SIGNATURES

Examiner ___

Staff JE Classé O.D.

(10/82)

Figure 16.1. *Continued*.

vary from patient to patient and from case to case but should include the chief complaint and all information essential to the proper evaluation of this complaint (patient profile, history, and examination findings).

The patient profile should include such data as age, race, sex, marital status, occupation, avocation, and special needs.

The history should include the chief complaint, ocular history, past medical history, and family health history.

Examination findings should include all pertinent tests and observations necessary to satisfy the standard of care.

Various forms may be employed to record this information, and many practitioners have developed personalized forms to enable them to inscribe patient data efficiently and thoroughly. Because there is no perfect form that can serve the needs of all optometrists, the forms that are used here are to be considered samples of a problem-oriented format and not examplars of a flawless nature. Thus, in Figure 16.1 one means of recording the data base for a common chief complaint, blurred vision, is illustrated.[4]

Problem List

The use of a problem list enables the practitioner to review past and current problems at a glance, thereby assuring thoroughness and continuity of care. The list is based on positive examination findings and is an ongoing account of the problems that require management. The list is added to as old problems are resolved or as new problems develop and forms the basis for the diagnostic or therapeutic efforts undertaken by the practitioner. An example problem list is included as Figure 16.2.

PROBLEM NO.	DATE ENTERED	PROBLEM LIST	PROBLEM RESOLVED	DATE RESOLVED
1.	17-7-87	CMA OD/OS	Yes	17-7-87
2.	17-7-87	Presbyopia	Yes	17-7-87
3.	17-7-87	Choroidal nevus OS		
4.				
5.				
6.				
7				
8.				
9.				
10.				
11.				
12.				
13.				
14.				

PROBLEM LETTER	TEMPORARY PROBLEM LIST (ACUTE-LIMITED)	DATES OF OCCURRENCES

Figure 16.2. Sample Problem List. (Courtesy UAB School of Optometry)

Initial Plans

A plan must be developed for each problem, whether the problem is to be managed by the practitioner, co-managed in consultation with another health-care provider, or referred to another practitioner for specialized care. The plan may consist of further diagnostic testing, the use of specific treatment, or educational efforts directed at the patient. In formulating plans for specific problems, the practitioner should consider each of these components and note them in the patient record (see Fig. 16.3).

The importance of patient education should not be overlooked. In some cases the practitioner will have a clinical and legal obligation to communicate with the patient concerning examination findings (see Chapter 22), to inform the patient of meaningful symptoms (see Chapter 25), or to warn of the risks associated with the use of certain ophthalmic products (see Chapter 27). Better understanding may be achieved in many cases through the use of printed forms, which can also serve to remind the patient of the importance of timely care. An example of such a form can be found in Figure 16.4.

Progress Notes

A practitioner may use progress notes to monitor any efforts to solve a particular problem, and when so used the notes should be numbered and titled to correspond to the complete problem list for the patient (Fig. 16.5). Progress notes can also be employed for the evaluation of a specific chief complaint or for episodic care (Fig. 16.6). In both instances the progress notes should follow a specific format, which requires a four-step evaluation, often referred to by the mnemonic SOAP:

1. **S**ubjective complaint or updated case history
2. **O**bjective findings or observations
3. **A**ssessment of findings or progress of case
4. **P**lan for the problems listed in the assessment

The SOAP format is well understood by the medical profession and is readily accepted in legal proceedings.

The use of the problem-oriented record system is further illustrated in the Appendix.

A vital part of any optometrist's care is the decision to refer a patient to another health-care provider or to reschedule the patient for a return appointment. For clinicolegal purposes it is preferable to manage referrals and recalls in the manner described below.

Referrals

The optometrist must decide to whom the referral will be made. The more specific the selection, the more likely that patient compliance can be assured.

S - Subjective
O - Objective
A - Assessment
P - Plan

DATE	Prob. No.	INITIAL PLAN
7-17-87	1	Prescribe M_1 for FTW.
7-17-87	2	Prescribe +1.75 add
7-17-87	3	Monitor in 1 yr. at next exam. Photodocument.

Figure 16.3. Sample Plans for Treatment. (Courtesy UAB School of Optometry)

Patient Education Form: CATARACTS

The human eye is built much like a camera. Light enters through the pupil and is brought to focus on the retina by a lens inside of the eye in much the same way that the lenses of a camera focus the image on the film. To work well the eye must have a healthy retina just as a camera must have good film. In addition to that the lens of a camera must be clean and clear to form a good image or the camera must be taken apart to clean the lenses. A dirty lens in a camera will produce a poor picture just as if you were trying to look out of a dirty window.

The eye can change in many ways to produce a poor image. One of those ways is for the lens of the eye to become cloudy and distorted. This happens to all eyes with age. It just seems that some get cloudy a little bit sooner than others. This clouding and distortion of the normally clear crystalline lens is called a **cataract.** When you have a cataract, it is like looking through a dirty window. Even if the prescription for your glasses is changed, vision may still be cloudy. The figure illustrates the location of a cataract and how it blocks the light to the retina.

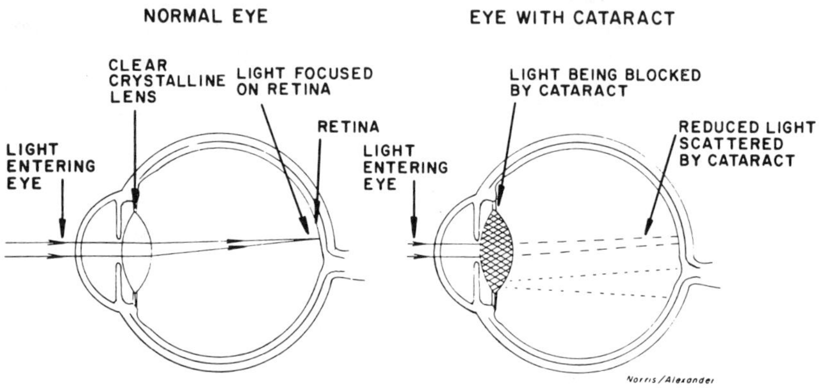

There are many forms of cataracts and not all of them must be removed immediately. Your doctor will advise you of the status of your cataract and how often you must have an eye examination. The repeat eye examinations are for your benefit to keep you advised of the progress of the cataract.

Cataracts don't get "ripe" before they can be removed. Cataracts are usually removed after the vision drops below 20/60 with glasses. This varies, however, depending on your individual needs. For example, if you were a truck driver, excellent stereo vision or 3-dimensional vision would be very important. This means that you need two good eyes and you may decide to have surgery before the vision drops below the 20/60 level.

Most cataract surgery today is performed at an outpatient facility under local anesthesia. A small incision is made in the eye and the cloudy crystalline lens is removed through the pupil which has been dilated. In well over 90 percent of the procedures a plastic lens implant similar to a contact lens is then placed behind the iris. Usually you have some vision back the next day.

Cataracts have become more prevalent in today's society because we are all living longer. Remember that cataract surgery is not to be taken lightly. The procedure is, however, fairly pain-free and should not be delayed if cataracts are clouding your vision. All of us will get cataracts if we all live to a ripe old age.

Remember! Your return appointment is in ______ months.

Please call sooner (1-205-934-5161) if you have problems or if you have questions.

Figure 16.4. Sample Patient Education Form. (Courtesy Larry J. Alexander, O.D.)

DATE: Sept. 12, 1987 **PROGRESS NOTES**

NAME W.C. Jones HOME PHONE 123-4567

ADDRESS 123 Main Street BIRTHDATE Sept. 12, 1901

REFERRAL SOURCE

OCCUPATION Retired WORK PHONE

S Complains of gritty, sandy eyes; particularly crusty at awakening. Onset 3 weeks ago. Takes artificial tears for relief, which is temporary. No other complaints.

O VA: OD 20/60+ @ 6 M w/W 20/40+ @ 40 cm w/W W: OD -4.50 -1.00 x 095
OS 20/50- 20/40+ OS -4.00 -0.50 x 085
add +2.50

Ret: OD -4.75 -1.00 x 090 20/50-
OS -5.00 -0.75 x 090 20/40-

MVA: OD -4.75 -1.00 x 095 20/50- Trial Frame: patient appreciates
OS -4.50 -0.50 x 085 20/40- improved VA w/MVA but does not want to change W

SLE: OD 2+ conjunctival injection; marginal blephritis; anterior chamber clear; corneal SPK w/fluorescein; 1+ papillae of bulbar conjunctiva; 3+ cataract
OS as noted for the OD

Ophthal: OD disc oval, no pallor, margins distinct, C/D= .1/.1
1 gt Myd 1% A/V is 2:3, no crossing changes
BIO drusen in macula; no hemorrhages or exudates
MDO GRA unremarkable
OS as noted for OD

A 1.Cataract OD/OS
2.Age-related maculopathy OD/OS
3.Bacterial keratoconjunctivitis OD/OS

P 1.Discussed surgical consult with patient; does not wish to see surgeon at present
2.Discussed significance with patient; follow at next exam
3.Rx Garamycin 1 gt q 4 hrs; hot compresses qid; RTC 2 days

J O'Dee
John O'Dee, O.D.

Figure 16.5. Sample Progress Notes. (Courtesy UAB School of Optometry)

Referral to a class of practitioners (e.g., ophthalmologists, family practitioners, and neurologists) or a choice of practitioners within a specialty (more than one doctor recommended) are less preferable than a specific doctor.

In making the referral, it is advisable for the optometrist (or the optometrist's assistant) to telephone the specialist's office and actually make the appointment for the patient, determining a date and time for the examination. This information should then be entered into the patient's record, along with other pertinent data about the referral. To ensure that the

PROGRESS NOTES

DATE: 25 March 1987

NAME Joe Parker | HOME PHONE 987-6543

ADDRESS 100 Residence Street | BIRTHDATE August 10, 1957

REFERRAL SOURCE

OCCUPATION Computer programmer | WORK PHONE 111-2222

S Complains of discomfort immediately following insertion of contact lens for OD. Wearing time 16 hrs a day. Current lenses 1½ years old. LEE 1½ yrs ago. Ocular and general health unchanged since last exam. Taking no meds.

O VA: OD 20/20 @ 6 M w/W W: OD -3.00 CSI lenses
OS 20/20 OS -3.25

SLE: OD lens is torn at edge; superficial staining of corneal epithelium
OS good centration and movement; no lens deposits

A 1. Torn lens edge OD; superficial abrasion of epithelium
2. No ocular health assessment in 1½ yrs

P 1. Replace lens for OD; re-check cornea
2. Schedule for eye health assessment

J O'Dee
John O'Dee, O.D.

GC20A

Figure 16.6. Sample Progress Notes—Episodic Care. (Courtesy UAB School of Optometry)

referral information is placed in the record, in some offices it may be useful to establish a fail-safe system of review that will double-check records at the end of the day to ensure the entries have been made.

Recalls

If an examination yields insufficient patient data, certain tests need to be repeated, or other follow-up must be instituted, then the optometrist will need to schedule the patient for a recall appointment. Recalls should be scheduled for a specific date and time before the patient leaves the office, even if the date of the recall is weeks or months in the future. The practitioner should note on the patient record the reason for recall and the tests to be performed and should be certain that the recall examination addresses the clinical problem for which the patient is being followed. If a patient fails to return as scheduled, in some cases it may be wise to communicate with the patient in order to determine the cause of the missed appointment (Fig. 16.7).

Record Entries

Another important clinicolegal issue concerns the completeness of record entries. Since the patient records of optometrists are generally admissible in legal disputes (to be discussed), the absence of appropriate entries in the record—or the inclusion of inaccurate information—can have a significant effect upon the outcome of litigation. Any inaccurate information or data that needs to be changed should be corrected in a proper and timely fashion. Erasures or marks that totally obliterate pertinent information should never be used. Instead, the person making the change should draw a line through the original entry, leaving the writing legible, and should then authenticate the correction by signing or initialing the corrected entry. It may also be appropriate to include the date and reason for the change (Fig. 16.8).

Care should be taken to avoid the appearance of unauthorized alteration of records in cases where the records will be used in litigation, since grave consequences may result (discussed later in this chapter). The completeness and accuracy of the patient record

Dear Mr./Ms. ____________________,

Your failure to appear at your scheduled appointment on ________ is a matter of concern for me and my staff. In my opinion, your condition is one that requires continued care, and it is for that purpose that we scheduled your follow-up appointment.

We feel that it is important that you receive further care, and we suggest that you call this office to reschedule the appointment, or, if you prefer, that you call another doctor to obtain the proper follow-up.

Please understand that the purpose of this letter is to stress upon you the importance of receiving further treatment, and is written out of concern for your visual welfare.

Sincerely,

____________________ O.D.

Figure 16.7. Letter to a Patient Who Has Missed a Recall Appointment.

BIOMICROSCOPY Angle OD 1:1 (T) 1:1 (N) OS 1:1 (T) 1:1 (N) Method: SLE

OD ~~cornea~~ 31Oct87, media, lens, iris unremarkable. Anterior adnexa unremarkable. Punctate corneal staining with fluorescein noted after tonometry.

OS as noted for OD.

T OD 17 mm Hg ANESTH. Fluress %

OS 16 ~~18~~ mm Hg 31 Oct 87 Erroneous entry. APPREHENSION (L) M H

(TAP) (NCT) MM TIME: 9 (a.m.) p.m.

Figure 16.8. Sample Corrections—Patient Record. (Courtesy UAB School of Optometry)

is of vital importance in any litigation but is of special significance in malpractice litigation. A well-kept record offers convincing evidence that the patient received reasonable care, whereas a poorly kept or inaccurate record can have the opposite effect altogether.

Although it is appropriate for practitioners to use abbreviations and other forms of notation to shorten the time spent recording, it is advisable for optometrists (or others making entries in the record) to employ clinical terms that are generally recognized and to avoid personal terms that require subjective interpretation.[5] It is also advisable to utilize descriptive terminology (e.g., the C/D is .5) rather than general terms that do not convey much information (e.g., fundus normal).

If persons other than the optometrist customarily make entries in the patient record, the optometrist should be certain to manually authenticate these entries by signing or initialing the record or by using another form of signature, such as a printed or stamped name or initials (seen most frequently in hospital records, such as the VA). Authentication may be important should litigation ensue.[6]

Ownership and Control

The ownership of patient records in a solo practice vests with the individual practitioner who maintains them.[7] Consequently, an associate who is employed by an optometrist has no claim to ownership of the records of patients seen by him or her in the private practice, such records being the property of the employer.[8] Of course, the two doctors could agree that the associate would retain the records of those patients examined by him, if they so desire. The ownership of patient records in a partnership will depend upon the provisions of the partnership agreement. Ordinarily, the agreement will specify some form of co-ownership between the partners. If the agreement is silent, the state's Uniform Partnership Act or case law will control.[9]

A corporation will customarily own the records of the patients seen by the employee-doctors, but if the state board of optometry has promulgated a regulation that the patient records of a commercial practice are the property of the examining optometrist and not of the corporate employer, such a regulation is valid and the employee-optometrist may take possession of the records should the employee-optometrist leave the business.[10] Where an optometrist is the employee of a hospital, all records are the property of the hospital and the doctor has no right to claim them.[11]

The owner of patient records has the right of physical possession and control.[12] As a general rule, such owners should not permit removal of the record from their control, except by court order. Therefore, neither the patient nor the patient's authorized representative has a right to possession of the record, but the doctor's right of physical control does not mean that the patient and variously interested third parties have no legal right of access to the record and the information it contains. Indeed, over the past several years the clear trend—both legislatively and judicially—has been to recognize that patients have the right to view and copy their records or to appoint authorized representatives to examine them.[13] Of course, since the publication of the Federal Trade Commission's Eyeglasses I rule in 1978,[14] all optometric patients have had the unquestioned right to a most important part of their record, the prescription, a requirement that was left unchanged by Eyeglasses II.[15] For this reason, entries in the patient record should be made with care and according to recognized professional standards. Furthermore, extraneous comments that reflect poorly upon the patient or are unrelated to the care being given should be avoided, and the doctor or assistant wishing to make personal entries should reserve these for personal notes that, although maintained with the patient record, do not reflect the care rendered and thus do not have to be shared with the patient or future eye-care providers.

Optometrists who have sold their practices or retired from practice, or whose patients have turned to successor doctors, are morally and ethically obligated to transfer the patient record or copies of it to the current optometrist when the patient so requests.[16] So also are the estates of deceased optometrists. But instead of delivering the entire original record to the new doctor, the former optometrist may wish to transfer a copy of the record or to send excerpts or summaries that will be adequate for the patient's care under the new doctor. In general, whenever patient information is to be divulged, it should only be as much information as is necessary to comply with the request. The full patient record must be released only on rare occasions (such as when there is a statutory obligation to do so or the doctor has received an order to do so due to litigation).[17] In most instances, a letter containing a summary will be sufficient, and the doctor should resist the temptation to copy the entire record verbatim and should transmit only the information actually requested, retaining a copy of the summary for inclusion in the original record.

When an optometrist requests patient information from a doctor or institution, the optometrist should be certain to have a signed, current release from the patient directing the doctor or institution to send the record—or a summary—to the optometrist.

Compliance with requests for patient information is a complex subject that involves a *potpourri* of statutory and case law, both federal and state.

The Patient's Right to Information

In increasing numbers the various jurisdictions, both federal and state, have recognized that patients have a legal right to the information in their doctors' records, even in the absence of pending litigation such as a malpractice case.[18] This right has been established in some jurisdictions by statute;[19] in others it has been authorized by judicial decision.[20] The leading federal and state laws are summarized below.

FTC Eyeglasses I Rule

Doubtless the leading example of this trend, as far as the profession of optometry is concerned, is the FTC's Eyeglasses I rule, which the FTC Commissioners declined to change during the Eyeglasses II proceedings.[21] Under the Eyeglasses I rule the patient has been granted a federally recognized right to obtain information related to the patient's prescription for spectacles or contact lenses.[22] The provisions of the Eyeglasses rules are discussed in Chapter 17.

Federal Freedom-of-Information Act

This statute[23] requires federal facilities to release copies of their medical records when requested by patients. Optometrists who are employed by Veteran's Administration hospitals, public hospitals, and possibly health maintenance organizations that have obtained their initial financing from the federal government, may find that their facilities' patient records are subject to this act.

State Freedom-of-Information Acts

A total of twenty-nine states[24] have enacted statutes that require the release of copies of patient records upon demand by the patient. Some of these laws expressly include optometrists, and the likelihood is good in many states that the definition of medical records will be broad enough to encompass optometric records. Thus, in these twenty-nine states an optometrist's duty to release a copy of his records to a patient may be substantially expanded to include any occasion that a patient makes a proper request. In five of these states,[25] the law requires the release of the patient's contact lens prescription (see Chapter 17), but in about half the states the duty to release records is applied only to hospitals (described below).

State Optometry Practice Acts

In ten states[26] the optometry practice acts provide for disciplinary actions to be instituted against practitioners—based upon allegations of unprofessional conduct—if they refuse to comply with requests for information or copies of records. In these states optometrists should respond appropriately to proper requests to avoid conflicts with state boards.

State Optometry Board Rules

In ten other states,[27] optometry board rules or regulations have been enacted that require optometrists to release patient information when presented with a valid request. Again, failure to comply subjects the optometrist to the possibility of disciplinary action.

State Statutes Requiring Hospital Records Release

Fourteen states' Freedom-of-Information Acts require hospitals[28] to permit patients to enjoy access to their medical records, and so optometrists working in or affiliated with hospitals may find their records subjected to these release requirements.

A summary of these various laws is provided as Tables 16.1, 16.2, and 16.3.

The effect of these statutes is to require optometrists in many jurisdictions to release copies of records or other patient information. Therefore, practitioners should be certain that refusals to provide requested information are not arbitrary and can be justified.

In addition to these statutory provisions, the courts have been active in defining the rights of patients to medical information. Although decisions have recognized that health-care practitioners have a right to withhold information from patients, the circumstances under which this right may be exercised are generally limited to life-threatening conditions and psychological dysfunctions.[29] In these cases the courts have weighed the patient's right to obtain the information and the doctor's right to keep what is be-

Table 16.1. State Freedom-of-Information Acts: 1987

State	Statute
Alaska	Alaska Stat. §18.23.065
California	Cal. Health and Safety Code, §25250
Colorado	Colo. Rev. Stat. §25-1-802
Connecticut	Conn. Gen. Stat. Ann. §4-104 (hospital records only)
Florida	Fla. Stat. Ann. §455.241
Georgia	Ga. Code Ann. §31-33-1
Hawaii	Hawaii Rev. Stat. §622-57 (not applicable to optometrists)
Illinois	Ill. Ann. Stat. §8-2003 (physicians only)
Indiana	Ind. Code Ann. §34-3-15.5-4 (hospital records only)
Louisiana	La. Rev. Stat. Ann. §40:2014.1 (hospital records only)
Maine	Me. Rev. Stat. Ann. titl. 22, §1711 (hospital records only)
Maryland	Md. Health Occ. Code Ann. §4-302 (hospital records only)
Massachusetts	Mass. Gen. Laws Ann. ch. 111, §70 (hospital records only)
Michigan	Attorney General's Opinion No. 5125 of May 30, 1978
Minnesota	Minn. Stat. §144.335
Nebraska	Neb. Rev. Stat. §84-712 (hospital records only)
Nevada	Nev. Rev. Stat. §629.061 (patient may inspect record)
New Jersey	N.J. Rev. Stat. Ann. §2A-82-41 (hospital records only)
New York	N.Y. Pub. Health Law §17 (McKinney)
Ohio	Ohio Rev. Code Ann. §3701.74 (hospital records only)
Oklahoma	Okla. Stat. tit. 76, §19 (not applicable to optometrists)
Oregon	Or. Rev. Stat. §192.525 (public hospital records only)
Pennsylvania	Pa. Stat. Ann. tit. 63, §390-2 (Purdon 1983) (hospital records only)
South Dakota	S.D. Comp. Laws Ann. §34-12-15 (hospital records only)
Tennessee	Tenn. Code Ann. §68-11-304 (hospital records only)
Texas	Tex. Rev. Civ. Stat. Ann. art. 5547-44 (hospital records only)
Virginia	Va. Code §8.01-413 (not applicable to optometrists)
West Virginia	W. Va. Code §16-29-1
Wisconsin	Wis. Stat. Ann. §146.83

Source: American Optometric Association, 1987.

lieved to be harmful relevations from the patient. The situation under which an optometrist could invoke such a defense would be extraordinary, to say the least. Thus, if litigation should be instituted by a patient seeking records or information, the defendant optometrist may be unable to justify a refusal to the court.

In any jurisdiction where the patient requesting information can show a legitimate need and purpose—where it can be shown that the information will facilitate further health care or is needed for the proper evaluation of a contemplated legal action—an optometrist should consider carefully before issuing a refusal.[30] Arbitrary refusals can only cause conflict with patients and their bona fide representatives, especially their attorneys.[31] In most cases it would be advisable to adopt a policy that the patient record will be made available to a patient's attorney upon written authorization from the patient.[32] This consent should be checked to be certain that it is current and genuine (see Fig. 16.9).

Optometrists should be familiar with the statutory and judicial authority that establishes the legal requirements for the release of patient information within their state or jurisdiction. In many states optometrists will need to consult legal counsel in order to determine specific statutory or judicial requirements. State board attorneys or counsel for state associations are probably the most knowledgeable sources to consult when attempting to secure this information.

Privileged Communications

The concept of confidentiality or privileged communication implies that private information entrusted to a doctor will not be divulged to a third party without the consent of the patient.[33] The Code of Ethics of the American Optometric Association demands that optometrists regard all patient information as confidential, and in some states the legislatures have enacted privileged communication statutes, which doubtless has led some practitioners to believe that the release of information to a third party will generally constitute a civil wrong giving the patient a cause of action for damages unless the release is specifically ordered by a court or authorized by the patient.[34] However, the ethical and legal issues surrounding a privileged communication cannot be so easily summarized.

First of all, there are some circumstances under which a doctor has a positive legal duty to disclose patient information, whether or not the patient has consented (an example is revealing the presence of a communicable disease to a spouse).

Secondly, a valid court order directing that the records of a doctor be made available to a third party or turned over to the court must be honored (such as

Table 16.2. Optometry Statutes or Board Regulations Requiring Release of Patient Records: 1987

State	Applicable Statute or Board Regulation	Comments
Arizona	Optometry Board Rule R4-21-212D and E	Requires release upon patient request
Arkansas	Ark. Stat. Ann. §72-822	Includes spectacle prescriptions; contact lens prescriptions excluded
Florida	Fla. Stat. Ann. §463.012(2)(b) Florida Board Rule 455.241	Copy of examination findings must be furnished upon request.
Idaho	Optometry Board Rule XV	
Indiana	Ind. Code Ann. §§16-4-8-1 and 16-4-8-2	Requires release upon written request. Contact lenses may be described in general terms.
Maryland	Md. Health Occ. Code Ann. §10-312	Failure to provide records to another doctor at patient's request may result in disciplinary action.
New Jersey	Optometry Board Rule 13, §38-6.1(c)	Records must be released upon patient request; includes prescriptions.
New Mexico	N.M. Stat. Ann. §61-2-14(E)	
New York	Optometry Board Rule 29.2	Requires release upon patient request
North Carolina	N.C. Gen. Stat. §90-127.3	Requires release upon patient request
North Dakota	Optometry Board Rule 10	
Ohio	Ohio Rev. Code Ann. §4725.17	Prescriptions must contain sufficient information to allow the patient to obtain the prescribed item from the provider of his choice.
South Dakota	Optometry Board Rule 20:50:04:06	Requires release upon patient request
Tennessee	Tenn. Code Ann. §63-822 and 63-8-120 (10)	Refusal to provide a spectacle prescription may result in charge of unprofessional conduct.
Texas	Tex. Rev. Civ. Stat. Ann. art. 4552-5.15(e)	
Utah	Optometry Board Rule §§1606 and 1607	
Vermont	Vt. Stat. Ann. tit. 26, §§1719(7) and 1719(12)(A)	Failure to make records available upon patient request constitutes grounds for charge of unprofessional conduct.
Virginia	Optometry Board Rule §3.1.F	Failure to release prescriptions for spectacles or contact lenses may be basis for charge of unprofessional conduct.
Washington	Optometry Board Rule WAC 308-53-250	Upon request, records must be provided to optometrist or physician in state.

Source: American Optometric Association, 1987.

Table 16.3. States Requiring Hospital Record Release: 1986

State	Act
Connecticut	Conn. Gen. Stat. Ann. §4-105
Florida	Fla. Stat. Ann. §458.16
Hawaii	Haw. Rev. Stat. §622.57
Illinois	Ill. Ann. Stat. ch. 51, §71
Indiana	Ind. Stat. Ann. §34-3-15.54
Louisiana	La. Rev. Stat. Ann. §40.2014.1 (applies to state hospitals only)
Massachusetts	Mass. Gen. Laws Ann. ch. 111, §70 (but hospital may destroy records after 30 years)
Minnesota	Minn. Stat. Ann. §144.335
Nevada	Nev. Rev. Stat. §629.061
Tennessee	Tenn. Code Ann. §53-1322 (access on good cause)
Virginia	Va. Code §8.01-413

Source: American Optometric Association, 1987.

when a patient is involved in an automobile accident and the patient's vision is a legal issue). We will discuss the use of optometric records in litigation presently.

But if it is a case in which information from a patient's record is disclosed by the doctor without the patient's express consent and in the absence of an affirmative statutory or common law duty to do so, the patient may seek to institute legal proceedings against the doctor, claiming damages for this violation of confidentiality. If this does occur, what is an optometrist's liability?

As previously mentioned, there are ethical obligations that require an optometrist or other health-care provider to respect the confidentiality of information obtained in the course of care and treatment, but at common law there was no doctrine of confidential or privileged communication between doctor and patient.[35] The common law recognized the doctrine of privileged communication only in three relationships: attorney-client, husband-wife, and priest-parishioner. Accordingly, a physician had no obligation under common law to hold medical information about a patient secret or confidential. To correct this situation, and to better establish a confidential relationship between physician and patient, the legislatures of approximately three fourths of the states have enacted laws known as the privileged communication statutes.[36] Only one state (Washington), however, has statutorily applied the privilege to optometrists, and in other states the courts have been divided as to whether or not optometrists should be included within the statutory privilege as physicians.[37]

In states where these laws have been enacted, medical practitioners are not allowed in legal proceedings to disclose information necessary to the care and treatment of the patient that was acquired while attending the patient in an official capacity. The privilege may be waived by the patient, however, thereby allowing the practitioner to provide the information to a third party or to testify concerning the communication in a court of competent jurisdiction. These statutes apply only to disclosures made in the course of judicial or quasijudicial proceedings and do not regulate private, out-of-court disclosures of patient information. Therefore, an aggrieved patient cannot institute a cause of action for the out-of-court release of confidential information based upon a violation of these statutes; rather, the patient must rely upon three other theories of civil action: defamation of character, invasion of privacy, or breach of an implied contract to respect confidentiality. Under the appropriate circumstances, claims alleging these causes of action may successfully be brought against optometric practitioners.[38]

Records as Evidence in Litigation

Because the common law did not recognize the doctor-patient relationship as privileged, patient information entrusted to or acquired by a doctor was not confidential and could be divulged in a court of law. Thus, in states without privileged communication statutes, medical records are generally admissible as evidence as litigation, including the patient records compiled by optometrists. These records can be examined by the attorneys or the court or even introduced into evidence so that they can be scrutinized by the jury, and the optometrist can be compelled to answer questions under oath concerning entries or omissions.

Even in states where privileged communications statutes have been enacted, there may be no privilege for optometrists because optometrists may not be recognized by the courts as physicians for purposes of the statute. As a result, the patient records of optometrists have been open to legal scrutiny in virtually all jurisdictions, a fact that adds extra importance to the recordkeeping burden of optometric practitioners. Whenever optometric patients are parties to litigation—in any state—the likelihood

I hereby authorize ______________________________ O.D. to furnish

______________________ ______________________

(Recipient) (Address)

information from my optometric record concerning ______________________

____

for the purpose of ______________________________.

______________ ______________ ______________

Patient Birthdate Address

I understand that I may revoke this consent at any time. I further understand that this consent will automatically expire upon the satisfaction of the authorization described above, or six months after the date of this release, whichever occurs first.

No other information may be forwarded to other persons or agencies without my express consent.

______________________ ______________________

Date Signature

______________________ ______________________

Witness Signature of parent or guardian

Figure 16.9. Sample Release of Patient Information.

is great that the optometrist's records, if needed for the purposes of litigation, will be obtainable.

Attorneys will seek by means of pretrial discovery to obtain information from the records of patients who are parties to litigation or from documents that they believe will aid the preparation and trial of the lawsuit. Depositions and orders to produce will be the usual means of obtaining this information. If the attorney seeks to have such information entered into evidence at court, the attorney will serve the optometrist with a *subpoena duces tecum*, which orders the optometrist to appear with the record in a court or other duly constituted tribunal having jurisdiction over the pending litigation. In most instances the optometrist will not be a party to the lawsuit, merely the person in possession of records which may or may not be relevant to the case. Therefore, the fight over what is pertinent or admissible will be between the opposing attorneys, and the optometrist will rely on the rulings of the court as to whether or not to provide the information. If the optometrist is a party to the case then the dispute is of more immediate interest, and the optometrist should obey the instructions of his attorney in handling and discussing patient records. It should be mentioned that there is also no privilege of confidentiality under federal law, and so the Internal Revenue Service can obtain access to optometric records for tax purposes.[39]

Of course, the most worrisome type of litigation is a malpractice case in which the optometrist is the defendant. More likely than not, in such a lawsuit the patient record will either be the cornerstone of the optometrist's defense or his Achilles' heel. A leading legal authority describes the importance of recordkeeping in the following words[40]:

> The physician's medical records on the patient's case may be of critical importance in proving that no negligence occurred or in refuting the patient's factual allegations of improper diagnosis or treatment. While proper completion of all records on each patient is obviously time-consuming and probably an active nuisance, a physician who is sued by a patient some considerable time after treatment terminated will be in a much more favorable position when his records indicate clearly to the court that proper treatment had been given. On the other hand, records which disclose negligent treatment will materially benefit the patient's case. Records which have been altered for any reason, even the most innocent, should always include notations of the date and reason for the change. If a negligence suit is filed subsequent to alteration of a record, and that alteration is apparent, it will undoubtedly be construed as a dishonest attempt to avoid liability.

It is to this issue of alteration of the record that we now turn.

Liability for Alteration of Records

A doctor's records are usually of critical importance in refuting allegations that there was negligence in the diagnosis or treatment of a patient's condition. Properly kept records are often sufficient to enable a doctor to verify that due care was exercised in a given case. But records must be carefully maintained. If changes are to be made, both the date and the reason for the change should be carefully noted on the record contemporaneously with the change. Failure to do so increases the opportunity for misunderstanding should litigation arise later.

An optometrist examined a patient who presented with the complaint of "tired eyes," and he detected opacities of the lens in each eye. The patient alleged that she was told the spots were cataracts, and that she would be referred to a medical practitioner in two or three years. The doctor alleged that she was told to see an ophthalmologist immediately. There was a notation to this effect in his records, but it was made in a color of ink that was different from the other entries. The optometrist was sued for failure to refer the patient, who was subsequently seen by a physician, diagnosed as having uveitis, and hospitalized. At trial, liability hinged upon the doctor's records. He testified that it was his custom to make notes on his records after the patient visit was concluded and that he had a number of pens at his desk that he used for this purpose. The jury, however, believed the patient's assertion that she had not been referred and awarded her $80,000.[41]

Alteration of records that are under subpoena in a case can be punishable as a criminal offense. Under no circumstances should records be altered after a notice of subpoena is received.[42] Furthermore, records that are to be used in litigation should be carefully preserved and no effort to "improve" them should be made by either the doctor or his assistants.[43] When the summons and complaint of a lawsuit are received, the first thing that the doctor will want to do is look at the records to refresh his memory. Recollections of the examination that are not recorded are best left that way; to do otherwise unalterably weakens the doctor's defense.

A young boy who failed a school vision screening was examined (with some difficulty) by an optometrist. The boy was returned to school, again failed the vision test, and was subsequently examined by another practitioner, who diagnosed the boy as suffering from neurofibromatosis. The disease had progressed to such an extent that it was inoperable and would cause the boy to lose his sight altogether. The boy sued the optometrist for malpractice, alleging that the optometrist's failure to refer him at the time of examination (which was ten months before the diagnosis was made) had prevented him from receiving treatment which would have arrested the progress of the disease. The optometrist answered that he had referred the patient to a physician. Unfortunately, his records did not document this averral. After the suit was filed the optometrist made an entry in the boy's record to this effect in order to preserve his memory of the examination. Although the optometrist made no attempt to hide the fact that he had made the entry after the lawsuit had been filed, his defense was (obviously) considerably weakened. The case was settled for $500,000, with an additional sum being paid as an annuity to the boy for 20 years.[44]

The presentation of evidence to establish or refute that a doctor has been negligent not infrequently becomes a contest between experts for the plaintiff and defendant. It is not uncommon for these experts—all of whom profess to have a familiarity with the standard of care—to differ completely in their conclusions as to liability. For this reason, expert testimony is truly a sword that cuts both ways.

Expertise does not have to be limited to the issue of negligence; experts may be summoned to court to analyze the meaning of entries in a patient record or even to offer an opinion concerning the veracity of these same entries. Handwriting experts have been known to differ and do so with the same regularity found among liability experts (i.e., frequently). The result is a contest in which the jury must decide who is the more believable. Any alteration of the records once a malpractice claim has been filed opens the door for this kind of contest. The prudent practitioner will avoid making such changes no matter how certain he is of the truthfulness of the material that has been added.

A 39-year-old upholsterer complaining of a "dark cloud" over his vision and halos at night was examined by an ophthalmologist, who detected a retinal hemorrhage in the left eye. He performed no tonometry and used digital palpation to test the intraocular pressure. He referred the patient to a family physician, but all tests were negative and the patient was returned to the ophthalmologist, who performed two additional examinations three weeks and five weeks after the first visit, diagnosing the patient's condition as branch retinal vein occlusion.

About two months after the initial examination, and while the ophthalmologist was at a seminar, the patient experienced a sudden onset of intense intraocular pain and decreased acuity. He was seen by another physician, who found bilateral chronic open-angle glaucoma compounded by an acute attack of glaucoma in the left eye. The patient was treated but ultimately became blind in his left eye and had but 5 degrees of visual field in his right eye. The patient sued, alleging that tonometry had not been performed in an adequate and timely fashion.

At the trial the ophthalmologist's records of the second patient examination become a key issue. An expert for the patient testified that there was a typewritten entry of "T A 18 OU," but that it was at a slightly different position on the typewriter line than the other entries on the chart, which indicated the possibility of alteration of the record. In addition, the patient testified that tonometry had not been performed at all. The doctor's explanation was that he dictated his findings and the secretary transmitted them onto the record. Occasionally the secretary would be interrupted, remove the record card from the typewriter, and resume the transcription later after the other task had been completed. Despite this testimony the jury awarded the patient $600,000 as damages.[45]

A deliberate alteration of records can be construed by the trial court as an attempt to avoid liability.

A woman being treated for the thirteenth time by an eye, ear, nose, and throat (EENT) specialist for a blocked tear duct was injured when the instrument the physician was using struck her cornea. After the injury, her daughter—who was a nurse—asked to see her mother's records. Despite the best efforts of the EENT specialist, the woman suffered a permanent vision loss, and eventually she sued the physician for injuring her cornea. At the trial the daughter was asked to examine the records, and she testified that they had been materially altered since the time of her mother's injury. She was also able to establish that one of her mother's visits to the doctor right after the injury was not documented at all. The court held that the altered records created a presumption of negligence on the part of the physician.[46]

Because patient records are entered into evidence with great frequency, extraneous comments should be assiduously avoided. In particular, comments that denigrate the patient or members of the patient's family should be omitted since they convey the impression that the doctor is not interested in the patient's welfare.

Retention of Records

From the foregoing discussion, it should be evident that the optometrist who has well-kept files and thorough records that are up-to-date is in a much better position to testify at a deposition or in a trial than is the optometrist who has poorly organized files and sketchy patient records that omit vital information. But there is another aspect to recordkeeping that is most important, the retention of records. How long should they be kept?

Although optometrists collect the kind of information that is not as likely to be used in litigation as that which is collected by physicians, there is always a chance that an optometrist could be an important witness or party to litigation filed long after the patient has been dismissed. Ideally, no patient records should be thrown away, and there are ways to preserve records (such as through the use of microfilm) without incurring great expense or requiring copious amounts of space. But, if records are to be eventually discarded, there are some potential problems that the practitioner needs to consider.

Actions may be brought against an optometrist on the basis of contract (a dispute over the fee, for example) or on the basis of a tort, which is an action for personal injury (such as a malpractice suit). The optometrist should plan to retain his records at least as long as the statute of limitations for these actions. As might be expected, state statutes vary in the length of time under which a claim can be brought for either of these offenses. Because of the ongoing effort known as tort reform, it is likely that the statutes of limitation noted herein have undergone change.[47] Legal counsel should always be consulted whenever specific legal advice is needed.

The statute of limitations for contract actions varies from state to state, with the period within which a suit may be brought varying from three to fifteen years. A summary of the various state limits may be found in Chapter 19. The statute of limitations for malpractice actions is also variable; depending on the state, it is from one to eight years. A list of the various state statutes of limitation may be found in Chapter 19.

If the patient is a minor, however, the laws are different because a minor is allowed to bring suit after he has reached adulthood. State laws differ as to the period of time within which the suit must be

Table 16.4. States Requiring Retention of Medical Records: 1979

State	Requirement
Florida	Records must be retained for 1 year after doctor's death
Illinois	No statute specifically for medical records, but the Uniform Business Records Retention Act requires that records be retained for 3 years
Massachusetts	Medical Board rule requires that physicians retain records for 3 years
Nevada	Medical records must be retained for 5 years
New Jersey	State Board of Medical Examiners requires medical records to be retained for 7 years
New York	Medical records must be retained for 6 years under a ruling by the State Board of Regents

Source: Chapman, S., How Long Should You Keep Your Patients' Records?, *Legal Aspects of Medical Practice*, vol. 7, no. 8, 1979, pp. 19–38.

brought after adulthood is attained. (In fact, the age of adulthood itself varies from state to state.) Statutes of limitation for minors may also be found in Chapter 19.

As the rather confusing array of statutes demonstrates, the prudent doctor should consult with legal counsel before discarding any patient records. Most states do not require health-care providers to retain patient records for any minimum period of time (see Table 16.4). Therefore, it will be the state statutes of limitation that will dictate the length of time records should be preserved. Optometrists who are contemplating retirement should consider these matters before discarding their records.

One aspect of the patient record that has not been discussed is the obligation to give a copy of the prescription to the patient or to release prescription information to third parties. This complex issue will be discussed in the following chapter.

Notes

1. Louisell, D.W., and H. Williams, *Medical Malpractice*, Matthew Bender Co., New York, 1978, p. 185.
2. In a few states legal requirements establish the minimum examination that must be conducted by an optometrist. Since in these states a practitioner must be able to substantiate the procedures used for a given patient, it can be argued that recordkeeping is mandated by legal requirements in a few states. For an example, see the Utah Optometry Board Rules, §§1606 and 1607.
3. See Weed, L., *Medical Records, Medical Education,*

and Patient Care, Press of Case Western Reserve, Cleveland, 1970; and Weed, L., *Implementing the Problem-Oriented Medical Record*, Medical Computer Services, Seattle, 1976.

4. The use of the problem-oriented system in optometry is well illustrated by the handbook, *Scope of Practice: Patient Care and Management Manual*, American Optometric Association, St. Louis, 1986. The example records used in the Appendix are taken from this useful manual.
5. For a review of common abbreviations, see Berman, M., and T. Stelmack, Ophthalmic Clinical Abbreviations, *Journal of the American Optometric Association*, vol. 55, no. 8, 1984, pp. 601–604.
6. In the usual case the optometrist will make the entries in the patient record, but in many practices assistants will also enter data into the record, and in this event it is best for the optometrist to initial or sign the record so that the data can be authenticated. Otherwise, in a legal proceeding the optometrist may be precluded from testifying as to the accuracy of the information since it could be argued that to do so would constitute hearsay. For a discussion, see Classe, J., Recordkeeping and Documentation in Clinical Practice, *Southern Journal of Optometry*, vol. 5, no. 2, 1987, pp. 11–25.
7. See *McGarry v. J.A. Mercier Co.*, 272 Mich. 501, 262 N.W. 296 (1935).
8. Many disputes between associates and their employers have involved ownership of records or patient lists. For this reason it is recommended that the employment agreement specify who will own the records and the rights, if any, that the associate is to have in the records once the employment is terminated. A similar agreement should be entered into as to patient lists, addresses, and related information. In most, if not all, jurisdictions the unauthorized use of records and lists will give the injured party legal justification for an action for damages.
9. The ownership of patient records in a partnership can be a difficult issue to resolve if a partnership is dissolved on less-than-amicable terms. The Uniform Partnership Act holds that partnership property such as patient records belongs jointly to the partners, which may not adequately resolve the issue of ownership in many instances. Therefore, it is preferable for practitioners to specify in the partnership agreement how the patient records will be divided in the event of dissolution.
10. See *Albelson's, Inc. v. New Jersey State Board of Optometrists*, 5 N.J. 412, 75 A.2d 867 (1950).
11. See *Flaum v. Medical Arts Center Hospital*, reported in *New York Law Journal*, vol. 160, no. 36, 1968, p. 2.
12. Avery, M., *Medical Records in Ambulatory Care*, Aspen Systems Corp., Rockville, Md., 1984.
13. Statutory law has been enacted in numerous states to allow access to medical records by patients or their representatives. E.g., see *Wis. Stat. Ann.* §804.10 (West Supp. 1976), which requires all hospitals or physicians having possession of medical records to make them available for inspection and copying by the patient or the patient's representative. The federal government has enacted a freedom of information act, 5 U.S.C. §552(a), which requires copies of medical records compiled by federal health facilities to be released to requesting patients. Optometrists are often defined as medical providers for purposes of these types of statutes.
14. The Eyeglasses I trade regulation rule can be found in 16 C.F.R. §456 (1978).
15. The FTC published a staff report in 1980, *State Restrictions on Vision Care Providers: The Effect on Consumers*, and in December published an Advance Notice of Proposed Rulemaking in the Federal Register (45 F.R. 79,823). The FTC's intention to proceed with the rulemaking process was made public on January 4, 1985, when the agency's Notice of Proposed Rulemaking was published (50 F.R. 598).
16. See *Matter of Weiss*, 208 Misc. 1010, 147 N.Y.S.2d 455 (1955).
17. Avery, supra note 12 at pp. 157–181.
18. A summary of the evolving nature of laws increasing patient access to medical records can be found in Tucker, G., Patient Access to Medical Records, *Legal Aspects of Medical Practice*, vol. 6, no. 10, 1978, p. 15.
19. As to the evolving right of patients to obtain optometric information, an example statute can be found in *Cal. Health and Safety Code* §§25251 and 25252, which allow patients to obtain copies of their optometric records on written request with the payment of a nominal fee.
20. The case *American Optometric Association v. Federal Trade Commission*, 626 F.2d 896 (D.C. Cir. 1980) established that patients in all jurisdictions have the right to obtain certain prescription information.
21. 16 C.F.R. §456 (1978).
22. Ibid. The Eyeglasses I rule defined a prescription as sphere power, cylinder power and axis (if any), prism (if any), and the signature of the "refractionist."
23. 5 U.S.C. §552(a).
24. Alaska, California, Colorado, Connecticut, Florida, Georgia, Hawaii, Illinois, Indiana, Louisiana, Maine, Maryland, Massachusetts, Michigan, Minnesota, Nebraska, Nevada, New Jersey, New York, Ohio, Oklahoma, Oregon, Pennsylvania, South Dakota, Tennessee, Texas, Virginia, West Virginia, and Wisconsin. See *Bulletin from the Licensure and Regulation Committee of the American Optometric Association*, vol. 45, no. 97, June 16, 1987, and its supplement, vol. 46, no. 8, Aug. 6, 1987.
25. Alaska, Florida, Minnesota, West Virginia, and Wisconsin. See *Bulletin from the Licensure and Regulation Committee of the American Optometric Association*, note 24 supra.
26. Arkansas, Florida, Indiana, Maryland, New Mexico, North Carolina, Ohio, Tennessee, Texas, and Vermont. See *Bulletin from the Licensure and Regulation Committee of the American Optometric Association*, note 24 supra.
27. Arizona, Florida, Idaho, New Jersey, New York,

North Dakota, South Dakota, Utah, Virginia, and Washington. See *Bulletin from the Licensure and Regulation Committee of the American Optometric Association*, note 24 supra.

28. Connecticut, Indiana, Louisiana, Maine, Maryland, Massachusetts, Nebraska, New Jersey, Ohio, Oregon, Pennsylvania, South Dakota, Tennessee, and Texas. See *Bulletin from the Licensure and Regulation Committee of the American Optometric Association*, note 24 supra.
29. Tucker, supra note 18.
30. The patient's right to medical information is usually defined in language that specifically includes optometrists or is broad enough to include optometrists, and so the entire patient record may have to be copied, summarized, or made available for inspection. Since prescription information—for either spectacles or contact lenses—is an integral part of the optometrist's records, in many jurisdictions the patient's right to the entire record will make it mandatory that prescription information be released. However, a copy of a record or a summary of prescription information does not satisfy the requirements of a "prescription," which must meet certain legal requirements and be signed by a licensed practitioner. For a review of these laws, see Classe, J., Optometrist's Duty to Release Patient Information, *Southern Journal of Optometry*, vol. 5, no. 1, 1987, pp. 9–15.
31. For a discussion, see Matz, S.S., Why and When You Should Cooperate with a Lawyer, *Legal Aspects of Medical Practice*, vol. 8, no. 7, 1980, p. 23.
32. See Gerber, P.C., When Lawyer Calls, Don't Hang Up!, *Optometric Management*, vol. 18, no. 5, 1982, p. 71.
33. For a review of the general requirements of confidentiality as they pertain to physicians, see Bergen, R.P., Law and Medicine: Keeping the Patient's Secrets, *Journal of the American Medical Association*, vol. 195, no. 5, Jan. 31, 1966, p. 227; Morse, H.N., Law and Medicare: Physician's Liability for Improper Disclosure, *Journal of the American Medical Association*, vol. 198, no. 7, Nov. 14, 1966, p. 331; and Holder, A.R., Law and Medicine: Disclosure of Confidential Information, *Journal of the American Medical Association*, vol. 216, no. 2, Apr. 12, 1971, p. 385.
34. See Coblens, S.L., Privileged and Confidential Communications Between Optometrists and Patients, *American Journal of Optometry and Archives of American Academy of Optometry*, vol. 48, no. 12, 1971, pp. 1048–1052.
35. See Morris, R.C., and A.R. Moritz, *Doctor and Patient and the Law*, 5th ed., C.V. Mosby Co., St. Louis, 1971, pp. 271–291.
36. Ibid.
37. See *State v. Viola*, 82 N.E.2d 306 (1948), *appeal dismissed*, 148 Ohio St. 712, 76 N.E.2d 715, *cert. denied*, 334 U.S. 816, 68 S. Ct. 1070 (1948) (a licensed optometrist is a physician within the meaning of the statutory privilege); Contra: *People of the State of Michigan v. Baker*, 94 Mich. App. 365, 288 N.E.2d 430 (1980) (statutory physician-patient privilege does not apply to optometrists).
38. For a discussion, see Roach W.H., S.N. Chernoff, and C.L. Esley, *Medical Records and the Law*, Aspen, Rockville, Md., 1985.
39. See Peck, R.L., Open Season on Your Medical Records Is Here, *Medical Economics*, vol. 56, no. 7, Apr. 16, 1979, p. 29.
40. Holder, A., *Medical Malpractice Law*, Wiley and Sons, New York, 1976, pp. 294–295.
41. *Tempchin v. Sampson*, 262 Md. 156, 277 A.2d 67 (1971).
42. See Holder, A., supra note 40 at 394–399.
43. For an example of how altered records can affect the outcome of a malpractice case, see Rosenberg, C.L., How "Doctored" Records Added Up To $4,500,000, *Medical Economics*, vol. 56, no. 1, Jan. 8, 1979, p. 81.
44. An account of this case can be found in Gerber, P., How To Blow Your Own Malpractice Defense, *Optometric Management*, vol. 17, no. 7, 1981, p. 19.
45. This case is described in California Malpractice Topics, *Professional Liability Newsletter*, vol. 14, no. 3, Feb. 1983.
46. *James v. Spear*, 338 P.2d 22 (Cal. 1959).
47. For comments on tort reform, see Hunt, K., Is There Any Real Hope for Malpractice Reform?, *Medical Economics*, vol. 62, no. 8, Apr. 15, 1985, pp. 23–28; Brown, S., Malpractice Reform: Doctors 4, Lawyers 0, *Medical Economics*, vol. 62, no. 12, June 10, 1985, pp. 31–47; and Gold, A., Malpractice Reform, *Journal of the American Optometric Association*, vol. 58, no. 12, Dec. 1987, pp. 1000–1003.

Chapter 17

Prescriptions

Staff now recommends that the Commission modify the rule to require practitioners to release prescriptions only upon request of the patient, based on record evidence that consumers are generally knowledgeable enough to request eyeglass prescriptions if they want them and that practitioners release them upon request. For the same reasons, staff recommends that the Commission not modify the rule to require practitioners to offer a prescription to every patient regardless of whether the patient requests it. . . . The Commission also raised three additional questions regarding possible extensions of the prescription release requirement.

One, the Commission asked whether optometrists and ophthalmologists should be required to release to patients complete contact lens prescriptions. The record does not support a recommended rule in this area. It does not contain sufficient reliable evidence to permit a conclusion that refusal to release contact lenses is a prevalent practice or that there are no quality justifications for refusal to release.

Two, the Commission asked whether optometrists and ophthalmologists should be required to release duplicate copies of prescriptions to patients who lose or misplace their original copies. The record contains no evidence that practitioners refuse to release duplicate copies of eyeglass prescriptions to consumers who request and therefore provides no basis for a recommendation that practitioners should be required to release duplicate copies of prescriptions.

Three, the Commission asked whether eyeglass dispensers should be required to return the eyeglass prescription to patients after filling the prescription. The record contains no significant evidence that dispensers refuse to return prescriptions to patients. Therefore, such a requirement is not warranted by the record.

—From the report of the staff to the Federal Trade Commission, *Ophthalmic Practice Rules, State Restrictions on Commercial Practice* (Eyeglasses II)

Spectacle Prescriptions
Contact Lens Prescriptions
Prescription Release

Spectacle Prescriptions

The prescription requirements for spectacles and contact lenses described in this chapter were subject to change under the Federal Trade Commission's (FTC) proposed trade regulation rule known as Eyeglasses II.[1] Faced with a Hobson's choice, represented by the opposing views[2] of the FTC staff[3] and the Eyeglasses II hearings presiding officer,[4] the FTC Commissioners decided in 1988 not to implement the prescription release requirements of the rule. Therefore, the prevailing federal law regulating prescriptions and prescription release is still Eyeglasses I.[5]

Even though the Eyeglasses II proposals were not adopted, they are interesting in that they represent the point of view of the FTC staff, which is responsible for the enforcement of Eyeglasses I. For this reason, the provisions of Eyeglasses I that were subject to change under Eyeglasses II have been identified in the notes and discussed in some detail.

In addition to the requirements established by the FTC, the states may exercise regulatory authority over prescriptions and prescription release, and statutes or optometry board rules have been enacted in several states for this purpose. These laws may themselves be amended, and in silent jurisdictions new laws may be passed, further complicating the regulatory scheme. Therefore, practitioners will need to stay informed in order to remain up to date in this rapidly evolving area of the law.

All practitioners are currently required to comply with the prescription requirements of Eyeglasses I,[6] which is applicable in every jurisdiction. The basic provisions of the rule are:

- The doctor must offer a copy of the spectacle prescription to the patient at the conclusion of the examination.[7]
- If the doctor determines that there is no reason to prescribe spectacles, no prescription needs to be tendered to the patient.
- If the patient is wearing spectacles, and no change in the prescription is required, the prescription still must be offered to the patient even though there will be no change in the spectacles.[8]
- The prescription must contain a certain minimum of information: sphere power, cylinder power and axis (if any), and prism power and orientation (if any), and it must be signed by the doctor;[9] these requirements may be superseded by state laws or board regulations that require additional information to be included in prescriptions for spectacles (found in six states—see Table 17.1); in states where more information is necessary, the doctor must include the additional information on the prescription.
- A doctor can charge a fee for writing a prescription if all patients are charged a fee for this service (and not just those patients who choose to obtain their spectacles elsewhere).[10]
- An expiration date can be placed upon the prescription as long as it is reasonable (the expiration date may be regulated by statute or board rule in the jurisdiction).[11]
- A fee can be charged for verifying spectacles obtained from another ophthalmic provider.
- No disclaimers can be placed upon the prescription.[12]

Violations of the rule are punishable by a fine of up to $10,000 per offense. To date there have been no prosecutions of the rule by the federal government.

Although the Eyeglasses I rule only pertains to the release of prescriptions after an eye examination, there are other legal requirements that may necessitate a subsequent release of the spectacle prescription when requested by the patient or various third parties. These laws are discussed in the concluding section of this chapter.

Table 17.1. State Prescription Requirements for Spectacles: 1986

State	Requirements
Alaska	Sphere power; cylinder power and axis; prism power and position of base; interpupillary distance; name of the patient; date of the prescription; name and office location of the doctor; expiration date of the prescription
Arizona	Refractive power; reading addition and type of bifocal prescribed; interpupillary distance (far and near); signature of the doctor; date of the refraction
Idaho	Sphere power; cylinder power and axis; prism power; add power, if applicable; position of the optical centers; segment type, location, and size; tint; coating; type of lens material (glass or plastic)
Kansas	Sphere power, cylinder power and axis; prism power and base direction; size, type and power of the multifocal; interpupillary distance, far and near
Maine	Sphere power; cylinder power and axis; prism power and base direction; interpupillary distance; type and form of lenses; type and placement of multifocal segments; placement of optical centers (for distance and near)
Utah	Sphere power; cylinder power and axis; prism; add; interpupillary distance

Source: American Optometric Association, 1986.

Contact Lens Prescriptions

The Eyeglasses I rule also applies to prescriptions for contact lenses. Key provisions of the rule are:

- The contact lens prescription must be offered to the patient by the doctor.[13]
- The offer must be made at the conclusion of the examination.[14]
- The prescription for contact lenses only includes those requirements necessary to constitute a minimum prescription for spectacles (i.e., sphere power, cylinder power and axis (if any), prism (if any), and the signature of the doctor);[15] if the state law requires that more information be included in the prescription, the doctor must include the additional information (found in seven states; see Table 17.2).
- A fee can be charged for writing the prescription if all contact lens patients are charged the fee

Table 17.2. State Prescription Requirements for Contact Lenses: 1986

State	Requirements
Alaska	Issue date; expiration date; name and office location of the prescriber; name of the patient
Arizona	Type of contact lens; radius of inside curvature; power; optical zone diameter; peripheral curve; signature of the doctor; date of examination
Idaho	*Hard lenses*: base curve; peripheral curves, including radii and widths; overall diameter; optical zone diameter; power; center thickness; color; expiration date. *Soft lenses*: lens manufacturer; base curve; power; overall diameter; color; expiration date
Kansas	Lens material; base curve; back vertex power; prism power; overall diameter; optical zone diameter; peripheral curve radii and widths; center thickness; color; edge shape
Maine	Base curve; peripheral and intermediate curves; overall diameter; optical zone diameter; power; center thickness; edge shape; color; form
Ohio	Date; information sufficient to enable the patient to obtain the lens prescribed
Texas	*Hard lenses*: base curve; power; overall diameter; optical zone diameter; peripheral curves and widths; blend; center thickness; color; type of lens material; manufacturer. *Soft lenses*: base curve; power; overall diameter; manufacturer; type of lens and water content; color; sterilization procedures

Source: American Optometric Association, 1986.

(and not just those patients who wish to obtain their contact lenses elsewhere).[16]

- An expiration date may be included on the prescription as long as it is reasonable (the expiration date may be regulated by statute or board rule in the jurisdiction).[17]
- A fee may be charged to verify contact lens materials obtained from another provider.

Although violations of the rule are punishable by a fine that may be as much as $10,000 per offense, there have been no efforts on the part of the federal government to prosecute persons for failing to observe the requirements of the rule.

The obligation to give contact lens information to the patient may be expanded by federal and state laws or regulations. These important legal requirements are described in the following section.

Prescription Release

The FTC's Eyeglasses I rule is not the only legal requirement that pertains to the release of spectacle or contact lens information. Federal and state laws may also dictate when prescriptions—and other patient information—must be divulged by optometrists. Examples of statutes that may affect prescription release are federal and state freedom-of-information acts, state optometry practice acts, and regulations issued by state boards of optometry. But these laws affect more than just the prescription information included in patient records. They can compel the release of any or all patient information contained in optometrists' records, and they are not limited to the period immediately following the examination, but must be observed by practitioners whenever a valid demand for a copy of the record is made by the patient. Records release laws have been enacted in a sizeable number of jurisdictions, and it is necessary for optometrists who practice in these jurisdictions to be familiar with their legal obligation to supply information to patients (see Chapter 16).[18]

There is a distinction between a requirement to provide copies or summaries of patient records and a requirement to supply a prescription. A copy or summary of a record might include prescription information, but this information does not constitute a prescription for legal purposes. A prescription is an order on behalf of a patient to a third party, specifying the criteria that must be satisfied by any spectacles or contact lenses dispensed to the patient by the third party. In order to be valid it must be signed by a provider who is licensed within the jurisdiction and presented to the third party before the date of expiration.

The FTC's Eyeglasses I rule requires a copy of the contact lens prescription to be given to the patient at the conclusion of the examination. In fifteen states, however, the patient's right to obtain a contact lens prescription is enlarged by freedom-of-information acts, optometry practice acts, or optometry board rules (see Table 17.3). Even though an optometrist in these states may have complied with the Eyeglasses I rule, there may be a further obligation to provide a prescription to the patient or a third party. Failure to observe this requirement may subject the optometrist to disciplinary action by the state board of optometry.

Laws that obligate optometrists to provide copies of spectacle or contact lens prescriptions to patients create potential legal conflicts concerning responsibility for prescriptions filled by third parties. Determining who is at fault in such a case can be a most complex matter, but, in general, if the prescription is

Table 17.3. Record Release Requirements for Contact Lens Prescriptions: 1987

	Freedom-of-Information Act	Optometry Practice Act	Board Rule or Regulation
Alaska	Alaska Stat. §18.23.065		
Arizona			Rule R4-21-212D and E
Florida	Fla. Stat. Ann. §455.241	Fla. Stat. Ann. §463.012(2)(b)	
Indiana		Ind. Stat. Ann. §§16-4-8-1 and 16-4-8-2 (information may be given in general terms)	
Maryland		Md. Health Occ. Code Ann. §10-312 (only to other health care providers)	
Minnesota	Minn. Stat. Ann. §144.335		
New Jersey			Rule 13, §38-6.1(c) (only to another M.D., O.D., or other licensed ophthalmic dispenser in New Jersey)
New York			Rule 29.2
North Carolina		N.C. Gen. Stat. §90-127.3	
Ohio		Ohio Rev. Code Ann. §4725.17	
Vermont		Vt. Stat. Ann. tit. 26, §§1719(7) and 1719(12)(A)	
Virginia			Rule §3.1.F
Washington			Rule WAC 308-53-250 (to another O.D. or M.D. in Washington only)
West Virginia	W. Va. Code §16-29-1		
Wisconsin	Wis. Stat. Ann. §146.83		

Source: American Optometric Association, 1987.

appropriate and is filled incorrectly by a third party, the legal responsibility for any resulting injury will be borne by the third party. Therefore, optometrists should be certain that any information written on a prescription is correct.

Another important aspect of prescription writing is completeness. For example, if the optometrist gives the patient a contact lens prescription that contains refractive data only (i.e., it is in compliance with the minimum requirements of the Eyeglasses I rule), and a third party provides the patient with contact lenses based upon this prescription, the probability is great that the lens parameters (and even the lens manufacturer) will be different from those chosen by the optometrist. Yet the lenses will be in conformance with the prescription, for such a prescription will not include the lens parameters. If the patient suffers an injury while wearing these lenses, the apportionment of fault may be difficult to determine and, consequently, both parties will likely be named as defendants if there is a lawsuit.

Similarly, if an optometrist writes a spectacle prescription that satisfies only the minimum requirements of the FTC rule, and a third party fills the prescription as written but is allowed to determine the choice of lens material (because the prescription is silent), then once again both parties may be sued (and even jointly held liable) if the patient is injured by a shattered lens.

The FTC staff report for Eyeglasses II addresses this problem, stating that "it is not the Commission's intent to impose liability on an ophthalmologist or optometrist for the ophthalmic goods and services dispensed by another seller pursuant to the ophthalmologist's or optometrist's prescription."[19] Despite this declaration, there is ample opportunity for litigation and for this reason it may be advisable for the practitioner to place written limitations on the prescription.

One of the most important limitations is the designation of whether the prescription is for spectacles or for contact lenses. A prescription that is intended to be for spectacles may be noted as such, even if not required under state law,[20] and there is no duty to state that a patient's prescription makes him or her suitable for contact lenses, as was first required by the FTC rule.[21] If a contact lens prescription is written, the practitioner should specify that daily wear lenses are for "daily wear only," thereby precluding a third party from dispensing lenses for extended wear.[22]

Any prescription may be limited by using an

I, J. Doe, having been made fully aware of the potential risk of impairment to my eyes and visual health while wearing contact lenses, hereby accept full responsibility for obtaining periodic professional eye examinations.

It has been recommended to me that these examinations should be done every 6 months.

Flexible Contact Lens Specifications:

Date prescribed: ______

Manufacturer: ______

Expiration Date: ______

	BASE CURVE OR SERIES	LENS DIAMETER	LENS POWER
O.D.			
O.S.			

Hard Contact Lenses Specifications: Date Prescribed: ______ Laboratory: ______

	BASE CURVE	SECOND RADIUS	2nd CURVE WIDTH	THIRD RADIUS	3rd CURVE WIDTH	LENS DIAM	O.Z. DIAM	LENS POWER	THICK-NESS	EDGE	LENS TINT	ADD/PRISM
O.D.	7.38	8.2	.3	11.0	.3	8.8	7.6	-4.25	.12		Grn	
O.S.	7.34	8.2	.3	11.0	.3	8.8	7.6	-2.75	.12		Grn	

Date of latest contact lens examination: Feb. 1, 1988

JB Classé, O.D.

Date Feb. 1, 1988 Patient J. Doe

Witness ______

Figure 17.1. Sample Hard Contact Lens Prescription and Warning. (Courtesy UAB School of Optometry)

SCHOOL OF OPTOMETRY / The Medical Center
University of Alabama at Birmingham
1716 University Blvd.
BIRMINGHAM, ALABAMA 35294
Phone: 934-3303

Interpupillary Measurements:
Dist. 64 R.____ L.____
Near 60

RECORD # 12345

PATIENT: Charles Prentice DATE: Jan. 1, 1988

PHONE NUMBER: 123-4567 EXPIRES JAN. 1, 1989

Base Curve			Sphere	Cylinder	Axis	Prism	Base	Decentration In	Out
	Distance	R	-2.00	-1.00	005				
		L	-2.00	-0.75	180				

Special Instructions and Rx Use			Add	Seg. Hght.	Seg. Type	Seg. Width	Seg. Dec.	Total Dec.	Vert. MRP
For spectacles only	Addition	R							
Polycarbonate lenses only		L							

JB Classé, O.D.

PATIENT COPY License #409

Figure 17.2. Prescription for Spectacles. Prescriptions for spectacles may include any of the following information: refractive data (as required by federal or state law); statement "Spectacle Prescription Only;" lens material; expiration date; comment that a fee will be charged for the verification of materials obtained from another provider; special instructions ("safety glasses"); signature. (Courtesy UAB School of Optometry)

expiration date. If a prescription has expired, the patient may be required to undergo examination in order to obtain another copy, which is intended to protect the patient's vision and ocular health (a requirement that has received favorable review by our nation's highest court).[23]

Although waivers or disclaimers are generally not allowed, there are certain comments that the optometrist may include upon the prescription in order to put the patient on notice concerning ophthalmic materials that are to be obtained from another ophthalmic provider.

The optometrist can note on the prescription that, "This office is not responsible for prescription changes occurring since the date of this examination," which informs the patient of the possibility of

CONTACT LENS RELEASE

I, Charles Prentice, having been made fully aware of the potential risk of impairment to my eyes and visual health while wearing contact lenses, hereby accept full responsibility for obtaining periodic professional eye examinations. I also understand that neither my optometrist nor the UAB School of Optometry will be responsible for contact lenses dispensed outside of the practice. A professional fee will be rendered for subsequent verification and/or examination involving contact lenses which we have not dispensed.

Flexible Contact Lens Specifications:

Date Prescribed: Jan. 1, 1988
EXPIRES ON Jan. 1, 1989
Manufacturer: CSI

	BASE CURVE OR SERIES	LENS DIAMETER	LENS POWER
O.D.	8.6	14.8	-3.00
O.S.	8.6	14.8	-3.00

These lenses are for DAILY WEAR only

Hard Contact Lenses Specifications: Date Prescribed: ______ Laboratory: ______

	BASE CURVE	SECOND RADIUS	2ND CURVE WIDTH	THIRD RADIUS	3RD CURVE WIDTH	LENS DIAM.	O.Z. DIAM.	LENS POWER	THICK-NESS	EDGE	LENS TINT	ADD/ PRISM
O.D.												
O.S.												

Date of latest contact lens examination: Feb. 1, 1988

John G. O'Dee, O.D.

Date Feb. 1, 1988

Patient Charles Prentice

Witness Mary C. Smith

University Station / Birmingham, Alabama 35294
An Affirmative Action / Equal Opportunity Employer

Figure 17.3. Prescription for Soft Contact Lenses. Prescriptions for contact lenses may include any of the following information: refractive data (as required by federal or state law); lens parameters (as required by state law); limitation to daily wear; expiration date; comment that a fee will be charged for the vertification of materials obtained from another provider; special instructions ("monovision fit"); signature. (Courtesy UAB School of Optometry)

vision changes subsequent to the examination that may make even an unexpired prescription no longer appropriate for the patient.[24] Another comment that the optometrist may wish to include involves fees to be charged for the verification of ophthalmic materials obtained elsewhere:

> Lenses dispensed by your ophthalmic provider should meet or exceed ANSI Z-80 or Z-87 standards. I assume responsibility for the accurate fitting, fabrication, and dispensing of eyewear by this office. If verification of eyewear dispensed by another provider becomes necessary, a charge will be made.[25]

A related form of limitation that a practitioner may wish to consider for inclusion upon the prescription is the choice of lens material. The designation of ophthalmic lens material is clearly appropriate in those circumstances where the optometrist feels that impact resistance is an important clinical consideration. If the doctor specifies an impact-resistant lens material and a third party fills the prescription so that it does not satisfy this requirement, then the legal responsibility for any injury suffered by the patient as a result of the improper lens material will be borne by the third party. Likewise, special instructions (such as "safety glasses") may be placed upon the prescription and must be observed by the provider of the ophthalmic materials. If the complete contact lens parameters are listed on the prescription (i.e., lens specifications as well as refractive data), then the provider must dispense lenses according to these parameters or be responsible for any economic or physical damages suffered by the patient as a result of the provider's failure to do so[26] (see Fig. 17.1).

If the ophthalmic materials obtained from another provider do not conform to the prescription specifications, then the optometrist should inform the patient of the pertinent discrepancies so that the patient can obtain satisfactory redress.

Because of the growing willingness of the courts and legislatures to permit patients to have access to their medical records, including prescriptions for spectacles and contact lenses, conflicts can best be avoided by adopting a liberal attitude toward patient requests for prescription information. Whenever prescriptions are provided, it is in the best interests of both patient and practitioner to include as much information as possible, and in all cases to include at least the minimum amount of information specified by federal or state law. This most important aspect of practice should be given careful consideration by all practitioners (see Figs. 17.2 and 17.3). Only by describing the spectacle or contact lenses with great specificity can the optometrist minimize the opportunity for litigation.

Notes

1. Eyeglasses II is an effort to amend the trade regulation rule approved by the FTC in 1978. The FTC's intentions with regard to Eyeglasses II were first voiced in a report of the staff of the Federal Trade Commission, released in 1980 by the Bureau of Consumer Protection, entitled *State Restrictions On Vision Care Providers: The Effects On Consumers* (Eyeglasses II). For a review of the proposed rule's major components, see Cohn, S., Eyeglasses II: Commercial Optometry Set Free, *Optometric Management*, vol. 21, no. 3, 1985, pp. 30–37.
2. Commentary on the opposing views of the FTC staff and the presiding officer at the FTC hearings can be found in News Review, FTC Feuds Over Rule, *Review of Optometry*, vol. 123, no. 12, 1986, p. 5; and "'Eyeglasses II' Should Not Be Issued, Presiding Officer Says in Report to FTC," *AOA News*, Dec. 15, 1986.
3. Federal Trade Commission, *Ophthalmic Practice Rules, State Restrictions On Commercial Practice*, Federal Trade Commission, Washington, D.C., 1986.
4. Greenan, J., *Report of the Presiding Officer on Proposed Trade Regulation Rule: Ophthalmic Practice Rules 16 C.F.R. Part 456*, Public Record 215-63, Federal Trade Commission, Washington, D.C., 1986.
5. The Eyeglasses I rule can be found in 16 C.F.R. §456 (1978).
6. The requirements of the Eyeglasses I rule are described by Classe, J., The Effects of FTC Rulings on the Practice of Optometry, *Southern Journal of Optometry*, vol. 21, no. 5, 1974, pp. 347–350.
7. Under Eyeglasses I, a copy of the prescription has to be offered to the patient, but Eyeglasses II would have changed this obligation so that a copy of the prescription would have to be given to the patient only when requested. The patient's right to receive this copy of the prescription was specifically limited under Eyeglasses II: only one copy of the prescription had to be given to the patient and the right to receive the copy ended either one year after the fitting process was completed or when the prescription expired, whichever was sooner. See 16 C.F.R. §456.2(a) of the recommended rule.
8. Eyeglasses II would have changed this requirement so that an optometrist would be obligated to give the patient a copy of the prescription only when requested, even though no change in the old prescription was deemed necessary.
9. The minimum prescription requirements under Eyeglasses I are expressly listed in the rule, but under Eyeglasses II a prescription was defined as "the written specifications for spectacle lenses which are derived from an eye examination, including all of the information specified by state law, if any, necessary to obtain

spectacle lenses" (16 C.F.R. §456.1 (h)). This definition has two interesting implications: prescriptions for spectacles would no longer contain a federally mandated minimum of information; in the six states that specify the minimum requirements of a prescription for spectacles, optometrists would have to list these requirements to be in compliance with the rule.

10. Eyeglasses I allows an optometrist to charge a fee for writing a prescription, as long as all patients receive this charge. The Eyeglasses II staff report notes that less than 1 percent of optometrists are apparently charging such a fee (1986 staff report at 255). There are three "unfair acts" that are singled out as being prohibited: refusing to examine a patient unless he or she has agreed in advance to purchase any ophthalmic goods from the examiner; charging the patient an additional fee as a condition to releasing the prescription; and withholding release of the prescription until the patient has paid for the spectacles unless immediate payment would also have been required of patients not obtaining ophthalmic materials. See 16 C.F.R. §456.2 of the recommended rule.
11. In North Carolina, the optometry practice act provides that: "The prescriber shall state the expiration date on the face of every prescription, and the expiration date shall be no earlier than 365 days after the examination date." *N.C. Gen. Stat.*, Chap. 90, art. 6, §127.3. Where state law specifies the minimum period of time before expiration, practitioners must observe this provision.
12. Although the FTC has consistently argued that no disclaimers can be placed on the prescription, the 1980 staff report for Eyeglasses II makes it clear that an optometrist will be held responsible only for the examination and the prescription, and not for the ophthalmic materials provided by another party (1980 staff report at 269–270). The recommended rule itself proclaims that "it is not the Commission's intent to impose liability on an ophthalmologist or optometrist for the ophthalmic goods and services dispensed by another seller pursuant to the optometrist's or ophthalmologist's prescription" (16 C.F.R. §465.5(a)). Therefore, certain limitations may be placed upon the prescription in order to clarify this separation of responsibility (described in the concluding section of this chapter).
13. Under Eyeglasses I the requirement to provide the patient with a copy of the prescription is mandatory. Under Eyeglasses II the optometrist would have been required to give a copy of the prescription to the patient only upon request. There were two specific limitations to the patient's right to receive this copy of the prescription: only one copy had to be provided and the right to obtain it ended either one year after the fitting process was completed or "whenever the prescription expires," whichever was sooner. See 16 C.F.R. §456.2(a) of the recommended rule.
14. Under Eyeglasses I there was some ambiguity as to when the obligation to release a copy of the prescription actually arose: was it at the end of the initial fitting process or after trial lenses had been worn and the doctor was satisfied that the comfort, physiology, and acuity were satisfactory? The 1986 Eyeglasses II staff report clarifies this question, stating that "release of the contact lens specifications refers only to release after the fitting process is complete, and does not encompass release for the purpose of intitial fitting." (1986 staff report at 281.) Thus the FTC expressly recognizes that the fitting process may extend over several days or weeks, and that the obligation to honor the patient's request for a copy of the prescription does not arise until this fitting process has been completed. The determination of when this point has been reached is left to the judgment of the clinician.
15. Under Eyeglasses I the prescription for contact lenses was limited to those components that described the refractive properties of the lens, and there was no requirement to provide the lens specifications, such as base curve, lens diameter, lens manufacturer, or similar components. This distinction was continued under Eyeglasses II. The 1986 staff report discusses the merits of requiring lens parameters to be included on the prescription but comments that, "it cannot be concluded from the record that there are no quality justifications for refusing to release contact lens prescriptions" (1986 staff report at 296). This statement limits the application of prescription requirements under Eyeglasses II to the refractive properties of contact lenses. There are, however, currently seven states that define contact lens prescriptions in more comprehensive terms, and in these states a prescription for contact lenses should include those parameters that are specified by law. Of course, if a practitioner wishes to provide the patient with a more complete prescription, he or she is free to do so, and for liability reasons should do so.
16. Eyeglasses I specifies that, if a fee is charged for writing a prescription, it must be applied to everyone and not just to those patients who wish to use the prescription to obtain their lenses elsewhere. Under Eyeglasses II this same rule would have been applicable, with three "unfair acts" specifically prohibited: refusing to examine a patient unless he or she has agreed in advance to purchase any ophthalmic goods from the examiner; charging the patient an additional fee as a condition to releasing the prescription; and withholding release of the prescription until the patient has paid for the contact lenses, unless immediate payment would also have been required of patients not obtaining ophthalmic materials. See 16 C.F.R. §456.2 of the recommended rule.
17. Eyeglasses I does not mandate a specific period of time for the expiration date of a contact lens prescription, merely requiring that it be "reasonable." Neither Eyeglasses I nor Eyeglasses II prohibit a state from establishing a minimum expiration date for prescriptions (such as North Carolina has done; see note 11 supra). The 1980 FTC staff report comments that the rule is not intended to interfere with the professional judgment of practitioners and that an expiration date

would be considered to be unreasonably short only when it is "equivalent to an actual refusal to return the prescription" (1980 staff report at 263–264).

18. A description of the various legal requirements that pertain to the release of patient information may be found in Classe, J., Optometrist's Duty To Release Patient Information, *Southern Journal of Optometry*, vol. 5, no. 1, 1987, pp. 9–15.
19. 16 C.F.R. §456.2(d) of *Ophthalmic Practice Rules, State Restrictions on Commercial Practice*, Federal Trade Commission, Washington, D.C., 1986.
20. For example, in North Carolina the State Board of Examiners has made it clear that prescriptions for spectacles should be marked as such in order to reduce confusion on the part of the public:

    A patient is entitled, without equivocation, to a copy of his or her prescription following an eye examination at such time as the examining optometrist has determined what the prescription shall be. The law is very precise, however, in stating that any prescription that *does not* have a statement on its face that it is intended by the prescriber to be for contact lenses, is considered a spectacle lens prescription, and can only be filled and dispensed by a dispensing optician as such. . . . To further minimize the risks of misunderstanding between the optometrist and his patients, it is recommended that all prescriptions released to patients that are intended for spectacle lenses to so state by having the prescription blanks printed or stamped with words to that effect, i.e., "this is a spectacle lens prescription only," "not intended for contact lenses," etc.

    The Release of Prescriptions, the Fitting of Contact Lenses, and the Dispensing of Contact Lenses on Prescription, letter by John D. Robinson, O.D., Secretary of the North Carolina State Board of Examiners in Optometry, Oct. 8, 1981.
21. The FTC staff commented in its report, *State Restrictions on Vision Care Providers: The Effect on Consumers* at pp. 259–260, released in 1980, that:

    The definition (of prescription) has been amended to eliminate all references to contact lenses. This change will end the confusion that was generated by the original definition concerning the obligation of optometrists and ophthalmologists to place the wording, "OK for contact lenses" on prescriptions. The new definition eliminates any requirement that an optometrist or ophthalmologist include on the prescription the wording, "OK for contact lenses" or similar language.
22. The advent of product liability litigation over extended wear lenses raises the possibility of a new cause of action against optometrists based upon allegations that the lenses are unreasonably dangerous and not suitable for the purpose for which prescribed, even when worn as directed. A patient who is clearly not an extended wear candidate and who obtains a prescription permitting the purchase of extended wear lenses may be able to state a cause of action against the optometrist for failing to note this restriction upon the prescription. Under such a situation the patient may also allege negligence as a cause of action since the optometrist is under a duty to protect the patient against unreasonable risks of injury. See Classe, J., and M. Harris, Liability and Extended Wear Lenses, *Journal of the American Optometric Association*, vol. 58, no. 10, 1987, pp. 848–854.
23. In *Williamson v. Lee Optical of Oklahoma*, 348 U.S. 483, 75 S. Ct. 461 (1955), the U.S. Supreme Court noted that eye examinations are of such public concern that the state may implement regulations designed to promote proper vision care. The expiration date on a prescription can help to serve this purpose by protecting the patient from foregoing periodic eye examinations and thus increasing the likelihood of undetected eye disease.
24. Clinical problems include diabetic patients, whose refractive errors can change drastically if the disease is not under control, and contact lens patients, whose ability to see clearly through spectacles can vary significantly depending upon the physiology of the contact lens fit and when the spectacles are to be worn. For a discussion of these problems, see Amos, J. (Ed.), *Diagnosis and Management in Vision Care*, Butterworths, Boston, 1987.
25. The author is grateful to Dr. Donald Springer of Anniston, Alabama, for suggesting the language cited herein.
26. The more complete the prescription, the less likely that a patient will obtain an unsatisfactory replacement lens from another ophthalmic provider, because the provider must dispense a lens in compliance with the provisions specified in the prescription or be liable for any economic or physical injury suffered by the patient as a result of the substitution. See Classe, J., Liability in Contact Lens Practice, *Southern Journal of Optometry*, vol. 4, no. 3, 1986, pp. 52–57; and Classe, J., and M. Harris, Liability and Extended Wear Contact Lenses, *Journal of the American Optometric Association*, supra note 22.

PART SIX

PROFESSIONAL LIABILITY

Chapter 18

Legal Basis for Malpractice

He who knoweth the law and knoweth not the reason thereof, soon forgetteth his superfluous learning.
—Lord Coke, *Institutes: Commentary Upon Littleton*

The Law of Torts
Negligence
Legal Duty and the Standard of the Reasonable Person
Failure to Provide Due Care
Proximate Cause
Injury

The Law of Torts

The word *tort* is derived from the Latin *tortus*, which means twisted; in French, tort means wrong. From these antecedents, it would seem that a tort represents some conduct that is twisted, crooked, or wrong. For many decades legal scholars have struggled to define this word in a concise and intelligible way, not merely for law students but for lawyers and judges as well. Unfortunately, as one of this century's most pre-eminent U.S. legal scholars in the field of torts acknowledges, "a really satisfactory definition of a tort has yet to be found. . . . Broadly speaking, a tort is a civil wrong, other than a breach of contract, for which the court will provide a remedy in the form of an action for damages."[1]

As the quotation from Lord Coke points out, an understanding of the law is best achieved through an appreciation of the legal theory that forms its basis. There is little in the definition of tort, however, that indicates why it has been the subject of such intense legislative activity during the past decade.

The definition of tort that we have selected—which is from the famous textbook, *The Law of Torts*, by Professor William L. Prosser—states that[2]:

- A tort is a civil offense (not a crime).
- It is based upon a legal wrong other than breach of contract.
- If a tort is proven, damages can be awarded.

This definition recognizes two things that a tort is not: It is not a crime[3] and it is not an action that arises out of contract.[4] A tort comes into being when there is a breach of duty between two parties, the duty being fixed and imposed upon the parties by law, without their consent and even in the presence of efforts to evade it. For example, the driver of an automobile incurs certain legal duties to all persons on the street the moment his vehicle enters it even if he has not consented to them and even if he does not understand them. Much of tort law is occupied with this idea of breach of duty, which is described as an unreasonable interference with the interests of others. Consequently, liability in tort is imposed because the one causing the injury has acted with an unreasonable intention or has departed from a reasonable standard of care.

The historical evolution of tort law is interesting, for both the form and the principle of current-day U.S. tort law are inextricably linked to the court system that evolved in England after the Norman conquest in 1066. Beginning with the 1200s a system of courts began to develop throughout England, and as the courts grew in size and influence, there arose a variety of substantive and procedural rules that were intended to limit those offenses for which the courts could award a remedy. In order to be heard by the court, a plaintiff had to file a paper (a *writ*) with the court charging the defendant with a specific offense.[5] These writs were very formal and required rigidly stylized procedures. In order to summon a defendant into court, the plaintiff had to choose the writ that was most appropriate and apply it as well as possible to the facts in his particular case. If the facts could not sustain the writ, there could be no justice because there was no remedy allowable under the law.

In the beginning all wrongs were considered to be offenses against the crown and were classified as crimes, such as felonies (e.g., murder) or crimes of trespass; there was no separate court or category of offenses that were deemed to be civil offenses. Over the course of time, however, crimes of trespass were modified by ecclesiastical law into the offenses that resemble present-day torts. The two writs that are most important are the two 13th century writs known as the action of trespass and the action of trespass on the case.

The action of trespass was initially a criminal proceeding that provided for the trial and punishment before the King's Court of those persons who were guilty of serious and forcible breaches of the peace. The convicted defendant was subjected to a fine and, if the fine was not paid, to imprisonment. It was during these criminal proceedings for the action of trespass that damages first began to be awarded incidentally to the injured plaintiff.[6]

But the action of trespass was only a remedy for forcible, direct, and immediate injuries. It was not until some time later that a remedy for injuries that were not forcible or direct was devised, the action of trespass on the case. The often-quoted illustration of the difference between the two actions is that of a log thrown off of a wagon onto the road. A person who is struck by the log as it falls can maintain an action for trespass; a person who is injured later by the log as he stumbles over it in the road can maintain an action for trespass on the case.[7] This latter individual, upon proof of damages, could receive compensation from the wrongdoer for any injuries, even though they were indirectly received and not forcibly caused.

This distinction between the two offenses, which was based on the causal sequence of the wrong, i.e., whether the injury was direct or indirect, did not last. Over the next 600 years the courts began to look instead to the intent of the wrongdoer or to the wrongdoer's failure to adhere to some reasonable standard of care. The courts extended the action of trespass on the case to include unintentional injuries that were inflicted directly and immediately; trespass remained a remedy for intentional torts. In the 19th century, unintentional injuries that were direct and immediate emerged as a separate tort known as negligence.[8]

The torts based on intentional and negligent actions were both built on the idea that liability followed fault and that one who departed from a reasonable standard of care or intent should be held responsible for a resulting injury. Over the past century, however, this fault-oriented ideology has been supplanted to some extent in tort law by the principle of strict liability, e.g., that a person can be liable though the person is without fault. The idea began with the imposition of strict liability on the keepers of animals and spread to include situations that involved dangerous activities and dangerous products. Finally it evolved into a form of social policy, choosing to impose liability where there is blame on neither side upon the one who can best bear the loss.[9] In sanctioning the movement toward strict liability, the courts have stressed that the one being held liable is acting for his own purposes and is seeking to profit from his actions and that he is in a better position than the injured victim (i.e., the consumer) to administer the risk inherent in his activities (typically, by passing the cost on to the public). Liability is imposed on that element of society best able to shoulder it.[10]

One other interesting development within tort law has occurred in the past twenty-five years and has involved the healing arts exclusively. The new doctrine evolved in part from a concept developed by courts of equity, the fiduciary relationship.[11] Doctors and other professionals are fiduciaries who are sought by the public because of their special knowledge and skills and, as such, owe an affirmative duty of disclosure to those who come to them for advice or services. Conjoined with this concept of the fiduciary is another: that a person of sound mind has a right to determine what shall be done with his body and that no one has the right to compel him to accept treatment that he does not want.[12] These two ideas have developed into the doctrine of informed consent, which is a legal duty on the part of members of the healing arts to warn a patient of the possible hazards of an experimental or unusual course of treatment and to explain the usual complications or expected results of a standard course of treatment. Failure to do so can result in liability for the doctor, either on the basis of an assault and battery or for negligence.[13]

The historical evolution of tort law has led to the four major theories of liability that will be discussed within this textbook:

1. *Negligent Torts*—those torts based upon a duty to conform to a reasonable standard of conduct and that confer liability for injury caused by a failure to conform to the required standard. The negligent

torts that will be discussed in this text are malpractice (Chapters 19, 23–28), premises liability (Chapter 29), and liability for emergency care (Chapter 14). (Additional comments on negligence as an aspect of specialty practice may be found in Chapters 30–32.)

2. *Intentional Torts*—those torts based upon "an intent to bring about a result which will invade the interests of another in a way the law will not sanction."[14] The intentional torts that will be discussed in this text are defamation of character, disclosure of confidential information, invasion of privacy, and fraud (Chapter 20).

3. *Strict Liability*—those torts based neither upon intent nor upon negligence but rather upon the existence of an absolute duty to make safe, the breach of which results in liability. The strict liability torts that will be discussed in this text are products liability and vicarious liability (Chapters 21 and 27).

4. *Informed Consent*—a tort that bases liability upon the breach of a duty to explain adequately to a patient the course of treatment that is being proposed. Informed consent will be discussed in some detail (Chapter 22).

We begin with a description of the legal basis for negligence.

Negligence

Negligence is defined as "conduct which falls below a standard established by the law for the protection of others against an unreasonable risk of harm."[15] It is a relative latecomer to the law of torts, not being recognized as a separate tort until the early years of the 19th century, 1825 being the usual date given for its implementation as an independent basis for tort liability.[16] As compared to the intentional torts, negligence does not require an intent to bring about the consequences that follow a particular act, the knowledge that they are substantially certain to occur, or even a belief that they will occur. All that is required is a *risk* that the consequences will occur, a risk that is of sufficient magnitude to lead a reasonable person to anticipate the risk and to guard against it. For example, if an automobile driver fails to take notice of the icy condition of the highway and drives so fast that he loses control of his car and strikes someone, it is negligence. If he runs down someone in the street with the desire to do so (or the belief that he is certain to do so), it is an intentional battery. If he hits someone on the street because the brakes on his car were defectively made, strict liability can be imposed (and the one liable will not be the driver but rather the manufacturer of the brakes). Negligence is *conduct* rather than a state of mind or a social policy; it is behavior that involves an unreasonable risk to others.

Negligence has been found to apply to members of the healing arts.[17] In one of the well-known early decisions, the definition of medical negligence was expressed as follows:

> A physician and surgeon, by taking charge of a case, impliedly represents that he possesses, and the law places upon him the duty of possessing, *that reasonable degree of learning and skill that is ordinarily possessed* by physicians and surgeons in the locality in which he practices, and which is ordinarily regarded by those conversant with the employment as necessary to qualify him to engage in the business of practicing medicine and surgery. Upon consenting to treat a patient, *it becomes his duty to use reasonable care and diligence in the exercise of his skill*, and the application of his learning to accomplish the purpose for which he was employed. He is under the further obligation to *use his best judgment in exercising his skill* and applying his knowledge. The law holds him liable for an injury to his patient resulting *from want of the requisite skill and knowledge* or the omission to exercise reasonable care or the failure to use his best judgment [emphasis added].[18]

Courts have recognized that there are four distinct elements to medical negligence, all of which must be present in order for a doctor to incur legal liability[19]:

1. A duty—or obligation—recognizable in the law, such as that existing between doctor and patient, requiring that the doctor conform to certain recognized standards of conduct in order to protect the patient against unreasonable risks
2. A failure by the doctor to conform to the required standard
3. A reasonable and close causal relationship between the doctor's conduct and the resulting injury to the patient
4. Actual loss or damages suffered by the patient

In order to explain negligence fully, each of these four elements must be described and illustrated. By learning the theoretical framework on which negligence is based, a practitioner is better able to understand the practical application of the law to the day-to-day practice of his profession.

Legal Duty and the Standard of the Reasonable Person

The doctor and patient relationship is one that is based in contract (discussed in Chapter 13). The contract may be express or implied, for a consideration or gratuitous, but where the relationship is found to exist, the doctor is under a duty to conform to a certain standard of conduct in order to protect the patient against an unreasonable risk of harm. This standard of conduct, which is a fundamental aspect of the law of negligence, is expressed through the standard of the reasonable person.

The courts have devised as a standard a hypothetical ideal against which they can compare the actions of those charged with negligence. This ideal is a model of all the proper qualities demanded of the good citizen and is known as the reasonable person.[20] When negligence is at issue, the conduct of the one being charged is compared to the conduct of this reasonably prudent person: What would a reasonable person have done under the same or similar circumstances?

This reasonable person, however, must reflect the special abilities or attributes of the one to whom the comparison is being made. As a result, if an optometrist is being charged with negligence, then his conduct is compared to that of an ordinarily prudent optometrist acting under the same or similar circumstances. If he acted as an ordinarily prudent optometrist would have acted in treating the patient, there can be no negligence and hence no malpractice.

Note that this standard requires than an optometrist's conduct be measured by that of a hypothetical optometrist and not necessarily by that of a hypothetical ophthalmologist. Cross-profession comparisons have historically not been allowed when establishing standards of conduct.[21]

The following case, which occurred in 1931, illustrates how the courts use the reasonable person standard.

A workman with a foreign body lodged in his eye came to an EENT specialist for treatment. The physician examined the eye and removed a piece of glass. For the following three to four days the patient returned to the doctor, complaining of pain and a foreign body sensation in the eye; he also began to experience decreased acuity. Finally the physician took X-rays, found a piece of steel that had penetrated the cornea, and removed it. Unfortunately, the eye had become so infected that it was eventually lost. The workman sued the EENT specialist for malpractice, and at the trial an expert witness for the worker testified that the reasonable, standard practice was to use X-rays to locate an intraocular foreign body and that each day and hour that the steel remained in the eye increased the chance of blindness. The defendant doctor was found to have been negligent in delaying so long before taking the X-rays to locate the steel.[22]

Observe that the court required expert testimony to be given in order to establish the standard of care that would be expected of an EENT specialist. The defendant EENT specialist's actions were then compared to this standard and found to be below it. Using an expert witness to establish the standard of conduct is an inherent part of medical negligence litigation. The expert witness in this case was another EENT physician; had the defendant been an optometrist, the appropriate expert would have been another optometrist. The healing arts, like other professions, set their own minimum acceptable level of conduct, at or above which all practitioners are expected to perform. Failure to adhere to the standard creates liability.

Failure to Provide Due Care

Once the doctor-patient relationship has been established, the doctor is obligated to diagnose and treat the patient's anomaly. The words *due care* are used to describe the legal requirement that a practitioner adhere to some established minimum of care after a course of treatment has been chosen. A doctor may choose a highly reasonable course of therapy, but if he performs the therapy in a negligent manner, causing injury to the patient, he has not performed his duty to treat the patient with due care. Of course, he can fail to provide due care at any stage of the therapeutic process: in arriving at a diagnosis, while prescribing or initiating therapy, or in follow-up care. He may even fail to act at all. Failure to adhere to the hypothetical standard at any stage may lead to liability.

As to the standard itself, it is often stated that a doctor is expected to exercise reasonable care in the treatment of his patients and to possess a standard minimum of special knowledge and ability. The level of ability he is expected to display is often described as being that degree of skill and learning commonly possessed by members of the profession in good standing, and he will be liable if any harm results to a patient from his failure to maintain this standard.[23] The expected level of ability is frequently referred to as that of the average member of the profession. Using the word average in this context, however, is inappropriate since only those in good professional standing are to be considered in establishing the standard, and of these it is not the middle but the *minimum* common skill that is used as the lowest level of performance, below which liability is incurred.[24]

In summary, an optometrist is expected to treat a patient with at least reasonable skill, care, and diligence and to possess a minimum degree of knowledge and ability that he will employ in the course of the treatment he gives. Although the demands of due care seem logical and eminently fair and, therefore, simple to apply, such is not always the case. Due care can be difficult to define in a rapidly changing profession such as optometry and can be expected to evolve with time into a more stringent standard that reflects the increased knowledge and technical skill of scientific advancement. Two cases involving general practitioners can be used to illustrate the evolutionary nature of due care and the inherent difficulty of trying to establish liability under such a shifting standard.

In a 1903 case, a patient sought the services of a general practitioner (GP) for the treatment of an eye condition. Despite the GP's efforts, the patient gradually lost his sight. Thereafter the patient brought suit against the physician for malpractice, alleging that the physician had misdiagnosed his condition and that the misdiagnosis had constituted a lack of due care. At the trial it was established that the patient had been suffering from glaucoma, which the GP had diagnosed as being conjunctivitis. Expert testimony for the physician, however, established that glaucoma was a rare disease, one that could only be diagnosed with special instruments and skills not expected of a general practitioner, that glaucoma could easily be mistaken for conjunctivitis by a general practitioner, and that the treatment given, although incorrect, was not below the standard of care expected of a GP. The general practitioner was found to have not been negligent.[25]

In another case occurring twenty years later, a general practitioner who examined a woman's eye misdiagnosed a detached retina. The patient relied upon the GP's diagnosis and assurances that her eye would be all right, and so she sought no further medical aid. Some time later, realizing that her vision had not improved, she consulted an eye specialist, but her vision loss had become permanent. She sued the GP for malpractice, alleging that the misdiagnosis had been below the standard of care. At the trial expert testimony established that special instruments and knowledge were required to make a proper examination of the eye and that they were not expected of a general practitioner. But the expert testimony also established that a GP should realize, given the presenting symptoms, that it was incumbent on him to refer the patient to a specialist with the instruments and knowledge necessary to make a proper diagnosis and achieve a cure. The general practitioner was found to be negligent for not making the referral.[26]

Note once more that expert testimony was needed to define the minimum common skill expected of the defendant doctors under the circumstances of the two cases. In the first, and older, case the physician was found to have prescribed a reasonable course of therapy, even though it was incorrect, and to have acted with due care. In the second case, the doctor was held to be negligent for doing virtually the same thing because his peers testified that the patient's condition required referral to a specialist, and he failed to adhere to this minimally acceptable standard of conduct.

Before leaving the subject of due care, there is one important corollary that must be discussed, the *locality rule*. Early decisions by the courts relegated the standard of care expected of a doctor to the degree of care that other doctors exercised in the community, in the same general neighborhood, or in the same or a similar locality, all being phrases that had the effect of limiting a doctor's liability by restricting the area from which an injured patient could obtain an expert witness.[27] This doctrine also used to be known as the horse and buggy rule because —at least at its inception—it was used to avoid the application of big city standards to a rural doctor.

Over the intervening decades the accessibility of modern medical techniques and equipment has become widespread, and the locality rule has slowly been eroded away by the advent of progress within the healing arts.[28] Today, the New York expert and the Philadelphia lawyer can try a case in any jurisdiction where the rule is no longer extant, and the majority of states have abolished or modified the rule. But in those few states where the rule is still applied, malpractice is much more difficult to prove against optometrists, physicians, and other healthcare providers.

Proximate Cause

The third element of medical negligence is proximate cause. The law demands that there be some reasonable connection between the act or omission of the doctor and the damages that are suffered by the patient. This relationship, which is referred to as proximate cause (or legal cause) is one of the most widely discussed, confusing, and disagreed-on concepts in the entire field of law.[29] The basic idea is that a doctor's conduct is a cause of the injuring event if his conduct was a material element and a substantial factor in bringing it about. At first glance this legal relationship between cause and effect may not seem difficult, but the correlation between the injury and the act (or failure to act) cannot always be made sufficiently clear so as to satisfy the requirements of materiality and substantiality. In a trial the burden of showing this relationship is on the injured patient, and he must do so by a preponderance of the evidence in order to prevail.[30] It is often difficult to meet this burden, as the following case illustrates.

A patient was examined by an ophthalmologist, who prescribed glasses, but the patient experienced headaches while wearing the glasses and eventually went to a nearby school of optometry, where he was given another examination and another pair of glasses was prescribed. The patient's headaches subsided, and he thereafter sued the ophthalmologist, alleging malpractice. The trial court awarded the patient $55, and the doctor appealed. On appeal, it was noted that no expert testimony had been introduced at the trial by the plaintiff-patient. The ophthalmologist had testified on his own behalf, however, and had stated that the glasses he prescribed were of the proper strength to correct the patient's vision and that the patient had suffered from high blood pressure, which could have been the cause of his headaches. The appellate court reversed the decision, stating that not only had the patient failed to offer any expert testimony to establish that the defendant physician had breached his duty of due care but also that the patient had failed to establish any causal relationship between the headaches and the glasses prescribed by the ophthalmologist.[31]

The mere fact that the patient experienced headaches while wearing one pair of glasses and none while wearing a different pair did not meet the burden of proof needed to establish the materiality and substantiality requirements of proximate cause. Again, it was expert testimony—or, in this case, the absence of expert testimony—that was the deciding factor. An expert witness is needed to prove proximate cause just as an expert is needed to prove a breach of the duty of due care. Even though an expert may be incompetent to testify as to the standard of care, he may be allowed to testify concerning proximate cause.[32] He may also be permitted to testify as to the last element of medical negligence that must be discussed, the injury suffered by the plaintiff.

Injury

For a plaintiff to receive compensation from a court of law he must show the court not only that there was a breach of the duty of due care but also that the breach of duty was the proximate cause of an actual, physical injury. This term, as applied to malpractice, includes all the forms of injury that the mind can conjure up, whether temporary or permanent, petty or disabling, hidden or evident. But an actual injury must occur.[33]

A patient is compensated for his injury through the award of damages, which is that amount of money that the jury or the court feels is appropriate under the circumstances. There are two basic types of damages that can be awarded to an injured plaintiff: compensatory (also called actual) damages and punitive damages.

Compensatory damages are intended to do just that, to compensate those who are injured so that they are placed in as good a position as they would have been in had the malpractice never occurred. Examples of compensatory damages include hospital and doctor bills, lost income, pain and suffering, and like matters.[34] Compensatory damages are the usual outcome of a malpractice trial that is decided in favor of the plaintiff. In some cases, however, nominal damages are awarded; they are small amounts of money that are granted when the jury perceives the doctor as only being slightly wrong or the injury as minor. In cases where there is significant injury (e.g., quadriplegia), compensatory damages can mount into the millions of dollars. Fortunately, the exposure of optometrists to this magnitude of injury is minimal.[35] As to eye injuries in general, compensatory damages for the loss of an eye have already reached the $1 million mark, and compensation for ocular injuries—particularly blindness—can only be expected to escalate in future years.[36]

Punitive damages are intended to punish or to set an example of the offender in order to deter others. They are a rare phenomenon, relatively speaking, in tort law.[37] In order for punitive damages to be awarded, something more than the mere commission of a tort must be present: there must be circumstances of aggravation or outrage, or a fraudulent motive, or a conscious and deliberate disregard of the interests of others that amounts to conduct that could be called wilful or wanton. Punitive damages have been awarded in malpractice cases involving physicians, but these cases are rare. The opportunity for an optometrist to participate in the kind of conduct that would result in a verdict against him for punitive damages is virtually nonexistent.[38]

Even though injury would seem to be the easiest element of malpractice to prove, that is not always true, as is demonstrated by the following case.

A workman was involved in an industrial accident in which sulfur dioxide gas was expelled into his face. Although he suffered no immediate pain, he began applying wet bandages to his eyes. About ten minutes after the accident occurred a doctor arrived, gave the workman a cursory examination, and left without prescribing any treatment. For several days after the accident the patient experienced great pain in his eyes, and ultimately he suffered some permanent vision loss. He brought suit against the doctor for failing to institute or recommend treatment for the injury. At the time of the trial (1940), expert testimony was divided as to whether or not any treatment could have been undertaken by the doctor to alleviate the pain and damage that was caused by the expelled acid. Consequently, the court held that, where there was substantial disagreement between medical experts as to the proper treatment required, a jury could not accept one theory to the exclusion of the other since the issues in controversy were beyond the knowledge of laymen. Because the plaintiff was unable to prove that the doctor's failure to act had caused him any injury, the doctor was granted a verdict in his favor.[39]

The burden to prove negligence is upon the plaintiff, and a failure to do so will result in a decision in favor of the defendant (see Chapter 33 for a discussion of the civil trial process).

Notes

1. Prosser, W.L., *Law of Torts*, 4th ed., West, St. Paul, Minn., 1971, p. 1.
2. Id. at 2.
3. A tort is not an action on behalf of the public, as is a criminal prosecution, and cannot result in the loss of liberty, as in a criminal case. The same act, however, can be both a crime against the state and a tort against an individual. For a discussion, see id. at 7–14.
4. Contracts are entered into by the exercise of free will between competent and consenting parties; torts arise by action of law where there is a breach of duty that is the legal cause of an injury. See id. at 4–7.
5. For a brief discussion of the historical development of tort law, see id. at 19–23 and 28–31.
6. Id. at 28.
7. Id. at 29.
8. For another review of the evolution of negligence, see Reed, E.A., Understanding Tort Law: The Historic Basis of Medical-Legal Liability, *Legal Aspects of Medical Practice*, vol. 5, no. 10, 1977, pp. 50–52.
9. Prosser expresses the development of strict liability theory as follows: "The courts have in effect recognized a new doctrine, that the defendant's enterprise, while it will be tolerated by the law, must pay its way." Prosser, supra note 1, at 494.
10. For a trial lawyer's view of strict liability, especially as it is applied to defective products (a category that includes defective ophthalmic lenses), see Belli, M., *My Life On Trial*, Popular Library, New York, 1977.
11. One who enjoys a relationship of trust and confidence with another is in the position of a fiduciary and owes a duty to the other to make no misrepresentations either by misstating known facts or by withholding information necessary for the formulation of an informed decision. For a discussion, see Holder, A., *Medical Malpractice Law*, Wiley & Sons, New York, 1975, pp. 225–234.
12. For an enuciation of this policy, see *Schloendorff v. Society of New York Hospital*, 211 N.Y. 125, 105 N.E. 92 (1914).
13. Informed consent has been widely discussed in various medical journals. A review can be found in the Law and Medicine series of the *Journal of the American Medical Association*. See the following editions of the journal: Informed Consent, Part I, vol. 214, no. 6, Nov. 9, 1970, pp. 1181–1182; Informed Consent, Part II, vol. 214, no. 7, Nov. 16, 1970, pp. 1383–1384; Informed Consent, Part III, vol. 214, no. 8, Nov. 23, 1970, pp. 1611–1612; More on Informed Consent, Part I, vol. 224, no. 13, June 25, 1973, pp. 1831–1832; and More on Informed Consent, Part II, vol. 225, no. 1, July 2, 1973, pp. 95–96.
14. Prosser, supra note 1, at 31.
15. *Black's Law Dictionary*, 4th ed., West, St. Paul, Minn., 1968.
16. Prosser, supra note 1, at 30.
17. The application of negligence and other tort law to optometry comes long after cases involving physicians and other members of the healing arts. Medical malpractice law has a direct influence upon optometry and is the source of many legal principles that affect the profession. For an excellent background text on medical malpractice law, see Holder, supra note 11.
18. *Pike v. Honsinger*, 49 N.E. 760 (N.Y. 1898).
19. Prosser, supra note 1, at 143.
20. Prosser, supra note 1, at 149–150, describes the reasonable person in the following terms:

    The whole theory of negligence presupposes some uniform standard of behavior. Yet the infinite variety of situations which may arise makes it impossible to fix definite rules in advance for all conceivable human conduct. The utmost that can be done is to devise something in the nature of a formula, the application of which in each particular case must be left to the jury, or to the court. The standard of conduct which the community demands must be an external and an objective one, rather than the individual judgment, good or bad, of the particular actor; and it must be, so far as possible, the same for all persons, since the law can have no favorites. At the same time, it must make proper allowance for the risk apparent to the actor, for his capacity to meet it, and for the circumstances under which he must act.

21. The rules of evidence have traditionally required testimony to be limited to those individuals who are from the same "school" as the defendant, which has served as a potential barrier to physician testimony concerning optometric standards of care. See *Sims v. Callahan*, 112 So.2d 776. (Ala. 1959) for an example case. In many jurisdictions, however, the rules of evidence have become increasingly liberal, and cross-profession testimony is much more likely today than in the past. For example, an osteopath was permitted to testify as to the standard of care expected of a physician in *Harris v. Bales*, 459 S.W.2d 742 (Mo. App. 1970). But if an expert witness is not familiar with the standards applicable to another profession, then the expert's testimony as to the standard of care may be barred. See *Botehlo v. Bycura*, 320 S.E.2d 59 (S.C. App. 1984), in which an orthopedic surgeon was held to be unqualified to testify concerning the standard of care expected of a podiatrist. For an example case in which physician testimony was allowed to establish the standard of care expected of an optometrist, see *Fairchild v. Brian*, 354 So.2d 675 (La. App. 1977).
22. *Hoffman v. Houston Clinic*, 41 S.W.2d 134 (Tex. Civ. App. 1931).
23. Prosser, supra note 1, at 162–163.
24. Ibid.
25. *Wohlert v. Seibert*, 23 Pa. Super. 213 (Pa. 1903).
26. *Smith v. Mallinckrodt Chemical Works*, 212 Mo. App. 158, 251 S.W. 155 (1923).
27. For a general discussion of the locality rule and its effect on medical malpractice cases, see Holder, note 11 supra, pp. 53–55.
28. For example, in Alabama after more than seventy years of observance, the locality rule was discarded in favor of a national medical community. See Classe, J., *Zills v. Brown*: A New Standard for Doctors in Alabama?, *Alabama Trial Lawyers Journal*, vol. 8, no. 2, Fall 1980, pp. 4–11.
29. Professor Prosser, supra note 1, at 236–237, describes the concept of proximate cause in part as follows:

"Proximate cause"—in itself an unfortunate term—is merely the limitation which the courts have placed upon the actor's responsibility for the consequences of his conduct. In a philosophical sense, the consequences of an act go forward to eternity, and the causes of an event go back to the discovery of America and beyond. "The fatal trespass done by Eve was cause of all our woe." But any attempt to impose liability upon such a basis would result in infinite liability for all wrongful acts, and would "set society on edge and fill the courts with endless litigation." As a practical matter, legal responsibility must be limited to those causes which are so closely connected with the result and of such significance that the law is justified in imposing liability. Some boundary must be set to liability for the consequences of any act, upon the basis of some social idea of justice or policy.

30. The evidence offered by the plaintiff must carry the greater weight compared to the evidence offered by the defendant in order for the jury to grant a judgment in favor of the plaintiff. This is a far less stringent burden than in a criminal case, where the evidence against the accused must be so strong that jurors must not harbor even a reasonable doubt in order to return a verdict of guilty.
31. *Hawkins v. Richardson*, 29 Ill. App. 3rd 597, 331 N.E.2d 201 (1975).
32. Physician testimony is routinely found in malpractice cases involving optometrists since expert testimony is required to establish the injury suffered by the plaintiff patient. Such a physician may also be asked the standard of care applicable under the circumstances, which establishes the contestable legal issue as to whether the physician's testimony on this question is admissible. For a discussion, see "Competency of Physician or Surgeon of School of Practice Other Than That to Which Defendent Belongs to Testify in Malpractice Case," 85 A.L.R.2d 1022.
33. Nominal damages, to vindicate some technical right, will not be permitted if no actual injury has occurred. Similarly, the threat of a future injury is not sufficient to satisfy the proof of damages. In a few cases, iatrogenic disorders (psychiatric disorders caused by the doctor) have been recognized as valid causes of action. See *Ferrara v. Galluchio*, 5 N.Y.2d 16, 152 N.E.2d 249 (1958). Contra: *Morgan v. Aetna Casualty Company*, 185 F. Supp. 20 (D.C. La. 1960); *Kraus v. Spielberg*, 37 Misc. 2d 519, 236 N.Y.S.2d 143 (1962); and *Winik v. Jewish Hospital of Brooklyn*, 31 N.Y.2d 936, 293 N.E.2d 95 (1972).
34. In the past few years various states have enacted statutes that limit the amounts that juries may award for noneconomic injuries, i.e., for pain and suffering. Judicial review has upheld the right of legislatures to limit this type of injury in malpractice cases. See Gold, A.R., Malpractice Reform, *Journal of the American Optometric Association*, vol. 58, no. 12, Dec. 1987, pp. 1000–1003.
35. For optometrists, the most significant type of malpractice case—in terms of damages—involves allegations of failure to diagnose a tumor. See Gerber, P., How to Blow Your Own Malpractice Defense, *Optometric Management*, vol. 17, no. 7, 1981, pp. 19–25.
36. The value of an eye has already reached seven figures. An award of more than $1 million resulted from an on-

the-job injury to a 23-year-old railroad worker in 1977. See "Worker Who Lost Eye Wins $1 Million Award," *St. Louis Post-Dispatch*, June 30, 1981.

37. For a discussion, see Prosser, supra note 1, at 9–14.
38. The author is unaware of any case in which punitive damages have been awarded against an optometrist for an act of malpractice. For a case involving punitive damages awarded against an ophthalmologist, see *Graham v. Whitaker*, 321 S.E.2d 40 (S.C. 1984).
39. *Peddicord v. Lieser*, 105 P.2d 5 (Wash. 1940).

Chapter 19

Optometric Malpractice

The first thing we do, let's kill all the lawyers.
—William Shakespeare, *King Henry VI, Part II*

Current Status

One of the most perplexing aspects of being a professional is embodied in the word *malpractice*. The word has a stigma that is well captured by the following definition: "Any professional misconduct, unreasonable lack of skill or fidelity in professional or fiduciary duties, evil practice, or illegal or immoral conduct."[1]

The connotations of words like evil, illegal, and immoral are of something that verges on criminality, but medical malpractice is *not* a criminal offense; it is a tort—the tort of medical negligence—and, therefore, it is an aspect of the civil law.

Malpractice has a long history. The first recorded case occurred in England in 1374 and involved a physician[2]; the first recorded U.S. case occurred in 1794 in the state of Connecticut.[3] (It is arguable whether Shakespeare's advice, if taken at that time, would have prevented the subsequent developments in American jurisprudence that culminated in the 1970s with the much-discussed malpractice crisis. In any event, Shakespeare's comment was manifestly impractical.)

Optometry did not achieve legal recognition in the United States until the 20th century; as a result, allegations of malpractice against optometrists have been a recent legal phenomenon. The first precedent-setting case against an optometrist occurred in 1939 in Alabama, at a time when the law of medical malpractice was well settled, and resulted in optometrists being treated like other practitioners within the healing arts by the courts.[4] In the half a century that has followed, both the number and the sophistication of claims have increased steadily with each passing decade. The underlying cause has been the profession's technological advancement and change in philosophy.

Optometric liability over the past four decades is directly related to these developments: In the 1940s optometrists were still concerned solely with the fitting of glasses; there were no instruments that touched the patient's eye and there was little opportunity for injury outside of an incorrect prescription, a defective lens, or a poor spectacle fit. A survey of malpractice claims that was conducted in the latter part of the decade (1948) revealed that the largest paid claim was a mere \$1,859.[5] The reported claims themselves reflect the limited exposure to malpractice afforded the practitioners of the day (see Table 19.1).

The latter three claims in Table 19.1 are representative of the undercurrent of liability for misdiagnosis and failure to refer that has grown in importance with each passing decade to become the leading cause of professional liability within optometry.

By the 1950s, contact lenses had begun to emerge as a satisfactory alternative to spectacles for a significant portion of the U.S. population, and optometrists began to provide contact lens services, which for the first time required the use of objects that came

Table 19.1. Survey of Malpractice Claims Against Optometrists: 1948

Claims that a fall downstairs resulted from improper lenses having been furnished
Claims that the glasses produced dizziness
Claims that the patient's nose was injured when struck by an examining instrument
Claims that the delay in having the prescription for the glasses made up caused injury
Claims that the patient's temples and ears were infected by the eyeglass frames
Claims that the patient was unable to read the papers on a desk while standing erect
Claims that the acid used in soldering glasses blistered the patient's eyes
Claims that the optometrist failed to recognize the presence of ocular pathology
Claims that the optometrist, having recognized the presence of ocular pathology, failed to advise the patient to seek other professional care and advice
Claims that the optometrist, having recognized the presence of ocular pathology, failed to inform the patient and, instead, furnished glasses to improve vision, so that the patient was unaware that his pathological condition was becoming worse under the false security that the improved vision furnished

Source: Hofstetter, H.W., *Optometry: Professional, Economic, and Legal Aspects*, C.V. Mosby, St. Louis, 1948.

in physical contact with the eye. A survey of claims in 1960[6] found that, although more than one half of all optometric malpractice claims were still related to errors in refraction and to spectacle lens breakage, 10 percent of claims were due to contact lenses. Contact lens claims fell into three categories[7]:

CLAIM	PERCENT
Injuries incurred from wearing the lenses	47
Injuries incurred from fitting the lenses	32
Other injuries (patient dissatisfaction, lost time from work, and similar causes)	20

Another persistent source of injury—patient falls—accounted for 4 percent of the claims surveyed in 1960.[8]

During the 1960s, the number of claims filed against optometrists increased by one-third, with the average cost per claim escalating by an even greater 52 percent (from $1,565 to $2,375).[9] There were two reasons for this upward trend: contact lenses, which accounted for 37 percent of the total number of cases by the decade's end (compared to 10 percent at the start)[10] and tonometry, which launched optometry on the road to becoming a health-care profession and which further increased the opportunity for ocular injury since the technique required touching the patient's eyes with an instrument. Tonometry—although not historically an aspect of optometry—was clearly needed by the public, and optometrists, due to their numbers and distribution, were the appropriate ones to perform the service.

Tonometry claims began to assert themselves as a source of litigation in the 1960s. Claims did not arise merely because of an injury received during the performance of tonometry but also because of failure on the part of optometrists to perform the test at all.[11]

Other, less consequential, causes of injury were patient falls, shattering lenses or flammable frames (e.g., product liability claims), incorrect spectacle corrections causing alleged visual impairment, and laceration of the eyes from optometric equipment or while fitting frames to the patient's face.[12]

The passage of diagnostic and therapeutic drug laws signaled a new direction for optometry and a new source of liability for optometrists. The decade of the 1970s was a tumultuous period in many respects, and the issue of professional liability was one of the most hotly contested problems of the era,[13] with even optometrists drawn into the *angst* of defending malpractice cases.[14] Professional liability insurance premiums and liability claims for physicians escalated at an unprecedented rate, engendering an acrimonious debate among the legal and medical professions and the insurance industry.

During the 1970s a number of important surveys were performed to investigate the extent of the malpractice problem,[15] and for the first time comprehensive statistics were compiled for study. States enacted a variety of legislation that was intended to afford physicians more protection from malpractice claims and to limit the size of malpractice awards, but claims continued to proliferate despite these efforts.[16]

Perhaps the most comprehensive and unbiased of the studies undertaken during the 1970s was performed by the National Association of Insurance Commissioners (NAIC). Malpractice claims against optometrists were miniscule compared to the judgments and settlements that accumulated against physicians; claims against optometrists averaged about one fourth in terms of dollars compared to those filed against ophthalmologists ($6,640 compared to $23,171).[17] The malpractice studies clearly indicated that litigation initiated against physicians based upon allegations of improper diagnosis increased substantially during the 1970s[18] (see Table 19.2). Although errors related to treatment (surgical

Table 19.2. Errors Alleged in Malpractice Claims: 1970–1978

Study	% Claims Due to Errors in Diagnosis	% Claims Due to Errors in Treatment	% Claims Due to Drug Side Effects	% Claims Due to Other Causes
Malpractice Commission (1970)	14	86	—	—
St. Paul Insurance Company (1973–1978)	25	50	3	22
National Association of Insurance Commissioners (1975–1978)	27	45	10	18

errors primarily) remained the largest category of claims, diagnostic errors had doubled by the decade's end.

This trend was also reflected in malpractice claims involving optometrists. The most commonly alleged error for optometrists was misdiagnosis.[19] Even so, optometry's posture is quite good when seen in context, compared to that of its sister profession, ophthalmology, and other health-care professions (Table 19.3).

The study conducted by the National Association of Insurance Commissioners reviewed 71,788 malpractice claims reported by 128 insurors during a $3\frac{1}{2}$ year period (1975–1978). The claims reported to the NAIC included those filed against physicians, dentists, optometrists, and virtually every other category of health care practitioner (including ancillary personnel). The statistical findings of the study are interesting in several respects, particularly those pertaining to indemnity paid, comparisons of claims by specialty, distribution of claims, final disposition of claims, and time required to close claims. These findings are summarized in Table 19.4.

Table 19.3. Comparison of Malpractice Claims by Profession: 1975–1978

Profession	No. of Claims	Average Indemnity per Claim ($)	Average Expense per Claim ($)
Dentists	329	7,523	2,162
Chiropractors	114	14,396	4,083
Podiatrists	46	11,327	2,064
Optometrists	40	6,627	2,249
Ophthalmologists	354	23,171	4,395

Source: National Association of Insurance Commissioners, 1980.

The total amount of indemnity paid during the study—$876 million—was recouped by insurers through the escalation of professional liability insurance premiums. Despite the upward trend of premiums, optometrists fared considerably better than did ophthalmologists. Statistics compiled during the years of the NAIC study illustrate the significantly different premiums paid by the two professions: Ophthalmologists paid twenty-two times the amount that optometrists did for professional liability insurance premiums in 1975; by 1978 this figure had become nearly twenty-five times as large. As a result, malpractice insurance premiums for ophthalmologists were considerably higher in terms of percent of gross expense (3 to 5 percent of gross income) than were the corresponding premiums for optometrists (less than 1 percent of gross income) (see Table 19.5).[20]

These trends have continued into the 1980s. A review of malpractice claims filed against optometrists during the period 1977 to 1986 determined that errors of diagnosis—particularly failure to detect open-angle glaucoma, ocular tumors, and retinal detachment—have become the leading source of large claims.[21] Contact lenses and ophthalmic pharmaceutical agents constituted additional important sources of litigation. Although the cost of professional liability insurance coverage for optometrists has continued to increase, the cost of insurance as a percentage of gross income has remained well below 1 percent, and thus has continued to be far less expensive than the premiums paid by ophthalmologists.[22]

Despite the upward trend of professional liability premiums, they cost no more for optometrists who practice in states that permit the use of therapeutic pharmaceutical agents than for optometrists who practice in states that allow diagnostic drug use only[23] (see Table 19.6).

Table 19.4. Summary of Findings—National Association of Insurance Commissioners: 1980

Indemnity Paid

There were 71,788 claims, which resulted in the payment of $876 million in indemnity by the reporting insurors. During the $3\frac{1}{2}$ years of the study (1975 to 1978), the average award per injury increased 70 percent, from $26,565 to $45,187, and even after adjustment for inflation the average indemnity showed an increase of 42 percent. In 1975 only five awards of $1 million or more were reported, in 1978 there were 23 paid claims equal to or surpassing the $1,000,000 mark (three out of every one thousand paid claims). These statistics indicate a definite upward trend in the dollar amount of paid claims.

There were 47 reported claims against optometrists; the total indemnity paid on these claims was $312,000, an average of $6,640 per claim. Only two of the paid claims involving optometrists were in excess of $50,000.

Comparisons of Claims by Speciality

Interestingly, optometrists incurred a far smaller number of claims (47) than did ophthalmologists (354), despite the fact that there are more than twice as many optometrists rendering eye care in the United States. The average indemnity paid by ophthalmologists ($23,171) was 3.5 times the average indemnity paid by optometrists ($6,640). Even for common nonsurgical procedures that the two professions share there was an important difference: the average indemnity paid by ophthalmologists ($12,779) was almost double that of optometrists ($6,640). The total indemnity of $8,203,000 resulting from the 354 claims against ophthalmologists was more than 26 times the total indemnity of $312,000 resulting from the 47 claims against optometrists.

Distribution of Claims

The distribution of claims for all years, when broken down into types of allegation, showed that the most commonly cited error was an improperly performed procedure, followed by diagnostic errors, drug injuries, falls, and other events or causes. For optometrists the most common claim was misdiagnosis.

Final Disposition of Claims

The percent of claims paid increased over the $3\frac{1}{2}$ years of the study from 37 to 39 percent. Therefore, greater than 6 out of every 10 cases filed were resolved in favor of the defendant.

Of the less than four out of every ten claims that were resolved in favor of the plaintiff, 94 percent were settled, and only 4 percent actually resulted in court dispositions. (The 4 percent of these claims that were resolved in court resulted in payments to plaintiffs that were 2.8 times higher than the claims that were settled by the parties themselves.)

Litigation was, for the most part, a minor part of the disposition of the 71,788 claims reported during the course of the study. In 1975, at the beginning of the study, only 7 percent of all medical malpractice claims were disposed of in courts of law; this percentage did increase each year, until by 1978 the percent of claims resolved by litigation had risen to 18 percent. The reason for this rise was the remarkable success of defendants who chose to go to court: in 1975 defendant doctors won 8 out of every 10 (82%) of reported court cases, and by 1978 this percentage had risen even higher, to 9 out of every 10 (89%). Once a doctor went to court his chances of receiving a verdict in his favor were quite good.

Time Required to Close Claims

The time required to close a claim depended upon whether it was one in which indemnity was paid or one which was closed without payment. For paid claims, at the outset of the study 37 months were required in order to close the claim; by the end of the study this period had increased to 46 months. For claims in which there was no indemnity paid to the plaintiff, the period of time from initiation of the claim to closure was 26 months at the start of the study and 38 months by the study's conclusion.

Source: National Association of Insurance Commissioners, 1980.

Table 19.5. National Average for Malpractice Premiums by Specialty for a Standard Policy: 1975–1978

Specialty	1975 ($)	1976 ($)	1977 ($)	1978 ($)
Ophthalmology	2,290	3,109	3,578	4,160*
Optometry	104†	124†	148†	168†

Source: Health Care Financing Administration, 1979.
*Source: *Medical Economics*, January 22, 1979.
†Source: Aetna Life and Casualty Company, 1980.

Sources of Cases and Claims

Allegations of malpractice involving optometrists have risen in the 1980s, and there are certain areas of practice in which optometrists are clearly most at risk to incur a claim. The most frequent source of large claims against optometrists involves allegations of misdiagnosis of disease.

Misdiagnosis

Liability for misdiagnosis can arise under either of two circumstances: failure to detect a disease that the patient actually has or diagnosis of a disease that the patient does not have. In making a diag-

Table 19.6. Costs of Professional Liability Policies for Optometrists for $1,000,000 of Coverage: 1986

State	Cost ($)
"Diagnostic" States	
Alabama	360
Arizona	540
Arkansas	360
California	450
Colorado	450
Connecticut	450
Delaware	450
District of Columbia	540
Georgia	360
Hawaii	360
Idaho	450
Illinois	450
Kansas	360
Louisiana	360
Maine	450
Massachusetts	360
Michigan	450
Minnesota	450
Mississippi	360
Montana	450
Nevada	450
New Hampshire	540
New Jersey	540
New York	540
North Dakota	450
Ohio	360
Oregon	450
Pennsylvania	540
South Carolina	360
Tennessee	360
Texas	450
Utah	450
Vermont	360
Virginia	360
Washington	450
Wisconsin	450
Wyoming	360
"Therapeutic" States	
Florida	450
Indiana	360
Iowa	450
Kentucky	360
Missouri	450
Nebraska	360
New Mexico	540
North Carolina	360
Oklahoma	360
Rhode Island	450
South Dakota	450
West Virginia	450
"Drugless" States	
Alaska	450
Maryland	450

Source: Poe and Associates, 1986.

nosis of a patient's condition, a doctor is expected to possess and employ the same degree of skill, care, and knowledge that a reasonable, prudent doctor would have used under the same or similar circumstances. This means that a patient is entitled to an ordinarily careful and thorough examination, given the particular circumstances, the condition of the patient, and the doctor's opportunity to examine the patient. A duly careful doctor will use the degree of thoroughness that is appropriate and possible under the circumstances, and as long as he has complied with recognized standards that would be exercised by like doctors under the same or similar circumstances, he will not be held liable merely because he failed to discover something during the course of his examination.[24] Determining the recognized standards, however, may be a difficult and complex task.

If a doctor, as an aid to reaching a diagnosis, does not seek to make use of the scientific means and facilities available to him for the assimilation of an adequate data base, then the result is no longer an error of judgment but rather a negligent failure to secure an adequate factual basis upon which to support his diagnosis. This opens up a veritable Pandora's Box of legal problems for optometrists in states where diagnostic pharmaceuticals are permitted and where there are optometrists who choose not to avail themselves of their use. What would be the outcome in a case where the optometrist misdiagnoses a condition that he otherwise could have correctly identified had he used the appropriate diagnostic agent? A physician has the responsibility to keep up with the advances in medicine; would not an optometrist have a similar obligation to keep up with the latest advances in optometry?

The principle of due care (which is discussed in Chapter 18) requires that a doctor possess that degree of skill and learning that is ordinarily possessed by members of his profession in good standing. One important aspect of this standard is the requirement that the doctor keep up with the latest advances within the profession.[25]

A patient being treated by a physician began to experience difficulties with his vision. Despite these difficulties the doctor continued to prescribe the medication. The medical literature was replete with references to the medication's visual side effects and indicated that use of the medication should be terminated if vision problems began. The patient eventually lost the sight of one eye and sued the physician. The jury ruled in his favor and the doctor appealed. In upholding the verdict against the physician, the appellate court observed, "A physician impliedly represents that he is keeping abreast of the literature and that he has adopted those techniques which have become standard in his line of practice."[26]

There are two areas of applicability: (1) failure to keep up with the degree of knowledge that is ordinarily possessed by members of the profession and (2) failure to adopt those standard techniques that are performed by members of the profession.

It seems illogical that this concept would not also apply to optometrists, and it is certainly feasible that, under the appropriate factual situation, a court would rule that an optometrist is under a legal obligation to render treatment to his patients based upon an adequate understanding of new developments in the profession.

A possible defense to such a situation would be that even though the treatment given was not in line with new developments, it was in conformity with the customary and approved practice of the particular locality. Hence the optometrist would try to show that he was following the practices and treatment methods commonly utilized by his peers. This defense may not be sufficient, however, because in recent years the courts have held that if the local custom is in fact negligent, the argument that is widespread offers no defense from liability.[27] By example, if no optometrists in a particular locality test for glaucoma, that custom would not be sufficient of itself to avoid liability if an individual patient suffered vision loss due to the optometrist's failure to detect the disease because he did not test for it.

Another defense that could be offered would be the argument that the failure to offer the test or technique was in keeping with the standard of care exercised by a respectable minority of practitioners within the profession. Whether or not this defense would supercede the obligation to use all available diagnostic tests (e.g., to keep up with the latest advances) is debatable.[28]

To date there have been no cases involving optometrists' failure to keep up with professional advances, but as more sophisticated instrumentation is adopted for use in private practice, and as more practitioners employ ophthalmic pharmaceutical agents, the possibility that failure to keep abreast of new developments will become a legal issue increases.

Misdiagnosis claims against optometrists most frequently arise from a failure to determine that the patient has a condition which requires referral. If the condition is a serious one the damages can be substantial.

A patient complaining of "tired eyes" was examined by an optometrist, who detected "spots or opacities" in the lens of each eye. The patient alleged the optometrist told her there was evidence of incipient cataract and that he would refer her to a physician when it was appropriate, in two or three years. The optometrist prescribed glasses and the patient purchased them, but they did not alleviate her symptoms and so she consulted an ophthalmologist eleven days later. The physician diagnosed uveitis and hospitalized and treated the patient, but she ultimately suffered a bilateral loss of visual acuity. She sued the optometrist for malpractice, alleging misdiagnosis. The physician testified at the trial that, had he seen the patient at the time of the optometrist's examination, he could have averted much of the patient's vision loss. The optometrist defended the claim by asserting that he had told the patient she should be seen by an ophthalmologist, but the patient denied the optometrist's averral and the jury awarded her $80,000.[29]

The leading cause of large claims alleging misdiagnosis is failure to diagnose open-angle glaucoma (discussed separately in Chapter 23). Other large claims involve failure to diagnose ocular tumors (Chapter 24), and failure to diagnose retinal detachment (Chapter 25). Other sources of claims involve ocular foreign bodies (Chapter 26), ophthalmic materials (Chapters 27 and 30), and ophthalmic drugs (Chapter 28).

Misdiagnosis is inextricably linked with failure to refer; the two causes of action are virtually always alleged together.

Failure to Refer

An optometrist who has performed an examination that is in compliance with the recognized standards expected of a reasonable practitioner (see Chapter 18), and who does not detect any pathology, may be absolved from any responsibility for negligence even though pathology is in fact present.[30] But an optometrist who recognizes pathology and does not refer the patient to the appropriate specialist will almost certainly be found liable for negligence.[31]

A patient came to an optical shop to purchase some glasses. Because the optometrist who usually worked there was on vacation, the optician in charge sent the patient to a nearby optometrist for refraction and examination. The optometrist detected a small tumor about the size of a pea in the patient's eye but told only the optician of this finding. The patient returned to the optician, who sold him some spectacles but failed to inform him of the tumor. The patient subsequently suffered blindness in the eye and sued the optometrist, the optician, and the optical shop for malpractice. All were found liable for his injury.[32]

Another obvious area of potential litigation involves the timeliness of the referral. If the doctor waits too long to refer, allowing some permanent injury to result, then he will be found liable for the resulting visual loss.

A 12-year-old boy was hit in the eye by a small metal object shot from a rubber band by a playmate. An optometrist examined the boy and allegedly advised his parents either to see a physician or to return to him the following day. The next day the boy returned and was seen by the optometrist's partner, who detected a corneal opacity, contacted an ophthalmologist, and sent the boy to him. The boy suffered a vision loss nevertheless, and the optometrists were sued for failure to refer the patient promptly. The boy's parents refuted the optometrist's contention that they were told to consult a physician, and the doctor's records were void of information and hence of little value on this key point. The suit was settled in favor of the patient for $86,500.[33]

Note that more adequate recordkeeping could have been of great help in defeating this claim. All referrals should be adequately documented so as to leave no room for uncertainty. Poor recordkeeping can of itself so cripple a doctor's defense that he is in essence defeated before the trial even begins. The prudent optometrist will leave nothing to chance and will personally (or through ancillary personnel) contact the doctor to whom the patient is being referred to communicate the reason for referral and to arrange an appointment, document the referral in the patient's record, and request a follow-up communication from the doctor to whom the patient was referred. (For a further discussion of recordkeeping, see Chapter 16.)

Duty to Follow

Just because a doctor has concluded his immediate treatment of a patient, that does not mean his responsibility has ended. In order to terminate his relationship with a patient, the optometrist must obtain the consent of the patient, give the patient sufficient notice of termination so that the patient can obtain another doctor, or determine that the patient is no longer in need of treatment. If information received by the doctor after the patient has been released indicates that further diagnosis or treatment is needed, then the doctor is required to contact the patient and so advise him. And if further treatment is necessary, the patient should be adequately and properly informed by the doctor (and this communication should be documented). In a 1963 case involving an ophthalmologist, this was the key issue.

A patient with a foreign body in one eye went to a hospital emergency room for treatment. He was seen by a general practitioner, who called in an ophthalmologist. X-rays were taken of the patient's eye, but nothing was found. The patient left and was not seen by the two physicians again. The eye became infected and the patient consulted another doctor, who found a piece of steel in the eye and removed it. The patient, however, ultimately went blind in the eye as a result of the infection. He sued the first ophthalmologist who had examined him, alleging insufficient follow-up. The ophthalmologist answered that he had asked the patient to return the next day so that he could again try to locate the foreign body, but the patient denied this allegation and maintained that he had specifically asked the ophthalmologist if it was necessary for him to return and the physician had said it was not.[34]

If a patient is scheduled for re-examination, the doctor's daily appointment logbook and—if possible—the patient's record should reflect this fact. Often a busy practitioner does not have the time to make these entries. In this event the doctor may delegate the responsibility to an office assistant.

Doctors who are to be absent from their offices for a lengthy period of time need to arrange for a substitute to see those patients requiring follow-up. A doctor should carefully document all instances in which follow-up has been delegated to another practitioner.[35]

Failure to follow-up can, in rare cases, lead to a claim of abandonment (see Chapter 13).[36]

Claims Procedure

Every optometrist should be aware of the procedures that will be followed by his insurer in the event a claim is filed (or if there is the possibility that a claim will be filed). Since insurers differ with respect to the manner in which they manage claims, individual optometrists should consult with their agents to inquire about company policy; the following comments are intended to serve as a general description of the liability claims process.[37]

If an optometrist is served with a summons and complaint, he should immediately notify his insurer that a lawsuit has been filed against him. If an incident occurs that could potentially form the basis for a claim, the optometrist should likewise contact his insurer and report the incident. In either case, the report should be given either to the agent from whom liability insurance was purchased or to the nearest claims office operated by the insurer.

The insurer will be obligated to investigate the claim or potential claim, and an investigator will be assiged to collect all the available facts and to assemble them into a report. While conducting this investigation the patient record will be examined and the optometrist will be interviewed. The investigator's report will be reviewed by the insurer's claims staff and, in most cases, by a specialist consultant, and ultimately the insurer will decide whether the claim states a cause of action for which there may be liability. If the insurer feels that the optometrist may be liable, the case will be discussed with the optometrist and a decision concerning settlement of the claim will be sought. The optometrist can retain his own personal counsel to participate in these discussions and to advise him as to the advisability of settling the claim.

If the decision is to settle the claim, the insurer will negotiate with the plaintiff over the amount to be paid as damages. If the insurer and the plaintiff do not reach agreement, the claim will have to be litigated. Even if a claim does go to court, that is no bar to settlement. The lawsuit can be settled at any time during the trial; it can even be settled after the jury has returned a verdict (for example, a case that is likely to be appealed or has been appealed).

If the claim is such that the insurer feels it has no merit, a decision will be made to defend the case. In this event there is a strong likelihood that the claim will end up in court, particularly if the optometrist is strongly opposed to any settlement (even for nuisance value). Although professional liability policies have traditionally required the consent of the policy holder in order to settle a claim, most insurance companies no longer include this provision in their policies. Consequently, an optometrist cannot prevent the settlement of a claim under such a policy by demanding to have his day in court.

At the trial, the optometrist will be represented by attorneys who are paid by the insurer. The optometrist may also wish to have his own personal attorney represent him in court, but he must pay for his attorney's services himself. When an optometrist is sued for an amount that is in excess of his professional liability coverage (which should not occur given the relatively inexpensive umbrella coverage currently available), he should strongly consider retaining his own attorney, since the insurance company represents his interests only up to the limits of his policy and any excess judgment or settlement must be paid from his own personal resources.

Defenses

If an optometrist decides to go to court, it will be necessary to plead and establish a defense. The first (and most common) way to defeat the claim is to show that one of the elements of malpractice cannot be proven: that there was no negligence, no compensable injury to the patient, or no legal relationship between the treatment given and the injury alleged by the patient. The burden is on the plaintiff-patient to prove his case beyond a reasonable probability. If he can do so, then the defendant doctor attempts to rebut the case by offering a defense. (The progression of a civil lawsuit through the legal process is discussed in Chapter 33.)

There are several defenses that can be used by a defendant doctor. The following paragraphs focus on four of them: contributory negligence, assumption of risk, statutes of limitation, and *res judicata*.

Contributory Negligence

In some cases a defendant doctor in a malpractice suit may be able to show that a patient contributed to his own injury, and when such conduct can be proven, it is termed *contributory* negligence. The conduct must contribute as a legal cause to the injury that the patient suffers and must be such that it falls below the standard to which the patient is required to conform for his own protection.[38] In some states, even though a doctor was in fact negligent, contributory negligence on the part of the patient will prevent him from recovering damages and so defeat the malpractice suit. In the eyes of the law, both parties are considered to be at fault.

Contributory negligence is governed by the very same set of standards as is negligence. A patient is expected to conform to the same hypothetical standard of conduct that is applied to the doctor, e.g., that of the reasonable person of ordinary prudence under like circumstances.[39] Contributory negligence can consist of a failure to discover or appreciate a risk that would be apparent to a reasonable person, a mistaken or inadvertent means of dealing with the mistake, or an intentional exposure to a known danger. In those states where contributory negligence can be claimed, the negligence of the patient—no matter how slight the departure from ordinary standards of conduct—constitutes a complete defense for the doctor. Thus, if contributory negligence is proven, the patient is completely barred from recovering damages.

For contributory negligence to be successful, the defendant doctor must show that the patient's negligence occurred at the same time as his own. If this is established, the patient can recover no damages. But if the patient's negligence occurs *after* the doctor's and is additive so that it serves to worsen the doctor's negligence, then the doctor may still be held liable, but the subsequent negligence of the patient will lessen the amount of damages to be awarded.[40] As a practical matter, negligence concurrent with medical treatment is extremely rare.

A patient was to be given an injection by a physician who was obviously intoxicated. The patient allowed the injection to be given and was injured. He sued the physician for malpractice and the doctor pleaded contributory negligence. The court held that the patient could not recover because a reasonably prudent person would have refused to permit a drunken physician to administer an injection unless it was under dire circumstances, such as an emergency. The concurring negligence of both parties barred recovery of damages.[41]

Although a patient has a duty to follow the reasonable instructions and treatment of his doctor, if a doctor has been negligent the patient may terminate the relationship and seek other care. In fact, it may be contributory negligence on the part of the patient to fail to consult another doctor after negligence has occurred.

A workman got some cement particles in his eyes and sought the services of a physician, who was able to remove some, but not all, of them. The patient was instructed to return to the physician's office, but he was unhappy with the way he had been treated by the doctor and failed to keep the follow-up appointment. His eyes became infected, but he failed to consult another practitioner for three months, at which time he finally sought additional care. Despite the second physician's efforts, he suffered a permanent vision loss. He sued the first doctor for malpractice, alleging that the physician's failure to remove all the cement particles was negligence. The doctor responded by stating that the patient was contributorily negligent in failing to follow his advice to return for further evaluation and in failing to seek any medical care for the three months. The court ruled in favor of the physician, thus precluding the patient from recovering any damages.[42]

For contributory negligence to be proven, the patient's conduct must not only meet the criteria discussed in this section, but also the patient's mental and physical capacity must be such that he is able to understand instructions and to look out for his own safety. His mental and physical conditions are important factors to be weighed heavily by the courts whenever contributory negligence is at issue.[43]

A majority of states[44] have adopted a different principle: *comparative* negligence. The hardship inherent in contributory negligence, in which the entire burden of loss can fall upon the injured party, has been the driving force that has led many states to devise a means of dividing the damages between both parties. The first efforts in this regard were general apportionment statutes,[45] which held that, if a defendant's fault was found by the jury to be twice as great as that of the plaintiff, then the plaintiff—although admittedly negligent himself—could receive two thirds of his damages. Following these early laws, special statutes began to be enacted, holding that the plaintiff could recover where his negligence was not as great as that of the defendant.[46] These statutes and the judicial decisions that followed became known as the partial or modified comparative negligence rules; although they differed slightly from state to state, each was alike because it permitted a plaintiff to recover as long as his share of the fault was not 50 percent or greater.

Finally, the pure form of comparative negligence—in which the relative misconduct of the two parties was truly apportioned—began to appear in various jurisdictions. It permitted a plaintiff as much as 99 percent at fault to recover 1 percent of his damages against a defendant who had negligently injured him.[47] This trend toward liberality in state statutes and decisions permitting comparative negligence can be expected to continue.[48] The effect will be to eradicate gradually a defense that has been successfully used in many professional liability cases, the defense of contributory negligence. It is highly likely that comparative negligence, in one of its forms, will be the law in every jurisdiction in the not-too-distant future.

Assumption of Risk

The nature of the doctor-patient relationship is such that the law places upon the doctor an affirmative duty of disclosure, in order that the less knowledgeable patient may make an intelligent and informed decision as to whether he wishes to undergo the prescribed treatment. This requirement is the doctrine of informed consent, which will be discussed in Chapter 22. As a result of this doctrine, every doctor is under an obligation to explain to his patient the hazards, the possible complications, and both the expected and the unexpected results of treatment, so that the patient can understand the nature of the proposed treatment as well as its inherent risks. A patient who wishes to proceed in the face of an adequate informed consent that some risk is involved is said to have assumed the risk of treatment.[49]

But assumption of risk is rarely used since the patient must be notified of *all* the risks of a treatment plan (even unpreventable results), understand them, and knowingly consent to the plan. To use the defense, all risks must not only be explained but also there must be no negligence on the part of the doctor (no patient assumes the risk that his doctor will be negligent).[50] The doctrine is of obviously limited usefulness but could be applicable in certain circumstances (e.g., against patients who agree to wear experimental contact lenses after a full explanation of possible results have been given to them; see Chapter 30).

Statutes of Limitation

To prevent stale claims and to avoid unduly burdening the courts, limits have been established for the period of time after injury that a malpractice suit may be brought.[51] These limits are obviously needed in malpractice cases since delay seriously affects a court's ability to evaluate a claim fairly. Just as optometry practice acts vary remarkably from state to state, statutes of limitations differ significantly from state to state, depending upon the legal basis for the malpractice claim and the time at which the statute begins to run.

The great majority of malpractice claims are based in tort, for which limitations as short as one year may be imposed, with the most common statute allowing two years before suit will be barred. The following cases illustrate how these statutes are subject to interpretation by the courts.

A 47-year-old man who complained of headaches and sensitivity to bright lights was examined by an optometrist who found no need to change the patient's glasses and dismissed him without treatment. The patient, complaining of the same symptoms, was seen again by the optometrist sixteen months later, at which time bifocals were prescribed, but the patient delayed ordering them for a month. Because the bifocals did not alleviate his complaints, the patient consulted an ophthalmologist. The physician diagnosed the patient as having open-angle glaucoma, and estimated that the disease had been present for eight years. Less than two years after being fitted for the bifocals, but more than two years after the date of the examination, the patient sued the optometrist, who defended on the basis that the claim was barred by the statute of limitations. The court, in applying the two-year statute for malpractice within the state (Idaho), held that the period for filing the suit had expired one month before the suit was filed, using the date of the second examination rather than the date the bifocals were chosen as the day that began the running of the statutorily permissible period.[52]

A patient who complained of difficulties with her vision was examined by an optometrist employed by an optical shop, and the doctor prescribed spectacles and informed her that her visual difficulties would disappear in two weeks. She wore the spectacles for five months but continued to have complaints. She consulted another doctor, who found that she had a detached retina secondary to diabetic retinopathy. She subsequently sued the optometrist and optical shop for failure to diagnose her condition and failure to refer. The complaint was filed fifteen months after the optometrist's examination. The defendants pleaded the statute of limitations as a defense, arguing that she did not bring the case within one year of the examination, as required by the state statute. The state supreme court, however, held that negligence by optometrists did not fall within the one year statute of limitations for medical malpractice actions and applied a two-year statute that pertained to bodily injury instead. The case was remanded to the trial court for further disposition.[53]

Differences among the states as to interpretations of when the statute begins to run can make the period become much longer (see Table 19.7).

An alternative theory of liability is *breach of contract* (see Chapter 13 for a discussion of the con-

Table 19.7. State Statutes of Limitation for Malpractice: 1979

State	Statute of Limitation for Malpractice Actions	Statute of Limitation for Malpractice Actions Brought by Minors
Alabama	2 years from occurrence, or 6 months after discovery, if no more than 4 years after occurrence	If under 4, until 8th birthday; otherwise, adult law applies
Alaska	2 years from occurrence	2 years from discovery
Arizona	3 years from occurrence	If under 7, period begins at 7 or on death, whichever is first; otherwise, adult law applies
Arkansas	2 years from occurrence	Until 18 plus 1 year
California	1 year from discovery, but no more than 3 years from occurrence	3 years from occurrence or prior to 8th birthday, whichever is longer
Colorado	2 years from discovery, but no more than 3 years from occurrence	If under 6, then 2 years after the minor turns 6; otherwise, 2 years from discovery
Connecticut	2 years from discovery, but no more than 3 years after occurrence	2 years from discovery, but no more than 3 years after occurrence
Delaware	2 years from occurrence, if not reasonably discoverable then 3 years from occurrence	If under 6, then 3 years from occurrence, or until age 6; otherwise, adult law applies
Florida	2 years from discovery, but no more than 4 years from occurrence	2 years from discovery
Georgia	2 years from occurrence	Until 18 plus 2 years
Hawaii	2 years from discovery, but no more than 6 years from occurrence	Until 18 plus 2 years
Idaho	2 years from occurrence	6 years from occurrence
Illinois	2 years from discovery, but no more than 4 years from occurrence	Until 18 plus 2 years
Indiana	2 years from occurrence	If under 6, until 18th birthday; otherwise, adult law applies
Iowa	2 years from discovery	Until 18 plus 1 year
Kansas	2 years from occurrence; if not reasonably discoverable, then 4 years from occurrence	Until 18 plus 1 year
Kentucky	1 year from discovery, but no more than 5 years from occurrence	Until 18 plus 1 year
Louisiana	1 year from occurrence; if not reasonably discoverable, then 3 years from occurrence	Same as for adults, regardless of age
Maine	2 years from occurrence	Until 18 plus 2 years
Maryland	5 years from occurrence or 3 years from discovery, whichever is sooner	Adult limitation period begins at age 16
Massachusetts	3 years from occurrence	If under 6, until 9th birthday; otherwise, adult law applies
Michigan	2 years from occurrence, or 6 months from discovery, whichever is later	Until 18 plus 1 year
Minnesota	2 years from occurrence	Until 18 plus 2 years
Mississippi	2 years from discovery	Until 21 plus 2 years
Missouri	2 years from occurrence	If under 10, until 12th birthday; otherwise, 2 years from occurrence
Montana	3 years from occurrence, or 3 years after discovery, if no more than 5 years after occurrence	Same as for adults, regardless of age
Nebraska	2 years from occurrence; if not reasonably discoverable, then 6 years from occurrence	2 years from occurrence
Nevada	4 years from occurrence	4 years from occurrence
New Hampshire	2 years from occurrence	Until age 8 plus 2 years
New Jersey	2 years from discovery	Until age 23
New Mexico	3 years from occurrence	Until age 6 plus 3 years; otherwise, adult law applies

Table 19.7. *Continued*

State	Statute of Limitation for Malpractice Actions	Statute of Limitation for Malpractice Actions Brought by Minors
New York	30 months from occurrence	10 years from discovery
North Carolina	3 years from occurrence, or 1 year from discovery, if no more than 4 years from occurrence	Until 18 plus 1 year
North Dakota	2 years from discovery, if no more than 6 years after occurrence	Until 18 plus 1 year
Ohio	1 year from discovery, if no more than 4 years after occurrence	If under 10, until 14th birthday; otherwise, adult law applies
Oklahoma	2 years from discovery, if no more than 3 years after occurrence	Until 18 plus 2 years
Oregon	2 years from discovery, if no more than 5 years after occurrence	Until 18 plus 1 year
Pennsylvania	2 years from discovery	2 years from discovery
Rhode Island	2 years from occurrence, or 1 year after discovery, whichever is later	Until 16 plus 1 year
South Carolina	3 years from occurrence, or 3 years from discovery, if no more than 6 years after occurrence	Until 18 plus 1 year
South Dakota	2 years from occurrence	3 years from occurrence unless child is under 6; if under 6, then 2 years after 6th birthday
Tennessee	1 year from occurrence, or 1 year after discovery, if no more than 3 years after occurrence	Until 18 plus 3 years
Texas	2 years from occurrence	If under 12, until 14th birthday; otherwise, adult law applies
Utah	2 years from discovery, if no more than 4 years after occurrence	2 years from discovery
Vermont	7 years from occurrence	Until 18 plus 7 years
Virginia	2 years from occurrence	Until 18 plus 2 years
Washington	3 years from occurrence, or 1 year from discovery, if no more than 8 years after occurrence	Until 18 plus 3 years
Washington, D.C.	3 years from discovery	Until 18 plus 3 years
West Virginia	2 years from discovery	2 years from discovery
Wisconsin	3 years from occurrence	3 years from occurrence or until age 10, whichever is later
Wyoming	2 years from occurrence, or 2 years from discovery, whichever is longer	Until 8th birthday or 2 years from occurrence, whichever is longer

Source: Chapman, S., How Long Should You Keep Your Patients' Records?, *Legal Aspects of Medical Practice*, vol. 7, no. 8, Aug. 1979, pp. 19–38.

tractual nature of the doctor-patient relationship). A breach of contract action offers a plaintiff some advantages: negligence no longer has to be proven, expert testimony is no longer required, and the statute of limitations is much longer. The usual time within which an action for breach of contract must be brought is five to seven years. Each state statute will have to be consulted to know the exact period (see Table 19.8).

Most practitioners think of contracts as written agreements signed by the parties, but implied contracts can form the basis for an action against a doctor by a patient. In some states treatment of a patient by an optometrist, even where there is no express (written) agreement, creates an implied contract in which the doctor impliedly warrants that he possesses the requisite skill to perform the treatment undertaken and that he will exercise ordinary skill and care. This implied contract can be used as the basis of a patient's claim for damages.[54]

Another type of action that can be brought against an optometrist is an action for *wrongful death*,

Table 19.8. State Statutes of Limitation for Contracts: 1976

State	Limitation for Actions Brought for Written Contracts (yrs)
Alabama	6
Alaska	6
Arizona	6
Arkansas	5
California	4
Colorado	6
Connecticut	6
Delaware	3
District of Columbia	3
Florida*	5
Georgia	6
Hawaii	6
Idaho	5
Illinois	10
Indiana	15 (money)
Iowa	10
Kansas	5
Kentucky	15
Louisiana*	10
Maine	6
Maryland	3
Massachusetts	6
Michigan	6
Minnesota	6
Mississippi	6
Missouri	10
Montana	8
Nebraska	5
Nevada	6
New Hampshire	6
New Jersey	6
New Mexico	6
New York	6
North Carolina	3
North Dakota*	10
Ohio	15
Oklahoma	5
Oregon	6
Pennsylvania*	6
Rhode Island	6
South Carolina	6
South Dakota	6
Tennessee	6
Texas	4
Utah	6
Vermont	6
Virginia	5
Washington	6
West Virginia	10
Wisconsin	6
Wyoming	10

*The Uniform Commercial Code provides a 4-year statute of limitations for sales contracts, which is applicable in all states but those marked with an asterisk.

Source: *Credit Manual of Commercial Laws*, 1976.

which is brought by the personal representative of a patient who dies as a result of treatment (or lack of treatment). Wrongful death actions may be permitted even though the statute of limitations for tort might bar a standard malpractice suit.[55] In most cases, however, actions for wrongful death must be brought within one to two years after death or they will be barred by the statute.

Once the correct statute of limitations is known, the key question becomes: When does the statutory period actually begin to run? The states are divided on this question. Some hold that the statute of limitations begins to run on the date of the injury to the patient, while others hold that a later time can start the running of the statute.

A number of courts have held that the statutory period begins to run on the date that the patient is injured, whether or not the patient was put on notice of the malpractice. Other courts have refused to start counting the time until the patient discovered or by the exercise of reasonable diligence should have discovered the doctor's conduct was negligent, which can significantly extend the time limit. In one case, for example, the claim was allowed twenty-three years after the injury.[56] A few courts have held that the statute of limitations does not begin until the course of treatment that includes the wrongful act or omission and that is related to the original condition or complaint is terminated. Therefore, continuing treatment of a patient past the time of the malpractice may not start the statute running.[57]

Fraud (see discussion in Chapter 20) that conceals a negligent act or injury will also delay the running of the statute of limitations.[58]

A relatively recent development may provide a means of clarifying the problem of when a malpractice claim should be barred. At least eleven states[59] have adopted a new type of statute that permits all actions for injury or death brought against health-care practitioners to be filed within a stated period after the date of the discovery of the injury or within another, i.e., longer, stated period after the date of the act that caused the injury.

For example, California law[60] allows a one-year period beginning from the date of the discovery of the malpractice or a three-year period beginning with the date of the act complained of, with the court to apply the period that runs out first. The statute is tolled by only three specific events: fraud, intentional concealment, or foreign objects left within a patient's body. The California law, in effect, imposes an absolute limit of three years on actions for medical malpractice. These statutes might well become the majority in the future.

Res Judicata

Res judicata is Latin for "the thing has been decided." As with other Latin phrases, it has come to represent a doctrine of the law, namely that a legal controversy, once litigated to completion, cannot be the subject of a subsequent suit. For example, once a malpractice case has been adjudicated, the plaintiff cannot reopen the case by filing another suit in a separate jurisdiction or base a second suit between the same parties on the same facts even though a separate cause of action is used (e.g., product liability, warranty).

The usual application of *res judicata* to medical malpractice litigation occurs when a doctor sues a patient to collect an unpaid bill. In such a suit, a patient may claim negligence on the part of the doctor as a defense. If the patient loses the case, he cannot later assert a second malpractice claim against the doctor because "the thing has been decided."[61] If the patient does not plead negligence as a defense, however, he may later bring a suit for malpractice against the doctor.[62]

The converse situation is also upheld. If the patient sues a doctor for malpractice, and the doctor does not—in defending the action—claim the amount of the unpaid bill, when the doctor is awarded a judgment in his favor he cannot later bring a suit to collect the unpaid fee because of *res judicata*. The doctor must claim the amount owed for his services at the time the malpractice claim is litigated.[63]

Res judicata can be applied only if both the parties and the facts in the first action are identically the same as those in the second suit. This rule is usually expressed in terms of evidence: If the evidence necessary to support the first action is the same as the evidence necessary to support the second action, then the second action is barred.

It has been reported by some authorities[64] that a dissatisfied patient who is sued by a doctor for an unpaid bill may assert negligence as a defense or even file a separate malpractice suit in response. Dissatisfied patients who have not paid their bills require careful management by the doctor; litigation should be employed only when clearly appropriate and preferably in those cases in which the prospects of retaliatory legal action are remote.

Countersuit

Much has been written of the success enjoyed by a few doctors who, angered by being unfairly prosecuted in a malpractice case, succeeded in countersuing their former patients and the attorneys who represented them. Indeed, verdicts have escalated quite dramatically since the first such case, *Berlin v. Nathan*, in 1976.

A radiologist took X-rays of a woman's finger, injured during a tennis match. The X-rays did not show a fracture, and so he treated her for a dislocation. She later sued him for $250,000, alleging that his failure to find the fracture created a permanent impairment. The doctor successfully defended on the basis that X-rays were taken correctly, but no fracture was revealed, and that even had a fracture been detected, his treatment would have been the same. The doctor then countersued the patient and her attorney, contending that the malpractice suit had been brought against him without reasonable cause and that the attorney was legally negligent in bringing a suit that had no basis. The jury awarded the doctor $8,000.[65]

The wide publicity given this case created a flood of countersuits nationwide. In the year following the *Berlin* decision more than 100 suits were filed by physicians.[66] Some of them resulted in substantial verdicts.

A patient treated by a doctor after an accident had to return to the hospital two months later for further treatment and suffered bed sores and other minor ailments during his stay in the hospital. A malpractice suit was brought against the physician who had originally treated the patient. The doctor successfully defended the suit and then countersued the lawyer representing the patient, alleging legal negligence in the bringing of the malpractice suit. The doctor was awarded $85,000.[67]

An orthopedic surgeon was sued for malpractice, the suit alleging that he had set the patient's broken arm incorrectly by employing a steel rod implant that was one inch too long. On the day the case was to go to trial, the patient's lawyer dropped the

Table 19.9. Key Points in Avoiding Malpractice

Key Points
Misdiagnosis is the most likely cause of malpractice. Do not permit reduced acuity, visual field loss, diplopia, or other signs or symptoms to go unexplained.
If the case is not one that a practitioner wishes to handle, the patient should be referred to a practitioner who will provide the necessary care. If further diagnostic testing is required (including a dilated fundus examination), be certain that the referral is made before the patient has left the office.
When making a referral, schedule the appointment for the patient and record the doctor, date, and time of the referral. In a busy office, this may best be accomplished by a telephone call by the assistant. If referral is suggested, this fact should always be documented in the patient record.
Document all recall appointments (and patient failures to return as scheduled) in the patient record.
Maintain clear, accurate, contemporaneous patient records at all times.
Obtain written permission before initiating any experimentation with a patient or before releasing any patient information to a third party.
When appropriate, discuss examination findings with the patient, as required by the doctrine of informed consent.
Test for glaucoma on all patients, regardless of age.
Warn all patients with reduced or impaired vision who can be expected to encounter difficulty while driving a vehicle or operating dangerous machinery of the increased risk of injury they face when performing these tasks.
Prescribe polycarbonate plastic when impact resistance is a key clinical consideration, and warn patients of the limited impact resistance of glass and allyl resin lenses.
Verify all orders of ophthalmic materials to ensure that they comply with impact-resistance standards, particularly orders for safety eyewear. Verify all contact lenses prior to dispensing to ensure they are correct.
Select the appropriate ophthalmic drug and adhere to generally accepted standards as to dosage and concentration. Warn of the side effects of drug use as required by the doctrine of informed consent.
Supervise employees adequately and do not permit them to perform duties that they are not qualified to perform.
Routinely inspect equipment and premises to ensure that they are not hazardous to patients and personnel.
Obtain adequate professional liability insurance coverage.

case. The physician countersued for malicious prosecution. The jury awarded him $175,000.[68]

Despite these highly publicized successes, countersuits soon hit a snag. The traditional form of countersuit, which is based upon malicious prosecution, is hampered by a number of legal obstacles. A minority of states require special damages to be proven in malicious prosecution cases, and even states with more liberal laws require that malice be proven, which effectively prevents these suits from being brought there also.[69] The cases cited in this section—and numerous others—although successfully tried, were later reversed by higher courts, which rejected the legal theories on which they were based. To date few appellate courts have upheld decisions in favor of doctors who claimed that they were maliciously prosecuted for malpractice.[70]

But the countersuit movement has probably had some short-term effect, in spite of these reversals in the appellate courts. One study of malpractice cases in the Chicago area showed that 1,499 doctors were defendants in malpractice cases in 1975, before *Berlin* and its progeny, and that this number had declined to 628 by 1977, a reduction of 58 percent.[71] Even so, these highly touted countersuits, plus the many "tort reform" laws enacted during the latter part of the 1970s,[72] have done little to ease malpractice litigation, which has continued to grow during the 1980s.

Avoiding Malpractice

It is hoped that the foregoing discussion of professional liability will be useful to optometrists by enabling them to better understand the intricacies of malpractice law. Awareness of the areas of practice most likely to produce a claim is also valuable because this knowledge enables optometrists to construct a set of guidelines intended to prevent the possibility of injury (see Table 19.9). It should always be remembered, however, that no one is immune from suit. Consequently, optometrists should be certain to obtain the appropriate professional liability insurance (see Chapter 54).

Notes

1. *Black's Law Dictionary*, 4th ed., West, St. Paul, Minn., 1968.
2. Reed, E.A., Understanding Tort Law: The Historic Basis of Medical-Legal Liability, *Legal Aspects of Medical Practice*, vol. 5, no. 10, 1977, pp. 50–52.
3. Ibid.

4. *Hampton v. Brackin's Jewelry and Optical Co., Inc.*, 237 Ala. 212, 186 So. 173 (1939).
5. Hofstetter, H.W., *Optometry: Professional, Economic, and Legal Aspects*, C.V. Mosby Co., St. Louis, 1948, p. 84.
6. Elmstrom, G.P., *Optometric Practice Management*, Chilton, Philadelphia, 1963, p. 217. Also reported in the *Journal of the California Optometric Association*, vol. 28, no. 6, Dec. 1960–Jan. 1961, p. 372.
7. Ibid.
8. Elmstrom, supra note 6, at 214.
9. Morgan, E.H., The Professional Liability Problem and Optometry, *Journal of the American Optometric Association*, vol. 42, no. 2, 1971, pp. 160–164.
10. Ibid.
11. Example tonometry claims are reported in Elmstrom, G.P., *Advanced Management For Optometrists*, Professional Press, Chicago, 1974, p. 402.
12. Morgan, supra note 9.
13. The mounting number of claims prompted the federal government to conduct a study of malpractice in 1971 and resulted in *Medical Malpractice: Report of the Secretary's Commission on Medical Malpractice*, Department of Health, Education and Welfare, Washington, D.C., DHEW publication number (OS) 73-88, released in 1973. This publication describes the issues then confronting the medical profession, issues that—more than a decade later—have not been adequately resolved.
14. An optometric perspective of the malpractice crisis can be found in My Malpractice Nightmare, *Review of Optometry*, vol. 119, no. 12, Dec. 15, 1982, pp. 28–34.
15. Studies were performed by the federal government (*Medical Malpractice: Report of the Secretary's Commission on Medical Malpractice*, Department of Health, Education and Welfare, Washington, D.C., DHEW Publication No. (OS) 73-88, 1973); by St. Paul Fire and Marine Insurance Co. (reported in the *New England Journal of Medicine*, vol. 300, no. 1, Jan. 1979, p. 26); and by the insurance industry at large (National Association of Insurance Commissioners, *Malpractice Claims*, vol. 2, no. 2, Sept. 1980, Madison, Wis.).
16. The legislative effort that began in the late 1970s is discussed by Chapman, S. and F. White, Are the New State Malpractice Laws Working to Protect You?, *Legal Aspects of Medical Practice*, vol. 8, no. 5, 1980, pp. 40–46.
17. *Malpractice Claims*, National Association of Insurance Commissioners, vol. 2, no. 2, Madison, Wis., Sept. 1980.
18. Ibid.
19. Ibid.
20. See Elmstrom, G., Malpractice: What Can O.D.'s Expect?, *Optical Journal and Review of Optometry*, vol. 114, no. 1, 1977, pp. 42–52; and Greenspan, N.T. Medical Malpractice Insurance Premiums, *Group Practice Journal*, vol. 29, no. 6, 1980, pp. 17–25. The *AOA News*, Feb. 15, 1979, reported that optometrists—paying $138 for malpractice coverage—expended only 0.15 percent of median gross income for malpractice coverage. By comparison, the January 22, 1979, issue of *Medical Economics* reported the average premium of $4,160 for ophthalmologists to represent 3.1 percent of gross income; the study by Greenspan cited *supra* maintained that ophthalmologists paid 5 percent of gross income for malpractice coverage.
21. Classe, J., Malpractice and Optometry: A Personal Commentary, *Southern Journal of Optometry*, vol. 5, no. 3, 1987, pp. 26–31. By 1986, the cost of professional liability insurance for AOA-affiliated optometrists was about $450 for a million dollars of coverage, according to a study performed by Poe and Associates. On the other hand, premiums for ophthalmologists had escalated to $7,630. See *Medical Economics* of Nov. 9, 1987, at pp. 190–191.
22. Ibid.
23. Ibid.
24. *Adkins v. Ropp*, 14 N.E.2d 727 (Ind. 1938).
25. See Failure to "Keep Up" as Negligence, in the Law and Medicine series of the *Journal of the American Medical Association*, vol. 224, no. 10, June 4, 1973, p. 1461.
26. *Reed v. Church*, 8 S.E.2d 285 (Va. 1940)
27. *Incollingo v. Ewing*, 444 Pa. 263, 282 A. 2d 206 (1971); *Morgan v. Sheppard*, 188 N.E.2d 808 (Ohio 1963); and *Favalora v. Aetna Casualty Co.*, 144 So. 2d 544 (La. 1962).
28. For an example case involving an ophthalmlogist, see *Sims v. Callahan*, 112 So. 2d 776 (Ala. 1959).
29. *Tempchin v. Sampson*, 262 Md. 156, 277 A.2d 67 (1971).
30. See Misdiagnosis Without Fault: Part I, *Journal of the American Medical Association*, vol. 219, no. 7, Feb. 14, 1972, pp. 967–968; and Misdiagnosis Without Fault: Part II, *Journal of the American Medical Association*, vol. 219, no. 8, Feb. 21, 1972, pp. 1127–1128.
31. For a discussion of misdiagnostic errors in general, as they apply to all forms of medical practitioners, see Holder, A.R., *Medical Malpractice Law*, Wiley and Sons, New York, 1975, pp. 65–96.
32. *Evers v. Buxbaum*, 253 F.2d 356 (D.C. Cir. 1958).
33. Reported in the *AOA News*, June 15, 1976.
34. *Barnes v. Bovenmeyer*, 122 N.W.2d 312 (Iowa 1963).
35. See *Browning v. Hoffman*, 111 S.E. 492 (W.Va. 1922); and Abandonment: Part III, *Journal of the American Medical Association*, vol. 225, no. 11, Sept. 10, 1973, p. 1429.
36. The claim of abandonment is one that does not occur except under exceptional circumstances. In the study of malpractice claims against physicians performed by St. Paul Fire and Marine Insurance Company, the claim of abandonment accounted for only 0.8 percent of claims compiled over a five year period. For a discussion, see Curran, W.J., Malpractice Claims: New Data and New Trends, *New England Journal of Medicine*, vol. 300, no. 1, Jan. 1979, p. 26.
37. See Gerber, P.C., What to Do When a Patient Plans to Sue, *Optometric Management*, vol. 23, no. 5, 1987,

pp. 36–42.

38. For a discussion of contributory negligence as it pertains to malpractice claims, see Holder, supra note 31, pp. 298–306; and the *Journal of the American Medical Association*, Contributory Negligence: Part I, vol. 218, no. 5, Nov. 1, 1971, pp. 785–786; Part II, vol. 218, no. 6, Nov. 8, 1971, pp. 933–934; and Part III, vol. 218, and no. 7, Nov. 15, 1971, pp. 1109–1110.
39. See Prosser, W.L., *Law of Torts*, 4th ed., West, St. Paul, Minn., 1971, pp. 416–427.
40. See Negligence of Patient Subsequent to That of Physician, *Journal of the American Medical Association*, vol. 205, no. 2, July 8, 1968, p. 161.
41. *Champs v. Stone*, 58 N.E.2d 803 (Ohio 1944).
42. *Hanley v. Spencer*, 115 P.2d 399 (Colo. 1941).
43. *Flynn v. Stearns*, 145 A.2d 33 (N.J. 1958); *Steele v. Woods*, 327 S.W.2d 187 (Mo. 1959); *Kent v. County of Hudson*, 245 A.2d 747 (N.J. 1968); *Clark v. Piedmont Hospital*, 162 S.E.2d 468 (Ga. 1968); *Bennett v. New York*, 59 Misc. 2d 306, 299 N.Y.S.2d 288 (N.Y. 1969); and *Our Lady of Mercy Hospital v. McIntosh*, 461 S.W.2d 377 (Ky. 1970).
44. As of 1982, a total of thirty-eight states had adopted at least some form of the comparative negligence doctrine. For a review, see Miller, L.J., Comparative Negligence, in the Law and Medicine series of the *Journal of the American Medical Association*, vol. 248, no. 12, Sept. 24, 1982, p. 1443.
45. See Prosser, supra note 39, at 433–439.
46. Ibid.
47. Ibid.
48. Ibid.
49. Ibid.
50. See Holder, supra note 31, at 225–245.
51. For a discussion of statutes of limitation, see id. at 319–326, and Meotti, M.P., Your State's Cutoff Date on Malpractice Suits May Not Be Cut and Dried, *Legal Aspects of Medical Practice*, vol. 7, no. 8, 1979, p. 34.
52. *Holmes v. Iwasa*, 104 Idaho 179, 657 P.2d 476 (1983).
53. *Whitt v. Columbus Cooperative Enterprises*, 64 Ohio St. 2d 355, 415 N.E.2d 985 (1980).
54. For a discussion of implied contracts and warranties involving health-care practitioners, see Lane, B.J., and H.L. Hirsh, The Broken Promise: Physician's Breach of Warranty, *Case & Comment*, Sept.–Oct. 1984, p. 3.
55. *Smith v. McComb Infirmary Association*, 196 So. 2d 91 (Miss. 1967); and *Klema v. St. Elizabeth's Hospital of Youngstown*, 170 Ohio St. 519, 166 N.E.2d 765 (1960).
56. *Ruth v. Dight*, 453 P.2d 631 (Wash. 1969).
57. New York and Washington are examples. See Meotti, supra note 51.
58. *Toal v. United States*, 438 F.2d 222 (2d Cir. 1971).
59. California, Colorado, Connecticut, Florida, Idaho, Illinois, Montana, Navada, Oregon, Utah, and Washington. This list could be changed by ongoing legislative efforts at tort reform, which affects statutes of limitation. See Meotti, supra note 51.
60. *Cal. Cir. Proc. Code* §340.5 (as amended 1975).
61. *Gates v. Preston*, 41 N.Y. 113 (1869); *Blair v. Bartlett*, 75 N.Y. 150 (1878); and *Lawson v. Conaway*, 16 S.E. 564 (W. Va. 1892).
62. *House v. Hanson*, 72 N.W.2d 874 (Minn. 1955). If a default judgment is obtained by the optometrist in an effort to recover an unpaid bill, the courts have held that the patient has not waived his right to sue the optometrist for negligence at a later time. See *Gwynn v. Wilhelm*, 360 P.2d 312 (Ore. 1961).
63. *Black v. Dillon*, 213 Cal. App. 2d 295, 28 Cal. Rptr. 678 (1963).
64. Elmstrom, G., supra note 11 at 389.
65. *Berlin v. Nathan*, 21 Ill. 682, 64 Ill. App. 3d 940, 381 N.E.2d 1367 (1978). Optometric commentary on the *Berlin* case can be found in Green, D., You Can Fight That Malpractice Suit!, *Optometric Management*, vol. 12, no. 12, 1976, p. 89.
66. Berlin, L., Countersuit, in James, A.E., (ed.), *Legal Medicine*, Urban and Schwarzenberg, Baltimore, 1980, pp. 117–133.
67. Reported in News Briefs, *Journal of Legal Medicine*, vol. 5, no. 6, 1977, p. 57.
68. Reported in News Briefs, *Journal of Legal Medicine*, vol. 5, no. 8, 1977, p. 55.
69. For a discussion of the legal obstacles to be overcome in order to prevail in a countersuit, see Rhem, S.D., and N.L. Trusch, Malicious Prosecution Suits as a Counterbalance to Medical Malpractice Actions, *Journal of Legal Medicine*, vol. 5, no. 8, 1977, p. 43.
70. There have been few exceptions to the trend against countersuits. See Reed, B., Don't Count Out the Countersuit Movement Yet, *Legal Aspects of Medical Practice*, vol. 8, no. 8, 1980, p. 34.
71. Berlin, supra note 66, at 121.
72. See Chapman, S., and F. White, note 16 supra; and Rosenberg, C.I., Why a New Malpractice Crisis Is Coming, *Medical Economics*, vol. 56, no. 22, Oct. 29, 1979, p. 109.

Chapter 20

Intentional Offenses

It's the same old story
Everywhere I go,
I get slandered,
Libeled,
I hear words I never heard
In the Bible.
And I'm so tired,
I'm oh so tired,
But I'm trying to keep my customers satisfied,
Satisfied.
—Paul Simon and Art Garfunkel, "Keep the Customer Satisfied," from *Bridge Over Troubled Water.* © 1970 Paul Simon. Used by permission.

Although the intentional torts do not seem similar at first glance, they are alike in that each requires an intent to perform the act that results in the injury. Unlike negligence, which is concerned with actions that must be measured by a reasonable standard of conduct, the intentional torts use intent as the standard against which conduct is measured.

The most commonly encountered offense in this category is defamation.

Defamation

A written or oral communication that is made by one person to another person about a third person and that injures the reputation of the third person by diminishing the esteem, respect, goodwill, or confidence in which the person is held or by exciting adverse or derogatory feelings against the person, constitutes the personal tort of defamation. In order for defamation to be proven a plaintiff must show that the communication was published, sufficient to identify him, reasonably understood to be defamatory, and caused injury to his reputation. Institutions may claim damages as well.

The Tennessee Academy of Ophthalmology hired a sociologist to write a report on the practice of optometry within the state. The report was highly critical of the ethical and professional standards of Tennessee optometrists and claimed that the Southern College of Optometry had knowingly contributed to the situation. The school sued the Academy, the sociologist, and several individual ophthalmologists for defamation, alleging that the study was false, that it had been published in reckless disregard for the truth, and that it had caused the school economic injury. The trial court dismissed part of the claim, but the Tennessee Court of Appeals reversed the trial court and ordered the case to proceed to trial. Subsequently, the jury awarded the school more than two million dollars in compensatory and punitive damages.[1]

When the defamatory words are directed at a group or class of persons rather than an individual, the possibility of group defamation arises. For any individual member of a group to sustain an action against the publisher, the individual must establish that he is a member of the group or class and that there is some reasonable personal application of the words to himself.[2] Only where the members of the group or class are small have the courts been willing to permit an action by an individual who alleges that the defamation was directed at him.[3] References to portions or subsets of a group or class are usually not actionable since all members are not defamed and those who are cannot be identified. As a result, the civil remedy of group defamation has been successful only in rare instances.

For the optometrist in private practice, care must be exercised whenever the following communications are made: doctor to patient, doctor to third party (when transmitting patient information), and staff to third party.

Oral communications between doctor and patient are, in the usual case, made face-to-face outside the presence of others. Since publication is a necessary element of defamation, there can be no defamation where no third party hears the communication. Written communications to a patient from an optometrist do not customarily contain the kind of information that constitutes defamation of character; rather, the communications from an optometrist to a third party concerning the patient represent the greater opportunity for defamatory publication.

In some instances communications to third parties may not be defamatory but may create liability for disclosure of confidential information or invasion of privacy. Optometrists must be sure that written comments about patients are factual and proper. Remarks about a patient's character should be omitted; only pertinent information should be communicated. When patient data is being divulged, a written release should always be obtained beforehand.

As to communications from patients, every optometrist has encountered those situations in which another doctor's prescription or treatment plan has resulted in a dissatisfied patient. As the doctor's conduct is explained by the unhappy patient, it is easy to draw the conclusion that the diagnosis and treatment were wrong and easier still to remark about it later to a colleague or friend. But basing an opinion of another doctor's competency upon the remarks of a disenchanted patient is a risky business. A letter to the doctor, chiding him for his "mistake" is riskier still. Any written or oral comments to other practitioners should be of the "I thought you would want to know" variety and not an attempt to excoriate the practitioner (no matter what his state or persuasion).

An optometrist serving as head of an army eye clinic was the subject of several letters written by a local ophthalmologist who was a consultant to the clinic. The letters were written to army officials, state medical authorities, and practicing physicians and alleged that the optometrist had committed malpractice at the eye clinic and had entered into the practice of medicine because of the diagnosis and treatment he performed. The optometrist sued for libel, maintaining that the allegations were false and that they had injured his reputation. Eventually the ophthalmologist's services were discontinued at the eye clinic, and the case was settled in favor of the optometrist for $20,000.[4]

If the doctor is the object of comments that injure his reputation and must defend his conduct, under some circumstances he may be able to recover damages.

A physician examined a 92-year-old Medicaid patient who had been referred to him by another doctor and recommended that the patient be hospitalized. The family refused, and the doctor afterward submitted a bill to Medicaid for $85, eventually being compensated in full by the payment of $44. The patient's brother therafter telephoned the county medical society complaining that the physician's treatment was superficial and that the $85 fee was outrageous, despite the fact that he was not present at the time of the examination. The physician was required to defend himself before the society and was formally cleared of these allegations, after which he sued the brother for $625, as compensation for the six hours he was forced to spend in defense of his reputation. The small claims court in which the case was heard awarded him a judgment for $632.[5]

There is one other potential issue that deserves mention: communications made by the optometrist to his staff and by his staff to the patient. Communications by a doctor to his staff are privileged under the law of defamation when they are made in connection with patient care, but remarks that injure the reputation of an assistant (such as an accusation of embezzlement) are never subject to a claim of privilege and, if untrue, are actionable. Comments of a personal nature about employees are best made face-to-face behind closed doors; under these circumstances there is no opportunity for defamation since there is no publication. Communications made by a doctor's staff to his patients constitute a special problem for the doctor because, if they are made during the course of the staff member's employment, the doctor is liable for what was said due to vicarious liability (this problem is discussed in Chapter 21).

Defenses

There are several defenses available to a defendant who has been accused of publishing a defamatory communication. At common law, proof that the publication was true constituted a complete defense to a suit for defamation even if the publication was made without a legitimate motive or reason. This rather broad protection has been modified in some states so that truth is a defense only if the publication is made with a proper motive or for a justifiable end.[6]

Another complete defense is available to some defendants under certain circumstances, even if the communication is untrue and demonstrably has the effect of injuring the plaintiff's reputation: The defense of absolute privilege can be claimed by persons making otherwise actionable oral or written publications in judicial proceedings, legislative proceedings, executive proceedings, and political broadcasts.[7] Absolute privilege can be asserted by a wide range of persons who are involved in any of these proceedings including judges, lawyers, witnesses, parties to litigation, legislators, witnesses at legislative hearings, executive officers of government (federal and state) and many of their subordinates, and political candidates.

A qualified privilege can be claimed as well, principally by those who publish with a proper motive and who exercise reasonable care in determining the veracity of the publication. Such persons are entitled to publish information that is offered in good faith to protect or advance their own legitimate self-interests. Thus one may publish information that is reasonably necessary to defend one's reputation or to protect other areas of importance, such as a business. Similarly, a person may publish in order to protect others or the public good, but the publication must be justified by the importance served, it must be necessary to satisfy a legal or moral duty, and it must meet generally accepted standards of conduct.[8]

The qualified privilege extends to situations in which the publisher and the recipient of the publication have a common interest, such as those who have business dealings with one another or who are common members of a professional, educational, or social organization. It also extends to those who are under a moral or social duty to act in the public interest or to make "fair comment" on matters of public concern. News reporting is included within this qualified privilege, but constitutional protection has increased the privilege enjoyed by the press beyond that traditionally granted under common law.[9]

The qualified privilege can be claimed by optometrists under the appropriate circumstances. For example, the patient records of an optometrist can be used for purposes of research, education, or for peer review or quality assurance, and an optometrist sued for defamation with regard to the use of information released for any of these purposes could claim a qualified privilege to do so as a defense. Another use of the qualified privilege would be its application to the communications between doctors who are jointly treating a patient (usually due to referral of the patient to a specialist for diagnosis or treatment).

A family physician treating a patient for a swollen arm referred the patient to a specialist after a week of unsuccessful therapy. The specialist examined the patient, withdrew some blood, and had the blood sent off for analysis. Based on the blood analysis, the specialist diagnosed the patient as being syphilitic and described his findings in a letter to the family physician. The diagnosis was wrong. The patient subsequently sued the specialist, but the appellate court, in upholding the trial court's ruling, held that the communication between two doctors, since it pertained to the diagnosis and treatment, was privileged.[10]

Communications made by a doctor to his office assistants are subject to the claim of qualified privilege, but unauthorized communications made by the office personnel to third persons may create liability for defamation if the communications are false and cause injury.

A woman who ran a catering business was being treated by a doctor for a false positive reaction to the Wasserman test, a matter that caused her some embarrassment. The doctor's assistant told a number of persons that the woman was being treated for syphillis, which was not true. The false remarks had a deleterious effect on the woman's business, and so the woman sued the assistant for slander. The court held that she had a valid cause of action.[11]

Another type of communication that can create liability is an ill-phrased collection effort.

A doctor who had tried for six years to collect a $15 fee finally turned the unpaid account over to a lawyer for litigation, but the patient successfully pleaded the statute of limitations and avoided payment. The doctor then wrote the patient's employer, for whom the doctor provided services, stating that "having no other defense, (the patient) cowardly slinks behind that of statutory limitation" and that the doctor no longer wished to be associated with the firm. The employer responded to the letter by firing the patient-employee. The patient thereupon sued the doctor for libel and was awarded a judgment of $633.[12]

Communications made by doctors to attorneys who are representing patients involved in litigation, as long as they are relevant to the legal controversy, will be held to be privileged even if untrue and otherwise actionable.[13] But communications to attorneys representing parties whose interest is adverse to that of a patient are not privileged and are actionable in themselves.[14] Of course, there are times when records are requested under legal process, and these requests must be complied with (see Chapter 16).

One other partial defense that can be claimed by a defendant in a defamation suit is mitigation of damages, which is most commonly established through the publication of a retraction or through evidence establishing that the defamatory material was published with a proper motive and with the reasonable belief that it was true.[15] But the effect of this defense is merely to reduce the damages that a plaintiff can receive and not to bar them altogether.

Defamation may be distinguished from two other intentional torts, breach of the duty not to disclose confidential information, and invasion of privacy. Optometrists can incur legal liability for these actions as well.

Disclosure of Confidential Information

An optometrist enjoys a fiduciary relationship with his patients (see Chapter 13), and because of this relationship an optometrist can be held liable for disclosing confidential information about a patient even though the information is true and accurate. Note the distinction between defamation—in which the communication is alleged to be untrue—and this tort, in which there does not have to be an allegation that the communication was not true. It has long been held that physicians have a duty not to disclose information of a confidential nature revealed by their patients during the course of an examination,[16] and the same principle is applicable to optometrists. The Code of Ethics of the American Optometric Association expressly holds that optometrists have an ethical obligation to keep the personal or business matters of their patients confidential.[17] As a result, optometrists should refrain from freely discussing their patient's habits, symptoms, business activities, or financial status. It is important for optometrists to obtain their patients' confidence and trust and for patients to feel that their secrets and personal matters will not be divulged without their consent. Therefore, the duty of confidentiality is one that works to the benefit of both optometrist and patient.

There are many matters that an optometrist may discover during the course of history-taking, diagnosis, and treatment that are of a confidential nature, e.g., physical infirmities suffered by the patient, diseases for which the patient is undergoing treatment, and limitations or deficiencies of the patient's visual system. As long as these matters are not communicated to a third party, there can be no breach of the duty not to disclose confidential information. (A "third party" does not include the optometric technician or office assistant, who may share in the information without there being a disclosure; but the sharing of such information with aides creates a problem of itself, the possibility that the aide will make the improper disclosure.) There will be instances in which an optometrist may find it necessary to communicate his findings to others. The most common instances are reports to agencies, insurance reports, communications to the patient's spouse, and findings of communicable disease.

Reports to Agencies

Many optometrists perform developmental testing on students in an attempt to ascertain whether or not a visual problem is contributing to the student's poor academic performance. These examinations are performed on request, which may come from the parents of the student, the school that the student attends, or a state, county, or city agency. The results of the optometrist's examination may be communicated not only to the student but also to the source referring the student. Reports often influence the classification of students into the learning disabled (LD) category by the school or agency. A good faith report to a school or agency that has a legitimate interest in the student does not breach the duty of confidentiality owed by the optometrist.[18]

If a report is incorrect, the doctor issuing the report has a duty of correcting the mistake within a reasonable period. Failure to do so implies a malicious intent that may create liability.

A 13-year-old student developed a foot infection so severe that she required a home teacher. The treating physician was asked to certify the medical cause for her absence from school and mistakenly attributed it to pregnancy. Despite several requests from the student's parents to change the report, the physician made no effort to contact the school or to correct the mistake. The physician was sued and a judgment was returned against him for $7,000 ($5,000 of which was for punitive damages). The physician appealed, but the appellate court upheld the decision, stating that the physician had a duty to correct the mistake and that his failure to do so constituted a breach of the duty.[19]

A common problem faced by optometrists involves patients who continue to drive despite reduced visual acuity or visual fields.[20] The usual situation occurs when an optometrist examines a patient whose acuity or visual field loss has made it not only personally dangerous but also legally impermissible for the patient to continue to operate a motor vehicle. Admonishments to the patient that he or she should no longer drive, repetition of this advice to family members, and notations in the record that these warnings have been communicated to the patient or the family member are necessary for proper patient management (this problem is discussed in more detail in Chapter 32). But such steps do not ensure that the patient will actually refrain from driving. Should the optometrist do more, such as notifying the appropriate state agency that the patient is no longer legally eligible to possess a driver's license? Or would a unilateral release of patient information constitute a breach of the duty to refrain from disclosing confidential matters?

Several states have adopted physician reporting statutes that permit doctors to report those patients that they believe are unable to drive safely.[21] Seven states[22] require doctors to submit these reports; three states[23] provide for permissive reporting. These compulsory statutes vary in their exact provisions but are all intended to serve the same purpose: A doctor who believes that a patient has a reportable disorder that would interfere with safe driving may report the patient to the appropriate state agency without incurring a breach of the duty to respect confidentiality. Unfortunately, only one of the state laws includes vision disorders within the category of reportable conditions; however, this same state includes optometrists within the named occupations eligible to submit these reports.[24]

There are no reported cases establishing the responsibility of optometrists for disclosure of confidential information, but there have been several cases involving physicians[25] that would probably be applicable to optometrists. These cases have held that a physician has a qualified privilege to divulge confidential information about a patient where the patient's life is in jeopardy or "necessity" exists.[26] Such a criterion would seem to be somewhat difficult for an optometrist to satisfy. Necessity implies that a desperate or serious or threatening condition must exist before the information can be released. And there are further limitations to the qualified privilege: the disclosure must be done in good faith, reasonable care must be exercised as to its truth, only necessary information should be conveyed, and the disclosure should be limited to only those persons who out of necessity should receive the information.

The burden of satisfying all these legal requirements would probably discourage most optometrists from disclosing patient information except under the following circumstances: with the consent of the patient, pursuant to a court order, or as required by statutory enactments.

Insurance Reports

Optometrists are frequently required to supply patient information for insurance reports. Although it would be a rare situation in which an optometrist would be held liable for the unconsented release of patient information to an insurer, such a circumstance is possible. For example, the release of false information without the patient's knowledge to an insurer who is investigating the patient's condition could create liability. A disclosure that is within the patient's interest or the public interest, however, will not be held to constitute a breach of confidentiality.

The father of a newborn child purchased an insurance policy on the infant's life. The infant subsequently died of a congenital heart defect, and the father filed a claim. The insurance company investigated the cause of death and, after learning of the heart defect from the infant's pediatrician, refused to pay the claim. The father sued the pediatrician, alleging that the physician had never told him of the heart defect and that the doctor had breached the duty of confidentiality. The court held that a patient has a legal right to confidentiality unless his own best interest or the public interest required disclosure and that an insurance case constituted a public interest that waived the patient's right to nondisclosure.[27]

The most careful policy that an optometrist could adopt would be to require patient (or parental) consent before releasing any information requested by the patient's insurance carrier. Of course, any form that the patient has signed and asked the optometrist to complete and submit to the insurer will not create liability since it contains the patient's consent (i.e., signature).

If an optometrist is in possession of patient information that is wanted by the patient's insurance carrier because there is pending litigation, the optometrist should require the carrier to obtain the written consent of the patient before releasing the information. (Of course, patient records that are under subpoena must be delivered to the court ordering them.) Practitioners should beware of verbal inducements by insurance investigators and should not release patient information because of verbal allegations made by investigators or terminate the doctor-patient relationship based solely upon these allegations.[28]

Communications to Spouses

During the course of history-taking or examination, an optometrist may obtain information about the patient that should be reported to the patient's spouse. (In particular, the presence of a communicable disease—discussed below—should be reported to a spouse who is unaware that the patient has the disease.) An optometrist may report to one spouse the medical condition of the patient-spouse without breaching the duty to refrain from disclosing confidential information.[29]

An optometrist who discovers that a patient's acuity is below that legally necessary to operate a motor vehicle should inform the patient's spouse of this finding. The appropriate entry should also be made in the patient's record.

Findings of Communicable Disease

Physicians have a legal obligation to report certain communicable diseases (especially venereal diseases); they also have a legal right to warn those who may come in contact with the person carrying the disease.[30] Optometrists would not ordinarily diagnose communicable diseases affecting the eye because the usual procedure would be to refer the patient for the appropriate diagnostic tests. Should an optometrist make such a diagnosis, however, there would probably arise an obligation to warn those who come in close contact with the patient of the risk of infection. Ocular manifestations of sexually transmitted diseases (e.g., gonorrhea, pediculosis, syphilis, chlamydial infections, acquired immune deficiency syndrome (AIDS), herpes) should be carefully investigated and, where the prospect of contagion is found, appropriate warnings should be given.

The optometrist-patient relationship is one that requires the doctor to be most circumspect in discussing information of a confidential nature that is revealed during the course of examination or treatment. Optometric ethics also demand confidentiality. Since remarks made during social occasions are sufficient to give rise to a cause of action, a practitioner should take pause when tempted to indulge in gossip or idle conversation about patients. Some professional liability insurance policies exclude disclosure of confidential information as a covered eventuality.[31] Only when an optometrist is required to produce documents in a legal dispute, or the optometrist's records are under subpoena by a court of competent jurisdiction, is the release of confidential information absolutely justified.

Invasion of Privacy

There are circumstances under which the unauthorized publication of patient information can constitute a civil offense for which damages may be awarded. The rationale for such a law is that a patient has a right to be free in his personal affairs from unreasonable and serious interference that transcends the limits of decent conduct and that offends a person of ordinary sensibilities.[32] This right to privacy protects patients from unwanted commercial exploitation in four seemingly unrelated ways that are, nevertheless, united under the broad legal category of invasion of privacy. These four separate causes of action that constitute invasion of privacy can be applied to the doctor-patient relationship.

Appropriation of the Patient's Name or Likeness

The unauthorized commercial appropriation of a patient's name, photograph, or likeness can be construed as an invasion of the patient's right to privacy.

A patient had plastic surgery performed on her nose by two surgeons, who took before and after photographs. Without her permission, the photographs were published in a medical journal, where they were featured as part of an article entitled "The Saddlenose." The patient sued the physicians, alleging that they had invaded her privacy. In deciding in her favor, the court noted that the article could not be said to have been written purely for scientific purposes and that, even in a scientific publication, such an article may be no more than "an advertisement in disguise."[33]

Publication of pictures that identify a patient by name or appearance—without the patient's consent—can create liability even if they appear in a scientific journal for legitimate scientific purposes. The optometrist who takes a facial photograph to document the patient record should not publish the photograph without obtaining the patient's consent, making a reasonable effort to disguise the patient's identity, and ensuring that the patient's name is not included with the picture or article. Unidentified fundus photographs or slit-lamp photographs of a patient may be published in scientific journals or used for educational purposes without the necessity of patient consent, since the name or appearance of the patient cannot be ascertained from the photographs alone. Even so, it is always advisable to obtain consent if it is anticipated that some publication of patient data will eventually occur.

Even if the patient gives the necessary consent, if the purpose for which the consent was given is violated, the patient may have a cause of action for invasion of privacy. A patient who consents to publication in a scientific journal and who later discovers that the publication has been made for commercial purposes may successfully sue for damages.[34]

Intrusion on the Patient's Privacy

There have been cases in which a physician allowed a layman or other nonessential person to be present while the physician was conducting an examination or treating the patient. The presence of such a person, without the patient's consent, has been held to constitute an invasion of the patient's privacy in some instances.[35]

Although it would be a most atypical situation in which an optometrist in private practice could be found liable for this type of violation, optometry clinics could conceivably be held responsible for permitting unauthorized persons to observe or participate in patient care. Nonessential persons should not be allowed to intrude upon the privacy of patients.

Public Disclosure of Private Facts

An optometrist should never consider disclosing patient information to the popular press without ensuring that the patient understands the exact use and publication of the information and without acquiring the written consent of the patient.

A physician treating a woman with an unusual ailment that caused her to eat ten times that of a normal person allowed the woman's picture and name to be published in a daily newspaper. The woman sued for invasion of privacy and received a judgment in her favor.[36]

An optometrist who diagnoses a child as learning disabled should be cautious that this information does not find its way into the press. Even apparently innocent disclosures can create liability.

A newspaper story on a special education class in a public school contained photographs that were labeled "retarded" and "trainable mentally retarded" and that included the children's names. The newspaper was found to be liable for an invasion of the children's privacy.[37]

In dealing with the press, an optometrist must aspire to protect a patient's right to privacy and should refrain from disclosing any information that could potentially embarrass the patient. Queries by the press should be addressed to the patient unless the optometrist has been given the patient's consent to reveal the information.[38]

Another fertile area of litigation involves public notice of debts. Since a debt or account is a private matter, any public disclosure of a debt owed could constitute an invasion of privacy.[39] Debt collection is a complex legal problem that requires caution and judgment on the part of the optometrist (see Chapter 51 for a discussion of the legal difficulties inherent in debt collection efforts).

Publicity Placing the Patient in a False Light

A public disclosure by an optometrist that places a patient in a false light creates a cause of action against

I, ______________________, hereby consent to have the eyes and associated areas of ______________________________ photographed for the documentation and/or diagnosis of an eye condition and/or disease that may be present.

I also understand that these photographs may be used to document my ocular status as well as for future use in publications, video tapes, or other educational presentations that may or may not be of benefit to me.

Signed: ______________________
Date: ______________________
Witness: ______________________

Figure 20.1. Informed Consent for Eye Photography. (Courtesy of the UAB School of Optometry)

the optometrist for invasion of privacy. Examples of such disclosures would be: attributing to the patient some spurious comment or opinion, using the patient's name in a petition or document without authorization, or employing the patient's photograph to illustrate an article with which the patient has no reasonable connection.

No matter which variety of invasion of privacy is asserted against an optometrist, consent will always be a complete defense. If the patient has consented to the specific publication, then the consent will bar the patient from recovering damages. Therefore, it is essential that an optometrist acquire the knowledgable and written consent of a patient whenever information about a patient is to be released under circumstances such as those described in this section. A consent form permits the optometrist to retain a permanent record of the information transmitted to the patient in seeking his consent and provides evidence of the patient's authorization (a sample form is enclosed as Fig. 20.1).

Fraud

Fraud can arise under a variety of circumstances:

- If a doctor assures a patient that there is no risk in the treatment plan, knowing full well that this assertion is untrue, then the doctor is liable for fraud and any forseeable consequences of the treatment (e.g., experimental contact lenses or solutions are used without the patient's knowledge or consent).
- If a doctor makes a misrepresentation as to the progress of results of a treatment plan, concealing poor results, the doctor is probably liable for fraud (e.g., the patient is told that a corneal ulcer is healing when it is in fact getting worse).
- If the doctor recommends treatment without reasonable medical or scientific justification, and solely for economic advantage, the doctor is subject to an action for fraud (e.g., spectacles are prescribed for a patient who has no need of them).

An active misrepresentation, by words (oral or written), demonstration, or exhibition, can create liability. If a patient reports discomfort or pain, such being the result of negligent treatment, and the doctor falsely reassures him that all is well, then the doctor is liable for fraud.

An ophthalmologist performed cataract surgery on a patient who was an attorney. Despite the patient's repeated visits to the doctor's office after the surgery and his complaints that he could not see out of the eye, the ophthalmologist kept reassuring him that "everything was fine" and that his vision would improve. After the passage of a considerable period of time the patient consulted another ophthalmologist, who told him that half of his iris had been removed. The patient thereupon sued the surgeon for negligence and deceit and both causes of action were upheld by the court.[40]

A doctor who actively attempts to prevent the patient from discovering that a mistake has been made merely compounds his problem. Although an admission that negligence has occurred may be used against the doctor, efforts to conceal the mistake will double the doctor's liability to include both the negligence and the fraud. Under such circumstances, punitive damages are a genuine possibility. A doctor has the absolute obligation to tell his patient the truth and not to make any misrepresentations.[41]

A passive misrepresentation is also actionable since a doctor, as a fiduciary, has an affirmative duty to divulge all material facts to his patients. Thus, silence—if used to conceal a mistake—may be sufficient to support an action for fraud.

A patient sought the services of an ophthalmologist for the removal of some dirt that had blown in his eye. The ophthalmologist told the patient that the intraocular pressure in the eye was elevated and performed "simple surgery" on the eye. The patient thereafter lost his sight in the eye, which the surgeon attributed to progression of the patient's glaucomatous condition. The patient sought a second opinion from another ophthalmologist and described the first ophthalmologist's diagnosis and treatment. The second doctor told the patient that his loss of sight was due to glaucoma and not due to negligence during the surgery and that sight could not be restored in the eye.

Eight years later, the patient was examined by a third ophthalmologist, who found that he did not have glaucoma and that the vision in the eye could have been saved had the appropriate surgery been performed at the time of the second ophthalmologist's examination. Almost two years later, the patient sued the first two doctors and they pleaded the statute of limitations. The trial court dismissed the action but, on appeal, the appellate court held that the affirmative misrepresentations on the part of the two doctors had failed to commence the running of the statute of limitations and that the patient had a cause of action against both physicians even though the suit was filed ten years after they had examined him.[42]

Thus, an active misrepresentation can significantly extend the statute of limitations.

Each of the causes of action described in this chapter, although not accorded the attention given to malpractice, can be the source of liability. The prudent optometrist will understand the basis for each of these torts, be aware of those circumstances under which they are most likely to occur, and take the appropriate steps to prevent their occurrence in clinical practice.

Notes

1. *Southern College of Optometry v. Tennesse Academy of Ophthalmology*, __ S.W.2d __ (Tenn. App. 1986). An account of the trial's outcome is reported in the *AOA News*, Jan. 1, 1988.
2. Group defamation has been difficult to prove. A statement that "Many optometrists are incompetent" is not actionable because the "many" could not be identified by a reasonable person based upon this statement. See Prosser, W.L., *Law of Torts*, 4th ed., West, St. Paul, Minn., p. 750.
3. According to Professor Prosser, the largest group was a football team that consisted of sixty to seventy members. Other groups included twenty-five salesmen in a department store, a twelve member jury, and a family. Id. at 750.
4. An account of this case can be found in Eye-Treating Dispute Stirs Libel Suit, *The Indianapolis Star*, Sept. 15, 1978.
5. This case is recounted by J.E. Scott in Turning the Tables, *Private Practice*, vol. 13, no. 10, 1981, p. 33.
6. Prosser, supra note 2, at 796.
7. Id. at 776–785.
8. Id. at 785–796.
9. A constitutional privilege has been enjoyed by the press since the decision of the U.S. Supreme Court in *New York Times v. Sullivan*, 376 U.S. 254, 84 S. Ct. 710, 717 (1964), which held that the First Amendment of the U.S. Constitution conferred a qualified privilege upon the press that extended even to *false* statements of fact, as long as they were not motivated by malice, or made with the knowledge that they were false, or published in reckless disregard of the truth. As a result, fair comment by the press on matters of concern has been constitutionally protected by this court-mandated qualified privilege. For application to optometry, see *Gaynes v. Allen*, 339 N.W.2d 678 (Mich. App. 1983).
10. *Thornburg v. Long*, 101 S.E. 99 (N.C. 1919).
11. *Schessler v. Keck*, 125 Cal. App. 2d 827, 271 P.2d 588 (1954).
12. *Hollenbeck v. Ristine*, 86 N.W. 377 (Iowa 1901).
13. *Mickens v. Davis*, 294 P. 114 896 (Kan. 1931), and *Hagler v. Major*, 186 S.W.2d 564 (Mo. 1945).
14. *Alexander v. Knight*, 197 Pa. Super 79, 177 A.2d 142 (1962).
15. Prosser, supra note 2, at 799–801.
16. *Boyd v. Wynn*, 286 Ky. 173, 150 S.W.2d 648 (1941).
17. The Code of Ethics of the AOA specifies that an optometrist should "Hold in professional confidence all information concerning a patient and use such data only for the benefit of the patient." See Chapter 4.
18. The prevailing opinion is that the breach of confidentiality must be done with malice in order for there to be liability on the part of the doctor. See *Iverson v. Frandsen*, 237 F.2d 898 (10th Cir. 1956); *Morris v. Rousos*, 397 S.W.2d 504 (Tex. Civ. App. 1965); and *Clark v. Geraci*, 208 N.Y.S.2d 564 (N.Y. 1960).
19. *Vigil v. Rice*, 74 N.M. 693, 397 P.2d 719 (1964).
20. See Classe, J., Optometrist's Duty to Warn of Vision Impairment, *Southern Journal of Optometry*, vol. 4, no. 1, 1985, pp. 66–69; and Gold, A., Failure to Warn, *Journal of the American Optometric Association*, vol. 57, no. 4, 1986, pp. 317–319.
21. Garfinkel, P.E., and Shlensky, R., Should You Be Required to Report Potentially Dangerous Drivers?,

Legal Aspects of Medical Practice, vol. 8, no. 1, 1980, p. 17.

22. Ibid. California, Connecticut, Indiana, Delaware, Nevada, New Jersey, and Oregon.
23. Ibid. Georgia, Maryland, and North Dakota.
24. Ibid. Connecticut.
25. *Barry v. Moench*, 8 Utah 2d 191, 331 P.2d 814 (1958); and *Hague v. Williams*, 37 N.J. 328, 181 A.2d 345 (1982).
26. For more information, see Disclosure of Confidential Information, in the Law and Medicine series of the *Journal of the American Medical Association*, vol. 216, no. 2, Apr. 12, 1971, pp. 385–386.
27. *Hague v. Williams*, 37 N.J. 328, 181 A.2d 345 (1962). Contra: *Felis v. Greenberg*, 15 Misc. 2d 881, 273 N.Y.S.2d 288 (1966).
28. Insurance carriers have been found to be liable for interrupting the doctor-patient relationship. See *Panko v. Consolidated Mutual Insurance Co.*, 423 F.2d 41 (3rd Cir. 1970); and *Hammond v. Aetna Casualty Co.*, 237 F. Supp. 96 (D.C. Ohio 1956).
29. *Pennison v. Provident Life Insurance Co.*, 154 So. 2d 617 (La. 1963); and *Curry v. Corn*, 52 Misc. 2d 1035, 277 N.Y.S.2d 470 (1966).
30. *Simonsen v. Swenson*, 104 Neb. 224, 177 N.W. 831 (1920); *Cochran v. Sears Roebuck and Co.*, 34 S.E.2d 296 (Ga. 1945); and *Shoemaker v. Friedberg*, 183 P.2d 318 (Cal. 1947).
31. Where the policy does not expressly exclude disclosure of confidential information as a covered eventuality, it has been held that the disclosure is included within the policy provisions. see *Hammer v. Polsky*, 36 Misc. 2d 482, 233 N.Y.S.2d 110 (1962).
32. *Griswold v. Connecticut*, 381 U.S. 479, 85 S. Ct. 1678 (1965). It should be noted that not all states have been forced to consider the matter, and in some of the states that have ruled on the tort the right to privacy has been carefully limited.
33. *Griffin v. Medical Society of the State of New York*, 11 N.Y.S.2d 109 (1939); see also *Clayman v. Bernstein*, 38 Pa. D.&C. 543 (1940).
34. See *Feeney v. Young*, 191 A.D. 501, 181 N.Y.S. 481 (1920), in which a film of a patient's cesarean section delivery was shown in public theaters after the patient had consented to the film's use at a medical society meeting.
35. *DeMay v. Roberts*, 9 N.W. 166 (Mich. 1881); and *Carr v. Shiflette*, 82 F.2d 874 (D.C. Cir. 1936).
36. *Barber v. Time, Inc.*, 159 S.W.2d 291 (Mo. 1942).
37. *Deaton v. Delta Democrat Publishing Co.*, 326 So. 2d 471 (Miss. 1976).
38. *Horne v. Patton*, 291 Ala. 701, 287 So. 2d 824 (1973).
39. *Brents v. Morgan*, 221 Ky. 765, 299 S.W. 867 (1927).
40. *Hundley v. Martinez*, 158 S.E.2d 159 (W. Va. 1967).
41. *Keen v. Coleman*, 20 S.E.2d 175 (Ga. 1942); *Haskins v. Howard*, 16 S.W.2d 20 (Tenn. 1929); *Garlock v. Cole*, 199 Cal. App. 2d 11, 18 Cal. Rptr. 393 (1962); and *Baum v. Turel*, 206 F. Supp. 490 (D.C. N.Y. 1962).
42. *van Bronckhorst v. Taube*, 341 N.E. 2d 791 (Ind. App. 1976).

Chapter 21

Strict Liability

You stand behind your product. If 999,999 people trust and buy your product, you take their money. If one person trusts and buys your product, you take his money too. If your product benefits those 999,999, that is as it should be. If your product hurts that one, then by God you had better make it good to him the best way you can—because he trusted you to stand behind your goods.
—Melvin Belli, *My Life on Trial*

Product Liability
Vicarious Liability

The development of the legal theory of strict liability has been not only a matter of legal concern but also a social phenomenon, an attempt to replace the legal concept of fault with liability without fault, and to shift the responsibility for injury upon those members of society best able to suffer the financial consequences (an idea well described by Melvin Belli). In the context of optometry, there are two major areas of application: product liability and vicarious liability.

This chapter discusses product liability theory; however, the application of product liability law to the dispensing of ophthalmic materials is described in Chapter 27.

The other topic of this chapter is vicarious liability, which pertains to the responsibility of optometrists for employees, agents, and partners, and which is a well-established legal concept with wide application to everyday optometric practice. The prudent optometrist will understand the legal ramifications of this form of strict liability.

Product Liability

The early law of torts was distinguished by a slow progression toward the recognition of fault as the basis for legal redress. But over the past century there has been a growing movement toward liability without fault. The most rapid development of what is in essence a policy of social justice has occurred in the field known as product liability, to which strict liability has only recently been applied.[1]

Product liability refers to the liability of a seller of a product to a consumer who is injured by it, even though the seller had no direct involvement with the injured consumer (e.g., the seller was the manufacturer or wholesaler of the product, not the retailer). Up to the 19th century, the general rule was that an original seller of goods was not liable for damages caused by their defects except to the immediate purchaser.[2] In the early 1900s there began a prolonged and hotly debated legal struggle in the United States over the marketing of defective food and drink; it was during this battle that the movement toward strict liability began. In a 1913 case involving a seller of bad food a court held that there was an *implied warranty* of fitness and that by placing goods on the market there was a representation to the consumer who purchased them that they were safe for use.[3] This implied warranty, founded in strict liability, made the manufacturer liable for the first time to the ultimate user instead of to the middleman.

Twenty years later, another blow was struck for strict liability when it was held that representations about goods, whether written or spoken, created an *express warranty* that the product would comply with the representation.[4] Another victory for strict liability theory came in 1960, when a court held that implied warranty would be extended to include a product other than food[5]; thereafter, a flood of products were held to an implied warranty of safety to the user or consumer of the product, including ophthalmic lenses and contact lenses.[6]

But warranties on the sale of goods also were governed in part by the Uniform Commercial Code (UCC), which was intended to regulate transactions between commercial dealers but had an unfair influence on the sale of products to consumers. Problems with the UCC ultimately led to the decision to jettison the idea of warranty altogether and to define the consumer's right to relief exclusively on the basis of strict liability, a result[7] that automatically conferred liability on any seller of a defective product that caused injury to a user, even though the user had not bought the product from the seller (see Chapter 27 for a further discussion). This principle was widely adopted by the courts[8] and is the law in the majority of jurisdictions today.

A consumer using a product in a reasonably foreseeable and intended manner who is injured by the product has a cause of action if it can be shown that[9]:

- the product is defective, and
- the seller is engaged in the business of selling the product (either as manufacturer, distributor, or retailer) and
- the product reaches the consumer without substantial change in the condition in which it was sold

The importance of product liability law is that it is applicable to that most ubiquitous product of the optometric service, the ophthalmic lens.[10]

An optical laboratory or optometrist can be liable as a matter of law for the marketing of defective ophthalmic lenses if:

1. the lab (or doctor) is ordinarily engaged in the business of selling (or dispensing) such lenses
2. the lab (or doctor) placed the lenses on the market with the expectation that they would reach consumers without undergoing substantial change
3. the lenses are—at the time of the injury—in substantially the same condition as when they left the optical laboratory's (or doctor's) possession and control
4. the lenses are defective, e.g., they do not meet the reasonable expectation of an ordinary consumer as to their safety (or, alternatively, defective can be defined as that which renders a product unreasonably dangerous and hence not fit for the ordinary purpose for which it was intended)
5. there is injury to the plaintiff (patient) as a proximate consequence of the defective condition of the lenses, and despite the fact that they were being used in a reasonably foreseeable and intended manner

Lenses found to be in noncompliance with impact resistance standards would satisfy the requirement that they be defective, thereby establishing—from an evidentiary standpoint—the most difficult of the five elements to prove. Once the plaintiff has offered proof of each element, the defendant must rely on a defense.

A defendant in a product liability case can rely on any of four defenses: (1) lack of causal relation, (2) abnormal use of the product, (3) assumption of risk, and (4) contributory negligence. None of these defenses are very useful to a defendant optometrist.

Lack of Causal Relation

The optometrist or optician who actually dispenses defective lenses can assert as an affirmative defense that there was no causal relationship between his activities and the defect that caused the injury. Although the optical laboratory fabricating the lenses would seemingly bear the entire burden of responsibility in this event, such is not always the case. Assuming that the dispenser of the lenses can successfully demonstrate that he received the defective lenses from the optical laboratory in the usual and customary course of business, that he did not contribute to the defective condition, and that in fact he did not have any knowledge of the defective condition, he still will probably fail to carry the burden of this affirmative defense since he must also show that he did not have the opportunity to inspect the lenses. For example, industrial strength lenses must be no thinner than 3 mm. Failure to inspect safety lenses to ensure that they satisfy this criterion could not be used as a defense, since the dispenser has the opportunity (and the responsibility) to verify all ophthalmic materials sold to patients.

Abnormal Use of the Product

The patient is not expected to alter the lens materially or to use it in some unforeseeable way. Similarly, the patient is expected to heed the warnings and instructions of the doctor or laboratory. When lenses are shattered, however, it is difficult to determine the presence of any alterations. And unless patient instructions or warnings are documented, proving them usually ends up being a matter of one person's word against the other's. But if a patient suffers injury due to some susceptibility or idiosyncracy that is peculiar to him, there can be no recovery.[11]

Assumption of Risk

It would be highly unusual for the average consumer to discover that a lens was defective, assume the risk of continued use, and thereby proceed to make an unreasonable use of it. Also, this defense is an affirmative one, requiring that the optical laboratory carry the affirmative burden of establishing a patent or obvious defect.

Contributory Negligence

Negligence on the part of the patient can be averred in some circumstances and can provide a complete defense in some states. For example, if the patient fails, when asked during the history, to inform the doctor or dispenser that the glasses are to be worn for some extrahazardous activity, there is a possibility that this omission on the part of the patient would constitute contributory negligence and hence could be used as a defense. In the usual case, however, the patient relies on the doctor to prescribe the type of lenses or frames most suitable for a described purpose, which obviates the utility of contributory negligence for the overwhelming majority of patients.

Since the defenses available to a defendant optometrist will most likely be of limited usefulness, the case often hinges on whether a lens is actually defective, which in turn depends on compliance or noncompliance with impact resistance standards. Successful product liability lawsuits have been brought alleging defective design, defective warnings or directions, and defective inspection. Cases illustrating the liability of optometrists under these circumstances can be found in Chapter 27.

Vicarious Liability

Under certain circumstances, an optometrist can be liable for the conduct of partners, employees, opticians, technicians, and office assistants. In fact, an optometrist can be financially responsible for the negligence or intentionally wrongful acts of such persons, even though the optometrist's personal conduct is without fault. The negligent or intentional act is imputed to the optometrist, who is held to be vicariously liable for the resultant damages. For vicarious liability to be found, however, a special relationship must exist between the optometrist and the one actually negligent or intentionally causing injury: The negligent or intentional act must be committed by the *servant* or *agent* of the optometrist.

The relationships of master and servant and principal and agent are central to understanding vicarious liability. The underlying theory of the law can be found in the Latin phrase *respondeat superior*, which means "let the master answer." The following paragraphs discuss those cases in which a master will be held responsible for the wrongful acts of his servant, and a principal for the acts of his agent.

Master and Servant

A servant is a person who is employed to perform services in the affairs of another, and whose physical conduct in the performance of these services is controlled, or is subject to the right of control, by the other (the master).[12] Control is not interpreted to mean that the master has the actual right to control every physical activity of the servant. Rather, it refers to the master's right to direct the manner in which services are to be performed by the servant. The master and servant relationship is most commonly found between employers and employees in sole propietorships, and an optometrist-employer can occupy the position of master with regard to a number of employees: other optometrists (as long as they are paid wages and hold no ownership interest in the practice); optometric technicians (even if they do not perform their duties under the direct supervision of the optometrist); office assistants (whether physically inside or outside the office, as long as they are acting within the line and scope of their duties); and opticians (if they are salaried-in-house employees).

The liability of masters for the torts of servants is, in essence, a form of strict liability. But a master will not be held responsible for the criminal act of his servant unless the master in some way directed, participated in, or approved the act. Liability is limited to negligence and intentionally wrongful acts (such as defamation).[13]

That liability is successfully imputed to the master does not absolve the servant from legal responsibility for the wrongful act.[14] Should a lawsuit be filed, the injured party has the option to include the servant as a co-defendant or to sue the master alone.[15] If included, the servant will be responsible for any judgment for damages rendered against him. And, if the master becomes the sole defendant and is compelled to pay damages for the servant's wrongful act, the servant is liable to the master for the amount paid as damages. But a plaintiff is not allowed to recover twice. A legal action against either the master or the servant that results in the recovery of damages precludes a subsequent suit by the plaintiff against the other party.[16]

There is one important limitation to the imposition of vicarious liability: the wrongful conduct of the servant must be within the scope of employment before the master can be held vicariously liable. A servant who is on a frolic of his own,[17] e.g., who is acting outside the line and scope of his duties on some personal business or task that is not connected with his employment, will be held solely liable for his conduct. There will be no responsibility on the part of the master for the servant's tortious acts, whether negligent or intentional.[18]

There are many circumstances under which an optometrist can fall victim to vicarious liability, and a common situation involves the optometrist-associate of an individual proprietor in private practice. Even though the associate may perform examinations, make diagnoses, and recommend courses of treatment without consultation with or supervision by the employer-optometrist, the associate is still a salaried employee whose services are directed by the employer. If the associate is negligent or commits an intentional tort while acting within the line and scope of his employment, the rationale of *respondeat superior* can be applied to impute the associate's liability to the employer.[19] An associate who runs a branch office and is free from supervision of any kind will similarly create liability for his employer.

An unlicensed optometrist who is an employee (such as an intern or an optometrist who has failed to pass the state optometry board examination) creates a special problem. If the unlicensed optometrist is negligent and the employer is sued, a judgment against the employer may not be covered by his professional liability insurance if the insurance policy only provides indemnification for the negligence of *duly qualified* assistants. The insurer may maintain that the unlicensed optometrist is not duly qualified, thus precipitating a lawsuit over insurance coverage.[20] To avoid conflict with one's insurer (and to satisfy the provisions of one's state optometry law), the unlicensed optometrist should take care not to "practice optometry" as would a licensed optometrist. The employer should supervise the unlicensed optometrist's duties and should take care to avoid any appearance of impropriety.

Depending upon the right to control, a commercial outlet may or may not be responsible for the torts of an associated optometrist. Some commercial optometrists lease space from the optical corporation and are lessees only, while others are paid a salary for services by the corporation; the former example would not typically create sufficient control for *respondeat superior* to be applied, whereas the latter example probably would.

The employee with the greatest opportunity to create liability for an optometrist is the aide (technician or assistant).[21] Individual optometrists vary in the number and complexity of the duties that they delegate to their aides, but regardless of the amount of supervision an aide receives, any wrongful act that is within the scope of the aide's employment can impose liability.

An 18-year-old man requested safety glasses from his optometrist, and the glasses were dispensed. Later the patient was in an automobile accident during which a lens shattered, causing the patient to lose sight in one eye. The patient filed suit, alleging that the lens was not a safety lens and that the failure to provide him with the lens he had ordered had proximately caused his injury. It was discovered that, when the original order was turned over to the optometrist's technician, she had failed to mark the order as one for safety glasses. Therefore, the patient had erroneously been given dress-strength lenses. The case was settled against the employer-optometrist for $42,100.[22]

Many malpractice cases are won or lost on the quality of the patient records. A vigilant optometric aide can be of enormous value, particularly to busy practitioners, in double-checking patient records to be sure that entries are complete and correct. Optometrists should document all patient recalls and referrals in the patient record at the time the recall appointment is made or the referral arranged. An optometric aide whose duties include verifying these entries provides a useful service.

A young boy, hit in the eye by a small metal object, was examined by an optometrist. The following day, he returned, was reexamined by the optometrist's partner, and was sent to an ophthalmologist for treatment. Despite the physician's efforts he suffered a vision loss in the injured eye and sued the optometrists for failing to refer him in a timely manner. In defense the optometrists alleged that, at the time of the first examination, the boy's parents had been advised either to take him to an ophthalmologist or to return the following day for a follow-up examination. The parents denied that they had been advised to seek a physician's care at the first visit. The optometrists' records did not contain any supporting documentation for their assertion that referral had been recommended. The suit was settled for $86,500.[23]

The ability of optometric aides to communicate with patients is of obvious importance. Telephone requests for information, advice, and assistance are answered—at least initially—by the aide. In-person requests are also fielded by aides, many times to shield the beleaguered doctor. Financial arrangements and bill collection efforts are usually managed by the aides. Many comparable communications are routinely conducted each working day by optometric aides, and it is the employer who bears the ultimate responsibility for what is said. All optometric aides should be warned against making guarantees or warranties, releasing patient information without the proper authorization, making potentially defamatory statements, and soliciting unpaid bills through improper collection efforts. In each of these instances, the optometrist could end up paying for the aide's mistake.

One area of optometry that requires a particularly well-trained aide is contact lens practice. Office procedures should be reviewed periodically and any opportunity for inadvertence or mistake should be eliminated.

A patient's soft contact lenses caused a servere reaction on his corneas, and he sued the optometrist who had fitted him with the lenses. It was subsequently discovered that the optometrist kept the containers for both the contact lens cleaning solution and the saline solution—which were of identical color—in the same area of the office. The technician had gotten them confused and had inadvertently soaked the lenses in the cleaning solution, causing the injury to the patient's eyes. The suit was settled in favor of the patient.[24]

In every practice there are occasions during which the optometrist is absent from the office. During these occasions, the aide is the one in charge. Patient problems do not cease because the doctor is absent.[25] Frequently, patients will solicit information or seek to obtain ophthalmic products from the aide. Diagnosis and treatment are not within the scope of an aide's legally allowable duties. An aide who practices optometry faces a complex and difficult situation: Since the aide is acting outside the scope of employment, there may be no liability imputed to the master and the aide may be solely responsible. Furthermore, the aide could be held to the standard of care of an optometrist in the event that negligence is alleged. For these reasons, aides should be cautious whenever imparting advice or performing duties in an employer's absence.[26]

Optometric technicians and office assistants are an important source of manpower for optometry; they are a vital and necessary adjunct to the profession. But proper utilization of their skills requires that they be given adequate training and supervision.[27]

Opticians are employed by a small percentage of optometrists in private practice. Since their patient contact is usually limited to dispensing ophthalmic materials, there is reduced opportunity for wrongdoing. But a tort committed by an optician during the course of employment can be imputed to an optometrist-employer. Likewise an optician in charge of an optical shop can create liability for an optometrist owner.[28] The most likely causes of claims against opticians would be product liability or negligence.

A patient went to an optical shop to purchase some glasses. The optician in charge sent the patient to a nearby optometrist for refraction and examination. The optometrist detected a small tumor in the patient's eye but told only the optician of this finding. The patient returned to the optician, who sold him some spectacles but failed to inform him of the tumor. The patient subsequently suffered blindness in the eye and sued the optometrist, the optician, and the optical shop for malpractice. All were found liable for his injury.[29]

The master and servant relationship is not the only one to which the doctrine of *respondeat superior* is applied. Principals and their agents also have interrelated responsibilities that, under certain circum-

Principal and Agent

An agent is defined as one who acts for, or in place of, another person (the principal) by authority from him and who is appointed by the principal to act as a substitute, with the power to do the things that the principal may do.[30] Therefore, an agent differs from a servant by being invested with the capacity to act for another person in a representative fashion. (A common example of this power is the capacity of an agent to bind a principal to a contract.) An agent has more independence than a servant and is not subject to the right of direct control inherent in the master and servant relationship. But because the agent's activities are for the benefit of the principal and are at the appointment of the principal, it has long been held that the principal is liable under the doctrine of *respondeat superior* for the wrongful acts of the agent. The position of a principal is, in essence, that of surety for the agent, and should the agent commit a negligent or intentionally wrongful act, the principal will be liable to the injured party. The agent, in turn, will be liable to the principal for any damages.

The principal and agent relationship is an inherent characteristic of a professional association or corporation. The professional association (PA) or professional corporation (PC) is a legal entity that serves as the principal for its agent-employees. For example, the corporate officers as agents are typically empowered to perform certain acts on its behalf, such as signing contracts. Once ratified, the contract becomes the responsibility of the corporation and not of its officers. Employees of the corporation who perform services are also acting as agents, and so any negligent or intentionally wrongful act committed by them is imputed to the principal.[31] For corporate employees, the benefits are obvious: The wrongful act of one employee does not create individual liability for any others. Only the corporate assets can be used to pay a judgment rendered against the PA or PC on the basis of *respondeat superior*; the assets of the officers and employees cannot be used to satisfy the judgment.

One interesting application of the principal and agent relationship can be found in those situations in which optometrists and ophthalmologists work together for a common business entity. Whenever practitioners from the two disciplines share facilities, care should be taken to identify individual doctors as either OD or MD.

A woman with reduced vision in one eye called a medical clinic for an appointment. She was seen by a doctor (who was not identified as an optometrist) and was diagnosed as having a cataract, told to maintain her usual activities, and advised to return periodically for reevaluation. The patient's pupils were not dilated because the state law (Louisiana) did not then allow optometrists to use diagnostic pharmaceutical agents. About two months later the patient realized that she could not see out of the eye, and made another appointment at the clinic. She was seen by an ophthalmologist, who dilated her pupils and diagnosed her as having a retinal detachment. She was referred to a surgeon, who reattached the retina and treated her for the underlying cause of the attachment, an ocular tumor caused by von Hippel-Landau disease. The patient sued the medical clinic, alleging that the optometrist's name was improperly displayed, that she had been misled into believing that a physician had examined her, and that this deception had prevented her from receiving adequate care. Although the trial court ruled in favor of all defendants, the appellate court reversed the decision and rendered a $25,000 judgment against the optometrist and his employer, the medical clinic.[32]

Optometrists should always take care to identify themselves by the academic title OD or Doctor of Optometry and not by the vague moniker doctor.

Technically, the owners of a professional association or corporation, the stockholders, may be separate from the management, the officers; in actuality, the ownership and the management of a PA or PC are merged because only professionals can be stockholders, and it is these same professionals who also serve as the corporate officers. Despite this variation from the usual situation encountered in corporations, the general rule pertaining to liability still prevails: The stockholders are not personally liable for a judgment obtained against the professional association or corporation; only the corporate assets can be used to satisfy the judgment. It is this insulation from liability (plus a few tax advantages) that makes a professional association or corporation desirable as a form of business.

A partnership also creates a principal and agent relationship, but it differs significantly from the one found in professional associations or corporations. Since both the ownership and the management of the partnership reside in the partners, each partner is held to be the agent of the other. For example, one partner can bind the other partners to a partnership contract. Similarly, the negligent or intentionally wrongful act of one partner that is committed while conducting partnership business will create liability for all other partners.[33] Partners are said to be *jointly and severally* responsible for their tortious acts.

An ophthalmologist in a medical partnership fitted a patient for contact lenses. Over a period of almost ten years the patient returned with complaints about her eyes. Finally her intraocular pressures and visual fields were tested, and she was found to have open-angle glaucoma. She sued all the partners for negligence, and the case was eventually decided in her favor against them.[34]

Typically, a partnership will be sued along with the individual partners. If a judgment is returned against them all, who must bear the brunt of payment? When a partnership and its individual partners are held to be liable, the judgment usually must be satisfied out of the assets of the partnership and the negligent partner before the personal assets of the other partners can be used to pay any unpaid balance or judgment. Thus, adequate professional liability insurance is essential. As with other business entities, the partnership—and its partners—incur responsibility for the tortious acts of employees under the doctrine of *respondeat superior*.

Because of the unique aspects of partnership law, the decision to enter into a partnership arrangement is not one that should be taken lightly. In addition to the generally prevailing concepts of liability law described in this section, there are numerous provisions in the *Uniform Partnership Act* (UPA) concerning the rights and responsibilities of partners to one another and to the people they serve. The UPA will be held to control the rights and responsibilities of the partners if the partnership agreement is silent (see Chapter 38 for a further discussion).

Consultations can create an agency relationship and joint liability. A consultation is regarded as a joint enterprise, which is a limited undertaking that is entered into by two or more individuals under such circumstances that all have an equal voice in directing the conduct of the undertaking; each is considered to be the agent of the other, and any act committed by one that is within the scope of the undertaking is to be charged vicariously against the others.[35] Consultations may be distinguished from referrals by this joint effort at participation.

In general, an optometrist who is unable or unwilling to continue the treatment of a patient, and who refers the patient to a practitioner other than his employee, agent, or partner, is not liable for the negligence of the other practitioner unless the optometrist did not exercise due care in making the recommendation or substitution.[36] But the optometrist must take no further part in the case, leaving the patient care solely in the hands of the practitioner to whom the patient was referred. If the optometrist continues on the case, either as a consultant or as a participant, the result can be a joint enterprise that creates joint liability if there is negligence. While serving with one another, all practitioners must answer for their individual conduct and also for the conduct of each of the others that was observed or, in the exercise of reasonable vigilance, should have been observed.[37] For example, an optometrist who performs the postoperative care of a patient referred to an ophthalmologist for surgery, may be held to participate in a joint enterprise with the surgeon for this aspect of the patient's care.

Independent Contractors

The tort of an independent contractor, as distinguished from that of a servant or agent, cannot be imputed to a master or a principal.[38] An independent contractor is one who contracts to do a piece of work according to his own methods and without being subject to the control of his employer, except as to the result of the work.[39] An example of an independent contractor is a substitute doctor.

A doctor who uses a substitute to manage his patients is not liable for the tortious acts of the substitute unless the substitute was in fact the agent of the doctor[40] or the doctor did not employ due care in the selection of the substitute.[41]

In determining whether or not a substitute is an agent, there are two key considerations: (1) whether the substitute agreed to carry out a certain course of treatment for the doctor (agency) or chose to do the work according to his own methods (independent contractor) and (2) whether the source of payment for the substitute's services was from the doctor (which infers agency) or from the patient (which infers that the substitute was an independent contractor).

In selecting a substitute, the doctor must choose a competent and qualified practitioner.[42] Notice of the substitution may have to be given to patients in some cases,[43] so that they will have the opportunity to consult with a doctor other than the substitute if they so wish. Failure to give a timely notice, if it results in an adverse effect on the patient's condition, can lead, in rare cases, to a claim of abandonment.[44]

There is one other form of business arrangement that can create joint liability: office sharing. Optometrists who merely share an office without any provision for sharing the responsibility for each other's patients do not incur any liability for one another's professional negligence. But if they consult with one another in the care of a patient, a joint liability exists for those actions that they undertake together.

Notes

1. The development of this legal theory, in the words of Roscoe Pound, shows "a strong and growing tendency,

where there is blame on neither side, to ask, in view of the exigencies of social justice, who can best bear the loss and hence to shift the loss by creating liability where there has been no fault." Pound, The End of Law as Developed in Legal Rules and Doctrines, *Harvard Law Review*, vol. 27, no. 3, 1914, p. 195.

2. Prosser, W.L., *Law of Torts*, 4th ed., West, St. Paul, Minn., p. 641.
3. *Mazetti v. Armour & Co.*, 75 Wash. 672, 135 P. 633 (1913).
4. *Baxter v. Ford Motor Co.*, 168 Wash. 456, 12 P.2d 409, *affirmed*, 15 P.2d 1118 (1932).
5. *Henningsen v. Bloomfield Motors, Inc.*, 32 N.J. 358, 161 A.2d 69 (1960).
6. For ophthalmic lenses, see *Filler v. Rayex Corp.*, 435 F.2d 336 (7th Cir. 1970); for contact lenses, see *Barbee v. Rogers*, 425 S.W.2d 342 (Tex. 1968).
7. Section 402A of the *Second Restatement of Torts.*
8. The first case to apply it was *Greenman v. Yuba Power Products*, 59 Cal. 2d 57, 27 Cal. Rptr. 697, 377 P.2d 897 (1963).
9. This language is taken from Section 402A of the *Second Restatement of Torts.*
10. It should be noted that some states hold that one who uses a product in the performance of a service cannot be held liable under strict liability theory or implied warranty, and instead must be charged with negligence. For the application of this logic to optometry, see *Barbee v. Rogers*, 425 S.W.2d 342 (Tex. 1968).
11. For an example case involving ophthalmic products, see *Walstrom Optical Co. v. Miller*, 59 S.W.2d 895 (Tex. Civ. App. 1933).
12. Professor William L. Prosser, in his textbook, supra note 2, at 459 et seq., describes the vicarious liability of a master as follows:

    A multitude of very ingenious reasons have been offered for the vicarious liability of a master: he has a more or less fictitious "control" over the behavior of the servant; he has "set the whole thing in motion," and is therefore responsible for what has happened; he has selected the servant and trusted him, and so should suffer for his wrongs, rather than an innocent stranger who has had no opportunity to protect himself; it is a great concession that any man should be permitted to employ another at all, and there should be a corresponding responsibility as the price to be paid for it—or, more frankly and cynically, "In hard fact, the reason for the employers' liability is the damages are taken from a deep pocket."
13. The master is liable not only for negligence but also for "any intentional tort committed by the servant where its purpose, however misguided, is wholly or in part to further the master's business." Id. at 464.
14. For a discussion, see 99 A.L.R. 408, "Personal Liability of Servant or Agent to Third Person for Injuries Caused by the Performance or Nonperformance of His Duty to His Employer."
15. The decision of whom to sue is a matter of tactics; an employee without insurance or whose testimony is essential to establishing liability against the employer is often not named as a defendant or, if named, is dropped from the suit before trial (but after a deposition or other form of testimony has been taken).
16. Prosser, supra note 2, at 380.
17. For a discussion of all of the ramifications of this phrase, see id. at 464.
18. These situations can involve very fine distinctions. For example, an office assistant who takes her car to "run to the bank" will be solely responsible for any injury she negligently causes while on this personal "frolic." But what if the employer asks her to make a deposit for the practice and she negligently causes an injury? Vicarious liability could be imposed under the latter set of facts, causing the employer to be responsible for damages. See id. at 461–464.
19. See Bergan, R.P., Use of Irregular Paramedical Personnel, *Journal of the American Medical Association*, vol. 207, no. 5, Feb. 3, 1969, pp. 1027–1028; and Bergen, R.P., Irregular Assistants and Legal Risks, *Journal of the American Medical Association*, vol. 207, no. 6, Feb. 10, 1969, pp. 1231–1232.
20. See O'Hern, V.M., Physicians Employed by Physicians, *Journal of the American Medical Association*, vol. 204, no. 1, Apr. 1, 1968, p. 257; and Holder, A.R., Unlicensed Treatment, *Journal of the American Medical Association*, vol. 214, no. 1, Oct. 5, 1970, pp. 209–210.
21. See Classe, J., How Your Helper Can Help You Get Sued, *Optometric Management*, vol. 16, no. 11, 1980, pp. 61–65.
22. Reported in the *AOA News*, Sept. 15, 1976.
23. Ibid.
24. Reported in the *AOA News*, June 15, 1975.
25. A vacationing or out-of-town doctor can be liable for an employee's negligence that is committed while the doctor is out of town. See *Moulton v. Huckleberry*, 46 P.2d 589 (Or. 1935).
26. The author is aware of a case in which the optometrist was attending a continuing education seminar and the contact lens technician was permitted to see patients during his absence. A patient alleged that the technician was negligent and a lawsuit resulted, with the optometrist ultimately being held liable by the jury for the patient's injuries. Unsupervised aides can create a serious liability issue for practitioners. See Classe, J., Optometrist's Liability for Contact Lenses, *Southern Journal of Optometry*, vol. 4, no. 3, 1986, pp. 52–57.
27. See Holder, A.R., *Medical Malpractice Law*, Wiley and Sons, N.Y., 1977, pp. 200–224.
28. The type of business entity that employs the optician (individual proprietorship, partnership, or corporation) determines which master will be liable for the optician's negligence. If an optician works in a dispensary located inside an optometrist's office (and that is a part of the optometrist's practice), the optometrist will be liable if the optician is acting within the line and scope of his duties when the negligent act

occurs. For a discussion of vicarious liability as applied to optometry, see Gabel, W., Vicarious Liability, *Journal of the American Optometric Association*, vol. 58, no. 7, 1987, pp. 599–601.

29. *Evers v. Buxbaum*, 102 App. D.C. 334, 253 F.2d 356 (D.C. Cir. 1958).
30. For a review of the law of agency, see Henn, H.G., *Agency and Partnership*, West, St. Paul, Minn., 1972.
31. See Morris, R.C., and A.R. Moritz, *Doctor and Patient and the Law*, 5th ed., C.V. Mosby, St. Louis, 1971, p. 377.
32. *Fairchild v. Brian*, 354 So. 2d 675 (La. App. 1977).
33. *Hess v. Lowery*, 122 Ind. 225, 23 N.E. 156 (1890); and *Wolfsmith v. Marsh*, 337 P.2d 70 (Cal. 1959). A partnership arrangement must be distinguished between an employee-employee relationship, for co-employees are generally not responsible for one another's negligence. See *McGray v. Cobb*, 152 N.W. 262 (Minn. 1915).
34. *Helling v. Carey*, 83 Wash. 2d 514, 519 P.2d 981 (1974).
35. Prosser, supra note 2, at 475.
36. For the application of the law to physicians, see *Graddy v. New York Medical College*, 19 A.D.2d 426, 243 N.Y.S.2d 940 (1963).
37. *Rogers v. Canfield*, 262 N.W. 409 (Mich. 1935). Most of these cases involve surgical consultation and participation by two or more doctors after the referral, but optometrists could incur similar liability while treating a patient with another doctor or participating in some type of joint patient management. See O'Hern, V.M., Liability of Referring Physician, *Journal of the American Medical Association*, vol. 204, no. 3, Apr. 15, 1968, pp. 273–274; and Holder, A.R., Duty to Consult, *Journal of the American Medical Association*, vol. 226, no. 1, Oct. 1, 1973, pp. 111–112.
38. Prosser, supra note 2, at 468.
39. A more detailed discussion may be found in Morris and Moritz, supra note 31, at 374.
40. *Wilson v. Martin Memorial Hospital*, 232 N.C. 362, 61 S.E.2d 102 (1950).
41. *Stohlman v. Davis*, 220 N.W. 247 (Neb. 1928).
42. Only if the doctor has failed to employ due care in the selection process and if the substitute is not duly qualified does the prospect of liability arise. See *Beauchamp v. Davis*, 309 Ky. 397, 217 S.W.2d 822 (1948). This duty can extend to third parties, such as opticians who fabricate spectacles or supply contact lenses for the doctor's referrals. An optometrist who works in close association with or for an optical outlet would seem to run a legal risk if the optometrist knew or should have known that prescriptions were being filled improperly.
43. Notice to patients depends upon the seriousness of the patient's case and the length of time the doctor is going to be away. A doctor is expected to provide a competent substitute, give the patient timely notice of his absence, and not absent himself when the patient is in a critical condition. See 57 A.L.R. 2d at 417, "Liability of Physician for Lack of Diligence in Attending Patient."
44. See Holder, supra note 27, at 375–387.

Chapter 22

Informed Consent

Any human being of adult years and sound mind has a right to determine what shall be done with his own body; and a surgeon who performs an operation without his patient's consent commits an assault, for which he is liable in damages.
—From the opinion of Judge Cardozo, *Schloendorff v. Society of New York Hospital,* 195 N.E. 92 (1914)

Legal Basis

Doctors and certain other professionals are *fiduciaries,* persons who occupy a relationship of trust and confidence with those who seek their services. Fiduciaries owe an affirmative duty of disclosure to persons who come to them for advice or services, and thus may not make misrepresentations, either by misstating known facts or by withholding necessary information. Consequently, a doctor is legally obligated to make a full and complete disclosure of the pertinent facts relating to a recommended procedure in order to obtain the patient's informed consent.

A fundamental precept of Anglo-American law is that an individual's person is inviolate and that the unconsented touching of one person by another (even if the touching is beneficial) constitutes a battery per se for which damages may be awarded. Consent to medical procedures is based upon this principle.[1]

The failure to obtain consent for a diagnostic or therapeutic procedure has been held by the courts to be a clear-cut case of assault and battery. There has evolved, however, a difference of opinion concerning those instances in which consent was actually given by the patient but was based on an inadequate disclosure of the risks involved or the alternative forms of therapy available. Assault and battery, which was an intentional tort, did not seem to fit this situation as well. A solution was reached in 1960, when the Kansas Supreme Court held for the first time that failure to inform a patient adequately of the risks and alternatives to a medical procedure was negligence and that actions brought against a doctor for inadequate disclosure should be based on the negligent tort of malpractice rather than on the intentional torts of assault and battery.[2] Although this decision proved to be popular and was widely accepted, there remained the very substantial problem of how to determine whether a given disclosure was adequate. The solution to this second problem created a schism among the courts, as their decisions rapidly became divided into two camps, the so-called professional community and reasonable patient rules.

The *professional community rule*[3] adopted the usual requirements necessary to establish negligence: A doctor had to conform to the standard of care expected of like doctors acting under the same or similar circumstances; negligence could only be proven by expert testimony establishing that the defendant doctor had not met the prevailing professional standard in disclosing the risks and alternative procedures to the patient.

A series of decisions contra to this rule propounded a markedly different standard.[4] The *reasonable patient rule* held that the scope of disclosure should not be determined by the standards of the medical profession but by the patient's need to know information that would be material to his ability to make an informed decision. To make an intelligently reasoned

Table 22.1. Jurisdictions Applying the "Professional Community" Rule: 1980

Alabama	*Roberts v. Woods*, 206 F. Supp. 579 (1962)
Arizona	**Shetter v. Rochelle*, 2 Ariz. App. 358, 409 P.2d 74, *modified* 2 Ariz. 607, 411 P.2d 45 (1965)
	**Hales v. Pittman*, 118 Ariz. 305, 576 P.2d 493 (1978)
Arkansas	*Pegram v. Sisco*, 406 F. Supp. 776, *affirmed* 547 F.2d 1172 (8th Cir. 1976)
Colorado	**Mallett v. Pirkey*, 171 Colo. 271, 466 P.2d 466 (1970)
	Mudd v. Dorr, 574 P.2d 97 (1977)
Delaware	*DiFilippo v. Preston*, 53 Del. 539, 173 A.2d 333 (1961)
	* *Wagner v. Olmedo*, 365 A.2d 643 (1976)
	Del. Code Ann. tit. 18, §6852 (1978 Cum. Supp.)
Florida	*Bowers v. Talmadge*, 159 So.2d 888 (1963)
	Russell v. Harwick, 166 So.2d 904 (1964)
	Fla. Stat. Ann. §768.46 (1978 Supp.)
Georgia	*Young v. Yarn*, 136 Ga. App. 737, 222 S.E.2d 113 (1975)
	Ga. Code Ann. §§88-2901 to 2907 (1971)
Hawaii	*Nishi v. Hartwell*, 52 Haw. 188, 473 P.2d 116 (1970)
	Hawaii Rev. Stat. §671-3 (1976)
Idaho	*Reidinger v. Colburn*, 361 F. Supp. 1073 (1973)
	Idaho Code, §§39-4301 to 4306 (1975)
Illinois	*Green v. Hussey*, 127 Ill. App. 2d 174, 262 N.E.2d 156 (1970)
Indiana	*Lloyd v. Kull*, 329 F.2d 168 (7th Cir. 1964)
	Joy v. Chau, 377 N.E.2d 670 (1978)
Kansas	*Natanson v. Kline*, 187 Kan. 186, 354 P.2d 670 (1960)
	* *Yeates v. Harms*, 193 Kan. 320, 393 P.2d 982 (1964)
Massachusetts	*Schroeder v. Lawrence*, 359 N.E.2d 1301 (1977)
Michigan	*Roberts v. Young*, 369 Mich. 113, 119 N.W.2d 627 (1963)
	**Shulman v. Lerner*, 2 Mich. App. 705, 141 N.W.2d 348 (1966)
	Marchlewicz v. Stanton, 50 Mich. App. 344, 213 N.W.2d 317 (1973)
Mississippi	*Ross v. Hodges*, 234 So.2d 905 (1970)
Missouri	*Aiken v. Clary*, 396 S.W.2d 668 (1965)
Montana	*Negaard v. Estate of Feda*, 152 Mont. 47, 446 P.2d 436 (1968)
	Doerr v. Movius, 154 Mont. 510, 463 P.2d 477 (1970)
Nebraska	*Neb. Rev. Stat.* §§44-2816, 2820 (1978)
New Hampshire	*Folger v. Corbett*, 394 A.2d 63 (1978)
	N.H. Rev. Stat. Ann., §507-C (1977 Supp.)
New Jersey	*Gleitman v. Cosgrove*, 49 N.J. 22, 227 A.2d 689 (1966)
	Kaplan v. Haines, 96 N.J. Super 242, 232 A.2d 840 (1967), *affirmed* 51 N.J. 404, 241 A.2d 235 (1968)
New York	*Karlsons v. Guerinot*, 57 A.D.2d 73, 394 N.Y.S.2d 933 (1977)
	N.Y. Pub Health Law (McKinney) tit 44, §2805-d (1976-77 Supp.)
North Carolina	**Butler v. Berkeley*, 25 N.C. App. 325, 213 S.E.2d 571 (1975)
	N.C. Gen. Stat., §90-21.1 (1977 Cum. Supp.)
North Dakota	* *Walker v. North Dakota Eye Clinic, Ltd.*, 415 F. Supp. 891 (1976)
	* *Winkjer v. Herr*, 277 N.W.2d 579 (1979)
	N.D. Cent. Code Ann., ch. 26-40.1
Oregon	*Getchell v. Mansfield*, 260 Or. 174, 489 P.2d 953 (1971)
	Holland v. Sisters of St. Joseph of Peace, 270 Or. 129, 522 P.2d 208 (1974)
	Or. Rev. Stat. §677.097 (1977)
Tennessee	*Longmire v. Hoey*, 512 S.W.2d 307 (1974)
	Tenn. Code Ann., §23-3417
Texas	*Gravis v. Physicians and Surgeons Hospital of Alice*, 415 S.W.2d 674 (1967)
	Marsh v. Arnold, 446 S.W.2d 949 (1969)
	Gaut v. Quast, 505 S.W.2d 367 (1974)
	Karp v. Cooley, 493 F.2d 408 (5th Cir. 1974)
	Tex. Code Ann., art. 4590 (1978 Cum. Supp.)
Utah	*Ficklin v. MacFarlane*, 550 P.2d 1295 (1976)
	Utah Code Ann., §78-14-1 et seq. (1977)

Table 22.1. *Continued*

Vermont	*Small v. Gifford Memorial Hospital*, 133 Vt. 552, 349 A.2d 703 (1975)
	Vt. Stat. Ann., tit. 12 §1909 (1979 Cum. Supp.)
Virginia	*Bly v. Rhoads*, 216 Va. 645, 222 S.E.2d 783 (1976)
Wyoming	*Govin v. Hunter*, 374 P.2d 421 (1962)
	Stundon v. Stadnik, 469 P.2d 16 (1970)

*Indicates cases involving eye care

Source: Rosoff, A.J., *Informed Consent: A Guide for Health Care Providers*, Aspen, Rockville, Md., 1981.

choice regarding consent to a procedure, a patient had to receive information concerning the inherent and potential hazards of the procedure, alternative methods of treatment, and anticipated conditions that would result if the patient refused to give his consent.

In divulging this information, a doctor is expected to observe several general guidelines[5]:

- If a procedure inherently involves a known risk of death or serious bodily harm, it has to be disclosed.
- Complicated procedures have to be explained in lay terms.
- The relatively minor risks inherent in common procedures do not have to be disclosed when it is common knowledge that such minor risks are of very low incidence.
- In common procedures a remote possibility of death or serious bodily harm does not have to be disclosed.
- No disclosure has to be made if the patient requests that he not be informed, if the patient already knows of the risk, or if to inform the patient would cause him to be unable to make a rational decision.

To maintain a successful cause of action under the reasonable patient rule, a patient has to show that an adequate disclosure would have resulted in his refusal to undergo the procedure. The test is whether a prudent person in the patient's position would have consented to the procedure if he had been adequately informed.

The decisions establishing the reasonable patient rule were widely followed by both the medical and the legal professions.[6] The most controversial aspect of the rule was the liberal evidentiary change that allowed a completely different means of determining the scope of the required disclosure. Since materiality of risk was to be determined by the significance a reasonable person would attach to a given risk, the scope of disclosure prevalent in the medical profession was no longer a determinative factor (as it was under the professional community rule). The upshoot of the reasonable patient rule was that a patient could recover damages from a doctor despite having received a nonnegligent diagnosis and treatment, as long as the disclosure given by the doctor was inadequate. Tables 22.1 and 22.2 list those jurisdictions in which the professional community and reasonable patient rules have been adopted.[7] In a few states no rule has been established by courts or legislatures (see Table 22.3). The debate and discussion that has attended the development of these rules has made informed consent the most widely taught legal subject in medical schools (even more popular than malpractice).[8]

Informed consent has even crept into optometry, but there are few occasions when informed consent may be necessary, such as prior to dilation of an eye that has an extremely narrow anterior chamber angle. A sample consent form for diagnostic procedures is included as Fig. 22.1.

The brouhaha over informed consent has been somewhat ironic because a comprehensive study of malpractice claims conducted by the National Association of Insurance Commissioners (NAIC) in the late 1970s revealed the number of reported claims based on informed consent to be a paltry 2.8 percent of all the malpractice claims filed during the $3\frac{1}{2}$ years of the study.[9] One explanation offered for this low percentage of claims is that informed consent, by itself, is a weak claim for relief and that it is resorted to only in those cases that have a marginal chance of prevailing.

There has been virtually no comment about informed consent in the optometric literature because there have been no reported cases involving optometrists.[10] The preponderance of cases have involved surgeons; only a minority of cases have been concerned with medical procedures (such as the use of therapeutic pharmaceutical agents that resulted in unwarned-of side effects). But the potential application of the doctrine of informed consent to the use of ophthalmic drugs should not be disregarded. Therapeutic agents, in particular, are amenable to claims based on lack of an informed consent, and ophthalmic drugs have been the cause of many claims against

Table 22.2. Jurisdictions Applying the "Reasonable Patient" Rule: 1980

Alaska	*Patrick v. Sedwick*, 391 P.2d 453 (1964)
	* *Poulin v. Zartman*, 542 P.2d 251 (1975)
California	*Salgo v. Stanford Univ. Board of Trustees*, 154 Cal. App. 2d 560, 317 P.2d 170 (1957)
	Cobbs v. Grant, 104 Cal. Rptr. 505, 502 P.2d 1 (1972)
District of Columbia	*Canterbury v. Spence*, 464 F.2d 772 (D.C. Cir. 1972)
Kentucky	* *Holton v. Pfingst*, 534 S.W.2d 786 (1975)
	Bennett v. Graves, 557 S.W.2d 893 (1977)
Louisiana	*Percle v. St. Paul Fire and Marine Ins. Co.*, 349 So.2d 1289 (1977)
	Reynier v. Delta Women's Clinic, Inc., 359 So.2d 733 (1978)
	Hanks v. Drs. Ranson, Swan and Burch, Ltd., 359 So.2d 1089, *writ denied*, 360 So.2d 1178 (1978)
	Steele v. St. Paul Fire and Marine Ins. Co., 371 So2d 843 (1979)
	La. Rev. Stat. Ann. §40:1299.40 (1975)
Minnesota	*Cornfeldt v. Tongen*, 262 N.W.2d 684 (1977)
	Minn. Stat Ann. §144.651
New Mexico	*Demers v. Gerety*, 92 N.M. 396, 589 P.2d 180 (1978), *reversed* 92 N.M. 749, 595 P.2d 387 (1978)
Ohio	*Congrove v. Holmes*, 37 Ohio Misc. 95, 308 N.E.2d 765 (1973)
	Bruni v. Tatsumi, 46 Ohio St.2d 127, 346 N.E.2d 673 (1976)
	Ohio Rev. Code Ann. §2317.54 (1978 Supp.)
Oklahoma	* *Lambert v. Park*, 597 F.2d 236 (10th Cir. 1979)
Pennsylvania	*Cooper v. Roberts*, 220 Pa. Super. 260, 286 A.2d 647 (1971)
	Jeffries v. McCague, 242 Pa. Super. 76, 363 A.2d 1167 (1976)
	Pa. Stat. Ann., tit. 40, §1301.101 et seq. (1976)
Rhode Island	*Wilkinson v. Vesey*, 110 R.I. 606, 295 A.2d 676 (1972)
	R.I. Gen. Laws §9-19-32 (1976)
Washington	*Keogan v. Holy Family Hospital*, 22 Wash. App. 366, 589 P.2d 310, *cert. denied* 601 P.2d 1303 (1979)
	* *Gates v. Jensen*, 92 Wash. 2d 246, 595 P.2d 919 (1979), *reversing*
	20 Wash. App. 81, 579 P.2d 374 (1978)
	Wash. Rev. Code Ann., §§7.70.050-.060 (1978 Supp.)
Wisconsin	*Trogun v. Fruchtman*, 58 Wis. 2d 596, 207 N.W.2d 297 (1973)
	Scaria v. St. Paul Fire and Marine Ins. Co., 68 Wis. 2d 1, 227 N.W.2d 647 (1975)

*Indicates cases involving eye care.

Source: Rosoff, A.J., *Informed Consent: A Guide for Health Care Providers*, Aspen, Rockville, Md., 1981.

ophthalmologists.[11] Although a minority of optometrists can legally utilize therapeutic agents, these optometrists encounter the same legal risks under the doctrine of informed consent as do ophthalmologists and need to be cognizant of these risks (see Chapter 28 for a discussion).

In addition to liability for pharmaceutical agents, there are other applications of the doctrine of informed consent that have potential application to optometrists, even though, as yet, only ophthalmologists have been litigants in these cases. Testing for glaucoma is one example of an area of practice common to both professions that has become a significant testing ground for the expansion of informed

Table 22.3. Jurisdictions with No Definitive Rule: 1980

Connecticut	*Ruby v. Massey*, 452 F. Supp. 361 (1978)
Iowa	*Grosjean v. Spencer*, 258 Iowa 685, 140 N.W.2d 139 (1966)
	Iowa Code Ann. §147.137 (1979-80 Cum. Supp.)
Maine	*Downer v. Villeux*, 322 A.2d 82 (1974)
Nevada	*Corn v. French*, 71 Nev. 280, 289 P.2d 173 (1955)
	Nev. Rev. Stat. §§41A.110, 41A.120
South Carolina	*Walker v. Pierce*, 560 F.2d 609 (4th Cir. 1977)
South Dakota	*Cunningham v. Yankton Clinic*, 262 N.W.2d 508 (1978)
West Virginia	No applicable case law or statute

Source: Rosoff, A.J., *Informed Consent: A Guide for Health Care Providers*, Aspen, Rockville, Md., 1981.

I hereby authorize Dr. _______ to perform upon (myself or name of patient) the following diagnostic procedure: ______________________________

____

I have been fully informed of the risks, possible alternative methods of treatment, and possible consequences of this procedure.

I fully understand the nature of this procedure and authorize its administration.

Signed ______________________________
(Patient or person authorized to sign for patient)

Witness ______________________ Date ______________________

Figure 22.1. Sample Consent for Diagnostic Procedure

consent (discussed infra). Since the application of informed consent varies from state to state, it is imperative that optometrists be familiar with the interpretation (i.e., professional community or reasonable patient rule) that is the law in their particular jurisdiction. In addition, it is important that optometrists obtain a basic understanding of informed consent's impact upon the daily practice of the profession.

It is to the application of the doctrine to clinical practice that we now turn.

Application to Clinical Practice

There are three basic categories under which liability for failure to obtain an informed consent can be incurred by an optometrist:

1. Failure to disclose the risks of a proposed treatment
2. Failure to disclose alternatives to therapy
3. Failure to disclose abnormalities

Failure to Disclose the Risks of a Proposed Treatment

A doctor is under a duty to disclose the severity and probability of risks in a proposed procedure. For optometrists, the most obvious application of this duty is when testing experimental ophthalmic products.

An optometrist fitted a young patient with an experimental flexible contact lens and dispensed an experimental accessory solution. The patient suffered damage to his corneas from chemical burns and sued the optometrist for malpractice. The optometrist had neither made a full disclosure of the experimental nature of his work to the patient nor had he secured the consent of the patient's parents (e.g., a written release). The optometrist was held to be liable for the patient's damages.[12]

Optometrists who serve as investigators for the purpose of conducting clinical trials of a particular ophthalmic product for a manufacturer typically receive detailed instructions and a copious set of patient consent forms, the intent of which is to assure an adequate and documented informed consent. Careful documentation should always accompany the performance of clinical trials, and any experimentation conducted by an individual optometrist on his patient population should likewise be carefully documented in the records of those patients who agree to participate in the study. A signed form is the most consistent means of assuring that each patient receives the necessary information (see Chapter 30 for an example).

A second application of this duty is limited to those practitioners who use therapeutic pharmaceutical agents.[13] Patients must be advised of the risk associated with the use of drugs. For example, topical steroids have adverse side effects (e.g., cataracts, glaucoma) that are a known risk of use; systemic steroids can cause severe side effects, including death.[14] The *Physicians Desk Reference* (PDR) and the package inserts that accompany each medication should be consulted, as necessary, to advise the patient properly. Of course, the risks that must be disclosed to the patient are determined by the law (professional community or reasonable patient rule) of the state in which the doctor practices.

Since it is not necessary to disclose a remote possibility of injury for common procedures, in the ordinary case there is no duty to disclose the statistically remote possibilities of the use of diagnostic pharmaceutical agents.[15] (This caveat applies both to professional community and reasonable patient rule states.) Informed consent and ophthalmic pharmaceutical use is described in Chapter 28.

Regardless of the status of the law, an optometrist should always fully understand the risks associated with any optometric procedure and should be prepared to discuss these risks with any inquiring patient.

Failure to Disclose Alternatives to Therapy

A patient must be advised of the alternative procedures available, including—in reasonable patient rule states—those alternatives that the doctor regards as undesirable for the patient.[16] The doctor must avoid making the choice of therapy for the patient because the patient should always have the right to veto any proposed course of treatment.

There are many circumstances under which an optometrist could be charged with failing to advise the patient of alternatives to therapy. Consider the following list:

- Failure to disclose the alternative of referral for a cataract patient with reduced visual acuity
- Failure to disclose the alternative of referral for a patient with elevated intraocular pressure but no visual field loss (i.e., ocular hypertension)
- Failure to disclose the alternative of treatment by a low vision specialist for a patient with profound loss of visual acuity or markedly restricted visual fields
- Failure to disclose the alternative of referral for an infant with strabismus
- Failure to disclose the alternative of referral for a patient suffering from learning disability
- Failure to disclose alternatives to extended wear contact lenses
- Failure to disclose alternative choices for impact-resistant ophthalmic lens materials when prescribing for athletes, children, monocular patients, or adults in physically active occupations
- Failure to disclose alternative forms of therapy available to patients afflicted with hereditary diseases

Doubtless there are numerous other circumstances that could be imagined. Because optometrists have a legal responsibility to refer patients who they feel are in need of a specialist's care, the issue of when a patient should be referred is of obvious significance. Even though an optometrist might consider referral undesirable under a particular set of circumstances, in the reasonable patient rule states this decision will be a jury matter because it is the patient's need to know and not the standard of care within the profession that determines whether the alternative to therapy should have been disclosed to the patient. Remember that the optometrist does not have to be negligent in his diagnosis and treatment of the patient; he can be liable if it is shown that a fully informed, reasonable patient would have chosen the alternative choice of treatment (whatever it might be).

Failure to Disclose Abnormalities

Although failure to disclose abnormalities is not within the traditional scope of informed consent, a case involving open-angle glaucoma has expanded the scope of the tort to include this cause of action.[17]

A 56-year-old woman was examined by an ophthalmologist, who performed Schiotz tonometry and obtained readings of 23.8 mm Hg for each eye. He performed no visual field examination and did not tell the patient of the elevated intraocular pressures. Two years later, at another examination, she was found to be functionally blind due to open-angle glaucoma. She sued the ophthalmologist for negligence, but the trial court found in his favor. She appealed the decision, and the state supreme court held that, under the doctrine of informed consent, the ophthalmologist had a duty to tell her of any abnormal findings and to inform her of any diagnostic procedures that could be undertaken to determine the significance of the findings. The ophthalmologist was found to be liable for breach of the doctrine of informed consent.[18]

The gist of the ruling is that the doctrine of informed consent can be applied to borderline intraocular pressure readings obtained during tonometry, and that a prudent doctor will always inform a patient of suspicious findings and perform further diagnostic tests (e.g., dilated fundus examination, gonioscopy, and visual fields). There are four other aspects of this ruling: (1) the duty to disclose arises at the time the doctor encounters the abnormality; (2) the duty to disclose may arise before the doctor has made a diagnosis or has recommended a course of therapy; (3) tests that might lead to the discovery of disease are material facts that must be disclosed to the patient; and (4) the fact that the doctor has complied with the standard of care within his profession (in satisfying himself that the patient does not suffer from disease) will not insulate him from liability.

Testing for glaucoma is a fertile area for litigation, either on the basis of negligence in failing to diagnose its presence (malpractice) or on the basis of failing to disclose an abnormal diagnostic finding (informed consent).[19] Whether other courts in other jurisdictions will apply this expanded application of the doctrine of informed consent cannot be predicted. Likewise, the liability of optometrists for informed consent can only be the subject of speculation, given the current state of the law. But the trend over the past several years has been one of expansion of the doctrine in the few landmark cases that have been decided, and there is no reason to suspect that this trend will change.

Notes

1. Informed consent has been the subject of several papers appearing in the Law and Medicine series of the *Journal of the American Medical Association*. See the following: Informed Consent, Part I, vol. 214, no. 6, Nov. 9, 1970, pp. 1181–1182; Part II, vol. 214, no. 7, Nov. 16, 1970, pp. 1383–1384; and Part III, vol. 214, no. 8, Nov. 23, 1970, pp. 1611–1612.
2. *Natanson v. Kline*, 187 Kan. 186, 354 P.2d 670 (1960).
3. Ibid.
4. *Woods v. Brumlop*, 71 N.M. 221, 377 P.2d 520 (1962); *Cooper v. Roberts*, 220 Pa. Super. 260, 286 A.2d 647 (1971); *Cobbs v. Grant*, 8 Cal. 3d 229, 502 P.2d 1, 104 Cal. Rptr. 505 (1972); *Canterbury v. Spence*, 464 F.2d 772 (D.C. Cir. 1972); and *Wilkinson v. Vesey*, 110 R.I. 606, 296 A.2d 676 (1972). Because of the influence of the California and District of Columbia courts, *Cobbs* and *Canterbury* have received the most attention. See Rosoff, A.J., *Informed Consent: A Guide for Health Care Providers*, Aspen, Rockville, Md., 1981, for a state-by-state listing of cases.
5. For a discussion, see Johnson, B.A., An Overview of Informed Consent, in James, A.E. (ed.), *Legal Medicine*, Urban and Schwarzenberg, Baltimore, 1980, p. 281.
6. See the Law and Medicine series in the *Journal of the American Medical Association*. More about Informed Consent, Part I, vol. 224, no. 13, June 25, 1973, pp. 1831–1832; and Part II, vol. 225, no. 1, July 2, 1973, pp. 95–96.
7. Adapted from Rosoff, note 4 supra.
8. As of 1987, the Association of Schools and Colleges of Optometry and the American Optometric Association have proposed a model curriculum for legal aspects of practice. See *A Curriculum Model for Practice Management*, published jointly by ASCO and the AOA. For a review of the state of the art of legal education in schools of medicine, see Grumet, B.R., Legal Medicine in Medical Schools: A Survey of the State of the Art, *Journal of Medical Education*, vol. 54, no. 9, Oct. 1979, p. 755.
9. Reported by Curran, W.J., Malpractice Claims: New Data and New Trends, *New England Journal of Medicine*, vol. 300, no. 1, Jan. 1979, p. 26.
10. Harris, M.G., and R.E. Dister, Informed Consent in Contact Lens Practice, *Journal of the American Optometric Association*, vol. 58, no. 3, 1987, pp. 230–237.
11. See Bettman, J.W., A Review of 412 Claims in Ophthalmology, in Medicolegal Aspects of Ophthalmology, Bettman, J.W. (ed.), *International Ophthalmology Clinics*, vol. 20, 1980, pp. 131–142.
12. Reported in the *AOA News*, June 15, 1976.
13. See Drug Reactions, *Journal of the American Medical Association*, vol. 197, no. 8, Aug. 22, 1966, p. 221; Physician's Liability for Drug Reactions, *Journal of the American Medical Association*, vol. 213, no. 12, Sept. 21, 1970, pp. 2143–2144.
14. Bartlett, J.D., and S.D. Jaanus, *Clinical Ocular Pharmacology*, Butterworth, Boston, 1984.
15. Keller, J.T., The Risk of Angle Closure from the Use of Mydriatics, *Journal of the American Optometric Association*, vol. 46, no. 1, 1975, pp. 19–21.
16. See *Archer v. Galbraith*, 18 Wash. App. 369, 567 P.2d 1155 (1977).
17. For a review of this new application of the tort, see Ravzi, E., Informed Consent in Washington: Expanded Scope of Material Facts that the Physician Must Disclose to His Patients, *Washington Law Review*, vol. 55, 1980, p. 655.
18. *Gates v. Jensen*, 92 Wash. 2d. 246, 595 P.2d 919 (1979). For commentary, see Thal, L.S., *Gates v. Jensen*: Another Precedent for Glaucoma Testing, *Journal of the American Optometric Association*, vol. 52, no. 4, 1981, pp. 349–353.
19. Glaucoma as the basis for malpractice is reviewed in 67 A.L.R. 3d 175.

PART SEVEN

CLINICOLEGAL ASPECTS OF PRACTICE

Chapter 23

Optometrist's Duty to Detect Glaucoma

Although the incidence of glaucoma in the range of the plaintiff is approximately one in 25,000, this alone should not be enough to deny her a claim. Where its presence can be detected by a simple, well-known harmless test, where the results of the test are definitive, where the disease can be successfully arrested by early detection and where its effects are irreversible if undetected over a substantial period of time, liability should be imposed upon defendants even though they did not violate the standard existing within the profession.
—From the concurring opinion of Judge Utter, *Helling v. Carey,* 591 P.2d 981 (1974)

Necessity to Test for Glaucoma

There is a perception both within and without the profession that optometry is part of the health-care system and that optometrists represent an important line of defense in that system against ocular and systemic disease. One of the most important diseases in this regard is glaucoma, and one of the most important clinicolegal issues facing optometrists today concerns the responsibility of clinicians for the detection or diagnosis of glaucoma. Failure to detect glaucoma is the leading cause of large malpractice claims against optometrists.[1]

Persons in the United States who suffer some degree of vision impairment (without being legally blind) constitute a sizable portion of the population, an estimated 11.4 million, most of whom are male and between the ages of twenty-five and sixty-four.[2] The leading cause of all degrees of vision impairment is cataract, but glaucoma is an important source as well, constituting 9 percent of cases and affecting over a million persons.[3] Open-angle glaucoma, the primary disease, has an incidence in the general population of 0.5 percent,[4] but this statistic varies with different age-population groups.

A screening performed by the National Society to Prevent Blindness in 1973 of almost 72,000 persons across the United States diagnosed glaucoma in the following age groups and percentages[5]:

AGE	PERCENT
Over 65 years	1.1
35-44 years	0.2
Under 35 years	0.03

Therefore, as a clinical entity, glaucoma is a disease that occurs with sufficient frequency for optometrists to pay it heed, but there is also the issue of severity to be considered.

In its open-angle form, glaucoma is an insidious disease that, if untreated, can progress to severe vision loss, including blindness. Because of technological advances the measurement of intraocular pressure is a relatively quick, painless, and accurate means of testing for the disease. When combined with ophthalmoscopy, evaluation of the visual field, and gonioscopy, the clinician is able to arrive at a definitive diagnosis and to initiate treatment. Both medical and surgical management of glaucoma are available, and these remedies are effective in arresting the progress of the disease. Thus glaucoma is particularly suited to early detection: If discovered in the beginning stages, the injury is minimal; if undetected over a relatively lengthy period of time, there is severe injury. Furthermore, the basic test—tonometry—is neither expensive nor time-consuming. For these reasons, there is compelling clinical evidence for optometrists to examine for the disease.

But what of the legal obligation? How have the courts interpreted the clinical evidence and expressed the legal duty expected of practitioners?

For the most part, the cases that have established liability for detection of glaucoma have involved the medical profession. Perhaps the leading case is *Helling v. Carey*,[6] which was based upon the following facts: Ms. Helling sought the services of Dr. Carey, an ophthalmologist, in order to be fitted with contact lenses; she was in her early twenties and myopic. She was fitted for lenses and seen numerous times over the course of nearly a decade for various complaints that seemed to be associated with lens wear. Finally her intraocular pressure and visual field were tested, and she was found to have open-angle glaucoma. She was 32 years of age, and her visual field was reduced to 5° vertical and 10° horizontal, a severe impairment. She filed suit, alleging negligence on the part of the defendants for failing to test her for glaucoma in a more timely fashion.

At trial, evidence offered by the defendant physicians and by expert witnesses testifying on their behalf established that glaucoma was a relatively rare disease in the below-40 age population, with an incidence of approximately one in 25,000, and that for this reason it was not the standard of care to test routinely in this age bracket for the disease. Consequently, the trial court awarded a judgment in favor of the doctors. Ms. Helling appealed the decision, arguing that the standard of care was inadequate to protect her from injury, and the state Supreme Court, in reversing the trial court, made the following observation:

> *The incidence of glaucoma in one out of 25,000 persons under the age of 40 may appear quite minimal. However, that one person, the plaintiff in this instance, is entitled to the same protection as afforded persons over 40, essential for timely detection of the evidence of glaucoma where it can be arrested to avoid the grave and devastating result of this disease.* The test is a simple pressure test, relatively inexpensive. There is no judgment factor involved, and there is no doubt that by giving the test the evidence of glaucoma can be detected. The giving of the test is harmless if the physical condition of the eye permits. The testimony indicates that although the condition of the plaintiff's eyes might at times have prevented the defendants from administering the pressure test, there is an absence of evidence in the record that the test could not have been timely given [emphasis added].[7]

This decision engendered an unusual amount of publicity in both the legal and the medical professions, and the deluge of commentary undoubtedly reached the ears of optometrists.[8] In fact, a study of tonometry at two colleges of optometry revealed that, by 1978, the percentage of patients in the 11–20 age bracket being given tonometry had risen significantly, to approximately 80 percent of patients as compared to less than 10 percent of patients five years earlier (in 1973, before the *Helling* decision was rendered).[9] The clear message transmitted to practitioners by this case was to test for glaucoma routinely, regardless of the patient's age. Emphasis was added by another legal issue emerging in the 1970s: the doctrine of informed consent.

The doctrine of informed consent permits a patient to recover damages for nonnegligent diagnosis and treatment and is based on the duty imposed on doctors to disclose information prior to initiating treatment of the patient.[10] Legal protection is granted to the patient because of the unequal status of the parties, and because the patient has the right to consent to or to veto any proposed procedure, a decision-making process that relies on the information received from the doctor. As a result, the courts have imposed a duty upon doctors to supply information so that an informed consent to treatment can be obtained from the patient.

The leading case applying the doctrine to the testing of glaucoma is *Gates v. Jensen*.[11] Mrs. Gates was 54 years old and "severely myopic" at the time she was first examined by the defendants. She complained of difficulty in focusing, blurred vision, and gaps in her vision. Her intraocular pressures were 23.8 mm Hg in each eye as determined by Schiotz tonometry, and direct ophthalmoscopy was unremarkable through an undilated pupil. Visual fields were not evaluated. In response to Mrs. Gates' inquiry about her intraocular pressure, she was told that she had been checked for glaucoma and that she was all right. Her complaints were diagnosed as being due to the contact lenses she wore and she was treated accordingly.

Over the next two years Mrs. Gates was seen on twelve occasions at the defendants' clinic, during which her condition, including her visual acuity, worsened. When the diagnosis of open-angle glaucoma was eventually made, Mrs. Gates' best corrected visual acuity was reduced to 20/200, and she ultimately became functionally blind. She sued, alleging negligence and a breach of the doctrine of informed consent, arguing that the physicians had a duty to inform her of abnormalities discovered during a routine examination and of diagnostic procedures that may be taken to determine the significance of the abnormalities. The trial court found for the defendant doctors, and Mrs. Gates appealed.

The state Supreme Court, in reversing the trial court, described the application of the doctrine of informed consent to the facts in the case:

> The basis of this duty is that the patient has a right to know the material facts concerning the condition of his or her body, and any risks presented by that condition, so that an informed choice may be made regarding the course which the patient's medical care will take. The patient's right to know is not confined to the choice of treatment once a disease is present and has been conclusively diagnosed. Important decisions must frequently be made in many non-treatment situations in which medical care is given, including procedures leading to a diagnosis, as in this case. These decisions must all be taken with the full knowledge and participation of the patient. The physician's duty is to tell the patient what he or she needs to know in order to make them. *The existence of an abnormal condition in one's body, the presence of a high risk of disease, and the existence of alternative diagnostic procedures to conclusively determine the presence or absence of that disease are all facts which a patient must know in order to make an informed decision on the course which future medical care will take* [emphasis added].[12]

The principle established by *Gates* has obvious application to those occasions in which a clinician finds patients with borderline intraocular pressures. The clinician is obligated either to inform the patient of the findings—so that the patient can determine if he or she wishes to undergo further testing—or to undertake such tests as are necessary to arrive at a diagnosis of the patient's condition. Failure to disclose elevated ocular pressure, even in the absence of visual field loss (i.e., ocular hypertension) may create liability under the doctrine, should the patient later suffer some measurable loss of the visual field. Therefore, not only is it necessary to test routinely for glaucoma, it is advisable to communicate borderline findings to the patient and to initiate any additional testing that is appropriate. (This is discussed in more detail subsequently.)

The *Helling* and *Gates* decisions have established theories of liability that are applicable to the clinical practice of optometry. It is noteworthy to point out in each of these cases that the patient was a contact lens wearer whose disease was undiagnosed for a period sufficient to create significant damages. And there are other opportunities in clinical practice for liability, as the cases in the next section illustrate.

Liability for Failure to Diagnose Glaucoma

There are two basic types of glaucoma that a clinician must be able to detect: open-angle glaucoma and angle-closure glaucoma. The following cases describe circumstances under which legal action has been initiated for alleged misdiagnosis of both forms of the disease.

Open-Angle Glaucoma

Open-angle glaucoma is defined as elevated intraocular pressures occurring in the presence of an open angle associated with a characteristic field loss and changes in the optic nerve head; it is painless and slowly progressive. Studies have shown that relatively few patients with ocular pressures between 20 and 29 mm Hg develop characteristic glaucomatous field loss within five years, and that the usual progression of the disease should be measured in terms of decades rather than years.[13] Since the patient is rarely aware of the disease, it is most commonly discovered during a routine examination. But if tonometry, visual fields, ophthalmoscopy, and gonioscopy are not performed, the diagnosis of the disease may be missed (as the *Helling* and *Gates* cases illustrate).

Although glaucoma detection is most readily associated with elevated intraocular pressure, *low-tension* glaucoma is a rare disease that manifests in visual field loss despite intraocular pressures that are within the range of normal. It has been reported that the prevalence of low-tension glaucoma is from 0.3 to 4 percent of all open-angle glaucoma patients, but this percentage may be misleadingly low because studies reveal a higher relative prevalence and incidence in the normal patient population than in those persons found to have open-angle glaucoma.[14] The primary characteristic of the disease is that visual field loss occurs despite an open angle and intraocular pressures that are below 21 mm Hg by applanation. For the optometric clinician, the difficulty in detecting low-tension glaucoma is compounded by the fact that intraocular pressures, even if measured, will not indicate the presence of disease. Careful ophthalmoscopy and a sensitive visual field examination will be necessary or the diagnosis will be missed.

A 52-year-old laborer was examined by an optometrist, who did not test the patient for glaucoma. One and one-half years later, the optometrist examined the patient again and performed tonometry, which revealed intraocular pressures of 19 and 20 mm Hg. The optometrist detected macular changes and recommended that the patient see a physician, which he did. Shortly thereafter the patient was admitted to a hospital, complaining of severe headache and sudden visual loss. The patient was found to have a retinal branch vein occlusion, diabetes mellitus, and open-angle glaucoma with visual field loss. The patient received a trabeculectomy to control the intraocular pressure, but ultimately the patient's vision declined to the extent that he was unable to work. He sued the optometrist for failure to diagnose glaucoma and refer him to a specialist for treatment.[15]

When performing a routine eye health assessment of patients, it is advisable to test visual fields as well as intraocular pressures in order to detect the presence of low-tension glaucoma.

If an examination reveals elevated intraocular pressures, visual field defects, anomalies of the anterior chamber, or optic nerve changes, referral of the patient may be indicated in order for medical treatment to be initiated. Whenever referrals are necessary, it is best to contact the doctor to whom the patient is being referred and make the appointment for the patient. Merely suggesting to the patient that another doctor be seen may not be adequate in the absence of supporting documentation in the patient record concerning the referral. Furthermore, poor communication may itself lead to the possibility of liability.

A woman who had difficulty understanding English was examined by an optometrist. He alleged that he told her to see an ophthalmologist, but she later denied being told this. In any event, some time later she was examined by a physician and found to have a severe vision loss due to open-angle glaucoma. She thereafter sued the optometrist for malpractice and was awarded $350,000 in damages by the trial court.[16]

Adequate documentation of referrals is essential. All optometrists should institute careful record controls so as to minimize the opportunity for poor communication and inadequate documentation.

An alternative form of open-angle glaucoma is *pigmentary* glaucoma, which may be defined as ocular hypertension associated with an open angle that is excessively pigmented in all quadrants, with characteristic changes in the optic disc and visual field loss.[17] Segmental peripheral iris atrophy of the posterior pigment layer and Krukenberg's spindle is usually associated with this form of glaucoma, which is most commonly found in males, myopes, and persons between 30 and 50 years of age. Failure to detect this condition may create the potential for liability.

A young female patient in her early 20s being fitted for contact lenses by an optometrist was found to have pigment deposits on her corneal endothelium. The doctor requested that the patient return for gonioscopy and visual fields at a follow-up examination (after the lenses had been dispensed), but the patient cancelled the appointment and did not return until nearly twelve months had passed. At this examination the optometrist noted that the patient's optic cup had increased from .2 to .4 in size, and that her intraocular pressures were 39 and 26 mm Hg. She was referred to an opthalmologist, who made the diagnosis of pigmentary glaucoma. Subsequently the patient sued the optometrist for failing to diagnose the condition at the first examination.[18]

Suspicious findings discovered during an examination need to be communicated to the patient, and follow-up must be instituted in an expeditous manner. In many states, even though the patient is negligent, if the doctor is also negligent then the negligence of the patient will merely be compared to that of the doctor, thereby decreasing the amount of the damages to be awarded to the patient rather than barring them altogether (known as comparative negligence).[19] Therefore, noncompliance on the part of the patient may not be sufficient to prevent a malpractice case from being successfully waged if the doctor's conduct is also deemed to be below the standard of care. Patients who require further diagnostic testing (or referral) for glaucoma should be warned in writing if they fail to keep scheduled appointments, and copies of these letters should be retained in the patient record as documentation.

Another problem for clinicians involves patients who are at low risk for glaucoma. Although the presence of open-angle glaucoma in the below-40 age population is very low (.03 percent according to the 1973 survey by the National Society to Prevent Blindness, which is three out of every 10,000 persons screened),[20] failure to detect the disease, even in this low-risk population, may result in a legal dispute alleging negligence on the part of the clinician.

A 15-year-old was examined by an optometrist, who performed Mackay-Marg tonometry and found the intraocular pressures to be "high normal." The youngster was asked to return in two weeks, at which time the tonometry was repeated, but the results were of poor quality and uncertain as to their interpretation. Visual fields were not assessed. The patient was not seen again for two years, at which time it was discovered that intraocular pressures were elevated and the optic cups were enlarged. Visual fields demonstrated a field loss. The youngster was referred for treatment but soon thereafter brought suit against the optometrist, alleging failure to diagnose and refer in a timely fashion.[21]

It is advisable to test routinely for glaucoma in all age brackets and to follow-up on all suspicious findings.

Angle-Closure Glaucoma

There is another form of the disease that practitioners must be able to detect, angle-closure glaucoma, which can be found in three clinical forms[22]:

- Acute—a dramatic, violent attack in which the entire angle is usually closed
- Subacute—intermittent, milder attacks that involve closure of part of the angle
- Chronic—silent, gradual closure of the angle that can be confused with open-angle glaucoma

The primary symptoms of the *acute* form of angle-closure glaucoma are ocular pain, nausea, vomiting, and rapid loss of vision. There is markedly elevated intraocular pressure (typically 60–90 mm Hg), epithelial edema, a mid-dilation of the pupil, and usually complete closure of the angle. If misdiagnosed, there is obvious potential for significant injury, and so optometric clinicians should be careful to rule out the disease if patients have any of the appropriate signs and symptoms.

A woman suffering from extreme eye pain, blurred vision, and nausea went to the emergency room of a hospital and was examined by an intern, who was unable to see the fundus due to corneal edema. He consulted an ophthalmological resident by telephone, and the resident diagnosed conjunctivitis, prescribed an antibiotic, and told the intern to release the patient. Consequently, the patient was not examined by an ophthalmologist for two weeks, at which time her condition was diagnosed as acute angle-closure glaucoma. Despite nine surgeries, the patient lost vision in both eyes. In addition, she developed diabetes due to prednisolone reaction. The case was settled for $2.1 million.[23]

One important consideration when discussing angle-closure glaucoma is the possibility of initiating an attack secondary to mydriasis during the optometric examination. Although the prevalence of significantly narrow angles susceptible to closure in the general population has been estimated to be 2–6 percent,[24] the risk of angle closure due to the application of a mydriatic pharmaceutical agent is extremely low. For the general population, the risk is estimated to be only 1 in 183,000, and for persons over 30 years of age, only 1 in 45,000.[25] Furthermore, it is suggested that there is a greater danger of overlooking significant retinal disease by failing to dilate the pupil than there is of inducing angle closure.[26] Therefore, the use of mydriatics by optometric clinicians is both necessary and desirable. Perhaps the most significant legal problem faced by optometrists who use mydriatic pharmaceutical agents is the failure to respond promptly to an angle closure suffered by a patient or the failure to recognize that an angle closure has, in fact, occurred. In this regard, telephone diagnoses of patient complaints should be avoided when the possibility of angle closure exists. It is always advisable to make a physical examination of the patient to rule out the possibility of an angle closure. Failure to do so can create liability.

An ophthalmologist used a mydriatic during the course of an examination. Some hours after the examination, the patient called the doctor and complained of headache and discomfort. The physician prescribed an analgesic and rest but did not see the patient. The patient's condition did not improve, and so she consulted another physician the following day. She was found to have an acute angle closure. Suit was instituted against the physician who had failed to examine her.[27]

Angle closure does not have to be as dramatic as in these cases, and in fact the *subacute* form of the disease is more common than the acute form and results in milder, recurrent attacks in which the angle closes intermittently and partially, causing a rise in intraocular pressure that is proportional to the amount of the angle closed. Symptoms include episodes of blurred vision and of colored halos around lights, but these typically subside spontaneously. Gonioscopy is necessary in order to make the diagnosis with certainty, but slit-lamp examination, ophthalmoscopy, and tonometry are also necessary. Failure to detect the disease can result in significant damages.

A 39-year-old upholsterer complaining of a "dark cloud" over his vision and halos at night was examined by an ophthalmologist, who detected a retinal hemorrhage in the left eye. The physician performed no tonometry and used digital palpation to test the patient's intraocular pressure. He referred the patient to a family physician, but all tests were negative and the patient was returned to the ophthalmologist, who performed two additional examinations three and five weeks after the first visit, diagnosing the patient's condition as branch retinal vein occlusion. About two months after the initial examination, and while the ophthalmologist was at a seminar, the patient experienced a sudden onset of intense intraocular pain and decreased acuity. He was seen by another physician, who found bilateral chronic open-angle glaucoma compounded by an acute attack of glaucoma in the left eye. The patient was treated but ultimately became blind in his left eye and had but five degrees of visual field in his right eye. The patient sued the ophthalmologist, alleging that tonometry had not been performed in an adequate and timely fashion. The trial court awarded the patient $600,000.[28]

The *chronic* form of angle-closure glaucoma occurs over a period of several months or more, without symptoms, due to a gradual closure of the angle that results in a progressive increase in the intraocular pressure. It is often mistaken for the open-angle form of glaucoma and can be confirmed by gonioscopy that reveals angle closure and by findings of elevated intraocular pressure, visual field defects, and cupping of the optic disc. At with the other forms of angle-closure glaucoma, referral should be prompt, preferably by scheduling the appointment for the patient.

It should be added that glaucoma can occur as a toxic effect of diagnostic or therapeutic drugs administered by clinicians. As previously described, the use of mydriatics for dilation of the pupil, in rare instances, can precipitate an attack of angle-closure glaucoma (see Chapter 28). Certain ophthalmic pharmaceutical agents used for therapeutic purposes can cause open-angle glaucoma. The most common cases result from the prolonged application of topical steroids.

A 13-year-old girl was taken to a pediatrician for a minor eye infection, which the physician diagnosed as conjunctivitis and treated with an ophthalmic ointment (Neodecadron®) containing a corticosteroid component. The patient was able to fill the prescription seven times over a two-year period, after which time it was discovered she had a steroid-induced glaucoma that left her with virtually no visual field in one eye and but 75 percent of the visual field in the other eye. She sued the pediatrician, alleging that the side effects of topical steroids were well reported and that the physician was negligent in permitting her to use the drug over such a lengthy period. The pediatrician defended the claim by alleging that the pharmacy had continued to fill the prescription without authorization, but pharmacy employees testified that the doctor's office was called each time the prescription was presented for refill. The jury awarded the young girl $1.5 million.[29]

The potential for drug-induced glaucoma should not be overlooked by optometrists.

Management of Ocular Hypertension

Another difficult clinical and legal issue concerns those patients whose intraocular pressures and optic nerve heads are suspicious but whose visual fields are full. The management of ocular hypertensives, glaucoma suspects, or preglaucoma patients has been a source of continuing controversy within the medical profession,[30] a debate that continues unresolved.[31]

Optometrists face the same difficulties as physicians in making the clinical decisions regarding management of these patients. Does an optometrist have a legal duty to refer glaucoma suspects or patients with suspicious findings because of the unsettled state of medical opinion? There are no cases that touch upon the legal responsibility of optometrists for these patients, but it must be remembered that the standard of care expected of optometrists is based upon what a reasonable optometrist would have done under the same or similar circumstances, and so expert testimony will be required to establish the necessary conduct (discussed in Chapter 35).[32] Although the automatic referral of these patients to physicians will relieve the referring optometrist of responsibility, such management may be expensive, unjustified, and not in the patient's best interests. If an optometrist decides to monitor a glaucoma suspect, the clinical management must be within the standard of care. An informed consent must be obtained, and the patient must be examined at periodic intervals for the purpose of measuring intraocular pressure and visual fields. Because of their greater sensitivity and reliability, visual fields measured at threshold should be obtained.[33] If a patient does suffer some determinable visual field loss, then referral (or treatment) is mandatory. Although it is arguable that the patient's field loss, no matter how slight, constitutes an injury for which damages could be awarded by a court, as long as the optometrist has explained all relevant findings to the patient, informed the patient of alternative treatment options, and obtained the patient's consent to monitor the IOP and visual fields, there will be no liability.

Clinical Application

The preceding review of cases and claims concerning an optometrist's duty to test for glaucoma enables us to construct a few general guidelines applicable to clinical practice.

- Perform an ocular health examination on all patients, and include the measurement of intraocular pressures as a routine procedure. Do not omit health testing because patients are seeking contact lenses, binocular vision therapy, or other services.
- A routine ocular health examination should include an assessment of the patient's visual field, even in the absence of elevated intraocular pressure or significant patient visual complaints.
- In difficult or ambiguous cases, recall the patient for further testing. Serial intraocular pressure measurement or visual field evaluation should be employed as necessary to rule out or confirm the presence of disease.
- Discuss findings—even if they are only suspicious—with the patient and emphasize the importance of recall and follow-up to ensure patient compliance; document patient failure to comply with scheduled recall or referral appointments.
- When referring glaucoma patients, make the appointment by telephone for the patient and document the referral in the patient record.
- Do not delay examination of any patient who may possibly be suffering from angle-closure glaucoma.

Although the precedent-setting cases cited in this chapter have primarily involved ophthalmologists, several cases involving optometrist defendants have been the subject of appellate review.[34] Optometrists must consider the attitude of the courts in assessing their duty to patients and must be cognizant of the special risk that glaucoma poses as a subject for litigation.

Notes

1. Based on the author's communications with Aetna Life & Casualty, Inc., which for many years served as the provider of group professional liability coverage for optometrists.
2. National Society to Prevent Blindness, *Vision Problems in the United States*, N.Y., 1980. Data is based on 1977 cases.
3. Ibid.
4. Duke-Elder, S., and B. Jay, Diseases of the Lens and Vitreous, *System of Ophthalmology*, vol. 11, C.V. Mosby, St. Louis, 1969, pp. 392–398.
5. National Society to Prevent Blindness, *National Screening 1973 Project Summary*, N.Y., 1974.
6. 83 Wash. 2d 514, 519 P.2d 981 (1974). A review of this case and annotations on glaucoma testing as the basis for malpractice can be found in 67 A.L.R. 3d 175.
7. See 519 P.2d at 982.
8. For an account of this case, see Classe, J., and S. Wechsler, *Helling v. Carey*: Caveat Medicus (Let the Doctor Beware), *Journal of the American Optometric Association*, vol. 48, no. 12, 1977, pp. 1526–1529.
9. Godio, L., J. Ruskiewicz, and W. Chao, The Impact of a Court Decision on the Actual Practice of Eye Care, *American Journal of Optometry & Physiological Optics*, vol. 59, no. 3, 1982, pp. 267–270.
10. The legal basis for informed consent has been enunciated by Justice Cardozo in the case of *Schloendorff v. Society of New York Hospital*, 211 N.Y. 125, 195 N.E. 92 (1914), in which he stated, "Every human being of adult years and sound mind has a right to determine what shall be done with his own body."
11. 92 Wash. 2d 246, 595 P.2d 919 (1979). See Thal, L.S., *Gates v. Jensen*: Another Precedent for Glaucoma Testing, *Journal of the American Optometric Association*, vol. 52, no. 4, 1981, pp. 349–353.
12. 595 P.2d at 922, 923.
13. Schwartz, B., Primary Open-Angle Glaucoma, in T.D. Duane (ed.), *Clinical Ophthalmology*, vol. 3, chap. 52, p. 3, Harper & Row, New York, 1976.
14. See Levene, R., Low Tension Glaucoma: A Critical Review and New Material, *Survey of Ophthalmology*, vol. 24, no. 6, 1980, pp. 621–664.
15. Based on a personal communication with the author.
16. Ibid.
17. Schwartz, B., in T.D. Duane (ed.), supra note 13.
18. Based on a personal communication with the author.
19. In a minority of states, the standard of contributory negligence still remains, which bars *all* recovery on the part of the patient if the doctor can show that the patient was negligent (and this is so even if the doctor was also negligent). The clear trend in the law, however, is toward comparative negligence, which makes documentation of recalls and referrals a necessary aspect of clinical practice. For a discussion, see Prosser, W.L., *Law of Torts*, 4th ed., West, St. Paul, Minn., 1971, pp. 416–427.
20. Testimony offered in the *Helling* case maintained that the incidence (number of new cases in a population over a period of time) of glaucoma in the below-40 age category was 1 in 25,000. See 519 P.2d at 983.
21. Based on a personal communication with the author.
22. Simmons, R.J., and R.L. Dallon, in T.D. Duane (ed.), *Clinical Ophthalmology*, vol. 3, chapter 53, Harper & Row, New York, 1976.
23. *Kim v. New York Hospital*, reported in 25 *ATLA Law Reporter* 328, 1982.
24. Cockburn, D.M., Prevalence and Significance of Narrow Anterior Chamber Angles in Optometric Prac-

tice, *American Journal of Optometry & Physiological Optics*, vol. 58, no. 2, 1981, pp. 171–175.
25. Keller, J.T., The Risk of Angle Closure from the Use of Mydriatics, *Journal of the American Optometric Association*, vol. 46, no. 1, 1975, pp. 19–21.
26. For a discussion of the risks and benefits concerning the use of mydriatics by optometrists, see Bartlett, J.D., and S.D. Jaanus (eds.), *Clinical Ocular Pharmacology*, chap. 15, Butterworths, Boston, 1984.
27. See Bettman, J.W., A Review of 412 Claims in Ophthalmology, in Medicolegal Aspects of Ophthalmology, Bettman, J.W. (ed.), *International Ophthalmology Clinics*, vol. 20, Winter 1980, p. 132.
28. See California Malpractice Topics, *Professional Liability Newsletter*, vol. 14, no. 3, Feb. 1983.
29. *Thurston v. Ninio*, reported in 23 *ATLA Law Reporter* 428, 1980.
30. For a review of the debate within ophthalmology, see Kirsch, R.E. and D.R. Anderson, Clinical Recognition of Glaucomatous Cupping, *American Journal of Ophthalmology*, vol. 75, 1973, p. 442–454; Drance, S.M., Correlation Between Optic Disc Changes and Visual Field Defects in Chronic Open-Angle Glaucoma, *Transactions of the American Academy of Ophthalmology and Otolaryngology*, vol. 81, 1976, p. 224–226; Schwartz, B., J.C. Rieser, and S.L. Fishbein, Fluorescein Angiographic Defects of the Optic Disc in Glaucoma, *Archives of Ophthalmology*, vol. 95, 1972, p. 95; Chandler, P.A., and W.M. Grant, Ocular Hypertension Versus Open-Angle Glaucoma, *Archives of Ophthalmology*, vol. 95, 1977, pp. 585–586; Kolker, A.E., and B. Becker, Ocular Hypertension Versus Open-Angle Glaucoma: A Different View, *Archives of Ophthalmology*, vol. 95, 1977, pp. 586–587; Shaffer, R., "Glaucoma Suspect" or "Ocular Hypertension"?, *Archives of Ophthalmology*, vol. 95, 1977, p. 588; Phelps, C.D., Ocular Hypertension: To Treat or Not To Treat?, *Archives of Ophthalmology*, vol. 95, 1977, p. 588; and Chandler, P.A., and W.M. Grant, Further Comments on Ocular Hypertension (letter), *Archives of Ophthalmology*, vol. 95, 1977, pp. 1083–1084.
31. The debate continues: Johnson, T.D., and T.J. Zimmerman, A Revisit: Ocular Hypertension, Glaucoma Suspect, Preglaucoma, or Glaucoma?, *Annals of Ophthalmology*, vol. 17, no. 7, 1985, pp. 390–391; Shields, M.B., A Revisit: Ocular Hypertension, Glaucoma Suspect, Preglaucoma, or Glaucoma?, *Annals of Ophthalmology*, vol. 17, no. 8, 1985, p. 456; Schwartz, B., A Reply to Johnson and Zimmerman, *Annals of Ophthalmology*, vol. 17, no. 9, 1985, p. 518; Phelps, C.D., in Response to Johnson and Zimmerman, *Annals of Ophthalmology*, vol. 17, no. 10, 1985, pp. 598–600; and Henry, C., and T. Krupin, Management of Ocular Hypertension, *Annals of* Ophthalmology, vol. 17, no. 11, 1985, pp. 672–674.
32. As to the standard of care expected of optometrists, in several states there are rules of evidence that hold that if a practitioner adheres to a course of therapy that is supported by a respectable minority of like practitioners, then there can be no liability on his part as a matter of law because a practitioner will not be held negligent merely because his therapy differs from that espoused by the majority. For a sample case, see *Sims v. Callahan*, 112 So. 2d 776 (Ala. 1959).
33. See Harrington, D.C., *The Visual Fields*, 5th ed., C.V. Mosby, St. Louis, 1987, pp. 18–26.
34. For cases involving allegations of failure to diagnose glaucoma in which optometrists were defendants, see *McMahon v. Glixman*, 393 N.E.2d 875 (Mass. 1979); *Whitt v. Columbus Cooperative Enterprises, Inc.*, 64 Ohio St. 2d 355, 415 N.E.2d 985 (1980); *Collins v. American Optometric Assn.*, 693 F.2d 636 (7th Cir. 1982); and *Holmes v. Iwasa*, 104 Idaho 179, 657 P.2d 476 (1983).

Chapter 24

Optometrist's Duty to Detect Ocular Tumors

A quick tally of specialists involved in the case would list: three ophthalmologists, one pediatrician, one team of medical doctors at an army medical center, one pathology laboratory, three ophthalmic pathologists, and one parasitologist. That collection of medical heavyweights was not only unable to come up with a definitive, differential diagnosis, but also made outright contradictory opinions, and, when they agreed, they larded their opinions with "possibly," "probably," and "maybe." Yet, a lone optometrist was blamed for the tragic course of events [because] the judge concluded that referral was made too late to save the eye, an eye for which there never was a definitive diagnosis, and for which the consensus indicates there was no effective treatment.
—William Baker, O.D., commenting on the case, *Steele v. United States*, in *Oregon Optometry*, Fall 1980

Unlike other eye diseases, ocular tumors can pose a threat to life, and for this reason they deserve special consideration. The appropriate clinical techniques must be employed because the estimated prevalence of ocular tumors is but 12 per 100,000 and the number of new cases annually is less than 1 per 100,000, both small figures that reflect the rarity of neoplastic disease.[1] Optometrists must be cognizant of the clinical steps necessary to recognize the presence of malignant neoplastic disease because the survival rate for patients with localized ocular tumors is almost 80 percent when treatment can be initiated early in the disease process.

Unfortunately, the spectre of litigation looms menacingly over this aspect of optometric practice because failure to detect an ocular tumor can result in substantial injuries that are compensable in a court of law. The responsibility of optometrists for the detection of tumors is well established legally, due in no small part to the increasing health orientation of the profession, a development that has exerted a profound effect on the standard of care applicable to the clinical practice of optometry. An argument on behalf of a defendant optometrist that he or she should not be held liable for failure to detect an ocular tumor can be persuasive only when it can be established that a skillful optometrist, performing an examination that complies with recognized standards, would not have detected the disease. Given the rather extensive array of instruments and diagnostic tests available to optometrists, this is an argument that will, in most cases, have difficulty being persuasive. It should be pointed out, however, that the law does not place a duty upon the optometrist to discover everything that is wrong. Rather, the optometrist is expected to exercise reasonable care and to possess a standard minimum of knowledge and ability (see Chapter 18). For that reason, routine examinations of asymptomatic patients may not require a dilated fundus examination with the binocular indirect ophthalmoscope, which is the most likely means of detecting an intraocular tumor.

Even so, when a patient has signs or symptoms that would indicate to a reasonable optometrist the necessity for further or more detailed testing, then the legal requirement for appropriate examination (and, where necessary, for referral) must be satisfied or the practitioner faces the prospect of liability.

A military optometrist examined a 4-year-old boy whose mother had noticed his eyes were crossing. The optometrist diagnosed accommodative esotropia and prescribed spectacle lenses but noted an old, inactive hemorrhage in the child's right eye. At a follow-up examination one month later, the mother reported that the child's eye was not crossing as frequently. The optometrist changed the prescription, but noted that the reflex in the right eye was not good. He instructed the mother to bring the child back in four months, but the child was not seen until six months later, at which time the optometrist found the acuity in the right eye to be limited to light perception. The child was referred to a physician and eventually examined by a number of specialists, who found a retinal detachment secondary to possible retinoblastoma or *Toxocara canis*. The eye was eventually enucleated and the optometrist was sued for misdiagnosis and failure to refer in a timely fashion. The trial court awarded $250,000 in damages.[2]

This case illustrates the difficulty in determining the cause of vision loss before the injury has progressed past the point where meaningful intervention may be possible[3] (a point emphasized in the epigraph).

The proof of failure to provide due care is based on expert testimony, which is weighed by the jury in deciding whether the defendant optometrist was negligent.[4] In most cases, medical testimony will also be allowed.[5]

Now let us turn to a review of cases in which the courts have imposed liability upon optometrists for failure to adhere to the standard of care.

Duty to Detect Ocular Tumors

The earliest reported case[6] discussing the responsibility of optometrists for detection of ocular tumors arose out of the following facts: A patient went to an optician for glasses, but because the optometrist who worked for the optician was on vacation, the patient was sent to a nearby optometrist for examination. The optometrist detected a small intraocular tumor about the size of a pea, but instead of informing the patient of this finding, the optometrist telephoned the optician, recommending that the patient be sent to an ophthalmologist for consultation. The optician, however, dispensed glasses to the patient and said nothing of the possible pathology, and this lack of disclosure led to a failure on the part of the patient to seek further care, which ultimately resulted in total vision loss in the affected eye. Assessing the responsibility of the optometrist in this case, the court held that although the optometrist was not required by law to make a correct diagnosis, professional standards necessitated disclosure and referral. Therefore, even in commercial settings it is clear that the duty of the optometrist is to inform the patient fully and to see that proper referral is obtained. Detected ocular pathology that goes untreated presents an almost certain opportunity for liability.

But what of *failure* to detect a tumor? A more recent case[7] points out the necessity for thorough examination and careful follow-up in the presence of suspected ocular disease. A patient of a health-care clinic received an eye examination from a staff optometrist, who found her to have best corrected visual acuities of 20/40 and 20/25, the reduced vision being attributed to cataracts.[8] The optometrist did not perform a dilated fundus examination, because the state law at the time did not permit optometrists to use drugs for diagnostic purposes, nor did the optometrist refer the patient to the ophthalmologist on the clinic staff because they had an understanding that patients would not be referred to the physician until visual acuity dropped to 20/50 or 20/60.

About two months later the patient suddenly realized that she could not see out of one eye and returned to the clinic, where the diagnosis of retinal detachment was made. The patient was referred for surgery, and it was found that the detachment was secondary to von Hippel-Lindau disease (retinal angiomatosis), an uncommon disease that can manifest in retinal tumors (angiomas). The tumor classically presents early as a smooth dome-shaped mass fed by an enlarged tortuous artery and drained by an arterialized vein, and as it enlarges, it can cause retinal detachment.[9] These tumors are most commonly found in the midperiphery of the retina, and thus in most cases cannot be detected without dilation and examination with a binocular indirect ophthalmoscope.

Although the trial court found in favor of the defendant optometrist, upon appeal the decision was reversed, the appellate court finding that "the evidence is overwhelming that (the plantiff's) eye should have been dilated, and the only reason this was not done was because of (the optometrist's) negligence in not referring her to a qualified ophthalmologist."[10] Unfortunately, the court also held that the optometrist's actions in examining the patient for disease transcended the bounds of optometry and entered the practice of medicine, which permitted the optometrist to be held to "the same rules relating to the duty of care and liability as ophthalmologists."[11] Thus physicians were allowed to testify as to the standard of care expected of optometrists, a development that has profound implications in negligence cases involving optometrists.[12] The court reversed the decision of the trial court and awarded the patient $25,000 in damages.

The preceding case illustrates the necessity for dilation in cases where disease is suspected and slit-lamp and ophthalmoscopic examinations are required. Practitioners who do not utilize dilation are under a legal obligation to refer these patients to doctors who can perform a dilated fundus examination to rule out pathology. Failure to observe this rule can lead to liability.

Another view of optometric responsibility has been enunciated in a 1984 case[13] that concerned allegations of an undiagnosed brain tumor. The patient had been on hypertensive therapy for more than two years when he was examined by an optometrist, who was not aware of the therapy but who discovered that the patient's blood pressure was elevated and suggested that he see a physician. According to the patient, the optometrist also detected papilledema but did not tell him what to do about it. About a month after the examination the patient returned to the physician, who detected papilledema and referred the patient to an ophthalmologist, who confirmed the finding but instituted no treatment. Eight months thereafter a neurosurgeon diagnosed a brain tumor, subsequent to which the patient sued the physician, the optometrist, and the ophthalmologist for negligence.

The optometrist filed a motion to remove himself as a defendant, and the trial court granted the motion. The patient appealed, however, arguing that the optometrist had failed to inform him of the consequences of his condition or to refer him to the appropriate specialist for treatment. In reversing the trial court (thereby reinstituting the optometrist as a defendant), the state supreme court rejected the optometrist's argument that the patient was already under the care of a physician and that no further referral was necessary, observing that "in our view... it is clear that the duties and responsibilities of an optometrist would not be relieved under these circumstances."[14]

This case points out the need for a careful history that documents the health problems of the patient and the treatment being rendered for them. It also demonstrates the responsibility that the courts are willing to impose on optometrists for the detection of diseases (such as brain tumors) manifesting themselves through ocular signs or symptoms. Clearly, a careful ophthalmoscopic examination is a necessity, and the fact that a patient is being treated by a physician for a condition observable by the optometrist does not relieve the optometrist of the obligation to explain the findings and to see (under the appropriate circumstances) that referral is made to the proper specialist.

These precedent-setting cases have established several important clinical guidelines:

- An optometrist has a legal duty to detect pathology, even pathology as rare as an ocular tumor, if a reasonable optometrist possessing the minimum degree of skill and learning common within the profession and performing an ordinary examination would have detected the pathology.
- Detection of disease requires referral to a competent specialist for treatment.
- Failure to refer for a dilated fundus examination and other appropriate testing can create liability if disease is in fact present and the failure to refer results in injury to the patient.
- When examining for disease an optometrist may be held to the standard of care expected of ophthalmologists, and physician testimony may be permitted as to the standard of care expected under these circumstances.
- An optometrist should take a thorough health history and ascertain the treatment being rendered for any health problems detected.
- Co-existing ocular or systemic disease should be ruled out when a pathological condition is detected.

With these guidelines in mind, let us review some clinical situations in which optometrists may be charged with the legal responsibility for detection of tumors.

Failure to Detect Ocular Tumors

Malignant neoplastic disease is an uncommon finding, and for this reason it is important for optometrists to understand the mechanism of disease.

In the normal eye there are three groups of cells that can give rise to melanoma,[15] and they may be found in the pigment epithelium, the conjunctiva, and the uvea. The most important for our purposes are those of the uvea (iris, ciliary body, and choroid). A *nevus* is composed of uveal cells that have benign characteristics, whereas *melanoma* refers to cells that have malignant characteristics. The number of persons with choroidal nevi may be as high as 30 percent of the adult population.[16] The number of new cases annually is estimated to range from 1 to 2 percent in the general population,[17] whereas the prevalence of ocular malignant melanoma is estimated to be 14 per 100,000 and the incidence about 5 to 7 per million per year.[18] Studies have shown that malignant tumors have a predisposition for Caucasians (175:1 ratio of Caucasians to nonCaucasians)[19] and for persons over 50 years of age (3 per million in those under 50 and 21 per million in those over 50).[20] As these statistics indicate, the possibility is quite low that a practitioner will encounter a patient with malignant melanoma during his or her clinical career. Even so, a doctor must be prepared for this unlikely eventuality.

An optometrist who worked for an optical company examined a Caucasian woman in her early 60s who complained of decreased vision in one eye. The best corrected visual acuity was 20/40 in the affected eye and 20/25 in the other. Although the optometrist performed ophthalmoscopy and tonometry, he did not perform a dilated fundus examination or a test of the visual field, attributing the decreased acuity to cataracts, which were present in both eyes. About nine months later the patient's continued difficulties with her vision caused her to seek another examination from a different doctor, and the diagnosis of ocular malignant melanoma was made. Because of the size of the tumor, the eye had to be enucleated. The optometrist was sued for negligence, with the allegation being that a timely diagnosis of the tumor would have spared the patient's eye and decreased the risk of metastatic disease.[21]

It is essential to perform an examination that is within the standard of care, i.e., one that a reasonable optometrist would have performed under the same or similar circumstances. In so doing, the optometrist should consider the following aspects of clinical diagnosis.

History

Age, race, and state of health are important indicators. For example, a history of mastectomy or pulmonary or gastrointestinal symptoms should increase the suspicion of the doctor as to the possibility of metastatic tumor. Epidemiological factors should also be considered.

Dilated Fundus Examination

An examination with the binocular indirect ophthalmoscope is essential because of the advantages of stereopsis and a wide field of view. Both the posterior pole and the peripheral fundus can be examined, even through hazy media, and flat lesions such as RPE hyperplasia or choroidal nevi can be differentiated from tumors, which are usually pigmented, domed, or mushroom-shaped, with orange (lipofuscin) pigment on the surface and an occasional halo at the margin. The examination should be conducted in both white and red-free illumination.

Biomicroscopy

Examination of the dilated pupil with the slit lamp is important and can be most valuable in the detection of iris and ciliary body tumors. The three mirror fundus lens can be used to supplement ophthalmoscopy, permitting magnification and binocularity both at the posterior pole and in the periphery.

Transillumination

This is a necessary test for some types of tumors (e.g., reflex in the pupil, is often overlooked by clinicians. A pigmented tumor can cast a dark shadow that is observable within the reflex by the examiner.

Visual Field Assessment

This is a necessary test for some types of tumors (e.g., pituitary adenomas) but can also be helpful for the detection of malignant melanomas, which usually produce field defects.

Fundus Photography

Monocular or stereoscopic views of the fundus and comparison over time (useful for periodic follow-up of suspicious nevi, discussed below) are valuable adjuncts to direct observation.

Specialized Testing

Patients can be referred for ultrasonography or fluorescein angiography or other specialized testing to determine the presence of disease.

The determination of the diagnostic tests that should have been performed in any given case will, of course, depend on the testimony of expert witnesses.

In the great majority of cases, the eye is *not* the

primary site of the tumor. A comprehensive study[22] found that only 12 of 92 malignant melanoma cases involved a primary site that was ocular. If there is metastasis from the eye, however, the damages can be consequential.

A patient was seen by his optometrist over a two-year period, and at the last visit the optometrist diagnosed the patient as having a cataract. The patient was referred to an ophthalmologist, according to the doctor; the patient maintained that he was merely told to return in six months. In any event, the patient did not see an ophthalmologist but was examined by a general practitioner four months later. The physician sent the patient to a retina specialist, who diagnosed malignant melanoma and removed the eye. The specialist stated that, had he examined the eye earlier, he could possibly have removed it before the melanoma had an opportunity to mestastasize. The patient subsequently died of cancer and a suit for wrongful death was filed, alleging that the optometrist failed to correctly diagnose what was wrong with the eye and to consult specialists who would have made a full and correct diagnosis.[23]

If the plantiff in the lawsuit is deceased, the claim —as in the case above—will be for wrongful death, the only circumstance under which an optometrist would have to defend such a charge based on allegations of clinical negligence.

One other clinical factor that optometrists should consider is the possibility that a choroidal nevus may evolve into a malignant melanoma, a rare development but one that is made more possible if the nevus is larger than five disc diameters in size.[24] General clinical guidelines are as follows[25]:

- For nevi smaller than two disc diameters, periodic examination is all that is necessary.[26]
- For nevi between two and five disc diameters in size, specialized tests (e.g., ultrasonography and fluorescein angiography) should be considered at periodic intervals in addition to the regular examination.[27]
- For nevi greater than five disc diameters, specialized tests are mandatory and periodic follow-up must be instituted at regular intervals.[28]

In all cases, it is wise to photodocument the nevus so that changes over the course of time will be detected.

Optometrists may be charged with negligence for failure to detect a brain tumor that manifests itself through ocular signs or symptoms. Suspicious or unresolved findings (such as decreased visual acuity, headaches, and diplopia) merit thorough examination and periodic recall to rule out the presence of an underlying tumor.

A 5-year-old kindergarten student failed an eye test and was taken by his mother to an optometrist for an examination. The optometrist noted that the fundus was "normal" and that the visual field was "full". Although the youngster complained that vision in one eye was blurry, no glasses were prescribed. After the examination, the mother allegedly informed the doctor that the child complained of headaches, and the optometrist recommended that the boy be seen by the family physician. About three months later the youngster complained of problems seeing the television and of falling over chairs, and about five months after the optometrist's examination the mother took the child to a physician, who noted optic atrophy of one eye and papilledema of the other and referred the child to a hospital for a diagnostic evaluation. The child was diagnosed as having astrocytoma and hydrocephalus and underwent surgery for removal of the tumor. He subsequently received twenty-five radiation treatments. Suit was filed against the optometrist for failure to diagnose the brain tumor and for failure to refer to a specialist.[29]

One essential test that must not be omitted when examining for a tumor is assessment of the visual field. In many cases field changes will be present early in the course of the disease and timely detection will permit successful therapy to be instituted. In particular, optometrists should be aware of the possibility of tumor of the pituitary gland, the most common intracranial neoplasm that produces symptoms affecting vision.[30] Patients complaining of chronic headache, fatigue, and vision loss require careful visual field assessment to rule out the presence of such a tumor, which often begins as a monocular vision loss in the form of a central scotoma, followed by an asymmetrical superior bitemporal hemianopia that is due to compression on the chiasm.[31] Failure to detect pituitary tumor in the presence of signs and symptoms of disease may result in litigation.

A patient was examined by an optometrist and found to have reduced visual acuity. The patient was referred to another optometrist for evaluation, and the doctor noted that there was a significant amount of corneal astigmatism present with best corrected visual acuity being 20/60, also commenting that the patient "appears to have lenticular complications. No pathology front or back of eye. Ks are not changed. Might try anterior toric lens to correct." The patient was returned to the referring optometrist. Five months later the patient complained of double vision, and three months afterward, the patient was unable to count fingers at a distance of two feet, at which time it was found that the patient was suffering from a pituitary tumor that was compressing the optic nerve. Suit was instituted against the optometrists for failure to diagnose the patient's condition and refer the patient to a specialist for treatment.[32]

Therefore, optometrists should consider the value of periodic testing of the visual field, either through the use of the tangent screen or through the use of automated perimetry, and should incorporate visual field assessment into ocular health examinations given to patients on a periodic basis.

Tumors are also present within the anterior adnexa, and optometric clinicians should examine the adnexa carefully to rule out the presence of disease. The most common lid tumor is basal cell carcinoma, which accounts for about one fifth of all lid tumors,[33] more than 90 percent of all malignant tumors of the lid,[34] and is more common than squamous cell carcinoma by a ratio of 40:1.[35] Basal cell carcinoma is usually a darkly discolored, raised area with pearly, rolled edges and a central depression that—with the passage of time—may become progressively eroded or ulcerated.[36] These tumors erode into the orbit if untreated, causing the destruction of soft tissue and resulting in potentially fatal cellulitis or sepsis.

Failure on the part of an optometrist to determine that an external tumor is present can lead to liability.

During an examination a patient was found to have a lesion on her left eyelid that was diagnosed by the optometrist as being a blocked oil gland. The optometrist noted that the patient should "use warm compresses for one week, return if not open, call if place on lower lid gets worse—would need to refer." Almost two years later the patient was examined by a physician, who detected a lesion in the left lower eyelid that, on biopsy, was found to be basal cell carcinoma. The size of the lesion was determined to be 13 × 5 mm, and two operations were required to remove the affected area and repair the eyelid. The patient sued the optometrist, alleging failure to diagnose and refer in a timely fashion.[37]

Optometrists should use gross and slit-lamp examination of the anterior adnexa to detect external tumors and should refer suspicious cases to a specialist for differential diagnosis. Patients who are undergoing treatment of anterior segment pathology should be carefully observed, and under some circumstances it may be wise to follow-up on patients who do not keep recall appointments.[38]

If a practitioner fails to detect ocular disease such as a tumor, it is the failure to refer that initiates the cause of action, and it is the degree of injury that is suffered by the patient from the time the referral should have been made to the time that therapy is initiated to arrest the disease that determines the damages for which the patient may claim compensation. If a practitioner does recommend referral, it is necessary to document the referral in the patient record[39] (see Chapter 16).

Notes

1. The data on incidence, prevalence, and survival rates is from Kleinstein R.N. and H.F. Lehman, Incidence and Prevalence of Eye Cancer, *American Journal of Optometry & Physiological Optics*, vol. 54, no. 1, Jan. 1977, pp. 45–51. The risk of developing malignant neoplastic disease is greater in whites than in blacks and increases with age. About 31 percent of malignant tumors of the eye occur in people under the age of fifteen; 4 percent between the ages of fifteen and thirty-four; 21 percent between the ages of thirty-five and fifty-four; 17 percent between the ages fifty-five and sixty-four; and 26 percent over the age of sixty-five. The highest regional incidence rate for white males is in the south.
2. *Steele v. United States*, 463 F. Supp. 321 (D.C. Alas. 1978).
3. Baker, W., My Two Cents Worth, *Oregon Optometry*, vol. 47, no. 3, Fall 1980, p. 2.
4. The purpose of expert testimony is to assist the jury in understanding technical terms, principles, and standards that are not within the common knowledge of laypersons. Expert testimony is routinely used in negligence cases to establish the standard of care, the relationship between what the doctor did or did not do and the injury (proximate cause), and the damages suffered by the plaintiff. Thus, expert testimony is an essential (and often deciding) factor in a negligence case, especially with regard to the most important element to be proven, the standard of care. For a discussion of the proof of negligence, see Prosser, W.L., *Law of Torts*, 4th Ed., West, St. Paul, Minn., 1971.
5. In general, only an expert from the same "school" as the defendant doctor is competent to testify as to the standard of care expected of the doctor, i.e., a dentist may testify as to the standard of care expected of a dentist, a physician may testify as to the standard of care expected of a physician, and an optometrist may testify as to the standard of care expected of an opto-

metrist, etc. But this rule has been liberalized in many jurisdictions to permit testimony of experts from different schools where it can be shown that the subject of the testimony is common to both professions. Because virtually all optometric malpractice cases will involve physician testimony on behalf of the patient as to the injury suffered and proximate cause, the trend toward increasing liberality means that physicians may be permitted to testify as to the standards expected of optometrists. In some instances, the opposite may also be allowed, i.e., optometric expert testimony as to the standard of care expected of ophthalmologists. See Classe, J., Liability and the Primary Care Optometrist, *Journal of the American Optometric Association*, vol. 57, no. 12, 1986, pp. 926–929.

6. *Evers v. Buxbaum*, 102 App. D.C. 334, 253 F.2d 356 (D.C. Cir. 1958). An annotation of this and other malpractice cases can be found in 51 A.L.R. 3d 1280.
7. *Fairchild v. Brian*, 354 So. 2d 675 (La. App. 1977).
8. The optometrist did not make the diagnosis of cataract on the basis of a slit-lamp examination but rather on the basis of the refraction and direct ophthalmoscopy. 354 So. 2d at 676.
9. For a description of the disease, see Reese, A.B., *Tumors of the Eye*, 3d ed., Harper & Row, Hagerstown, Md., 1976, pp. 266–269. A very early retinal angioma is a flat, reddish papule that can easily be overlooked, but as the mass grows, the feeding and draining vessels become more prominent and hard exudates may form a circle around the angioma. Further growth will result in a total exudative retinal detachment. Ultimately, neovascularization, shallowing of the anterior chamber, and glaucoma can result.
10. *Fairchild*, supra note 7, at 680.
11. Id. at 679.
12. If an appellate court interprets the acts of the defendant optometrist to be outside the scope of optometry as defined by state statute or judicial decision, the court can justify using physician testimony to set the standard of care expected of the optometrist, the rationale being that the optometrist is practicing medicine rather than optometry. See Classe, supra note 5.
13. *Wills v. Klingenbeck*, 455 So. 2d 806 (Ala. 1984).
14. Id. at 807.
15. These cells, melanocytes, are melanin-producing and melanin-containing cells. Uveal melanocytes are distributed throughout the stroma of the iris, ciliary body, and choroid. The most frequent malignant neoplasm of the eye is malignant melanoma of the uvea; 85 percent of these melanomas are found in the choroid, 9 percent in the ciliary body, and 6 percent in the iris. See Scheie, H.G., and D.M. Albert, *Adler's Textbook of Ophthalmology*, W.B. Saunders Co., Philadelphia, 1977. About 1,000 cases of uveal malignant melanoma are estimated to be diagnosed each year. See Young S.E., and J.K. Shields, Malignant Tumors of the Uveal Tract, *Current Problems in Cancer*, vol. 5, no. 1, 1980, pp. 3–35.
16. Gass, J.D.M., Problems in the Differential Diagnosis of Choroidal Nevi and Malignant Melanomas, *American Journal of Ophthalmology*, vol. 83, no. 3, 1977, pp. 299–323.
17. Gantley, J.P., and G.W. Comstock, Benign Nevi and Malignant Melanomas of the Choroid, *American Journal of Ophthalmology*, vol. 76, no. 1, 1973, pp. 19–25.
18. Dorn, H.F., and S.J. Cutler, *Morbidity from Cancer in the United States*, Public Health Monograph No. 56, U.S. Government Printing Office, Washington, D.C., 1959; and Cutler, S.J., and J.L. Young, *Third National Cancer Survey: Incidence Data*, National Cancer Institute, Monograph No. 41, U.S. Government Printing Office, Washington, D.C., 1975.
19. Hogan, M.J., and L.E. Zimmerman, *Ophthalmic Pathology: An Atlas and Textbook*, W.B. Saunders, Philadelphia, 1962.
20. Wilkes, S.R., D.M. Robertson, L.T. Kurland, and J.R. Campbell, Incidence of Uveal Malignant Melanoma in the Resident Population of Rochester and Olmstead County, Minnesota, *American Journal of Ophthalmology*, vol. 87, no. 5, 1979, pp. 639–641.
21. Based on a personal communication with the author.
22. Zakka, K.A., R.Y. Foos, C.A. Omphroy, and B.R. Straatsma, Malignant Melanoma. Analysis of an Autopsy Population, *Ophthalmology*, vol. 87, no. 6, 1980, pp. 549–556. In this study of 12,383 consecutive cases, eyes were available for autopsy in 8,345 cases (65 percent). The results were as follows:
    - Ninety-two of 12,383 cases had malignant melanoma
    - In 12 cases, the primary site was ocular
    - In 76 cases, the primary site was nonocular
    - In 4 cases, the primary site was unknown

    Therefore, only 12 of 8,345 patients had ocular malignant melanomas where the eye was the primary site of the neoplasm, and metastatic disease was present in 75 percent of these cases.
23. Reported in the *AOA News*, Sept. 15, 1976.
24. A good review of optometric management of choroidal nevi can be found in Brown, F.T., The Choroidal Nevus: Guidelines for Management, *Southern Journal of Optometry*, vol. 1, no. 4, 1983, pp. 12–16.
25. A discussion of the difficulties attendant to clinical management of nevi and melanomas can be found in Gass, J.D.M., Problems in the Differential Diagnosis of Choroidal Nevi and Malignant Melanomas, supra note 16.
26. These nevi are considered to be benign. The clinician should be certain to examine with binocular indirect ophthalmoscopy in both white and red-free light. See Brown, supra note 24.
27. These nevi should be regarded with suspicion, and the clinician should be careful to examine for elevation, disruption of the overlying RPE (drusen), and subretinal fluid. The examination should include binocular indirect ophthalmoscopy, visual field analysis, and fundus photography. Follow-up should be instituted every four to six months. See Brown, supra note 24.
28. These nevi should be considered melanomas until studies establish otherwise and should be examined thoroughly for elevation, disruption of the overlying

RPE, and subretinal fluid. Referral for specialized testing is mandatory. See Brown, supra note 24.

29. Based on a personal communication with the author.
30. A discussion of pituitary tumors is contained in Duane, T.S. (ed.), *Clinical Ophthalmology*, vol. 2, chap. 6, Harper & Row, Hagerstown, Md., 1984, pp. 7–8.
31. For an interesting account of a case involving delayed diagnosis of pituitary tumor, see Donin, J.F., The Chiasm: A Medicolegal Locus Minoris Resistantiae, *Survey of Ophthalmology*, vol. 26, no. 6, 1982, pp. 334–336.
32. Based on a personal communication with the author.
33. Aurora, A., and F. Blodi, Lesions of the Eyelids: A Clinicopathologic Study, *Survey of Ophthalmology*, vol. 15, no. 2, 1970, p. 94.
34. Ferry, A., The Eyelids, in Sorsby, A. (ed.), *Modern Ophthalmology*, vol. 4, Lippencott, Philadelphia, 1972, pp. 833–853.
35. Aurora, A., and F. Blodi, supra note 33.
36. For a discussion of basal cell carcinoma and other lid tumors, see Reese, A.B., *Tumors of the Eye*, supra note 9 at 38–62.
37. Based on a personal communication with the author.
38. Although the responsibility to return for follow-up care rests with the patient, it is advisable in many cases for the doctor to contact the patient to determine why a recall appointment has been missed. In states where comparative negligence is used to determine the damages to be awarded to the plaintiff, the fact that the patient has been negligent in delaying or failing to return as scheduled will not bar the negligence claim altogether and will serve only to reduce the amount of damages the plaintiff may receive. Consequently, documentation of efforts to contact the patient or of patient refusal to return for recall appointments becomes most important and should not be overlooked by the practitioner. See Classe, J., Record-Keeping and Documentation in Clinical Practice, *Southern Journal of Optometry*, vol. 5, no. 2, 1987, pp. 11–25.
39. A discussion of how failure to document can affect the outcome of a large claim for damages can be found in Gerber, P., How to Blow Your Own Malpractice Defense, *Optometric Management*, vol. 17, no. 7, 1981, pp. 19–25.

Chapter 25

Optometrist's Duty to Detect Retinal Detachment

Defendants have averred that [the defendant optometrist] has exercised his optometric skills in a good and reasonable manner. This is probably correct insofar as his optometric skills are concerned. However [he] transcended the bounds of optometry [by diagnosing an ocular disease] and, in so doing, is subject to the same rules relating to the duty of care and liability as the ophthalmologist. . . . Further, the standard of care among ophthalmologists would be to dilate the eye. . . . Thus, the Court has no alternative but to conclude that [the] defendant was negligent.

—From the opinion of Judge Chaisson, *Fairchild v. Brian*, 354 So. 2d 675 (1977)

Legal Basis for Liability
Cases Involving Primary Retinal Detchment
Cases Involving Predisposing Conditions
Clinical Examination and Duty to Follow

One of the most difficult clinicolegal problems facing optometrists is the diagnosis of retinal detachment. The alchemy of this problem is a complex mixture of technological advances in instrumentation, legal changes in the optometric standard of care, and clinical subtleties in the decision-making process. Before the advent of drug laws that permitted optometrists to dilate the pupil, the ability of optometric clinicians to examine for retinal detachment was limited to an examination of the posterior pole, typically through the use of direct ophthalmoscopy (or, less frequently, monocular indirect ophthalmoscopy). Optometrists could not examine the periphery and could not enjoy the benefits of stereopsis (i.e., by using binocular indirect ophthalmoscopy or fundus contact lenses). Consequently, in many cases optometrists were obligated to refer patients to ophthalmologists for dilated fundus examination, which resulted in numerous negative referrals and in unnecessary expenses for the patient (e.g., travel costs, lost time from work, and physician's fees). In some cases optometrists were even blamed by individual ophthalmologists for adopting this conservative philosophy, which called for referral without positive findings but when signs or symptoms were suspicious.

Legislative modification of the optometry practice acts, to permit the utilization of diagnostic pharmaceutical agents, has exerted a significant effect on this decades-old pattern of referral. Almost universally, optometrists now have the right to effect dilation to rule out retinal detachment, even when the retinal periphery is involved. Indeed, such an examination (i.e., into the periphery) may be a duty in some cases because of the standard of care expected of optometric practitioners certified to use diagnostic drugs.[1] Thus it would seem that optometrists should be prepared to use the binocular indirect ophthalmoscope because it is the instrument of choice for an examination of the peripheral retina.

For those optometrists who are not certified to use diagnostic pharmaceutical agents, or who decide not to use them in a given case, there remains a legal obligation to refer the patient to a practitioner who can perform the necessary tests. Failure to examine the patient—or to refer for examination—if signs or symptoms of retinal detachment are present or if the patient is significantly at risk for retinal detachment can lead to liability.

There is a surprisingly large pool of patients with whom optometric clinicians must be concerned as to the likelihood of retinal detachment. Various studies have found that the incidence of nontraumatic retinal detachment in phakic persons is approximately 5 to 10 per 100,000 population per year.[2] When traumatic retinal detachment is considered, this figure is even higher. Because males are more likely to suffer trauma than females, the incidence of detachment in males is higher (61 percent compared to 39 percent in females). In selected patients, however, the risk is much higher. For *primary retinal detachment*, in which a spontaneous break occurs in the retina, the detachment is usually preceded by posterior vitreous detachment (PVD). The finding of PVD is quite common in persons older than 65 years of age, being reported in approximately 80 percent of aphakic eyes and 31 percent of phakic eyes.[3] Between 8 and 15 percent for all patients with acute symptomatic PVD have a retinal tear.[4] Other risk factors that are predisposing conditions are aphakia, glaucoma, lattice degeneration, myopia, trauma, and the proliferative retinopathies[5] (to be discussed).

Since, taken as a whole, these patients represent a significant portion of the population seen by optometrists, it is important for optometric clinicians to develop a proper means of managing them. Proper management requires that optometrists adhere to the applicable standard of care in the following areas of practice:

- Recognition of the patient who is at risk or has a retinal detachment
- Examination to rule out the presence of retinal detachment
- Diagnosis of the retinal detachment, if present, and referral on a timely basis

The importance of observing the standard of care in each of these areas of practice becomes evident when malpractice claims are considered. Claims alleging failure to diagnose retinal detachment are an important source of large claims against optometrists,[6] and in a study of malpractice claims among ophthalmologists it was reported that failure to diagnose retinal detachment was a leading cause of claims against these physicians.[7]

In reviewing the liability of optometrists and ophthalmologists for failure to diagnose retinal detachment, there is a common thread that runs through all the cases: failure to perform a dilated fundus examination. Despite the presence of suspicious symptoms such as decreased acuity, spots, and large floaters, patients were not given a retinal examination through a dilated pupil. If a dilated fundus examination is made, there may be no liability even though a detachment is present, since the detection of detachment may be beyond the legal standards applicable under the circumstances. As one leading ophthalmological commentator has described it:

> The. . .retinal detachment cases often were associated with failure to diagnose. Every ophthalmologist has missed, or will miss this diagnosis and hence this is not below standard. Failure to look for the detachment in a patient with suggestive symptoms may very well be below standard. In a surprisingly large number of cases, the physician did not dilate and carefully examine the. . . eye, and the detachment was missed.[8]

Let us now turn to a discussion of the legal basis for the liability of optometrists for failure to diagnose retinal detachment.

Legal Basis for Liability

The leading case that discusses optometric liability for retinal detachment is *Fairchild v. Brian*, which arose out of the following facts.[9] The plaintiff, Mrs. Fairchild, made an appointment at a health clinic to have an eye examination because she realized she was having difficulty seeing out of her right eye. She was examined by on optometrist, Dr. Brian. The pertinent findings of this examination were that she had best corrected visual acuity of 20/40 in the right eye and 20/25 in the left eye and that he attributed the reduced vision to "lens changes". Although ophthalmoscopy was performed and no retinal pathology was noted, it was done through an undilated pupil. Applanation tonometry, retinoscopy, and refraction constituted the remainder of the examination. The optometrist did not dilate the patient because the state law did not permit the use of mydriatics by optometrists. He discussed his findings with Mrs. Fairchild, advised her of the availability of a surgical consultation for the cataracts, and released her without further treatment.

About two months later, while watching television one evening, Mrs. Fairchild suddenly realized that she could not see out of her right eye. She was subsequently examined by an ophthalmologist at the clinic, who informed her that she had a detached retina that required immediate surgery. The detachment was on the temporal side of the right eye and involved the macula. There were fixed folds, which indicated the detachment had been present for some time. Two surgical procedures were required to reattach the retina, but a completely successful outcome was not obtained.

Mrs. Fairchild then brought suit, alleging as one cause of action the failure of the optometrist to diagnose the detachment in a timely manner and attributing the poor outcome of the surgery to the two-month delay in receiving treatment. The trial court found in favor of the optometrist, concluding that Mrs. Fairchild had failed to prove by a preponderance of the evidence that she in fact had a retinal detachment at the time of Dr. Brian's examination. Mrs. Fairchild appealed this decision, and the appellate court reversed, awarding her $25,000 in damages.

In discussing the duty owed the patient by the optometrist, the appellate court stressed the importance of an examination for disease, holding that—under the facts of this case—the optometrist could be held to a medical standard of care.

> The testimony and evidence have clearly established that early senile cataract is an eye disease. Further, the reasonable standard of care among ophthalmologists would be to dilate the eye subsequent to an initial determination that a cataract exists. Thus, the court has no alternative but to conclude that defendant Brian was negligent and that such negligence is imputed to his employer.[10]

The court reasoned that the existence of cataract required a dilated examination, and that this failure to dilate *for the cataract* contributed to the failure to diagnose the retinal detachment. It is not difficult to imagine a court that could reach a similar conclusion if a patient had PVD (or the symptoms of PVD) or a predisposing condition for retinal detachment (or a predisposing condition that, through a reasonable examination, should have been discovered).

Nor was the court deterred by the speculative nature of imposing liability for a disease that could not be conclusively proven to be present at the time of the examination. Noting that the optometrist's failure to dilate the eye was the reason for the uncertainty, the court went on to conclude that this breach of the standard of care was of itself sufficiently related to the injury suffered by the patient to satisfy the legal requirements of proximate cause.[11]

The lesson of this case is that, where retinal detachment is concerned, failure to examine may be used by the courts as sufficient justification to impose liability when allegations of delay in diagnosis can be used to substantiate claims of injury. Under the appropriate clinical circumstances, it is manifestly important for the optometrist to perform a dilated fundus examination to rule out the presence of disease.

Cases Involving Primary Retinal Detachment

A retinal detachment occurs when fluid accumulates in the potential space between the sensory retina and the retinal pigment epithelium. In a *rhegmatogenous* detachment the fluid accumulates in this space through a break in the retina. We will consider a *break* to be a full-thickness retinal defect, a *tear* to be a break caused by vitreous traction, and a *hole* to be an atrophic, round break.[12] A *primary retinal detachment* is a rhegmatogenous break that is spontaneous and not due to an antecedent event (e.g., trauma) or a predisposing condition (e.g., proliferative retinopathy). Primary detachments are typically preceded by PVD.

Between 8 and 15 percent of patients who complain of acute symptomatic PVD have a retinal tear,[13] (but perhaps as many as one half of patients with retinal detachments will have no antecedent symptoms).[14] As the vitreous collapses it can tear away glial tissue from around the optic disc, causing the appearance of a floater. Traction by the vitreous on the retina can cause photopsia, the flashes of light or colored lights that are reported by about one third of patients with PVD.[15] Hemorrhage can result if peripapillary or retinal vessels are torn by vitreous traction or when vessels crossing retinal tears are compromised. In these cases patients may report a shower of floaters or blurred vision. Vitreous hemorrhage is found in 13 to 19 percent of patients with acute PVD[16] and is an ominous sign since acute PVD with vitreous hemorrhage has a 70 percent incidence of retinal tears.[17] Because almost all patients with retinal detachment have PVD, failure to adequately examine a patient presenting with PVD may not satisfy the standard of care.

A 55-year-old woman who had been the patient of an optometrist for several years complained of the sudden onset of a large floater. The optometrist found her visual acuity in the affected eye to be 20/20 and performed direct ophthalmoscopy. Because the state law did not permit the use of mydriatics by optometrists, he did not dilate the patient's eyes. The optometrist attributed the sudden onset of the floater to PVD, and discussed this finding with the patient, warning that she should return if she experienced a sudden decrease in vision. Two weeks later, she noticed a sudden drop in visual acuity in the affected eye and a shower of floaters. She returned to the optometrist, who referred her to an ophthalmologist for presumed retinal detachment. Despite the surgery, she suffered some permanent impairment and filed suit against the optometrist, alleging that he was negligent in not referring her at the time of the first examination so that a dilated fundus examination could have been performed to rule out the presence of a detachment.[18]

All patients with symptoms of PVD of recent onset should be given a dilated fundus examination, preferably with the binocular indirect ophthalmoscope and the Goldmann three-mirror contact lens. If no hemorrhage and no detachment are present, the patient should be reexamined in one to two weeks and at periodic intervals thereafter for six months, following which the development of retinal detachment will be unlikely.[19] Patients should also be instructed to return for further examination if they notice an increase in floaters (which could be due to increased vitreous traction and a possible retinal tear) or a "curtain" or "shadow" (which could be due to retinal detachment).

Patients who complain of the symptoms of acute PVD and who are found to have reduced visual acuity should be given a dilated fundus examination. Failure to do so may lead to liability.

A 52-year-old construction worker who was a long-time patient of an optometrist complained of seeing spots in front of his left eye. The optometrist examined the patient, finding the best corrected vision to be 20/40 in the eye. Ophthalmoscopy was performed, but the patient's eyes were not dilated because the state law did not permit the use of drugs for diagnostic purposes by optometrists. The optometrist noted "media clear" and "fundi normal" for both eyes and advised the patient that new glasses were not needed. The patient desired to have reading glasses, however, and received these glasses two weeks later. Subsequently the patient called the optometrist, expressing dissatisfaction, and went to another doctor, who referred him to a physician. The patient was diagnosed as having a retinal detachment and had surgery about a month after the initial visit to the optometrist's office. Suit was instituted against the optometrist for misdiagnosis and failure to refer.[20]

Because of potential clinical and legal ramifications, reduced visual acuity should never be permitted to go unexplained.

Another source of cases involves those patients in which a predisposing condition exists, thereby putting the patient more at risk for retinal breaks and subsequent detachments. These cases are discussed in the following section.

Cases Involving Predisposing Conditions

There are several predisposing conditions to retinal detachment that are of clinical significance (see Table 25.1), including aphakia, glaucoma, lattice degeneration, myopia, trauma, and the proliferative retino-

Table 25.1. Predisposing Conditions to Retinal Detachment

Finding	Importance
Myopia	Myopes have 42% of all retinal detachments; the lifetime risk of detachment for a myope greater than 5 diopters who lives to the age of 60 years is forty times greater than the risk for an emmetrope living to that same age.
Lattice degeneration	The direct cause of 21% of all retinal detachments; 70% of these cases are in patients younger than 40 years of age; most are slowly progressing detachments caused by atrophic holes posterior to or at the end of the lattice.
Aphakia	Between 2%–5% of patients who have cataract surgery will have a subsequent retinal detachment; bilateral detachment is much higher in aphakic eyes; intracapsular and extracapsular extractions have about the same incidence of subsequent detachment.
Glaucoma	Between 4%–7% of patients with retinal detachment have open angle glaucoma, compared to less than 1% in the general population; miotic drugs used in glaucoma therapy can cause detachment.
Blunt trauma	Most common tears are linear tears along the posterior border of the vitreous base and dialyses (separation of the retina from the nonpigmented epithelium of the pars plana at the ora serrata); most common locations are superonasal and inferotemporal; the interval between trauma and detachment exceeds 8 months in 50% of cases.
Proliferative retinopathies	
Diabetes	Usually due to nonrhegmatogenous retinal detachment caused by traction from the adhesion of the vitreous to the retina or fibrovascular proliferations.
Branch retinal vein occlusion	Rare cause of rhegmatogenous detachment due to adhesion of vitreous to proliferative vessels that can tear the retina if the vitreous collapses, causing traction.
Sickle-cell retinopathy	Rhegmatogenous detachment may be caused by vitreous traction on proliferative fronds.

pathies. Since patients with these conditions are more likely to suffer retinal detachment, optometric clinicians should be cognizant of the risk these conditions pose and should manage these patients accordingly. Failure to recognize the presence of detachment in patients with predisposing conditions creates the likelihood that liability will be imposed.

A 21-year-old laborer who was a six-diopter myope complained of decreased vision in one eye. The optometrist examined him with a biomicroscope but did not take visual acuities and did not perform ophthalmoscopy. Based on the external examination, the optometrist diagnosed conjunctivitis and initiated treatment. The patient returned about a month later and was examined by the optometrist's partner, who performed acuities and detected severely decreased vision in one eye. The partner scheduled the patient for a comprehensive eye examination the following week. Instead of following this advice the patient consulted another doctor that same day, who diagnosed retinal detachment and referred the patient for surgery. Following the surgery, the patient sued the optometrists for malpractice, alleging that the optometrists had not performed an adequate examination and that the delay in diagnosis of the detachment had decreased the chances of success in reattaching the retina.[21]

Myopes suffer 42 percent of all retinal detachments.[22] Investigators have found that 18 percent of eyes with 6 diopters of myopia or higher have full-thickness retinal breaks.[23] The reasons for this substantial number of detachments is threefold: Myopes have an increased incidence of lattice degeneration; they have a higher incidence of PVD; and the thin retina of myopic eyes is more prone to develop breaks.[24]

Other predisposing conditions that place a patient substantially at risk to develop retinal detachment are aphakia and lattice degeneration (see Table 25.1). But the presence of certain diseases—glaucoma and the proliferative retinopathies—can also increase the chances of detachment and thereby create the opportunity for litigation.[25]

A woman who was diabetic made an appointment to see an optometrist for difficulties she was experiencing with her vision. The optometrist prescribed glasses and advised her that the visual difficulties would disappear in two weeks. She obtained the glasses at the adjoining optical shop and wore them for five months, at which time she consulted another doctor, who found that she had a detached retina and diabetic retinopathy. She sued the optometrist and the optical shop, alleging that the defendant's failure to diagnose and recommend appropriate medical attention proximately resulted in the loss of vision in one eye and accelerated the deterioration of vision in the other.[26]

Although retinal detachment is a rare consequence of diabetes, optometrists should be certain to perform a dilated fundus examination on these patients to rule out the existence of retinal complications that could exert a deleterious effect on vision. Other diseases that present some risk and, therefore, merit careful fundus examination are branch retinal vein occlusion and sickle cell retinopathy (see Table 25.1).

Another important predisposing condition is blunt trauma, which is a nonpenetrating direct injury to the eye and is the leading cause of retinal detachment in children and adolescents.[27] Since blunt trauma causes rapid compression of the eye, the relatively inelastic vitreous cannot stretch quicky enough to prevent severe traction at the vitreous base, usually at the posterior border, resulting in a linear tear.[28] In severe cases the anterior border can also be torn, resulting in avulsion of the vitreous base.[29] The most common retinal tears are dialyses (separation of the retina from the nonpigmented epithelium of the pars plana at the ora serrata), located either superonasally or inferotemporally.[30] Detachments due to blunt trauma are not always immediately evident; eight months after the trauma, only 50 percent of detachments will have been detected, and after two years 20 percent of these detachments will still be undiagnosed.[31]

Because the most common retinal breaks are in the periphery, binocular indirect ophthalmoscopy is necessary in order to perform an adequate examination. Due to the lengthy interval that may occur between the time of the trauma and the diagnosis of the detachment, follow-up of the patient is necessary in order to ensure a timely diagnosis. Failure to warn the patient of the likelihood of complications may constitute a breach of the legal duty owed these patients.

A 47-year-old woman was struck in the eye with a fist and suffered a black eye, with a 3-mm hyphema and a depressed fracture of the orbit. The ophthalmologist treated the patient conservatively and two months after the trauma found that the muscle balance was acceptable and that ophthalmoscopy and gonioscopy were normal. The patient was released but ten months after the trauma experienced the symptoms of a retinal detachment. Fol-

HOME MONITORING OF VISION DR. ALEXANDER HOME PHONE:

Instructions:

1. If you wear glasses or contacts for reading, wear them for these two tests.
2. Hold the sheet of paper 16 inches from your eyes (estimate or measure with a tape). We suggest that you cut a piece of string 16 inches long and keep it in the fold of the sheet as a quick check.
3. It is very important that you ***test each eye separately every time. NEVER*** do these tests with both eyes open/uncovered at once. They are strictly "one-eyed" tests! So, cover your left eye with your hand when you are checking your right eye and cover your right eye when you check your left eye.
4. You should be able to read the paragraph marked with a check and then look at the center dot of the little checker board and see if ***any*** of the lines are wavy or if any portion of the checker board is missing. Do the test just like we did it in the office.

TEST NUMBER ONE IS TO SEE IF YOU CAN READ SMALL PRINT AT NEAR:

Card is held in good light 14 inches from eye. Record vision for each eye separately with and without glasses. Presbyopic patients should read thru bifocal segment. Check myopes with glasses only.

6 3 9 2 5 ᗰ E Ǝ X O X 8 5 20/50

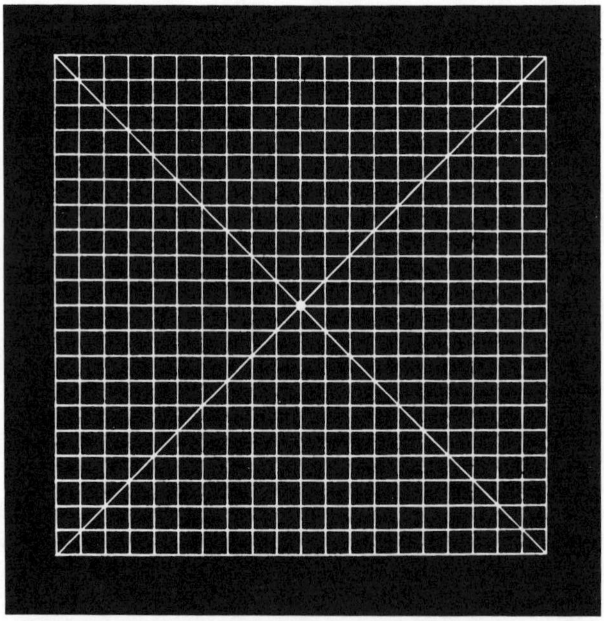

Figure 25.1. Home Monitoring of Vision. (Courtesy of Larry J. Alexander, O.D.)

lowing surgery to reattach the retina the patient sued the ophthalmologist for negligence, alleging that she had not been warned of the possibility of detachment and of the importance of immediate examination if the symptoms of detachment occurred.[32]

Patients with predisposing conditions should be periodically examined to rule out the existence of detachment. These patients should also be warned of the symptoms of detachment so that immediate examination can be instituted. These two responsibilities are discussed in the next section.

Clinical Examination and Duty to Follow

The standard of care expected of optometrists in the evaluation of patients with suspected retinal detachment involves two factors: using proper clinical techniques and instrumentation during the examination and utilizing appropriate communication and follow-up in negative cases.

Clinical Examination

Patients who have the signs and symptoms of retinal detachment must be given a dilated fundus examination. The instruments of choice are the direct ophthalmoscope, the binocular indirect ophthalmoscope, and the Goldmann three-mirror contact lens. Visual acuities should be taken in every case (even routine examinations).

Patients who complain of the symptoms of acute PVD should also be given a thorough dilated fundus examination, preferably with the binocular indirect ophthalmoscope and the Goldmann three-mirror contact lens. The clinician must identify the cause of any reduced acuity and must be certain to examine carefully for vitreous hemorrhage.

Patients who have predisposing conditions that put them at risk for retinal detachment must be given a thorough dilated fundus examination to rule out the presence of retinal breaks, including binocular indirect ophthalmoscopy and, where appropriate, the Goldmann three-mirror contact lens.

In all three categories of patients, adequate counseling and follow-up must be maintained.

Duty to Follow

The optometrist's responsibility to the patient is not ended because the examination turns up only negative findings. There is an obligation to affirmatively disclose all findings and to explain the risks the patient faces with regard to a subsequent detachment. Furthermore, it is necessary for the optometrist to describe the symptoms of retinal detachment and to stress the necessity for vigilance on the patient's part so that immediate examination can be undertaken in the event the patient's visual status changes abruptly. One excellent means of ensuring adequate patient understanding and compliance with instructions is through the use of printed materials (see Fig. 25.1). A "home" Amsler Grid can be given to the patient and, if used in accordance with the printed instructions accompanying the grid, can serve as a sensitive measure of any macular changes affecting the patient's vision. Printed materials can be of valuable assistance to clinicians who have an obligation to monitor specific cases.

As with other areas of optometric practice, documentation of findings, instructions, and recall should not be overlooked. Printed materials can assist in this responsibility as well.

Notes

1. The standard of care expected of optometrists can be summarized by the general statement: What would a reasonable optometrist, using the minimum acceptable degree of skill and learning, have done under the same or similar circumstances? Where a patient is at risk for retinal detachment, it will certainly be arguable that the minimum standard will require examination of the periphery. The same argument can be made for signs or symptoms that indicate the possibility of detachment. Therefore, if an optometrist is to undertake an examination of at-risk or suspicious patients, it would seem that binocular indirect ophthalmoscopy may be a necessity. For a discussion of how dilation is a necessary aspect of the standard of care, see Alexander, L.J., and J. Scholles, Clinical and Legal Aspects of Pupillary Dilation, *Journal of the American Optometric Association*, vol. 58, no. 5, 1987, pp. 432–437.
2. For a sample review, see Ashrafzadeh, M.J., C.L. Schepens, I.T. Elzeneing, R. Moura, P. Morse, and M.F. Kraushar, Apakhic and Phakic Retinal Detachment, *Archives of Ophthalmology*, vol. 89, no. 6, 1973, pp. 476–483.
3. See Jaffee, N.S., Vitreous Detachments, in *The Vitreous in Clinical Ophthalmology*, St. Louis, C.V. Mosby, 1969, pp. 83–98.
4. See Tasman, W.S., Posterior Vitreous Detachment and Peripheral Retinal Breaks, *Transactions of the American Academy of Ophthalmology and Otolaryngology*, vol. 72, no. 2, 1968, pp. 217–224; and Lindner, B., Acute Posterior Vitreous Detachment and Its Retinal Complications, *Acta Ophthalmologica*, vol. 87, (Suppl. 1), 1977, pp. 1–108.
5. For a concise discussion of the various risk factors that constitute predisposing conditions for retinal detachment, see Benson, W.E., *Retinal Detachment, Diagnosis and Management*, Harper & Row, Hagerstown, Md., 1980, pp. 27–39.
6. This statement is based upon data provided at the symposium, "Professional Liability, Optometry, and the Public Health," Section on Public Health and Occupational Vision, Meeting of the American Academy of Optometry, St. Louis, Mo., Dec. 10, 1984. The leading cause of large malpractice claims against optometrists is misdiagnosis. The most commonly misdiagnosed conditions are the glaucomas, ocular tumors, and retinal detachments.

7. See Bettman, J.W., A Review of 412 Claims in Ophthalmology, in Medicolegal Aspects of Ophthalmology, Bettman, J.W. (ed.), *International Ophthalmology Clinics*, vol. 20, Winter 1980, pp. 131–142. Retinal detachment claims ranked third, behind only drug complications and cataract cases in frequency, constituting 11.4 percent of claims (fifty-one cases) in the series.
8. Id. at 136.
9. 354 So. 2d 675 (La. App. 1977). This case has been discussed previously by the author. See Classe, J., Optometrist's Duty to Detect Retinal Detachment, *Southern Journal of Optometry*, vol. 3, no. 2, 1985, pp. 7–13.
10. 354 So. 2d at 679.
11. In order to establish liability, a plaintiff must show a causal relationship between what the defendant did or did not do and the injury suffered by the plaintiff. This link between the alleged negligence and the injury is called proximate cause. In this case the majority of the members of the court felt that the failure to dilate of itself created the relationship necessary to satisfy this legal requirement. In a vigorous and well-reasoned dissenting opinion, however, Judge Covington points out that Mrs. Fairchild's testimony at the trial was that she told Dr. Brian the loss of vision in her right eye was in the temporal field, the same location as the detachment. Since a temporal detachment in the right eye would lead to a nasal field defect, one must agree with the judge that the testimony of four experts (three ophthalmologists and one optometrist) to this effect raises a substantial question as to whether the blurred vision complained of by the plaintiff was in fact due to the cataract and not to the retinal detachment. Despite this evidence, the majority opinion held that there was sufficient cause to find the optometrist liable! See id. at 681.
12. For a discussion see Benson, supra note 5, at 2–12.
13. See Linder, supra note 4; Jaffe, supra note 4; and Tasman, supra note 4.
14. See Morse, P.H., and H.G. Scheie, Prophylactic Cryotherapy of Retinal Breaks, *Archives of Ophthalmology*, vol. 92, no. 3, 1974, pp. 204–207.
15. See Morse, P.H., H.G. Scheie, and A. Aminlari, Light Flashes as a Clue to Retinal Disease, *Archives of Ophthalmology*, vol. 91, no. 3, 1974, pp. 179–180.
16. See Jaffe, supra note 3.
17. Ibid. See also Lindner, supra note 4; and Tasman, supra note 4.
18. Based upon a personal communication with the author.
19. For a succinct discussion of the management of PVD, see Benson, supra note 5, at 4.
20. Based upon a personal communication with the author.
21. Ibid.
22. See Ashrafzadeh, supra note 2.
23. See Hyams, S.W., E. Neumann, and Z. Friedman, Myopia-Aphakia; Vitreous and Peripheral Retina, *British Journal of Ophthalmology*, vol. 59, no. 9, 1975, pp. 483–485.
24. For a review of the various factors that put myopic eyes at risk for retinal detachment, see Byer, N., Clinical Study of Lattice Degeneration of the Retina, *Transactions of the American Academy of Ophthalmology and Otolaryngology*, vol. 69, no. 6, 1965, pp. 1064–1081; and Jaffe, supra note 4.
25. See Benson, supra note 5, at 33–38.
26. *Whitt v. Columbus Cooperative Enterprises*, 64 Ohio St. 2d 355, 415 N.E.2d 985 (1980).
27. See Cox, M.S., C.L. Schepens, and H.M. Freeman, Retinal Detachment Due to Ocular Contusion, *Archives of Ophthalmology*, vol. 76, no. 5, 1966, pp. 678–685; and Winslow, R., and W. Tasman, Juvenile Rhegmatogenous Retinal Detachment, *Transactions of the American Academy of Ophthalmology and Otolaryngology*, vol. 85, no. 3, 1978, p. 607.
28. For excellent illustrations of the retinal breaks found in blunt trauma, see Schepens, C.L., *Retinal Detachment and Allied Diseases*, W.B. Saunders Co., Philadelphia, vol. 1, 1983, pp. 68–87.
29. This injury is pathognomonic of ocular contusion. See Cox, supra note 27.
30. There have been two large studies investigating the location of peripheral retinal breaks due to blunt trauma; one study found the superonasal tears to be the most common, the other study found the inferotemporal to be the most frequent site for tears. See ibid.; and Hagler, W.S., and A.W. North, Retinal Dialysis and Retinal Detachment, *Archives of Ophthalmology*, vol. 79, no. 4, 1968, pp. 376–388.
31. The long-term effects of blunt trauma should be understood by all optometrists. There is a latent interval between the ocular contusion and the clinical appearance of the detachment:
    - 12 percent of detachments occur immediately
    - 30 percent of detachments will be detected in one month
    - 50 percent of detachments will be detected in eight months
    - 80 percent of detachments will be detected in two years

    Thus long-term follow-up of these patients is a necessity. See Cox, supra note 27.
32. A report of this case can be found in Bettman, J.W., A Retrospective Look at Twenty-two Medicolegal Claims. How They Might Have Been Avoided, *Survey of Ophthalmology*, vol. 28, no. 1, 1983, pp. 55–60.

Chapter 26

Liability for Ocular Foreign Bodies

It is the proper practice,. . .that when a patient comes. . .with a laceration on his eyeball, that some examination should be made to determine whether there is any steel. . .or other foreign substance that has entered the eye through such laceration and lodged therein,. . .[and] one of the well-recognized methods for making such determination is the use of the X-ray. . .[which] should be used under such circumstances to make such determination.
—From the opinion of Judge Lane, *Hoffman v. Houston Clinic*, 41 S.W.2d 134 (1931)

Injuries to the eye are—unfortunately—a common occurrence and are second only to cataracts as a cause of visual impairment.[1] There are an estimated 938,000 persons with vision impairment due to eye injury; the incidence of such impairments is estimated to be 40,000 cases. These persons are most likely to have suffered an injury-producing accident in and about the home, and the most common type of eye injury is one due to a foreign body.[2] A study of more than 1,000 eye accidents revealed that 69 percent were caused by flying or falling objects—58 percent of which were objects of less than one-half millimeter in diameter—and that 60 percent of those injured were not wearing eye protection.[3] Consequently, foreign bodies pose a significant clinical problem for optometrists.

Because of the frequency of injury and the potential for visual impairment, it is not surprising to discover that ocular foreign bodies have often been the subject of litigation. In a survey of malpractice claims against ophthalmologists, it was found to rank fifth (8.7 percent of cases) as a source of claims,[4] occurring with about the same frequency as claims involving glaucoma. There are no statistics concerning foreign body–related claims against optometrists, and, even more importantly, there are no appellate cases involving optometrists that can be used to establish legal guidelines,[5] and so we must look to the experiences of physicians in attempting to determine the legal responsibilities that may be imposed on optometrists for the diagnosis and management of ocular foreign bodies.

And there is yet another aspect of this problem that requires mention. At present no state law authorizes the performance of surgery by optometrists, and only a few state laws expressly list removal of foreign bodies as within the definition of the practice of optometry.[6] Thus a certain degree of legal ambiguity exists over the entire issue, for optometric clinicians may rightfully wonder when—or if—removal of ocular foreign bodies constitutes surgery and thereby becomes a procedure that is outside the scope of optometry.[7] Again, there is little precedent to provide guidance for practitioners, but this question will be explored in an effort to make optometrists aware of the issues that may be considered if a legal dispute should arise.

Cases Involving Liability for Ocular Foreign Bodies

Numerous decisions have been rendered on the *failure* to remove an ocular foreign body.[8] In these cases the physician's liability has been due to inadequate examination, principally the failure to take X-rays.

A workman who had been hit in the eye with a broken spring consulted an eye, ear, nose, and throat specialist, describing the manner in which he was injured and complaining that his eye felt as though something was in it. The acuity in the injured eye was 20/40, and the physician noted a central corneal abrasion of such character as to cause the reduced acuity. He examined the iris, lens, and the interior of the eye with a direct ophthalmoscope but did not observe a foreign body and concluded that there was no corneal perforation. He saw the patient on several occasions during the next $2\frac{1}{2}$ months, during which period the patient complained persistently of a foreign body sensation. The patient eventually consulted another physician, who ordered X-rays, and a piece of steel was found to be embedded in the patient's lens. The foreign body was removed, but a cataract resulted and the lens also had to be removed. The patient sued the physician who had failed to take X-rays, and the trial court found him to be liable.[9]

In discussing the liability of the physician, the state supreme court made the following observation:

> The evidence shows that the X-ray is sometimes necessarily employed for the purpose of locating foreign substances in the eye. Although the X-ray is used in not to exceed 4 percent of the cases, according to the testimony in this case, it does indicate that the ophthalmoscope cannot be infallibly relied upon for that purpose.... Whether it (X-ray) should be used depends upon the satisfaction which the ophthalmoscopic examinations give to the examiner.... We think that...the exercise of ordinary care and skill, under the circumstances of this case, require the use of the X-ray to ascertain the nature of the injury to plaintiff's eye.[10]

The necessity for X-rays (or ultrasound or other diagnostic tests) exists whenever the circumstances of the injury are such that a reasonable clinician would suspect the possibility of an intraocular foreign body.

An employee was working in a machine shop when a piece of metal flew off the machine and struck his eye. He was taken to an eye, ear, nose, and throat specialist, who removed a piece of brass from the eye but ordered no X-rays. The patient returned the next day, complaining of pain, but the physician assured him nothing was wrong. The patient returned the next two days complaining of pain and blurred vision in the eye, but the physician told him that there was nothing in the eye and that he imagined the pain. Finally, five days after the injury, the physician took X-rays and discovered that a piece of steel had been embedded in the patient's cornea. Although he removed the steel, a serious infection had set in and the eye was eventually enucleated. The patient sued the physician, alleging negligence in the failure to obtain X-rays in a timely manner so as to prevent the infection. The doctor was held to be liable.[11]

The detection of a superficial foreign body does not automatically rule out the possibility that an intraocular foreign body could be present as well.

A worker who had been hammering some metal was hit in the eye by a foreign body. He went to the emergency room, where a metallic particle was found to be embedded in the corneal epithelium. The foreign body was removed without difficulty, the patient was treated, and thereafter the eye healed without incident. Five months later, however, the patient was found to have the signs and symptoms of siderosis. An intraocular metallic foreign body was found and removed. The attending physician was sued for failure to examine for and detect the intraocular fragment at the time of the injury.[12]

Although X-rays are not indicated on every occasion that a patient has a corneal foreign body, whenever the history indicates an injury caused by metal striking metal, it is advisable to consider X-rays (or ultrasound or other appropriate diagnostic tests) to rule out the presence of intraocular foreign body.

Another aspect of care for corneal foreign bodies concerns adequate follow-up of the injury. Once a corneal foreign body is removed, it may be necessary to cycloplege the eye and to employ an antibiotic to ensure healing without complications. Appropriate follow-up will necessitate rescheduling the patient so that the course of healing can be monitored by the practitioner. Failure on the part of the patient to return as scheduled can be a key factor in determining the liability of the doctor should complications occur.

A patient who had gotten several cement particles in his eye was seen by a physician, who removed some of them and instructed the patient to return if difficulties were encountered. The patient did not feel that he had been treated appropriately by the physician, and so he did not return. By three months later his eye had become severely infected due to particles that had not been removed, and he sought the services of another physician. Despite the second physician's treatment, he suffered some permanent vision loss. He sued the first physician, alleging that the doctor was negligent in failing to remove all of the cement particles. The physician answered that the patient was contributorily negligent in failing to return as instructed. The court held that the patient could not recover, even if the physician had been negligent.[13]

Because documentation is essential if a doctor is going to establish that the patient was negligent in failing to heed instructions or to return for recall appointments, it is important that the record reflect these communications. Practitioners should ensure that vital information is written in the record so as to constitute a contemporaneous account of the care rendered the patient.[14]

In some cases the injury may be such that the loss of vision is unavoidable and thus there can be no liability on the part of the clinician. For example, there are reported cases involving sympathetic ophthalmia,[15] severe injuries for which no intervention could spare vision,[16] and delays in diagnosis that did not contribute to vision loss.[17]

In the next section, the clinical presentation of ocular foreign bodies and the potential liability of optometrists for misdiagnosis or mismanagement will be discussed.

Optometrist's Liability for Ocular Foreign Bodies

There are no precedent-setting cases that pertain to the liability of optometrists for the removal of foreign bodies, but a clinician will be held to that minimum degree of skill and learning that is ordinarily possessed by members of the profession in good standing. What is the standard of care that will be applied by the courts in foreign body cases?

Complaints of pain, a foreign body sensation, tearing, photophobia, or ciliary injection, or a history of injury (especially while striking metal on metal) should alert the optometrist to the possibility of a corneal or intraocular foreign body. Visual acuity should always be determined in the affected eye, even if acuity is markedly impaired (such as finger counting, hand motion, or light perception).

The use of the slit lamp is indicated, as is the instillation of sodium fluorescein to stain the corneal epithelium and to demarcate the extent of the foreign body. Linear corneal scratches may indicate that the foreign body is embedded in the upper tarsal conjunctiva. In this event the lid should be everted and the conjunctiva inspected.

Foreign bodies embedded in the cornea should be removed completely in order to relieve pain and to permit epithelial cell growth over the affected area. An attempt to remove the foreign body by irrigation—directing a stream of fluid (saline solution) against the foreign body so as to wash it off the cornea—should be used first, and if this is unsuccessful, a topical anesthetic may be instilled to prepare for dislodging the foreign body by other means. Although a moistened, cotton-tipped applicator is frequently used by clinicians to remove corneal foreign bodies, this technique usually results in the removal of surrounding corneal epithelium and may be less desirable than lifting the foreign body gently from the corneal surface with a sharp instrument. A sterile spud or needle may prove to be a better choice,[18] although the use of such an instrument may raise legal issues pertaining to surgery (see infra). The instrument is held tangent to the cornea and moved in a sideways fashion to lift or gently scrape off the foreign body.

If a ferrous metal foreign body has been embedded for several days, a rust ring may remain even after the foreign body has been removed. If it cannot be removed easily, it frequently can be lifted off a day or so later when the surrounding corneal epithelium has softened. A hand-held rust ring remover burr may be employed for this purpose,[19] although again the issue of surgery emerges when such a technique is used.

If a large or painful abrasion results following the removal of the foreign body, a broad spectrum antibiotic ointment effective for *Pseudomonas* (e.g., gentamicin, tobramycin, polymixin B) should be instilled and a short-acting cycloplegic (cyclopentolate 1 percent or homatropine 5 percent) used to decrease the patient's discomfort. A pressure patch may also be needed to immobilize the eyelid and prevent the irritation caused by blinking.[20]

No patient with a foreign body or resultant corneal abrasion should be maintained on topical anesthetics (due to the inhibition of healing and possibility of corneal opacification) or topical steroids (because of the increased chance of secondary bacterial, viral, or fungal infection).[21]

Since a foreign body may introduce microorganisms to the cornea, the eye should be examined the next day and be monitored until the affected area no longer stains with fluorescein and healing is completed.

The optometric clinician should be aware of the possibility of an intraocular foreign body that has penetrated the cornea or sclera. Lowered intraocular pressure may be one indication of a penetrating injury. Or the Seidel test may be employed, in which fluorescein is applied to detect a small or subtle flow of aqueous humor.[22] Intraocular foreign bodies can cause marked disruption of the intraocular structures or may produce a severe purulent panophthalmitis, and so timely detection is most important. Signs of global penetration by a foreign body include the following[23]:

- Decreased visual acuity
- Hypotony
- Shallowing or flattening of the anterior chamber
- Alteration in pupil size, shape, or location
- Marked conjunctival chemosis
- Corneal or scleral laceration

Even if the appearance of the eye is normal, a penetrating foreign body may be present. If the history of the injury is suspicious (such as while striking metal on metal), the clinician should consider the advisability of referral for X-ray, ultrasound, or other diagnostic tests. If not detected and removed, retained foreign bodies can cause loss of vision, especially those of iron (which can oxidize within the eye [siderosis] to form an irreversible ferrous compound that causes gradual loss of vision) or copper (which rapidly reacts with ocular tissues [chalcosis], but this condition is reversible if the particle is removed).[24]

A 29-year-old heavy equipment mechanic was injured at work when a foreign body entered his eye. He immediately consulted a general practitioner, who did not order X-rays or refer him to a specialist. Six months later, after visits to two general practitioners and a specialist, the patient consulted an ophthalmologist, who took an X-ray, discovered an intraocular foreign body and removed it. The patient sued the two general practitioners, alleging they were negligent in failing to locate the foreign body or to refer him, and he also sued the specialist, alleging that he was negligent in failing to X-ray the eye or to examine him with a slit lamp. He maintained that the failure to diagnose the iron intraocular foreign body led to siderosis, which caused him to lose vision in the eye. The physicians contended that the standard of care did not require an X-ray under the circumstances, that the patient gave an incomplete history, and that the loss of vision suffered by the patient was caused by the initial trauma rather than by the alleged negligence. The jury awarded the patient $120,000.[25]

In examining a patient with ocular foreign body, it is important to use the appropriate instrumentation (e.g., slit lamp, ophthalmoscope, tonometer), to consider the possibility of intraocular penetration, and to refer the patient for X-ray, ultrasound, or other diagnostic tests where appropriate.

If an optometrist has complied with the standard of care, a claim for damages based on allegations of negligence will be defeated, even if the standard is established by physician testimony.[26] But the optometrist is still susceptible to the allegation that removal of the foreign body is surgery or outside the practice of optometry as defined by state statute. We will examine this possibility in the concluding section of this chapter.

Defining Surgery

The optometry practice acts vary with regard to proscriptions against surgery. Whereas no state law lists surgery as an act within the definition of optometry, in the statutes of twenty-eight states there is an express prohibition against the performance of surgery by optometrists. In twenty-two other states, the law is silent, i.e., it does not list surgery as an act prohibited to optometrists. In only a few state optometry practice acts is the removal of ocular foreign bodies specifically listed as an act within the definition of optometry.[27] Nevertheless, it is reasonable to assume that corneal foreign bodies are removed by optometrists in every state in the nation. When, if at all, could such conduct become surgery or otherwise be considered as outside the definition of optometry?

The definition of surgery is generally broadly interpreted. A leading legal encyclopedia defines it as follows:

> *Surgery.* Surgery is a branch of medical science. More specifically, it is that branch of medical science which treats of mechanical operative measures for healing diseases, deformities, or injuries; the art, practice, or work of treating diseases, injuries, or deformities by manual operation or mechanical appliances, or the branch of medicine that is concerned with such treatment; therapy of a distinctly operative kind, such as cutting operations. In its primitive and broadest sense the term includes adjustment of bones, muscles, ligaments and nerves by manual operation.[28]

When the courts have been called upon to define surgery, they have likewise tended to express the term in broad language.[29]

Apparently there is but one case in which the appellate courts have determined whether or not the removal of an ocular foreign body is within the practice of optometry, and this case occurred half a century ago.[30] The facts of the case are as follows.

A woman went to the office of an optometrist for the purpose of obtaining a replacement for a broken lens, but the optometrist's examination revealed that one eye had become irritated due to a foreign substance lodged in the eye. The optometrist allegedly anesthetized the eye, removed the foreign substance, and "prescribed medicines to be placed in her eye at regular intervals." He removed a foreign substance from both eyes four days later, and she was seen regularly by him over the following week, after which period she alleged that he told her "she was going blind and would lose her entire sight of both eyes." She sued the optometrist for negligence in the treatment of her condition, and he answered that he had removed some dirt and dust particles from her eyes and asked that the suit be dismissed. His insurance company, however, refused to defend him against the claim.

The case went to trial, and a jury awarded the patient $3,000. The optometrist thereafter settled the case with the patient for $2,500, and then brought suit against the insurance company, asking to be indemnified for the $2,500 and for $600 in attorney's fees. The insurance company defended on the basis that the optometrist's removal of the foreign substance from the patient's eyes was not within the statutory definition of optometry and that—since the policy of insurance indemnified him against claims arising from the practice of "optometry only"—there was no legal obligation on the company's behalf to pay the demanded amount. The appellate court upheld the insurance company's position and denied the optometrist's claim for reimbursement.[31]

Although the court held that the insurance company did not have a legal obligation to defend the optometrist or to pay the claim, the principal reason cited for this decision was the optometrist's settlement of the case, which required the court to accept the plaintiff-patient's version of the facts. As expressed in the words of the court:

> The trial. . . resulted in a verdict in favor of Mrs. Rowell for $3,000, in which Kime acquiesced by the payment to her of $2,500 and the court costs. Thereby he admitted the facts pleaded in her amended petition as the basis of her cause of action, and he cannot now deny the issuable facts therein alleged, especially since it is clear from the evidence in the instant case that what he did in removing from her eyes the foreign substance was outside of and not included in the practice of optometry as defined by the statute. *Had Kime successfully contested the claim of Mrs. Rowell, a far different question would be presented, but on the record, not only of the verdict in her favor but on the admitted facts, Kime has no claim against the appellant insurance company* [emphasis added].[32]

Because of the age of this case, and the peculiar circumstances of the decision, it does not provide guidance of a useful nature to contemporary practitioners of optometry. It does point out, however, one important factor: the possibility that an optometrist will not be afforded liability coverage by his insurer should the insurance company decide that the optometrist's actions are outside the scope of practice.[33] Furthermore, an optometrist who has been held to be acting outside the scope of practice by a state board of optometry is subject to disciplinary measures by the board.[34]

Because of the broad definition of surgery, differences that exist from state-to-state in the optometry practice acts, and lack of legal precedent with regard to the liability of optometrists for removal of foreign bodies, this issue must be viewed as one that is at present legally undecided. Indeed, should claims arise to test this question, because of these differences they will almost certainly be decided on a case-by-case basis, which is to say that these cases will themselves be of limited applicability. Consequently, a certain degree of uncertainty can be expected to loom over this issue for years to come.

In deciding foreign body–related cases, there are two factors that the courts will probably consider in determining if removal of a foreign body constitutes surgery or is an act that is outside the definition of the practice of optometry:

1. *Degree of penetration*—It would seem evident that a foreign body that has penetrated through the cornea (or sclera) would require surgery in order to be removed. A foreign body embedded in the cornea, however, does not present so clear-cut a situation. Obviously a foreign body lodged in the corneal epithelium offers the least degree of penetration and thus is most amenable to removal by means other than "mechanical operative measures," but the problem of penetration becomes more difficult as Bowman's membrane, the corneal stroma, and Descemet's membrane are involved. It is arguable that any foreign body that has not penetrated the corneal endothelium is merely embedded and that removal consists of doing no more than extracting an object without resort to "manual operation" or "mechanical appliances." The degree of penetration during this procedure may not be determinative: For example, acupuncture—which requires manual operation and the use of penetrating mechanical appliances—has been determined not to be surgery.[35]
2. *Instrumentation*—If a stream of liquid is used to dislodge the foreign body, it is difficult to perceive that such an action constitutes the performance of a "manual operation"; and if a cotton-tipped applicator is used for the same purpose, the selection of

this instrument does not conjure up the image of a "mechanical device." But the use of a spud or a needle (which is often more desirable than a cotton-tipped applicator) creates an impression that is more in keeping with the definition of surgery. Furthermore, the use of a burr (to remove a rust ring) is probably even more illustrative of therapy of an operative kind and thus more possibly an act of surgery. But the practice of optometry in most states permits acts such as tonometry, which requires flattening of the cornea with a mechanical appliance; the use of orthokeratology, which requires treatment with a mechanical appliance (not unlike a splint) in order to alter the contour of the cornea[36]; lacrimal dilation and irrigation, procedures that are performed with a mechanical device; and diagnostic tests that require mechanical devices such as finger pricks (for blood glucose evaluation), ophthalmodynamometry, scleral indentation (in conjunction with binocular indirect ophthalmoscopy), and posterior pole examination with a fundus contact lens.

Obviously, the question of what constitutes surgery is a complex one that must be regarded with concern in those states where acts of surgery are outside the statutory definition of optometry. In states where surgery is not expressly prohibited to optometrists, the question of whether or not a given act—such as the removal of an ocular foreign body—is within the scope of optometry will likewise require careful consideration by the courts. Since there are no decisions to provide guidance, optometrists should be certain to observe the standard of care applicable under the circumstances.

Despite the paucity of case law on this issue, the problem may be solved, in some states, by clarifying rulings from state boards of optometry, or in all states by amendments to the optometry practice acts to expressly include this procedure. By example, the Florida statute (amended in 1983)[37] states that "Optometrists are prohibited from performing surgery; provided, however, that optometrists may remove extraocular foreign bodies from the eye and its appendages and perform similar or related acts." Because of the uncertainty that attends all litigation, legislation would be a preferable means of addressing this problem and should be considered in those states seeking modification of the optometry practice act.

Notes

1. Eye Injuries, *Vision Problems in the United States*, National Society to Prevent Blindness, N.Y., 1980.
2. Ibid. Eye injuries are estimated to be 2.4 million cases per year. Foreign bodies account for 35 percent of these cases and are the most common cause of injury.
3. Reported in *Trades and Services Safety News*, vol. 2, no. 2, 1983, State Compensation Insurance Fund, and based on a survey conducted by the U.S. Department of Labor, reported in the *Journal of the American Optometric Association*, vol. 54, no. 12, 1983, p. 1097.
4. Bettman, J.W., A Review of 412 Claims in Ophthalmology, in Medicolegal Aspects of Ophthalmology, Bettman, J.W., (ed.), *International Ophthalmology Clinics*, vol. 20, Winter, 1980, p. 132. The leading sources of claims were drug complications (14 percent), cataracts (12.8 percent), retinal detachment (11.4 percent), and glaucoma (9 percent).
5. Although there are no cases in the law reporters, claims involving ocular foreign bodies have been filed against optometrists. None of these claims, however, has evolved into a precedent-setting case. In a study of 36 optometric malpractice claims conducted by the author, there were 2 foreign body claims involving optometrists, but both were dropped by the plaintiff. See Classe, J., Malpractice and Optometry: A Personal Commentary, *Southern Journal of Optometry*, vol. 5, no. 3, 1987, pp. 26–31.
6. As of 1988, those states expressly permitting the removal of foreign bodies are Arkansas, Florida, Iowa, Kansas, Kentucky, Missouri, Montana, North Dakota, South Dakota, and Tennessee.
7. The definition of the practice of optometry must be consulted in order to determine the scope of practice permitted in the state. If an act is outside the scope of practice, the optometrist has technically entered into the practice of medicine, for which the optometrist may be subjected to discipline (and the loss of professional liability insurance coverage). See Classe, J., Liability and the Primary Care Optometrist, *Journal of the American Optometric Association*, vol. 57, no. 12, 1986, pp. 926–929.
8. For a review of leading cases involving physicians, see Holder, A., Foreign Bodies in the Eye, Law and Medicine Series, *Journal of the American Medical Association*, vol. 218, no. 3, Oct. 18, 1971, pp. 495–496.
9. *Kosak v. Boyce*, 201 N.W. 757 (Wis. 1925).
10. 201 N.W. at 759, 760.
11. *Hoffman v. Houston Clinic*, 41 S.W.2d 134 (Tex. Civ. App. 1931).
12. Bettman, J.W., A Retrospective Look at Twenty-two Medicolegal Claims. How They Might Have Been Avoided, *Survey of Ophthalmology*, vol. 28, no. 1, 1983, pp. 55–60.
13. *Hanley v. Spencer*, 115 P.2d 399 (Colo. 1941). The concept of contributory negligence is discussed by Holder, A.R., *Medical Malpractice Law*, Wiley and Sons, New York, 1976, pp. 298–306.
14. The importance of documentation has been discussed by Classe, J.G., Record-Keeping and Documentation in Clinical Practice *Southern Journal of Optometry*, vol. 5, no. 2, 1987, pp. 11–25.

15. *Stuhr v. Barkwill*, 332 P.2d 603 (Or. 1958).
16. *Lippold v. Kidd*, 269 P. 210 (Or. 1928); *Marian v. Carroll*, discussed in *The Citation*, vol. 23, 1971, p. 33.
17. *Henderson v. Mason*, 386 S.W.2d 879 (Tex. Civ. App. 1964); and *Barnes v. Bovenmeyer*, 122 N.W.2d 312 (Iowa 1963).
18. Newell, F.W., and J.T. Ernest, *Ophthalmology: Principles and Concepts*, 3d ed., C.V. Mosby, St. Louis, 1974, pp. 157–158.
19. Terry, J.E., in Bartlett, J.D., and S.D. Jaanus (eds.), *Clinical Ocular Pharmacology*, Butterworth, Boston, 1984, pp. 698–700.
20. Ibid.
21. Ibid.
22. Ibid. To detect a small leak, a moistened fluorescein strip or drop of Fluress is placed in the injured eye and the affected area observed. If pressure in the eye is low, it may be necessary to apply digital pressure in order to observe the leaking aqueous.
23. Langton, D.P., *Manual of Ocular Diagnosis and Therapy*, Little, Brown & Co., Boston, 1980, p. 38.
24. Newell and Ernest, supra note 18, at 158.
25. *Ayers v. Farinella*, reported in *The Citation*, vol. 28, 1974, pp. 119–120.
26. In order to establish negligence, the optometrist must be shown to have breached the standard of care. The standard of care that is expected under the facts of the case must be established by expert testimony. Ordinarily the courts require practitioners of the same "school" to qualify as experts, but if the optometrist is acting outside the scope of practice, a medical expert may be permitted to testify, since it can be argued that the applicable standard is a medical standard. Even so, an optometrist who has complied with the standards described herein will satisfy the legal duty expected under the law, since the optometric and medical standards have little, if any, difference in foreign body cases. See Classe, J., Liability for Ocular Urgencies and Emergencies, *Southern Journal of Optometry*, vol. 4, no. 4, 1986, pp. 51–58.
27. Interestingly, both the Florida and the Iowa optometry practice acts prohibit surgery, yet expressly allow the removal of superficial foreign bodies. Thus there is some legislative authority for the position that the removal of corneal or other nonperforating foreign bodies is not surgery. See *Fla. Stat.* §463.014(3) and *Iowa Code Annot.* §154.1.
28. C.J.S.2d, Physicians and Surgeons, §1, p. 817.
29. Typical court definitions include the following:

    The word "surgery" comes from two Greek words signifying the hand and work. Originally, it was part of the profession of barbers, but later was taken up by physicians and now is recognized as that branch of medical science, and more specifically, that branch of medical science which treats of mechanical or operative measures for healing diseases, deformities, or injuries. [*State of Kansas ex rel. Beck v. Gleason*, 148 Kan 1, 79 P.2d 911 (1938).]

    "Surgery" is that branch of medical science concerned with corrections of deformities, repair of injuries, diagnosis and care of disease, relief of suffering, and prolongation of life by manual and instrumental operations. [*Hartford Acc. & Indem. Co. v. Barfield*, 89 Ga. App. 562, 80 S.E.2d 84 (1954).]

    "Surgery" is therapy of a distinctly operative kind, such as cutting operations, the reduction and putting up of fractures and dislocations and similar manual forms of treatment. [*Napier v. Greenzweig*, 256 F. 196, 197 (2nd Cir. 1919).]

    "Medicine" and "surgery" as used in provision of Chiropractice Act declaring that license to practice chiropractice shall not authorize practice of "medicine" and "surgery", denies chiropractors the use of drugs and medical preparations and the severing or penetrating of tissues of human beings. [*People v. Fowler*, 32 Cal. App. 2d Supp. 737, 84 P.2d 326 (1938).]
30. *Kime v. Aetna*, 66 Ohio App. 277, 33 N.E.2d 1008 (1940).
31. The definition of optometry in Ohio at this time was "the application of optical principles, through technical methods and devices in the examination of human eyes for the purpose of ascertaining departures from the normal, measuring their functional powers and adapting optical accessories for the aid thereof." Quoted in *Kime v. Aetna*, 33 N.E.2d at 1010.
32. Id. at 1011.
33. It will be left to each individual insurer to determine whether the optometrist will be defended and any judgment paid (to the limits of the policy). Under some circumstances the insurer may be willing to defend the optometrist but not to pay a judgment.
34. Even though an optometrist has complied with the standard of care and thus has treated the patient in a nonnegligent fashion, there is still the prospect of discipline by the board of optometry to contend with, should a complaint be filed with the board alleging that the optometrist has acted outside the scope of care permitted under the state statute.
35. *Acupuncture Society of Kansas v. Kansas State Board of Healing Arts*, 226 Kan. 639, 602 P.2d 1311 (1979).
36. At least one ophthalmological commentator considers orthokeratology to be surgery:

    Orthokeratologists apply rigid splints to the tissues in an effort to change their geometry either permanently or semipermanently. There are other circumstances in which practitioners press foreign substances against body parts with force sufficient to mold and change the shape of the tissues. Orthopedic surgeons apply nonliving splints to the limbs in order to change the shape of deformed bones and joints, and orthopedic surgeons apply mechanical splints to the teeth and jaws to alter the growth patterns and shape of those tissues. Surgery does not require the cutting of tissues or the letting of blood. Orthokeratology, putting splints on the cornea, is surgery.

Safir, A., *Ophthalmology*, vol. 86, no. 5, 1979, p. 711.

37. Senate Bill 168, which has had an interesting legal history, was adopted by the Florida legislature in 1983, vetoed by the governor, and brought before the courts on the basis that the veto was not timely. Although the circuit court upheld the veto, the First District Court of Appeals reversed the trial court (465 So.2d 1319), and in 1985 the case was appealed to the Florida Supreme Court, which upheld the veto. See *Florida Society of Ophthalmology v. Florida Optometric Association*, 489 So. 2d 1118 (1986).

Chapter 27

Liability for Ophthalmic Materials

(This state) has adopted the doctrine of strict liability by sellers of products "in a defective condition unreasonably dangerous to the user."...Here the thinness of the lenses made them unreasonably dangerous to users, so the doctrine of strict liability is applicable. However, the defendant argues against strict liability, on the ground that the sunglasses were "unavoidably unsafe products." Even assuming arguendo *that the state of the art is not capable of producing a shatter-resistant or splinter-free baseball sunglass [this defense] furnishes no shelter from liability [unless] the product is "accompanied by proper...warning," which the defendant's product lacked.*

—From the decision of Judge Cummings, *Filler v. Rayex Corporation*, 435 F.2d 336 (7th Cir. 1970)

Although professional liability for optometrists most often involves injuries related to misdiagnosis, a steady percentage of cases is due to injuries from ophthalmic materials. Among products causing ocular injury, the next-to-highest category—personal use items—includes ophthalmic products such as spectacle lenses and contact lenses.[1] Some of these injuries from ophthalmic products result in litigation. There are two types of legal theories used to establish liability: negligence and product liability. In both types of claims the most important factor has been the development of plastic lenses as a substitute for glass.

The superior impact-resistance of plastic has been the principal reason for its clinical use in lieu of glass, and in this regard polycarbonate plastic has proven to be the most desirable lens material by far.[2] Laboratory tests comparing the impact-resistance of polycarbonate to heat-tempered glass, chemically tempered glass, and allyl resin (CR-39®) plastic have demonstrated the remarkable difference between these materials (Tables 27.1 and 27.2).

The other major development has been the adoption by the federal government of impact-resistance requirements for ophthalmic lenses, an event that has established national standards for both dress and industrial use lenses. This shift to mandatory standards from what had previously been voluntary guidelines has significant legal ramifications for all optometrists.[3]

We begin with a review of cases alleging negligence.

Negligence as the Basis of Liability for Ophthalmic Lenses

Allegations of negligence require evidence that the defendant doctor did not conform to the standard of care expected of like practitioners acting under the same or similar circumstances. Optometrists are expected to exercise reasonable prudence and to demonstrate that minimum degree of learning and

Table 27.1. Lens Impact Data for Selected Glass and Plastic Ophthalmic Lenses

Type of Lens Material (2 mm. thick—avg. +2, plano, −2)	Energy (ft/lb.)	Miles per Hour: Steel BB (0.177 in.)	Miles per Hour: Steel Ball (0.217 in.)	Miles per Hour: Steel Ball (0.250 in.)	Breakage (%)
Polycarbonate dress eyewear	7.34	539	383	307	0
Allyl resin (CR-39®)	0.96*	193	137	110	50
Glass, chemically hardened	0.31*	110	78	63	50
Glass, heat/air hardened	0.18*	84	60	48	50

* Energy at which 50 percent of lenses will break.
Source: Gentex Corporation, 1984.

skill possessed by members of the profession in good standing, and failure to measure up to the standard of care can create liability. For optometrists who prescribe or dispense ophthalmic materials, there are three aspects of practice that have proven to be sources of claims alleging negligence: (1) failure to prescribe the lens material of choice, (2) failure to warn of the limited impact-resistance of glass, and (3) failure to inspect and verify lens orders.

Failure to Prescribe the Lens Material of Choice

The selection of ophthalmic lens material is usually left to the optometrist, and so negligence in making this selection will create liability. The most common type of claim alleges a failure by the optometrist to select the most impact-resistant material for the patient.

Table 27.2. Potential Impact Energy of Various Missiles

Missile	Potential Impact Energy (ft./lb.)
BB	0.5–1.5
22 caliber slug	100.0
Human fist	2.0–4.0
Pitched baseball	21.0
Stone, $1\frac{3}{4} \times \frac{3}{4} \times \frac{1}{2}$ in., thrown 30 ft.	8.9
Stone, $2 \times 1\frac{1}{2}$ in., thrown 30 ft.	7.9
3 lb. hammer dropped 10 ft.	30.0
Automobile crash at 20 m.p.h., head striking dashboard	67.2
Lawnmower blade throwing small stone 30 ft.	6.0–23.0
Grinding wheel throwing chips 2 ft.	0.7–28.0

Source: Gentex Corporation, 1984.

A policeman was struck by a drunk as he was entering a bar for a routine investigation. The blow shattered his spectacles, causing a piece of glass to be driven into an eye, thereby creating a permanent loss of acuity. He sued both the optical company filling the prescription and the optician dispensing the spectacles, alleging they were negligent for failing to provide him with lenses that were either more impact resistant or less likely to come out of the frame in sharp, jagged pieces (i.e., plastic lenses). A verdict of $180,000 was returned in his favor.[4]

Most cases in this classification involve the negligent selection of glass (rather than plastic) as the lens material. Since the impact-resistance of polycarbonate is vastly superior to glass, for some patients the selection of polycarbonate is virtually mandatory.[5] Monocular patients, athletes, children, and persons who are physically active and whose occupations make them more likely to be exposed to the risk of ocular injury are the leading candidates for polycarbonate lenses. Even industrial-strength glass lenses may not be an adequate choice when impact-resistance is a key consideration.

A myopic rancher who required spectacles for full-time wear was examined by an optometrist. Because the patient's activities required him to spend much of his time out of doors, he requested that photochromic lenses be prescribed. The optometrist ordered glass lenses, but specified that they were to be of industrial strength (i.e., a minimum of 3-mm center thickness). While wearing the glasses, the patient was struck in the face by a rope, which shattered one of the lenses, causing serious injury to his eye. He thereafter sued the optometrist, alleging that a more impact-resistant lens material, polycarbonate, should have been prescribed. The optometrist's defense was that polycarbonate was not widely available at the time of the examination and that industrial strength glass was the appropriate impact-resistant material under the circumstances. The jury found in favor of the optometrist.[6]

Although this case was defended on the basis that polycarbonate lenses were not available for use, it is unlikely that such a defense could be successfully waged today because of the improved distribution and versatility of polycarbonate. Furthermore, under the appropriate circumstances (such as prescribing for a worker who needs on-the-job eyewear), even industrial strength polycarbonate may be required in order to comply with legal standards. If an optometrist recommends polycarbonate and a patient disregards this advice in favor of glass (typically to enjoy the advantages of photochromic lenses), the optometrist should be certain to document the patient's decision.[7]

The doctrine of informed consent obligates the optometrist to explain the differences between the various lens materials, but if the patient chooses glass despite this warning, the clinician has fulfilled his responsibility and may dispense the less impact-resistant material. A practitioner may wish to draft a form to be used on these occasions, which is to be signed by the patient and which states that the patient is aware of the limited impact-resistance of glass and has voluntarily chosen to purchase the glass lenses despite the optometrist's warning. This form may be retained in the patient's record for as long as is necessary. Although such a declaration by the patient is not exculpatory in itself, it is compelling evidence in the event there is a legal dispute.

Because of the FTC's Eyeglasses I Rule, patients must be given a copy of the spectacle prescription at the conclusion of the examination. Optometrists would be wise to specify the lens material by incorporating it into the prescription so that the patient will be prevented from inadvertently purchasing a lens material of reduced impact-resistance from another ophthalmic provider[8] (see Chapter 17 for a discussion of prescription requirements).

Failure to Warn

An optometrist may be held liable for negligently failing to warn of the significant difference in impact resistance between glass lenses and polycarbonate lenses. The optometrist (or assistant) who dispenses ophthalmic materials should recognize those patients for whom impact resistance is of clinical importance and should discuss the selection of materials with them.

A worker at an automobile plant was required to wear safety glasses while at work, and selected some glasses sold to the plant by an optical shop for that purpose. While wearing them at work one of the lenses was shattered, causing a unilateral loss of vision. The worker sued the optical company that sold the plant the glasses, alleging that the company was negligent in failing to warn him of the difference in impact-resistance between safety glass and polycarbonate plastic. The company defended the claim on the basis that the frame and the lenses (which were made of glass) were in compliance with ANSI Z-87.1 standards. Despite this contention, the jury awarded the plaintiff over $1 million as damages for his injury.[9]

With the advent of polycarbonate, there is doubtless some temptation on the part of optometrists (and their ophthalmic assistants) to use the word shatterproof. Even polycarbonate will shatter, however, and so the word shatterproof is one that should be expunged from the lexicon of all ophthalmic providers.[10] When describing the risk of injury due to lens breakage, it is best to do so by using the words impact resistance. (See the concluding section of this chapter, which discusses guarantees and warranties.) Warnings may be advisable when there is reason to believe the patient is at risk for injury and the relative impact-resistance of the various ophthalmic materials is unknown to the patient.

Failure to Inspect

All optometrists have a legal obligation to inspect orders of ophthalmic materials to ensure that patients receive the lens material desired and to verify that the order is in compliance with the applicable standards.[11]

An 18-year-old man ordered safety glasses from his optometrist. Later the patient was in an automobile accident and suffered the loss of an eye when one of the lenses shattered. It was then discovered that when the original order was turned over to the optometrist's technician, she failed to mark the order as one for safety glasses. Hence, although the patient had ordered and paid for safety lenses, he had received dress lenses. The patient sued, alleging negligence, and the case was eventually settled for $42,100.[12]

The duty to inspect is especially important for industrial strength lenses and frames (safety glasses), but all orders for ophthalmic materials should be inspected to verify that they satisfy the applicable standards. (These standards are described in the section of this chapter that discusses product liability.) All offices should institute a verification system for orders of ophthalmic materials so as to minimize the risk of injury to the patient.

Liability for Frames

A second source of negligence claims for ophthalmic materials concerns injuries from frames. Although these claims constitute a relatively small percentage of cases, there is potential for liability. Types of cases may be classified as: idiosyncratic responses, improper safety frames, and improper sports frames.

Idiosyncratic Responses

Individual patients may develop allergic responses to frames or ophthalmic devices, but where it can be shown that such responses are idiosyncratic and thus unpredictable, there can be no negligence and hence no liability.

A patient purchased some frames from an optical shop, but shortly after she began wearing them she developed a rash where the frames came in contact with her face. She returned to the shop, where she was told that too much dye had been used on the frames. The dye was of a type commonly employed throughout the optical industry. She sued the shop, alleging negligence in the application of too much dye, and a jury awarded her $500. Upon appeal the judgment was reversed, the appellate court noting that all medical testimony in the case indicated that the cause of the patient's injury "was the idiosyncracy of her skin that made it susceptible to an eyeglass frame that would not, in any way, injure an ordinary person" and that the injury was not such as could reasonably have been anticipated.[13]

Frames that cause injury due to an improper fit or modification, however, may be the source of a meritorious negligence claim.

Improper Safety Frames

Standards for frames to be used in an industrial setting are more stringent than those for frames to be used for dress wear (discussed in the section on product liability). One important provision of these standards is the requirement that both a safety frame and safety lenses be dispensed to patients requesting safety glasses. Failure to provide an approved frame —even if safety lenses are prescribed—can create the potential for liability.[14]

A female industrial worker requiring safety glasses for wear while at her factory job was examined by an optometrist. After the examination was concluded, she was shown some approved industrial safety frames. She preferred to purchase dress zyl frames, however, and ordered these frames along with the industrial thickness lenses. Some time later she was working at a lathe when a bushing struck and shattered one of the lenses, injuring her eye. She sued the optometrist, alleging that the lenses and frame were not in compliance with the standards necessary for safety glasses.[15]

If an optometrist supplies safety glasses for a plant or an industrial program, they should be inspected to ensure that they are in compliance with the applicable standards.

Optometrists should be certain that all orders for safety glasses are composed of both approved frames and industrial strength lenses. (If assistants are responsible for the ordering, verifying, and dispensing of safety glasses, they should understand the applicable standards as well.)

Improper Sports Frames

Liability may ensue from failure to prescribe the appropriate frames for sports and recreational activities, if the risk of injury is significant. The racquet sports constitute the most likely source of claims, ocular injury arising either from balls that strike the frames at high rates of speed or from violent blows from the racquets themselves.[16] The improper frame, if struck by a ball or racquet, can cause serious damage to the patient's eye or adnexa and contribute to injury due to ophthalmic lens breakage.[17]

A patient who had lost one eye in a childhood accident was a racquetball player, and wished to have adequate eye protection while participating in the sport. He was examined by an ophthalmologist, who suggested that he consult an optician for the appropriate eye protection. The optician fit the patient with frames containing glass lenses, commenting that "it would take a Mack truck to cause them to break." While wearing the glasses during a racquetball game the patient was struck by the ball, which caused the lens to shatter into many fragments. After surgery was able to save some of the patient's sight, he sued the optician for negligence, alleging that a more impact-resistant lens and frame would have prevented the injury.[18]

Frames for athletes should be carefully selected and should offer reasonable protection for the sport. For participants of the racquet sports, a wrap-around polycarbonate frame with no hinges (and polycarbonate lenses) is the frame of choice. (Open frames are inadequate because they permit penetration of the ball.) Optometrists should dispense only those sports frames that meet established standards for impact-resistance.[19]

A 22-year-old manager of a racquetball club purchased a pair of Pro-Tec lensless safety goggles that were sold for the purpose of providing eye protection when playing squash, racquetball, and handball. While playing racquetball with a club member the ball penetrated the lensless opening in the goggles and struck his eye, causing external injury and traumatic cataract and significantly affecting his binocular vision. He sued the manufacturer of the goggles, alleging that they were improperly designed and tested. Evidence established that tests of the goggles conducted by the Canadian Sports Standards Commission revealed a high-velocity racquetball could penetrate the lens opening and strike the eye. The case was settled in favor of the plaintiff for $150,000.[20]

Since many patients seek one pair of frames and lenses for both work and leisure activities, optometrists should take careful histories and document instances in which patients choose frame designs that create a potential risk of injury. Without such documentation, clinicians face a much more difficult legal struggle in attempting to establish lack of culpability on their part.

Negligence and Contact Lenses

Contact lens practice is the leading source of negligence claims against optometrists. Liability may arise in the fitting or wear of lenses, but failure to monitor contact lens patients and to assess ocular health are the causes of large claims. Because of the numerous clinical and legal issues that must be considered by contact lens practitioners, this subject is considered separately in Chapter 30.

Product Liability and Ophthalmic Lenses

Although professional liability is most often associated with the concept of negligence, there is another important aspect of liability related to the practice of optometry: product liability.

Product liability is a legal issue for optometrists because practitioners of optometry not only render services, they also sell ophthalmic materials. Because glasses and contact lenses are sold by optometrists to the public, optometric practitioners are held to certain legal standards with regard to the safety of these products, and these standards are considerably different than those based on negligence.

Product liability law is based on the concept of strict liability, which is also referred to as absolute liability. As these terms infer, liability is conferred on a defendant despite the absence of negligence on his part, despite the fact that he observed the highest standards of care in preventing the possibility of negligence and despite the arguable contention that the defendant is "without fault." Liability is absolute and is really an application of social policy, namely that the designer, manufacturer, or seller of a product will be held responsible as a matter of law when a consumer is injured due to a defect in the product, the underlying social policy being that the designer, manufacturer, or seller is better able to bear the brunt of economic loss than is the consumer. Under this theory of law, optometrists may be held liable when patients are injured by ophthalmic materials that are found to be defective. (Product liability theory is reviewed in Chapter 21.)

Perhaps the most difficult aspect of the law—from the viewpoint of an injured consumer—is to establish that the product is defective, which is an evidentiary matter requiring expert testimony. In order to offer proof that an ophthalmic lens is defective, the expert must present evidence that establishes some standard upon which to base judgment. For ophthalmic lenses, the most important criteria have been the impact-resistance standards established through the American National Standards Institute. Therefore, a review of the development of these standards is necessary.

Standards for Ophthalmic Lenses

There are two types of standards that must be considered: those applicable to dress lenses and those applicable to industrial strength lenses.

The Z 80 Standard

The development of standards for the ophthalmic industry-at-large began in 1956, when the American Standards Association (ASA) undertook to establish the first national standard for ophthalmic lenses. The ASA Committee charged with this responsibility was known as the Z 80 Sectional Committee on Standards for Ophthalmic Lenses, and the AOA was one of the original organizations that participated in the committee's standard-making process.[21]

The ASA Committee began drafting standards in the early 1960s and in 1969 changed its name, becoming the American National Standards Institute (ANSI). Revisions of these standards were published in 1972 and 1979, the last revision occurring after the U.S. Congress enacted the Medical Devices Act in 1976, which gave the federal government power to oversee the safety and effectiveness of all medical devices.[22] These devices included (among 8,000 items) ophthalmic products such as spectacle lenses, contact lenses, and ophthalmic solutions. The law conferred regulatory authority on the Food and Drug Administration (FDA) and provided for the FDA to bring within its jurisdiction the responsibility for ensuring compliance of all covered medical devices with existing standards. The impact-resistance standards to which ophthalmic lenses were expected to conform were those established by ANSI and adopted by the FDA. ANSI ophthalmic subcommittees are listed in Table 27.3.

The current standards for dress lenses are expressed in *ANSI Requirements for First-Quality Pre-*

Table 27.3. ANSI Ophthalmic Subcommittees: 1988

Z 80.1-1987	Recommendations for prescription ophthalmic lenses
Z 80.2-1972	Prescription requirements for first quality contact lenses
Z 80.3-1986	Requirements for nonprescription sunglasses and fashion eyewear
Z 80.4-1974	Accessory solutions used with contact lenses made of conventional hard plastic materials such as PMMA
Z 80.5-1979	Requirements for dress ophthalmic frames
Z 80.6-1983	Physicochemical properties of conventional hard plastic contact lenses
Z 80.7-1984	Optical and physical requirements for intraocular lenses
Z 80.8-1986	Requirements for soft contact lenses
Z 80.9-1986	Low vision aids

Source: American National Standards Institute, 1988.

Table 27.4. American National Standards Institute Z 80.1-1987 Recommendations for Impact-Resistance of Prescription Ophthalmic Lenses

Section 4.8: Impact Resistance

4.8.1 **Prescription Impact-Resistant, Occupational, and Educational Corrective Lenses.** Tolerances for optical performance characteristics should be as outlined in this standard. Safety requirements shall comply with ANSI Z 87.1-1979 (or the latest revision thereof.)

4.8.2 **Prescription Impact-Resistant Dress Eyewear Lenses.** All lenses shall be capable of withstanding the impact test described in 4.8.4. Laminated, plastic, and raised-ledge multifocal lenses that may be damaged by impact test procedures may be certified by the lens manufacturer as conforming to the intial design testing or statistically significant sampling specified by Title 21, *Code of Federal Regulations*, 801.410.
All monolotihic (not laminated) glass lenses shall be treated to be resistant to impact.

4.8.3 **Special Corrective Lenses.** Certain lenses prescribed for specific visual needs are not suitable for the drop-ball technique of testing. Wherever possible, such lenses should be treated to be resistant to impact; however, impact-testing requirements are waived. These lens types include:

(1) Prism segment multifocals
(2) Slab-off prisms
(3) Lenticular cataracts
(4) Iseikonics
(5) Depressed segment one-piece multifocals
(6) Biconcaves, myodiscs, and minus lenticulars
(7) Custom laminates and cemented assemblies

4.8.4 **Test Procedure.** The impact resistance of lenses subject to individual tests shall be measured with a 15.9 mm (5/8 inch ± 0.0001 inch) diameter steel ball weighing not less than 15 grams (0.56 ounces) dropped from a height of not less than 127 centimeters (50 inches), or an equivalent impact. Steel balls shall comply with the requirements of American National Standard Specifications for Metal Balls, ANSI/AFBMA Standard 10-1975, or the latest revision thereof, for chrome alloy steel (ANSI Type E52100), of density 27.5 balls per pound, ball grade No. 25 or better.

Source: This material is reproduced with permission from American National Standard Z 80.1-1987, © 1987 by the American National Standards Institute. Copies of this standard may be purchased from the American National Standards Institute at 1430 Broadway, New York, NY 10018.

scription Lenses, Z 80.1-1987. For legal purposes, the most important aspect of Z 80.1 is the requirement for impact-resistance (see Table 27.4), which states that "all lenses shall be capable of withstanding the impact test" (a steel ball of 5/8 inches in diameter weighing not less than 15 grams is dropped from a height of fifty inches onto the lens).

Z 80.1 also describes standards for refractive power (sphere, cylinder, and cylinder axis), vertical and horizontal placement of the major reference points in a mounted pair of lenses, horizontal placement of reading segments, base curves of ophthalmic lenses, and other parameters. These are the standards that practitioners must grapple with today whenever they evaluate laboratory performance.[23]

Standards for nonprescription sunglasses and fashion eyewear have also been established under ANSI guidelines, and Z 80.3-1986 sets the applicable standards for impact-resistance, which are the same as those described above for prescription ophthalmic lenses. Therefore, whether prescription or nonprescription eyeglasses are dispensed by an optometrist, they will be held to the same legal standard for impact resistance, i.e., the drop ball test.

Table 27.5. Types of Eye Protection Required by ANSI Z 87.1-1979

Category	Type
Spectacles (with or without sideshields)	Plano Prescription Filter
Goggles	Cup Chipping Welding Laser Flexible-fitting Chemical-splash
Face shields	Wire screen Clear plastic Tinted plastic Absorptive plastic
Curtains	Opaque Transparent
Welding helmets	

Source: Sherr, A.E., Industrial Safety Glasses—An Update, *Journal of the American Optometric Association*, vol. 51, no. 2, Feb. 1980, p. 129.

The Z87 Standard

Concomitant with the concern for a national standard regulating dress eyewear was the parallel concern for a national standard applicable to industrial lenses, frames, and protective devices. This problem was first addressed in 1968 when industry-wide standards were issued for ophthalmic products used in the workplace. The standards were identified as the *Z 87.1-1968 Standards for Occupational and Educational Eye and Face Protection*, and, like their Z 80 counterpart, constituted a voluntary set of guidelines proposed by ANSI.[24] The Z 87.1 standards established minimum specifications for eye and face protectors, ophthalmic lenses of industrial strength, and frames and sideshields.

Industrial eye protection received a major boost in 1970 when the Occupational Safety and Health Administration (OSHA) adopted Z 87.1-1968 as its standard for industrial eyewear, thereby conferring legal legitimacy upon these previously voluntary guidelines. The Z 87.1-1968 standard was revised and reissued in 1979 as *ANSI Standard Z 87 Practice for Occupational and Educational Eye and Face Protection* (see Table 27.5). The types of devices covered by the standard can be classified into five categories: spectacles, goggles, face shields, welding helmets, and curtains.

Among the most important considerations of Z 87.1-1979 are those pertaining to safety spectacles. All safety spectacles (with or without side shields) must be marked with a permanent trademark to identify the manufacturer and a Z 87 logo to show that the spectacles comply with Z 87-1979 standards (see Table 27.6). Lenses, both glass and plastic, must contain the identifying trademark of the entity fabricating the spectacles and pass a lens impact test. In addition plastic lenses must pass a penetration resistance test (see Table 27.7). Industrial safety lenses must be a minimum of three millimeters in thickness (whether prescription or plano), regardless of type of lens material (glass, allyl resin, or polycarbonate). Therefore, lens thickness is a legal factor under Z 87.1, particular for minus lenses, which are thinnest at the center (see Table 27.8).

Product Liability as the Basis of Liability for Ophthalmic Lenses

Cases based on product liability theory must allege some defect in the lenses that makes them unreasonably dangerous for their intended purpose.[25] The most common means of establishing that a lens is defective is through the presentation of evidence that shows the lens is not in compliance with the applicable standards (either Z 80 or Z 87, as appropriate).

Table 27.6. ANSI Z 87.1-1979—Spectacles: Metal, Plastic, and Combination Metal and Plastic

6.1.2.1 General Requirements. Safety spectacles require special frames and lenses. Therefore, combinations of frames and lenses not meeting this standard are *definitely not in compliance.*

Plastic fronts should be so designed as to satisfactorily accept lens insertion through the frontal side only.

Spectacles shall consist of two lenses and a frame front which supports the lenses around their entire periphery, of suitable size and shape for the purposes intended, connected by a nose bridge, and retained on the face by temples or other suitable means. The spectacles shall be furnished with or without side shields, depending upon their intended use. The fronts, temples, and side shields can be of metal or plastic construction or a combination of metal and plastic. All parts shall meet the requirements of 6.2. Spectacles may be classified as Type I—Metal Front, Type II—Plastic Front, or Type III—Combination Metal and Plastic Front.

6.1.2.1.1 Protection. Spectacles without side shields shall provide frontal protection to the eye from flying objects and, when required, from glare and injurious radiations.

6.1.2.1.2 Marking. Spectacles shall be designed for industrial exposure and shall bear both a permanent trademark identifying the manufacturer and a "Z87" logo indicating compliance with this standard, on fronts and temples, as described in 4.8. The front shall also carry a designation of the eye size and bridge size (where applicable). Temples shall be marked as to overall length or fitting value, or both. Lenses shall bear only a single trademark to identify both the manufacturer and compliance with this standard; filter or absorptive lenses shall also be marked with the shade number. See 6.3.3.3.4 for special marking requirements for variable-tint lenses.

Corrective-protective (Rx) ophthalmic fixed-tint lenses such as Pink No. 1 and 2; Gray No. 1, 2, and 3; and Green No. 1, 2, and 3, need not have a shade marking. Such fixed-tint lenses shall carry only the manufacturer's monogram.

6.1.2.1.3 Front and Lens Sizes. The front lens container and the lenses shall be of identical shape and configuration and of such dimensions as to assure support of the lenses by the front *around their entire periphery.*

The fronts and lenses may be available in 42; 44; 46; 48; 50- and 52-mm eye sizes in S7, S10, or other symmetrical ophthalmic shapes, and the distance between the lenses (bridge size) measured at the nearest point of bridge gap may range from 18 mm to 26 mm and shall be specified.

A tolerance of the specified bridge size ±1 mm shall be permitted. These bridges are known as keyhole types.

A saddle or universal fitting bridge also may be used.

Plano lenses shall be flat or 6.0 ± 1/4 diopter curve. Corrective (Rx) lenses are to be as specified on the individual prescription.

6.1.2.1.4 Temples. Temples may be of the cable, spatula, or temple headband combination type, as specified, and shall be of such design as to permit adjustment and fit comfortably and securely on the wearer. The size of the temples shall be clearly marked, except on the temple headband combination type.

6.1.2.1.5 Hinges. Front and temple hinges shall be securely fastened, shall mesh in a suitable manner, and shall be joined in such a way as to eliminate accidental separation.

Source: This material is reproduced with permission from American National Standard Z 87.1-1979, © 1979 by the American National Standards Institute. Copies of this standard may be purchased from the American National Standards Institute at 1430 Broadway, New York, NY 10018.

The types of situations in which defective lenses have been demonstrated can be classified as follows:

- Defective design
- Defective warnings or directions
- Defective inspection

Defective Design

The most common cause of claims in this classification concerns prescription lenses alleged to be defective because they are not in compliance with Z 80 or Z 87 standards. Because current standards for dress lenses require that the drop-ball test be administered to assess impact-resistance, failure to meet this minimum standard as required by Z 80.1 can create the potential for liability.[26]

A prescription for glass spectacle lenses for a 6-year-old hyperope specified that they be tempered. The lenses were heat treated by the optical lab filling the prescription and dispensed to the child. Six months later one of the lenses was struck by a rock thrown by a playmate and shattered, two slivers penetrating the youngster's eye. He suffered a traumatic cataract, which necessitated surgery and resulted in a permanent vision defect. He thereafter sued the laboratory, alleging that the lenses had been improperly heat treated and that the drop-ball test had not been performed as required by ANSI Z 80.1 standards. Although the jury's verdict was in favor of the defendant, on appeal this judgment was reversed, the court holding that "the object of heat treatment was to reduce the dangers from the slivers when a lens fractured. A jury could find from

Table 27.7. ANSI Z 87.1-1979: Methods of Testing Spectacles

§6.1.2.3 The portion of the front that supports the lens shall be of sufficient strength to withstand, without breakage and without ejecting the lens completely, the impact-resistance test for lenses specified in 6.1.2.3.2.

§6.1.2.3.2 Lens in Frame Retention Test— All Types. The frame with inserted lenses convex side up, shall be supported, centered in relation to the mechanical center of the lens, on the text fixture shown in Fig. 5. To assure uniform test support, the bridge portion of the frame shall rest on the bridge support block. The temples shall be held between the knurled clamping knobs so that the frame is essentially horizontal.

A 25.4-mm (1-inch) diameter steel ball, weighing approximately 68 grams (2.4 ounces), shall be dropped in free fall from a height of 1.27 meters (50 in.) onto the outer surface of the lens, perpendicularly impinging the lens within a circular area of 10-mm ($\frac{5}{8}$-in) diameter centered at the lens mechanical center. Test each lens separately. Upon impact, the lens edge shall not be chipped, the lens shall not be inwardly dislodged from its seat and the lens shall not be completely ejected from the frame. Frame distortion is permissible.

§6.1.2.3.3 Lens Impact Test

(1) Lens on Block—Glass and Plastic: The lens shall be removed from the frame and placed mechanically centered, convex side up, on the test block of an anvil composed of the parts shown in Fig. 7, mounted in the hole of the base plate shown in Fig. 6, the whole assembly on a flat, horizontal work surface of convenient height.

A 25.4-mm (1-in) diameter steel ball, weighing approximately 68 grams (2.4 ounces), shall be dropped in free fall from a height of 1.27 meters (50 in) onto the horizontal outer surface of the lens, perpendicularly impinging the lens within a circular area of 16-mm ($\frac{5}{8}$-in) diameter centered at the lens mechanical center. The lens shall not fracture in this test.

(2) Penetration Resistance—Plastic Only. The lens shall be removed from the frame and placed mechanically centered, convex side up, on the test block of an anvil composed of the parts shown in Fig. 7, mounted in the hole of the baseplate shown in Fig. 6, the whole assembly on a flat, horizontal work surface of convenient height. This requirement shall be waived for corrective protective (Rx) lenses.

A pointed projectile of suitable size, consisting of a new Singer No. 25 or equal size 135 × 17 needle, fastened into a holder weighing approximately 44.2 grams (1.56 ounces), shall be freely dropped, point downward, from a height of 1.27 meters (50 in) onto the horizontal outer surface of the lens. The projectile may be guided, but not restricted, in its perpendicular fall by being dropped through a tube extending to within approximately 101.6 mm (4 in) of the lens. The lens shall not be pierced through by the impact.

Source: This material is reproduced with permission from American National Standard Z 87.1-1979, © 1979 by the American National Standards Institute. Copies of this standard may be purchased from the American National Standards Institute at 1430 Broadway, New York, NY 10018.

Table 27.8. ANSI Z 87.1-1979: Lenses for Persons Requiring Visual Correction

6.3.2.6 Lenses for Persons Requiring Visual Correction. Persons whose vision requires the use of corrective (Rx) lenses shall use protectors of one of the following types:

(1) Safety spectacles whose protective lenses provide the proper optical correction and withstand the drop-ball test specified in 6.1.2.3.3. (Such lenses are exempted from the requirements for parallelism of surfaces. Minimum thickness of prescription lenses shall be 3.0 mm (0.12 in), except in the case of lenses of strong plus power, when the edge thickness may be reduced to 2.5 mm (0.1 in), provided they meet the impact test specified in 6.1.2.3.3).

(2) Goggles that can be worn over corrective (Rx) spectacles without disturbing the adjustment of the spectacles.

Source: This material is reproduced with permission from American National Standard Z 87.1-1979, © 1979 by the American National Standards Institute. Copies of this standard may be purchased from the American National Standards Institute at 1430 Broadway, New York, NY 10018.

the evidence here that the lens, when used in a reasonably to be anticipated manner, failed to fulfill its purpose because of defects which might have been found to exist."[27]

The optometrist is particularly vulnerable when prescribing for young children, athletes, monocular patients, or persons who are physically active and whose occupations make them more likely to be exposed to the dangers of flying projectiles or the likelihood of ocular trauma.

A young man wearing spectacles prescribed by an optometrist was playing basketball when an elbow came in contact with one of the lenses, shattering it into many splinters that penetrated one eye. Ultimately he suffered a 25 percent vision loss in the eye and sued the optometrist, alleging that the lenses were dangerously thin and did not satisfy ANSI Z 80.1 standards since they had not been given the drop-ball test for impact resistance. The jury awarded him $30,000.[28]

The material of choice is polycarbonate for athletic patients. Glass lenses are contraindicated.

Nonprescription lenses, especially for sports activities, should be carefully evaluated before being recommended to a patient.

A high school baseball player was practicing for a varsity game when he misjudged a fly ball that tipped off his glove and struck his flipped-down plano baseball sunglasses. The lens shattered into sharp splinters that pierced his eye, necessitating the eye's removal nine days later. The sunglasses were advertised as "just perfect for active and spectator sports—world's finest sunglasses." They resembled ordinary sunglasses except for the flip feature. But their center thickness was only 1.5 mm, and they were not tempered for impact resistance. The youngster sued the manufacturer of the sunglasses under product liability law. The court held that the reduced center thickness made the lenses unreasonably dangerous and awarded the plaintiff $101,000.[29]

An optometrist selling nonprescription lenses to athletes should be certain that the lenses are of an appropriate impact-resistant material and that they are suitable for the activities for which they are purchased. Optical shops and dispensaries selling over-the-counter eyewear are particularly vulnerable to product liability claims.

A second form of defective design—improper modification—is of particular interest to optometrists who fabricate their own eyewear.

A 5-year-old child wearing glasses was playing with a young friend when she slipped and fell against a small, sharply pointed stake. The force with which she fell was so great that the stake shattered one of the spectacle lenses, driving a sliver of glass into her eye. As a result of the injury, she suffered a permanent vision loss, with the best vision obtainable in the affected eye being reduced to 20/40 (a 15 percent impairment). Her parents filed suit against the doctor who prescribed the lenses, the manufacturer of the lenses, and the optical company that edged and mounted the lenses based on the doctor's prescription. The case went to trial against the optical laboratory alone, based on product liability theory. Expert testimony for the plaintiff at the trial maintained that "shoddy work" by the optical company in edging the lenses had reduced the ability of the lenses to withstand heavy impact and had caused the shattering that injured the child. The laboratory's experts testified in turn that the force of the blow was sufficient to shatter the lenses, poor workmanship notwithstanding, and that, had the child not been wearing glasses, the injury would have been even more severe. The jury awarded the plaintiff $350,000 despite testimony.[30]

When ordinary glass receives a heavy blow on one surface, tension is produced in the glass on the opposite side, causing fracture in the opposite lens surface (and injury).[31] A safety lens under compression does not allow this opposite-surface tension to accumulate so rapidly, and so fracture of the lens surface is less likely to occur. Any surface cracks or edge flaws greatly reduce this effect, however, and so surfacing and edging of safety lenses must be carried out with great care. An optometrist supervising such work for an in-house laboratory must conduct a careful inspection of lens edges to insure that no lens compromise occurs.[32]

An optometrist who orders his lenses from an optical laboratory should inspect the fabricated lenses and should reject any lenses that are poorly edged (or otherwise unsatisfactory).

Defective Warnings or Directions

An optometrist has a duty to warn his patients of the limitations of the ophthalmic lenses that he dispenses. He also has a duty to explain to patients the safe and proper use of the lenses, including lenses that are impact-resistant.[33]

A medical social work supervisor was at bat in a baseball game when he checked his swing, causing a pitched ball to stike his glasses, breaking one lens and lacerating his cornea in three places. He sued the optometrist who had fitted him for the glasses, alleging a failure to warn that the lenses were not shatterproof. A jury awarded him $50,000.[34]

Not only should patients who are fitted with dress lenses be warned; patients for whom industrial thickness lenses must be prescribed should also receive the appropriate warning.

A 24-year-old lathe operator required safety glasses for his job. The glasses were delivered to his employer with a one-inch tab affixed to the nosepiece stating that the glasses were impact-resistant but not unbreakable, but this tab was routinely removed before the glasses were distributed to the workers. While wearing the glasses an object struck the lathe operator's right lens, causing it to shatter and lacerate the eyelid, cornea, and iris, resulting in permanent loss of visual acuity, headaches, and photophobia. The lathe operator sued the lens manufacturer under product liability theory, alleging failure to provide an adequate warning. The jury returned a verdict in his favor for $57,724 and the manufacturer appealed. In affirming the decision of the trial court, the court of appeals ruled that the warning of a potential product danger must be in a form reasonably expected to catch the attention of the user and must convey a fair indication of the nature and extent of the danger. In this case, the court observed, the package label lulled the user into a false sense of security by failing to inform the user that the lenses were not shatterproof.[35]

A careful in-office procedure of lens selection, prescription verification, and patient education should be an integral part of every optometric practice.[36]

Defective Inspection

An optometrist can be found liable for a failure to inspect lenses dispensed to patients, particularly orders for safety glasses.

A young man purchased what were allegedly safety glasses from an optical shop at a naval base exchange but was severely injured when a screw driver flipped up and struck a lens, shattering it and driving glass into his eye. He filed suit, alleging failure to provide lenses pursuant to his request (safety glasses) and failure to inspect the lenses to ensure they were correct. The lenses ordered for him were not safety glasses and they had not been inspected as required. The case was settled for $41,000.[37]

The responsibility for inspection rests with the ophthalmic dispenser, and every optometrist should institute a careful in-office verification procedure for all lens orders.

Under prevailing product liability law, optometric clinicians must be safety conscious at all stages of the optometric service:

- In the determination of the appropriate lens material
- In checking the lens order for correctness
- In inspecting the fabricated lens to ensure that it complies with ANSI standards
- In warning patients of the impact-resistance of lens materials
- In educating patients concerning the proper use and care of lenses and frames

Product Liability and Contact Lenses

Although the legal responsibility of optometrists for the fitting and dispensing of contact lenses is discussed in Chapter 30, product liability as it applies to contact lenses will be addressed here briefly.

Despite the formulation of ophthalmic standards that are applicable to contact lenses (through ANSI), there is no ready means of establishing the responsibility of doctors for contact lens injuries under product liability theory. Consequently, there have been few instances in which product liability has been at issue, even though the legal risks of prescribing contact lenses have often been described.[38] Although the defective character of spectacle lenses has been clearly established in product liability cases, a different result has been reached in the courts with regard to the defective nature of contact lenses. There has been but one reported case, involving hard contact lenses, and it held that the lenses could not be subjected to product liability theory.[39]

A patient who was fitted for hard contact lenses by an optometrist employed by an optical chain suffered pain and discomfort and, after sixteen months of wear, permanent corneal scarring. He sued under product liability law, alleging that the lenses were improperly fitted, that he had been given improper instructions for their use, and that they had caused the injury to his eyes. The jury found in his favor and awarded him $10,000 in damages. The case was appealed to the Texas Supreme Court, which held that the doctrine of strict liability would not be extended to include the fitting of contact lenses by optometrists since "a professional relationship is present in the fact that contact lenses are prescribed and fitted by a licensed optometrist after examination of the eyes and in the exercise of his judgment." The court maintained that the lenses were never a finished product offered to the public in regular channels of trade and that, because they required modification, were not of themselves a defective product. The decision of the trial court was reversed.[40]

There have been no precedent-setting cases testing the application of product liability law to soft or extended wear contact lenses. Therefore, we must await the judgment of the courts as to how the law will regard these ubiquitous products of optometric practice.

Guarantees and Warranties

It is generally held that a doctor is not a warrantor of cures or a guarantor of certain results,[41] and it has long been a tenet of the law of medical malpractice that a doctor will not be held liable merely because a poor result follows his efforts.[42] But if a doctor makes a guarantee of results, then he will be held to the guarantee.[43]

A little league baseball player fitted with glasses by an optometrist was hit in the eye with a ball. His glasses shattered and he developed a substantial vision loss as a result of the lacerations. His parents sued for damages, claiming they were told by the optometrist that the glasses were unbreakable. This was found to be in the nature of a guarantee, and the optometrist was held liable for the child's vision loss.[44]

A physically active young man sought the services of an optometrist, who performed an examination and prescribed standard, heat-treated dress glass lenses. While on a hunting trip the young man tripped and fell, and his head struck the ground. One of the prescription lenses shattered as a result of the impact and severely lacerated his eye. Although he sought treatment immediately, he suffered a series of complications and ultimately lost the use of the eye. He sued the optometrist who had performed the examination and the optical laboratory that had fabricated and heat-treated the lenses, alleging that the lenses were an unsafe product and that the optometrist had told him that the lenses were shatterproof. The jury found that the optometrist's remarks constituted a guarantee and awarded the young man $90,000 in damages.[45]

Guarantees can be established by the words of assistants or employees of the doctor as well as by the doctor himself. Careful instruction and supervision of office personnel is necessary to avoid ill-chosen remarks.

Warranties are promises that some proposition or fact is true.[46] There are two basic kinds of warranties that could have applicability for optometrists: *express* warranties are those that are explicitly and aptly stated by a seller to a buyer, whereas *implied* warranties are those that are derived by implication or inference from the nature of a transaction or the circumstances of the parties. Under those circumstances where the courts have held that the purchase of glasses or contact lenses is a sale of goods, the transaction is one that involves either express or implied warranties.[47] Such a result is more likely with side-by-side or independent dispensaries.[48]

Express warranties are created by an affirmation of fact ("these lenses are plastic"), any description of the product ("these are Hydrocurve contact lenses"), or any use of a model ("these are the frames that will be ordered for you"). Any stated fact that relates to the glasses or contact lenses is an express warranty; any description of the glasses or contact lenses is an express warranty that they will be as described; any sample creates an express warranty that the glasses or contact lenses will conform to the sample. An optometrist may be held legally accountable for any express warranties he (or those employed by him) might make.

Implied warranties do not require a spoken or written statement in order to exist; rather, they arise out of implication or inference.[49] There are two important implied warranties that can be inferred from the sale of ophthalmic goods: those of merchantability and of fitness for a particular purpose.[50]

A warranty of merchantability only exists for merchants who deal in the kind of goods being sold; an optical dispensary that sells glasses or contact lenses to a patient could qualify, including side-by-side dispensaries or other independent business arrangements in which the sale of ophthalmic goods occurs independent of the optometrist. Only when the transaction involves glasses or contact lenses is it of the type that could cause the warranty to come into play. To be merchantable, the glasses or contact lenses must "pass without objection" and be fit for the ordinary purpose for which they were intended.[51]

The second implied warranty, that of fitness for a particular purpose, also has potential applicability to optometrists who have commercial or side-by-side dispensaries in which ophthalmic goods are dispensed. The basic requirements for such a warranty are that the dispenser be aware of the purpose for which the glasses or contact lenses will be used and that the patient rely on the dispenser's superior knowledge and skill in their selection.[52] Under an implied warranty of fitness for a particular purpose, the dispenser—by selecting the glasses or contact lenses for the patient—guarantees that his selection will be suitable for the patient's needs, even if nothing to this effect is said. The following case will illustrate how liability may be imposed.[53]

A woman obtained an eye examination from an optometrist who worked for a department store. She relied on the optometrist's skill and judgment in determining the correct prescription and style of glasses for her needs. Two months later, while wearing the glasses, she fell down the steps of her home and was injured. She sued the optometrist and his employer, the department store, alleging that the improper fit of the glasses had caused her to be unable to gauge the distance of the steps at her home and had caused her injury. She further alleged that there was an implied warranty that the glasses should be fit for the purpose for which they had been purchased, i.e., to walk around her house. The court found in her favor against both the optometrist and his employer on the basis of implied warranty.[54]

Efforts to apply warranty theory to the sale and fitting of contact lenses have thus far been unsuccessful.[55]

A man who was fitted for hard contact lenses by an optometrist-employee of a large optical chain attempted to wear the lenses for sixteen months without success. At the end of this time he gave up on the lenses and sought the services of another practitioner, who found his corneas to be permanently scarred and who attributed the scars to the poor fit of the lenses. He thereupon sued the optical chain, alleging breach of the warranty of fitness for a particular purpose. The trial court found in his favor and awarded him $10,000, but the case was appealed by the optical chain to the state supreme court, which held that, since hard contact lenses were not products sold through ordinary channels of trade and since professional judgment was required for their fitting, warranty theory would be inapplicable. The decision of the trial court was reversed and a judgment was entered in favor of the optical chain.[56]

There have been no reported cases establishing the applicability of warranty theory to soft contact lenses fitted or dispensed by optometrists.

Notes

1. Personal use items include contact lenses, sunlamps, pencils, eyeglasses, hair brushes, and similar products. They accounted for 15 percent of eye injuries. National Society to Prevent Blindness, *Vision Problems in the United States*, New York, 1980.
2. See Davis, J.K., A Polycarbonate Ophthalmic-Prescription Lens Series, *American Journal of Optometry and Physiological Optics*, vol. 55, no. 8, 1978, pp. 543–552; Silberstein, I.W., The Fracture Resistance of Industrially Damaged Safety Glass Lenses, Plano and Prescription—An Expanded Study, *American Journal of Optometry and Archives of American Academy of Optometry*, vol. 41, no. 4, 1964, pp. 199–221; Peters, H.B., The Fracture Resistance of Industrially Damaged Safety Glass Lenses, *American Journal of Optometry and Archives of American Academy of Optometry*, vol. 39, no. 1, 1962, pp. 33–35; Duckworth, W.H., et al., Basic Principles of Lens Fracture Testing, *American Journal of Optometry and Physiological Optics*, vol. 55, no. 11, 1978, pp. 751–759; Kors, K., and R. St. Helen, Base Line Fracture Resistance Studies of Tempered and Non-tempered Glass Ophthalmic Lenses, *American Journal of Optometry and Archives of American Academy of Optometry*, vol. 50, no. 8, 1973, p. 632–640; Robson, P.M., Ophthalmic Lens Study: Impact Resistance of Chemically Tempered and Thermally Tempered Lenses, *Corning Glass Works Report M-185*, 1975; Chase, G.A., R.P. Krause, and T.R. Kozlowski, Chemical Strengthening of Ophthalmic Lenses, *American Journal of Optometry and Archives of American Academy of Optometry*, vol. 50, no. 6, 1973, pp. 470–476; Scaief, A.L., An Alternative to the Drop Ball Test for the Measurement of Ophthalmic Glass Fracture Resistance, *American Journal of Optometry and Physiological Optics*, vol. 52, no. 11, 1975, pp. 765–773; and Duckworth, W.H., et al., Strength of Thin Chemtempered Lenses: Drop-Ball Testing, *American Journal of Optometry and Physiological Optics*, vol. 55, no. 12, 1978, pp. 801–806.
3. The adoption of the previously voluntary Z 80.1 standards by the federal government was not greeted with enthusiasm by the ophthalmic industry. For a sample opinion, see Marks, R., Z 80.1 Standards—Can They Be Met?, *Optometric Weekly*, vol. 67, no. 46, Nov. 11, 1976, p. 1238.
4. *Newgent v. Toler*, reported in 21 *ATLA Law Reporter* 113, 1978.
5. In the opinion of the author, the selection of polycarbonate is not mandatory for each and every patient but rather is to be considered the lens material of choice in those cases in which impact-resistance is an overriding clinical concern. Sample situations in which impact-resistance is the paramount consideration include prescribing eyewear to be used as safety glasses, dispensing frames and lenses to be worn during athletic competition, selecting spectacles and lenses for children who are physically active, and recommending eye protection

for monocular patients. For an example rationale, see Classe, J., Legal Aspects of Prescribing for Athletes and Sportsmen, *Journal of the American Optometric Association*, vol. 58, no. 8, 1987, pp. 674–679.

6. Based on a personal communication with the author.
7. See Classe, J., and J. Scholles, Liability for Ophthalmic Materials, *Journal of the American Optometric Association*, vol. 57, no. 6, 1986, pp. 470–477.
8. Ibid. If an optometrist specifies the type of lens material to be used, the ophthalmic dispenser must comply with the written prescription or obtain the permission of the doctor before any changes can be made. Failure to fill the prescription as written will create liability for the ophthalmic dispenser if the change is the cause of the patient's injury (e.g., failure to dispense polycarbonate as prescribed leads to patient injury when the substitute lens is shattered by an impact that the polycarbonate lens would have withstood). In offices or dispensaries where ophthalmic technicians or opticians are engaged in dispensing services, employers should be certain to instruct these individuals as to the proper documentation of warnings and communications with patients who have no ophthalmic material specified on their spectacle prescriptions.
9. The judgment was reversed on appeal, with the court ruling that the manufacturer of the spectacles had no duty to warn the worker since the spectacles had been sold to a "sophisticated user of protective eyewear," the worker's employer. See *Rusin v. Glendale Optical Co., Inc.*, 805 F.2d 650 (6th Cir. 1986). This type of defense will not be available to optometrists who dispense eyewear directly to patients.
10. There are several cases in which the plaintiff's allegations involved the dispenser's failure to warn that the lenses were not shatterproof. See *Hayes v. Hamberg*, reported in 14 *ATLA News Letter* 372, 1971; *Corey v. Robinson*, reported in 19 *ATLA News Letter* 245, 1976; and *Weidenhamer v. International Harvester, et al*, reported in 20 *ATLA Law Reporter* 18, 1977. In each of these cases the plaintiff received a substantial award.
11. For commentary on the necessity for verification of ophthalmic lens orders, see Kirschen, M., Verifying Impact Resistance, *Optometric Management*, vol. 13, no. 9, 1977, pp. 55–59.
12. Reported in the *AOA News*, June 15, 1976.
13. *Walstrom Optical Co. v. Miller*, 59 S.W. 2d 895 (Tex. Civ. App. 1933).
14. For a review of the requirements for safety glasses, see Sherr, A.E., Industrial Safety Glasses—An Update, *Journal of the American Optometric Association*, vol. 51, no. 2, 1980, pp. 129–137.
15. Reported by Lynch, B.E., Are You Safe On Safety Glasses?, *Optometric Management*, vol. 2, no. 2, 1984, pp. 58–61.
16. For a discussion of ocular injuries in sports, see Vinger, P. (ed.), Ocular Sports Injuries, *International Ophthalmology Clinics*, vol. 21, no. 4, 1981.
17. For a review of the problems of providing vision care to athletes who participate in racquet sports, see Easterbrook, M., Eye Injuries in Racquet Sports, in Vinger, supra note 16.
18. See Kapan, P.J., Legal Aspects: Patient's Perspective, in Vinger, supra note 16.
19. Athletic eyewear dispensed by optometrists should meet or exceed the standards established by the American Society for Testing and Materials (ASTM), which include:

ASTM F910	Qualifications for faceguards in youth baseball
ASTM F803	Eye protection for use by players of racket sports
ASTM F659	Specifications for eye protective devices (alpine skiers)
ASTM F513	Eye and face protective equipment for hockey players

A copy of these standards may be obtained by writing ASTM, 1916 Race St., Philadelphia, PA 19103.

20. *Soutee v. Pro-Tec, Inc.*, reported in 25 *ATLA Law Reporter* 375, 1982.
21. The inclusion of the AOA among the committee's members was not only because optometrists were involved in the fabrication and dispensing of ophthalmic lenses but also because optometrists—through the AOA—had already set up a committee on standards (1945) and had promulgated standards to be used throughout the profession (1952). See Sherr, supra note 14.
22. See 21 U.S.C. §§351–360k.
23. A copy of the ANSI standards may be purchased from the American National Standards Institute, 1430 Broadway, New York, N.Y. 10018
24. See Sherr, supra note 14.
25. For a review of product liability theory as it applies to eyeglasses, see Classe, J., Eyeglasses as the Basis of a Products Case, *Alabama Trial Lawyers Journal*, vol. 6, no. 4, July/Aug./Sept. 1978, pp. 14–17.
26. The Z 80.1-1972 standards specified a minimum center thickness for dress lenses as the criterion for impact resistance. Lenses that were less than two millimeters thick were not in compliance with the standard and were the subject of several product liability cases. See *Filler v. Rayex Corp.*, 435 F.2d 336 (7th Cir. 1970). Because of the increased impact resistance of chemical tempering for glass lenses, the 2-mm center thickness was dropped in the 1979 version of ANSI Z 80.1, and the drop-ball test became the standard. The drop-ball test continues to be the appropriate standard, even after Z 80.1 was revised in 1987.
27. *Kopp v. C.C. Caldwell Optical Co.*, 547 S.W.2d 872 (Mo. App. 1977).
28. *Hayes v. Hamberg*, reported in 14 *ATLA News Letter* 372, 1971.
29. *Filler v. Rayex Corp.*, 435 F.2d 336 (7th Cir. 1970).
30. Reported by Marks, R., Product Liability: The New Malpractice Menace, *Optometric Management*, vol. 13, no. 1, 1977, pp. 26–27.
31. See Silberstein, I.W., The Fracture Resistance of Industrially Damaged Safety Glass Lenses, Plano and Pre-

scription—An Expanded Study, *American Journal of Optometry and Archives of American Academy of Optometry*, vol. 41, no. 4, 1964, pp. 199–221.

32. A 1976 study by the Optical Wholesalers Association tested the ability of thirty laboratories across the United States to fabricate ten glass and five plastic prescriptions in accordance with the ANSI Z 80.1-1972 standards. Only 54 percent were found to be in compliance. Reported by Marks, R., supra note 30.
33. See Kirschen, M., supra note 11.
34. *Corey v. Robinson*, reported in 19 *ATLA News Letter* 245, 1976.
35. *American Optical Co. v. Weidenhamer*, 404 N.E.2d 606 (Ind. App. 1980).
36. Unfortunately, there are some circumstances under which an optometrist may not be able to verify ophthalmic materials ordered through a plant or industrial safety glass program. Such a result occurs when the patient-employee must send the prescription to an ophthalmic dispenser to obtain the glasses, and the glasses are then mailed directly to the employee. Optometrists should endeavor to acquaint supervisors, managers, or others in authority with the importance of prescription verification.
37. *Westerman v. State Optical Co., Ltd.*, reported in 15 *ATLA News Letter* 458, 1972.
38. See Elmstrom, G., The Risks You Run with Contacts, *Optometric Management*, vol. 2, no. 6, 1965, pp. 7–9; Ullen, R., Legal Implications in Fitting Contact Lenses, *Journal of the American Optometric Association*, vol. 32, no. 11, 1961, pp. 288–291; Simmons, E.F., *Synopsis of Jurisprudence for Optometrists*, Burgess Publishing Co., Minneapolis, 1963; Elmstrom, G., and H. Kohn, *Legal Aspects of Contact Lens Practice*, Burgess Publishing Co., Minneapolis, 1964; Feld, L.P., The Optometrist and Contact Lenses: Legal Liability Without Fault!, *Optical Journal and Review of Optometry*, vol. 107, no. 9, 1970, pp. 32–35; and Lane, M.J., The Legal Risks You Run Prescribing Contacts, *Optometric Management*, vol. 13, no. 3, 1977, pp. 53–61.
39. For a report on the case, see Texas Appeals Court Reverses Jury Award in Contact Lens Case—Conflicting Views on Theory of Implied Warranty, *Optical Journal and Review of Optometry*, vol. 104, no. 8, 1967, pp. 49–50.
40. *Barbee v. Rogers*, 425 S.W.2d 342 (Tex. 1968).
41. *Custodio v. Bauer*, 251 Cal. App. 2d 303, 59 Cal. Rptr. 463, 470 (1967).
42. See *Staloch v. Holm*, 111 N.W. 264 (Minn. 1907); *Lane v. Calvert*, 138 A.2d 902 (Md. 1958); and *Teig v. St. John's Hospital*, 387 P.2d 527 (Wash. 1963).
43. *Bailey v. Harmon*, 74 Colo. 390, 222 P. 393 (1924); *Hawkins v. McGee*, 84 N.H. 114, 146 A. 641 (1929); *Seanor v. Browne*, 154 Okla. 222, 7 P.2d 627 (1932); *Robins v. Finestone*, 308 N.Y. 543, 127 N.E.2d 330 (1955); *Noel v. Proud*, 189 Kan. 6, 367 P.2d 61 (1961); *Camposano v. Claiborn*, 2 Conn. Cir. 135, 196 A.2d 129 (1963); *Sullivan v. O'Connor*, 363 Mass. 579, 296 N.E.2d 183 (1973); *Cirafici v. Goffen*, 85 Ill. App. 3d 1102, 407 N.E.2d 633, 637 (1980); and *Scarzella v. Saxon*, 436 A.2d 358 (D.C. App. 1984).
44. Reported in the *AOA News*, June 15, 1976.
45. Based on a personal communication with the author.
46. For a discussion of warranty, see Prosser, W.L., *Law of Torts*, 4th ed., West, St. Paul, Minn., 1971, pp. 650–656. For a review of cases involving breach of warranty by physicians, see Lane, B.J., and H. Hirsh, The Broken Promise: Physician's Breach of Warranty, *Case and Comment*, Sept.–Oct. 1984, pp. 3–14.
47. In general, the courts have rejected the notion that medical services give rise to the statutory warranties of the Uniform Commercial Code. See *Carroll v. Grabavoy*, 77 Ill. App. 3d 895, 396 N.E.2d 836 (1979), in which the court held that dentures were not goods within the meaning of the Uniform Commercial Code. Although there is a case in which the court held that the sale of eyeglasses by an optometrist created an implied warranty of fitness, *Gilbert v. Louis Pizitz Dry Goods Co.*, 237 Ala. 249, 186 So. 179 (1939), it was decided before the adoption of the Uniform Commercial Code. Under UCC §2-313, express warranties may be created by any affirmation of fact, a description of the goods, and any sample or model.
48. If eyeglasses are sold by an optical shop, upon the written prescription of an optometrist or physician, then the likelihood is much greater that a sale of goods under the Uniform Commercial Code will have been effected. Similarly, the purchase of over-the-counter (ready-made) eyewear from a drug store or a department store will lead to the creation of warranties as a result of the sale of goods by the merchant.
49. See *Vaughn v. Shelton*, 514 S.W.2d 870 (Tenn. App. 1974).
50. See Uniform Commercial Code (UCC) §2-314(b). Where a seller deals in goods of a particular kind, and a buyer relies upon the seller's judgment to select goods that are appropriate for the particular purpose described, then there is an implied warranty that they will be fit for the intended purpose. In order to be merchantable, goods must be at least such as will pass without objection in the trade or be fit for the ordinary purpose for which they will be used.
51. Ibid.
52. Ibid.
53. It should be pointed out that this case, which is used for purposes of illustration, was decided before the creation of the Uniform Commercial Code, and so it will be each individual state court's interpretation of the state UCC provisions that will determine whether a cause of action may be stated on the basis of a sale of eyeglasses.
54. *Gilbert v. Louis Pizitz Dry Goods Co.*, 237 Ala. 249, 186 So. 179 (1939).
55. A discussion of the application of implied warranty to contact lens sales may be found in Texas Appeals Court Reverses Jury Award in Contact Lens Case—Conflicting Views on Theory of Implied Warranty, *Optical Journal and Review of Optometry*, vol. 104, no. 8, 1967, pp. 49–50.
56. *Barbee v. Rogers*, 425 S.W.2d 342 (Tex. 1968).

Chapter 28

Liability for Ophthalmic Pharmaceutical Agents

A young man had an acutely inflamed throat. He went to his doctor, who gave him an injection of penicillin. The sore throat quickly got better.

Three days later, the young man began to itch. The itching got worse and he developed hives all over his body. The doctor made the correct diagnosis of an allergic reaction to penicillin. He prescribed antihistamines. The hives disappeared.

The young man, a machine operator, got drowsy from the antihistamines and cut his hand at work. The nurse in the dispensary gave him first aid and put on an antibacterial ointment containing penicillin. The hives returned and now the young man had swelling of the eyes and lips. The doctor recognized that a potentially dangerous allergic reaction was present; he ordered a course of corticosteroid treatment. Result—the itchiness, the hives, and the swellings disappeared, and the patient was well again.

Except that now he had pain in his belly plus heartburn, and he began to show signs of blood in his stools. The correct diagnosis of a peptic ulcer (induced by the corticosteroid) was made. The young man did not do well on medical treatment; he continued to bleed from his ulcer. His doctor, therefore, had a surgeon in consultation. The two doctors agreed that partial gastrectomy was necessary, an operation to remove the ulcer-bearing portion of the stomach. The operation was successful.

But because of the previous bleeding and the unavoidable blood loss at the operation, a transfusion of 1,000 milliliters (two pints) of blood was given. Hepatitis (inflammation of the liver) followed. The young man became intensely jaundiced; he vomited his food and had to be fed intravenously for a few days. His youth did him in good stead. He recovered from his hepatitis.

At the right ankle, where the intravenous needle and the plastic tube had been inserted into a vein exposed by cutting through the skin, a tender nodule appeared. It became red and inflamed, evidence of infection. Because of the bad experience the patient had had with penicillin, the doctor prescribed tetracycline. The inflammation promptly subsided.

Because of the antibiotic, diarrhea came on and the patient had severe colicky cramps. The doctor ordered a special diet and gave a new synthetic antispasmodic drug to control the cramps. The diarrhea stopped.

The new drug was in the belladonna class. It relaxed smooth muscle all over the body, and by its action on the iris, it caused dilation of the pupil.

The young man's vision was impaired. He drove his car into a tree. Exitus young man.

—Douglas Mackintosh, *Systems of Health Care*

The Standard of Care
Misuse of Diagnostic Drugs
Misuse of Therapeutic Drugs
Documentation
Use of Standing Orders

The evolution of ophthalmic drug use by optometrists has a relatively brief history, beginning in 1971 with the amendment of the Rhode Island Optometry Practice Act. As of 1988, forty-eight states and the District of Columbia authorize the use of ophthalmic pharmaceutical agents by optometrists, with twenty states specifically authorizing the use of these agents for therapeutic purposes.[1]

Although the drug amendments engendered a remarkable amount of political activity, they have been enacted at a faster rate than the original optometry practice acts that recognized the legal right of optometrists to pursue their calling.[2] Despite the negative pronouncements by some ophthalmologists concerning the use of ophthalmic pharmaceutical agents by optometrists, there have been no reported cases[3] alleging improper use by optometric clinicians of drugs for diagnostic or therapeutic purposes, and so the liability of optometrists for ophthalmic pharmaceutical use is legally untested. As a consequence, we must turn to the experiences of ophthalmologists in order to find legal precedent and case reports illustrating potential liability for the clinical use of these drugs.

In fact, optometric liability for large malpractice claims continues to be associated with misdiagnosis, with the overwhelming number of allegations involving *failure* to use ophthalmic drugs for diagnostic purposes, as a consequence of which ocular pathology goes undetected and untreated. Therefore, in terms of current optometric liability, an optometrist is far more likely to become embroiled in a legal dispute for failure to use an ophthalmic pharmaceutical agent (or to refer the patient to a practitioner who will use the appropriate agent) than for misuse of a drug. Nevertheless, liability can result from the misuse of ophthalmic drugs, as our colleagues in ophthalmology have demonstrated, and it is important for optometrists to be aware of the legal issues that drugs bring to clinical practice.

This chapter will describe the standard of care to be applied to an optometrist employing ophthalmic pharmaceuticals (including the doctrine of informed consent, which can be important in some cases). Then we will turn to those circumstances under which misuse of ophthalmic drugs have been alleged, utilizing cases and claims to illustrate those instances in which liability has been imposed. The chapter will conclude with a brief discussion of the documentation necessary whenever ophthalmic drugs are employed and with a description of the use of standing orders by optometrists.

The Standard of Care

An optometrist's liability for a pharmaceutical agent that has been administered or prescribed hinges upon the standard of care prevalent within the profession. As long as the optometrist uses the minimum degree of skill and learning ordinarily expected of a like practitioner under the same or similar circumstances, he will not be liable. In adhering to this standard of care, the doctor faces potential liability in five major areas:

1. The doctor is expected to understand the properties of the drugs that he administers or applies, including dangerous side effects.[4]
2. The doctor is expected to choose a drug that is suitable under the circumstances and is the proper pharmaceutical agent for the patient's condition.[5]
3. The doctor is expected to make a reasonable effort to determine if an allergic reaction will occur by making all necessary inquiries of the patient to learn if there is any evidence that would indicate the possibility of a reaction.[6]
4. The doctor is expected to warn the patient of side effects that may result from the patient's use of the drug, and the doctor is expected to comply with the doctrine of informed consent in this regard.[7]
5. The doctor is expected to monitor the patient adequately while the patient is taking a drug or under its effects and is expected to be able to manage any adverse side effects suffered by the patient as a result of the drug (or to refer the patient as necessary).[8]

Although these obligations emphasize knowledge and clinical skill, there is another legal requirement that influences the standard of care to be applied in these cases, and the source of this requirement can be found in the legal relationship that exists between an optometrist and his patients.

The nature of the doctor-patient relationship is such that the law places upon the doctor an affirmative duty of disclosure in order that the less knowledgeable patient may make an intelligent and informed decision as to whether he or she wishes to undergo the prescribed treatment. This legal requirement has given rise to the doctrine of informed consent, which makes it mandatory that the doctor explain to the patient the hazards, possible complications, and both the expected and unexpected results of standard treatment (see Chapter 22 for a discussion of informed consent in clinical practice). Thus the patient must understand the nature of the proposed treatment as well as its inherent risks. Without this understanding, the consent obtained by the doctor—even the patient's signature on a consent form—will probably be legally invalid.

Informed consent cases most often occur when the patient is generally aware of the nature of the treatment and has signed a consent form but is not aware of the risk of permanent damage inherent in the treatment. If a patient suffers an unfortunate result from the treatment (e.g., serious corneal scarring due to experimental or extended wear contact lenses), and the patient can establish that his doctor not only failed to warn him of this possible eventuality but also that a duly careful doctor would have done so, then the doctor may be sued for failing to obtain a valid consent even though no negligence is proven. How the doctor goes about the task of informing a patient is left to his individual judgment (and to the requirements of state law), but his efforts must be capable of engendering the patient's understanding. If a patient tells his doctor that he does not want to know about the risks, then the doctor has no further obligation. When drugs are being used, however, the patient often needs to be warned of side effects.

Medication prescribed by a physician (chloroquine) had serious and permanent effects on the patient's vision. The medical literature abounded with reports of the side effects of the medication, but the physician had not read any of the articles. The court found that he was negligent in failing to keep up with and be aware of new developments in the field.[9]

There are differences from state to state in the disclosure requirements necessary to comply with the doctrine of informed consent.[10] Optometrists in those states where drugs may be employed for therapeutic purposes should take the time to acquaint themselves with the minimum requirements under the law and should be careful not only to comply with legal requirements but also should document these requirements in the patient record as necessary.

In order to comply with the requirements of the doctrine of informed consent, an optometrist must be familiar with the correct utilization of therapeutic drugs and must understand both the toxic and the allergic responses to therapy. This information must be shared with the patient under some circumstances (depending on the requirements of state law) and places a burden on the optometric practitioner to understand fully both the expected and the unexpected results of therapy. We will now turn to a brief description of cases and claims in order to illustrate those circumstances under which an optometrist is most vulnerable to liability for use of ophthalmic pharmaceuticals.

Misuse of Diagnostic Drugs

Ophthalmic pharmaceutical agents have been employed by optometrists for diagnostic purposes for more than a decade, and several studies have determined the relative risk and incidence of adverse affects associated with their use. A study of more than 15,000 drug applications at six schools of optometry found no cases requiring urgent or emergency medical intervention and a low incidence of mild and transient side effects.[11] A report by the Department of Regulation and Licensing of the State of Wisconsin on the use of pharmaceutical agents for diagnostic purposes by optometrists in that state found that only 27 out of 195,842 patients who were administered these agents experienced adverse reactions and that all of these cases involved transient reactions that required no medical treatment.[12] And a study of 12,492 drug applications involving both private practitioners and a school of optometry teaching clinic found the incidence of adverse reactions to diagnostic agents to be less than .25 percent.[13] Therefore, optometric liability for the use of these drugs must be considered relatively low, assuming that the most appropriate agent is selected and that it is employed in the appropriate manner clinically. But if a drug is misused, liability can result, and the discussion that follows describes clinical situations under which this has occurred.

The most common diagnostic pharmaceutical agents used by optometrists are anesthetics, mydriatics, and cycloplegics.

Anesthetics

Anesthesia is necessary for some diagnostic tests, the most common being tonometry. There are several known adverse effects of topical anesthesia, but the risk is sufficiently small that informed consent is not necessary and negligence is not likely unless an inadequate history has been taken and an otherwise preventable adverse reaction is precipitated (i.e., application of the anesthetic despite a prior history of adverse reaction).

Repeated application of a topical anesthetic to a compromised cornea, however, can result in corneal opacity and incur liability for the doctor who has permitted this misuse of the drug.[14]

A boy was struck in the eye by the edge of a hat and suffered a corneal abrasion. He was examined by a physician, and placed in a hospital overnight for observation. The doctor prescribed a topical anesthetic (Ophthaine®) for the patient's ocular discomfort and permitted the nursing staff to leave the medication at the patient's bedside for further use as needed. A permanent corneal opacity resulted from the improper use of the anesthetic. The case was settled for $75,000.[15]

Corneal sloughing, which is the most common adverse effect experienced by patients, is transient and involves no permanent injury. Since it is an unpredictable response to the drug; there can be no liability, unless the doctor knows or should have known that an adverse response would occur.[16]

Mydriatics

If a mydriatic is to be used, a complete history should be taken prior to application to ensure that there has been no previous adverse reaction (e.g., a history of prior angle closure). It is also necessary to assess the depth of the anterior chamber angle prior to the instillation of the mydriatic. The prevalence of significantly narrow angles susceptible to closure in the general population has been estimated to be 2 to 6 percent,[17] and it has been suggested by some authors that there is a greater danger to the patient of overlooking retinal disease by failure to employ mydriasis than there is of inducing angle closure by this procedure.[18] Because the risk of angle closure is extremely remote (except in 2 to 6 percent of the population), in patients with unremarkable histories informed consent is not required.[19] A slit-lamp assessment, however, is advisable.

If it is known in advance of the appointment that the patient will undergo a dilated fundus examination, he should be advised of this fact so that appropriate transportation arrangements can be made. Reschedule appointments may be necessary in some cases so that alternative travel plans can be arranged. In all cases it is wise to ensure that patients have sunglasses to protect against glare, or to provide patients with disposable mydriatic sunglasses designed for this purpose.

A patient should be carefully monitored after a mydriatic has been applied and should be given careful instructions to follow in the event an adverse reaction occurs. The chances of the worst type of adverse reaction—an angle closure—are very small, about 1 in 45,000 in those above thirty years of age and about 1 in 180,000 for the general population.[20] Telephone requests for aid require thoughtful consideration and, on many occasions, reexamination, as the following case illustrates.

An ophthalmologist used a mydriatic during the course of his examination. Some hours after the appointment, the patient called the doctor, complaining of headache and discomfort. The physician prescribed an analgesic and rest but did not see her. The patient's condition did not improve, and so she consulted another physician the following day. She was found to have an acute angle closure. Suit was instituted against the physician who had failed to examine her.[21]

Patients may require assistance or special attention while under the effects of mydriasis, and this may necessitate careful management of the elderly, the impaired, or other persons likely to be handicapped by the drug.[22]

A 77-year-old woman who had come to an ophthalmologist's office for an examination had drops of a mydriatic (Mydriacyl®) placed in her eyes. She was not warned that the drops would affect her vision. When she was called by an assistant to be examined, she tripped and fell because her vision was so blurred. Despite the fall, the ophthalmologist conducted an examination, but she complained of stiffness in her leg and had to be taken to a hospital. She was found to have fractured her hip and required two operations and over 100 days in the hospital to repair the injury. She sued the ophthalmologist for failing to warn her of the mydriatic's effect on her vision and for leaving her unattended while under the effects of the drug. She was awarded $10,000 in compensatory damages and an additional $10,000 as punitive damages.[23]

There are circumstances under which a third party may institute a suit for damages against the doctor for failure to warn the operator of a motor vehicle of a visual impairment that causes the vehicle to injure the third party[24] (described in Chapter 32).

Cycloplegics

There will be occasions when cycloplegic refractions must be performed on certain patients. Young children, accommodative esotropes, latent hyperopes, and uncommunicative patients will be the usual cases that require cycloplegia. As with mydriasis, a history and an evaluation of the angle are necessary prior to instillation of the drug, and follow-up is a necessary aspect of proper management. The patient should be observed after the cycloplegic has been applied and the appropriate warnings should be given to minimize the risk of injury after the patient has left the office. Cycloplegics are especially toxic to children when administered in the inappropriate concentration or with the incorrect frequency.[25]

As with other diagnostic agents, the optometrist who decides not to use the drug as a necessary aspect of the patient examination may find himself in an untenable position legally.

An optometrist prescribed lenses for a young patient, but they gave him severe headaches, nausea, and a deep-seated pain in his eyes. The child's mother brought him back for reexamination, but the optometrist urged her to allow the boy to continue to wear the lenses. When the symptoms persisted, she consulted an ophthalmologist, who dilated the youngster's eyes, performed a cycloplegic refraction, and prescribed a new pair of glasses. The optometrist was thereafter sued for malpractice. At the trial the ophthalmologist testified that it was not possible to determine the correct prescription without cycloplegia and that the misprescribed glasses might retard the proper development of the child's eyes. The jury found the optometrist negligent.[26]

There are two cycloplegics that are commonly employed by optometrists: the drug of choice under most circumstances is cyclopentolate hydrochloride, but atropine sulfate is also used under limited circumstances (accommodative esotropes under four years of age).[27] The classic regimen for atropine of three drops a day for three days preceding the refraction has been modified by recent investigators to three drops on the day preceding the refraction. Using an ointment and a lower concentration of the drug are also recommended since they decrease the risk of an adverse reaction. When atropine is to be applied by parents, it is advisable for the optometrist to inform the parents of the risks and signs of atropine toxicity.

Because optometrists in many states have recently acquired the legal right to use drugs for diagnostic purposes, the tendency of practitioners in these states has been to apply them conservatively. Optometrists have been careful not to overuse these drugs, and this has proven to be in the public interest. Likewise, optometrists who employ ophthalmic pharmaceutical agents for therapeutic purposes have adopted a conservative attitude toward their use because there is risk of injury whenever therapeutic drugs are used, as numerous cases filed against ophthalmologists have shown.

Misuse of Therapeutic Drugs

The right to use drugs for therapeutic purposes has been enjoyed by optometry since 1976, when West Virginia became the first state to amend its optometry practice act to specifically declare that optometrists could utilize these agents. Following the enactment of the West Virginia law, the right of the state to permit the use of these agents by optometrists was challenged in a lawsuit filed by an ophthalmologist.[28] Ultimately, the state supreme court refused to review the trial court's determination that the use of therapeutic drugs by optometrists could be authorized by the legislature and that, therefore, the use of these drugs could lawfully be included within the definition of optometry.[29]

Since the history of optometric involvement with drugs used for therapeutic purposes is a limited one, the legal ramifications of their use must come from the experiences of ophthalmologists. Thus the case reports and statistics cited herein are based upon published cases and claims involving physicians.

A leading study involved a review of 412 claims against ophthalmologists[30] (see Table 28.1). Of

Table 28.1. Reported Malpractice Claims against Ophthalmologists

Basis for Claim	No. (and Percent) of Cases
Drug complications	58 (14)
Cataracts	53 (12.8)
Retinal detachment	51 (11.4)
Glaucoma	37 (9)
Intraocular foreign bodies and trauma	36 (8.7)
Medical retina	27 (6.5)
Retrolental fibroplasia	26 (6.3)
Intraocular infection	24 (5.8)
Intraocular lens implants	20 (4.6)
Anesthesia	20 (4.6)
Oculoplastic procedures	14 (3.2)
Motility	9 (2)
Neuroophthalmological procedures	9 (2)
Tumors	8 (1.9)
Contact lens	7 (1.7)
Preoperative antibiotics	7 (1.7)
Nasolacrimal procedure	3 (0.7)
Spectacles	2 (0.5)
Corneal transplant	1 (0.2)
Miscellaneous	29 (7)

Note: The total is more than 412 because some cases were included in more than one category.

Source: Bettman, J.W., A Review of 412 Claims in Ophthalmology, in Medicolegal Aspects of Ophthalmology, *International Ophthalmology Clinics*, Winter 1980, vol. 20, p.132.

the cases reviewed, fifty-eight involved drug complications, the leading category among all claims. (However, the author remarks that these may be disproportionate since he was a consultant for several pharmaceutical manufacturers.) The majority of the cases involved steroids, most frequently topical steroids that caused cataracts or open-angle glaucoma.

A second category of claims involved glaucoma therapy, particularly miotics that caused retinal detachment and carbonic anhydrase inhibitors associated with complications.

Another important cause of claims cited in the study concerned misdiagnosis, followed by the inappropriate therapeutic regimen. This may be the type of claim to which optometrists are most vulnerable. The jump from diagnosis to therapeusis is a significant one legally and offers an increased opportunity for litigation, even though it is arguable that drugs used for diagnostic purposes are more toxic and potentially more harmful than are drugs used for therapeutic purposes.[31] The reason for this increased risk is that therapeusis presupposes a correct diagnosis. It is uniformly agreed that the decision making necessary to reach a diagnosis is a more difficult undertaking than is the decision making required to initiate treatment. Therefore, failure to make a correct diagnosis is a more likely eventuality than is inappropriate management of a correctly diagnosed condition.

These three major categories of therapeutic drug litigation will be discussed in the following sections.[32]

Corticosteroids

The majority of cases reviewed in the study involved the use of steroids, most frequently topical steroids that caused cataracts or open-angle glaucoma.[33] The underlying cause of these lawsuits was that the prescribed steroids were used for a period sufficient to cause these complications. Claims typically allege negligence on the part of the doctor in prescribing or permitting the long-term use of the steroids and in failing to inform the patient of the adverse effects of such usage.

A hairdresser was allergic to dyes used in her work and consulted an ophthalmologist, who prescribed topical corticosteroids. This treatment alleviated her symptoms and was continued for almost two years, after which time it was found that she had bilateral cataracts, glaucomatous optic cups, and restricted visual fields. The patient sued, claiming that she should not have been permitted to use the corticosteroids for such a long period and that she had not been informed of the possible complications of cataract and glaucoma as a result of long-term steroid therapy.[34]

Many of these cases concern how or why the patient was able to obtain so many refills. In some cases, the receptionist was found to have given a verbal order to refill without consulting the doctor; in others, the pharmacist refilled the prescription under the claim of a telephone order; in still others the patient was found to have lied to the pharmacist about the doctor's orders for refills. In order to avoid this problem, it is advisable to have the following printed on prescription blanks, "The above instructions regarding refills may not be altered" and to retain a copy of the prescription in the patient's record.[35]

With all drugs, and especially the corticosteroids, the doctor should have reason to believe that their use is necessary and that the route of administration is appropriate. Systemic administration with the risk of systemic complications should not be used if a topical administration will suffice.

An obese 35-year-old man with a history of questionable diabetes was found to have a moderate uveitis in one eye. He was placed on systemic steroids (prednisone), and after three days the uveitis was improved, and so the steroids were continued. Seven days later the uveitis was cured, but the patient complained of increased thirst and urination and the steroids were tapered off. Within three days the patient developed severe polydipsia and polyuria and became comatose. He was hospitalized, but in spite of all efforts, he died. Suit was instituted for wrongful death, with one allegation being that topical rather than systemic steroids should have been prescribed.[36]

An optometrist should be familiar with the contents of the package insert (or its duplicate in the *Physician's Desk Reference*). The package insert is considered to be a part of the drug by the Food and Drug Administration, and it can be introduced into evidence at trial, allowing the defendant doctor to be questioned closely concerning its contents.[37]

A patient with mild iritis, mild diabetes, and hypertension was given both topical and systemic steroids for the iritis. She developed acute pancreatitis and died. There was nothing in the history to indicate that topical administration, in itself, might not have sufficed. Furthermore, acute pancreatitis was a known complication of systemic steroids. A suit was filed against the doctor and settled in the patient's favor.[38]

Many of the larger claims involving drug complications are due to the systemic administration of a therapeutic agent. Topical administration should always be considered first.

Antiglaucoma Agents

The cases involving glaucoma therapy fell into two general categories, those in which retinal detachment followed the initiation of miotic therapy and those in which carbonic anhydrase inhibitors were utilized without clear justification.

In several cases retinal detachment occurred shortly after the use of a miotic or after an increase in the strength of the miotic being administered.

A five diopter myope was examined by an ophthalmologist and diagnosed as having open-angle glaucoma, for which 2 percent pilocarpine was prescribed. Eight days later he was found to have a rhegmatogenous retinal detachment in one eye. Although the retina was reattached, there was a permanent loss of acuity because the macula was involved. The patient sued, claiming that nonmiotic antiglaucoma drugs should have been employed since the risk of detachment was significant for him.[39]

It is important to perform a dilated fundus examination prior to the initiation of antiglaucoma therapy. Patients who are at risk for retinal detachment because of high myopia, lattice degeneration, a prior history of detachment, or other predisposing factors should either be treated without miotics or should be warned of the possibility of complications so that an informed consent can be obtained. Such patients should also be given periodic and careful follow-up and should be taught the signs and symptoms of retinal detachment so that they can obtain immediate care if detachment occurs.

Carbonic anhydrase inhibitors have known side effects, and so the use of such a drug must be clearly necessary in order to avoid legal complications.[40]

A patient with bilateral glaucoma was treated with the usual topical glaucoma medications and with a carbonic anhydrase inhibitor, acetazolamide (Diamox®). The pressure was well controlled, but after prolonged therapy the patient developed kidney stones that had to be removed surgically. After the operation, the IOP was adequately controlled without the Diamox®. A lawsuit was initiated, with the key question being, "Was the carbonic anhydrase inhibitor necessary?"[41]

The optometrist should always carefully consider whether a lower dose of a drug would be sufficient, particularly if the recommended dosage in the package insert is to be exceeded. The package insert is there to guide the doctor. Unlike the manufacturing pharmaceutical company, the optometrist is not legally bound to follow its directions. There are times when good judgment indicates that the instructions not be followed exactly as worded or that the recommended dosage be exceeded, but the doctor who deviates from the instructions should be within the standard of care when doing so. It would be wise to document in the patient's record why the benefit-to-risk ratio indicated that a deviation from the recommended indication or dosage be made.

Misdiagnosis

One of the best opportunities for misuse of therapeutic drugs occurs in conjunction with misdiagnosis. The wrong therapeutic regimen is initiated because the doctor misinterprets the cause of the patient's eye problem. In these circumstances, a lawsuit for large damages is a distinct possibility.

A woman suffering from extreme eye pain, blurred vision, vomiting, and nausea went to the emergency room of a hospital and was examined by an intern, who was unable to see the fundus due to corneal edema. He consulted an ophthalmological resident by telephone, and the resident diagnosed conjunctivitis, prescribed an antibiotic, and told the intern to release the patient. Consequently, the patient was not examined by an ophthalmologist for two weeks, at which time her condition was diagnosed as acute angle-closure glaucoma. Despite nine surgeries, the patient lost vision in both eyes. In addition, she developed diabetes due to prednisolone reaction. The case was settled for $2.1 million.[42]

Another typical example of this type of case involves steroid therapy. An optometrist can encounter legal difficulty if steroids are prescribed when an ocular injury is due to organic material.

A patient who had been struck in the eye by a tree branch while horseback riding consulted an ophthalmologist for the resulting corneoscleral abrasion and laceration. The physician prescribed a topical antibiotic and corticosteroid and patched the eye. He examined the eye two days later, at which time it seemed better, and so the regimen was continued. Several days later, however, a gray infiltrate was observed, and subsequently a fungal corneal ulcer was diagnosed. Although the condition was cured after the appropriate therapy was initiated, a corneal scar remained that reduced the patient's acuity to 20/60. Suit was instituted, alleging misdiagnosis.[43]

The best defense against misdiagnosis is to adhere to the standard of care when assessing ocular disease or injury. If referral is indicated under the circumstances of the case, then it should be obtained without delay and appropriately documented in the patient record.

In summary, an optometrist should know the indications, precautions, warnings, and possible contraindications of any drug that is to be prescribed. If the recommendations regarding dosage or method of administration as indicated in the package insert are not to be followed, the doctor should be certain that such a regimen can be justified.[44]

Five other points that should be observed[45]:

- Be careful regarding refills and instruct all office personnel in this regard.
- If a drug might produce complications (such as a steroid) have the patient make a definite appointment for a follow-up visit.
- Contact the patient if such a follow-up appointment is not kept.
- Do not use a drug systemically if topical application will suffice; weigh the risks and benefits of systemic medication in each case; always use the route of administration in which the probability of benefit is great and the possibility of risk is low.
- Communicate with the patient; weigh the benefit-to-risk ratio of a given drug in open discussion with the patient.

Documentation

A key aspect of pharmaceutical use is adequate documentation in the patient record. It is essential to maintain a timely and accurate record of the following information:

- History of drug use, including those drugs taken for prolonged periods
- Current medications being taken and history of allergies
- Previous adverse reactions to any drugs, especially ophthalmic drugs
- Identification of the drug being used or prescribed, including concentration and dosage and appropriate information as to refills (see Fig. 28.1)
- Signs and symptoms of an adverse reaction to any drug administered or prescribed
- Required warnings to patients as to the possible side effects of drug use and of action to take in the event of an adverse reaction
- Management of the patient in the event there is an adverse reaction

Proper recordkeeping is of vital importance in the event there is litigation.

____________________ **O.D.**

Name of patient: ____________________

Address: ____________________

Rx: ____________________

Drug: __________ **Dose:** __________

Quantity: ____________________

Sig: ____________________

Label contents

☐ **May not be refilled**

☐ **May be refilled** __________ **times**

The above instructions regarding refills may not be changed.

____________________ **O.D.**

License Number ____________________

Figure 28.1. Sample Form for Drug Prescriptions. (After Bettman, J.W. A Review of 412 Claims in Ophthalmology, in Medicolegal Aspects of Ophthalmology, *International Ophthalmology Clinics*, Winter 1980; 20:133.)

Use of Standing Orders

In states where the optometry practice act does not permit using ophthalmic pharmaceutical agents for therapeutic purposes, or where the language permitting such drug use is limited, it may nevertheless be possible for optometrists to manage cases requiring the use of therapeutic agents, through the formulation of standing orders.

It has long been a standard practice in medicine for physicians to delegate certain responsibilities related to patient care to other health-care providers.[46] Perhaps the leading example of this practice can be found in hospitals, where a wide range of responsibilites—including the dispensing of therapeutic pharmaceutical agents—are routinely delegated to nurses. Another example, in which a less structured form of supervision is typically present, involves physicians' assistants and nurse practitioners. Although the use of standing orders by optometrists is a relatively recent phenomenon, standing orders have been utilized for years in hospitals, multidisciplinary clinics, and educational settings such as schools of optometry.

Standing orders may be employed by optometrists and physicians who wish to work in consultation through agreed upon protocols for the management of certain types of cases. The advantages of this type of arrangement are many: patients are spared the cost and inconvenience of travel, lost workdays, and extra office visits when physicians are not readily accessible; physicians who may not have the specialized equipment commonly possessed by optometrists or who may practice only in urban areas far removed from a sizeable portion of the patient population are still able to participate in patient care; and optometrists are able to contribute to the management of patients who would otherwise have to be referred for treatment.

Although standing orders may be created through a verbal agreement between the optometrist and physician, the preferable means of establishing the consultation relationship that forms the basis for standing orders is through a carefully drafted document listing detailed instructions for each clinical disorder to be treated. This document should include itemized steps for treatment, including the specific drugs or the general drug categories to be employed, and should provide for appropriate consultation with the physician, including the physician's verbal or written order for the drugs to be prescribed or dispensed (an example of how standing orders might be drafted is illustrated in Fig. 28.2).

Key elements in the formulation of a workable set of standing orders include the following:

- A thorough, detailed set of written orders to be followed by the optometrist when a described clinical disorder is diagnosed, the diagnosis of the disorder to be made in consultation with the physician (who does not have to be physically present)
- Treatment by the optometrist in accordance with the written orders (and the patient record should reflect this fact)
- Verbal or written orders by the physician for any drugs to be prescribed or dispensed (but no presigned prescriptions should be used)
- Authentication (i.e., review and signing or initialing of the patient record) by the physician within a reasonable period of time after treatment has been initiated
- Provisions for management in the event the patient does not respond to therapy within a reasonable period

Legal aspects of this arrangement affecting both practitioners include the possibility of professional liability lawsuits and the specter of disciplinary action by medical or optometry boards.

Generally speaking, when two practitioners act in consultation during the management of a patient's case, each is considered to be the agent of the other, and thus they bear legal responsibility for the acts or omissions of one another. If either practitioner is negligent then both may be held responsible for the patient's injury. When standing orders are used, if the optometrist is negligent in the diagnosis or treatment of the patient, then the physician may also be held liable under this theory. But if the optometrist exceeds the limits of the standing orders, or acts in contravention to their provisions, then the physician may be found not responsible since the optometrist has not acted in accordance with the agreed upon treatment. When standing orders are being considered, the practitioners' professional liability insurance carrier should be consulted in order to ensure that the appropriate coverage is obtained.

The use of standing orders by optometrists, being of recent origin, has been legally tested in very few jurisdictions, and so many legal questions concerning their utilization remain unanswered.[47] The extent to which certain duties can be delegated to optometrists, and the degree of supervision required by consulting physicians, are two of the many important issues that at present are legally undefined. As a result, optometrists and physicians must be certain that the standing orders do not constitute the unauthorized practice of medicine or other offenses for which a board of optometry or medical board could impose disciplinary sanctions. It may be advisable for the practitioners to consult with legal counsel, risk control personnel, or other advisors who may be of assistance in the drafting or implementation of the orders.

Standing Orders

I. Blepharitis
   A. Bacitracin or erythromycin lid scrub b.i.d.
   B. Selenium sulfide shampoo to hair several times weekly
   C. Johnson's Baby Shampoo lid scrub b.i.d. to cleanse lid margins of crusts
   D. Patient's clinical chart should be reviewed and signed by physician within one week of initial visit
   E. Return in 1 to 4 weeks for follow-up

II. Chemical Injury to the Eye
   A. Phone advice to patient (or at time of first contact): Wash eye(s) copiously with water or sterile saline solution, if available
   B. At time of examination, determine the etiologic agent
      1. Acid
         a) Instill topical ocular anesthetic drops in affected eye(s)
         b) Copiously irrigate affected eye(s) with sterile saline or irrigating solution
         c) Examine anterior chamber(s) for evidence of inflammatory response
         d) Instill sodium fluorescein
         e) Severity assessment
            (1) Superficial punctate keratitis involving less than 50% of the corneal surface with no evidence of inflammatory response in the anterior chamber(s):
            Proceed with standing orders— see C below
            (2) Severe keratitis (e.g., deep corneal insult involving greater than 50% of the corneal surface) and/or any evidence of anterior chamber inflammatory response:
            Either consult with physician or refer the patient for emergency medical treatment
      2. Alkali
         a) Instill topical ocular anesthetic drops in affected eye(s)
         b) Copiously irrigate affected eye(s) with sterile saline or irrigating solution
         c) Evaluate anterior chamber(s) for evidence of inflammatory response
         d) Instill sodium fluorescein
         e) Consult immediately with physician or refer the patient for emergency medical treatment
      3. Mild, non-acid, non-alkali chemical injuries (superficial punctate keratitis due to hair spray, shampoos, allergic reactions to topical ophthalmic medications, etc.)
         a) Irrigate as in A above
         b) Instill topical ocular anesthetic when indicated
         c) Topical ophthalmic antibiotic or antibiotic/steroid drops q.i.d.
         d) Patient's record should be reviewed and signed by physician within 48 hours of the initial visit (if therapeutic agent is used)
         e) Return in 2 to 3 days or sooner if symptoms worsen
   C. Standing Orders
      1. Instill cycloplegic (e.g., atropine 1%, homatropine 5%, scopolamine 0.25%) in affected eye(s)
      2. Instill topical ophthalmic antibiotic ointment in affected eye(s) (e.g., gentamicin, tobramycin, bacitracin/polymyxin B)
      3. Pressure patch affected eye(s)
      4. Return in 24 hours
      5. Determine appropriate course of action based on follow-up evaluation
      6. Patient's clinical chart should be reviewed and signed by physician within 48 hours of the initial visit

III. Bacterial Conjunctivitis
   A. Antibiotic ophthalmic solution (e.g., sodium sulfacetamide, gentamicin, or chloramphenicol) 1 gt O.U. q.i.d.

or B. Antibiotic/steroid combination (when associated with corneal marginal infiltrates)
   C. Warm compresses and appropriate lid hygiene instructions
   D. Patient's clinical chart should be reviewed and signed by physician within one week of the initial visit
   E. Return in one week or sooner

IV. Corneal Abrasion
   A. Instill topical anesthetic in affected eye(s)
   B. Biomicroscopic evaluation including anterior chamber evaluation
   C. Instill sodium fluorescein
   D. Instill cycloplegic
      1. Small abrasion—short-acting cycloplegic (e.g., cyclopentolate 1%)
      2. Large abrasion—long acting cycloplegic (e.g., homatropine 5%, scopolamine 0.25%)
   E. Instill antibiotic ointment (e.g., gentamicin, sodium sulfacetamide, bacitracin/polymyxin B)
   F. Pressure patch
   G. Recommend appropriate analgesic agent when indicated (e.g., aspirin or acetaminophen)
   H. Return in 24 hours
   I. Determine appropriate course of action based on follow-up evaluation
   J. Patient's clinical chart should be reviewed and signed by physician within 48 hours of the initial visit

V. Superficial Foreign Bodies
   A. Instill topical anesthetic in both eyes (2 drops in affected eye)
   B. Remove foreign body
      1. Attempt to irrigate foreign body from eye with sterile saline or irrigating solution
      2. If (1) is unsuccessful, then attempt to remove foreign body from eye with a sterile cotton-tipped applicator
      3. If (1) and (2) are unsuccessful, then attempt to remove foreign body from eye with a sterile hypodermic needle (approximately 25 gauge) or foreign body removal spud
      4. If possible, the removed foreign body should be attached to the patient's record
   C. After removal of the foreign body, continue with instructions for corneal abrasion beginning at (B)

VI. Anterior Uveitis
   A. Nongranulomatous
      1. Instill long-acting cycloplegic (e.g., homatropine 5%, scopolamine 0.25%) one (1) drop in affected eye(s) q.i.d.
      2. Topical steroid (e.g., prednisolone acetate 1.0%)
         a) Dosage depends upon severity
            (1) Mild: One (1) drop in affected eye(s) q.i.d.
            (2) Moderate: One (1) drop in affected eye(s) q.2h.
      3. Supportive therapy if indicated
         a) Warm compresses
         b) Systemic analgesic (e.g., aspirin or acetaminophen)
         c) Sunglasses
      4. Patient's clinical chart should be reviewed and signed by physician within 48 hours of initial visit
      5. Return in 24 to 48 hours
      6. Determine appropriate course of action based on follow-up evaluation
   B. Granulomatous
      1. See section A (1 through 6) above (non-granulomatous anterior uveitis) for appropriate therapy
      2. Refer patient to physician for systemic evaluation

Figure 28.2. Examples of Standing Orders. (Courtesy Jimmy D. Bartlett, O.D.)

Despite the uncertain legal questions surrounding the use of standing orders, they deserve consideration by optometrists serving in multidisciplinary health-care institutions, in hospitals or teaching clinics, in optometric referral centers, and perhaps even by optometrists in private practice who enjoy strong personal and professional relationships with physicians willing to collaborate in the management of ocular disease cases. It would seem that standing orders offer optometrists an opportunity to better serve the public and enables optometry to more completely achieve its stated goal of serving as a primary health-care profession.

Notes

1. As of 1988, the two states that have not yet amended their optometry practice acts to authorize the use of ophthalmic pharmaceutical agents by optometrists are Alaska and Maryland.
2. The original optometry practice acts were enacted from 1901–1924, a total of twenty-three years being required for all jurisdictions. To date, forty-eight states and the District of Columbia have added drug amendments to these laws over a period of seventeen years.
3. As of this writing there have been no precedent-setting cases published in the law reporters involving misuse of ophthalmic pharmaceutical agents by optometrists, nor is the author aware of any large malpractice claims based on such allegations. For a review of cases and claims, see Classe, J., Optometry and Malpractice: A Personal Commentary, *Southern Journal of Optometry*, vol. 5, no. 3, 1987, pp. 26–31.
4. See, e.g., *Reed v. Church*, 8 S.E.2d (Va. 1940) (failure of the prescribing physician to be aware of the side effects of prolonged use of chloroquine).
5. See, e.g., *Rotan v. Greenbaum*, 273 F.2d 830 (D.C. Cir. 1959) (injection of penicillin for mumps causing anaphylactic shock and death).
6. See, e.g., *Yorston v. Pennell*, 397 Pa. 28, 153 A.2d 255 (1959) (repeated applications of penicillin despite history of allergy, causing serious cardiovascular side effects).
7. See, e.g., *Trogun v. Fruchtman*, 58 Wis. 2d 596, 207 N.W.2d 297 (1973) (the court held that the physician must adequately advise the patient of the effects of the drug INH, which caused hepatitis).
8. See, e.g., *Thaggard v. Vafes*, 119 So. 647 (Ala. 1928). (Physician failed to examine patient suffering side effects of a drug containing arsenic.) An analysis of liability for drug reactions can be found in Physician's Liability for Drug Reactions, *Journal of the American Medical Association*, vol. 213, no. 12, Sept. 21, 1970, pp. 2143–2144.
9. *Reed v. Church*, 8 S.E.2d 285 (Va. 1940).
10. Disclosure requirements under the doctrine of informed consent have been discussed by Harris, M.G. and R.E. Dister, Informed Consent in Contact Lens Practice, *Journal of the American Optometric Association*, vol. 58, no. 3, 1987, pp. 230–237.
11. Yolton, D.P., J.S. Kandell, and R.L. Yolton, Diagnostic Pharmaceutical Agents: Side Effects Encountered in a Study of 15,000 Applications, *Journal of the American Optometric Association*, vol. 51, no. 2, 1980, pp. 113–118.
12. Report of Ann J. Haney, Secretary, Wisconsin Department of Regulation and Licenses, "Diagnostic Pharmaceutical Agents," January 26, 1982.
13. Applebaum, M., and S.D. Jaanus, Use of Diagnostic Pharmaceutical Agents and Incidence of Adverse Effects, *American Journal of Optometry and Physiological Optics*, vol. 60, no. 5, 1983, pp. 384–388.
14. See Lyle, W.M., and C. Page, Possible Adverse Effects from Local Anesthetics and the Treatment of Those Reactions, *American Journal of Optometry and Physiological Optics*, vol. 52, no. 11, 1975, pp. 736–744.
15. *LeMade v. Wilson*, reported in 20 *ATLA Law Reporter* 91, 1977.
16. Although photophobia, blurred vision, pain, and other symptoms of corneal sloughing would constitute an injury for which damages could be awarded, the injury is of a transient nature, resolving itself in the usual case within twenty-four to forty-eight hours, and so the damages in such a case would be nominal. Furthermore, corneal sloughing is an adverse response that is unpredictable, and negligence would be difficult to establish unless the clinician had failed to learn of the reaction during the history, thereby precipitating an otherwise preventable injury. The author is not aware of any malpractice claims alleging this type of injury. See Classe, J., Liability for Use of Ophthalmic Pharmaceutical Agents, *Southern Journal of Optometry*, vol. 2, no. 4, 1984, pp. 43–49.
17. Cockburn, D.M., Prevalence and Significance of Narrow Anterior Chamber Angles in Optometric Practice, *American Journal of Optometry and Physiological Optics*, vol. 58, no. 2, 1981, pp. 171–175.
18. For a thorough discussion of the benefits of mydriatic use by optometrists, see Bartlett, J.D., and S.D. Jaanus, (Eds.) in *Clinical Ocular Pharmacology*, Butterworths, Boston, 1984, chapter 15.
19. Alexander, L.J. and J. Scholles, Clinical and Legal Aspects of Pupillary Dilation, *Journal of the American Optometric Association*, vol. 58, no. 5, 1987, pp. 432–437.
20. Keller, J.T., The Risk of Angle Closure from the Use of Mydriatics, *Journal of the American Optometric Association*, vol. 46, 1975, no. 1, pp. 19–21.
21. Bettman, J.W., A Review of 412 Claims in Ophthalmology, in Medicolegal Aspects of Ophthalmology, Bettman, J.W. (ed.), *International Ophthalmology Clinics*, vol. 20, 1980, pp. 131–142.
22. The selection of the appropriate mydriatic in a given case is important both clinically and legally. For an excellent discussion, see Bartlett and Jaanus, supra

note 18, at 431–467.

23. *Graham v. Whitaker*, 321 S.E.2d 40 (S.C. 1984).
24. For an interesting application of the duty to warn, see *Kaiser v. Suburban Transportation System*, 65 Wash. 2d 461, 398 P.2d 14 (1965), in which a physician was held liable for injuries sustained by passengers of a bus when the driver fell asleep at the wheel due to medication prescribed by the physician. See also Classe, J., Optometrist's Duty to Warn of Vision Impairment, *Southern Journal of Optometry*, vol. 4, no. 1, 1986, pp. 66–69; and Gold, A.R., Failure to Warn, *Journal of the American Optometric Association*, vol. 57, no. 4, 1986, pp. 317–319.
25. The toxicity of cycloplegics is reviewed in the following papers: Hopkins, G.A., and W.M. Lyle, Potential Systemic Side Effects of Six Common Ophthalmic Drugs, *Journal of the American Optometric Association*, vol. 48, no. 10, 1977, pp. 1241–1245; Bartlett, J.D., Administration of and Adverse Reactions to Cycloplegic Agents, *American Journal of Optometry and Physiological Optics*, vol. 55, no. 4, 1978, pp. 227–233; and Gray, L.G., Avoiding Adverse Effects of Cycloplegics in Infants and Children, *Journal of the American Optometric Association*, vol. 50, no. 4, 1979, pp. 465–470.
26. *Kahn v. Shaw*, 65 Ga. App. 563, 16 S.E.2d 99 (1941). This case readily illustrates the necessity for pharmaceutical use by optometrists and the unnecessary circumstances under which litigation can ensue where pharmaceutical use is denied.
27. The use of cycloplegics is reviewed by Amos, D.M., in *Clinical Ocular Pharmacology*, supra note 16, Chapter 16.
28. *Esposito v. Shapero*, Sixth Judicial District, Division Two, C.A. 76 1214, Dec. 13, 1976. Review of the case was denied by the West Virginia Supreme Court on June 6, 1977.
29. Classe, J., The Right to Practice Primary Care, *Journal of the American Optometric Association*, vol. 57, no. 7, 1986, pp. 549–553.
30. Bettman, supra note 21, at 132.
31. For a review of the adverse effects of topical therapeutic pharmaceutical agents, see Wilson, F.M., Adverse External Ocular Effects of Topical Ophthalmic Medications, *Survey of Ophthalmology*, vol. 24, no. 2, 1979, pp. 57–88.
32. Another review of drug-related liability cases can be found in Bettman, J.W., A Retrospective Look at Twenty-two Medicolegal Claims. How They Might Have Been Avoided, *Survey of Ophthalmology*, vol. 28, no. 1, 1983, pp. 55–60.
33. *Aetna Casualty & Surety Co. of Illinois v. Medical Protective Co.*, 575 F. Supp. 901 (D.C. Ill. 1983).
34. Bettman, supra note 32, at 59.
35. Bettman, supra note 21, at 132–134.
36. Reported by Rubsamen, D.S., A $625,000 Verdict for Death from a Rare Illness, in California Malpractice Topics, *Professional Liability Newsletter*, vol. 12, no. 7, 1981.
37. For a discussion of the significance of the package insert, see Dixon, M.G., *Drug Product Liability*, Matthew Bender, New York, 1987, §6.10.
38. Bettman, supra note 32, at 59–60.
39. *Weaver v. Grace*, reported in 21 *ATLA Law Reporter* 64, 1978.
40. *Bacardi v. Holzman*, 182 N.J. Super. 422, 442 A.2d 617 (1981).
41. Bettman, supra note 32, at 60.
42. *Kim v. New York Hospital*, reported in 25 *ATLA Law Reporter* 328, 1982.
43. Bettman, supra note 32, at 54.
44. For a discussion, see Mindel, J.S. and J.I. Goldstein, Non-Approved Use of Food and Drug Administration Approved Drugs, *American Journal of Ophthalmology*, vol. 88, no. 3, part 2, 1979, pp. 626–628.
45. Bettman, supra note 21, at 133–134.
46. *Smith v. Wharton*, 154 S.E.12 (N.C. 1930).
47. The use of standing orders by optometrists has not been the subject of appellate review in any jurisdiction. But they have been upheld as valid by the Pennsylvania Board of Optometry in a case involving the use of standing orders by optometrists at the Pennsylvania College of Optometry. The orders were written by a Philadelphia ophthalmologist and were used by optometrists at the college to permit the co-management of patients with ocular disease. In the state of Texas the medical practice act was amended to provide for optometrists to administer drugs pursuant to a standing delegation order from a physician. The Attorney General of Texas has upheld the constitutionality of this amendment (opinion No. JM-454 of March 20, 1986, reported in *Bulletin from State Legislative Affairs Advisory Committee, Statutory Definition Committee*, vol. 44, no. 92, April 25, 1986, published by the American Optometric Association). Until an appellate court rules on the use and application of these orders, they will remain an uncertain aspect of clinical practice. Even so, they are an appropriate means of defining responsibilities whenever optometrists undertake the co-management of patients with physicians.

Chapter 29

Liability for Premises

Accidents will occur in the best regulated families.
—Charles Dickens, *David Copperfield*

Premises Liability

Malpractice is not the only application of negligence law. There are numerous other situations that may create liability for negligence; one of the most common involves the liability of doctors for their premises.

A person in possession of land has the privilege to make use of the land for his own benefit, but his privilege is qualified by a due regard for the interests of others who may be affected by it. Accordingly, there is a duty or obligation on the part of the one in possession of land (such as an optometrist who occupies an office building) to those who enter on the premises (such as patients or other visitors). An injury incurred by a patient while upon the premises can result in liability for the optometrist in possession.[1]

Premises Liability

A visitor to land is classified in accordance with his legal status: trespasser, licensee, or invitee. Visitors who enter on the premises of a health-care practitioner are considered to be invitees.[2]

Invitees are business visitors; because they enter on the premises at the invitation of the one in possession, they are owed the highest duty. In general, it is held to be an affirmative duty, under which the one in possession is obliged to protect the invitee against those dangers that he is aware of and those dangers which with reasonable care he should discover.[3] Thus, a doctor has an obligation to maintain the office premises in a safe condition, both for obviously dangerous conditions of which he is aware and for dangerous conditions, that, through the exercise of reasonable diligence, he should have discovered. Since premises refers to the office, the areas of ingress and egress, the furniture, the equipment, and any other items that present a hazard to the safety of the patient, the duty is not a small one.[4] A doctor who breaches this duty and, as a proximate result thereof, causes a patient to suffer an injury, may be held liable under negligence law for damages.

Injuries from equipment or premises have long been a source of consternation among optometrists. In fact, past investigators have found premises liability to be one of the constant causes of litigation against optometric practitioners.[5] Whether the optometrist practices in his own building, or as a tenant in a building that he does not own, he owes an affirmative duty to his patients to protect them against any dangers that he knows of or that through the exercise of reasonable care he should have known of. This duty constitutes the legal basis for premises liability.

Defective Premises

The premises of an optometrist's office includes not just the working area itself but an area of invitation, which incorporates into the definition of premises the office entrance, all parts of the office that may reasonably be expected to be used by the patient, and a safe exit from the office.[6]

The duty owed to patients is fourfold[7]:

1. The optometrist must take care to avoid negligently injuring the patient.
2. The optometrist must warn the patient of any latent dangers of which he is aware.
3. The optometrist must inspect the premises to discover any patently dangerous conditions.
4. The optometrist must take reasonable precautions to protect the patient from dangers that are foreseeable.

Dangers that are obvious or that are known to patients usually require no more than a warning, regardless of whether they are outside the office or inside.

A doctor's examination of a patient was not concluded until after dark, by which time sleet had begun to fall. The patient fell in the doctor's parking lot due to the slipperiness of the pavement. She sued the doctor for her injuries. In affirming a decision in favor of the doctor, the court held that the sleet and snow posed an obvious danger that patients are expected to protect themselves against.[8]

A patient who was walking from the reception room to the examination room in a doctor's office slipped and fell, injuring herself. She sued the doctor, alleging that the floor was slippery and had caused her to fall. The evidence established that the floor had been waxed eleven days previously and that no one else had suffered an accident during that period of time. In affirming a decision in favor of the doctor, the court noted that the patient had been wearing high heel shoes and had doubtless fallen due to her own carelessness.[9]

There may be instances, however, in which a warning will not be sufficient.[10] Falls inside the office are governed by a number of factors. The condition of the premises, the age and condition of the patient, and the patient's ability to take ordinary notice of surrounding and potential dangers are among the most common.

A patient who needed a crutch to get around went to an ophthalmologist for an eye examination and had his pupils dilated. When the patient left the office and entered the hallway, his crutch slipped on a spot mopped minutes before by a janitor, and he fell and was injured. He sued both the janitorial service and the landlord, and they were both held to be liable for his injuries.[11]

Patients should routinely be warned of the effects of pupillary dilation, and patients with infirmities should be assisted as necessary to prevent the chance of an unfortunate accident. For elderly patients who drive, it is reasonable to suggest that they have someone bring them to the office and take them home (if it is known that they will be subjected to dilation during the couse of the examination). Failure to warn a patient of the effects of pupillary dilation constitutes a potential source of litigation that is entirely preventable. Optometrists should be sure that all patients receive the appropriate warning, even those who have received a dilated fundus examination on previous visits.

A 77-year-old woman was to be examined by an ophthalmologist. To facilitate the examination, dilating drops (Mydriacyl®) were placed in the patient's eyes. She was left in a waiting room by herself, without supervision, and due to the blurred condition of her vision fell and broke her hip. She sued the doctor for her injuries, alleging that he had a duty to provide safe premises. The jury, finding that the woman had not contributed to her injuries by any negligent conduct on her own behalf, awarded $20,000 in damages, determining that the ophthalmologist and his staff had breached the affirmative duty to make the office premises reasonably safe.[12]

A patient who faints can fall and be injured, and syncope preceding or during certain diagnostic tests (tonometry for example) is not completely unexpected.[13] Where a doctor has no preliminary indication that the patient is susceptible to syncope or has previously suffered a fainting spell or a seizure, there is no liability. The risk of injury under such circumstances is not considered to be foreseeable.[14]

Defective Equipment

Faulty instruments or equipment can pose an unnecessary hazard to both doctor and patient. Optometrists have a duty to inspect their equipment, and the standard of care required of doctors is generally stated as follows: If a defect is apparent to ordinary observation, and, even if not, if it should have been discoverable through a reasonable inspection, then the doctor will be held liable for any injury suffered by the patient as a result of the defect.[15] Only when there is a latent defect that is not discoverable is the doctor held not to be liable for a failure to conduct the inspection.[16]

There are few opportunities for equipment-related injuries in optometric practice. The most common injuries are probably caused by instruments defectively attached to walls, stands, and tables; electrical defects in ophthalmic instruments and equipment; and office furniture either kept in poor repair or inherently dangerous.

A patient seated on a chair in a doctor's examination room was injured when the chair overturned. Because the nature of the chair's design made it likely that the chair would turn over, the patient was able to state a cause of action against the doctor.[17]

If an optometrist or his assistants suspect that an instrument or a piece of equipment is defective, it should be removed from service immediately and repaired. Continuing to use a defective instrument or piece of equipment that can cause injury creates certain liability.

Whenever equipment is used in a negligent manner, liability will be imposed for the negligence.

A physician who was attempting to measure the intraocular pressure of a patient used a Schiotz tonometer immediately after it has been sterilized. Instead of allowing it to cool properly, the doctor merely waved the instrument in the air for a couple of minutes; he did not determine the temperature of the instrument foot plate, which was later estimated to be 475 degrees Fahrenheit when the doctor applied it to the patient's eye. The patient was awarded $60,000 for the resulting loss of vision.[18]

As an aside, pharmaceutical agents that are defective can also become the basis of a suit for damages. For example, *Pseudomonas aeruginosa* can successfully multiply in a sodium fluorescein solution, and when the fluorescein is applied to the eye during tonometry, the *Pseudomonas* can cause a particularly severe bacterial infection of the cornea. The optometrist is under a duty to inspect pharmaceutical agents used in his practice and to maintain them in accordance with the manufacturer's instructions (e.g., certain drugs should be kept refrigerated). The expiration date of pharmaceutical agents should be noted, and, when reached, the drug should be discarded.[19]

Obligations of Optometrist-Lessors or Lessees

An optometrist who leases space to others in an office building (the lessor) incurs certain obligations; so too does an optometrist who occupies leased property (the lessee). The lessor must disclose to the lessee any dangerous condition of which he has knowledge that is in existence at the time the lessee takes possession.[20] Failure to do so confers liability upon the lessor for any injury to the lessee or his invitees that occurs due to the nondisclosure. The lessor is liable if he is aware of conditions from which a reasonable person would have concluded there was danger.[21]

This responsibility extends not only to dangerous conditions existing at the time the lessee takes possession but also to conditions that have the potential to become dangerous and are likely to become so during the course of the lease. If the leased property is used for a purpose that involves the admission of the public (e.g., a doctor's office), the lessor is required to employ reasonable care to inspect and repair the premises before transferring possession to the lessee.[22] But this requirement is limited to repairs before the lessee occupies the property; what about repairs that are needed later during the term of the lease?

An agreement by the lessor to keep the premises in repair will bind the lessor and will make him liable for breach of contract or for tort.[23] And if he is negligent in making these repairs, he is liable for any injuries resulting from the negligence.[24] Furthermore, if the lessor attempts to make repairs—although not bound to do so—he will still be held liable for any failure to exercise reasonable care that causes injury.[25] Even if the lessor entrusts the repairs to a third party (an independent contractor), the lessor can still be held liable for the third party's negligence.[26] Therefore, lessors may refuse to make repairs upon leased property (see Chapter 49 for a discussion of the contractual obligations common to lease agreements).

Notes

1. A summary of the law can be found in Holder, A.R., Medical Premises Liability, Part I, in Law & Medicine, *Journal of the American Medical Association*, vol. 226, no. 5, Oct. 29, 1973, pp. 597–598; and Holder, A.R., Medical Premises Liability, Part II, *Journal of the American Medical Association*, vol. 226, no. 6, Nov. 5, 1973, pp. 717–718.
2. Invitee is a legal term for those persons who enter on another's premises for purposes of business and on the invitation (express or implied) of the one in possession of the premises. See Prosser, W.L., *Law of Torts*, 4th Edition, West, St. Paul, Minn., 1971, pp. 385–398.
3. Id. at 385.

4. Id. at 391.
5. These and other professional liability claims are reported by Elmstrom, G., in *Optometric Practice Management*, Chilton, Philadelphia, 1963, p. 217.
6. Prosser, supra note 2, at 391.
7. A review of liability for injuries from premises and equipment can be found in Holder, A.R., *Medical Malpractice Law*, Wiley and Sons, New York, 1975, pp. 175–199.
8. *Jeswald v. Hutt*, 15 Ohio St. 2d. 224, 239 N.E.2d 37 (1968).
9. *Cullison v. Red*, 149 S.W.2d 153 (Tex. Civ. App. 1941).
10. For example, untended icy steps, which are dangerous even to someone fully aware of them, and which must be traversed in order to enter or leave the optometrist's office, can create liability if an injury occurs although a warning is given. The rationale behind this rule of law is that the patient can be expected to try and negotiate the steps regardless of the warning, and that, under such circumstances, the doctor has a duty to make the steps safe rather than merely issue a warning. See Prosser, supra note 2, at 385–398.
11. *Truxillo v. Gentilly Medical Bldg., Inc.*, 225 So. 2d 488 (La. 1969).
12. *Graham v. Whitaker*, 321 S.E. 2d 40 (S.C. 1984).
13. See Bergen, R.P., Patients Who Faint During Office Visits, *Journal of the American Medical Association*, vol. 195, no. 3, Jan. 17, 1966, pp. 261–262.
14. Ibid.
15. Holder, supra note 7, at 175–178.
16. Ibid.
17. *Walker v. Rynd*, 280 P.2d 259 (Wash. 1955).
18. *Dean v. Dyer*, 64 Cal. App. 2d 646, 149 P.2d 288 (Cal. 1944).
19. According to Angela Holder, supra note 7, at 154–165, "Drugs constitute the overwhelming majority of therapeutic agents which are the subject of suits."
20. For a discussion of the obligations of lessors and lessees, see Prosser, supra note 2, at 399–412.
21. Ibid.
22. Ibid.
23. Ibid.
24. Ibid.
25. Ibid.
26. An independent contractor is defined as "One who, exercising an independent employment, contracts to do a piece of work according to his own methods and without being subject to the control of his employer except as the result of the work." *Black's Law Dictionary*, 4th ed., West, St. Paul, Minn., 1968.

PART EIGHT

CLINICOLEGAL ASPECTS OF SPECIALTY PRACTICE

Chapter 30

Clinicolegal Problems in Contact Lens Practice

The insertion, fitting and adjusting of contact lenses involves the introduction of foreign material into a most delicate orifice of the body and is a process which concerns the health and welfare of the public and requires the exercise of professional skill and judgment.
—From the decision of Judge Sloan, *State of Oregon ex rel. Reed v. Kuzirian,* 365 P.2d 1046 (1961)

Fitting Agreements
Prepaid Service Agreements
Experimental or Nonapprovad Use of Lenses
Extended Wear Lenses
The Contact Lens Prescription
Malpractice and Contact Lenses
Product Liability

Legal problems confront the contact lens practitioner on a daily basis. Lens fitting agreements, prepaid service agreements, FDA protocols for experimental lenses (i.e., clinical trials), informed consent documentation, compliance with FTC prescription requirements, extended wear lenses, and the specter of malpractice are but a few of the commonly occurring matters that concern the doctor who decides to enter the realm of contact lens practice. How should this formidable array of potentially vexatious legal issues be managed by a private practitioner? The following discussion suggests some ways to approach these problems.

Fitting Agreements

Fitting agreements are no longer just for the busy contact lens practitioner, they are for everyone who fits, prescribes, and dispenses contact lenses. There are three basic reasons for utilizing a fitting agreement:

1. To provide a signed contract that serves as a legal manifestation of the agreement between doctor and patient
2. To ensure that the patient fully understands all costs and how such costs are to be paid
3. To educate the patient so that the patient realizes the agreement with the doctor includes services as well as materials

A well-written fitting agreement not only spells out the dollars and cents involved but also prepares the patient for his or her responsibilities as a contact lens wearer by emphasizing that the patient is entering into a comprehensive treatment plan, one that requires long-term cooperation. By putting the patient on notice from the outset that the fitting of lenses is only the first step, that immediate follow-up is an integral part of the contractual agreement, and that even a preventative system for avoiding future problems is available (e.g., prepaid service agreements), doctors who use fitting agreements have clearly separated themselves from other contact lens providers in the ophthalmic marketplace. Emphasis on services and adequate follow-up is a distinguishing sign of the competent contact lens practitioner.[1] The formality of a contractual agreement discussing these very points—which must be agreed to and signed—is not lost upon the patient. The contract reinforces an idea that doctors must promote, namely that the purchase of contact lenses is not the same as the purchase

Hard Contact Lens Fitting Agreement

Fitting you with contact lenses places a joint responsibility on both of us. Therefore, you must understand what our contact lens fitting program includes. Please read this over carefully, and if you have any questions, feel free to discuss them with us.

Our contact lens patients receive the following materials and services:

1. Examination of ocular health
2. Vision analysis and spectacle prescription
3. Examination for contact lenses
4. Dispensing of contact lenses, patient care kit, and instructional materials; education and instruction in handling, care, and maintenance of your contact lenses;
5. Evaluation of lens fit with the lenses on the eye.
6. Progress evaluations and follow-up care for a period of __ months.

Since there are many variables to contact lens fitting, there is no guarantee that you will become a successful contact lens wearer. However, we will use up to __ lenses in the fitting procedure and will work with you and follow-up for __ months without additional charge. Any lenses used thereafter will be billed to you as an additional charge.

Contact lenses are made by many laboratories employing various materials and designs. As a result, costs vary. And on occasion we will fit a patient with lenses from one laboratory and, after several weeks or months, will feel that better results might be obtained with lenses from another laboratory. Whenever this situation occurs, you will be advised, and the fee structure will be adjusted to reflect any differences in costs.

If the fitting of your lenses is discontinued within the __ month fitting period, a refund of __% of all fees paid will be made upon return of all lenses and the patient care kit. After the __ month fitting period, no refunds will be made.

We agree to fit ______________ with contact lenses as per the above, using ______ lenses, for a fee of $____, the fitting period commencing on the day the contact lenses are dispensed. Contact lenses are not dispensed until payment is received in full.

During the fitting period, lost lenses will be replaced at a cost of $____ per lens, damaged lenses at a cost of $____ per lens when the damaged lens is returned to this office, and additional lenses, if required, at $____ per lens.

I have read and understood the above agreement.

______________________   __________   ______________

Patient   Date   Witness

Figure 30.1. Sample Head Contact Lens Fitting Agreement. (Courtesy of the UAB School of Optometry)

of other consumer items, despite the *caveat emptor* approach of some ophthalmic providers. A properly composed agreement will assist doctors in their efforts to make patients receptive, cooperative, and understanding of the fitting and follow-up process.

What should such a fitting agreement contain? Figs. 30.1, 30.2, and 30.3 are sample agreements that incorporate the basic ideas expressed in the preceding paragraph.[2] All such agreements should contain a common minimum of information:

1. The agreement should emphasize that the contact lens fitting places a joint responsibility on both parties to conform to the requirements of the contract, and that the patient is expected to live up to his end of the bargain (especially important with patients obtaining extended wear lenses).
2. There must be a list of the covered materials and services, which may include:
   - assessment of ocular health
   - refraction and spectacle prescription
   - fitting of contact lenses
   - dispensing of the lenses, a care kit, and instructions
   - education and instruction in the care, handling, and maintenance of the lenses
   - evaluation of the lens fit as necessary (a period of time may be specified) to ensure that the fit is satisfactory
   - a limited number of progress checks

3. The agreement should specify the policy for refunds if the lens fit is unsuccessful.
4. The cost of replacing lost or damaged lenses during the fitting period should be specified.
5. The fee to be paid and how it is to be paid should be described.
6. A statement that "a successful fit cannot be guaranteed" should be included in the agreement.
7. The contract should be signed and dated by the patient, and the original should be retained in the patient record.

Such an agreement will promote understanding, reduce the potential for disagreements over fees, assist the staff in communicating with patients, and provide legal documentation in the event a dispute does arise.

Prepaid Service Agreements

A study of the contact lens population at a university teaching clinic[3] found that the first twelve months after dispensing was the period of time during which the majority of contact lens patients were at risk to discontinue lens wear and become dropouts. The key findings of the study were:

- For hard lens wearers, 81 percent of all those who terminated lens wear were found to drop out during the first twelve months after the initial fitting.
- For soft lens wearers, 68 percent of all those who terminated lens wear were found to drop out during the first twelve months after the initial fitting.
- The principal reasons given for discontinuing lens wear were discomfort (43 percent) and poor vision (16 percent), which intimates that 60 percent of these patients were not happy with the initial lens fit.

These results indicate that the first year of lens wear is a most vital period, one that the doctor should monitor closely if patients are to remain satisfied and to continue as contact lens wearers. One way to approach this problem is to offer the patient a prepaid service agreement.[4] If the doctor's services have already been paid for, the patient is motivated to return to the doctor for assistance if difficulties are encountered. Many contact lens practitioners offer these plans and are satisfied that they met a very genuine patient need by stressing prevention, a concept that is missing from the armamentarium of some segments of the ophthalmic marketplace. Truly, these plans help fortify the idea that the doctor offers much more than materials, and that in fact the doctor offers

Soft Contact Lens Fitting Agreement

Fitting you with contact lenses places a joint responsibility on both of us. We must attempt to fit your individual needs and you must follow our instructions exactly.

The basic soft contact lens fee will be $____ for the supplemental contact lens examination and diagnostic lens fitting. If lenses are ordered this is applied to the total fee. The fee for standard design contact lenses is $____ to which an educational credit is applied resulting in a fee of $____. The fee includes one pair of lenses, an initial supply of accessories, and all necessary services during the initial fitting period (the first six months from the date you receive the lenses). At least one half of the fee must be paid before the lenses can be ordered and the full fee must be paid before the lenses are dispensed to you. Fees for nonstandard lenses are determined on an individual basis.

Your MINIMUM fitting program will be as follows:
1st Visit—This initial fitting visit consists of a one-hour examination during which eye measurements and an evaluation of eye health for contact lens wear will be made. An evaluation of diagnostic lenses will be made, and lenses may be ordered at this time.

2nd Visit—Placement and removal procedures will be reviewed. If successful in learning these procedures, you will be allowed to take the lenses with you at this time. You will be given a wearing schedule that must be followed exactly. YOU MUST BRING WITH YOU A SUITABLE PAIR OF GLASSES THAT CAN BE WORN HOME AFTER EVERY VISIT.

Figure 30.2. Sample Soft Contact Lens Fitting Agreement. (Courtesy of the UAB School of Optometry)

3rd Visit—Based on the schedule you were given, you will come to the clinic having worn your lenses for at least four hours. The fit of the lenses and your adaptation to them will be evaluated and you will be advised of the prognosis for successful wear. If you elect not to continue, or if it is determined that you will not be a successful contact lens wearer you may stop at this point. If the lenses are returned to the clinic one half the basic fitting fee will be refunded. If you discontinue at any time subsequent to this visit it is understood that no part of the fee will be refunded.

Subsequent Visits—These will be scheduled as indicated to insure that your eyes are adapting properly to the lenses. You will be given a tentative discharge when we are satisfied with your adaptation to the lenses. A 30-day check-up will be scheduled at this time. Following the 30-day check-up, you will be given a tentative discharge if we are satisfied with your adaptation. However, subsequent visits will be required every six months thereafter.

It is imperative to your visual welfare that you be examined at least every six months after the date of your tentative discharge. The present fee for this progress evaluation is $_____ and is subject to change. Patients requiring care in the general optometry clinic and the contact lens clinic will be required to pay the prevailing fees in both clinics.

There is no way of foretelling how often or when your lenses will have to be refitted or replaced due to wear, improper handling, or changes in the refractive state of your eye.

During the initial fitting period there will be no additional charge for office visits or lens reorders necessary to obtain a satisfactory fit. After the initial fitting period you will be charged the usual fees for office visits and lens replacements. At the present time these fees are $_____ and $_____ per lens, respectively, for standard design lenses. Charges for nonstandard design lenses will vary according to the lens type.

If lenses are lost or damaged *at any time* there will be a charge for replacement.
If the lenses are insured with _____ or equivalent insurance the replacement fee is $_____ per lens. The replacement fee for uninsured lenses is $_____ per lens.
Signed this ___ day of ______ 19__.
Clinician's Signature ______________________________
Instructor's Signature ______________________________

PERMISSION FORM

CONTACT LENS SERVICE

This is to acknowledge that I have read the information contained on this consultation form, and I recognize that it is my responsibility to follow all instructions exactly, to report for periodic progress examinations every six months and to advise you of any change in my name, address, or phone number.

Signed this ___ day of ______ 19__.

____

(Patient's Signature)

This is to acknowledge that I have read the information contained on this consultation form and the above statement signed by ________. This is to advise you that my daughter/son/ward, ________ has my permission to be fitted by you with contact lenses.
Signed this ___ day of ______ 19__.

____

(Parent or Guardian's Signature)

NOTE: One copy of this form is to be given to the patient and the signed copy is to be placed in the patient's record.

Figure 30.2. *Continued.*

Fitting Agreement for Toric Soft Contact Lenses

After several years of working with many patients using various soft contact lens designs for the correction of astigmatism, we have reached the conclusion that we will fit all of our future patients who require a correction for astigmatism, and who wish to use soft contact lenses, in a one-year program that has the following features:

1. The program has a duration of 12 months. It begins the day the patient receives the lenses.
2. All fees must be paid in full at the time of delivery of the lenses.
3. Lenses will not be ordered from the laboratory until a nonreturnable deposit in the amount of $____ is made.
4. Lenses may be either investigative or FDA- approved.
5. Average delivery time of lenses is ______ days after the date of order.
6. We will use a total of ____ lenses at no additional charge as follows: we will begin with a pair of lenses (one lens for each eye). For each lens change required, the lens being replaced must be returned to us at the time the new lens is dispensed. If the lens has been lost, then a charge of $____ will be made for the new lens.
7. If more than ____ lenses are required, each additional lens will be charged to the patient at $____ per lens when the old lens is returned to us, or $____ per lens if a lens is not returned to us.
8. In the event that the fitting is unsuccessful at the end of the one-year fitting period, no refund will be made. However, if the patient will return the lenses and patient care kit to us, we will then fit the patient with either hard contact lenses or eyeglasses, whichever they may select, at no additional charge.

We agree to fit ________ with contact lenses as per the above, using ________ lenses, for a fee of $____, the fitting period commencing on the day the contact lenses are dispensed. Contact lenses are not dispensed until payment is made in full.

I have read and accept the above.

______________________________ ______________________________

Witness Patient

Date dispensed ______________

Figure 30.3. Sample Fitting Agreement for Toric Soft Contact Lenses. (Courtesy Drs. C.L. McEachern, W.M. Cannon, and M.C. McClay)

a comprehensive program of fitting, dispensing, adequate follow-up and problem prevention. Such emphasis on services is evident to the patient.

A suitable prepaid service agreement must explain the purpose of the contract, cost, and services and materials that are included and must provide for renewal. The actual provisions of the contract will vary among practitioners, but a representative agreement is enclosed as Fig. 30.4.[5]

Provisions that should be considered include the following:

1. A statement of purpose should be used to inform the patient that the agreement is intended to allow appropriate follow-up after the lenses have been dispensed and to encourage the patient to be seen promptly should difficulty be encountered.
2. The services and materials should be specified; for example, a daily wear soft lens agreement might provide for:
   - semi-annual progress checks
   - examinations whenever difficulty is encountered
   - cleaning of lenses whenever it is necessary
   - exchange of lenses if a re-fit is needed (including costs)
   - costs of purchasing replacement lenses
3. The period to be covered by the contract should be specified (generally one year).
4. Renewal of the contract should be provided for; usually renewal is available only to patients who have actually returned for a progress check prior to the expiration of the agreement.
5. The agreement may be limited only to patients who have actually been fitted with lenses by the optometrist.

Contact Lens Service Agreement

Our policy is to examine contact lens wearers at least twice a year, in order to evaluate their eyes and the lenses themselves. At all examinations we review care and cleaning of the lenses, evaluate the patient's progress in general, and try to prevent problems from occurring. We want our patients to have the freedom to call upon us whenever they experience difficulty or have questions, and to replace contact lenses or get additional ones at the lowest cost possible.

For these reasons we utilize a Contact Lens Service Agreement, which includes the following:

1. Semiannual examination of eyes and contact lenses.
2. Periodic checkup of eyes and contact lenses whenever difficulty is encountered.
3. Purchase of contact lenses at laboratory costs plus a minimum handling charge.
4. Cleaning of contact lenses when needed.
5. Minimum charges for the exchange of contact lenses.

Although we cannot extend the Contact Lens Service Agreement to patients we have not examined, we are happy to examine, establish, and maintain a patient record for persons now wearing contact lenses, and who wish to use our services.

Our Contact Lens Service Agreement covers a period of one year. Renewal may be accomplished annually, provided we make an examination of the patient during the twelve-month period. The Contact Lens Service Agreement may be renewed anytime within thirty days of expiration. It may be reinstated thereafter if we have examined the patient within the preceding twelve months, for a $__ fee, or upon completion of a current examination of eyes and lenses.

We agree to provide ________ with the following services:

1. Perform two contact lens examinations per year.
2. No charge for office calls during the year.
3. Purchase of additional lenses at $__ per lens.
4. Exchange of lenses for any reason at $__ per lens.
5. Cleaning of lenses as required at no charge.

I have read and understood the above agreement. I agree to pay $__ as consideration for the services enumerated above.

Patient	Date	Witness

Figure 30.4. Sample Contact Lens Service Agreement. (Courtesy Drs. C.L. McEachern, W.M. Cannon, and M.C. McClay)

6. The fee to be paid by the patient must be listed.
7. The agreement must be signed and dated by the patient and retained in the patient record; a copy is given to the patient.

Before establishing such a plan, it would be wise to determine the status of prepaid service agreements under state law. In a few states it has been argued that agreements have been written in such a way as to constitute policies of insurance,[6] particularly when it has not been made clear that they are intended to be contracts for services rather than for the replacement of materials.

Key aspects of prepaid service agreements include[7]:

- use of a single document to describe the services and materials available under the plan
- language that avoids insurance terminology
- emphasis upon services rather than upon materials (which should be regarded as incidental to the services)
- enforceability of the contract against successor doctors

If a plan is deemed to be a contract for insurance, the optometrist will find it necessary to meet state insurance requirements such as bonding and licensure,[8] and so it is appropriate to consult legal counsel or other knowledgeable sources before instituting a plan.

Despite these potential problems, in the great majority of states optometrists may utilize prepaid service agreements with minimal legal risk. The benefits to be derived from well-written agreements are several: patients are motivated to return without delay if complications are encountered; periodic visits allow the optometrist to check on the patient's care and handling procedures; the opportunity for financial disputes is reduced; and patients are encouraged to return to the optometrist's practice rather than seeking care elsewhere.

Optometrists should give careful consideration to instituting these plans, especially those practitioners who have a sizeable contact lens population.

Experimental or Nonapproved Use of Lenses

Special problems arise whenever a practitioner decides to embark upon the adventure of being a clinical investigator for experimental contact lenses, because there are remarkable legal obstacles to be overcome whenever clinical trials employing an experimental drug or product are performed. The Food and Drug Administration (FDA) has promulgated stringent guidelines for the clinical evaluation of proposed contact lenses or accessory solutions, and a relatively cumbersome administrative procedure has been formulated to regulate investigators.[9] A proposed change of "reliable" gas permeable hard lens materials from Class III to Class I was supposed to create an environment more responsive to alternative methods of approval, but, unfortunately, such has not been the case.[10] Although lenses made of PMMA have been moved to Class II, the FDA quashed its proposal to deregulate gas permeable lens materials, and it is expected that soft lens materials will remain in Class III in the foreseeable future (a discussion of the classification of contact lens materials can be found in Chapter 8).

Despite these well-understood difficulties, which seemingly are an inherent aspect of contact lens trials, several dozen types of soft lenses now glut the market, and professional interest and investigations continue. The advent of extended wear lenses presages a new era in contact lens practice, one that will require further clinical investigation. Therefore, optometrists will continue to become involved in investigatory efforts, and doctors will continue to confront the legal problems that clinical trials present. The legal principle that haunts experimental studies is informed consent[11] (see Chapter 22). This legal doctrine requires a doctor who is performing experimental trials to acquire the consent of participating patients, after first explaining the various factors necessary to make the patient's decision an enlightened and voluntary one. Failure to comply with the law can create liability for the doctor.

An optometrist fitted a young patient with experimental flexible contact lenses and dispensed an experimental accessory solution. The patient suffered chemical burns to the corneas in both eyes due to the solution and sued the doctor for his injuries. The doctor had not explained to the young patient or to his parents the experimental nature of his work nor had he obtained written consent to perform such a study. The lawsuit was settled in favor of the patient.[12]

These cases are rare today, however, because lens manufacturers commonly supply investigators with written materials that are designed to elicit an informed consent. But consent forms do *not* always contain the minimum amount of information deemed to be legally necessary. The points that must be discussed by such materials are:

- Purpose of the investigation
- Procedures (including examination schedule)
- Risks to the patient
- Benefits to the patient
- Alternate therapy available
- Withdrawal policy

A sample Information Sheet containing the minimal requirements listed above is enclosed as Fig. 30.5.[13]

After the patient agrees to participate in the investigation, the Informed Consent and Release should be signed. This document summarizes the consent being given and is signed by the patient and the investigator. If a minor is being asked to participate in clinical trials, then the child's parents or guardian should be included in all explanations and be required to sign as well. A copy of the Informed Consent and Release must be retained in the patient record. Otherwise, without the supporting documentation that the Informed Consent and Release represents, if there is a lawsuit it becomes a matter of one party's word against that of the other, which is not a very enviable position for a doctor. A sample Informed Consent and Release is included as Fig. 30.6.

Extended Wear Lenses

A potential problem for contact lens practitioners involves the current state of the art for extended wear lenses. At the moment, there have been no precedent-setting lawsuits, but there is evidence that *Pseudomonas* infections and other sources of corneal ulceration are more likely for extended wear patients.[14]

A young woman was fitted with extended wear lenses by an optometrist and told to return twenty-four hours post-dispensing for follow-up. The ex-

Information Sheet for ______ Contact Lens
Clinical Evaluation Program

PURPOSE: This program involves the clinical use of a new soft contact lens designed for those patients who have nondiseased eyes. The purpose of this study is to determine the usefulness of this new lens in terms of patient comfort, ease of handling the lens, visual acuity, and lens durability. If expectations are met, this lens design will provide comfort equal to those soft contact lenses presently available, but will provide better vision and durability. This means less frequent replacement of the lenses will be required, resulting in decreased cost to the patient. Also, the sterilizer used does not require distilled water as some of the other soft lenses do. This makes it easier to take proper care of the lenses without the added risk of electrical shock.

PROCEDURES: The procedures to be utilized involve the normal evaluations and established clinical techniques used in any contact lens fitting. The only variation from a noninvestigational lens involves the number of follow-up visits required.

Following the initial eye examination and lens fitting, the patient will be required to have check-ups at the following intervals from the dispensing date: (ATTACH SCHEDULE HERE)

This would complete the investigational program, but the patient should continue to have contact lens evaluations every six months. It should be pointed out that the above fitting and follow-up schedule is a minimum schedule; actual fitting may require a longer period of time.

RISKS: The risks involved in this study are no greater than those risks with soft contact lenses presently available. The patient will be provided with written instructions on the care and handling of ______ lenses. Provided the instructions are followed, there are no risks to the patient. If the instructions are not followed, the patient would be at risk to suffer transient eye irritation and pain.

BENEFITS: The patient benefits are a decreased cost in solutions needed and reduced lens replacement costs due to lens damage (compared to the soft lenses presently available).

ALTERNATE THERAPY: The patient does not have to participate in this study to obtain treatment. There are both soft lenses and hard lenses available.

WITHDRAWAL: Any patient participating in this study may withdraw at any time without fear of prejudice. In such an event, the patient would be treated with the best possible lenses presently available.

Figure 30.5. Sample Information Sheet for a Soft Contact Lens Clinical Evaluation Program. (Courtesy of the UAB School of Optometry)

amination revealed no problems and so she was rescheduled for reevaluation three days later. She did not return until a week had passed, and the optometrist's examination determined that the patient's lenses were unclean and that a small area of epithelial loss had developed in the cornea of one eye, causing the patient to complain of irritation in the eye. The optometrist prescribed Garamycin® drops and told the patient to return the next day, but the patient failed to keep the appointment and instead consulted a physician about a week later. The physician discovered a corneal ulcer about two to three millimeters in size, hospitalized the patient, and took cultures, which revealed that the patient suffered from a *Pseudomonas* infection. The patient sued the optometrist, alleging negligence in the management of her case.[15]

Informed consent requirements are important, and when prescribing extended wear lenses the clinician should prepare the patient for the increased responsibilities and risks of extended wear.[16] The clinician should also select the appropriate lenses; obtain an adequate lens fit; recommend the appropriate care system and regimen; institute a reasonable wearing schedule; and evaluate the patient with sufficient frequency to detect complications.[16]

Thus proper management of extended wear contact lens patients requires a more vigilant attitude on the part of optometrists. Because patients often do

_______ Contact Lens Informed Consent and Release

Name of Patient: ____________________
Investigation Project: ____________________
Investigator: ____________________

I, the undersigned patient (parent or guardian if patient is a minor), hereby attest that the Investigator, whose signature appears below, explained the following:

1. That I am being asked to voluntarily consent to participate in a clinical investigational project
2. The nature and purpose of the Investigation Project
3. That the lenses are prescribed and dispensed for investigational use only
4. That problems may arise in wearing lenses of this type
5. That I can withdraw from this Investigation Project at any time without prejudice to me.

I understand the above and consent to participate in the Investigation Project.

____________________ ____________________
Patient Date

____________________ ____________________
Signature of Parent or Guardian Date
if Patient is a Minor

I certify that I have defined and explained this study to the patient.

____________________ ____________________
Investigator Date

Figure 30.6. Sample Contact Lens Informed Consent and Release. (Courtesy of the UAB School of Optometry)

not comply with instructions, adequate follow-up of patients is desirable. Documentation allows optometrists to substantiate instructions and to increase patient awareness of the necessity for follow-up examinations. Patients need to be informed that the responsibility for care is a joint undertaking and that follow-up appointments are an integral part of the necessary management of extended wear cases. Of course, failure by the patient to keep scheduled follow-up examinations may absolve the doctor of liability should the patient suffer an injury related to lens wear that is due to this contributory negligence (see Chapter 19). Doctors may find that written agreements can improve patient compliance with instructions. A sample extended wear agreement and instruction sheet can be found in Figs. 30.7 and 30.8.

Although the specific provisions of these agreements will differ from practitioner to practitioner, there are certain matters that will probably be common to all, including the following:

1. Extended wear patients incur responsibilities that are more extensive than daily wear patients, and these responsibilities are a part of the written agreement.
2. Lens care procedures must be adhered to.
3. Periodic progress checks are a necessary aspect of extended wear.
4. Extended wear lens life is unpredictable.
5. A return to daily wear lenses may be necessary.
6. Certain symptoms will require clinical evaluation and, in some circumstances, cessation of extended wear.
7. The patient understands these responsibilities and agrees to abide by the requirements of the agreement.
8. The patient's dated signature represents agreement to all provisions of the contract.

The original agreement is retained in the record and a copy is given to the patient. Any noncompliance with the provisions of the contract should be noted in the record, particularly clinical matters such as changes in the wearing schedule or the lens care regimen, instructions to modify or discontinue extended wear, or warnings concerning complications or contraindications. Adequate record-keeping is of invaluable assistance if there is any legal dispute concerning the optometrist's management of the patient's case.

The Contact Lens Prescription

Ever since the Federal Trade Commission published its Eyeglasses I Rule, there has been more than a little

Follow-up Care Agreement for Extended
Wear Contact Lenses

With extended-wear contact lenses come additional care requirements. You must adhere to the recommended lens care procedures and you must return to this office for periodic progress evaluations.

We require the following progress evaluation schedule:

- After 24 hours of extended wear
- After 3 days of extended wear
- After 1 week of extended wear
- After each month of extended wear for the first 6 months
- After each 6-month period of extended wear

It is impossible to determine, in advance, whether you will become a successful user of extended-wear contact lenses. Certain personal, physiological, and environmental factors may adversely affect the success of extended-wear contact lenses and may necessitate a change in the recommended wearing schedule or termination of lens wear. These factors include:

- Poor lens hygiene
- Inability or unwillingness to return for follow-up visits
- History of allergic reactions
- Manual dexterity problems that would prevent periodic lens removal and cleaning
- Severe emotional stress
- Use of certain medications

If you experience discomfort, redness, extreme sensitivity to light, or blurry vision, remove your contact lenses at once and call this office. Do not ignore these symptoms.

If a lens accumulates deposits such as protein, calcium, nicotine, etc., that cannot be removed, that lens must be replaced. In rare instances a lens may dislodge from the eye and be lost or damaged, requiring a replacement. Lens life is unpredictable; frequent lens replacements should be expected.

Your cooperation is vital to your success with extended-wear contact lenses.

I understand the importance of periodic follow-up examinations and agree to keep scheduled appointments and follow the doctor's advice for continued safe extended wear. Noncompliance will be grounds for termination of my extended-wear program.

______________________	______________________	______________________
(Patient's signature)	(Date)	(Witness)

Figure 30.7. Sample Follow-up Care Agreement for Extended Wear Contact Lenses. (Courtesy of the UAB School of Optometry)

controversy generated by the ruling's applicability to contact lenses[17] (see Chapter 17). The most debated aspect of the rule has been the requirement that a doctor give to the patient a copy of the contact lens prescription at the conclusion of the examination. The two key elements are the prescription itself and the actual time at which it must be tendered to the patient. The FTC states that a prescription "must contain all information necessary for the patient to obtain the glasses or contact lenses from the dispenser of his choice."[18] If contact lenses are prescribed, however, the prescription must include "only those measurements and directions which would be included in a prescription for spectacle lenses. All prescriptions shall include all of the information specified by state law, if any."[19] To satisfy the rule (where the state law is silent), the prescription must contain only the following information:

- spherical power
- cylindrical power and axis (if any)
- prismatic power (if any)

Extended Wear Lens Care and Handling

Proper care is necessary for successful wear, normal lens life, and good eye health. You will be provided with products to clean, disinfect, and store your extended wear lenses. Use them as instructed.

Your lens cleaner is ______________________

Your lens disinfectant is ______________________

Your soaking solution is ______________________

Your rinsing solution is ______________________

Eyedrops to use before sleep and upon waking ______________________

NOTE: These products have been prescribed specifically for your lenses and eyes. Do not change or substitute brands unless you check with us first. Use of improper solutions may result in lens damage or eye irritation.

SPECIAL INSTRUCTIONS: ______________________

____

____

____

____

Please note that although certain brands of lenses may be FDA approved for 7, 14, or even 30 days of wear, the adaptability of your eyes is the key factor in determining wearing time. Trust us to recommend a schedule suited to your individual needs. And remember, like any medical device, contact lenses must be monitored on a regular basis. Professional follow-up care is the most important element in successful long-term lens wear.

IN THE BEGINNING IT IS NORMAL IF:

1) Your lenses itch or feel funny.
2) One lens is more noticeable than the other.
3) Your vision seems fuzzier than with glasses.
4) One eye sees better than the other.
5) You have trouble handling your lenses.

REMOVE AND DO NOT SLEEP IN YOUR LENSES IF:

1) You develop unusual pain or redness.
2) You develop unusually cloudy or foggy vision.
3) You experience a decrease in vision that does not clear up.
4) You suspect something is wrong.

WEARING SCHEDULE

______________________	Date ______________________
______________________	______________________
______________________	Clinician
______________________	______________________
______________________	Dispensed By
Next appointment: ______________________	______________________
	Patient

Figure 30.8. Sample Instructions for Extended Wear Lens Care and Handling. (© 1984 HMI, Vicksburg, MS. Reproduced with permission. All rights reserved.)

The prescription must be signed by the examining doctor and given to the patient at the conclusion of the examination.[20] Thus, a contact lens prescription needs to contain only these requirements, plus the examiner's signature, in order to satisfy the FTC rule. There are, however, some states that have more stringent requirements for a contact lens prescription, thereby superseding the FTC rule.[21] Furthermore, for liability reasons the prescription should be as complete as possible rather than merely list the minimum requirements needed to comply with the FTC rule (see Chapter 17).

The doctor must offer the prescription to the patient immediately after the examination is completed.[22] The time at which the contact lens examination is completed occurs when the optometrist can with confidence hand the patient a copy of the lens prescription and state that the patient can wear contact lenses and that the prescription tendered will provide the patient with proper visual acuity, comfort, and freedom from injury if it is correctly filled and if the patient follows the recommended cleaning and wearing instructions. Until the information from the actual fitting of the diagnostic contact lenses has been ascertained, and until the examination has been completed (including a trial wearing period), there is no obligation to provide the patient with a contact lens prescription.

If the optometrist gives the patient a copy of the prescription at the conclusion of the examination, there is no further obligation under the rule to comply with third party requests for prescription information. But there may be other statutory requirements that will compel the optometrist to release the requested information (see Chapter 17). If the patient requests that the prescription be sent to a third party, and the optometrist decides to comply, the best procedure is to require a written release from the patient before supplying the information.

Doctors should always write an expiration date on the prescription form, because an expiration date is an effective way to control potential contact lens abuse. The doctor may use his judgment in selecting an expiration date as long as the date is reasonable.[23]

If a patient loses the original prescription (given at the conclusion of the examination), under the FTC rule the doctor is under no duty to provide another copy, but if another prescription is to be given to the patient:

- the doctor may use the original expiration date
- the doctor may include contact lens information and instructions not written on the original prescription

Contact lens information that should be placed on the prescription includes the refractive data, lens parameters, lens manufacturer, and the notation that it is "for daily wear only," if in fact that is the case. Recording this information provides clinical and legal protection for both patient and practitioner (see Chapter 17).

Because federal or state laws may broaden the duty owed to release information to the patient, optometrists need to be familiar with the provisions applicable to their clinical setting (see Chapter 16).

Malpractice and Contact Lenses

It is only during the past few years that malpractice claims involving optometrists have resulted in substantial settlements or judgments. Claims involving contact lenses have constituted a growing percentage of these cases, with the number of claims amounting to about 10 percent of all malpractice cases in the early 1960s, rising to almost 40 percent of all cases by the early 1970s, and to nearly 50 percent of claims by the 1980s.[24] Although the majority of these claims have been due to the complications of daily wear lenses, the growing use of extended wear lenses can only be expected to add to the number of legal disputes. Because daily wear claims differ from those caused by extended wear lenses, we will consider the two types of lenses separately.

Daily Wear Lenses

Allegations of negligence in the fitting process and in the follow-up of complications are the most often-cited bases for claims involving daily wear lenses. Inadvertence is often the culprit in cases involving the fitting process.

A patient's soft contact lenses were rinsed in a solution that caused severe erosion of his corneas. Subsequently, it was discovered that the containers for both the contact lens saline solution and for the cleaning solution were the same color and were kept in the same area. The optometrist's technician had gotten them mixed up and had inadvertently given the patient the wrong one for his lenses, causing the damage to his eyes. The claim against the doctor was settled in favor of the patient.[25]

An important point illustrated by this case is that a doctor will be held liable for the negligence committed by an office assistant or optometric technician, due to the legal doctrine of *respondeat superior* ("let the master answer"). A doctor is well advised to review prevailing office procedures to ensure that misadventure and mistake are not the unwelcome invitees of current conditions or practices. Supervision of employees who clean, dispense, or otherwise handle contact lenses is advisable.[26]

A patient who had been fitted with soft contact lenses by an optometrist visited the doctor's office complaining about her lenses. The optometrist was out of town, but one of his assistants (who worked with contact lens patients) cleaned and returned the lens to the patient. Three days later the patient, complaining of reduced acuity and ocular discomfort, was examined by the doctor and found to have a central corneal abrasion. Despite the doctor's best efforts, the patient suffered recurrent corneal erosion and a permanent loss of acuity. She sued the optometrist, alleging negligence on the part of the assistant. In awarding damages to the patient, the jury found the doctor liable for failure to directly supervise the duties of his assistant.[27]

Practitioners should also be aware of the potential for large claims based on allegations of misdiagnosis.

A 20-year-old patient was fitted for contact lenses by two ophthalmologists. During the next nine years she was examined on numerous occasions by the doctors, but her intraocular pressure was never tested. When her IOP was finally taken and her visual fields measured, she was found to have open-angle glaucoma, with her field of vision reduced to ten degrees. She sued the physicians for malpractice, and they defended on the basis that the reasonable and ordinary standards of ophthalmology did not require routine testing for glaucoma in patients under forty years of age, due to the low incidence of glaucoma in that age group (1 in 25,000). The state supreme court held that the standards of the profession were too low to adequately protect the patient from malpractice and ruled against the defendant doctors.[28]

It is advisable to examine the ocular health of all contact lens patients prior to initiating contact lens fitting procedures. In particular, ophthalmoscopy, biomicroscopy, tonometry, and visual fields would seem to be an advisable aspect of every new patient's contact lens prefitting workup. Otherwise, the practitioner increases the risk that he will not detect a problem that may later result in a lawsuit alleging negligence for failure to diagnose ocular pathology.

Extended Wear Lenses

The development of extended wear lenses creates new opportunities for contact lens malpractice claims, in which the patient and the doctor are at odds over the instructions given for appropriate wear and maintenance of the lenses.[29] Follow-up and recall instructions, especially in states where there are comparative negligence statutes, are a necessary aspect of patient care. Proper recordkeeping is most important when managing patients who fail to keep appointments, tend to abuse their lenses, or disregard instructions concerning the appropriate cleaning or disinfecting regimen to follow. Clinicians should recognize that extended wear patients face risks that are different from patients who wear daily wear lenses.

A young woman was fitted with extended wear lenses by an optometrist. On the first night that she slept with the lenses in, she awoke at 3 A.M. with pain in her left eye. Although she removed the lens, the pain persisted, and so she returned to the optometrist later that day for examination. He found that she had suffered a corneal abrasion, and when her symptoms persisted he referred her to an ophthalmologist the following day. Despite the ophthalmologist's efforts, she continued to experience pain and after a week had to be hospitalized. A culture of her ulcer found that it was infected with *Pseudomonas aeruginosa*. She ultimately brought suit against the optometrist and the ophthalmologist, alleging that they were negligent in the management of her case.[30]

Optometrists should comply with the requirements of the doctrine of informed consent in communicating with extended wear patients. Lenses and solutions should be used properly; even the use of approved lenses or solutions in a nonapproved manner may result in legal difficulties.

An ophthalmologist prescribed gas-permeable contact lenses for a young patient. Although the lens material was approved for daily use only, the ophthalmologist prescribed the lenses for extended wear. The patient's mother subsequently discovered that the lens material had not been approved for use as prescribed, and although the patient had suffered no actual injury from the lenses, she filed a complaint with both the state board of medicine and the U.S. Food and Drug Administration.[31]

Failure to conform to manufacturer or governmental guidelines may be difficult to defend in light of patient injury and subsequent legal action. Optometrists should seek to use lenses and solutions appropriately, especially those intended for extended wear.

Monovision Lenses

A potential malpractice issue involves the prescribing of monovision lenses for presbyopic patients. Although this mode of correction reduces stereopsis and distance visual acuity, it is an accepted alternative to conventional fitting techniques and is not outside the standard of care. But patients who are fitted with monovision lenses must be adequately informed of the risks they face even when performing daily activities.[32]

In particular, activities that may create the risk of harm, such as operating a motor vehicle, participating in sports, and working around dangerous machinery deserve a word of warning. Patients should be advised to become accustomed to their lenses before attempting potentially dangerous activities while wearing them. Some activities are in fact sufficiently dangerous that the patient should be precluded from performing them while corrected by monovision (e.g., operating a motor vehicle at night). While the determination of those activities to be avoided by monovision patients is a matter of judgment, the obligation to discuss potential risks is not. The duty to warn is a legal requirement that must be observed by all clinicians.[33]

For activities that pose a significant risk of injury, alternative means of correction must be made available to the patient, such as lenses that correct the patient fully for distance (either contact lenses or spectacles). The wise clincian will document warnings and instructions in the patient record and will note those circumstances when alternative forms of correction are to be employed.

As with other aspects of contact lens practice, optometrists should be certain to adhere to established standards when prescribing contact lenses for special activities such as work, leisure activities, or sports.

Product Liability

Product liability law holds that if a product is so ill-designed or ill-constructed that it injures a consumer while the product is being used for its customary and intended purpose, then its designer, manufacturer, or seller (a category that may include optometrists) should, as a matter of law, bear the legal consequences for the injury (see Chapters 21 and 27). Unlike malpractice law, negligence is not the key issue. Instead, the product must be shown to be defective (unreasonably dangerous for the purpose sold or unable to meet the reasonable expectation of an ordinary consumer as to its safety). If this can be established, then liability will be imposed. Although the major impact of product liability law is upon manufacturers, there have been numerous cases applying product liability law to optometrists who have dispensed defective spectacle lenses (see Chapter 27). To date, optometrists have not been held responsible under product liability theory for injuries caused by contact lenses.

A patient who was fitted for hard contact lenses by an optometrist employed by an optical chain suffered pain, discomfort and corneal scarring as a result of the poor lens fit. He sued under product liability law and was awarded $10,000, but on appeal it was held that there could be no liability where there was no claim that the lenses were defective in themselves and where the lenses were not a finished product offered to the general public in regular channels of trade. The appellate court reversed the judgment, thereby establishing that product liability theory could not be applied to contact lenses.[34]

This case is about two decades old and involved hard lenses only. With the advent of extended wear soft lenses, sold as a finished product out of stock, the opportunity for the application of product liability theory to the contact lens practitioner would appear to be more genuine.[35]

A 15-year-old boy purchased extended wear soft lenses from an optical shop, and after three weeks of wear "in compliance with the instructions given," one eye became red and painful due to a corneal ulcer. The boy sued the optical shop, its parent company, and the lens manufacturer, citing—among other causes of action—that the lenses were unreasonably dangerous and defective and would cause injury even if worn as the instructions directed. The lawsuit also alleged that advertising claiming the lenses were safe for thirty days of continuous wear created an unreasonable risk of injury without including a warning of the dangers of wearing lenses for this period of time.[36]

Product liability may become a future legal issue for contact lens specialists.

Notes

1. The importance of adequate follow-up has received much attention in the professional literature. Nowhere is this concept more noteworthy than in the management of extended wear contact lens patients. For a review, see Masden, T.L., and R.W., Everson, What We Now Know About Extended Wear Risks, *Review of Optometry*, vol. 120, no. 10, 1983, p. 69.
2. The forms used in this chapter are based on fitting agreements developed by the University of Alabama at Birmingham School of Optometry for the school's contact lens clinic. Although they may not be appropriate for a practitioner in private practice, they offer a starting point for the optometrist who wishes to design his own. See Classe, J., Contractual Considerations in Contact Lens Practice, *Journal of the American Optometric Association*, vol. 57, no. 3, 1986, pp. 220–226.
3. Broome, P.W., and J.G. Classe, Long Term Success in Contact Lens Wear, *Contact Lens Forum*, vol. 4, no. 9, 1979, pp. 15–18.
4. Prepaid service agreements must not be insurance in disguise and should emphasize services to the patient, with the opportunity to obtain replacement lenses or other materials at reduced cost being incidental to the services. For a discussion, see Bailey, N.J., The 'Service Contract' Debate, *Contact Lens Spectrum*, vol. 1, no. 10, 1986, pp. 17–21.
5. The author is grateful to Drs. C.L. McEachern, W.M. Cannon, and M.C. McClay of Columbia, South Carolina, for providing the author with information on the use of fitting and prepaid service agreements in contact lens practice and for sharing the agreements used in their office.
6. Minnesota, Washington, and Wisconsin. See Bailey, supra note 4.
7. Ibid.
8. Ibid.
9. All contact lenses except those made of polymethylmethacrylate (PMMA) are classified as Class III under the FDA classification plan for ophthalmic medical devices, which means that premarket approval must be obtained before the lenses can be sold to the public. The FDA's stance has been interpreted as being in favor of large contact lens manufacturers. See Guerrein, R.L. (editorial), *Review of Optometry*, vol. 121, no. 11, 1984, p. 15, and the accompanying article, Paperwork Jam Hinders FDA, p. 3.
10. In 1982 the FDA issued a proposal to reclassify gas permeable daily wear hard lens materials from Class III to Class I, but in 1984 the agency withdrew the proposal. See FDA Quashes Deregulation Effort, *Review of Optometry*, vol. 121, no. 2, 1984, p. 8.
11. See Harris, M.G., and R.E. Dister, Informed Consent in Contact Lens Practice, *Journal of the American Optometric Association*, vol. 58, no. 3, 1987, pp. 230–237.
12. Reported in the *AOA News*, June 15, 1976.
13. The author thanks Dr. Norman Leach, formerly of the University of Alabama at Birmingham School of Optometry faculty, for his assistance in developing this form and the consent and release agreement discussed in this section of the chapter.
14. Weissman, B.A., B.J. Mondino, T.H. Pettit, et al, Corneal Ulcers Associated with Extended Wear Soft Contact Lenses, *American Journal of Ophthalmology*, vol. 97, no. 4, 1984, pp. 476–481; Hassman, G. and J. Sugar, Corneal Ulcers in Patients with Cosmetic Extended Wear Contact Lenses, *Archives of Ophthalmology*, vol. 101, no. 10, 1983, pp. 1549–1550; Cohen, E.J., P.R. Laibson, J.J. Arentsen, et al, Corneal Ulcers Associated with Cosmetic Extended Wear Soft Contact Lenses, *Ophthalmology*, vol. 94, no. 2, 1987, pp. 109–114; Wilson, L.A., R.L. Schlitzer, and D.G. Ahearn, Pseudomonas Corneal Ulcers Associated with Soft Contact Lens Wear, *American Journal of Ophthalmology*, vol. 92, no. 4, 1981, pp. 546–554; Margolies, L.J., and M.J. Mannis, Dendritic Corneal Lesions Associated with Soft Contact Lens Wear, *Archives of Ophthalmology*, vol. 101, no. 10, 1983, pp. 1551–1553; Chalupa, E., H.A. Swarbrick, B.A. Holden, et al, Severe Corneal Infections Associated with Contact Lens Wear, *Ophthalmology*, vol. 94, no. 1, 1987, pp. 17–22; and Mondino, B.J., B.A. Weissman, M.D. Farb, et al, Corneal Ulcers Associated with Daily Wear and Extended Wear Contact Lenses, *American Journal of Ophthalmology*, vol. 102, no. 1, 1986, pp. 58–65.
15. Based on a personal communication with the author.
16. See Classe, J., Optometrist's Liability for Contact Lenses, *Southern Journal of Optometry*, vol. 4, no. 3, 1986, pp. 52–57; and Classe, supra note 2.
17. The emphasis on shopping for contact lenses has had deleterious effects on consumers naive enough to believe that even replacement lenses can be purchased at bargain rates. See Pavlichko, J.L., Contact Lenses By Mail—What Does The Law Say?, *Review of Optometry*, vol. 116, no. 12, 1978, p. 16; and The Sale of Contact Lenses through Pharmacies and Mail Order Businesses, *Bulletin from the Licensure and Regulation Committee of the American Optometric Association*, vol. 45, no. 97, June 16, 1987.
18. The FTC's Eyeglasses I Rule was promulgated in 1978 and can be found in 16 C.F.R. §456. For commentary on the rule, see Swallowing the FTC's Bitter Pill, *Review of Optometry*, vol. 115, no. 12, 1978, p. 41; and Classe, J., The Effects of FTC Rulings on the Practice of Optometry, *Southern Journal of Optometry*, vol. 21, no. 5, 1979, pp. 20–24.
19. This provision of the rule would have been relaxed if the FTC had adopted the prescription release requirements of Eyeglasses II. See *Ophthalmic Practice Rules, State Restrictions on Commercial Practice*, Federal Trade Commission, Washington, D.C., 1986.
20. Ibid.
21. Ibid. The states that have more stringent requirements for contact lens prescriptions are Alaska, Arizona, Idaho, Kansas, Maine, Ohio, and Texas. See Classe, J., Optometrist's Duty to Release Patient Informa-

tion, *Southern Journal of Optometry*, vol. 5, no. 1, 1987, pp. 9–15.

22. Ibid. The FTC's Eyeglasses II proposal clarifies the time element as to when the prescription must be offered to the patient, specifying "the completion of the contact lens fitting process."
23. Ibid. The FTC rule permits states and practitioners to establish expiration dates for prescriptions as long as they are reasonable.
24. See Scholles, J., Malpractice—Watch Your Step, *Review of Optometry*, vol. 123, no. 4, 1986, p. 26.
25. Reported in the *AOA News*, June 15, 1976.
26. See Classe, J., How Your Helper Can Help You Get Sued, *Optometric Management*, vol. 16, no. 11, 1980, pp. 61–65.
27. Based on a personal communication with the author.
28. *Helling v. Carey*, 83 Wash. 2d 514, 519 P.2d 981 (1974).
29. See Classe, J., and M.G. Harris, Liability and Extended Wear Contact Lenses, *Journal of the American Optometric Association*, vol. 58, no. 10, 1987, pp. 848–854.
30. *Beaman v. Schwartz*, 738 S.W. 2d 632 (Tenn. App. 1986); reported in *Bulletin from the Office of Counsel of the American Optometric Association*, vol. 45, no. 100, June 19, 1987.
31. See Classe, supra note 16.
32. For a description of the duty to warn, see Gold, A.R., Failure to Warn, *Journal of the American Optometric Association*, vol. 57, no. 4, 1986, pp. 317–319; and Classe, J., Optometrist's Duty to Warn of Vision Impairment, *Southern Journal of Optometry*, vol. 4, no. 1, 1986, pp. 66–69.
33. Ibid.
34. *Barbee v. Rogers*, 425 S.W.2d 342 (Tex. 1968).
35. See Classe and Harris, supra note 29.
36. The author is aware of lawsuits in New York and Wisconsin that allege that a patient was injured by an extended wear contact lens that was designed, manufactured, and sold "in such a way that the lenses were capable of causing injuries when used in the manner intended and for a purpose expected or in a reasonably foreseeable manner." The case cited here, from Wisconsin, is described in News Review: Patient Sues Sterling, B&L, *Review of Optometry*, vol. 122, no. 12, 1985, p. 3.

Chapter 31

Clinicolegal Problems in Binocular Vision Practice

He had but one eye, and the popular prejudice runs in favor of two.
—Charles Dickens, *Nicholas Nickleby*

Patient's Right to Binocular Vision Therapy
Informed Consent and Contractual Obligations
Professional Liability

Binocular vision practice inevitably causes interaction with several aspects of the law:

- Legal rights on the part of patients to receive binocular vision therapy
- The doctrine of informed consent, which requires doctor-patient communication prior to the institution of therapy
- The standard of care applicable to the diagnosis and management of binocular vision patients

In this chapter we will address these considerations and their influence on clinical practice.

Patient's Right to Binocular Vision Therapy

Although binocular vision therapy is an accepted application of optometric science, there exists occasional difficulty in obtaining this acceptance from certain entities outside optometry, particularly those entities involved in the reimbursement of vision-care services through third-party health benefit plans. Patient rights to receive these services have had to be vigorously fought for by members of the profession, a fight that has even involved the argument that vision therapy is not a service within the scope of practice of optometry.

Blue Cross/Blue Shield of Maryland instituted an internal review of its reimbursement procedures for optometrists providing vision therapy to insureds and ruled that such procedures would no longer be reimbursable because "vision therapy, to the extent that it involves treatment, is not within the optometrist's scope of practice." The basis for this ruling was a modification of the state optometry practice act, which Blue Cross/Blue Shield interpreted as prohibiting optometrists from treating conditions of the eye. Thereafter, optometrists were denied reimbursement for vision training. The State Board of Examiners in Optometry was petitioned for a declaratory ruling as to the scope of practice and, after a lengthy evaluation, held that vision therapy was within the practice of optometry. Consequently, Blue Cross/Blue Shield revised its policy and provided reimbursement for these services to optometrists.[1]

Under Title 7 of the Social Security Act,[2] however, vision-care services are available for assisting the severely handicapped. Under Part A (Comprehensive Services), vocational rehabilitation is available to patients "whose disabilities are so severe that they do not presently have the potential for employment but may benefit from vocational rehabilitation services which will enable them to live and function independently."[3] Vocational rehabilitation[4] covers a full scope of optometric services, including:

> Visual training, and the examination and services necessary for the prescription and provision of eyeglasses,

contact lenses, microscopic lenses, telescopic lenses, and other special visual aids, as prescribed by a physician skilled in diseases of the eye or by an optometrist, whichever the individual may select.[5]

Each state adopts a plan for vocational rehabilitation in order to qualify for federal funds. The plan is administered through local or state rehabilitation departments and on a case-by-case basis by rehabilitation counselors. Under certain circumstances, vision training may be required as an educationally related service for the handicapped.

It was recommended by a school perceptual testing team that a handicapped child receive vision training, the cost of the training to be paid for by the school district. Upon district review it was held that vision training was not an educationally related service as determined by the state standards for educationally handicapped individuals. The parents of the child appealed to the state hearing board, which ruled that vision training was related to the child's educational program and had to be continued at school expense until it was no longer effective.[6]

Under the federal Education of the Handicapped Act,[7] optometrists may provide services for children with visual problems that interfere with the children's educability. The program includes "specific learning disabilities," which are defined as problems not primarily the result of sight but which have a physiological primary origin.[8] State and local educational agencies who have adopted plans under the federal program must assure that, among other things, a child with a suspected disability is evaluated by a multidisciplinary team and that vision is included where appropriate.[9] Parents must be involved in the process and give their consent before assessment begins. They also have the right to request an independent evaluation if they are dissatisfied with the school's assessment.[10]

In some instances, it may be appropriate to maintain that visual training must be performed under the direct supervision of an optometrist.

A school hearing officer ruled that vision training was required for a student and that the school was required to provide such training, either within the school setting or outside the school. The program was initiated at the school by an occupational therapist and the student's parents appealed, arguing that the training should be conducted under the direct supervision of an optometrist. The reviewing officer accepted the parent's argument, holding that due process had not been offered to the child and her parents since the appropriateness of the vision training program and the personnel chosen to administer it had not been established by the school.[11]

A detailed individualized education program must be written and followed for each handicapped child. The parent or school may request an optometrist to assist in drafting the program for a child with vision problems.[12]

A related issue involves the legal standards to be applied when there is a failure to diagnose learning disability. This is an unsettled part of both optometric and ophthalmological practice. Any claim that actually proceeds to trial will rely heavily on the opinion of experts as to what tests the ordinarily prudent eye doctor should perform to detect such an anomaly. Obviously, an important part of such a case would be a timely consultation with another practitioner, or, where necessary, referral to the proper professional for therapy. Optometrists are quite capable of assisting these types of patients, but physicians have historically been reluctant to refer their patients to optometrists for treatment. Failure to refer has been the subject of a lawsuit involving vision training.[13]

A student who was performing poorly in school was examined by two ophthalmologists, who did not detect a visual learning disability. The student was later examined by an optometrist and treated for the disability, and his performance at school improved. He sued the ophthalmologists, the Board of Education, and several school district employees and consultants for failing to identify and treat his visual learning disability, or to refer him to an optometrist. But the trial court held that there was no cause of action compensable under the state law and awarded no damages.[14]

Although this case has established no precedent, the publicity engendered by the trial has doubtless reduced the probability that like cases will be brought in the near future.[15]

Informed Consent and Contractual Obligations

About three decades ago, a California court held that a patient had to understand the procedure to which he or she had consented and the risks inherent in the procedure or the consent would be legally invalid.[16] In the years that have followed, both the courts and the legislatures have attempted to set standards that determine when consent is informed, but a clear-cut answer has not emerged. Instead, a gradual shift has taken place, from a standard based upon customary practice in the medical community to a standard that is based upon what a reasonable patient would consider material in order to make a decision (see Chapter 22 for a discussion).

The early informed consent cases limited the duty of the doctor to those disclosures that a reasonable practitioner would make under the same or similar circumstances, thereby defining the standard in terms of what professional colleagues would do. Over the course of years, however, a number of states have adopted a substantially different rule, focusing on the information necessary to inform an average, reasonable patient of the risks and outcomes of a proposed therapy. In these states, a practitioner can be held liable if the court finds that the patient did not receive the information necessary to reach an informed decision as to the treatment proposed. Although the degree of disclosure expected of a doctor depends on the provisions of state law, there is a commonality as to the types of items requiring disclosure.[17] These basic items are:

Diagnosis—The patient must be informed of the condition or problem diagnosed, but a diagnosis represents an inference from symptoms, test results, and other findings, and these indicators may be misleading. When significant reservations about the diagnosis exist, they should be candidly stated, and the steps leading to diagnosis, including the choice among alternative diagnostic techniques, should be discussed. Without proper testing, diagnosis of binocular vision anomalies can be an ambiguous exercise, and open communication with the patient as to results of testing and alternative techniques should be a regular part of any diagnostic workup.

Nature and Purpose of the Proposed Treatment—The explanation of the proposed treatment must be explained in nontechnical terms that the patient can reasonably be expected to understand. Where binocular vision therapy is concerned, this can be the most nettlesome aspect of informed consent.

Risks and Consequences of the Proposed Treatment—All risks do not have to be disclosed; those that are very remote and improbable can generally be omitted from the disclosure as not material to the patient's decision. The obligation to disclose extends only to risks that the doctor knows or reasonably should know are inherent in the proposed treatment. Binocular vision therapy poses few risks that are of the variety requiring extensive disclosure.

Probability of Successful Treatment—The doctor must make a truthful assessment of the likelihood that the proposed treatment will accomplish the intended result. In particular, a doctor must be careful when emphasizing positive projections that attempt to foster a posiive outlook as to the proposed therapy. While creating confidence is not to be discouraged, realism is essential to an informed consent. Thus the anticipated results of binocular vision therapy must not be unrealistically promoted by the doctor.

Feasible Treatment Alternatives—The patient must be aware of alternative forms of treatment in order to reach a truly informed decision. In making this disclosure, the doctor should consider those alternatives that would be generally acknowledged as feasible in the patient's case. Although the doctor is expected to counsel the patient and does not have to shrink from the use of persuasion, coercion should be avoided, and the patient's right to veto the proposed treatment presented. Doctors should be careful to discuss alternative forms of therapy in nontechnical terms.

Prognosis if Proposed Treatment Is Not Given—A last important consideration is a projection of what will happen without the proposed treatment. This is frequently used as a reason to guide the patient toward acceptance of the proposed treatment but should not be used to coerce the patient into acceptance of treatment that has a speculative prognosis. Only realistic expectations should be presented.

Failure to apply the principles of informed consent can lead to misunderstanding between doctor and patient and increase the risk of dissatisfaction. With regard to binocular vision therapy, most problems result from inadequate disclosures as to the nature or extent of the therapy and from disagreements as to the mode and cost of payments for the services rendered.[18] Therefore, it is in the best interest of both doctor and patient to ensure that these matters are described so that the risk of misunderstanding is minimized. The best means of accomplishing this is by using a written agreement.

A contract can achieve several goals:

- Explain the nature of the proposed therapy
- Describe patient obligations as participants within the program of therapy

The Visual Training Patient

It has been determined that you will benefit most by a program of visual training. The diagnosis of your visual problem and expected results of visual training have been discussed in full. The following is a summary of the significant points of this discussion.

A. Seeing is Learned
   1. Visual Training is a process of learning to see more efficiently.
   2. You must always be consciously aware that you are doing the learning—not us.
   3. A visual problem is *not* a disease; therefore, *we* cannot *cure* your problem. We can only guide you in the proper direction of learning. *You must do the learning.*
   4. The responsibility for the success of your case is yours—not ours.
   5. The two most important factors for adequate learning are:
      a) Motivation—You must have strong motivation; you must have the desire to learn.
      b) Practice Effect—A definite schedule must be strictly adhered to. Lack of adequate practice will hinder your progress.
   6. A successful visual training patient can expect to attain maximum visual achievement.

B. Materials: Single vision training lenses will be supplied and charged as necessary during the training period. In addition, supplementary training material and appropriate texts will be provided. There will be a $__ fee covering the cost of materials and lenses supplied. Preventive lenses necessary at the conclusion of visual training are dispensed at the patient's expense, as are any bifocals and other temporary lenses that may be required during visual training.

C. Visual Training Hours
   1. Winter Schedule:
      Tuesday, Wednesday, and Friday at 12:00
      Tuesday and Thursday at 3:30 and 4:30
      Wednesday and Friday at 3:00, 4:00, and 5:00
      Saturday at 9:00, 10:00, and 11:00
   2. Summer Schedule:
      Monday, Wednesday, and Friday at 9:00, 10:00, 11:00, 12:00, 3:00, 4:00, and 5:00

D. Schedule: Your schedule for Visual Training Sessions is:
   1. Orientation: ________ at 9:00 A.M.
   2. Office Training: ________
      a) The regular schedule for office visual training includes 12 sessions per month. If you miss an appointment, it is your responsibility to make this up.
      b) Orientation is considered the first two office training sessions.

E. Fees: Your fee per month will be:
   1. Multiple Visual Training Program
      a) Regular schedule: (12 office visits) $______
      b) Special schedule: (1) 8-session month $______;
         (2) 4-session month $______
   2. Individual Vision Development Guidance Program
      a) 8-session month $______ (grouped $______)
      b) 4-session month $______
   3. Strabismic Program $______
   4. Other: $____________________ Note: The monthly fee is customarily payable in advance

F. Progress Case Studies
   1. During vacations from active visual training, monthly progress examinations are scheduled. The fee for each is $______
   2. When active visual training and/or guidance is concluded, under ordinary circumstances, you will return for progress case studies as follows
      a) "one-month"—Fee $______
      b) "three-month"—Fee $______

c) "six-month"—Fee $______
d) "one-year"—and thereafter each year for complete visual analysis and programming of vision care for the purpose of maintenance, control and protection of the developed visual abilities. Regular annual reevaluation examination office visit fee prevails.

Insurance for Visual Training Patients

I. Coverage
   A. Presently, most (but not all) major medical health insurance policies cover visual training services.
   B. Fees for diagnostic examination and evaluation related to visual training are sometimes covered.
   C. Generally, visual training is not listed specifically as one of the services covered, but unless it is specifically *excluded*, it is usually covered.
   D. Since it is generally not listed specifically as a service covered by the policy, usually it is impossible to inquire in advance as to potential coverage by the insurance company and obtain a definite answer.
   E. Further, it has been our experience that since it is not listed as a specific covered service, claims for visual training services have been initially turned down and it has been the responsibility of the insured to go back to the company at a higher level until either the claim is acknowledged or appropriate acceptable reason is given for not honoring the claim.
      1. It must be noted that this is the responsibility of the insured, not ours.
      2. However, if any problem does arise, this should be brought to our attention so that we may offer you advice based upon past experience.
      3. State laws governing health care insurance exist that specifically protect the rights of the citizens of a state relative to coverage.
      4. If visual training is specifically excluded, this is a legal limitation of the policy and the patient should not expect coverage.

II. Procedure
   A. The insured will submit to the office an appropriate claim form.
   B. Following the first month of visual training, the claim form will be filled out and returned to the patient to be submitted; if the insured wishes the office to submit the form directly to the insurance company, *include an addressed and stamped envelope.*
   C. If the claim is honored, thereafter, each month, included in the monthly statement, will be an insurance receipt covering the past month's visual training that is to be submitted to the insurance company; there will be no need for us to fill out an additional company form.
   D. On the initial claim form and on the insurance receipts sent you monthly thereafter, we shall list all scheduled office visits (cancelled or not); as always, you will receive make-up sessions for cancelled visits but no insurance receipts for make-up sessions since this will have already been paid by the company.

III. Fees Paid
   A. Visual training is billed in advance and customarily is payable monthly in advance by the patient upon receipt of our statement.
   B. Insurance companies will pay the claim upon receipt of the claim form or monthly insurance receipt *to the insured, not to us, since you have paid us in advance.*
   C. It is NOT the policy of this office to accept payments from the insurance company— *you pay us, the insurance company reimburses you.*
   D. An insurance form will NOT be filled out and submitted unless payment is up to date.

Figure 31.1. Sample Visual Training Contract and Explanation of Insurance Policy. (Courtesy of Drs. R.A. Kraskin, J.D. Myers, and J.L. Kraskin)

- Determine cost and payment policy for the therapy
- Assist the patient in understanding vision insurance provisions for therapy.

A sample contract[19] that illustrates these typical provisions is attached as Fig. 31.1.

Even if a patient's condition is amenable to training, there is still the question of motivation that must be explored before a training plan is instituted. A written agreement can help reinforce the necessity for dedication and conscientiousness on the part of the patient.

Since training often requires a number of patient visits, the written agreement can incorporate a schedule into its provisions, informing the patient of how often, when, and how long the training sessions will be. The agreement can also specify the nature and cost of any materials that will be required to be purchased or rented.

Perhaps the most important feature of a written agreement for training services is the opportunity it offers to classify the fees that the patient will be expected to pay. Since visual training is a long-term arrangement, the fees for diagnostic workup, in-office training, and progress reports can be summarized in a manner that reduces the chances of misunderstanding. Third-party insurance coverage can be explained as well.

Binocular vision training can be expected to remain a topic of controversy, and the diligent practitioner will make careful use of the written contract in order to educate the patient and reduce the opportunity for conflict. (A careful practitioner will also be certain that his training techniques are reasonable and necessary.) If home training is recommended, patient understanding and compliance with the recommended regimen can be a concern for the doctor. Again, using printed forms that describe the therapy can be a valuable means of ensuring patient compliance.

Written forms are an inexpensive way to document communications between doctor and patient and should be considered by any practitioner who utilizes vision therapy on either an in-office or at-home basis. Failure to communicate these basic requirements of therapy can—and has—led to doctor-patient conflicts before state boards of optometry and in the courts.

Professional Liability

An important aspect of binocular vision practice concerns liability for negligence. As in other areas of optometry, failure to conform to the standard of care in examination, diagnosis, or treatment can lead to liability for malpractice. The potential for liability is relatively limited because of the unique nature of the binocular vision system. In order for malpractice to be established, the patient must suffer some actual, physical injury.

Acquired anomalies of binocular vision that are of adult onset (e.g., muscle palsies, paresis, and strabismus) do not typically increase in degree of injury in the absence of therapeutic intervention (surgery, prism therapy, or muscle exercises).

Infantile binocular vision anomalies, or the onset of problems during the critical period (birth to around age six), may require diagnosis and management in order to ensure that there is no permanent functional loss. For example, infantile strabismus—in the absence of therapy—may lead to permanent loss of fusion due to amblyopia and suppression.[20]

A six-year-old patient was examined by an optometrist employed by an indigent clinic and found to have anisometropic amblyopia and esotropia of the right eye with best VA of 20/200. The optometrist prescribed glasses but made no effort to treat the amblyopia. The patient was seen almost two years later (at age eight) by another optometrist at the clinic, who also made no effort to treat the amblyopia, finding that the best corrected acuity in the eye was still 20/200. A year and a half later, the patient (who was two months short of his tenth birthday) was examined by a physician, who maintained that the optometrists should have employed amblyopia therapy (i.e., patching) during the period the child was six to nine years of age and that the child's acuity could have been improved to 20/40 with the appropriate therapy. The child subsequently sued the optometrists, alleging that they were negligent in failing to institute amblyopia therapy on a timely basis.[21]

Failure to diagnose and treat (or refer for treatment) may lead to damages that could be awarded on the basis of negligence. Despite this possibility, there are few instances in which allegations against optometrists have established liability. When liability has been awarded, the allegations have most frequently centered around misdiagnosis, followed by the improper therapeutic regimen.

An optometrist prescribed plus lenses for a young patient, but they gave him severe headaches, nausea, and a deep-seated pain in his eyes. His mother brought him back for reexamination, but the optometrist urged him to continue to wear the lenses. When the symptoms persisted, she took the youngster to an ophthalmologist, who dilated his pupils, performed a cycloplegic refraction, and prescribed a new pair of glasses. The youngster thereafter sued the optometrist for malpractice. At the trial the ophthalmologist testified that it was not possible to examine the patient's eyes without dilation and that the misprescribed glasses might retard the proper development of his eyes. The jury found the optometrist negligent.[22]

This case also illustrates the necessity of pharmaceutical use for diagnostic purposes (cycloplegic refraction in this instance) within optometry.

The greatest possibility for negligence does not arise out of misdiagnosis of conditions affecting binocular vision but rather out of failure to diagnose pathological conditions co-existing in patients suffering from binocular vision problems. Since these patients exhibit symptoms that can mask underlying pathology (e.g., reduced acuity, asthenopia, diplopia, and headaches), the pathological condition can go undiagnosed by the doctor, creating serious injury and substantial damages. Strabismus is one such binocular vision anomaly.

A military optometrist examined a 4-year-old child whose mother had noticed his eyes were crossing. The optometrist diagnosed accommodative esotropia and prescribed spectacle lenses but noted an old, inactive hemorrhage in the child's right eye. At a follow-up examination one month later, the mother reported that the child's eye was not crossing as frequently. The optometrist changed the prescription but noted that the reflex in the right eye was not good. He instructed the mother to bring the child back in four months, but it was six months before the next examination was performed, at which time the doctor found the acuity in the eye to be limited to light perception. The child was referred to an ophthalmologist and was eventually examined by a number of physicians, many of whom disagreed as to the cause of the child's vision loss. The eye had to be enucleated, and the optometrist was sued for misdiagnosis and failure to refer in a timely fashion. The trial court awarded $250,000 in damages to the child.[23]

Reduced visual acuity is another condition that can mask underlying pathology.

A patient was examined by an optometrist and found to have reduced visual acuity that was believed to be due to refractive amblyopia. The patient was referred to another optometrist for evaluation, and his examination found that there was a significant amount of corneal astigmatism present, with best corrected visual acuity being 20/60. He commented that the patient "appears to have lenticular complications. No pathology front or back of eye. Ks are not changed. Might try anterior toric lens to correct," and returned the patient to the referring optometrist. Five months later the patient complained of double vision, and three months afterwards he was unable to count fingers at two feet, at which time it was found that he was suffering from a pituitary adenoma that was compressing the optic nerve. Suit was instituted against the optometrists for failure to diagnose the tumor and refer the patient to a specialist for treatment.[24]

When assessing patients for complaints related to binocular vision problems, it is necessary to perform a thorough health examination so as to rule out the possibility of occult or co-existing pathology. Periodic eye health examinations should be conducted on patients who are being treated on a long-term basis for binocular vision problems.

If pathology is detected and referral is necessary, the referral should be documented in the patient record. The best method to employ in making referrals is to contact the doctor to whom the patient is being referred, schedule the patient's appointment, and note the date, time, and purpose of the referral in the patient's record (see Chapter 16).

Notes

1. Maryland Board of Examiners in Optometry Declaratory Ruling re: Scope of Practice of an Optometrist-Vision Training and/or Vision Therapy and/or Orthoptics, Oct. 31, 1983.
2. Rehabilitation Act, 29 U.S.C. §§701 et seq.
3. See id. at §701.
4. Id. See 34 C.F.R. §361.1 for the definition of visual services.
5. See 45 C.F.R. §1361.1(dd).
6. *Gagne v. Concord Union School District*, State Department of Education hearing, May 1, 1981, reported in *Bulletin from the Office of Counsel of the American Optometric Association*, vol. 43, no. 46, Dec. 28, 1984.
7. Education of the Handicapped Act, 20 U.S.C. §§1400 et seq.
8. See 45 C.F.R. §121a.5 (b)(9).
9. See id. at §§121a.340 et seq. and 45 C.F.R. §§121.504 et seq.

10. See id. at §§121a.345 and 121a.504.
11. *In the Matter of Michelle Mills*, administrative hearing before the United School District #418 (1980), reported in *Bulletin From the Office of Counsel of the American Optometric Association*, vol. 43, no. 46, Dec. 28, 1984.
12. See 45 C.F.R. §§121a.340 et seq.
13. The author is grateful to Dr. Moses B. Gross of South Orange, N.J., for sharing information concerning the case that appears in this text.
14. Reported in the *News-Record*, Maplewood and South Orange, N.J., Oct. 9, 1975; and the *Star-Ledger*, Apr. 5, 20, 26, and 27, 1978.
15. See Swartwout, J.B., Optometry's Latest Malpractice Time Bomb!, *Optometric Management*, vol. 14, no. 6, 1978, pp. 69–73.
16. *Salgo v. Stanford University Board of Trustees*, 154 Cal. App. 2d 560, 317 P.2d 170 (1957).
17. For a review of disclosure requirements, see Rosoff, A.J., *Informed Consent: A Guide for Health Care Providers*, Aspen Systems, Rockville, Md., 1981, pp. 33–63.
18. See Luttjohann, L., Informed Consent and Release of Patient Records, *Kansas Optometric Journal*, vol. 51, no. 3, Mar./Apr. 1984.
19. The example contract used here is courtesy of Robert A. Kraskin, O.D., Jerry D. Myers, O.D., and Jeffrey L. Kraskin, O.D., of Washington, D.C.
20. Vereecken, E.P., and P. Brabant, Prognosis for Vision in Amblyopia After the Loss of the Good Eye, *Archives of Ophthalmology*, vol. 102, no. 2, 1984, pp. 220–224.
21. Based on a personal communication with the author.
22. *Kahn v. Shaw*, 65 Ga. App. 563, 16 S.E. 2d 99 (1941).
23. *Steele v. United States*, 463 F. Supp. 321 (D.C. Alas. 1978).
24. Based on a personal communication with the author.

Chapter 32

Clinicolegal Problems in Low Vision Practice

Eventually Monet painted nothing but the water lilies on his pond, finding more than sufficient inspiration in the patterns of their growth and movements. . . all these works seem like the records left by a man disappearing into his dreams—a dream of colour, and nothing but colour.

Monet once remarked that he would like to see the world as a blind man might if his vision were suddenly restored—as a brilliant play of colour on unrecognizable forms. This dissolving of the solidities of the world represents an unmistakable long-term tendency of Monet's art, though its final phase may owe something to the purely physical phenomenon of his failing sight. . . . Monet was suffering from a double cataract, and seemed doomed to total blindness. His old friend Clemenceau finally succeeded in convincing him that it was worth undergoing an operation; this was successful, and enabled him to work until the end of his life three years later—years devoted to the inexhaustible subject of water lilies.
—Nathaniel Harris, *The Impressionists*

The practitioner of optometry often must evaluate patients with severely reduced visual acuity or significantly restricted visual fields. In so doing, the optometrist incurs both clinical and legal obligations to these patients, for the proper management of low vision patients hinges upon the standard of care prevalent within the profession, which is described as that minimum degree of skill or learning necessary to render a reasonably thorough and accurate examination under the circumstances (see Chapter 19). Clinicians should always remember that their duty to the patient is to do what a reasonable optometrist would have done under the same or similar circumstances, and in some situations this will require referral of the patient to a specialist for such diagnosis or therapy as is appropriate. Optometrists who do not wish to manage low vision problems should keep in mind the obligation to refer and should identify competent practitioners to render these services just as certainly as they would practitioners skilled in the treatment of ocular disease.

Profound vision loss does not have to result in profound loss of enjoyment of life. Vision may be enhanced by a skillful practitioner knowledgeable in the use of low vision aids, and optometrists have a duty to monitor low vision patients to ensure that ocular health assessments are performed on a timely basis. Many progressive ocular diseases, once untreatable, are now amenable to therapy. Like the cataract-plagued painter, Claude Monet, whose visual impairment was an integral part of his art, and whose rehabilitation led to some of the best known paintings of the impressionist era, low vision patients require encouragement, skill, and assistance in order to deal with their impairment and to continue gainful lives. Optometrists offer the leading source of expertise to assist these patients.

Legal Obligations to Low Vision Patients

Low vision is a special application of optometric practice and reasonably may be expected to exist when there is an impairment of vision that prevents the patient from satisfactorily performing common visual tasks with a conventional optical correction. In terms of visual acuity, the most common criteria suggest that vision in the better eye should be 20/70 or less.[1] By comparison, the principal definition of legal blindness states that vision in the better eye should be 20/200 or less, or that the visual fields should be constricted to 20 degrees or less (see Chapter 15). The prevalence of those who suffer from low vision is about 1 percent, or 1,000 per 100,000, a total of approximately 4.7 million people nationally.[2] Legal blindness is conservatively estimated to be about 200 per 100,000, or .2 percent—about 500,000 persons nationally—with approximately 30,000 new cases per year.[3] Estimates of the most handicapped—those deemed to be legally blind—reveal that the great majority of these patients, about 70 or 80 percent, have some useful vision that would be likely to significantly gain from low vision care.[4]

The causes of visual impairment are most strongly associated with aging: macular disorders (mainly age-related macular degeneration), cataract, glaucoma, degenerative myopia and vascular retinopathies.[5] Many of these patients will have received regular vision care from optometrists only to have undergone a period of intensive ophthalmological attention for the pathological condition that caused the reduced acuity, followed by a period of no care after the possibilities for medical treatment have been exhausted and the patient has been informed that "no more can be done." Patients may have periodic ophthalmological assessments of ocular health, but rehabilitative treatment by optical or other means is typically totally neglected, an unfortunate eventuality that is especially true for the elderly. It may take years before the patient seizes the initiative and seeks attention from a knowledgable optometrist or low vision specialist. This failure to refer on the part of ophthalmologists has never been tested legally but offers interesting possibilities when the duty to refer for specialized treatment is considered.[6] Failure to refer for vision rehabilitation may in fact constitute a breach of the standard of care for which damages may be awarded. To date there have been no precedent-setting cases establishing the standard to be applied in such circumstances.

In any event, optometrists who do not consider themselves low vision practitioners should recognize that the great majority of low vision patients may benefit from rehabilitative treatment by optical or other means and that these patients should be referred to low vision specialists for evaluation. Failure to do so may not conform to the minimum standards expected of a reasonable optometrist under the circumstances.

Duty to Warn of Vision Impairment

Because low vision patients by definition suffer serious impairment of visual acuity or visual fields, optometrists have a particularly compelling duty to these patients to warn them of their visual impairment. Although, strictly speaking, we are concerned in low vision practice with severe vision loss, this duty is also present under conditions that affect vision to the extent that the conditions create a risk of injury. Failure to observe this duty can lead to liability.

Physicians have a legal duty to warn patients of conditions that create a risk of injury, and this duty has long been upheld by the courts when failure to warn of the condition is the proximate cause of an injury to the patient.[7] The typical case involves a medical condition that the patient does not realize will impair his or her operation of a motor vehicle or dangerous machinery and that causes the patient to lose control of the vehicle or to be involved in an accident with the machinery, resulting in injury to the patient. There is, however, a relatively recent series of cases that broaden the physician's liability to include third parties injured by the impaired patient.[8]

A diabetic patient with a long history of disease-related complications was hospitalized by two physicians during her third pregnancy. She was discharged from the hospital with her diabetes unstabilized, and at an office examination one week later, no fetal heart tones could be heard by the physicians. At a follow-up examination there were also no fetal heart tones discernible, and so the patient was advised to undergo surgery to have the dead fetus removed. The patient was instructed to drive to the hospital and while operating her car suffered a "diabetic attack," lost control of the vehicle, and struck a pedestrian standing by the side of the road. The injured pedestrian sued the patient and also the two physicians, alleging that the doctors had been negligent in failing to warn the patient not to drive in an irrational and uncontrolled diabetic condition. The doctors defended these allegations on the basis that they had no duty to the pedestrian that would subject them to an action for his injuries. The California Supreme Court held that the pedestrian stated a valid cause of action against the physicians.[9]

Other cases have involved a failure to warn the patient of the influence of drugs, especially those drugs whose effects could impair the patient's ability to operate a motor vehicle.

A patient with a long history of drug abuse was given Quaalude® by a physician who was treating her for depression. While under the influence of the drug, the patient lost control of her automobile and struck another vehicle, injuring its occupants. The patient was sued for negligence. During discovery proceedings, she alleged that she had not been warned by her physician of the hazards of operating a motor vehicle while under the influence of Quaalude®, and so the plantiff modified the complaint to include the doctor as a defendant as well. The physician answered that there was no doctor-patient relationship between himself and the injured motorists, and since he owed them no duty, there could be no responsibility on his part for their injuries. The Texas Court of Civil Appeals held that the injured motorists could maintain an action against the physician for damages.[10]

There have been other cases involving accidents caused by impaired driving ability in which the right of a third party to sue the physician has been recognized:

- A pedestrian struck by a motorist who suffered an epileptic seizure while operating his vehicle was found to state a cause of action against the motorist's physician.[11]
- A passenger on a bus who was injured when medication taken by the bus driver caused him to fall asleep and wreck the vehicle was found to be in the "general field of danger" caused by the failure of the physician to warn the bus driver not to drive, and thus was permitted to bring an action against the prescribing physician.[12]
- A company that employed a truck driver after a physician certified him as fit during a pre-employment physical was allowed to bring an indemnity action against the physician for damages paid by the company to third parties who were injured by the driver in an accident caused by the driver's "numerous physical disabilities."[13]

Although none of these cases involve impaired vision, it is not difficult to imagine circumstances under which an optometrist could become the defendant in such a suit. Clearly, patients whose vision no longer legally qualifies them to operate a motor vehicle should be warned not to drive, and a notation to this effect should be entered in the patient record. Patients who suffer some vision impairment (such as reduced acuity or restricted visual fields), who may be under the influence of an ophthalmic drug (mydriasis or cycloplegia being the usual problems), or who may have reduced binocularity (e.g., monovision contact lenses or one eye dilated or patched) are also persons to whom the duty to warn should be observed. In these instances it is advisable to note in the patient record that the appropriate warning has been given.

In no states are optometrists under a duty to report to the state government those persons whose vision no longer qualifies them to operate a motor vehicle, and an optometrist who volunteers to do so enters on legally untested waters.[14] But optometrists can discuss the matter fully with patients, and—when appropriate—with family members, and should do their best to secure a full understanding on the part of patients as to the hazards of continuing to operate a motor vehicle. Consequently, it is incumbent upon all optometrists to keep abreast of state requirements related to the operation of motor vehicles and to convey this information to the patient when it is in keeping with the standard of care expected within the profession.

States differ rather markedly in their determination of the minimum visual acuity, visual field, and other vision screening standards necessary to operate a motor vehicle. A study by the U.S. Department of Transportation (1980) compares these requirements in the various categories, but state statutes should be consulted to ensure that the data being cited to patients is in fact correct[15] (see Tables 32.1 and 32.2.).

Another aspect of vision and driving involves the use of bioptic telescopes. The U.S. Department of Transportation has ruled that "all driver license applicants, whether or not they wear bioptic lenses, should be provided the opportunity to take tests of vision, knowledge, and driving skill"; applicants who pass these tests may be issued licenses "subject to whatever reasonable restrictions on the privilege to drive that the state deems necessary."[16] Although only fourteen states currently have statutes recognizing the right of bioptic telescope wearers to have driver's licenses (Alaska, California, Idaho, Louisiana, Massachusetts, Maryland, Michigan, Maine, Missouri, Nevada, New York, South Dakota, Vermont, and Wyoming), applicants in all states should enjoy the opportunity to receive consideration on an individual basis for licensure as a bioptic

Table 32.1. Vision Screening Standards: United States, 1980

	Vision Screening Standards—Passenger Car/Pick-up Truck/Motorcycle/Motorscooter												
	Visual Acuity				Depth Perception	Field of Vision (in degrees)			Eye Coordination	Luminance Contrast	Dynamic Visual Acuity	Color Perception	Bioptics
	Both Eyes w/o Glasses	Both Eyes with Glasses	One Blind Eye w/o Glasses	One Blind Eye with Glasses		Left Eye	Right Eye	Both Eyes					
Alabama	20/70	20/70	20/60	20/60	—	—	—	—	—	—	—	—	—
Alaska	20/40*	20/40	20/40	20/40*	NR	NR	NR	NR	NR	NR	NR	NR	NR
Arizona	20/60	20/60	20/60	20/60	—	—	—	—	—	—	—	—	—
Arkansas	20/40	20/50	20/30	20/40	*	*	*	*	*	*	*	*	*
California	20/40	20/40	20/40*	20/40*	—	—	—	—	—	—	—	—	*
Colorado	20/40	20/40	20/40	20/40	*	*	*	*	*	*	*	—	*
Connecticut	20/40	20/40	20/30	20/30	NR	NR	NR	NR	NR	NR	NR	NR	NR
Delaware	20/40	20/40	20/40	20/40	—	—	—	—	—	—	—	—	—
District of Columbia	20/40	20/40	20/40	20/40	—	—	—	130	—	—	—	R,G	—
Florida	20/70	20/70	20/40	20/40	—	—	—	—	—	—	—	—	—
Georgia	20/60	20/60	20/60	20/60	—	140	140	140	—	—	—	—	No*
Hawaii	20/40	20/40	20/40*	20/40*	Yes	70	70	140	Yes	—	—	R,G,A	*
Idaho	20/40*	20/40	20/40	20/40	NA	—	—	—	—	—	—	—	—
Illinois	20/40	20/40	20/40	20/40	—	—	—	—	—	—	—	—	—
Indiana	20/40	20/50	20/30	20/50	—	—	—	—	—	—	—	—	—
Iowa	NR	20/70	NR	20/70	—	—	—	—	—	—	—	—	NR
Kansas	20/40	20/40	20/30	20/30	—	NR	NR	NR	NR	NR	NR	NR	NR
Kentucky	20/45	20/60	20/45	20/33	—	—	—	—	—	—	—	—	—
Louisiana	20/40	20/40	20/40	20/40	—	—	—	—	—	—	—	—	—
Maine	20/40*	20/40*	20/40*	20/40*	NR	NR	NR	NR	NR	NR	NR	NR	NR
Maryland	20/70*	20/70*	20/70*	20/70*	NA*	70	70	140	—	—	—	—	—
Massachusetts	20/40	20/40	20/40*	20/40*	—	90	90	120	—	—	—	Yes	20/40
Michigan	20/40	20/40	20/40	20/40	—	70	70	140	NR	NR	NR	NR	NR
Minnesota	20/40	20/40	20/40*	20/40*	NR	NR	NR	NR	NR	NR	NR	NR	NR
Mississippi	20/40	20/40	20/30*	20/30*	*	60	60	120	—	—	—	*	—
Missouri	20/40	20/40	20/40	20/40	—	—	—	—	—	—	—	—	—
Montana	20/40	20/40	20/40	20/40	NA	NA	NA	140	NA	NA	NA	NA	NA
Nebraska	20/40	20/40	20/40*	20/40*	NR	70	70	—	NR	NR	NR	NR	NR
Nevada	20/40	20/40	20/30	20/30	—	—	—	—	—	—	—	—	—
New Hampshire	20/40	20/40	20/30	20/30	NR	NR	NR	NR	NR	NR	NR	NR	NR
New Jersey	20/50*	20/50*	20/50*	20/50*	*	*	*	—	—	—	—	R,G,A	20/50
New Mexico	20/40	20/40	NR	NR	NR	NR	NR	NR	NR	NR	NR	NR	NR
New York	20/40*	20/40*	20/40*	20/40*	—	—	—	—	—	—	—	—	—
North Carolina	20/40	20/50	20/29	20/33	—	—	—	70	—	—	—	Yes	—
North Dakota	20/40	20/40	20/40	20/40	—	—	—	—	—	—	—	—	—
Ohio	20/40	20/40	20/30*	20/30*	NR	NA	NR	NR	NR	NR	NR	Yes	NA
Oklahoma	20/40	20/60	20/30	20/50	*	*	*	*	*	NR	NR	*	NR
Oregon	20/40	20/40	20/40	20/40	*	—	—	110	*	—	—	*	—
Pennsylvania	20/40	20/60	20/40	20/60	—	—	—	—	—	—	—	—	—
Rhode Island	20/40*	20/40*	20/40*	20/40*	NR	NR	NR	NR	NR	NR	NR	NR	NR
South Carolina	*	*	*	*	*	*	*	*	*	*	*	*	*
South Dakota	20/40*	20/40*	20/40*	20/40*	—	—	—	—	—	—	—	—	—
Tennessee	*	*	*	*	*	*	*	*	*	*	*	*	*
Texas	20/40	20/50	20/25	20/50	NR	—	—	—	—	—	—	*	—
Utah	20/40	20/40	20/30	20/30	Yes	—	—	—	NR	NR	NR	Yes	NR
Vermont	20/40	20/40	20/40	20/40	*	60	60	120	*	—	—	—	—
Virginia	20/40*	20/40*	20/40*	20/40*	NA	100	100	100	NA	NA	NA	NA	*
Washington	20/40	20/40	20/40	20/40	—	—	—	140	—	—	—	R,G,A	NR
West Virginia	20/40	20/40	20/40	20/40	NA	NA	NA	NA	NA	NA	NA	NA	NA
Wisconsin	20/40	20/40	20/30	20/30	NR	70	70	140	—	—	—	—	*
Wyoming	20/40	20/40	20/40	20/40	*	—	—	—	—	—	—	*	—

Symbols/Abbreviations: * = see Table 32.2 for clarification; — = no standard; R,G,A = red, green, amber; NA = not applicable; NR = no response.

Source: *Comparative Data, State and Provincial Licensing Systems*, U.S. Department of Transportation, Washington, D.C., 1980, pp. 17–20.

Table 32.2. Explanation of Vision Screening Standards

State	Explanation
Alaska	Applicants for school bus licenses must have 20/30 to 20/200 both eyes without spectacles; 20/30 to 20/20 both eyes with spectacles.
Arkansas	Examiner's judgment.
California	Applicants who are monocular may not operate Class 1 or 2 vehicles transporting passengers or materials requiring placards or markings on vehicle. Applicants using bioptic or telescopic lenses are given a special test by a driver improvement analyst.
Colorado	Depth and color perception tests given, not standard; other tests not given.
Georgia	Bioptics not permitted for bus/ truck/tractor-trailer license.
Hawaii	Applicants who are monocular or who use bioptics cannot obtain school bus/bus/truck/tractor-trailer license.
Idaho	At least 20/40 in one eye without spectacles; 20/40 in sighted eye with or without spectacles.
Kentucky	Telebioptic lenses not allowed.
Maine	Applicant must have vision in both eyes; 20/40 in one eye, 20/60 in the other eye for school bus/truck/tractor-trailer license.
Maryland	Applicant for passenger car/pickup truck/motorcycle/motorscooter license referred to a vision specialist for failure to meet 20/40 in each eye. For an unrestricted license, applicant must have at least 20/40 in each eye, at least 140 degree field of vision, and have binocular vision.
Massachusetts	Applicants who are monocular are not eligible for school bus licenses.
Minnesota	Applicants who are monocular are not eligible for school bus licenses.
Mississippi	First-time applicants for passenger car/pickup truck/motorcycle/ motorscooter license given depth and color perception tests; no denials made, applicant advised. Monocular applicants or those who fail depth perception test denied a license for school bus/truck/tractor-trailer operation.
Nebraska	Monocular applicants denied school bus licenses; visual acuity standards indicated in chart are not applicable for bus/truck drivers.
New Jersey	Applicants who are monocular denied school bus licenses; for bus drivers, acuity must be at least 20/40 and field of vision 70 degrees in each eye.
New York	School bus and bus driver applicants have the same requirements as are listed in the chart.
Ohio	Monocular applicants denied school bus licenses.
Oklahoma	Depth and color perception, field of vision, and eye coordination tests given for information only; applicants cannot fail based on these tests. Luminance contrast test given to applicants for bus/truck/tractor-trailer licenses.
Oregon	Depth and color vision screened, no minimum standards. Eye coordination checked for lateral and vertical imbalance.
Rhode Island	Applicants for school bus licenses must be binocular and have acuity of 20/30 in one eye and 20/70 in the other.
South Carolina	Data not available; minimum vision standards implemented July 1, 1976.
South Dakota	No minimum visual acuity standard indicated for tractor-trailer applicants.
Tennessee	Operator and motorcycle licenses; 20/70 or better using both eyes, and a doctor's statement. Regular chauffeur: at least 20/50 or better using both eyes, and a doctor's statement. Special chauffeur: 20/40 in the better eye and better than 20/100 in the poorer eye with a doctor's statement that it is the best possible correction. Cannot be color-defective.
Texas	Color perception checked for school bus applicants.
Vermont	Depth perception not applicable; however, referral to eye specialists will be made for reduced depth perception or eye coordination.
Virginia	A license restricted to daylight only may be obtained with a minimum visual acuity of 20/70 except for classified licenses. Applicants receiving a classified license—except for motorcycles—must have 20/40 or better visual acuity in both eyes. Bioptics are not permitted.
Wisconsin	Bioptics are not allowed.
Wyoming	Depth perception and color vision are checked; no minimum standard.

Source: *Comparative Data, State and Provincial Licensing Systems*, U.S. Department of Transportation, Washington, D.C., 1980, pp. 17–20.

telescope user while operating motor vehicles.[17] Optometrists should be capable of advising low vision patients as to this opportunity and should ensure that patients desirous of using bioptic telescopes are examined and advised by a competent low vision practitioner.

Genetic Counseling

Although not strictly an aspect of low vision practice, genetic counseling is an application of optometry that is conveniently discussed as a conclusion to this chapter. Genetic counseling has become a specialized branch of medicine that is most commonly conducted in medical institutions, either by physicians or by persons trained specifically in genetics. Optometrists, however, have a considerable interest in this subject due to the large number of ocular problems in which heredity plays an important role. In some cases the optometrist will refer the patient to a medical specialist for specific diagnosis and counseling, but the responsibility for referral and for follow-up care will many times rest upon the optometrist, and for this reason an understanding of the genetic counseling process will be beneficial to all practitioners.

The most important objectives of genetic counseling are to prevent blindness in individual families and reduce the incidence of blindness due to genetic disease.[18] Counseling requires knowledge sufficient to enable the practitioner to explain the disease, its prognosis, and the statistical probability of its occurrence in future offspring. For pregnant patients, prenatal diagnosis, carrier screening (if possible), or both may be advisable. Failure to ensure that the patient is advised of these alternatives can lead to liability.[19]

Malpractice claims arising from negligent genetic counseling can, for our purposes, be considered as consisting of two categories: those alleging a failure to inform the prospective parents of the risks of having a genetically diseased child in a given pregnancy and those alleging that the parents have been informed of the risks involved but that the tests performed to determine the presence or absence of disease have not been performed adequately.[20] For optometrists, the greatest concern is the first category, failing to inform the patient of the risk of having a genetically diseased child. This issue has taken on greater importance with the advent of *Roe v. Wade*, the U.S. Supreme Court decision that gives a woman an unrestricted right to an abortion in the first trimester of pregnancy.[21] Legal duties of a genetic counselor include the following:

- A duty to advise the parents correctly about the risks of occurrence of the specific genetic disorder in question; recognizing the parents' ethnic background as well as their family's medical history (Thus, a doctor should advise a Jewish couple about the possibilities of Tay-Sachs disease, a black couple about sickle-cell anemia, and an Italian couple about thalassemia. Likewise, if any of the parents' relatives have given birth to children having genetic defects, this should be considered.)
- A duty to see that the results of the test are provided before the third trimester
- A duty to communicate all results of prenatal genetic studies to parents

Thus a counselor who is involved with a couple desiring a child should obtain a complete family history, with special focus being placed on any genetic disease in either the father's or mother's family. In addition, the age and ethnic background as well as any diseases afflicting the mother should be considered. If the information obtained indicates a higher than normal risk in the pregnancy, the counselor should advise the couple of the possible complications discerned as well as the availability of amniocentesis and other prenatal screening procedures. This information should be conveyed to the couple while an abortion is still available, with the extent of the information conveyed depending on the standard of care applicable within the jurisdiction.[22]

Optometrists may not consider genetic ocular problems to be commonly encountered clinical situations, but such is not the case. An overwhelming number of patients are affected with these problems. Some examples are listed below[23]:

- Albinism
- Cataracts
- Color vision defects
- Corneal dystrophies
- Dyslexia
- Glaucoma
- Hypertensive retinopathy
- Macular dystrophies
- Nystagmus
- Optic atrophy
- Refractive errors
- Retinitis pigmentosa

Under the appropriate circumstances, an optometrist may find that the standard of care requires counseling or referral to the appropriate specialist for counseling and that failure to do so can create the prospect of liability. Although to date there are no reported cases involving optometrists, as the standard of care within the profession evolves toward a more medical orientation the likelihood of such a case becomes greater.

Notes

1. Bailey, I.L., A Profile of the Low-Vision Population, *Optometric Monthly*, vol. 69, no. 2, 1978, pp. 137–145.
2. Ibid.
3. Ibid.
4. Ibid.
5. Ibid.
6. For a consideration of the duty to refer low vision patients, see Low Vision Referrals: A Moral Issue, *Optometric Management*, vol. 19, no. 6, 1983, p. 93.
7. For example cases, see *Whitfield v. Daniel Construction Co.*, 83 S.E.2d 460 (S.C. 1954); and *Welke v. Kuzilla*, 144 Mich. App. 245, 375 N.W.2d 403 (1985).
8. For a review of the physician's duty to warn, see Tennenhouse, D.J., The Physician's Duty to Warn: A New Twist, *Survey of Ophthalmology*, vol. 28, No. 4, 1984, p. 339. For application to optometrists, see Gold, A., Failure to Warn, *Journal of the American Optometric Association*, vol. 57, no. 4, 1986, pp. 317–318; and Classe, J., Optometrist's Duty to Warn of Vision Impairment, *Southern Journal of Optometry*, vol. 4, no. 1, 1986, pp. 65–69.
9. *Myers v. Quesenberry*, 144 Cal. App. 3d 888, 193 Cal. Rptr. 733 (1983).
10. *Gooden v. Tips*, 651 S.W.2d 364 (Tex. Civ. App. 1983).
11. *Freese v. Lemmon*, 210 N.W.2d 576 (Iowa 1973).
12. *Kaiser v. Suburban Transportation System*, 65 Wash. 2d 461, 398 P.2d 14 (1965).
13. *Wharton Transport Co., Inc. v. Bridges*, 606 S.W.2d 521 (Tenn. 1980).
14. For a discussion of the duty to report persons whose vision no longer qualifies them to drive, see Garfinkel, P.E., and R. Shlensky, Should You Be Required To Report Potentially Hazardous Drivers?, *Legal Aspects of Medical Practice*, vol. 8, no. 1, 1980, p. 17. In the author's home state of Alabama, there is no vision examination required after the driver obtains a driver's license. Renewals of the license may be obtained merely by the payment of a fee. Thus there is ample opportunity to encounter patients whose vision makes them no longer legally eligible to operate a motor vehicle. The State Department of Public Safety, recognizing this problem, in response to an inquiry by the author made the following statement: "In the event you encounter an individual whose eyesight could cause problems in safe driving, please bring this to our attention. A letter indicating this person's name, address and date of birth with a brief description of the problem will be sufficient. We will then cite this person to a re-examination. This information will be kept confidential and your name will not be available to the person cited." Similar attitudes on the part of law enforcement officials in other states can be expected.
15. *U.S. Department of Transportation, and American Association of Motor Vehicle Administrators, Comparative Data—State and Provincial Licensing Systems*, U.S. Government Printing Office, Washington, D.C., 1980.
16. A discussion of the controversy over the licensing of persons using bioptic telescopes can be found in U.S. Department of Transportation and American Association of Motor Vehicle Administrators, *Functional Aspects of Driver Impairment: A Guide for State Medical Advisory Boards*, U.S. Government Printing Office, Washington, D.C., 1980.
17. For a case report of how low vision patients may use bioptic telescopes, see Ketteher, D.K., E.B. Mehr, and M.J. Hirsch, Motor Vehicle Operation by a Patient with Low Vision: A Case Report, *American Journal of Optometry and Archives of American Academy of Optometry*, vol. 48, no. 9, 1971, pp. 773–776.
18. For a review of genetic counseling for optometrists, see Fatt, H.V., and J.R. Griffin, *Genetics for Primary Eye Care Practitioners*, Professional Press, Chicago, 1983, pp. 45–80.
19. See Schulman, R.M. Genetic Screening and the Law, *Medical Trial Technique Quarterly*, vol. 29, no. 1, 1983, pp. 295–303.
20. Ibid.
21. 410 U.S. 113, 93 S. Ct. 705 (1973).
22. See Rogers, T.D., Wrongful Life and Wrongful Birth: Medical Malpractice in Genetic Counseling and Prenatal Testing, *South Carolina Law Journal*, vol. 33, no. 1, 1981, pp. 713–757.
23. Fatt and Griffin, supra note 18, at 61–97.

PART NINE

THE OPTOMETRIST IN COURT

Chapter 33

Civil Procedure

"Dr. Radcliff, I'm an attorney," Mason said. "I'm trying to get certain facts. I want..."

The man was shaking his head even before Mason had finished the question. "Information about a patient or a customer I don't give out. No."

"But," Mason said, "this is information which may be important. It might mean that as a witness..."

"As a witness, yes. You are a lawyer, you know the law. I am only an optometrist, a jeweler and a watchmaker. I do not know law. But this I think I know. I think that as a witness you give me a paper and I come to court, then you put me on the witness stand, I take an oath to tell the truth and I tell the truth. Then I answer questions. Then the judge will tell me I have to answer questions. Now I do not answer questions. I do not have to. Do we understand each other?"

There was a smiling courtesy in the man's eyes but an inflexible something in his manner which was hard as a granite cliff.

"We understand each other. Thank you just the same," Mason said.

—Erle Stanley Gardner, *The Case of the One-Eyed Witness.* (Reprinted with permission.)

Every optometrist faces the very good likelihood that, at one time or another, he will have to appear in court, either as plaintiff, defendant, witness, or juror.[1] Although the legal process is complex and can be confusing to the uninitiated, it is neither so large nor so complicated that an optometrist cannot grasp the basic substantive and procedural rules of court. A fundamental understanding of these rules is not just advantageous, it is necessary, especially if the optometrist enters the courtroom as a litigant. The following discussion focuses on several interrelated aspects of the civil trial process:

- Procedural conduct of a case
- Basic rules of evidence (especially those pertaining to expert witnesses)
- Depositions
- The optometrist as expert witness
- Courtroom testimony

The type of legal controversy with which an optometrist will most likely become involved is a civil lawsuit for damages. The usual case is one that is based either in contract or in tort; examples of such cases would be a dispute over the purchase price and mode of payment for an optometric practice (contract action) or a suit by a patient for damages arising out of alleged negligence on the part of the optometrist (tort action). The following sections describe the legal considerations involved in the determination of these kinds of cases, beginning with the procedural aspects of a case, which are initiation of the lawsuit, discovery, trial procedure, and appellate procedure.

Initiation of the Lawsuit

A civil case commences with the filing of the complaint.[2] The complaint is served on the defendant, along with a summons,[3] by the appropriate governmental official (the sheriff if the complaint is filed in a state circuit court or the U.S. Marshal if the complaint is filed in a federal district court) and is intended to notify the defendant of the nature of the claim being made against him and of the type of relief that is being demanded. The nature of the claim and the type of relief being sought depends on the party who is bringing the action; a state board of optometry would file an action seeking an injunction or based on *quo warranto*, whereas a patient alleging negligence on the part of a doctor would sue for damages.[4] No matter what relief is being sought, the complaint must contain the allegations that constitute the factual basis for the lawsuit and must state a cause of action for which relief can be granted.

The defendant is permitted a set period in which to answer the complaint. In answering the allegations of the complaint, the defendant can admit to some of the allegations and deny others. In order to deny liability for the plaintiff's injury, however, the defendant must deny the truth of some of the allegations (otherwise, there is no controversy). Proof of the disputed facts must be demanded by the defendant in the answer. Thereafter, the case will center around the proof offered by both parties to substantiate the disputed facts. Not surprisingly, the side that is the more believable usually sways the trier of fact (which can be either a judge or a jury) to grant a verdict in its favor.

The defendant may answer by claiming an affirmative defense such as the statute of limitations, *res judicata*, contributory negligence, or assumption of risk. These defenses bring new issues into the case. Since the statute of limitations and *res judicata* are strictly legal issues, they can be ruled on by the judge prior to trial. If the judge finds for the defendant on either issue, the case does not continue, because the plaintiff will not be permitted to bring a claim after the statute of limitations has run or the controversy has already been decided. In contrast, assumption of risk and contributory negligence are defenses that the defendant will have to prove at trial after the plaintiff puts on his case. In effect, they say "the plaintiff assumed the risk and so I am not responsible for his injury" and "even if I was negligent, the plaintiff was also negligent and therefore the plaintiff is not legally permitted to recover damages." In this eventuality it will be up to the trier of fact to determine if the defendant's proof of these defenses is more believable than the evidence offered in contravention by the plaintiff.

One additional option available to the defendant is the right to assert a claim against the plaintiff or another defendant or a nonparty. A claim by the defendant against the plaintiff is called a counterclaim (for example, a doctor counterclaims against a patient who is suing him for malpractice, asking the court to award him unpaid fees for professional services); a claim made by a defendant against another defendant is called a cross-claim (for example, in a product liability suit brought by a patient against both the doctor and the manufacturer for an injury received from a defective product, the doctor may file a cross claim against the manufacturer); a claim by the defendant against a nonparty is called a third-party claim (for example, a patient sues an optometric aide for negligence, and the aide files a third-party claim to bring her employer, the optometrist, into the case as a defendant). The effect of any of these claims is to broaden the issues to be adjudicated within the case.

If the defendant fails to answer the complaint within the allowed time, the plaintiff may move for a default judgment. Once granted by the court, it is as valid as a jury verdict. But most courts are quite liberal in permitting a defendant to have a default judgment set aside and to reopen the case as long as the motion to do so is filed within the allowable period of time.[5]

Once the defendant has answered the complaint, a long and extremely important period begins—the period that is preparatory to the trial or settlement of the case—known as the period of discovery.

Discovery

Discovery is a set of procedures and techniques used by the courts so that the opposing attorneys can assess the relative strengths and weaknesses of each other's cases. Discovery is intended to reduce the opportunity for concealment of pertinent facts and to eliminate surprise, thereby reducing the number of issues to be decided and minimizing artifice or cunning on the part of the litigants. There are several ways by which discovery can be conducted:

Oral or Written Depositions—Testimony taken under oath outside of court from a party or parties to a controversy, reduced to writing, authenticated, and intended for use at the trial of a case.

Written Interrogatories—Questions propounded of a party by the opposing party, requesting him to provide written answers that are given under oath.

Inspection or Production of Documents or Property—A physical inspection of documents or other property that is pertinent to the factual allegations of the lawsuit will be allowed; many times, the party asking for the inspection will also copy the documents for further examination later.

Physical and Mental Examinations—When the physical or mental condition of a party is in controversy, the adverse party may request that the party submit to examination by an expert selected either by the adverse party or by the court.

Requests for Admissions of Facts—Either party may request of the opposite party an admission as to the truth of statements, opinions of fact, or applications of law to facts that are germane to the case.

Each of these discovery techniques is available to plaintiffs or defendants, at their discretion. Which of them will be selected for use in a particular case depends on the nature and the seriousness of the controversy, for discovery is both time consuming and expensive. But discovery is inevitably necessary because it is the only way that a party can go to court completely prepared, knowing fully the factual basis for the adverse party's case. The most important discovery technique is the oral deposition (which is discussed separately in Chapter 34).

The process of discovery can stretch over a period of many months, and it is not unusual for a case to come to trial years after the occurrence of the incident that caused the case to be filed. This slow process of understanding the facts—both favorable and unfavorable—of a controversy allows the parties to review their positions and to arrive at a determination as to whether to proceed to court or to propose settlement of the matter. Settlement between the parties occurs in the overwhelming majority of cases and can result in the payment of damages to the plaintiff by the defendant, performance of some act by the defendant in favor of the plaintiff (or the performance of acts by both parties), or agreement to end the legal controversy without any further action by either party. There will be, however, a small percentage of cases in which agreement cannot be reached and these cases will be set for trial.

Prior to the trial most courts provide for a pretrial conference, which is used to acquaint the judge with the facts and legal issues of the case and which serves the additional function of settling many of the procedural matters expected to come up during the trial. Settlement of the case itself can also occur at the pretrial conference.

A case that is placed on the docket for trial can be specially set, which means that a specific time and place is established for the litigation of the case, or it can merely be placed on the trial docket, which means that it will be called only when the cases set before it are concluded.[6]

In preparing for trial the attorneys will meet with the party or parties that they represent and with the witnessess to be called in order to discuss the anticipated evidence and the trial procedure. Subpoenas[7] may be issued to assure that certain witnesses are in fact present at trial or that certain documents are brought to the courtroom with the witness. The quotation at the beginning of this chapter offers an illustration of a witness who requires a subpoena in order to be brought to court.

When the case is finally called for trial, the process becomes one of advocacy between opposing counsel, with the judge serving to rule on questions of law and to instruct the jury in the law for the purposes of evaluating the evidence, and the jury serving to resolve questions of fact. If neither party demands a trial by jury, the judge will serve as both the trier of law and the trier of fact; such an occasion is rare.

The trial process begins with the selection of the jury.

Trial Procedure

Prospective jurors undergo a process known as *voir dire*,[8] which is a period of questioning to determine prejudices and opinions. In some states the judge performs the questioning process; in others the attorneys may participate in or conduct the *voir dire* exclusively. After the questioning process is concluded, the attorneys alternately strike the prospective jurors until the appropriate number remains; the prospective jurors who are struck last serve as alternates. This jury is called a struck jury. The process may vary from state to state. An oath is then administered to the jurors and the trial begins.

Witnesses may be excluded from the courtroom during the trial on motion from attorneys for either party. If no such motion is made, witnesses may remain in the courtroom while testimony or arguments are being given. Since attorneys are by nature a cautious lot, witnesses are usually excluded so that they cannot hear the testimony of those who precede them.

The plaintiff's attorney begins the trial by presenting his opening statement to the jury, which is a description of the facts that the plaintiff expects the evidence will prove and an explanation of the cause of action that is being brought. The attorney for the defendant then presents his opening statement, which is a description of the facts that the defendant expects the evidence to prove and a denial that the defendant is legally responsible for the plaintiff's injuries. Following these opening arguments, the plaintiff presents his witnesses.

The plaintiff has the burden of proof in a civil case, which means that the plaintiff must produce evidence establishing the allegations of his complaint and that he must prove each disputed fact necessary to establish his claim by a preponderance of the evidence. For example, in a malpractice case, the plaintiff-patient must present his case first, during which he must offer proof that there was a breach of the standard of care owed the patient by the doctor; that the patient suffered an injury; and that the breach of the standard of care was the proximate cause of the injury. If the plaintiff fails to offer evidence of any of these legal elements, he has not met the burden of proof and the judge, upon proper motion, can direct a verdict in favor of the defendant.[9] Even if the plaintiff offers evidence on each of these elements, his evidence must carry the greater weight (a preponderance) compared to the evidence offered in defense by the defendant, in order for the jury to grant a verdict in his favor.

After the plaintiff closes his case (and if he is able to satisfy the evidentiary requirements just discussed), the defendant may—but does not have to—present a defense. For example, if the defendant has alleged contributory negligence in his answer to the complaint, he will offer evidence to this effect. In most cases, the defendant will take to the stand to assert his lack of culpability, but he does not have to. After the defendant has concluded his defense, the plaintiff may, by way of rebuttal, present evidence contradicting the proof offered by the defendant. Thereafter, the defendant may, by way of surrebutal, present facts in contradiction to the plaintiff's rebuttal. This exchange can continue as necessary until all the evidence is exhausted.

After the presentation of evidence is concluded, either attorney may make a motion for a directed verdict; however, if evidence has been presented by both parties in substantiation of the disputed facts in the case, the case will be allowed to go to the jury.[10] If the motion for a directed verdict is granted, the trial ends; if it is denied, the final arguments will be presented. The plaintiff is permitted to argue his case first, followed by the defendant, and finally the plaintiff is allowed to make the last remarks. The closing statements are used by counsel to review the evidence for the jury; in addition, the plaintiff sums up his damages while the defendant asserts his defenses.[11]

Upon the close of the final arguments, the judge instructs the jury in the applicable law, and the jury retires to consider its verdict. If the jury finds that the plaintiff's evidence has met the necessary burden, the verdict for damages will be in his favor; if not, the verdict will be for the defendant. In some jurisdictions, the jury does not have to reach a unanimous decision in order to render a verdict; the parties may agree by stipulation to a majority verdict as well. Once the verdict of the jury is read in court, the judge enters a judgment (a written order) according to the jury's decision. But the controversy is not always concluded by the verdict and judgment.

Appellate Procedure

Although the jury is the trier of fact and makes the ultimate decision as to liability, the trial judge has considerable discretion in granting posttrial motions for a new trial[12] or in directing a judgment that reverses the jury's verdict.[13] The trial judge may, upon proper motion by counsel, and where justice demands that he do so (i.e., where the judge feels that the jury's verdict was not supported by the evidence), grant either of these motions. In addition to these options, the parties may appeal the case to an appellate court by alleging a prejudicial error of law on the part of the judge.

If there is an appeal, the jury's decision as to the facts in the case will not constitute the reason for the appeal. Rather, it is the judge's decisions as to the law that form the basis for appeal. If the judge erroneously permitted evidence to be heard in the case, erroneously barred the presentation of evidence, or misstated the law when charging the jury at the conclusion of the trial, there is cause for appeal on the part of the injured party. The error must be substantial (i.e., have a prejudicial effect on the appellant's case) in order for the appellate court to order a new trial or reverse the judgment.[14] The legal issues raised by the appeal are ruled on by the appellate court, and, in so doing, the court creates a precedent for the point of law within that jurisdiction.[15] The appellate court may affirm the decision of the trial court, reverse the trial court and remand the case for re-trial, or reverse the trial court and award a judgment.[16] There is a hierarchy among appellate courts (see Chapter 7); in some states there is an inferior appellate court (such as a state court of appeals) from which one may appeal to the highest appellate court in the jurisdiction (usually called the supreme court of a state). The ultimate arbiter—and the only court that can set a law that affects every state and jurisdiction—is the U.S. Supreme Court. (It should be mentioned that the U.S. Supreme Court only hears appellate cases that involve a constitutional point of law; the cry "I'll appeal it all the way to the Supreme Court" is an empty one unless the litigant is arguing a constitutional issue that the nation's highest court is interested in deciding.)[17]

If a jury awards damages against a defendant, and the defendant appeals but loses the appeal, in many jurisdictions there is a penalty added to the damages that the defendant must pay in addition to the jury award.

Within this legal framework exists another set of rules and procedures that must be understood, those of the rules of evidence.

The Rules of Evidence

An optometrist is not expected to understand all the rules of evidence as a prerequisite to offering testimony in a case. But a basic knowledge of some of the fundamental considerations of this most technical aspect of trial law will enable the optometrist to avoid the usual pitfalls that await the unsuspecting witness and detract from testimony that otherwise could be complete and effective. An optometrist who must testify at either a deposition or a trial should be aware of the following general considerations.

The Firsthand Knowledge Rule

The rules of evidence are intended to ensure the fair and orderly presentation of facts that are material and relevant to the resolution of the legal controversy under consideration. In the ordinary instance, it is held that a witness will be allowed to testify only to facts that are within his own knowledge and perception. Thus, a witness is limited to those facts that he perceives through the use of his senses (e.g., sight, hearing, smell, touch, or taste) and is not allowed to testify as to what he thought, believed, inferred, or otherwise determined through the use of a mental operation[18]; opinions are not permitted (except during the testimony of experts, discussed in a subsequent chapter). The facts are to stand by themselves, and it is left for the jury to draw such inferences as are appropriate from the presentation of these facts. This rule of evidence is known as the firsthand knowledge rule, and it is the cornerstone of all legal testimony.

Materiality and Relevancy

Evidentiary rules are necessary to determine whether a given set of facts that are to be testified to by a witness are admissible. The first consideration is whether or not the evidence is material and relevant. In order to be material, the evidence must be offered to prove a proposition that is in issue; in order to be relevant, the evidence must have some reasonable relationship to the issues of the case or must tend to prove or disprove a material issue in such a way as to allow the jury to draw a logical inference concerning the issue for which the evidence is offered.[19] One of the trial judge's most important functions is to rule on the admissibility of evidence, and judges are given wide discretion in performing this task. Otherwise relevant evidence that the trial judge feels would unfairly prejudice the jury against one of the parties, unduly prolong the trial, raise unnecessary corollary issues, or whose probative value would be outweighed by some factor similar to the foregoing can be denied admission. For example, in a malpractice case an offer on the part of the plaintiff to introduce evidence that the defendant doctor had been sued for malpractice on a prior occasion would routinely be denied by the trial judge[20] because its effect would be to create an impression in the jury's mind that, since the doctor had been negligent before, he must have been negligent on this occasion as well.[21]

For this same reason, evidence offered by the defense of the doctor's reputation for skill or care is not admissible[22]; no matter how skillful or learned the defendant has been on prior occasions, it is his conduct on the occasion in question that is relevant to the controversy and evidence of his earlier skill and knowledge would not be allowed.

Another example applicable to malpractice cases involves the introduction of evidence that the defendant doctor is protected by professional liability insurance. Under most circumstances it will be held that, since such evidence is highly prejudicial to the defendant on the question of damages, it is not admissible.[23] (Furthermore, the majority view of the courts is that, during the discovery period, although a plaintiff may learn that the defendant is covered by liability insurance, the defendant does not have to divulge the amount or extent of coverage that he has.) Thus a doctor who "goes bare" (i.e., is not insured) will be found out if he does not volunteer this information to the opposing counsel (although most "bare" doctors do volunteer this information). It is doubtful that being uninsured has helped to avoid liability because plaintiff's attorneys have by and large indicated that they will not drop a suit merely because a doctor has no insurance.[24]

Hearsay

Since a necessary prerequisite to the admission of any evidence is the already discussed requirement that the facts must be within the knowledge and perception of the witness, an important body of law pertains to the problem of identifying hearsay evidence. Hearsay is defined as "a statement, other than one made by the declarant while testifying at the trial or hearing, offered in evidence to prove the truth of the matter asserted."[25] Hearsay evidence frequently consists of nothing more than a repetition of the words, writing, or conduct of another person, with this repetition by the witness of the other person's statement being used as an attempt to offer the words, writing, or conduct of the other person into evidence. Hearsay evidence is not admissible, however, because the statement that is being offered into evidence by the witness was not within the witness's personal knowledge or experience.[26]

Hearsay frequently crops up in connection with the testimony of doctors. For example, if a doctor examines a patient, the results of his examination are clearly admissible as evidence.[27] But if the patient, in describing his injury, says, "I hurt my neck when my car was hit from the rear," the repetition of this information in court by the doctor would be hearsay; the doctor might know that the patient has a neck injury, but he does not know that it occurred as the result of an automobile accident, and his statement to that effect would be hearsay. Thus most courts do not permit declarations by the patient to the doctor as to the cause of the condition being treated to be entered into evidence.[28] Of course, the patient may testify to the cause of the injury himself.

As with many rules of law, there are a number of exceptions to the general rule that hearsay will not be admitted. Several of these exceptions are applicable to optometric testimony.

Former Testimony Taken at a Hearing or in Another Action

The testimony of a witness that was recorded at another action (such as a trial or deposition) may be used if it was given under oath, the witness was subject to cross examination, there was identity of the parties and the issues, and the witness is no longer available to testify at the subsequent trial. For example, the deposition of an optometric aide who is no longer employed by the optometrist and who is no longer within the jurisdiction of the court could be used in evidence at the optometrist's trial. (The deposition would be read to the jurors by counsel, with one lawyer reading the questions and the other reading the answers.)

Admissions of a Party-Opponent

Statements made by an adverse party may be allowed into evidence if they were admissions, such as an expression of liability ("I'm sorry, it was all my fault"). Conduct can also be used as evidence (even silence in the face of an accusation) but offers to settle or compromise a legal dispute are not admissible because the courts wish to encourage parties to a legal action to settle their case without the time and expense of trial.

Declarations Against Interest

Like admissions, statements that are made in contravention to the pecuniary interests of the person making them are an exception to the hearsay rule. In order for the statement to be admissible, however, the person who made it must not be available to testify at the time of trial. An example would be an entry of "payment received" in a patient account book maintained by a doctor who is deceased and whose estate is suing to collect the account from the patient.

Spontaneous Declarations

These statements are one of the most widely applied exceptions to the hearsay rule; they are generally grouped into four categories: declarations of present bodily condition, declarations of present mental states and emotions, excited utterances, and declarations of present sense impressions. Statements concerning a present condition that are made by a patient to an optometrist constitute a very common exception; the rationale for their admission is that the courts assume a patient will be truthful in relating his condition to a doctor who is attempting to treat him.[29] For example, a patient's complaint, "I have a stabbing pain in my eye," would be admissible as a hearsay exception. Some courts will admit a patient's description of past symptoms or conditions that are related to a doctor for the purpose of diagnosis and treatment, as long as they pertain to the injury or illness for which the patient is obtaining treatment and are relevant to the legal issue under inquiry.[30] Therefore, a patient's comment, "I was told I had glaucoma a year ago," would be admissible if it pertained to the patient's current treatment by the doctor. Statements made to a doctor who is employed solely for the purpose of testifying on the patient's behalf are not admissible.[31] Nor is the testimony of a doctor who bases his opinion of a patient's condition exclusively on the findings of another doctor.[32]

Records of Past Recollection

This category of hearsay exceptions has wide applicability to optometric testimony. A doctor who testifies with the use of notes either will no longer remember the facts to which he is testifying (*past recollection recorded*) or will need to consult notes to refresh his recollection while testifying (*present memory refreshed*). Past recollection recorded requires that a proper foundation be established before the testimony will be admitted. To establish such a foundation, it must be shown that:

- the doctor recorded the information contemporaneously with the occurrence at a time when the information was fresh in his memory
- the information, if not recorded by him, was made in his presence, examined by him, and found to be correct
- the doctor lacks a present recollection of the information
- he had firsthand knowledge of the information that was recorded

Records qualified as past recollection recorded may be entered into evidence.[33]

Present memory refreshed permits a witness with an incomplete recollection to use notes made at the time of treatment in order to refresh his memory at the trial. The doctor recalls the occurrence because of the notes, which create an independent recollection of the information to be entered into evidence through the doctor's testimony. The notes may be inspected by the adverse party, used to cross-examine the doctor's memory, and even submitted to the jury.[34]

Regularly Kept Records

Regular entries in business books can be entered into evidence as an exception to the hearsay rule (although the admission of these records is now largely a matter of statutory law[35]). Records kept in the ordinary course of business are considered to be accurate and, in case of necessity, can be used as evidence of the matter recorded. Thus a wide range of records, including hospital records,[36] can qualify for admission as evidence at the time of trial.

Treatises and Professional Literature

Books, papers, treatises, and professional literature, when offered to prove the truth of the matters asserted in them, are hearsay.[37] Virtually all courts, however, allow such materials to be used for purposes of cross-examination of an expert.[38] The latitude allowed varies from state to state: some only allow the witness to be examined on a book or an article in the professional literature if he has relied on it specifically in forming an opinion[39]; others extend the rule to include the situation in which the expert admits to having relied on some general authority, although not the particular material to be used during questioning[40]; still other courts require the expert to acknowledge that he recognizes the material being used for examination as written by a recognized authority in the field[41]; and a few courts even allow an expert to be questioned on material that, although it is established as being written by a general authority in the field, was neither relied on by the expert in forming an opinion nor recognized by him as authoritative.[42] The significant difference between courts makes it necessary for an optometrist appearing in court as an expert witness to understand the law within his state or federal circuit, so that he can adequately prepare for trial.

These and other exceptions to the hearsay rule are important because the quality of an optometrist's testimony will depend on the admissibility of what he has to say. The problem of admissibility is particularly acute for the optometrist who serves as an expert witness because in most lawsuits the proof or disproof of liability often hinges on this witness's testimony.

Expert Testimony

Although the ordinary witness is prohibited from expressing an opinion and is limited to facts perceived through his senses, there is another category of witness to whom this limitation does not apply: the expert.[43] An expert witness is called to testify for the very purpose of expressing an opinion. For expert opinion to be admitted into evidence, the subject matter must be such that it is beyond the knowledge of the ordinary lay juror, and the expert witness must possess such knowledge, skill, or experience that his opinion will assist the jury in arriving at a decision.[44] The determination as to whether expert opinion will be admitted is left to the trial judge.[45]

The expert must be *qualified* before the trial judge will permit him to give opinion evidence. The process of qualification is performed at the outset of the expert's testimony and is a series of questions intended to establish that the expert possesses the requisite knowledge, skill, or experience related to the subject matter concerning which he will be offering his opinion. The types of questions asked of an expert relate to professional education, experience within the profession, and special skills or recognition (see Fig. 33.1 for a representative direct examination to establish that the expert is qualified to testify).

Occasionally, an opposing attorney will stipulate to the expert's qualifications without the necessity for this testimony.[46] On the other hand, if the opposing attorney wishes to test the competency of the expert, he can request permission from the judge to

Q. Please state your name and address.
A. James O'Dee, 123 Residence Street, Los Angeles, California.

Q. What is your profession?
A. I am an optometrist.

Q. Are you licensed to practice optometry within California?
A. Yes I am.

Q. When were you so licensed?
A. In 1979.

Q. Of what optometry school are you a graduate?
A. School of Optometry, the University of California, Berkeley.

Q. In what year did you graduate?
A. 1979.

Q. Did you perform a residency after graduation?
A. Yes I did.

Q. Where were you a resident?
A. The School of Optometry, University of Alabama at Birmingham.

Q. What was the specialty area of the residency?
A. Family practice optometry.

Q. Following completion of the residency, did you enter into private practice?
A. Yes, in Los Angeles, California.

Q. Where do you maintain an office?
A. 100 Main Street, Los Angeles.

Q. Are you a member of any optometric societies?
A. Yes, I am a member of the American Optometric Association, a fellow of the American Academy of Optometry, and I am also president of the California Optometric Association.

Q. Have you had occasion to teach in the field of your specialty?
A. Yes. I am an assistant clinical professor of optometry at the Southern California College of Optometry, and have been since 1986.

Q. Have you written and published any literature in the field of your specialty?
A. Yes, I have written articles that have appeared in the *Journal of the American Optometric Association*, the *American Journal of Optometry and Physiological Optics*, and the *Journal of Optometric Education*, and I have contributed a chapter to a textbook by a colleague, *The Clinical Practice of Optometry*.

Q. Approximately how many vision examinations have you performed on patients?
A. An estimate would be approximately 15,000.

Figure 33.1. Qualification of an Expert Optometric Witness

question the expert on *voir dire*, which is performed outside the presence of the jury. If the expert's qualifications are compromised by the attorney's inquiry, the trial judge may sustain an objection to the expert's testimony and prohibit him from offering opinion evidence.[47]

Optometrists may be qualified as experts and may express an opinion concerning matters that are within the scope of their training and experience.[48] In rendering this testimony, an optometrist usually cannot withhold information concerning the patient on the basis of the doctor-patient privilege because in most states this statutory obligation does not extend to optometrists (see Chapter 16). The particular types of cases in which optometric expert testimony may be useful are discussed in Chapter 35.

The opinion of an expert may be based on facts that he has acquired through his own observation or facts that he is asked to assume as being true. The second type of opinion testimony is presented through the use of a hypothetical question posed of an expert (discussed infra). Most courts do not permit an expert to base his opinion on the opinion of another expert or on facts that are reported by other witnesses; such an opinion would be founded on hearsay. Rather, there must be some evidentiary basis for the expert's opinion, founded either on his own observations or on a hypothetical situation that incorporates facts that are already in evidence.

Expert opinion does not have to be limited to the evaluation of a present condition. For example, the probable future consequences of an injury may be the subject of opinion testimony as long as the expert can state his opinion with reasonable medical certainty[49] and the testimony concerns reasonable probabilities[50] and not possible or speculative results.[51]

The majority of courts will not permit an expert to testify as to the ultimate fact to be determined by the jury.[52] An expert in most jurisdictions cannot state, "In my opinion Dr. X's conduct amounted to malpractice." The testimony must be phrased in terms of the standard of care, "In my opinion the described treatment was not within the exercise of ordinary care." An opinion that touches on the ultimate fact is said to invade the province of the jury. Since the answer to the question is to be settled by the jury—and not by the witnesses—for the expert to go further would be to answer the ultimate question of liability.

Q. Doctor, I'm going to ask you to assume that a 57-year-old woman complaining of blurred vision at distance and near and of bilateral ocular pain was examined by an optometrist located in Anytown, Oklahoma, or in a community similarly situated, in November of 1980. She has no previous history of ocular disease; her general health is good; she is taking no medications; and she has a pair of bifocal glasses that are five years old that she wears full-time. The results of your examination are as follows:

Refractive error −3.00 DS OD corrected to 20/20
−3.50 DS OS corrected to 20/20

Add +2.00 DS OD and OS, both eyes corrected to 20/20

Ophthalmoscopy is unremarkable

Intraocular pressures by applanation tonometry are 28 mm Hg OD and 27 mm Hg OS

Current spectacle prescription is
−2.50 DS OD with VA of 20/25
−3.00 DS OS with VA of 20/25

Do you have an opinion, based upon a reasonable degree of medical certainty, as to whether or not a reasonably prudent optometrist, based upon the facts that have been stated, would have performed further testing on this patient?

A. Yes, I have an opinion.

Q. What is that opinion?

A. In my opinion, the significant findings of 28 and 27 mm Hg during applanation tonometry, the bilateral pain, the patient's age, and the lengthy period since her last eye examination would cause a reasonably prudent optometrist to perform further testing on this patient.

Figure 33.2. Sample Hypothetical Questions Involving an Optometrist Expert

In any event, an expert's opinion is supposed to be advisory only, and the jury is free to give it whatever weight it wishes, including wholehearted acceptance or outright rejection.

The Hypothetical Question

Despite the majority rule, the expert often expresses an opinion that, hypothetically at least, does invade the province of the jury. Through the use of a masterful legal fiction known as the hypothetical question, the attorney describes a hypothetical situation (using the facts that have been testified to or entered into evidence)[53] and asks the expert to base his opinion on those facts (see Fig. 33.2 for an example hypothetical question). The expert is then able to express an opinion that, although it does not touch on the ultimate fact of the liability of defendant Dr. X, does touch on the ultimate fact of the liability of a hypothetical defendant Dr. X. Although thinly disguised as a hypothetical situation, the use of the same facts that have been introduced into evidence makes the analogy to the defendant clear to the jury. These questions are usually long and complicated, and whether a hypothetical question is proper and admissible is left to the discretion of the trial judge.

Despite the legal difficulties inherent in expert testimony, attorneys have increasingly relied on the opinion of experts, especially in professional liability cases (where a plaintiff can virtually never prevail without the supporting evidence of an expert). Malpractice claims require expert assessment on both sides, and the strength of the plaintiff's case and the theory of the defendant's defense usually hinge on the opinion of their respective experts. In the typical case, the attorneys learn these matters during discovery, principally through oral depositions. The oral deposition permits the attorneys to size up the opposition's expert and to probe his theory of the case. The determination to settle a case or to continue on to litigation often depends on the results of the deposition. Of course, in civil cases, the parties to the litigation will be deposed[54] as well as the experts and other important witnesses. The oral deposition may be conducted early in the progression of the case or it may be postponed until much later (when the witness's memory has faded). It is of such importance that it will be discussed as a separate chapter.

Notes

1. Although many states have enacted statutes that exempt professionals from jury service, there has been a trend in recent years to end all exemptions, even for attorneys, judges, politicians, and others intimately involved in the legal system itself. Therefore, although it is not discussed within this chapter, jury service is a very real possibility for the average optometrist. See Coblens, S., *Optometry and the Law*, American Optometric Association, St. Louis, 1976.
2. Of course, a considerable amount of preparation is required in order to file a lawsuit. For example, in a malpractice case the lawyer must interview the patient, examine the medical records, obtain an expert evaluation of the medical evidence, and determine the economic worth of the patient's claim for damages. The attorney bringing the legal action on behalf of the plaintiff may be paid a flat fee for his services or may receive payment based on the number of hours spent on the case (payment being based on an agreed-to hourly rate), or the attorney's fee may be a percentage of the award received by the plaintiff, a contingency fee. In personal injury actions, including malpractice cases, the usual arrangement is on a contingency basis. The attorney may advance all the costs of preparing the case for trial, trying the case, and appealing an adverse decision of the trial court. These amounts will be deducted from the plaintiff's award, of which the attorney receives a percentage as well, usually ranging from 25 to 50 percent (the percentage depending on the complexity of the case and the likelihood of victory). Defense attorneys are usually paid on an hours-worked basis; the hourly amount is scaled, being less for mundane matters such as legal research and higher for more difficult matters, such as taking a deposition or appearing in court.
3. A summons is a writ, usually directed to a specified official, requiring him to notify a named person that an action has been commenced against the person in the court from which the writ has been issued and demanding that the person appear at a specified time and place to answer the complaint in the action.
4. Before the days of the malpractice crisis in the mid-1970s, complaints alleging medical negligence commonly stated the amount of damages to which the plaintiff thought he was entitled. The amount of money demanded was contained in the so-called *ad damnum* clause. In the aftermath of the malpractice crisis, virtually every state struck the *ad damnum* clause or established a maximum amount of stated damages that could not be exceeded in the complaint. For an account of these and other legislative changes, see Chapman, S., and F. White, Are the New State Malpractice Laws Working to Protect You?, *Legal Aspects of Medical Practice*, vol. 8, no. 5, 1980, pp. 40–46; and Gold, A.R., Malpractice Reform, *Journal of the American Optometric Association*, vol. 58, no. 12, 1987, pp. 1000–1003.
5. Many default judgments are obtained against persons who have no intention of coming to court and who can be located only with great effort and skill. Once a judgment is obtained against such a person, the search

for justice has just begun; after the time in which the case can be reopened has passed, the problem becomes one of locating assets of the defendant that are subject to levy and execution (seizure and sale) to satisfy the judgment. There are many procedural matters that make this process time-consuming and frustrating.

6. Cases are numbered sequentially as they are called for trial; the case clerk of the court keeps track of all cases as they are disposed of by the courts and puts the attorneys whose cases are next on notice that they are about to be called. The attorneys, in turn, notify their parties and witnesses.
7. A *subpoena ad testificandum* is a command by the court for a witness to be present at a particular place and time for the purpose of giving testimony. A *subpoena duces tecum* commands the witness to bring documents that are in his possession or control to court and to produce them when called to testify.
8. *Voir dire* is French for "to see, to speak." As used in the courtroom, however, it means "to question," a form of examination permitted by the court to assess a witness's competency.
9. A directed verdict can come at the close of the plaintiff's case on motion by the defendant that the plaintiff has failed to offer evidence necessary to establish a *prima facie* case; in this event, since there is nothing to be decided by the jury (the elements of proof are strictly a legal matter), the defendant is entitled to a verdict in his favor as a matter of law. The award of such a directed verdict ends the trial.
10. For procedural reasons, such a motion may have to be made by counsel, even though counsel is certain that the judge will not grant it.
11. Since the *ad damnum* clause in malpractice litigation has been struck in virtually all states (in order to prohibit banner headlines or news stories that unfairly publicize large claims against doctors), the jury must rely on the plaintiff's proof of damages and the concluding arguments in order to determine the amount that should be awarded to the plaintiff so as to compensate him adequately for his injury.
12. Either party may make a motion for a new trial; the judge, as a condition to refusing the motion for a new trial, may require the plaintiff to agree to a reduction in the amount of damages awarded by the jury (called a *remittitur*) or may require the defendant to agree to an increase in the amount of damages awarded by the jury (called an *additur*).
13. A motion for a judgment notwithstanding the verdict, if upheld by the judge, causes a directed verdict to be entered for the party bringing the motion, thereby reversing the decision of the jury. By granting such a motion, the judge is saying, "I should not have let the case go to the jury for deliberation; rather, I should have granted the directed verdict at the conclusion of the presentation of the evidence." Thus, the party that had received a jury verdict in its favor now has lost the case and must appeal the judge's decision to an appellate court, hoping that the appellate court will reverse the trial court.
14. For a contemporary and entertaining discussion of the appellate process, as seen through the eyes of a well-known trial lawyer, read Bailey, F.L., *The Defense Never Rests*, Stein and Day, New York, 1971.
15. Adherence to the principle of *stare decisis*—"to abide by the rule of decided cases"—is a fundamental aspect of the Anglo-American legal system. A legal point, once decided, is to be adhered to in like cases unless social policy, legislative reform, or other compelling reasons dictate a change.
16. For an example of how an appellate court can reverse the decision of a trial court and award damages, see *Fairchild v. Brian*, 354 So. 2d 675 (1977), in which the Louisiana Court of Appeals reversed the dismissal of a suit against an optometrist and held that he was negligent, awarding $25,000 to the plaintiff.
17. The U.S. Supreme Court ultimately hears less than 1 percent of the cases that are appealed to the court. For an interesting account of the inner workings of the court and the court's decision rendering process, see Woodward, R., and S. Armstrong, *The Brethren*, Simon & Schuster, New York, 1979.
18. For example, a witness may testify, "I saw the defendant pick up the phone and heard him say, 'Hello, Martha,'" but the witness cannot testify, "The defendant got a call from Martha." There are certain judgmental matters, however, that are commonly allowed to be entered into evidence, such as "He was six feet tall" or "We were going fifty miles an hour," even though they are opinions and not matters of fact.
19. For a discussion of the relevancy of evidence, see *Am. Jur. Evidence*, vol. 20, §247.
20. See id. at §302 for a review of this issue.
21. Testimony given in a previous malpractice case, however, if it pertains to the same point that is disputed in the latter case, could be used by a plaintiff to impeach the doctor's testimony.
22. See, e.g., *Degnan v. Ransom*, 31 N.Y.S. 966 (1894); *Alexander v. Menefee*, 64 S.W. 855 (Ky. 1901); *Hackler v. Ingram*, 196 S.W. 279 (Tex. Civ. App. 1917); *Green v. Shaw*, 136 S.C. 56, 134 S.E. 226 (1926).
23. The controversial question of insurance against liability is discussed in Cleary, E.W. (ed.), *McCormick on Evidence*, 2d ed., West, St. Paul, Minn., 1972, pp. 479–483.
24. See, e.g., Carlova, J., Hell Yes, We'll Sue Doctors Who Go Bare!, *Medical Economics*, vol. 57, no. 8, Apr. 14, 1980, pp. 45–59; and Carlova, J., What Going Bare Means When the Patient Gets $200,000, *Medical Economics*, vol. 57, no. 18, Sept. 1, 1980, pp. 92–100.
25. *Federal Rules of Evidence* §801(c).
26. A discussion of some of the types of problems involving hearsay evidence that can crop up during the testimony of a medical expert can be found in Morris, R.C., and A.R. Moritz, *Doctor and Patient and the Law*, 5th ed., C.V. Mosby, St. Louis, 1976, pp. 249–254.
27. And this includes the subjective refraction, in which

the patient's responses determine the prescription for glasses. See *Hinds v. Johnson*, 347 P.2d 828 (Wash. 1959).

28. See, e.g., *Kramer v. John Hancock Mutual Life Ins. Co.*, 336 Mass. 465, 146 N.E.2d 357 (1957); *Mott v. Clark*, 146 A.2d 924 (R.I. 1958); *Brewer v. Henson*, 96 Ga. App. 501, 100 S.E.2d 661 (1957).
29. The question of privilege and its exceptions is described in *McCormick on Evidence*, supra note 23, at 212–228.
30. See *Peterson v. Richfield Plaza, Inc.*, 252 Minn. 215, 89 N.W.2d 712 (1958); *People v. Brown*, 49 Cal. 2d 577, 320 P.2d 5 (1958); *Gaines v. Schneider*, 323 S.W.2d 401 (Mo. App. 1959).
31. Declarations made to physicians employed only to testify in a case are described in the following annotations of the American Law Reports: 130 A.L.R. 977; 80 A.L.R. 1527; 67 A.L.R. 10; and 37 A.L.R. 3d 788, 816–826.
32. See *Muro v. Houston Fire & Gas Ins. Co.*, 329 S.W.2d 326 (Tex. Civ. App. 1959).
33. For a discussion, see *Am. Jur. Witnesses*, vol. 58, §§588–593.
34. See *McCormick on Evidence*, supra note 23, at 14–19.
35. Both the federal and the state courts have provided for using records as evidence. See The Commonwealth Fund Act, 28 U.S.C. §1732 and the Uniform Business Records as Evidence Act, enacted by the majority of states. The regularly kept records of professionals such as optometrists are included within the provisions of these statutes.
36. The admissibility of regularly kept records is discussed in *McCormick on Evidence*, supra note 23, at 717–734. Cases on this point include: *Globe Indemnity. Co. v. Reinhart*, 152 Md. 439, 137 A. 43 (1927); *Kirkpatrick v. Wells*, 319 Mo. 1040, 6 S.W.2d 591 (1928). See also *Edsall v. Rockland Paper Co.*, 38 Del. 495, 194 A. 115 (1937); *Tucker v. Tucker*, 222 Ala. 595, 133 So. 714 (1931); *Doane v. Doane*, 238 Mass. 106, 130 N.E. 484 (1921); *Radtke v. Taylor*, 105 Or. 559, 210 P. 863 (1922); *Dameron v. Harris*, 281 Mo. 247, 219 S.W. 954 (1920).
37. See *Am. Jur. Evidence*, vol. 20, §797, 22 C.J. §210.
38. See 60 A.L.R. 2d 77 for a discussion of the cross examination of experts through the use of treatises and professional literature.
39. See *McCormick on Evidence*, supra note 23, at 743–744.
40. Ibid
41. Ibid.
42. Ibid.
43. For an easy-to-read description of how an expert is qualified (with illustrative examples), see Morrill, A.E., *Trial Diplomacy*, Court Practice Foundation, Chicago, 1975, pp. 127–133.
44. The types of persons who are deemed to have special training or experience include optometrists, physicians, architects, accountants, plumbers, mechanics, and any other persons possessing specialized knowledge.
45. The decision of the trial judge will normally not be reversed unless it is clearly in contravention to law. Most disputes over this point occur in states where the locality rule remains in effect, which concerns the qualification of an expert to testify as to the standard of care expected of a practitioner within a community, neighborhood, or other limited geographical area. For a discussion, see Classe, J., *Zills v. Brown*: A New Standard for Doctors in Alabama?, *Alabama Trial Lawyers Journal*, vol. 8, no. 2, 1980, pp. 4–11.
46. Such occurrences are restricted to those instances in which an expert's qualifications are so outstanding that the opposing counsel would prefer that the jury not hear them out of concern that the jury will give the expert's testimony undue significance.
47. For an example case, see *People v. Singh*, 136 Cal. App. 233, 28 P.2d 416 (1934).
48. Cases involving optometrists as experts include *Bowser-Briggs v. Bennett*, 224 Tenn. 565, 458 S.W.2d 792 (1970); and *State of Oregon ex rel. Sisemore v. Standard Optical* Co, 188 P.2d 309 (1947).
49. See *Derrick v. St. Paul City Ry. Co.*, 252 Minn. 102, 89 N.W.2d 629 (1959).
50. See *American General Ins. Co. v. Florez*, 327 S.W.2d 643 (Tex. Civ. App. 1959).
51. See *Head v. Russell*, 307 S.W.2d 557 (Ky. 1958).
52. See *Johnston v. Order of United Commercial Travelers of America*, 182 Ark. 964, 39 S.W.2d 375 (1930); *De Groot v. Winter*, 261 Mich, 660, 247 N.W. 69 (1933); and *Miller v. Hooper*, 94 S.W.2d 230 (Tex. Civ. App. 1936).
53. Most courts hold that the facts contained in the hypothetical question should be substantially all those that relate to the issue on which the expert is giving his opinion. For an example case, see *Sanitary District of Chicago v. Industrial Commissioner*, 343 Ill. 236, 175 N.E. 372 (1931).
54. The Fifth Amendment, which bestows the privilege against self-incrimination upon witnesses, is applicable only to criminal offenses and thus has no applicability to civil matters, the details of which must be divulged to an examiner. A judge can order the witness to answer a question, turn over requested documents, or undergo a physical examination, all of which will be entered into evidence in the case.

Chapter 34

The Deposition

A good performance by a medical witness while giving a deposition can keep a case from ever going to trial. The plantiff's lawyer may see that his case isn't as good as he thought, or the defense lawyer may be reluctant to take on such a formidable witness before a judge and jury. Negotiations may then result in a settlement and again the medical witness is spared a time-consuming date in the courtroom.
—Jack E. Horsley, J.D., *Testifying in Court: The Advanced Course*

For the parties, the deposition and the trial are the most significant events of a lawsuit. Although motions filed by attorneys and arguments in favor of these motions can (and often do) profoundly affect the ultimate decision rendered in a case, these are matters outside the experience and assistance of the party bringing or defending the controversy. The giving of testimony, however, is a different matter, and a deposition is a vital means of obtaining testimony. The one being deposed, called the *deponent*, is questioned outside of court, under oath, before a stenographer who records the questions posed by the examining attorneys and the deponent's answers. The end result of the deposition is a typed transcript that is usable as evidence at the trial of the case.[1] The deposition is the most important form of discovery.[2] It allows for a full investigation of the controversy by fulfilling a number of important discovery objectives:

Discovery of Facts—Facts that cannot be obtained by investigation, from the client, or by other means can be obtained through the deposition; disputed facts can be corroborated, additional facts revealed, previously unknown witnesses identified, and important issues narrowed or clarified.

Evaluation of Witnesses—Witnesses are scrutinized and evaluated by the examining attorneys during the deposition process, with both the witnesses' demeanor and testimony being assessed in terms of their effect on the trial.

Preservation of Testimony—A witness who would be unavailable at the time of trial may be deposed and the transcript of his testimony thereby preserved for use later.

Admissions of Evidence—Examining attorneys will use the deposition to elicit factual admissions (or inadvertent misrepresentations) from witnesses, thereby "locking in" the witnesses' testimony (or misstatements) before trial. In particular, a witnesses' version of disputed facts can be closely questioned and his documentary evidence examined.

Impeachment—Since a deposition serves to preserve a witnesses' testimony, if a witness testifies at trial differently than at the deposition, the contradictory statement in the deposition can be used during the trial to reduce the witnesses' believability. Using prior inconsistent testimony to reduce the effectiveness of a witness at trial is termed impeachment.[3]

The effect of the deposition on the litigation process can be considerable.[4] Facts that were unknown prior to the deposition can have a significant influence on a litigant's decision to settle a dispute prior to trial. Of course, an unimpressive witness or ineffective testimony can have the reverse effect. Depositions are particularly useful when expert testimony is to be given in a case because liability and damages are the usual subjects testified to by experts, and both must be evaluated by the opposing attorneys before settlement can be discussed. Since the great majority of cases are settled before trial, in most instances the deposition is the only opportunity a litigant will have to offer his side of the dispute. For an expert witness, it will be his only chance to present his opinion of the facts. Therefore, the deposition must not be regarded as a preliminary matter of limited importance.

Key aspects of the deposition process are:

- Preparation
- The deposition procedure
- Examination by the opposing attorney
- Examination by the friendly attorney
- Review of the deposition transcript
- Use of the transcript for trial

Optometrists should be familiar with each of them.

Preparation

Attorneys usually hold a predeposition conference with deponents prior to the deposition date. The deponent should carefully prepare for this conference by reviewing the history of the incident that caused the lawsuit. Notes, letters, documents, or other evidence should be examined and brought to the conference for the benefit of the attorney. If there are key matters or questions that the deponent wishes to discuss with the attorney, he should write them down so that they will not be forgotten. As with trial testimony, the deponent should carefully review in his own mind the information that he expects to be questioned about and should rehearse those answers that are of the most significance.

The attorney may wish to conduct a dry run with the deponent, during which he poses the questions that he anticipates the opposing attorney will ask. This rehearsal permits the deponent to consider the substance and wording of his responses, thereby avoiding ambiguity and the opportunity for a misstatement of fact later.

In preparing the deponent, the attorney may review the answers given by the deponent to written interrogatories, the documents produced on request for the adverse party, or the results of a physical or mental examination. Although the review may seem to be tedious and time-consuming, it is the best way for a deponent to ensure that his version of the facts will be given a clear and thorough presentation.

Deposition Procedure

Deposition testimony is given under circumstances that are significantly different from those found at a trial. Generally, the deposition is a rather one-sided affair that favors the examining party because the deponent is obliged to answer all questions posed to him, including questions that could be inadmissible at trial.[5]

Since there is no judge present, the attorneys will have agreed prior to the initiation of questioning as to what objections must be made immediately and what objections will be reserved. The stipulations are intended to streamline the questioning process; the actual legal arguments over the admissibility of questions and answers will be conducted later, if there is a trial, before the judge.

The deposition may be taken anywhere. The usual location is the office of the examining counsel, but an expert witness is frequently examined in his own office. The setting is rather informal, with only the witness, the attorneys representing the parties, and a stenographer being present. The parties to the lawsuit may also attend the deposition, but usually they do not. If the attorneys know one another, a certain amount of conviviality may exist.

The examination process is initiated by the administration of the oath to the deponent by the stenographer. After the oath the opposing attorney questions the deponent, usually in considerable detail. During the examination process the attorney may introduce into evidence papers, notes, records, or other documents and may question the deponent concerning them. After the opposing attorney (or opposing attorneys if there is more than one opposing party) has concluded this direct examination the friendly attorney will be allowed to ask questions of the deponent. In the usual case, no questions are asked or the questions are limited to establishing a few key points. The opposing attorney can then pose further questions, followed by the friendly attorney, until each has concluded his examination. During the interrogation of the deponent, disputes may arise that require an off-the-record discussion. When comments are made off the record they are not recorded in the deposition transcript by the stenographer.

After the deposition is concluded, the deponent and the friendly attorney will usually discuss the results of the deposition, and the attorney will arrange to send the deponent a copy of the transcript so that he can review it for accuracy. After the transcript has been reviewed and any necessary corrections made, it is certified by the stenographer and the final copies are distributed.[6]

Examination by the Opposing Attorney

The first questions posed by the examining attorney may be intended to establish that the deponent understands the purpose of the deposition and the importance of the testimony that is to be taken. Thus if the deponent later gives contradictory testimony, he cannot resort to the plea that he did not understand the nature or significance of the deposition.

The tenor and substance of the examining attorney's questions will reveal his intent in posing a question: Broad questions that are intended to disclose new evidence will encourage rambling, far-reaching answers that the attorney hopes will lead to the discovery of new facts, whereas precise, specific questions are intended to produce succinct replies that the attorney can use against the deponent at trial. An examiner who is attempting to lock in a deponent's testimony will repeatedly ask, "Have you told us everything?" or "Did anything else occur?" These questions force the deponent to answer fully or to risk impeachment at trial. The examiner may ask leading questions, which are statements of fact that contain the answer and merely require an agreement from the deponent.[7] Such questions are an attempt to put words in the deponent's mouth through a yes or no response and must be carefully answered lest the wrong impression be created.[8] The attorney may ask a question in several different ways, either to ensure that the question receives a full response or to trap the deponent into making inconsistent statements. The sequence of questions will vary from examiner to examiner and from case to case. The questioning may proceed chronologically through the events of the lawsuit or may skip from point to point, delving into great detail at places and barely touching on some issues at all. There are certain pitfall questions, however, that usually crop up during the examination of an expert witness and that require careful responses.

Questions that Concern the Patient Records

The deponent should always review the entire patient record and should be familiar with the chronology of the doctor-patient relationship. In particular, the deponent should review the earliest entries concerning the facts that form the basis for the lawsuit.

Questions Concerning Communications with the Patient

The deponent should concentrate on such matters as what information the patient received, how it was communicated to the patient, why it was disclosed to the patient, and—of great importance in many cases—what was not communicated to the patient.

Questions about the Extent of Knowledge of the Treating Doctor

If the expert witness being deposed is the defendant in a professional liability case, the plaintiff's attorney will inquire into the particular situation that gave rise to the lawsuit. He will want to determine the knowledge of the doctor with regard to his diagnosis of the patient's condition, his understanding of the condition, why he ruled out other possible conditions, his treatment plan, his provisions for follow-up, and other pertinent issues. The deponent needs to answer these questions truthfully, but his answers should be to the point lest he educate the attorney or even go so far as to become the expert for the adverse party.[9] The deponent should try to avoid the use of treatises, texts, or other authorities to bolster his opinion because the attorney would be almost certain to question him about them in detail at trial. If testimony is later given in the courtroom before the jury, the introduction into evidence of supporting authorities is a less hazardous undertaking.

Questions that Are Intended as Catch-alls

An inquiry that begins, "Tell us everything you can about. . ." should be answered carefully and accurately but with an effort to achieve brevity. Long, complicated answers often beget difficulties at trial when the same questions are repeated and the answer is different (as it inevitably is to some degree).

Questions Asking Why

Although an opposing attorney rarely asks a "why" question at trial,[10] he will frequently ask such a question at the deposition, and the deponent must be prepared to explain why a certain piece of information was or was not given to a patient, why a diagnosis was or was not made, why a course of treatment was or was not pursued, and like questions that plumb the motivation and reasoning of the deponent through the course of his management of a patient. The answers to these questions will often be used by the opposing attorney to plan his approach to the presentation of the case at trial.

Questions Posing the Hypothetical Question

One way in which the opposing attorney can use a defendant doctor as his expert is by asking the doctor to assume that certain facts are true and then questioning the doctor concerning the proper diagnosis and treatment based on these facts.[11] For the unsuspecting doctor, this exercise can become one in which he ends up being an expert witness against himself. The deponent should be cautious in responding to hypothetical questions, and before venturing a response should be certain that he understands the hypothetical basis for the answer.

To avoid incorrect or misleading answers, the deponent may ask the attorney to supply additional facts, state that the question is not complete enough for an opinion to be stated, or maintain that he cannot give an opinion based merely on a hypothetical situation and must actually examine a patient in order to answer questions about diagnosis and treatment. If a deponent is uncertain about the correct manner in which to respond to a hypothetical question, he should consult with the friendly attorney prior to the taking of the deposition.

Questions Seeking Recognized Authorities

The opposing attorney will use the deposition of an expert witness not only to determine the expert's opinion of the case but also to learn the identity of the authorities that the expert relied on in reaching his opinion or that the expert recognizes as being authoritative in the field. The expert should be cautious in answering these questions since the examining attorney will review them for any information *contra* to the expert's testimony and will use such information at trial in an effort to impeach the expert. Treatises, texts, and professional journals that are specifically identified by the expert should be reviewed if the case goes to trial and the expert is to be called to testify.

When responding to the opposing attorney's questions during the deposition, the way in which a deponent answers can be as important as what is actually said. The expert witness, in particular, must seek to create a favorable impression upon the examiner because in the usual case his testimony will exert a considerable influence on its outcome. The deponent can improve his performance by observing serveral key points (applicable whenever testimony must be given) (see Table 34.1).

Examination by the Friendly Attorney

Since the purpose of a deposition is to serve as a discovery tool for the adverse party, the friendly attorney will ask very few, if any, questions. If the deponent is an optometric expert, the friendly attorney may inquire into his or her professional qualifications; pose questions related to the standard of care, proximate cause, or injury suffered by the plaintiff; or ask questions that are intended to clarify or counteract points made by the opposing attorney during his examination.

In posing his questions, the friendly attorney may ask leading questions, thereby assisting the deponent in getting the point across. The deponent may wish to expand on some answers given to questions posed by the attorney for the adverse party; the friendly attorney's examination gives him a chance to do so (provided the appropriate questions are asked). The deponent's responses may be phrased so as to be helpful to the attorney in this regard.

Review of the Deposition Transcript

After the stenographer has reduced the testimony to writing, the deponent will be given an opportunity to review the transcript for accuracy. Improperly spelled technical terms, incorrect book titles, and misnamed authors or journals are the usual errors requiring correction. The deponent will also be able to review the effect of his testimony, which can be quite different when seen on the printed page compared to the impression that seemingly was created at the time of the deposition itself.

The deponent will probably receive a copy of his testimony from the friendly attorney, especially if it is anticipated that the case will go to trial. The deposition should be kept in a convenient place, along with the answers to interrogatories, documents produced for the adverse party, and other materials that will be used by the expert to prepare for the trial itself.

Table 34.1. Conduct of the Witness During the Deposition

Do not answer a question that is not clear; rather, request that examining counsel repeat or rephrase it. All answers should be clearly expressed verbally, since the stenographer cannot record a shrug or hand movement.
Do not volunteer information that is not asked for merely because it could be relevant. If the examining counsel does not ask for "all you know," a restricted response is appropriate.
Do not feel that every question must be answered merely because it was asked. If you do not know the answer, you should not speculate but rather should respond, "I don't know."
Answers should be based upon facts, not upon hearsay information. If specific facts are asked for, and you have first hand knowledge of them, then you should answer fully but without volunteering extraneous information.
When a question of fact is asked, before giving a response you are permitted to consult any records that you might have, and you should do so, even if you are certain of the answer.
A response must be given to a question if you know the answer. If friendly counsel makes an objection, you should withhold your answer until instructed by the friendly attorney to continue. An instruction not to answer the question should be observed.
Do not argue with the examining counsel, and resist the temptation to use sarcasm, off-color remarks, or other inappropriate responses that, when read to a jury, will create an unfavorable impression.
Although an attorney may insist upon a "simple yes or no answer" to a question, you can state for the record that the question requires an explanatory answer. The friendly attorney may then, during his examination, bring out the further information that you wished to divulge.
Testimony can only be given to the extent of a witnesses' best memory. If you are uncertain about an answer and have no supporting documentary evidence, you should state the fact that you are uncertain. If you have no clear recollection of performing a certain act, but it was your standard practice to do such an act on a routine basis, then you may testify that it is your best memory that you did the act as a matter of routine.
Your dress, conduct, ability to express yourself, and potential impact on a jury will be under constant assessment by the opposing attorney. You hould enunciate clearly, dress neatly, and exercise courtesy to all the parties.
If you are uncertain about the response to a particular question, you can request an off-the-record discussion with the friendly attorney before answering.
If you become fatigued, you can request a recess, or even an adjournment of the deposition to another day.

Use of the Transcript for Trial

If a case proceeds to trial and the deponent is to be called to testify, the deposition transcript should be carefully reviewed to ensure that the testimony given at the trial is consistent with that given at the deposition. Key points should be carefully reviewed and the factual justification for them checked for accuracy because these issues are certain to be brought up at the trial, either during direct or cross-examination. If the deponent's testimony is expected to be different from that given at the deposition, a clear and understandable reason for the difference must be offered to the jury.

An expert should carefully review any opinion stated in the deposition and the reasons for it. Authorities recognized by the expert at the deposition should also be reviewed because the expert can anticipate being cross-examined on them at the trial. Contrary views in the literature will have to be explained to the jury. One way to do so is to state that optometry is an art and a science, different viewpoints are common to every discipline,[12] and although expert *X* is entitled to express an opinion that he feels is correct, on this particular point the witness feels that his opinion is the better reasoned and better supported one.

Opinions offered at trial that are in direct conflict with those given at the deposition can be used to impeach the expert. Impeachment is the use of proof to establish that a witness is unworthy of belief, and an expert whose testimony at trial contradicts that which was offered during the deposition faces an uphill battle to persuade the jurors that he is to be believed. Testimony at trial must be carefully prepared so that any differences can be explained to the jury. The expert should keep this fact in mind when readying himself for the trial.

If a deponent cannot be present at trial, but the friendly attorney wishes to present his testimony to the jury, the deposition can be read into evidence. The judge and the attorneys meet in private before the deposition is to be offered into evidence in order to determine what questions or answers are improper, and, with the improper material deleted, the testimony is read in open court with the jury present, usually with one lawyer reading the questions and the other lawyer reading the answers. If the deponent's testimony was favorable, but the deponent himself created a poor impression, the attorney may prefer to present the evidence in this fashion (although it can become an exercise in boredom for the jury if done poorly). The facts and documentary evidence thus presented become part of the trial record.

The use of optometric expertise in the litigation process is a matter that is not well understood by trial attorneys or by the courts. The next chapter discusses the application of optometric science and knowledge to some of the more common types of cases requiring expert opinion for their determination.

Notes

1. There is a recent trend among trial lawyers to use the video deposition, in which the witness's testimony is recorded on film or videotape and shown to the jury on a television monitor in the courtroom. The opposing attorneys may agree to use the video deposition or one of the attorneys may make a motion to the court to be allowed to take the deposition in this manner. Objections to the deponent's testimony are preserved since an improper question or answer can be edited out of the film or tape before it is shown to the jury.
2. References describing the particulars of rendering testimony are rare in the optometric and medical literature. A general discussion of the problems of serving as an expert witness (including the deposition) can be found in Horsley, J.D., *Testifying in Court: The Advanced Course*, Medical Economics Co., Oradell, N.J., 1975.
3. The concept of impeachment based on prior inconsistent statements is an important one for expert witnesses. Counsel will look long and hard for proof that a witness has made statements that are inconsistent with present testimony, including articles, speeches, courses, books, or other sources of opinion published by the witness. It would be helpful to a witness to understand how impeachment can occur. For a discussion, see Cleary, E.W. (ed), *McCormick on Evidence*, 2d ed., Ch. 5, West, St. Paul, Minn., 1972.
4. The importance of deposition testimony is discussed by Horsely, supra note 2. For a step-by-step review of the deposition process (including video depositions), see Morrill, A.E., *Trial Diplomacy*, 2d ed., ch. 12–15, Court Practice Foundation, Inc., Chicago, 1975.
5. Attorneys may reserve their objections to questions posed at a deposition because the answer to an improper question can be deleted from the deposition transcript if it is offered as evidence at trial. There may be, however, some questions that the attorney will have to object to (a question that is posed in an improper form being a common example). The witness will then be instructed to answer the question after the attorney has preserved his objection for the record. In other instances, the attorney may object to a question as being inadmissible on any basis and instruct the witness not to answer it; in which case the witness gives no response to the question whatsoever.
6. The costs of the stenographer are paid for by the party requesting the deposition. A copy of the transcript may be purchased by the opposing party from the stenographer.
7. The difference between a direct question and a leading question is as follows:
   DIRECT: "When patient *X* was seen by you on the date in question, what was his condition?"
   LEADING: "When you examined patient *X* on the date in question, he was complaining of pain in the right eye, wasn't he?"
8. If a question cannot be answered with a yes or no, the deponent should state this fact and attempt to give an explanatory answer. If the examining attorney cuts his response short, the friendly attorney may object or may pose the question during his examination of the deponent so as to obtain a full and accurate answer to the question.
9. Since a plaintiff in a professional liability case must find an expert who is familiar with the standard of care expected of the defendant, a way for the plaintiff to circumvent this problem is to depose an unwitting defendant. The defendant, as a qualified expert, can be used to establish the standard of care, proximate cause, and the extent of injury suffered by the patient. An alert defendant can avoid this trap, however, by asserting that the standard of care was what he did in the case.
10. The reason for this aversion to "why" questions at trial is that "why" answers often become speeches in which the witness is able to justify his actions to the jury.
11. An example of how a hypothetical question could be foisted on a defendant doctor is as follows: The plaintiff's attorney asks the defendant doctor if it would be contrary to accepted optometric practice not to refer a patient with the classical signs and symptoms of glaucoma. The doctor would answer that the defendant did not have the classical signs and symptoms of glaucoma, to which the plaintiff's attorney would respond by describing a hypothetical situation in which the classical signs and symptoms of glaucoma were present and conclude by asking the defendant doctor if it would be contrary to accepted optometric practice to fail to refer such a patient. An acquiescence by the defendant doctor supplies the foundation needed by the plaintiff's attorney because the plaintiff can thereafter be expected to testify that he or she had each of the signs or symptoms. The doctor's testimony permits a case that could have been decided in his favor on the basis of a directed verdict to be sent to the jury for deliberation.
12. By analogy, the U.S. Supreme Court, where a five to four and a nine to zero decision have the same effect of law, features substantial disagreement between experts.

Chapter 35

The Optometrist as Expert

During the early morning hours of September 28, 1971, a police car was dispatched to a small house in the village of Romeoville, Illinois. When the officers arrived they found a young housewife lying in a pool of blood on the bathroom floor. She subsequently died of her wounds. A pair of eye glasses was found near the body. . . . The key testimony centered on the comparison of the pair of glasses found at the scene, and a pair which was taken from the defendant by Naval Intelligence. The two pairs of glasses were brought to two well known optometrists from the Chicago area . . . (who) carefully examined both pairs of eye glasses. At the trial, both doctors testified that after having examined the glasses, they found them to be identical in every possible way. In their opinion, these two pairs of glasses were made for, and worn by, the same individual, (and) . . . the mathematical probability that these two pairs of glasses could belong to two different individuals was one in four trillion . . . . After the jury deliberated for only three hours, the defendant was convicted of the offenses of rape and murder. The prosecutor . . . stated that the testimony of these two optometrists was the key in obtaining the convictions. Their testimony proved that a person's eye glasses are as unique to each individual as are his fingerprints. It showed that eye glasses can be used in future cases for purposes of criminal identification. The testimony concerning the identification of the eye glasses was so convincing that it overcame the defendant's presumption of innocence.

—From "Eye Glasses as Unique as Fingerprints," *Journal of the Wisconsin Optometric Association*, vol. 14, no. 5, Sept.–Oct. 1972

Optometric Expertise in the Legal Forum

An expert is a witness who possesses technical information of a kind that is outside the experience and knowledge of the average person. Optometrists, because of their education in vision science and experience as vision-care providers, qualify as experts and may testify as such where the trial court believes that their testimony will assist the trier of fact in understanding the evidence. Yet optometrists rarely appear as experts in legal matters.

There are two reasons for this lack of optometric testimony: a reluctance on the part of the members of the profession to become involved in legal matters and a lack of knowledge on the part of attorneys as to the utility of optometrists. This result is unfortunate because optometrists can be of substantial use to the courts in presenting expert evidence in a variety of causes. The types of cases that would benefit from expert evidence offered by optometrists include the following:

- Personal injury claims
- Worker's compensation claims
- Professional liability claims
- Products liability claims
- Certain forensic cases

Personal Injury Claims

The most frequent cause of personal injury litigation is injury arising out of accidents involving motor vehicles. (In fact, moving motor vehicles are the third most common location for ocular injuries.) In each and every accident the vision of the participants is a *bona fide* issue; the acuity and field of vision of each driver or pedestrian should be investigated, yet all too frequently vision is ignored or merely given a superficial examination. There are 11 million persons who possess a best corrected acuity below 20/20 or have restricted visual fields,[1] but these matters are seldom explored by attorneys, who usually inquire if the litigant was wearing his glasses or contact lenses and leave it at that. And although lawyers frequently employed), visibility of persons or objects (deter-what occurred at the scene of the accident, they less frequently inquire into *why* the accident occurred. Lighting conditions (for which photometry can be employed), visibility of persons or objects (determined through photometry or other measurements), visual idiosyncracies of participants (e.g., color vision defects, reduced acuity at night, or monovision contact lenses), and similar matters are many times neglected. Optometrists, because of their unique training in the measurement, psychology, and correction of vision are the ideal professionals to perform this service. That the determination of these matters could exert an important influence on the evidence in a case is obvious. But optometric expertise should not be limited exclusively to causation; optometrists can also assist in the assessment of injury.

In the usual case, persons who suffer some personal injury affecting their eyes require immediate medical care, followed by a period of follow-up and convalescence, before a relatively stable end result ensues during which they are customarily returned to their routine vision care provider. Although the immediate injury and the follow-up care are important elements of damages, it is the end result that determines the visual disability, if any, and forms the most substantial element of damages.

By the time of the deposition, or trial, many months will have passed, and it will be the testimony at this time that will have the most influence upon the size of a settlement or jury verdict. The patients of optometrists who are injured, receive medical care, and then are returned to their optometrists for a resumption of optometric services can benefit from their optometrists' analysis of their disability; after all, their optometrist was familiar with their vision before the injury and will have to assess their post-injury condition in order to continue to provide long-term care. Far too frequently the analysis of the injury's result on the patient is left solely to the medical provider, who does not have the benefit of the optometrist's "before and after" viewpoint. Optometrists can and should play a larger role in the assessment of visual disability, particularly within a category of personal injury that is most important, workman's compensation.

Worker's Compensation Claims

There are over 1 million people in the United States who have some type of visual impairment resulting from an eye injury.[2] Of these, 19 percent were injured in the workplace.[3] Although treatment of these injuries is most often a medical matter, the assessment of resulting disability can be performed by an optometrist just as readily as by a medical provider.[4] If the injured worker was the patient of an optometrist prior to the injury, there is an even more compelling reason for the optometrist to perform this service.

The assessment of visual impairment should be performed according to the guidelines established in *Guides to the Evaluation of Permanent Impairment*, published by the American Medical Association's Committee on Rating of Mental and Physical Impairment.[5] The guide rates an individual's diminished visual ability as a percent of impairment of the visual system and as a percent of impairment of the whole person. Visual impairment is evaluated in terms of three visual functions: (1) corrected visual acuity at distance and near, (2) visual fields, and (3) ocular motility with absence of diplopia. The equipment necessary to perform an evaluation is standard optometric equipment[6]: visual acuity charts for distance and near, standard perimeter with a radius of 330 mm, tangent screen, and refraction equipment.

The criteria and methods of evaluation necessary to determine impairment of both the visual system and the whole person are discussed in Chapter 15. Optometrists have the expertise and the equipment to determine ocular disability and should fulfill their responsibility to their patients and to the legal system by increasing their involvement in worker's compensation claims.

Professional Liability Claims

There are two routes by which optometrists can become involved in a malpractice case: as treating doctors who must be witnesses or as expert witnesses on behalf of one of the parties. The former category is the more likely because optometrists who treat patients may be brought into a lawsuit whether they wish to testify or not, whereas expert witnesses testify of their own accord on behalf of one of the parties to the controversy.

No matter which category the optometrist falls into, his testimony may be elicited to determine factual matters pertinent to: (1) the standard of care to which the defendant doctor should be held, (2) the type of injury suffered by the plaintiff, the extent thereof, and the degree of permanent disability, if any, and (3) the proximate relationship between the injury and the alleged breach of the standard of care. In a malpractice case involving an optometrist-defendant, there would probably be little argument that the witness-optometrist would be qualifed to testify to facts or to offer an opinion as to the issues of injury or proximate cause. The standard of care could be another matter, however, depending upon the mode of practice (e.g., professional or commercial), the time in practice (e.g., was he or she practicing at the time of the alleged negligence?), or the location (e.g., state and city) of the defendant optometrist compared to that of the witness. Any of these factors might serve to convince the trial judge that the witness optometrist's testimony should not be allowed.

There is another possible bar to an optometrist's testimony as to the standard of care, and it involves those instances in which the defendant doctor is an ophthalmologist or general practitioner. Although the general rule requires that a witness professing familiarity with the prevailing standard of care be from the same "school" as the defendant, the trend of the courts has been toward liberalizing this rule. Where the services or skills of two professions overlap, the courts have begun to allow testimony from either profession as to the standard of care for those areas of overlap where, ostensibly, the standard of care is identical.[7] Unfortunately, there is ample opportunity for abuse in this practice, as some cases have illustrated.[8]

One impediment to medical testimony that is not applicable to optometrists is the doctor and patient privilege; only one state statute confers this right on the patients of optometrists (Washington). Consequently, optometrists usually must answer those questions posed to them in deposition or at a trial concerning the communications they have had with their patients. (For further discussion, see Chapter 16.)

Professional liability claims against optometrists are an inevitable result of increased professional responsibility, and optometric involvement in legal actions of this nature can be expected to grow.

Product Liability Claims

Eye injuries from various products affect about a quarter of a million persons annually, with the most common cause of injury being intraocular foreign bodies.[9] Defective ophthalmic products constitute a leading cause of these injuries, and optometrists can play an important role by: (1) protecting patients against the likelihood of injury, (2) analyzing ophthalmic materials to determine if they are defective products for which liability should issue, and (3) assessing the extent of the patient's injury.

Since compliance with ANSI Z 80.1 and Z 87.1 impact-resistance standards is necessary to satisfy the legal requirements related to dress and safety eyewear, and since optometrists are the professionals most familiar with these standards (and with ophthalmic products in general), it would seem that optometric input into product liability litigation would be essential. Much of the law related to ophthalmic product liability litigation is at present unsettled, and optometric expertise may be of importance in determining the precedent-setting cases yet to come.

Forensic Cases

There is a developing body of knowledge that applies optometric techniques and principles to forensic matters and that promises to add substantially to the field of legal medicine. For example: Photometry has been applied to certain criminal cases in which the identification of a suspect depended on the ability of a witness to see the suspect in dim illumination[10]; ophthalmoscopy and extracts of aqueous or vitreous have been used to determine the time of death in unwitnessed homicides[11]; assay of the vitreous for ethanol level in the body (rather than assay of the blood) is employed in automobile fatalities in which alcohol abuse is suspected[12]; and ophthalmic lenses are used as a means of identifying or locating persons.[13]

Another application of optometric expertise is the Horizontal Gaze Nystagmus Test, part of the National Standardized Field Sobriety Tests used to determine the intoxication of drivers. Optometrists are often needed to establish the admissibility of this evidence at trial.[14]

This rather new field of forensic optometry is an interesting one that, hopefully, will increasingly manage to draw the attention and expertise of optometrists as the application of optometric science to the law continues to grow.

The Expert Witness

Optometrists constitute a new and, as yet, rarely used source of knowledge for lawyers, and so optometrists must seize the initiative and educate attorneys as to their capabilities whenever possible. If an optometrist is asked to assist in a case as an expert, there are three factors that must be discussed in order to determine if the use of the optometrist will be appropriate: the optometrist's qualifications to testify as to the matter in dispute, the degree of preparation necessary for both the optometrist and the attorney in readying themselves for the litigation, and the fee to be paid the optometrist for his time.

Qualifications

Attorneys are not familiar with either the length or the breadth of optometric education. An optometrist who will be giving testimony at a deposition or a trial or both will need to acquaint the attorney with his educational qualifications, in terms of both didactic training and clinical experience. A *curriculum vitae* is a necessity, but it can only serve as a list of accomplishments; the particular knowledge and experience that the optometrist can bring to a legal problem should be explained so that the attorney can emphasize the optometrist's qualifications to the judge or jury. Opposing counsel may attempt to diminish an optometrist's qualifications by such remarks as "You didn't go to medical school did you, doctor"? or "You are not a MD, are you doctor"? Optometry school is clearly superior to medical school in the scope of vision science and the extent of clinical exposure to vision problems. Furthermore, optometrists must pass a series of national or state examinations to prove their competency in vision science, which is something that only board-certified ophthalmologists have to do. Unless the friendly attorney is made aware of these facts, he cannot counteract the opposing attorney's attempts to detract from the optometrist's testimony. Therefore, it is essential that the optometrist communicate with the attorney and extensively review his qualifications for the testimony that it is anticipated he will give.

Preparation

A question that is not asked cannot be answered, and an attorney who is not adequately prepared cannot present an effective case. An optometrist must review the sum and substance of his testimony with the attorney before it is given so that the necessary and proper questions can be formulated by the attorney and the necessary and proper answers can be received into evidence. Consultation with the attorney is the best means of accomplishing the understanding between questioner and answerer. All too often the busy schedules of attorneys and experts—and the distances that separate them physically—combine to restrict communications to mail and telephone exchanges until the time that testimony must be given. Such a development is most disadvantageous and should be avoided if at all possible. A full exchange between the expert and the counsel seeking the expert's opinion can only occur when there is face-to-face communication. The optometrist should endeavor to meet with the attorney and review the case prior to the actual taking of testimony so that the attorney can be adequately prepared. The most important occasions for which the attorney must prepare are the deposition of the opponent's expert, deposition of the expert optometrist, and trial. The optometrist should assist the attorney in his preparation for each of these events because, as attorneys will freely admit, it is the best prepared lawyer who more frequently prevails.

Fees

If an optometrist who has treated a patient receives a request from an attorney representing the patient (accompanied by a patient release) seeking information about the patient's visual status and prepares a report summarizing the pertinent findings, he may charge a fee for the time spent in preparing the report. The fee charged should be commeasurate with similar fees charged by other health-care providers in the community.

An optometrist who is to appear as a witness at a trial (such as a treating doctor who must appear in a worker's compensation case) will be served with a subpoena. For this service the witness will be paid a fee, which is usually a nominal amount that is set by statute.[15]

In neither of these cases is the amount of compensation very sizable, but both represent instances in which the optometrist's involvement with the controversy is minimal. He is merely supplying information pursuant to the patient's request on the order of the court.

A different state of affairs exists for the expert witness. When an attorney solicits the services of an expert, he is expected to compensate the expert for the time that the expert puts into the case; yet there are variations in the way that compensation for experts is computed and paid. One method—which is illegal—is to base the expert's fee on a contingency basis. In this event, the expert has a clear interest in the outcome of the case, which establishes a bias on his part in favor of the party whom he represents. This type of arrangement is contrary to public policy and contemporary ethics.[16]

Experts are not expected to be advocates (although they sometimes come across that way). They are expected to render a fair and impartial opinion and to be compensated for their time rather than for their advocacy. An expert witness who is too partisan often loses his effectiveness before the trier of fact; an expert witness who is more interested in his fee than in the case loses the confidence of those with whom he is working. An expert, like Caesar's wife, should avoid even the appearance of impropriety. Obviously, his task is not an enviable one, which is why the role of expert witness is one that is eschewed by many professionals.

The fee for an expert witness, like the fee for any professional service, varies from person to person. The usual and customary method of payment is fairly uniform, however, and is as follows: the attorney sends the expert the pertinent records, affidavits, depositions, and other evidence and requests an evaluation. The expert performs an evaluation in accordance with the attorney's instructions, for which he charges either a flat fee or a fee computed on an hourly basis and determined by the amount of time spent in making the evaluation. The expert sends the attorney a report, which is an assessment of the evidence that he has been provided. The expert may find the client's position to be favorable or he may find it to be unfavorable, but based upon his findings he makes a recommendation to the attorney, and, based upon this recommendation, the attorney makes his decision as to how to proceed. If the case proceeds into litigation, the chances are that the opposing party will seek to depose the expert concerning his assessment.

The expert may charge a fee for the deposition. Again, it may be a stated amount or may be based on the amount of time required to prepare and give the deposition.

If the case goes to trial, the expert may again claim a fee for his services. If travel is involved on any of these occasions, the expert can expect the expenses of travel to be paid in addition to the fee for his time, which—as before—can be either a set amount or based upon the actual time spent at trial.

If the expert has rendered professional services to the party to the litigation, these fees should be kept separate from the fees discussed previously. Not only are they damages that can be claimed by the litigant, they may be reimbursable to the optometrist through an insurance plan. In any event, the expert should bill the patient or his attorney separately for these services.

Lastly, if an optometrist is a witness at a criminal trial, he can expect to be paid a witness fee, which is set by statute and is usually nominal.

Whether an optometrist serves as an ordinary or as an expert witness, there are common problems that are associated with testifying in court. Although the deposition is a most important aspect of any legal controversy being litigated, it is less in importance to and quite different from the trial itself. In the concluding chapter of this section, the unique problems associated with offering testimony in the foreign and intimidating environment of the courtroom will be discussed.

Notes

1. The leading causes of vision impairment are cataract (31 percent), ocular injury (9 percent), glaucoma (9 percent), general disease (4 percent), congenital impairment (3 percent), and other disease (28 percent). Unknown causes account for the other cases (16 percent). *Vision Problems in the U.S.*, National Society to Prevent Blindness, N.Y., 1980. Data are based on 1977 cases.
2. Ibid. The total number of people with visual impairment is approximately 1.1 million as of 1980.
3. Ibid. The home is the most frequent location for ocular injuries (45 percent), followed by the workplace (19 percent), and moving motor vehicles (8 percent). Other locations account for the remaining injuries (28 percent).
4. The assessment of impairment should be performed by an optometrist when the injured worker was the patient of the optometrist prior to the impairment. The visual status of the patient before the injury is an essential aspect of the determination of the degree of impairment, so the optometrist's data will be an integral part of the case. Optometric testimony has been allowed in worker's compensation hearings. See *Bowser-Briggs v. Bennett*, 224 Tenn. 565, 458 S.W.2d 729 (1970).
5. *Guides to the Evaluation of Permanent Impairment*, 2d ed., American Medical Association, Chicago, 1984. A copy of the section describing impairment of the visual system can be found in the *Physician's Desk Reference for Ophthalmology*.
6. Id. at Ch. 7. Determining permanent visual impairment requires an assessment of the injured worker's ability to perform the activities of daily life. Reduced visual ability is expressed as a percentage of impairment of the visual system. Reduced ability of the individual is

expressed as a percentage of impairment of the whole person.

7. The states are far from uniform in their rules of evidence regarding expert testimony from different "schools." For example, in *Forthofer v. Arnold*, 60 Ohio App. 436, 21 N.E.2d 869 (1938), two osteopaths were ruled incompetent to state the standard of care expected of a doctor of medicine; but in *Cassell v. Schofield*, 319 Mo. 1169, 85 S.W.2d 580 (1928), osteopathic testimony was permitted as to the diagnosis made by a physician; and in *Miles v. Meadows*, 309 S.W.2d 284 (Tex. Civ. App. 1958), doctors of medicine were permitted to testify concerning the liability of an osteopath. Other examples of the liberality of the courts: *Dorr v. Headstream*, 173 Ark. 1104, 295 S.W. 16 (1927) (chiropractor permitted to testify as an expert in a negligence action against a physician); *O'Connor v. Bonney*, 57 S.D. 134, 231 N.W. 521 (1930) (nondentist testimony admissible in liability case against a dentist); and *Lundgren v. Eustermann*, 356 N.W.2d 762 (Minn. App. 1984) (psychologist competent to testify in a negligence case against a family physician). Even so, this liberality is not uniform: see *Botehlo v. Bycura*, 320 S.E.2d 59 (S.C. App. 1984) (orthopedic surgeon unqualified to serve as expert witness in negligence case against a podiatrist). The author has been unable to find any appellate cases ruling directly on the admissibility of optometrist expert testimony against an ophthalmologist or ophthalmological testimony against a defendant optometrist.
8. The management of certain types of cases can differ from profession to profession, and this difference can be based on the legal restrictions found in individual state optometry practice acts. See, e.g., *Kahn v. Shaw*, 65 Ga. App. 563, 16 S.E.2d 99 (Ga. App. 1941), in which an optometrist was held liable for failing to perform a cycloplegic refraction in a state where the law prevented the optometrist from using the drug necessary to perform such a refraction.
9. The most common types of products causing injury are: home structures and construction products (17 percent), personal use items (such as contact lenses and eyeglasses) (15 percent), home and family maintenance products (14 percent), sports and recreation equipment (13 percent), and home workshops and supplies (10 percent). *Vision Problems in the U.S.*, supra note 1.
10. For an interesting account of such a case, see Buckout, R., Eyewitness Testimony, *Scientific American*, vol. 231, no. 6, Dec. 1974, pp. 24–25.
11. Kevorkian, J., The Fundus Oculi as a "Post-Mortem Clock", *Journal of Forensic Science*, vol. 6, no. 2, 1961, pp. 261–272.
12. Coe, J.I., and R.E. Sherman, Comparative Study of Postmortem Vitreous Humor and Blood Alcohol, *Journal Forensic Science*, vol. 15, 1970, pp. 185–190; Naumann, HN., Postmortem Chemistry of the Vitreous Body in Man, *Archives of Ophthalmology*, vol. 62, 1959, pp. 356–363; Ganther, G.E., et al., Ascorbic Acid Levels in the Post-Mortem Aqueous Humor, *Journal of Forensic Science*, vol. 9, no. 4, 1962, pp. 150–155; Jaffe, F.A., Chemical Post-Mortem Changes in the Intraocular Fluid, *Journal of Forensic Science*, vol. 7, no. 2, 1962, pp. 231–237; Adelson, L., et al., Vitreous Potassium Concentration as an Indicator of the Postmortem Interval, *Journal of Forensic Science*, vol. 8, no. 4, 1963, pp. 503–514; Sturner W.Q., and G.E. Gantner, The Postmortem Interval, *American Journal of Clinical Pathology*, vol. 12, no. 2, 1964, pp. 137–144; Hansson, L., et al., Potassium Content of the Vitreous Body as an Aid in Determining the Time of Death, *Journal of Forensic Science*, vol. 11, no. 3, 1966, pp. 390–394; Leahy, M.S., et al., Quantitation of Ethyl Alcohol in the Postmortem Vitreous Humor, *Journal of Forensic Science*, vol. 13, no. 4, 1968, pp. 498–502; Coe, J.I., Some Further Thoughts and Observations on Postmortem Chemistries, *Forensic Science Gazette*, vol. 4, 1973, pp. 2–6; Adjutantis, G., and A. Coutselinis, Estimation of the Time of Death by Potassium Levels in the Vitreous Humor, *Forensic Science*, vol. 1, 1972, pp. 55–60; and Henry, J.B., and F.A. Smith, Estimation of the Postmortem Interval by Chemical Means, *Journal of Forensic Medicine and Pathology*, vol. 1, no. 4, 1980, pp. 341–346.
13. For an account of the use of eyeglasses to identify a defendant in a murder case, see Optometrists Testimony Key to Murder Conviction, *Journal of the Wisconsin Optometric Association*, vol. 14, no. 5, Sept.–Oct. 1972, p. 12. The author is also aware of the identification of homicide victims through the use of contact lenses.
14. Described by Tiffany, D.V., Optometric Expert Testimony: Foundation for the Horizontal Gaze Nystagmus Test, *Journal of the American Optometric Association*, vol. 57, no. 9, 1986, pp. 705–708.
15. Another type of testimony that is regulated by statute is that given by experts at workman's compensation hearings or trials. Many states have a statistically set limit on the compensation that can be paid to a witness. This compensation is typically rather modest. For a discussion, see Morris, R.C., and A.R. Moritz, *Doctor and Patient and the Law*, 5th ed., C.V. Mosby, St. Louis, 1971, pp. 230–234.
16. *Clifford v. Hughes*, 124 N.Y.S. 478, 139 A.D. 730 (1910); *County of Campbell v. Howard*, 133 Va. 19, 112 S.E. 876 (1922); *Miller v. Anderson*, 183 Wis. 163, 196 N.W. 869 (1924); *State v. First Bank of Nickerson*, 114 Neb. 423, 207 N.W. 674 (1926); and *Von Kesler v. Baker*, 131 Cal. App. 654, 21 P.2d 1017 (1933).

Chapter 36

Upon Being a Witness

I tried a case where the defendant's expert had outstanding qualifications, having served as chief of several hospitals. As I started to cross-examine, the first question I asked was: "Aside from being an expert in your field of medicine are you also an expert on how to testify in court?" The witness said, "What did you say?," and the judge looked at me as if I had lost my marbles. "What was the question?" I repeated it and the witness hardily replied, "Of course not!" "Did you ever write an article that appeared in the medical publication Medical Economics, *entitled, 'How To Testify In Court,' and say in that article, "Having appeared as a witness in court more times than I care to remember. . . ."*
The witness started to squirm and replied, "Oh, yes. Now I remember that article."
"Doctor, the sub-title of that article is, 'How To Get Through To the Jury.' Doctor, do you think you are getting through to this jury?" The witnesses' answer was lost in the laughter of the jury.
—Charles Kramer, J.D., "Cross Examination of the Medical Expert" *Trial*, vol. 13, no. 12, Dec. 1977

Preparation for Trial
Creating a Favorable Impression
Direct Examination
Proper Use of Records
Use of Demonstrative Evidence
Cross-Examination
Impeachment

The responsibility of being a trial witness is not one that should be regarded lightly, nor is it one that should be looked upon with a sense of dread.[1] Trial testimony *is*, however, a far different proposition from the relatively low-key presentation of evidence during a deposition. Sitting in the witness chair is an altogether different experience, one that requires special considerations. (See Fig. 36.1 for an example examination.)

The first matter the witness will ponder is the problem of when he will be called to testify. A subpoenaed witness must appear in court at the designated place and time. Doctors are often given special consideration by the trial judge, who—upon request by one of the trial attorneys—often will interrupt the sequence of the trial in order to accommodate the schedule of a medical witness. Therefore, when an optometrist is served a subpoena to appear in court, he should contact the attorney issuing the subpoena to arrange a mutually agreeable time for his appearance. The lawyer may be able to arrange for the optometrist's testimony be given at a predetermined time, thus sparing the optometrist from having to wait in court.

But knowing where to go and when to be there is but a small part of the array of problems that attend an appearance in court. In order to be an effective witness, the optometrist should understand a few basic considerations relating to:

- preparation for trial
- creating a favorable impression
- direct examination
- proper use of records
- use of demonstrative evidence
- cross-examination
- impeachment

Judge Keith returned to the Bench, said to Mason, "Any defense?"

"Yes, Your Honor. I wish to call one witness."

The District Attorney's face lighted with anticipation at the idea of an opportunity to cross-examine Mrs. Fargo, but Mason said, "Dr. Carlton B. Radcliffe who is under subpoena by the defense. Will you please take the stand?"

A choking, almost strangled cry sounded loud in the silence of the courtroom.

Everyone turned to where Mrs. Maynard had started to get to her feet, "You can't do that," she shouted. "You can't dredge out my private life and hold it up. . . ."

Judge Keith pounded his gavel.

"Silence," he roared. "Order in the court. Spectators will be silent. The rights of the parties will be amply protected by respective counsel."

Mrs. Maynard swayed, was seized with a fit of coughing and then dropped back into her chair.

Mason was frowning thoughtfully as he asked Dr. Radcliff the usual preliminary questions, then said, "You are a duly licensed and qualified optometrist, Doctor?"

"I am. Yes, sir."

"And you are acquainted with Mrs. Newton Maynard, the witness who has recently testified?"

"I am. Yes, sir."

"It is part of your business to prescribe, grind and fit lenses?"

"It is. Yes, sir."

"Now did you see Mrs. Maynard on the twenty-first day of September of this year?"

"I did not. No. sir."

"You did not?" Mason asked.

"No, sir."

"On the twentieth?"

"No, sir."

"I thought she delivered some glasses to you to be repaired?" Mason said.

"She did. Yes, sir."

"When?"

"On the twenty-second day of September."

"The twenty-second!" Mason exclaimed.

Mason turned to the Judge. "I beg the indulgence of the Court. This witness is not exactly hostile, but he has refused to make statements on the ground that to do so would be betraying the interests of the patient, and he would only make such statements in answer to questions if he were subpoenaed and called to the witness stand."

"Very well," Judge Keith said, leaning forward and showing his interest.

"At what time on the twenty-second?" Mason asked.

"At about eight o'clock in the morning."

"Was your place of business open at eight o'clock?"

"No, sir, but I live over my store with a telephone extension from the store. She called me at eight o'clock and told me she had an emergency rush job and wanted to know how soon I could grind a pair of lenses."

"What did you tell her?"

"I told her that I could not possibly have the lenses ground before the next day, and she asked me to have the glasses delivered to her home the moment they were ready."

"And this was at eight o'clock."

"Yes—within a minute or two. I had just started my breakfast. I always eat breakfast at eight o'clock."

"And then she brought the glasses around to you personally?"

"She did not. They came by messenger a few minutes later."

"Who was the messenger?"

"A boy. I haven't seen him before. He had the glasses wrapped up in a package."

"The new glasses were delivered to Mrs. Mayners when?"

"On the twenty-third, as I had promised."

"As I understand it, then," Mason went on triumphantly, "Mrs. Maynard had her glasses delivered to you soon after eight o'clock in the morning of the twenty-second and did not receive them back until the next day. Therefore, if she didn't carry a spare pair of glasses she couldn't possibly have been wearing her glasses on the twenty-second. I think you may inquire, Mr. Burger."

"Just a minute," the witness said "I don't know whether you are asking me a question, but it was not at all impossible for her to have been wearing her glasses on the twenty-second. These weren't her glasses."

"Weren't her glasses!" Mason said.

"These were entirely different glasses."

"You're sure?"

"Of course, I'm sure. These were glasses for a person around sixty years old. They were not Mrs. Maynard's prescription at all."

"Do you mean," Mason asked, "that you know Mrs. Maynard's prescription?"

"I don't know her prescription, but I know that these were not her glasses."

"How can you tell that if you don't know what her prescription is?"

"Because I can take one look at her eyes and the general construction of the glasses and tell that these are an entirely different prescription. She has the characteristic large pupil and very clear sclera, or white of eye, which is associated with shortsightedness, or myopia. These are of the opposite type glasses and are for a person about sixty years old."

"You can tell a person's age from the prescription of glasses?"

"Generally, you can. In fact, you can tell a lot about a person from his glasses. These glasses were probably for a person of Slavic descent. I would say they were for a man rather than a woman because of the nose measurement. There was rather a bulbous nose and. . . ."

"Will you kindly tell us," Mason said, venting his irritation now that the triumph which had seemed in his grasp was slipping through his fingers, "how can you tell that a man was of Slavic descent simply by an inspection of his spectacles?"

"Well, I can't tell absolutely. I said probably," the witness stated.

"And what caused you to believe that he might be of Slavic descent?"

"A great deal can be told by glasses," Dr. Radcliff said. "There is not only the prescription of the lenses themselves, but there are the shape, style and construction of the frames. For instance, on the present glasses there was a very wide nose measurement which indicated a bulbous nose, there were very short 'temples, as we call them, the side pieces holding the frame on the ears, approximately three and a half inches from the hinge to the beginning of the curve of the bow. That indicated a person with the type of skull usually found in persons of Slavic descent.

"The average temple measurement is four, four and a half and even five inches. Other types have a greater distance from ears to eyes. Then in addition to that there were indications that the left ear was approximately half an inch higher than the right ear. Furthermore there were parallel scratches on the outside of the lenses indicating that the person who wore the glasses quite frequently took them off and placed them face downward on a desk. Ordinarily particles of grit will not scratch optical glass, but if the glasses are placed on a hard surface containing grit and particles of perhaps sand, the tendency will be for the lenses to be scratched. This is particularly true in the case of the present glasses which have an inside curvature of ten diopters giving an exceptionally deep- dish, so that these glasses when placed on a table with the lenses down would be quite apt to receive scratches. The average inside curvature is six diopters."

"And you noticed all of these things from the glasses?"

"Yes, sir. The glasses and the frames."

"Why did you take such a particular interest in them?" Mason asked.

"Because that's my business."

"And what did you do with these glasses?"

"I replaced the lenses with fresh lenses and had them delivered by messenger on the morning of the twenty-third to Mrs. Maynard's Los Angeles address."

"I guess that's all," Mason said,

"That's all," the District Attorney announced, grinning broadly. "No questions."

Figure 36.1. Perry Mason's direct examination of Dr. Carlton B. Radcliff in *The Case of the One-Eyed Witness.* (Reprinted with permission.)

Preparation for Trial

Just as preparation is necessary in order for a trial lawyer to present a persuasive case, it is likewise necessary in order for a witness to offer persuasive testimony. While readying himself for a case, the optometrist will want to observe the following preparatory steps.

1. *Review of the Evidence*—An expert witness should always review all pertinent records, documents, and other evidence that will be used during the presentation of the case. The deposition testimony of the expert as well as that obtained from opposing experts should be reexamined and significant quotations identified. The use of exhibits or demonstrative aids should also be reviewed. In short, the expert

should familiarize himself with both the factual and the opinion evidence that is expected to be presented by both parties and should be able to locate important extracts from the documentary evidence without difficulty.

2. *Review of Strategy*—The expert should be prepared to discuss the strategy of the case with the attorney for the party who has called him as a witness.[2] There is nothing unethical or illegal about doing so; indeed, it is a necessary part of preparing for court. Cross-examining attorneys often ask an expert witness, "Have you discussed this case with anyone?," hoping that the doctor will answer no and that this answer can be discredited. The proper answer—yes—usually brings a second question, "Whom did you talk to about it?" The appropriate answer would be to name the attorney. The examiner then attempts to discredit the doctor by stating, "And you talked about the testimony you were going to give today, didn't you?" The best answer to this sort of attack is to reply, "We discussed the various medical matters that are present in this case and how to explain them most clearly to the jury."

Another question of this type that is frequently asked by examining attorneys is, "And what did the attorney tell you to say?" A good rejoinder to the insinuation of this question is to say, "The truth." The witness should review the important questions that will be posed of the opponent's expert and should assist the attorney in determining a strategy for the cross-examination of the expert.

3. *Review of Testimony*—The testimony that the expert is expected to give should be reviewed carefully prior to the trial, preferably by having the attorney pose questions to the expert so that the expert can vocalize his answers. If the responses are too technical, better answers can be suggested. Also, the attorney can familiarize himself with the pronunciation of unfamiliar terms. Exhibits that the expert will be identifying or demonstrative aids that will be used to educate the jury can be examined and their most effective use determined. For some of the more technical and difficult questions (such as the hypothetical question),[3] the expert and the attorney may prepare the question in writing so that there will be no opportunity for mistake at the trial.

4. *Review of Authorities*—If it is anticipated that the expert will be questioned concerning quotations from textbooks or the literature, the expert should conduct a pretrial review of the pertinent authorities (particularly those that profess an opinion *contra* to that of the expert). The expert should also review his own writings to determine if they contain information that can be used against him during cross-examination.[4]

5. *Settling the Fee*—The expert should endeavor to settle the fee for his services prior to the giving of testimony because doing so eliminates the inference that the fee is contingent on a successful result in the case. The expert should discuss with counsel his answers to questions posed by the opposing attorney concerning the fee for services. One question that is often asked is, "What are you being paid for your testimony?" A hesitant reply, an evasive reply, or one that implies that the witness actually is "being paid for his testimony" may have an adverse effect on the jury. A suitable response is one that emphasizes the lack of bias on the part of the expert: "I am not being paid for my testimony. I am being paid for my time, in the hope that my knowledge concerning the facts in this case will assist the jury in understanding them and in reaching a fair and informed decision." Such a response dispels the notion that the attorney is trying to create, that the expert is biased.

There are doubtless many other items that the expert or legal counsel will consider important and that will require the expert's time and attention.

Creating a Favorable Impression

Although an expert's testimony is what he is in court to give, it is well understood that most communication is nonverbal, even in a question-and-answer forum such as the courtroom. The appearance of the expert may have as much or more influence than what he actually says or, conversely, may so detract from his testimony as to make it valueless. There are three important aspects to creating a favorable impression that the expert should consider: dress, mannerisms, and demeanor.

Dress

The expert who is dressed inappropriately can significantly reduce his credibility. Wearing ostentatious clothes or jewelry or clothes that are too formal or too casual creates an unfavorable impression that the expert's words may not be able to overcome. The expert should dress comfortably in garments that leave him at ease, but they should be appropriate, which means—in most jurisdictions—that they should be somewhat conservative. A suit and tie are the most often-recommended clothes for men; for women, a conservatively cut suit or dress.[5]

Mannerisms

A well-dressed individual can greatly diminish the positive effect of his appearance if he exhibits mannerisms that are distracting—or worse—that reflect adversely on his believability. Particularly offensive are witnesses who stare at the floor or off into space, squirm in the witness chair in discomfort, slouch in boredom, or mumble their answers inaudibly or preach as if from the pulpit. The expert should consider his conduct carefully, from the moment he enters the courtroom to be sworn in to the moment he is dismissed. Annoying personal habits such as biting fingernails, chewing gum, or like mannerisms should be consciously curtailed. The witness should take the oath in a firm voice, seat himself with both feet on the floor and his upper body slightly forward. Eye contact with the counsel when a question is being posed or a short answer is being given, and with the jury when a lengthy or explanatory answer is necessary, is generally preferred. The witness's answers should be loud enough that the juror furtherest away has no difficulty in hearing them.

Demeanor

The demeanor of the expert witness is important since it conveys to the jury information concerning the expert's affiliation to the parties in the case. An expert who is the picture of politeness under direct examination but who immediately reacts with sarcasm or dislike to the cross-examination comes across as a biased witness. The expert should not exhibit an obvious bias toward counsel and should avoid emotional displays toward anyone: judge, jury, counsel, or spectators. A dispassionate, reasoned, and firm response is one that registers well with the jury.

Direct Examination

Direct examination allows a plaintiff or defendant to present his version of the controversy to the jury. The examination is conducted by the party's own attorney, who is required to ask questions that are not leading so that the facts are first revealed by the witness and not by the attorney. Since the direct examination is usually reviewed prior to the trial, when a certain amount of rehearsal is conducted, it is easy to lose the spontaneity that a totally fresh examination would yield. In particular there is a tendency on the part of the eager witness to respond too quickly to the examiner's questions, a trait that can create a negative effect on the jury. Although the witness should not reluctantly ponder a question, responses should avoid being too pat.

The opposite type of behavior can be just as damaging; failure to review expected testimony is usually an egregious error, since the result is an unclear and confusing narrative that manages only to puzzle the jury. The witness should be sure to review the important questions that he will have to answer with the examiner, particularly complicated and difficult questions (such as the hypothetical question) that the jury may not be able to comprehend fully. The correlation of documentary evidence or exhibits with the testimony should also be reviewed because, in long or complicated trials, there is no quicker way to lose the attention of the jury than to be discussing a document or exhibit that they cannot see.

An expert witness spends the direct examination attempting to educate the jury in the factors of the case that he considers to be important. A careful explanation of technical terms, the use of demonstrative aids to illustrate key concepts, and an attempt to achieve a doctor and patient relationship with the jury (rather than lecturing to them) will create excellent rapport. An interested jury will be a more attentive jury and will be able to remember more of the evidence that was presented. The expert's role on the stand is usually more that of educator than of anything else.

The judge may, at his discretion, question a witness. Responses to the judge should be courteous; all things being equal, the judge has the most authority and the greatest believability in the courtroom and the jurors will be influenced by his attitude toward a witness and that of the witness toward him.

A witness called to testify on behalf of one of the parties cannot be cross-examined unless the witness is hostile, the testimony given by the witness is inconsistent with prior statements made by the witness, or the testimony of the witness surprises the examiner. In each of these instances, upon the appropriate motion by the examining attorney and the approval of the trial judge, the examiner will be able to ask leading questions and to cross-examine the witness. A defendant doctor in a malpractice case can be called to testify against himself by the plaintiff and can be subjected to cross-examination by the opposing attorney.[6]

The direct examination is the key part of a party's case, and it requires the same preparation that is lavished on that most storied part of the trial process, the cross-examination.

Proper Use of Records

When an optometrist testifies on his own behalf, it is most likely that his patient records will become an important part of the evidence he presents. Of course, records are used to substantiate testimony, particularly testimony concerning important and disputed facts. And the records can serve as evidence themselves, either when the optometrist has no independent recollection of the information contained within them or when they merely serve to refresh his memory concerning information that he has only temporarily forgotten. In any event, the records will be reviewed by the opposing attorney, entered into evidence, and viewed by the jury. They will be given the closest scrutiny and are frequently the difference between a successful or disastrous defense by the defendant doctor (see Chapter 16 for a further discussion).

Juries are disposed to conclude that a doctor who maintains his records in a relaxed manner is probably a less than accurate and reliable witness. Therefore, patient records should be carefully maintained. If they are demanded by the court under a *subpoena duces tecum*, the optometrist must provide them as they are, without change, at the time and place specified. Any faults within them will be taken right into the courtroom.[7]

There are several ways by which a doctor can negate the generally positive support that his records normally afford him:

- By making sloppy entries that omit vital information and thus are obviously inadequate
- By using abbreviations and shorthand notations that cause them to be virtually undecipherable
- By failing to initial entries made by others (such as a technician), thus causing them to be hearsay
- By making extraneous remarks about the patient or the patient's anomaly that are distinctly unprofessional

A doctor on the stand who must devote his testimony to defending his record-keeping has lost the assistance of one of his most valuable allies.

When documenting patient records, the optometrists should strive to include each of the following items at *every* patient visit:

- Date of examination
- Chief complaint
- Examination findings
- Diagnosis
- Treatment
- Referral, recall, or reexamination information

The optometrist should seek to keep accurate financial records as well because these records can be used as evidence in a dispute over a patient's nonpayment of the optometrist's fee for professional services.

Alterations or deletions to a patient record should include the date, reason for the entry, and—if appropriate—a line through the data being changed (rather than erasing or obliterating the entry altogether).

The optometrist who expects his records to be introduced into evidence at a deposition or trial should be prepared to spend some time with his attorney reviewing them beforehand.

Use of Demonstrative Evidence

One of the most effective ways for a witness to present his testimony is by using exhibits and demonstrations.[8] In fact, demonstrative evidence is often the only way to make an otherwise confusing point clear. Enlargements of documents or photographs, slides, charts, models, films, or actual demonstrations for the jury are but a few of the many ways by which a witness can improve the quality of his testimony.[9]

The admissibility of demonstrative evidence is within the trial judge's discretion. When some physical evidence—such as a photograph—is to be offered into evidence at a trial, the witness must first identify it as correctly and accurately portraying the facts that it purports to represent. The judge can then order it admitted into evidence, subject to objection by the opposing attorney. Experiments and other exhibitions conducted in the courtroom must first be granted approval by the judge.[10] Thus if an expert witness wishes to make use of a demonstrative aid, he must notify the attorney well in advance of the trial so that the attorney can prepare for its admissibility.

There are three basic principles that should be adhered to when presenting demonstrative evidence:

1. The jury must accept and believe the evidence.
2. The jury must understand the evidence.
3. The evidence must be portrayed in a way that makes the jury remember it.

The use of demonstrative evidence can be a powerful ally for the expert witness, who often must not only explain what happened but also how it happened. The expert serves as an educator, teaching the jury through the use of the aid about the point of evidence that he wishes to have the jury understand and remember. To be effective, the use of an aid must be rehearsed, and if possible, the rehearsal should be conducted in the company of the attorney who will be assisting in its presentation.

Whenever demonstrative aids are used during the presentation of testimony, the aid must be clearly identified in words, both for the benefit of the jury and for the trial transcript: "I am now looking at a photograph of the interior of the plaintiff's right eye, identified as plaintiff's exhibit five." When identifying the structures within the exhibit, the same verbal description should be used in order to remove the opportunity for doubt or confusion. Although this technique seems redundant at times, it is essential for a clear presentation.

When using demonstrative evidence, the witness may engage in a little showmanship by using emphasis on words, colored chalks or highlighters, pointers, and the like. The witness who uses demonstrative evidence can establish a rapport with the jury that is difficult to achieve in any other way; if the presentation of the witness's testimony lends itself to the use of demonstrative evidence, it should be strongly considered.

Cross-Examination

The purpose of cross examination is to test the truthfulness of the witness. Generally, the cross-examiner is given considerable leeway in the questions that he is permitted to ask, and, unlike direct examination, he can ask leading questions. The determination of the proper extent of cross-examination, and the appropriateness of individual questions—like other evidentiary matters—is within the discretion of the trial judge.[11]

The cross-examination of expert witnesses is far broader than that of ordinary witnesses, for the expert can be questioned on his qualifications, the extent of his knowledge, the basis for his opinion, and his possible bias. Most cross-examinations of expert witnesses concentrate on any or all of the following five areas:

1. *Inadequacy of the Expert's Qualifications*—An expert's qualifications can be shown to be inadequate for the testimony he wishes to give; for example, an ophthalmologist attempting to testify as to the standard of care expected of an optometrist may not be competent to do so if it can be shown that he or she is unfamiliar with the matter at issue (e.g., orthokeratology).
2. *Inadequacy of the Expert's Knowledge*—The expert can be questioned closely on textbooks and professional journals, on the basis of his deposition, and from many other sources in an effort to demonstrate that he does not have adequate knowledge of the disputed factual matter.
3. *Inadequacy of the Expert's Examination*—The fact that the expert conducted no examination or merely performed a cursory examination of the injured party can be used to limit the effectiveness of the expert's testimony.
4. *Fee for Testimony*—The amount of compensation that the expert is to receive is an obvious area of inquiry.
5. *Bias*—Experts who testify consistently for one side in litigation can expect to be subjected to the following type of questioning:

   QUESTION: Have you ever testified before in a malpractice case?
   ANSWER: Yes.
   QUESTION: On how many occasions, doctor?
   ANSWER: About twenty.
   QUESTION: Did you, on any of these occasions, ever testify that a doctor was guilty of malpractice?
   ANSWER: No.

The witness who remains calm and avoids a vituperative exchange with the cross-examiner is likely to survive the examination with less damage to his testimony than is the witness who is drawn into an argument or resorts to sarcasm. Knowing the tendencies of the cross-examiner can assist the witness in preparing his testimony; the friendly attorney often will be able to advise the witness on the eccentricities of the cross-examiner and should be consulted concerning this point whenever possible. If preparation time permits, the witness should undergo a sample cross-examination by the friendly attorney. Preparation is extremely important because a good cross-examiner will look carefully for the one matter that will allow him to discredit the opposing expert's testimony. The effort to discredit a witness—impeachment—is the most stringent and arduous form of cross-examination that a witness can undergo.

Impeachment

Impeachment is a deliberate, premeditated attempt to demonstrate that the testimony of a witness is not trustworthy.[12] It is permitted when a cross-examiner seeks to impair the credibility of a witness by:

- attacking the reputation of the witness for truthfulness
- showing that the facts in the case are other than the witness has stated them to be
- demonstrating that the witness made prior statements or gave prior testimony that was contradictory
- establishing that the witness is biased

Many attorneys do not attempt to impeach an expert witness, reasoning that anything less than a complete success may achieve little more than arousing feelings of dislike for the cross-examiner. Nevertheless, there may be times when an attorney feels that, for tactical reasons, he must undertake impeachment of the opposing expert witness. There is no way to predict with any degree of certainty that a given expert will or will not be attacked in this manner in any given case. An attempt at impeachment, however, will quickly become evident to the witness.

When a witness comes under attack, he should endeavor to remain calm, look his antagonist in the eye, respond with firm answers, and refrain from looking like he wished he were somewhere else.

The optometrist who wishes to learn more about the adversary process and the problems of participation in the U.S. legal system should take the time to visit his city, state, or federal court. More can be learned from the observation of a trial than from any other source.

Notes

1. There are not many references written for doctors on the difficult matter of giving expert testimony but one such reference is Horsley, J.E., and J. Carlova, *Testifying in Court: The Advanced Course*, Medical Economics Co., Oradell, N.J., 1975. Although written for physicians, the text is just as applicable to optometrists. Interestingly, the book begins with a discussion of how to overcome the fear of testifying, a matter not to be taken lightly because *The Book of Lists*, under the category called "The Fourteen Worst Human Fears," ranked speaking before a group as the number one fear most people faced. Other sources of information are Morris, R.C., and A.R. Moritz, *Doctor and Patient and the Law*, 5th ed., ch. 12, C.V. Mosby, St. Louis, 1971; and Morrill, A.E., Preparing the Witness, *Trial Diplomacy*, ch. 3, Court Practice Foundation, Chicago, 1975.
2. The necessity for preparation before testifying cannot be overemphasized. As a preeminent trial attorney has put it, "It is an elementary principle of trial practice, that a lawyer should thoroughly discuss the case with the witness whose testimony he is offering. This is particularly important in the case of a medical witness." Koskoff, T., A Primer for Medical Evidence, *Medical Trial Techniques Quarterly*, 1956, pp. 381, 383, 410.
3. For a discussion of the hypothetical question, see Morris and Moritz, supra note 1, at 256–257, and Morrill, supra note 1, at ch. 8.
4. A review of the legal issues surrounding the use of medical or other scientific works can be found in "Use of Medical or Other Scientific Treatises in Cross-Examination of Expert Witnesses," 60 A.L.R. 2d 77; and "Medical Books or Treatises as Independent Evidence," 65 A.L.R. 2d 1102.
5. The appearance of a witness can have a favorable or unfavorable outcome on the testimony being given. For an interesting analysis of the importance of dress, see Molloy, J.T., *Dress for Success*, Warner Books, New York, 1975.
6. For a discussion of cross-examination, see Morris and Moritz, supra note 1, at 259–262.
7. The importance of adequate recordkeeping has been discussed in Chapter 16. The author is aware of malpractice cases in which the defendant doctor received the complaint in the case and a subpoena for the records simultaneously, which resulted in the records being taken and held by the court at the onset of the case. For a description of the perils of poor recordkeeping, see Horsley and Corlova, supra note 1, ch. 8.
8. See id. at ch. 9.
9. For an interesting discussion of how to use visual evidence to make evidence more meaningful, see Perlman, P., Seeing is Believing: Making Proof More Meaningful, *Trial*, vol. 17, no. 6, June 1981, pp. 34–38. The "father" of demonstrative evidence among plaintiff's lawyers is Melvin Belli, whose seminal article on the proper use of this trial technique, Demonstrative Evidence and the Adequate Award, may be found in the *Mississippi Law Journal*, vol. 22, 1951, p. 284. For a legal discussion of the formalities of utilizing demonstrative evidence, see Cleary, E. (ed), *McCormick on Evidence*, 2d ed., ch. 21, West, St. Paul, Minn., 1972.
10. A discussion of the use of demonstrative evidence, with illustrations of the procedure and testimony involved, can be found in Morrill, supra note 1, at ch. 6.
11. Cross examination has been the subject of numerous treatises. For varying perspectives, see Horsley and Carlova, supra note 1, at ch. 12 and 13; Kramer, C., Cross Examination of the Medical Expert, *Trial*, vol. 13, no. 12, Dec. 1977; and Merrill, supra note 1, at ch. 4.
12. A general review, with illustrations, of the use of impeachment can be found in Morrill, supra note 1, at ch. 9.

PART TEN

BUSINESS ENTITIES

Chapter 37

Individual Proprietorship

Solo practice, a single practitioner engaged in a one-unit office location, has been the entrepreneural thrust in health care for more than a century. Certainly, it has been the backbone of optometric care for the entire period of the profession's life since its legal recognition. . . . Indeed, the solo practitioner model will remain alive and vibrant through the lifetime of everyone who reads this column. But, as in the other professions, it has reached its zenith. The extent of solo practice is, in my respectful opinion, on the decline. . . . Mounting evidence points in the direction of the group or clinical health services delivery model. Its growth can only be at the expense of the solo practitioner.

—Alden N. Haffner, O.D., Ph.D., "Critical Issues in Optometry," *Optometric Weekly*, Feb. 24, 1977

The practice of optometry is a business, just as the practice of medicine or law or any other profession is a business, and the successful conduct of a business relies on the generation of a profit. The profit motive is a necessary aspect of practice; without it, the undertaking becomes one that is more properly termed a hobby. Optometrists must regard their profession as a form of business enterprise for which the production of a profit is a desired and necessary result.

There are unique characteristics that elevate a profession such as optometry above the level of an enterprise strictly run for profit. First of all, the product of a profession is the skill and judgment of its practitioners. An optometrist provides *services* (just as would a physician, dentist, or podiatrist), and although an optometrist also provides materials, these are incidental to the services (in the same fashion as crutches, dentures, or orthopedic shoes are incidental to the services of the other enumerated professionals).

A second consideration involves the relationship between an optometrist and his patients, which—because of the specialized learning of the optometrist and its relationship to his patients' health—requires the optometrist to adhere to certain standards and to divulge his findings fully.[1] Although spectacles and contact lenses are products that are sold in the course of business, when handled by an optometrist incidental to the performance of professional services the transaction becomes one quite apart from the mere sale of merchandise. Consequently, the motto of the marketplace—*caveat emptor* (let the buyer beware)—has no application to optometry.[2]

A third characteristic of the professional nature of optometry concerns the requirement that nothing be permitted to interfere with an optometrist's obligation to his patients. This problem most frequently involves the employment of optometrists by businesses that rely on the sale of ophthalmic goods and materials for profit. The necessity to sell goods intrudes upon the optometrist-patient relationship, adversely affecting the ability of the optometrist to exercise an independent judgment, i.e., one that is in the patient's welfare rather than for the benefit of the business. Numerous legal decisions have cited this problem as justification for upholding statutes prohibiting the practice of optometry by corporations.[3]

Although optometry has evolved from a trade into a health care profession, it remains a form of business, and it must conform to the legal and tax requirements necessary to the conduct of a business. The most important consideration in this regard is the type of business organization used for the delivery of services. The basic distinction between the choices available to an optometrist is whether to be self-employed or employed.

Table 37.1. Modes of Practice for Optometrists: 1964–1987

	Percentage of Optometrists		
Type of Practice	1964	1979	1987
Self-employed			
Solo	71.0	61.7	53.8
Partnership	8.0	13.1	17.2
Group	—	2.5	5.3
Employed			
Professional corporation	—	4.1	7.2
By optometrists	1.0	5.5	4.2
By others	20.0*	8.9	12.3

* Includes miscellaneous category.

Source: American Optometric Association Annual Economic Surveys, 1964–1987.

Self-Employment

The decision to become self-employed creates numerous responsibilities and obligations. Virtually without exception, an individual who seeks to become self-employed should obtain some practical experience beforehand, or the role of employer can develop into an unhappy burden that weighs heavily upon the practice itself, affecting adversely its viability both as a business entity and as a means of delivering health care. The most ready means of acquiring this experience is by working for another practitioner. Not infrequently, newly graduated optometrists discover that the intricacies of self-employment are far more challenging than are the demands upon professional skills.[4] Therefore, the first rule of self-employment is to be prepared. Although educational training can provide some preparation, there is no substitute for practical experience.

A self-employed practitioner may choose between three basic forms of business organizations: individual proprietorship, partnership, and the professional association or corporation (PA or PC).[5]

Individual proprietorship (or sole proprietorship) can be described as a nonincorporated business organization, which is owned in its entirety by an individual. The individual proprietorship has been the mainstay of optometric health care delivery for more than a century, but—as Dr. Haffner points out in the quotation at the head of this chapter—events within optometry and U.S. health care have caused the initiation of a slow decline in this form of practice. Statistics compiled by the American Optometric Association (AOA) indicate that during the decade of the 1970s the number of solo practices declined from roughly 70 percent to 60 percent of all forms of practice.[6] This trend has continued during the 1980s. The AOA survey of modes of practice for 1964–1987 is included as Table 37.1. It clearly indicates the drop in solo practices and the gradual rise of partnerships and salaried positions for optometrists.

Partnership can be described as an association of two or more persons to carry on as co-owners a business for profit.[7] Inherent in this relationship is the joint ownership of the business and the sharing of profit or loss between these owners. Partnerships among optometrists have slowly increased over the past decades, and much has been written concerning the desirability of partnership arrangements between experienced practitioners and recently licensed optometrists.[8] We will discuss partnership in Chapter 38.

Professional associations (PAs) and professional corporations (PCs) are artificial entities that are endowed by law with the capacity of perpetual succession, consisting of either a single individual or a collection of individuals, and are accorded a legal status that is akin to that of a separate being.[9] Because ownership and management are merged in PAs and PCs, these business entities will be considered a form of self-employment. We will discuss their complexities in Chapter 39.

Employment

The decision to establish a private practice demands a commitment to a particular state and city, a sense of dedication and a willingness to sacrifice that will probably detract from other goals, a substantial financial obligation, and keen management skills.

Optometrists who are not prepared to meet these rigorous demands will probably not find fulfillment in self-employment. These individuals are better candidates for employment by others.

Optometrists can be employed by other practitioners, the military, the government, universities and schools, the ophthalmic industry, health maintenance organizations, and many similar entities. Nearly 25 percent of all optometrists are employees, according to the 1987 AOA survey (Table 37.1). When these statistics are compared to those of a decade ago, it becomes evident that optometrists are forsaking traditional forms of practice (such as individual proprietorship) for other opportunities, particularly salaried positions. Statistics compiled by the National Center for Health Statistics during the late 1960s and early 1970s indicate that the percent of optometrists in salaried forms of employment rose by more than 60 percent,[10] a trend that is expected to continue during the 1980s and 1990s. Economics have played no small role in the evolution of this development.

Although the spectrum of employment opportunities for optometrists is large, we shall limit this discussion to but one, the associateship. An *associate* is an employee, and as such holds no ownership interests in the business entity for which he works. An associate does not share in profit and loss but rather is salaried and may receive additional employee benefits if eligible. The ultimate responsibility for the business belongs to the employer; the associate is liable only for his own conduct. An associate may participate in management decisions only to the extent permitted by the employer and receives only a few of the tax breaks designed to assist the small businessman. Despite these limitations in responsibility and opportunity, associateship can be used very effectively as a steppingstone to partnership or individual proprietorship. For many newly graduated optometrists, it has proven to be an ideal means of making the transition from academics to the business world.[11] In Chapter 44 we will discuss the problems of determining the appropriate contractual relationships and obligations between employer-optometrists and their associates and how to reduce these contractual matters to writing.

In the subsequent sections of this chapter we will investigate the organization of the individual proprietorship, liability that can be incurred by a sole practitioner, financial benefits that can be realized in this form of business enterprise, and major tax issues that must be considered by the optometrist-businessman. The chapter concludes with a discussion of expense sharing.

Organization

The individual proprietorship is a business enterprise conducted by a person. Ownership vests in the individual, who has total management authority over the business: If the services of others are needed, they can be hired; if funds are required, they can be borrowed; if real estate or equipment has to be obtained, it can be leased or purchased; in each of these circumstances the individual is personally liable. If losses result, sole proprietors must bear them alone, to the extent of their resources; if there are profits, they are theirs to enjoy. The business and the person are associated with one another more intimately than in any other form of business organization.

This independence enjoyed by the individual proprietor is a two-edged sword: While it allows free rein in management and financial decisions, it limits the business to the resources, acumen, and skill of the individual owner, which may be more of a detriment than an advantage for a beginning practitioner.

To start an individual proprietorship requires a minimum of formality, yet there are certain legal steps that must be observed. The following list summarizes those that are generally most important:

- The optometrist must have a current state license, to be displayed as required by law.
- A federal tax identification number must be obtained from the Internal Revenue Service.
- A state tax identification number must be obtained from the appropriate state agency.
- A local business license will be required in most communities and must be purchased by the optometrist.
- The optometrist should open a business checking account with a local bank.
- If the optometrist wishes to participate in third-party vision service plans, the appropriate private and governmental agencies must be notified so that provider numbers can be issued to the optometrist.
- Several tax forms will have to be completed by employees so that the appropriate withholding for both state and federal taxes can be determined (see Chapter 41).
- An account in a federal bank must be established so that federal withholding taxes can be deposited quarterly as required by law.
- Sales or use tax forms or permits will be required in those states that tax ophthalmic goods.
- Insurance carriers should be notified so that the appropriate coverage can be put into effect.

Much of the reporting that is required of a proprietorship relates to tax matters. Federal and state taxation establishes a series of deadlines, usually quarterly or annually, that must be met by the proprietorship. The most important of these requirements are discussed in Chapter 41.

The individual proprietorship is the oldest, simplest, and most prevalent type of business enterprise, and—compared to partnerships and professional associations or corporations—can be organized relatively informally, is subject to less regulation, and involves fewer problems of management and control. The individual proprietorship, however, ends at the proprietor's death or retirement and is taxed in the same manner as an individual. Some of the advantages and disadvantages of this form of practice are summarized in Tables 37.2 and 37.3.[12]

One aspect of the law that is of particular importance to individual proprietors concerns professional liability. We will discuss this thorny problem in the following section.

Liability

The individual proprietor is legally responsible for the conduct of the practice. There are two key areas in which this legal responsibility can be applied: contractual obligations and injuries to others.

Contractual Obligations

The proprietor will customarily be the person authorized to negotiate and ratify contracts for the business, although this responsibility may be delegated to another, thereby creating the relationship of principal and agent (see Chapter 21 for a more detailed discussion). Any contracts entered into by the proprietor or his agent for the benefit of the business become the personal responsibility of the proprietor, for which the proprietor's personal assets (including the assets used in the business) are at risk. The reason for this personal liability is that the proprietor typically signs such contracts as an individual, and in the event of default on his part the injured party may proceed against him to collect damages. If damages are awarded, they may be taken from the personal assets of the proprietor.

Unlike partnerships and corporations, which may own assets in their own name, the title to property in an individual proprietorship must be held by a person or entity other than the proprietorship. Thus, of the three basic types of business organizations, the

Table 37.2. Advantages of Individual Proprietorship

The formalities of organizing the individual proprietorship are minimal, as are the fees to be paid to begin practice, and the proprietor may start the practice without the obligations of qualification.
The individual proprietor may make business decisions without delay or formality and without having to confer with others.
The individual proprietor is not subject to the same legal risks inherent in partnership and in professional corporations (when owned by more than one shareholder) either for contract actions or for torts.
The individual proprietorship is less encumbered with the regulatory and reporting requirements commonly demanded of other types of business organizations (especially corporations) and is not subject to the double tax that may be imposed on incorporated practitioners.
The financial posture of the individual proprietorship is not dependent solely on the economic status of the practice but is judged on the personal assets of the practitioner as well.
The dissolution or sale of an individual proprietorship is usually less complex and less difficult than that of a partnership or professional corporation.

Source: Elmstrom, G., *Advanced Management Strategies for Optometrists*, Professional Press, Chicago, 1982, pp. 25–38.

Table 37.3. Disadvantages of Individual Proprietorship

The resources of the practice are limited to those of the individual proprietor, or to the capital that can be raised by the individual proprietor, who is solely responsible for repayment.
The individual proprietorship does not enjoy the same tax advantages as an incorporated practice, either in terms of tax write-offs for certain business-related expenses or in terms of qualified retirement plans; in a partnership many expenses are shared, whereas in an individual proprietorship they are borne alone.
The individual proprietor is the sole source of revenue for the practice, and the absence or incapacity of the proprietor results in a cessation of income.
The individual proprietor is subject to unlimited personal liability for the obligations of the practice and for tort claims that arise out of the conduct of the practice.
The individual proprietorship ends at the death or incapacity of the proprietor.
The value of an individual proprietorship drops rapidly at the death or incapacity of the proprietor, and thus may not be a source of significant income for the proprietor's surviving spouse.

Source: Elmstrom, G., *Advanced Management Strategies for Optometrists*, Professional Press, Chicago, 1982, pp. 25–38.

individual proprietorship creates the most exposure to personal liability. But insurance may be obtained that provides indemnification in the event of loss (see Chapter 54).

Injuries to Others

The law relating to personal injury is complex, and an effort to summarize many of the legal problems faced by optometrists can be found in Chapters 18 through 32. Generally stated, the responsibility for injury in an individual proprietorship falls on the shoulders of the proprietor. If a person is injured on a proprietor's premises or is injured by a proprietor's act (or failure to act), and if there is legal fault on the proprietor's part, then the proprietor may be held solely liable for the injury and consequent damages. Furthermore, under certain circumstances the proprietor may be legally responsible for the conduct of his employees, when the conduct results in injury to a person by an employee who is acting in the line and scope of his or her duties. This responsibility results from the legal relationship of master and servant, which applies to situations such as those commonly found between optometrists and their employees (whether the employees are optometrists, assistants, technicians, receptionists, or opticians). See Chapter 21 for a further discussion.

Thus the liability of sole proprietors is not limited to their own acts but can result as well from the acts of certain others performing duties on their behalf. For this reason, adequate liability insurance is a necessity.

This exposure to individual liability is greater in a sole proprietorship than in other forms of business. But a proprietor generally has the opportunity to exercise stricter control over management of the business, an ability that can be used to great advantage by a prudent practitioner. The importance of efforts to minimize inadvertence or mistake cannot be overemphasized.

Benefits

The individual proprietor is a small businessman and may take advantage of the many tax laws that are designed to provide incentives for the establishment, maintenance, growth, and transfer of a small business. Since the proprietor is an individual, the law pertaining to individual income tax occupies a key position in all business planning. The income and profit or loss from a sole proprietorship is reported on Schedule C of IRS Form 1040, and this schedule has a most significant influence on the determination of individual income taxes.[13] If there is a profit, the proprietor must pay these taxes as an individual at the tax rates applied to individuals. These rates are lower than for PAs or PCs.[14] If there is a loss, the proprietor may claim it, thereby lowering his or her personal tax liability. Thus the financial success of the business is reflected on the tax return of its owner, an important consideration when the proprietor decides to sell the business to another (see Chapter 48).

Since the profit derived from business is usually the most important source of income for the proprietor, decisions must be made as to how this income will be allocated for personal purposes. One important consideration in this regard is retirement planning. There are numerous ways in which income can be set aside for retirement, but we will not consider here the multitude of options available to the contemporary estate planner.[15] Rather, this discussion will be limited to a brief review of two of the major tax benefits available to the self-employed individual who is considering retirement planning: the individual retirement account (IRA) — including the use of IRAs as Simplified Employee Pensions (SEPs) — and the Keogh Plan.

Both the IRA and the Keogh Plan are a means of sheltering income that would otherwise be taxable. Sheltering refers to a statutorily approved means of deferring tax on income. It is not a way to avoid tax altogether, but allows the tax to be paid when the sheltered income is withdrawn, which is typically many years after it has been earned and at a time when the taxpayer is in a lower individual income tax bracket.

The following description of these two plans is based on tax laws in effect at the time of publication of this text.[16] Since these laws are among the most ephemeral in all of government, consultation with tax advisors is necessary before initiating any personal financial or retirement planning.

Individual Retirement Accounts

The Economic Recovery Tax Act of 1981 (ERTA)[17] substantially broadened the appeal and applicability of IRAs by increasing the amount that could be tax-sheltered and by enlarging the group eligible to save under the plan. Consequently, sole proprietors (or partners or employees) who wish to participate in a tax-sheltered retirement trust may do so by contributing up to $2,000 per year ($2,250 if there is a nonworking spouse) to an IRA. The contributions are made to qualifying investment trusts or custodial accounts (usually managed by banks) or may be used to purchase approved annuities or retirement bonds (offered by insurance companies or banks). A sole proprietor may participate in an IRA even if he contributes to other types of retirement plans. Earnings are tax-free until retirement (which must be between the ages of $59\frac{1}{2}$ and $70\frac{1}{2}$), death, or disability. When received, the distributions from the IRA will be taxed as ordinary income, but since the recipient should be in a lower tax bracket at this time, a tax savings may be realized.

The Tax Reform Act of 1986 has limited the deductibility of IRAs for certain taxpayers. A full deduction can be claimed only by individuals who are not covered by an employer-maintained retirement plan. For those covered under such plans, a full deduction may be claimed by single persons whose income is less than $25,000 and by married persons filing jointly whose income is less than $40,000. A partial deduction may be claimed until the adjusted gross income exceeds $35,000 for single taxpayers and $50,000 for married couples (see Chapter 42).

Even though $2,000 a year does not sound like a sizable savings plan, if initiated early in a professional's career the IRA account can grow into a pleasant nest egg (see Table 37.4). Since the interest earned by the account accumulates tax-free, the quality of the IRA investment is of some importance and thus an IRA plan should be selected with great care.

The IRA can also be used by employees, partners, and optometrists in a professional association or corporation.

Simplified Employee Pension (SEP)

A SEP is an individual retirement arrangement that allows the employer to make tax-deductible contributions to an IRA or annuity that has been established for the benefit of each employee at a bank, insurance company, or other organization qualified to sponsor an IRA. A self-employed practitioner may also own a SEP-IRA.

The employer may contribute up to $30,000 or 15 percent of an employee's compensation to the SEP-IRA, whichever is less. Contributions made to the SEP-IRA by the employer are included in the employee's income in the calendar year for which the contributions were made and must be reported as income to the IRS by the employer. The employee deducts the amount contributed to the SEP-IRA on his or her federal tax return.

Employees may also make contributions to IRAs they own independently of the SEP-IRA. The deductibility of these other IRA contributions will depend on the adjusted gross income of the employee (discussed above and in Chapter 42).

Although SEP-IRAs are much easier to administer than qualified pension or profit-sharing plans, these latter qualified plans do offer some advantages and greater flexibility (see Chapter 39). Therefore, legal counsel should be consulted before instituting an SEP-IRA or any other type of retirement plan.

Table 37.4. Contributions to an Individual Retirement Account: Projected Growth

Period	At 5% Growth ($)	At 10% Growth ($)	At 15% Growth ($)
After 5 years	11,603	13,431	15,507
After 10 years	26,410	35,899	46,698
After 15 years	45,308	69,899	109,434
After 20 years	69,428	126,005	235,620
After 25 years	100,213	216,363	489,423

Keogh Plans

The Self-Employed Individuals Retirement Act of 1962 (often referred to as H.R. 10) permitted self-employed individuals to establish qualified pension or profit-sharing plans comparable to those allowed by corporate employees (see Chapter 39). But the amounts that could be set aside each year were limited, and so the benefits were far inferior to those available to the employees of corporations. In the more than twenty years that have passed since the initiation of these plans, the limit on contributions has been relaxed, and today the Keogh Plan can compare most favorably with the pension and profit-sharing plans available to incorporated practitioners.[18]

There are several tax advantages to Keogh Plans for individual proprietors:

- The contributions are tax deductible annually.
- The fund is tax-sheltered until retirement.
- Withdrawals can be made on a favorable income tax basis at the termination of employment, at disability, or at retirement.
- The self-employed individual may serve as trustee of the plan.
- Death benefits of up to $5,000 may be paid to

the beneficiary or estate of a self-employed individual and will be excluded from income.

- The fund may be used for loans under certain circumstances.
- The plan may be integrated with social security, thereby reducing the size of the contributions to be made on behalf of employees.

The most common form of a Keogh Plan is a *defined contribution plan*. Under this type of plan a sole proprietor is permitted to contribute and deduct up to 25 percent of earned income per annum, up to a maximum of $30,000.[19]

For those individuals who have different retirement goals, there is a *defined benefit plan*. It establishes the annual amount that the sole proprietor wishes to receive during retirement, rather than the contribution to be made each year. The individual deducts the amount that an actuary determines to be necessary to fund this annual retirement benefit, which may be as much as 100 percent of compensation or $90,000, whichever is less. The size of the annual deduction depends on the amount of the desired retirement benefit and the age of the individual when he begins to fund the plan.[20]

The Keogh Plan is composed of rules that are highly technical and strictly enforced. Among the most important that the proprietor should be aware of are the following[21]:

Employees Must Be Included—Any full-time employee who has been employed for three years or more must be included in the plan. To qualify as full time, an employee must work more than twenty hours weekly and more than five months annually.[22]

Vesting Is Assured—Full vesting must take place in five years or gradually over seven years (20 percent after three years and 20 percent a year for the next four years). The contributions made to the plan on behalf of employees, plus any earnings on these contributions, are irrevocably theirs once their interest has vested, even if the employees quit or are fired.[23]

The Percentage Deducted Must Be Fair—Under a defined contribution plan, the proprietor cannot deduct a higher percentage of compensation than his employees. But even for equal percentages, because the amount of compensation will be different, the actual contributions will be unequal. For example, if the proprietor earns $50,000 and the employee earns $20,000, at the maximum rate of 25 percent they may contribute $12,500 and $5,000, respectively. Despite the disparity in the dollar value of the contributions, the percentage is the same and so the plan is fair.[24] The plan may also incorporate social security benefits into the amount paid for employees, further reducing the amount actually contributed by the employer on the employee's behalf.

Understand All Requirements Pertaining to a Plan Transfer—A plan may be transferred unless expressly prohibited by the Keogh Plan agreement. Usually all that is required is an amendment to the first plan and a transfer agreement. Sometimes a transfer means termination or liquidation charges will be assessed, and in order to avoid them the proprietor must discontinue funding the plan and start up a new one altogether. Transfer rules should be understood before the plan is entered into.[25]

Withdrawals Must Be Made as Required—Since these plans are intended to be retirement shelters, withdrawals must be initiated no sooner than age $59\frac{1}{2}$ and no later than $70\frac{1}{2}$ or penalties will be incurred. In the usual case, these withdrawals are made over a period of years. Taxes are paid on this income as it is received. A lump sum withdrawal may also be made, although there are adverse tax ramifications to such a decision.[26]

Keogh Plans may be initiated by optometrists in partnership also (see Chapter 38). The retirement planning of optometrists in professional associations or corporations is somewhat different than that for proprietorships and partnerships. Although incorporated practitioners may initiate IRAs, there are other tax shelters that may be utilized to create retirement nest eggs (see Chapter 39).

The integration of IRAs and Keogh Plans into a proprietor's estate plan is a well-accepted aspect of professional life. Surveys of contemporary optometric practitioners have demonstrated the necessity for retirement planning[27] and have illustrated the utility of these tax shelters as a means of achieving financial security.[28] They should be given due consideration by the individual proprietor.

Tax Considerations

Tax reporting is the principal form of regulation to which the individual proprietor is subject. There are two basic types of tax reporting that must be observed in a sole proprietorship: that which is related to the financial status of the business and that which is related to the financial status of the individual.

Business Tax Reporting

There are federal, state, and local tax requirements that must be observed by the individual proprietorship.[29] The profit or loss of the practice is determined on Schedule C, and this amount is then entered on Form 1040 (see Chapter 41). Schedule C, however, is not the only federal tax reporting required of the individual proprietor because periodically the proprietor must remit taxes for social security and unemployment insurance and for federal income tax withholding, including self-employment taxes (described in Chapter 41). In addition to these obligations, the individual proprietor will have to comply with state and local tax withholding requirements. As a result, the individual proprietor faces a constant succession of tax deadlines that must be met or penalties will be incurred. Tax reporting requirements are among the most vexing problems facing young or inexperienced practitioners and must be well understood *before* the business venture is entered into.

A calendar that outlines the customary deadlines for these major tax reports may be found in Fig. 37.1.

Individual Tax Reporting

The tax obligations of the individual are determined on Schedule A, which is attached to the individual tax return (Form 1040). Although the majority of this tax reporting involves personal deductions such as those for medical expenses, interest, taxes (other than those that are business related), casualty losses, and similar expenditures, there are some business-related expenses that can end up on Schedule A (such as health insurance premiums paid by the individual proprietor). As with all other aspects of tax law, the wise individual will endeavor to learn many of the basic rules and will maintain good records in order to simplify the tax reporting process. Competent tax counsel will be required in most cases to report accurately individual income.[30]

Expense Sharing

Two individual proprietorships may find that there are financial advantages to the sharing of facilities, personnel, and other expenditures.[31] Or an eventual partnership may be envisioned, and this form of practice may be utilized as a means of assessing the potential for such a merger.[32] The arrangement falls short of a partnership, for neither practitioner has any ownership interest in the practice of the other; rather, it consists of two independent businesses that have found it advantageous to share certain common expenses. In creating such a relationship, there are certain legal matters that must be considered. The most important of these involve the formal agreement between the expense sharing proprietors.

The basic requirements for expense sharing are listed below[33]:

- Each practitioner is an individual proprietor.
- Overhead expenses, such as the office lease, utilities, salaries of employees, insurance, and other necessary expenditures are shared on a pro-rata basis.
- Ownership of equipment and furnishings is usually separate, although certain items may be purchased and owned jointly.
- A joint bank account is established for the payment of joint expenses, and each practitioner is required periodically to contribute a certain sum to the account, which is typically determined on the basis of a stated percentage of gross income.
- Records are separate and remain the property of the individual practitioners.
- Payment upon accounts, collections, and accounts receivable are independently maintained.
- Personnel are usually jointly supervised, but a sole personnel manager can be designated by the practitioners if they so desire.
- A maximum sum is commonly stipulated for joint obligations unless both practitioners agree to the expenditure in advance.
- Adequate liability insurance is required of all practitioners.
- Arrangements may be made for coverage during absences, including compensation to be awarded for such coverage.
- Certain ethical standards or membership in certain professional organizations may be required of all practitioners.
- Some provision for termination of the arrangement upon adequate notice will be included in the agreement.

An expense sharing arrangement will require a carefully drafted contract that reflects the agreement of the parties.[34] Such a document is best prepared by an attorney. Key clauses within the contract are those describing the manner in which expenses are to be shared; how and what payments are to be made out of the joint account; how large, nonroutine expenditures are to be managed; the procedure to be followed in the event the agreement is to be terminated; and a

You may be liable for	If you are:	Use Form	Due on or before
Income tax	Sole proprietor	Schedule C (Form 1040)	Same day as Form 1040
	Individual who is a partner or S corporation shareholder	1040	15th day of 4th month after end of tax year
	Corporation	1120 or 1120-A	15th day of 3rd month after end of tax year
	S corporation	1120S	15th day of 3rd month after end of tax year
Self-employment tax	Sole proprietor, or individual who is a partner	Schedule SE (Form 1040)	Same day as Form 1040
Estimated tax	Sole proprietor, or individual who is a partner or S corporation shareholder	1040-ES	15th day of 4th, 6th, and 9th months of tax year, and 15th day of 1st month after the end of tax year
	Corporation	1120-W	15th day of 4th, 6th, 9th, and 12th months of tax year
Annual return of income	Partnership	1065	15th day of 4th month after end of tax year
Social security (FICA) tax and the withholding of income tax	Sole proprietor, corporation, S corporation, or partnership	941 8109 (to make deposits)	4-30, 7-31, 10-31, and 1-31
Providing information on social security (FICA) tax and the withholding of income tax	Sole proprietor, corporation, S corporation, or partnership	W-2 (to employee) W-2 and W-3 (to the Social Security Administration)	1-31 Last day of February
Federal unemployment (FUTA) tax	Sole proprietor, corporation, S corporation, or partnership	940 8109 (to make deposits)	1–31 4-30, 7-31, 10-31, and 1-31, but only if the liability for unpaid tax is more than $100
Information returns for payments to nonemployees and transactions with other persons	Sole proprietor, corporation, S corporation, or partnership		Form 1099—to the recipient by 1-31 and to the Internal Revenue Service by 2-28
Excise taxes	Sole proprietor, corporation, S corporation, or partnership		See the instructions to the forms

Figure 37.1. Major Tax Reporting Requirements. (From *Tax Guide for Small Businesses*, Internal Revenue Service, 1986.)

Table 37.5. Advantages of Expense-Sharing

Overhead expenses are reduced compared to those faced by an individual practitioner.
Patient coverage is readily available whenever one of the practitioners is away.
Consultation is available; if practitioners offer specialized services these services may be offered to patients without having to send the patients to another office.
Because of reduced overhead, more capital is available for equipment and instrumentation.
Sharing of personnel can improve office efficiency, especially if financial and patient recordkeeping is standardized.

Source: Gregg, J.R., *The Business of Optometric Practice*, Advisory Enterprises, New York, 1975, pp. 30–31.

Table 37.6. Disadvantages of Expense-Sharing

Conflicts over scheduling of patients may occur if receptionist loyalty is biased.
Shared expenses must be divided in a fair and reasonable manner or conflict will result.
Decisions about furnishings, salaries, improvements, and other matters may be sources of disagreement, creating a strained relationship.
Personnel must be shared on an equal or fair basis or discord can result.
Differences in personal or clinical style can create friction between practitioners and disenchant patients.

Source: Gregg, J.R., *The Business of Optometric Practice*, Advisory Enterprises, New York, 1975, pp. 28–29.

mandatory requirement that periodic review of the arrangement be conducted by the parties.

There are distinct advantages and disadvantages inherent in the expense sharing mode of practice. Some of the major considerations are listed in Tables 37.5 and 37.6.[35]

This chapter has briefly described some of the legal problems that accompany individual proprietorship. Since solo practice represents the most independent form of business organization, requiring financial and management skills of a high order, it should not be entered into without adequate preparation and reasonable expectations for success.

Notes

1. As a fiduciary, an optometrist has a legal obligation to divulge clinical findings to patients. See Chapter 22. The Code of Ethics of the American Optometric Association also places a moral burden on practitioners to observe high standards and to divulge findings fully and in a timely fashion. See Chapter 4.
2. For an excellent discussion, see Hirsch, M., and R. Wick, *The Optometric Profession*, Chilton, Philadelphia, 1968.
3. For a review of cases discussing the corporate practice of optometry, see "Right of Corporation, or Individual Not Himself Licensed, To Practice Optometry Through Licensed Employee," 102 A.L.R. 343 and 128 A.L.R. 585.
4. See Classe, J., The Need for Relevant Practice Management in the Optometric Curriculum, *Journal of Optometric Education*, vol. 5, no. 2, 1979, pp. 16–18.
5. A beginning practitioner should be certain to obtain copies of the many tax guides published by the Internal Revenue Service and distributed free of charge to taxpayers on request. Some guides that would be of help include number 334, *Tax Guide for Small Business*; number 533, *Self-employment Tax*; number 15, *Employer's Tax Guide (Circular E)*; number 539, *Employment Taxes*; number 541, *Tax Information on Partnerships*; number 542, *Tax Information on Corporations*; number 589, *Tax Information on Subchapter S Corporations*; and number 583, *Recordkeeping for a Small Business*.
6. In 1964 the AOA Economic Survey revealed that 71 percent of optometrists were in individual proprietorships. See Economic Survey—Report No. 4, *Journal of the American Optometric Association*, vol. 37, no. 7, 1966, pp. 683–685. By 1979 the percentage of solo practitioners had dropped to 60.5 percent. See the August 1, 1981, edition of the *AOA News* for the results of the survey. The 1987 survey revealed a further decrease in sole proprietorships to 53.8 percent. Survey results were described in the March 1, 1988 edition of the *AOA News*.
7. For a discussion of partnership as a mode of practice for optometrists, see Milkie, G., *Partnerships and Professional Corporations*, Optometric Development Enterprises, St. Louis, 1972.
8. Ibid.
9. Ibid.
10. Ibid.
11. See Ready or Not for an Associate?, *Optometric Management*, vol. 16, no. 3, 1980, pp. 13–19.
12. Described by Gregg, J., *The Business of Optometric Practice*, Advisory Enterprises, New York, 1981.
13. See Tax Guide 334, *Tax Guide For Small Business*, published by the Internal Revenue Service annually.
14. Although the Tax Reform Act of 1986 instituted some major changes in the tax brackets for individuals and for corporations, in 1987 professional service corporations received a major tax increase. As of 1988 an individual is taxed at the rate of 15 percent on the first \$17,850 of taxable income, then is taxed at 28 percent up to \$43,150 of taxable income. By comparison, a professional service corporation must pay a 34 percent tax on all net income. Even so, in most professional corporations, there are few corporate earnings to tax,

and so the optometrist ends up being taxed on his earning as an employee of the corporation.

15. For a review of basic concepts and strategies, see Brosterman, R., *The Complete Estate Planning Guide*, Mentor, New York, 1987.
16. See Goldberg, M.A., What Tax Reform Means to You and Your Practice, *Optometric Management*, vol. 22, no. 11, 1986, pp. 22–26; and Goldberg, M.A., Year-End Tax Strategies Under Tax Reform, *Optometric Management*, vol. 22, no. 12, 1986, pp. 22–26.
17. An analysis of the Economic Recovery Tax Act of 1981 can be obtained from Prentice-Hall, Englewood Cliffs, N.J., as a supplement to the 1982 edition of the Prentice-Hall *Federal Tax Course.*
18. The Economic Recovery Tax Act of 1981, §167, doubled the deductions allowable for Keogh Plans, Self-Employed Plans (SEPs), and Subchapter S Corporations. The Tax Equity and Fiscal Responsibility Act of 1982 again increased the limits of these plans significantly. An analysis of the 1982 law can be obtained from Prentice-Hall, Englewood Cliffs, N.J., as a supplement to the 1983 edition of the Prentice-Hall *1983 Tax Course.*
19. Tax Equity and Fiscal Responsibility Act of 1982, §191.
20. See Gray, J., Pros and Cons of the "Maxi-Keogh" Plan, *Optometric Management*, vol. 17, no. 3, 1981, pp. 35–43.
21. Ibid.
22. Ibid.
23. Ibid.
24. Ibid.
25. Ibid.
26. Ibid.
27. See Gregg, J., Your Practice Profile: Retirement Income, *Optometric Management*, vol. 17, no. 10, 1981, pp. 25–31.
28. Ibid.
29. For a discussion of tax reporting requirements, see the following Internal Revenue Service publications: number 334, *Guide For Small Business*; number 15, *Employer's Tax Guide (Circular E)*; number 539, *Employment Taxes*; and number 533, *Self-Employment Tax.*
30. See the Internal Revenue Service tax guide number 17, *Your Federal Income Tax.*
31. A description of some of the advantages of an expense-sharing arrangement can be found in the practice management guide published by the California Optometric Association; other references are Gregg, supra note 12, and Milkie, supra note 7.
32. Pazen, R.L., An Office Sharing Plan that Works, *Optometric Management*, vol. 15, no. 9, 1979, pp. 61–65.
33. Adopted from Gregg, supra note 12.
34. For an example contract, see Milkie, supra note 7.
35. Adopted from id.

Chapter 38

Partnerships

"You'll never understand me, but I'll try once more and then we'll give it up. Listen. When a man's partner is killed he's supposed to do something about it. It doesn't make any difference what you thought of him. He was your partner and you're supposed to do something about it."
—Dashiell Hammett, *The Maltese Falcon*

Organization
Liability
Benefits
Tax Considerations
Merger

The agreement to enter into partnership creates legal and personal obligations that are probably unmatched outside of any relationship except marriage. As the fictional detective, Sam Spade—hero of *The Maltese Falcon*—points out, partners are responsible for one another and are expected to conduct themselves accordingly. The association between partners is professional, social, financial, and legal, and—in its contractual sense—is unlimited in terms of duration, being severed only by the death of the partners themselves. Because so many interrelated factors are involved, the partnership business organization is more complex than the individual proprietorship, which was discussed in the preceding chapter.

A partnership can be described as "an association of two or more persons to carry on as co-owners a business for profit."[1] From this description we can determine at least three necessary requirements for the formulation of a partnership:

1. Two or more "persons"[2]
2. Co-ownership among these persons
3. The intent to earn a profit through a mutual undertaking

Thus a partnership is an aggregate of persons rather than a separate entity. The reason for this can be found in the common law, which required partners to be sued separately, as persons, rather than as a partnership. Statutory law has managed to convert the status of partnerships into that of quasi-entities, capable of holding title to property and of enjoying certain other property rights but a nonentity for tax purposes and for the purposes of litigation.[3] This statutory law has been adopted in all states except Louisiana and establishes the legal rights of partners and partnerships and of these who interact with them. Because the law is uniform from state to state, the statute has been named the Uniform Partnership Act (UPA)[4] (see Table 38.1).

Although the UPA sets forth in detail the rights and responsibilities of partners, many of these provisions are qualified by the phrase "unless otherwise agreed," which permits some leeway to partners in terms of the conduct of the partnership's internal matters. Consequently, partners may agree among themselves as to how the affairs of the partnership are to be managed. These agreements are best committed to writing. We will discuss many of the contractual matters that are commonly found in partnership agreements in Chapter 45.

But these agreements cannot modify or avoid legal responsibilities under the UPA that pertain to relationships between the partnership and third parties. The liability of partners to injured third parties will be controlled by the UPA and by applicable common law. Because of its unique character, the liability of

Table 38.1. Jurisdictions Adopting the Uniform Partnership Act

Alabama	Code 1975, §§10-8-1 to 10-8-103.
Alaska	A.S. 32.05.010 to 32.05.430.
Arizona	A.R.S. §§29-201 to 29-244.
Arkansas	Ark. Stats. §§65-101 to 65-143.
California	West's Ann. Cal. Corp. Code, §§15001 to 15045.
Colorado	C.R.S. 7-60-101 to 7-60-143.
Connecticut	C.G.S.A. §§34-39 to 34-82
Delaware	6 Del. C. §§1501 to 1543.
District of Columbia	D.C. Code 1981, §§41-101 to 41-142.
Florida	West's F.S.A. §§620.56 to 620.77.
Georgia	O.C.G.A. §§14-8-1 to 14-8-43.
Hawaii	H.R.S. §§425-101 to 425-143.
Idaho	I.C. §§53-301 to 53-343.
Illinois	S.H.A. ch. 106½, ¶¶1 to 43.
Indiana	West's A.I.C. 23-4-1-1 to 23-4-1-43.
Iowa	I.C.A. §§544.1 to 544.43.
Kansas	K.S.A. 56-301 to 56-343.
Kentucky	K.R.S. 362.150 to 362.360.
Maine	31 M.R.S.A. §§281 to 323.
Maryland	Code, Corporations and Associations, §§9-101 to 9-703.
Massachusetts	M.G.L.A. ch. 108A, §§1 to 44.
Michigan	M.C.L.A. §§449.1 to 449.43n.
Minnesota	M.S.A. §§323.01 to 323.43.
Mississippi	Code 1972, §§79-12-1 to 79-12-85.
Missouri	V.A.M.S. §§358.010 to 358.430.
Montana	M.C.A. 35-10-101 to 35-10-615.
Nebraska	R.R.S 1943, §§67-301 to 67-343.
Nevada	N.R.S. 87.010 to 87.430.
New Hampshire	R.S.A. 304-A:1 to 304-A:43.
New Jersey	N.J.S.A. 42:1-1 to 42:1-43.
New Mexico	N.M.S.A. 1978, §§54-1-1 to 54-1-43.
New York	McKinney's Partnership Law, §§1 to 74.
North Carolina	G.S. §§59-31 to 59-73.
North Dakota	N.D.C.C. 45-05-01 to 45-09-15.
Ohio	R.C. §§1775.01 to 1775.42.
Oklahoma	54 Okl. St. Ann. §§201 to 244.
Oregon	O.R.S. 68.010 to 68.650.
Pennsylvania	59 Pa. C.S.A. §§301 to 365.
Rhode Island	Gen. Laws 1956, §§7-12-12 to 7-12-55.
South Carolina	Code 1976, §§33-41-10 to 33-41-1090.
South Dakota	S.D.C.L. 48-1-1 to 48-5-56.
Tennessee	T.C.A. §§61-1-101 to 61-1-142.
Texas	Vernon's Ann. Texas. Civ. St. art. 6132b.
Utah	U.C.A. 1953, 48-1-1 to 48-1-40.
Vermont	11 V.S.A. §§1121 to 1335.
Virginia	Code 1950, §§50-1 to 50-43.
Washington	West's R.C.W.A. 25.04.010 to 25.04.430.
West Virginia	Code, 47 8A-1 to 47-8A-45.
Wisconsin	W.S.A. 178.01 to 178.39.
Wyoming	W.S. 1977, §§17-13-101 to 17-13-615.

Source: West Publishing Company, 1986.

partners is discussed separately in this chapter. We will describe other important applications of the UPA in Chapter 45.

Economic and governmental factors have created a difficult environment for the entrepreneural solo practitioner who has been the mainstay of optometric practice, as evidenced by the rise in partnerships among optometrists and the corresponding decline in individual proprietorships (see Chapter 37). The number of partnerships has reached about 17 percent of all forms of practice, and the optometric literature is replete with references to the advantages of the partnership mode of practice, especially for the new optometry school graduate and the established practitioner who is looking ahead to retirement.[5] Despite the evident interest within the profession for such matches, there has been no large-scale widespread acceptance in the private sector.[6]

There are obvious advantages to creating a partnership, both professional and economic[7] (Table 38.2).

The disadvantages of partnership primarily weigh upon the shoulders of the individual proprietor who decides to assume the burden of another practitioner. What the new partner loses in independence, how-

Table 38.2. Advantages of Partnership

Mutual professional stimulation, with consultation readily available and more expansive areas of practice and specialized services available for patient care
Less capital outlay per partner required to commence practice compared to that required of an individual proprietor
Economic benefits for the partners; earnings greater than that for individual proprietors
Expanded office hours, greater efficiency in procedures and use of personnel, and standardized recordkeeping
More free time for the partners; coverage during periods of absence; expanded opportunities for leisure, continuing education, and community service
Practice growth, with increased equity at retirement and buy-sell insurance to cover the death or disability of a partner

Source: Milkie, G., *Partnerships and Professional Corporations*, Optometric Development Enterprises, St. Louis, 1972, pp. 54–55.

Table 38.3. Disadvantages of Partnership

Loss of independence
Conflicts between partners based upon personality differences or philosophical differences as to clinical practice
Partners are legally responsible for one another, both in contract and in tort
Complex contract negotiations, increased bookkeeping, greater formality in decision making and in running the practice
Differences between partners in living standards, levels of income, hours of work, and partnership benefits
Value for a partner's interest at death or disability established through buy-sell life insurance, formulas, or other artificial means that may not accurately reflect the partner's true equity in the practice

Source: Milkie, G., *Partnerships and Professional Corporations*, Optometric Development Enterprises, St. Louis, 1972, pp. 54–55.

ever, he generally gains in terms of security[8] (Table 38.3). Furthermore, economic surveys conducted by the American Optometric Association have uniformly found that partners achieve greater earnings than do individual proprietors.[9] Thus, where partnerships are successful, they offer an alternative to the traditional mode of practice that is most attractive.

New partnerships arise principally through merger, either between two established practitioners or between an established practitioner and a recent licensee (the so-called senior-junior partnership). Of the two types of merger, a partnership between established practitioners presents the fewer economic and legal problems. Typically, these partners are more equal in financial terms than are senior-junior partners and require less complex agreements to establish the relationship.[10] Senior-junior partnerships usually arise through associateship or through expense-sharing, both of which permit the established practitioner an opportunity to work with the younger optometrist before a commitment to enter into partnership is made. Because of their importance, senior-junior contractual arrangements will be discussed fully in Chapter 45. Mergers between established practitioners will be described in the concluding section of this chapter.

Organization

The decision to enter into partnership is a serious one that should be given thoughtful consideration. There are many factors to be weighed, and the decision-making process involved in senior-junior partnerships is reviewed in Chapter 44. The initiation of a partnership is only the beginning of a series of legal steps designed to provide guidance for the conduct of the partners and their joint undertaking. There are three phases to partnership that must be discussed: formulation, maintenance, and dissolution.

Each phase presents legal problems that should be addressed by the partners before the partnership has been formed. In most cases legal advice is not only advisable, it is necessary in order for the partners to acquire a full understanding of the problems facing them and of the options available to provide for their resolution. The end result of these discussions will be a series of decisions that will establish the organization of the partnership. These decisions will then be committed to writing, and a formal document will be signed by the partners as evidence of their agreement. This Partnership Agreement (or Articles of Partnership) will thereafter serve as a reference for the duties and obligations of the partners to one another as to the formulation, maintenance, and dissolution of the partnership. Some of the important legal issues that must be discussed by the partners when considering each of these phases are described in the following paragraphs.

Formulation of the Partnership

There are certain formalities that must be observed by a beginning partnership:

Legal and Tax Requirements—The partnership will need to obtain federal and state tax identification numbers, a business license, a partnership bank account and will have to comply with federal and state requirements for the documentation of employee tax withholding and other tax obligations.

Notification of Third-Party Providers—The partnership will have to comply with federal, state, and private third-party vision service plan requirements as to the acquisition of new provider numbers.

Insurance Coverage—The liabilities of partners are different from those of individuals, and insurance coverage must be obtained that will provide adequate protection for the partnership (discussed later in this chapter).

Partnership Name—State law and ethical considerations may limit the name of the partnership.[11] In most states, the partnership name will have to be registered with the state so that interested third parties can learn the identity of the principals.

Existing Legal Obligations—Individual partners may have preexisting legal obligations such as leases, contracts, insurance policies, loans, or other obligations that may need to be transferred or otherwise disposed of. When making such transactions, care should be exercised to ensure that individuals are clearly identified as such and not as agents of the partnership (discussed subsequently).

In addition to the formal steps necessary to institute the partnership, the partners will have to consider a number of organizational details:

Status of the Individual Partners—The percent of ownership of each partner and the individual share of partnership profit or loss must be determined. In addition, the duties, hours, and location of work, and numerous other details pertaining to individual obligations to the partnership must be delineated (see Chapter 45).

Duration of the Partnership—The partnership may continue for an indefinite period or a specific termination date can be required. In either event, because of the consensual basis of the partnership relationship, any partner may resign and thereby dissolve the partnership,[12] and guidelines will have to be established for this eventuality.

Partnership Capital—One of the major problems facing the partners is the funding of the partnership. Before the partnership can become operative some proportional sharing of cash, property, and services will have to be agreed to and these contributions used to create the partnership capital. Although contributions are not taxable events (being considered an exchange for an interest in the partnership), they will have significant tax ramifications when each of the partners terminates his partnership interest. Where there is inequality between the partners as to their capital contributions, and equality of ownership is contemplated (as in senior-junior partnerships), some provision should be made between the partners to allow for the equalization of capital. A policy must be agreed on concerning the right of a partner to withdraw any portion of his capital contribution from the partnership prior to termination of the partnership.

Benefits—Which benefits (automobile expenses, insurance premiums, continuing education expenses, professional fees) are to be paid by the partnership and which are to be borne by the individual partners must be decided at the outset of the partnership. Any retirement plans (such as a Keogh Plan) to be offered at the beginning of the partnership must be clearly understood by all partners. Insurance coverage for death and disability should also be considered; a discussion of partnership benefits can be found in a subsequent section of this chapter.

Income—The income to be paid each of the partners, and how it is to be determined, are among the most important topics that the partners must settle. There are many complexities to the sharing of income, and any agreement must reflect the special circumstances faced by the individual partners. A discussion of the division of partnership income can be found in Chapter 45.

Ownership of Records—Some method must be selected by the partners for identification of individual and partnership records. Ownership of records is of vital importance because a partner may choose to withdraw from the partnership and establish an independent practice.

The written agreement between the partners should reflect their decisions concerning these and related matters and should include provisions for the continued maintenance of the partnership.

Maintenance of the Partnership

Once the partnership has begun, a different set of considerations arise. If the partnership is financially successful, the partners may desire to alter their facilities, equipment, number of personnel (by adding additional partners), and partnership benefits. The division of partnership income also may undergo change. These matters should be provided for prior to the initiation of the partnership.

Alteration of the Partnership—The partners should contemplate the necessity for purchasing additional equipment, modifying their premises or moving to a different location, increasing or changing the benefits to the partners, and taking on additional assistants or partners.

Changes in Work Status—Over the passage of time the partners may wish to institute changes in the hours of work expected of each individual (of particular importance in senior-junior arrangements). Provisions for this eventuality, and its effect on the division of income, are best decided in advance.

Modification of Income—In senior-junior partnerships, the percent of ownership and the distribution of profit usually is shared unequally at the beginning of the arrangement and parity is achieved over a period of time. The agreement between the partners should express these decisions in unambiguous language; if there is an adjustment to be made in the event of disability of one of the partners, it should be set forth clearly. There are a number of factors that can determine the manner in which the income from the practice will be distributed, and the partners should thoroughly understand them (see Chapter 45 for a discussion of some of these factors).

The problems of maintenance are often happy problems that are associated with the growth of the partnership. Unfortunately, there is also the inevitable problem of dissolution of the partnership, a complicated undertaking that can create personal hardship for some partners if not adequately provided for at the beginning of the partnership.

Dissolution of the Partnership

There are three ways in which a partnership can be terminated: withdrawal, long-term disability, or death of the partners. (Financial failure can also terminate a partnership but will not be discussed.) Withdrawal, whether due to personal reasons or because of retirement, is the leading reason for the dissolution of partnerships. Long-term disability is the second leading cause, and death is the least likely possibility.[13] Life insurance is more often than not the eventuality that is best provided for, and disability is frequently the least-carefully considered. The partners should take the time and effort necessary to discuss these matters fully and should reach agreement on the conduct of the partnership affairs during the difficult period of dissolution.

In a senior-junior partnership, it is contemplated that the older partner will reach retirement within a reasonably definable period of time and will desire to sell his share of the partnership, either to the junior partner or to a successor. If possible, agreement as to how this transfer is to be accomplished should be reached at the initiation of the parthership.[14]

Because a partnership is a voluntary association, any of the partners may end his relationship with the partnership without the approval of the other partners. For this reason the partnership agreement should specify the procedure approved by the partners for withdrawal. Under certain circumstances the withdrawing partner may be liable to the other partners for damages, and provision can be made for the damages to be paid in this eventuality.[15]

Dissolution requires that a final accounting be made among the partners as to the various partnership assets. Property contributed to the partnership will be returned to the partners, and all debts and obligations will be satisfied. For the partners, dissolution can be an event of some tax consequence, and professional advice should be solicited prior to the institution of the partnership about the potential ramifications of dissolution.[16]

Another result of dissolution is the division of the partnership's patient records. Rights to records and the information contained in them can be a controversial issue when a partner withdraws, and it is advisable to ward off this potential problem at the time of the establishment of the partnership.

Dissolution, like the other important considerations of partnership, can be conducted in accordance with the provisions stated in the partnership agreement, and with so many important issues available to be settled by the partners themselves, it is obviously advisable to prepare a written, comprehensive document that reflects the decisions of the partners as to their agreement if dissolution occurs. Failure to provide for this eventuality will result in the application of the Uniform Partnership Act (UPA) or state common law in the event there is a legal dispute between the partners.

The UPA is an attempt to describe what most people would intend a partnership to be and codifies many common law concepts that pertain to partnerships. One of the most important of these concepts is the determination that partners are co-owners for the purpose of doing business and that—as such—every partner is the absolute agent of every other partner and is the principal of each of the other partners as well. An agent is defined as one who acts for or in place of another person (the principal) by authority from him and who is appointed by the principal to act as a substitute, with the power to do the things that the principal may do. The principal is in essence a surety for the agent and is responsible to those with whom the agent conducts his affairs for any misfeasance on the agent's part.[17] Since partners may act interchangeably as agents and principals (depending on the type of activity being performed), they are responsible for the conduct of one another. This provision of the UPA—which cannot be altered by the partnership agreement—is most significant when looked at from the viewpoint of liability (discussed *infra*). A more detailed description of the liability of principals and agents can be found in Chapter 21.

Table 38.4. Selected Provisions of the Uniform Partnership Act

Definition of partnership and evidence of partnership
Partnership property
Partners as agents of the partnership
Conveyances of real property by the partnership
Admissions of partners as evidence against partnership
Wrongful acts of partners
Nature of partner's liability
Liability of incoming partners and retiring partners
Rights and duties of partners
Rights of retiring partners or estates of deceased partners
Information between partners
Partners accountable as fiduciaries
Books and rights of access and inspection
Rights to an accounting by partners
Continuation of partnership beyond a fixed term
Property rights of partners and co-ownership of specific partnership property
Nature of partner's interest in the partnership
Dissolution of partnerships and right to wind up the partnership affairs
Distributions of assets and liabilities at dissolution

Source: Uniform Partnership Act.

The UPA establishes legal requirements for the conduct of partnerships that are quite comprehensive. A brief summary of the UPA provisions can be found in Table 38.4.

Liability

Individual proprietors are liable for their conduct and for the conduct of employees that occurs in the line and scope of the employees' duties. Partners have a like obligation, for each is individually responsible for his or her own conduct and collectively they are responsible for the conduct of their employees. Because of the common-law rule that each partner is the agent and principal of every other partner, however, partners have a responsibility for one another as well. This responsibility is expressed in the UPA in the following language:

> All partners are liable:
> (a) Jointly and severally for everything chargeable to the partnership under sections 13 and 14[18]
> (b) Jointly for all other debts and obligations of the partnership; but any partner may enter into a separate obligation to perform a partnership contract.

Joint and several liability allows an injured party to sue one or more of the partners separately, or all of them together, at the party's option. Thus partners are liable for one another's acts and may be sued individually or collectively, which increases their exposure to liability beyond that faced by the sole proprietor.

There are two types of situations in which partnership liability is most frequently expressed: contractual obligations and injuries to others.

Contractual Obligations

There are many opportunities for partners to enter into contractual arrangements: the purchase of automobiles, equipment, ophthalmic materials, furnishings and fixtures, and other necessities of doing business require a sales contract. Loans are often needed to make purchases, and agreements for the leasing of equipment or automobiles are binding documents that involve transactions occuring over the course of several years. Any partner may sign a contract binding the partnership (and hence the other partners) to these obligations, and under certain circumstances the partnership (and thus the partners) will be responsible for the contract even though the partner who executed the agreement was not granted the authority to do so.[19] Therefore, partners must zealously oversee the conduct of their contractual relations with third parties.

One means of limiting the opportunity for ill-considered obligations is to require the agreement of all partners whenever an expenditure in excess of a certain sum is contemplated. Another time-tested procedure is to require the signatures of at least two persons on partnership checks. A formal policy for the approval of partnership expenditures should be expressed in the partnership agreement.

Whenever a partner signs an obligation on behalf of the partnership, the partner should be careful to describe his or her representative capacity. The customary means of designating an official position is to write, after the signature, words that describe the subscriber's position (e.g., "John Jones, as agent for Jones Eye Clinic, a partnership"). By so doing, the partner is removed from individual liability for the debt in the event the partnership does not ratify the obligation.[20]

Injuries to Others

Partners are under a legal duty to conform to certain standards of conduct so as to minimize the risk of injury to others. (This duty, and its significance for practitioners of optometry, is discussed in

Chapter 18.) If a partner fails to conform to the standard, and in so doing injures another person, not only is the partner potentially liable but also each of the other partners and all the partners collectively may be liable as well. This joint and several liability allows the injured party some degree of choice as to whom to sue, and any or all of the partners may end up as defendants.

Furthermore, in the event the injured party receives a judgment for damages and is unable to satisfy it by proceeding against the assets of the partner causing the injury, the injured party may proceed against any of the other partners held liable as defendants in the case or against the assets of the partnership if it is also been held responsible as a defendant.

In order to protect against such an eventuality, partnerships purchase a special form of professional liability insurance that provides indemnification for any partner held liable (see Chapter 54).

Partners are liable for the conduct of their employees, and if an employee injures a person while acting within the line and scope of his or her duties, the partner may be held responsible for the damages suffered by the person. Insurance coverage can also be purchased to provide protection against this eventuality.

The liability of partners is rather broad, and unlike professional associations or corporations, partnerships afford no shield against the suits of creditors or injured persons (discussed in Chapter 39). Due to the potential for loss that liability suits represent, partnerships must obtain adequate liability insurance coverage.

Benefits

The benefits that are realized by partners are not unlike those obtained by individual proprietors. The reason for this similarity lies within the structure of the partnership, which is, in essence, an association of individual proprietors. The tax reporting of partnerships reflects this fact because the partnership merely serves as a conduit for tax purposes, paying no tax itself and merely serving to determine the profit or loss that will become each partner's distributive share of the partnership proceeds. The partners then report the profit or loss on their individual tax returns. As a result, benefits paid for by the partnership on behalf of the partners come directly from the pockets of the partners themselves, which is no different from the situation faced by an individual proprietor.

Nevertheless, partnerships are used for the payment of certain benefits, such as automobile expenses, costs of attending continuing education seminars, professional dues and licensure fees, subscriptions to professional journals, and insurance premiums, because by diverting the cost of these expenditures through the partnership account, the partners are effectively able to create an allowance for these items.[21] Each partner receives a certain sum to be applied toward the enumerated benefits, and any individual excess is paid for by the individual partner. Or the partnership may agree to reimburse the partner in full for the expenses incurred for specified activities or items. The determination of which benefits will be paid out of partnership funds is one that the partners must negotiate among themselves. (A discussion of the allocation of these benefits is included in Chapter 45).

One benefit that particularly draws the interest of partners is insurance. Premiums for life and disability insurance, if paid for out of partnership funds, are not a business-related expense for which a tax deduction will be permitted. Partners are often urged to purchase buy-sell life insurance, which is employed by surviving partners to pay for the partnership interest of a deceased partner, but the necessity for these policies is open to debate (see Chapter 45). Only the professional association or corporation can claim as a tax deduction the cost of certain life insurance premiums. In a partnership, the payment of insurance premiums is customarily borne by the individual partners and not by the partnership.

If a partnership wishes to establish a retirement tax shelter, the choice is the same as that for an individual proprietorship, the Keogh Plan (see Chapter 37). Individual partners may open Individual Retirement Accounts (IRAs) if they so wish because these plans do not have to be adopted by the partnership. A Keogh Plan is a different matter, however, since it requires the inclusion of certain employees who desire to participate and thus involves the payment of partnership funds into an employee fund. The agreement of the partners will be necessary before instituting a plan with such far-reaching financial effects. If a Keogh Plan is desired, it affords a means of sheltering income that is presently comparable to that allowed of incorporated persons.[22] Since the Tax Equity and Fiscal Responsibility Act of 1982 (TEFRA), nonincorporated self-employed individuals (whether in an individual proprietorship or a partnership) have been able to look forward to tax-deferred retirement planning that compares very favorably to that previously reserved to incorporated persons alone.[23] (The benefits available to these individuals are described in Chapter 37.) Thus Keogh

Plans have grown in popularity as a means of setting aside income for retirement.

Of course, the primary benefits derived from partnership are personal and professional. In terms of taxation, however, the tax benefits granted to a partnership are more like those of individual proprietorships than those of professional associations or corporations. Some of the fundamental considerations of the tax reporting of partnerships are examined in the following section.

Tax Considerations

A partnership is not a taxable entity, and partnership profits (and other income and gains) are not taxed to the partnership. The partnership, however, must determine its total income and file Form 1065, U.S. Partnership Return of Income, which provides basic information on partnership income or losses for the year and the partners' distributive shares of that income or loss.[24] Each partner's distributive share of partnership items must be included in determining the partner's individual taxable income, which is reported on IRS Form 1040 (see Chapter 41).

Every partnership must file a return. There is a penalty for failure to file that can be assessed against the partnership for each month that the return is late or incomplete.

Although the partnership is not a taxable entity, it is permitted to deduct certain expenses that are ordinary and necessary to the conduct of business. These deductions reduce the distributive share of partnership income that is to be allocated to the partners. Thus they are, in effect, borne by the partners themselves in a proportional fashion. Income to partners is frequently expressed in terms of a draw against profits, paid on a monthly basis and applied at the conclusion of the tax year to the partners' distributive shares of the partnership profit. Individual partners may claim many of the same tax advantages as individual proprietors, and so a working knowledge of the basics of tax law is essential.

Usually, neither the partners nor the partnership will recognize a gain or loss when property is contributed to the partnership in exchange for an interest in it. Thus capital contributions are usually not taxable to the partners or the partnership. When distributions of property are made by the partnership to the partners, however, a number of factors must be considered in determining the tax consequences, and so professional tax advice is required. And if a partner acquires an interest in the partnership as compensation for services rendered (often used in senior-junior partnerships to equalize the percent of ownership between the partners), the net value of this interest must generally be included as gross income for the recipient.[25] When payments are made by the partnership to a retiring partner or to the estate of a deceased partner in return for the complete relinquishment of that partner's interest in the partnership, the tax consequences will be quite significant.[26] Professional tax advice will again be required.

Merger

The growing acceptance of partnership among optometrists has led to the occasional merger of established practitioners. There are excellent economic reasons for such partnerships, and the personal rewards are equally good (assuming that an individual is prepared for the changes that come with a sharing of ownership and control). Since each optometrist has acquired assets, belongings, obligations, patient records, personnel, and habits, there are practical considerations associated with merger that are quite significant. Numerous legal and tax matters are involved, and it is essential that competent professional advice be procured at the outset of the decision to merge so that unfortunate and preventable consequences do not undermine the new business association.

The discussion below touches upon some of the more important considerations that must be settled by the merging practitioners. It is by no means an exhaustive list.[27]

Income Division—The most important decision that the merging doctors must make concerns the division of income. Patient volume, gross and net income, working hours, and percentage of ownership are only a few of the matters that have to be reviewed (see Chapter 45). Probably the best policy is to air fully all financial details, review the various alternatives available for the sharing of income, then hold an open and frank discussion as to the best means of reaching an equitable division.

Premerger Agreement—In some instances (as when the purchase of real estate or other substantial obligations are incurred) practitioners who are committed to merger should consider a signed premerger agreement. The purpose of the agreement is to protect each doctor from the unilateral withdrawal of the other after sizeable financial obligations have been made.

Side Agreement—The merging practitioners may wish to execute an agreement between themselves that protects an innocent doctor or practice from any pre-merger liabilities of which they were not a part and provides for a sharing of liability which arises as a result of the merger.

New Office Space—A merger may require relocation to a new office since the office space of the individual practitioners may prove insufficient for the partnership. In considering the options, the practitioners should be careful not to underestimate the new practice's needs and should take care to lay out the office as efficiently as possible. Appropriate use of space, ancillary personnel, and patient flow should be determined.

Assets—The practitioners should decide which equipment, furnishings, fixtures, and like items are to be used in the new practice. Between established doctors the assets will be of roughly equal value in the usual case, and so their capital contributions will be approximately the same. In those instances where there is a significant difference, the practitioner making the larger contribution can receive a higher capital account balance, equalizing contributions of cash, or additional income from the practice that is equal to the difference.[28]

Personnel—The doctors should meet with their aides promptly in order to inform them of the merger and to discuss their future roles in the partnership. Which aides are to be retained, their specific responsibilities, the income they are to receive, and similar matters must be decided by the partners before the merger is completed. In a newly merged office a jointly drafted office policy manual can be used to delineate rights and responsibilities of employment, a necessary undertaking when the doctors exercised different policies in their former offices.

Records—It is advisable for the merging doctors to develop a single new filing system rather than to work from separate files, especially since much of the work necessary to integrate records and files can be performed in advance of the merger. Color coding of the patient records is an excellent idea in this type of practice. Because the practitioners will be jointly responsible for patient care, they should discuss and consider uniformity in the way record entries are made and organized.[29]

Appointments and Scheduling—Coordination of office schedules requires that the practitioners agree on how patients are to be divided, which in turn has significance for the patient load to be managed by each partner and for the division of income (if it is based upon productivity rather than on a percentage basis). Office personnel who schedule patients must understand the doctors' policy, as must those who perform the filing and recordkeeping duties.[30]

Fee Schedule—The partners must review their fee schedules to determine the fee policy for the common practice. A uniform fee system is necessary and must be communicated to the office personnel so that billing errors can be prevented.

Third-Party Insurance Plans—New provider numbers may be required when practitioners merge and should be applied for well in advance so as to prevent delays in reimbursement. The merger may cause a change in the fee profile of one of the doctors if he charged lower fees than his new partner, resulting in an economic dividend to the partnership.

Billing and Bookkeeping Systems—The partners should establish a single billing system for the practice. It is advisable to use a system that can indicate the amount of income that is generated by each doctor, even if income is not to be divided on the basis of productivity, because this statistical information is important to the evaluation of the new relationship. At the outset of the partnership, the financial records should be reviewed at least monthly in order for the partners to assess the partnership's financial progress.

Collections—The procedures to be followed in pursuing delinquent accounts should be determined before the merger rather than left to the time at which collections problems have arisen.

Notice to Patients and Colleagues—An announcement should be drafted jointly by the doctors and sent to patients and colleagues informing them of the new joint practice. Receptionists in the premerger offices should be sufficiently informed so as to be able to answer questions posed by telephone queries.

Analysis of Legal and Tax Considerations—Prior to the merger the practitioners should have their consultant draw up an in-depth analysis of the tax matters that must be dealt with by the new partnership. Tax planning is advisable, particularly at the outset of the relationship, and the prospective partners should devote ample time to this facet of their business venture.

As with any partnership, the fundamental consideration is one of fairness to each of the partners. Because of the consensual nature of the relationship between partners, and because of the lengthy duration of the association that is contemplated in virtually all partnerships, an agreement that is unfair or dealings that are not above board can only serve to undermine the rapport—and, ultimately, the ties—that hold the individual partners together.

A discussion of contractual provisions that are commonly found in partnership agreements, and of some of the legal problems that attend their adoption, are included in Chapter 45.

Notes

1. *Black's Law Dictionary*, 4th ed., West, St. Paul, Minn., 1968.
2. For purposes of forming a partnership, the "persons" may be corporations or professional corporations. Although there are some legal obstacles to overcome, two optometrists who are incorporated as PAs or PCs may join in a partnership. In some states a like result may be obtained by a partnership of health-care practitioners, such as optometrists and ophthalmologists, whether incorporated or not.
3. Since the partnership may not, in some states, be permitted to hold title to property, it has no assets that could be used to satisfy a judgment or other legal claim against the partnership. Therefore, although the partnership may be named as a party to litigation, the partners will be ultimately responsible for any damages or financial obligations of the partnership.
4. The Uniform Partnership Act was approved by the National Conference of Commissioners of Uniform State Laws in 1914. It has been adopted in all jurisdictions except Louisiana.
5. Perhaps the most comprehensive discussion (although now somewhat dated) can be found in Milkie, G., *Partnerships and Professional Corporations*, Optometric Development Enterprises, St. Louis, 1972. Another source of current information is Baldwin, R., R. Christensen, and J. Melton, *Rx For Success*, Vision Publications, Midwest City, Okla., 1983.
6. Although partnership has not yet become the rule in optometry, it would appear that the era of individual proprietorship has passed its zenith and that group practice in various forms is the future for the profession. See Haffner, A.N., The Backbone May Not Be So Strong, *Optometric Weekly*, vol. 68, no. 8, Feb. 24, 1977, p. 9.
7. Adopted from Milkie, supra note 5.
8. Ibid.
9. Ibid.
10. For a discussion, see Gregg, J., *The Business of Optometric Practice*, Advisory Enterprises, White Plains, N.Y., 1981.
11. In some states legal requirements may necessitate the listing of the names of the doctors providing services, in addition to the partnership name. State law and optometry board regulations will have to be consulted in order to be in compliance with these requirements.
12. No member of the partnership can be forced to provide services and participate in the partnership if that individual wishes not to do so. But remedies are available to the partner or partners who suffer damages as a result of the individual's withdrawal from the partnership if such withdrawal constitutes a breach of the partnership agreement. The agreement may specify the damages to be awarded and the remedies available to the injured parties in the event of such a breach. If the agreement does not specify these remedies, then the Uniform Partnership Act or the common law will be looked to in the event of a legal dispute to determine the rights and responsibilities of the parties.
13. Statistically, disability is a greater likelihood than death, and in a partnership it is essential that some thought be given to how the partnership will manage the disability of a partner. For a discussion of disability insurance, see Kaufman, S., Why Your Disability Insurance Might Not Pay Off, *Medical Economics*, vol. 59, no. 11, 1982, pp. 251–259; Geier, A., Your Best Buy In Disability Insurance, *Optometric Management*, vol. 19, no. 2, 1983, pp. 75–83; and Disability Insurance, *Consumer Reports*, Mar. 1983, p. 122.
14. See Milkie, supra note 5, for a more detailed discussion.
15. If a junior partner decides to leave the partnership before he has become a full partner, i.e., during the buy-in phase (which may require several years), the partnership agreement may specify that the junior partner will pay damages to the partnership for the premature severance of the agreement, such damages being termed liquidated damages. These damages may be included in the contract as the specific sum to be paid by either party in the event of a breach by the other.
16. For a discussion of the basic tax problems of partnership, see IRS publication guide number 541, *Tax Information on Partnerships*.
17. The law of agency is quite complex, and legal counsel will be needed at the outset of the partnership arrangement to ensure that the partners are familiar with the approved methods of conducting themselves when performing partnership business.
18. Joint and several liability exists when a creditor or other party may sue one or more of the parties to such liability separately, or all of them together at his option. *Black's Law Dictionary*, supra note 1.
19. For example, a partner might have the apparent authority to bind the partnership to a contract, and the effect will be the same as if the partner had the actual authority to do so. Apparent authority is defined as that which, although not actually granted, the principal knowingly permits the partner to exercise, or which he

holds himself out as possessing. Legal counsel may be required at the initiation of the partnership in order to clarify some of the problems of agency.

20. As long as a partner signs as agent for the partnership, if for some reason the partnership disavows the contract, the partner will not be individually liable for the debt. For a more detailed discussion, see Henn, H.G., *Agency and Partnership*, West, St. Paul, Minn., 1972.
21. The partnership tax return includes deductions for business-related expenses, which has the effect of permitting the partnership to pay for these items. Of course, this allocation of funds for benefits reduces the income that is received by the partners and taxed at their individual rates.
22. Limits on Keogh Plans, as of 1988, are 25 percent of income for defined contribution plans, up to a maximum of $30,000 per year, and 100 percent of income for defined benefit plans, to pay a benefit of up to $90,000 per year. These limits may change if Congress continues to tinker with federal tax laws for pensions and annuities.
23. Under TEFRA, the advantages of professional corporations were significantly reduced. See Amaon, G.P., and F.J. Tuthill, Most Tax Advantages of Professional Service Corporations Eliminated, But Some Benefits Remain, *Taxation for Lawyers*, vol. 12, no. 4, July–Aug. 1983, pp. 10–14.
24. See Internal Revenue Service guide number 541, *Tax Information on Partnerships.*
25. Ibid.
26. Ibid.
27. For more details on partnership by merger, see Milkie, supra note 5.
28. Ibid.
29. Ibid.
30. Ibid.

Chapter 39

Professional Associations and Corporations

In response to recent decisions of the federal courts, the Internal Revenue Service is conceding that organizations of doctors, lawyers, and other professional people organized under state professional corporation acts will, generally, be treated as corporations for tax purposes.
—Internal Revenue Service, *Technical Information Release 1019 of August 8, 1969*

The right of professionals to enjoy the benefits of that artificial offspring of business law, the corporation, has traveled an arduous and uphill path to reach its present status under the law. The original federal revenue acts regarded personal service corporations as partnerships that were not entitled to receive the benefits of incorporation, although certain associations that resembled corporations were permitted to be taxed as corporations and thus to receive favorable tax treatment. In 1948, in a well-publicized case,[1] a group of physicians in Montana founded a practice that was organized and managed as if it were a corporation and established a retirement plan that qualified under IRS rules for corporate retirement plans. The IRS Commissioner contested the group's corporate tax status but was defeated in the courts, despite the fact that Montana did not permit the corporate practice of medicine. Subsequent cases obtained the same result,[2] and a movement was born.

In 1960 the IRS issued the so-called Kintner regulations,[3] which were intended to restrict the opportunity for unincorporated associations to qualify for corporate tax treatment. Consequently, several states enacted laws enabling professional corporations to be formed, but the IRS amended the Kintner regulations in 1965 so that state laws would not be able to create corporations that could automatically qualify for favorable federal tax treatment. A series of court defeats for the IRS ensued,[4] at the conclusion of which the IRS conceded that personal service corporations formed under state professional association or corporation statutes would be accorded the tax privileges of corporations. (The IRS capitulation is quoted in part at the head of the chapter.) Laws permitting the formulation of these corporations have been passed in all fifty states and the District of Columbia.[5]

Corporations composed of professionals have become an accepted means of doing business and have permitted these professionals to enjoy tax advantages otherwise unavailable to self-employed persons. The IRS, however, has remained vigilant and has required that such organizations adhere strictly to the technical rules applied to corporations. In another widely discussed case, a group of doctors who formed a corporation as a tax device only and conducted their practices in an independent fashion without conforming to required corporate formalities were denied corporate status and tax advantages by the IRS.[6] Those who incorporate their practices must be careful to avoid the appearance of not conforming to corporate formalities, even when the corporation is composed solely of one individual.[7]

Professional corporations have enjoyed more

popularity in medicine than in optometry. Probably the major reason for the incorporation of less than 10 percent of optometric practices[8] is the independent-minded individual practitioner who has been the backbone of the profession throughout its history. Whereas physicians have tended to form groups, optometrists traditionally have done just the opposite. The formalities necessary to form a corporation, the technical obligations required to maintain it, and the complicated financial transactions that must be performed in order to realize the favorable tax advantages have mitigated against widespread acceptance within optometry. And with the recent changes in federal tax laws that elevate the benefits available to nonincorporated, self-employed practitioners, it seems unlikely that professional corporations will experience a surge in popularity among optometrists. Nevertheless, these important business entities should be understood by contemporary doctors of optometry because there are unique characteristics found in corporations that are present in no other form of business enterprise.

A corporation is an artificial creature of the law that is endowed with certain characteristics. Among the most important is the right of perpetual succession, which allows the corporation to continue despite the withdrawal, disability, or death of those who compose its ownership or are employed by it to perform services. Unlike individual proprietorships, which end with the retirement or death of the proprietor, and partnerships, which likewise must be dissolved when the partners end their association with one another, corporations may continue for as long as it is profitable for them to do so.

Another important general characteristic of corporations is the separation of ownership and management. In a sole proprietorship the individual owner has sole authority over how the practice is run; in a partnership the same result is obtained because ownership and management are merged in the partners, who direct among themselves the conduct of the practice; in a corporation, ownership and management may be separated so that the owners will not have any direct responsibility for or any direct authority over the manner in which the practice is managed. In professional corporations, of course, this advantage will not be fully realized.

Ownership of a corporation is indicated through the purchase of shares of stock. The stock is issued by the corporation for a face value, and afterwards its value is set by the law of supply and demand; the more profitable the corporation, the more valuable the stock. The stock is freely transferrable, although in a professional corporation there will be certain restrictions for its sale established by the state law that regulates these corporations. The primary restriction limits ownership of stock to certain licensees who are eligible to incorporate. At the present time the majority of states will not permit licensed professionals who are of different disciplines to join together in ownership of a common personal services corporation. As of 1980, only California, Iowa, Kansas, Mississippi, New York, and Pennsylvania permit optometrists to form a professional corporation or association with physicians.[9]

Because a corporation is recognized as a separate entity by the law, it possesses several of the rights normally accorded only to persons. Among these rights are the ability to own property in its own name, sue or be sued, and claim tax advantages that are separate and apart from those accorded to individuals. This status as an artificial being is one of the most meaningful characteristics of a corporation.

Liability for the debts of the corporation is limited to the corporation itself. If the corporation defaults on a loan, the creditor must proceed against the assets owned by the corporation and not against the assets of the stockholders or employees of the corporation. If the corporation enters into bankruptcy, the owners of the corporation are not responsible for more than their respective shares of ownership, and so their personal assets cannot be invaded to satisfy the indebtedness of the corporation.

The tax advantages available to corporations are often cited as the primary reason for professionals to incorporate. We will discuss tax benefits presently, but the sheltering of income through pension and profit-sharing plans, the purchase of life and health insurance through the corporation, the more effective management of business-related expenses, and the use of voluntary death benefit plans, are all distinguishing features of the incorporated practice. The tax advantage held by corporations has been significantly reduced by changes in federal tax law (discussed subsequently).

These characteristics distinguish both professional associations (PAs) and professional corporations (PCs) (see Table 39.1). Although there are technical distinctions between the two, in practical effect there is so little difference that the two terms will be used synonymously here. Because the corporation is a separate business entity, those dealing with a corporation must be put on notice that it is the form of business organization being used. Thus professionals who are incorporated are required to place PA or PC (depending on whether their state law authorizes the formation of an association or a corporation) behind the name of their organization.

Table 39.1. Characteristics of Professional Corporations and Associations

Method of organization

One or more persons who perform professional services may form a professional corporation or association in order to practice the profession. The articles of incorporation or association will describe the profession to be practiced, the identities of corporate shareholders and directors, and will specify that each of the stockholders and directors is duly licensed to practice the profession. The corporate name must be followed by the identification P.A. or P.C. and may have to contain the name of one or more of the shareholders or other designations.

Scope of services

The corporation or association may be organized only for the purpose of rendering one type of professional service (in most states) and may render its services only through its officers and employees, who shall be duly authorized to render the service.

Professional liability

Employees of the corporation or association will be responsible for any liability arising out of personal services rendered by the employees, but no employee will be personally liable in tort for any act in which he or she did not personally participate. A director, officer, or employee of a professional corporation or association will be liable in contract for any contract executed on behalf of the corporation or association within the limits of his or her actual authority.

Restrictions on ownership and transfer of shares

Only persons licensed to perform the services for which the corporation or association was formed may hold membership interest or be shareholders, and so shares of stock in the corporation or membership interests in the association may not be transferred or sold except to persons so licensed. The personal representative or estate of a deceased member or shareholder may continue to hold the deceased individual's shares for a reasonable period after death but may not participate in decisions concerning the rendering of professional services. The articles of incorporation or association may provide for restrictions on the transfer of shares or membership interests and for the redemption or purchase of the shares or membership interests by the corporation, association, or its owners.

Termination of employment

If an officer, shareholder, director, or employee of the corporation or association becomes legally disqualified to render professional services, he must sever, within a reasonable period, all employment with or financial interest in the corporation or association. Severence pay or other compensation for past services may be authorized by the corporation or association upon termination of employment.

Annual statements

The professional corporation or association must file at the anniversary date of incorporation a statement with the secretary of state that lists the identities of all members, shareholders, directors, officers, and employees.

There are a number of well-recognized advantages to incorporation that are available for optometrists. Most of the more important ones relate to the financial and tax benefits of incorporated practice.

Tax Benefits—Contributions to corporate profit-sharing plans of up to 15 percent of the participant's salary, and contributions of up to 25 percent of the participant's salary for a combined profit-sharing and pension plan, are the major reasons that corporations are favored by tax advisors. The money earned on the tax-free contributions to a tax-deferred compensation plan is accumulated tax-free as well. Tax is paid only when the participant receives benefits at retirement, at which time he is usually in a lower tax bracket.

Medical Expenses Reimbursement Plans—A corporation can reimburse its employees for all medical expenses incurred by them; the corporation receives a tax deduction, the employee a tax-free benefit.

Employee Insurance Programs—A corporation may purchase group term life insurance, disability income insurance, and medical and hospitalization insurance. The premiums on group term life insurance policies are deductible by the corporation and are not considered income for the employees up to the first $50,000 of coverage. Group medical insurance premiums paid by the corporation are deductible and are not considered income for the employee.

Death Benefits—A corporation may pay a death benefit of up to $5,000 to the family of an employee, such a benefit being deductible for the corporation and tax free to the family.

Sick Pay—A corporation can agree to continue to pay wages to a sick employee for a specified period of time and receive a deduction for these payments; the employee will be able to exclude at least part of these payments from taxable income.

Administrative Benefits—A corporation may be easier to use as an administrative unit, particularly if there are a number of doctors in the practice and these doctors withdraw or are hired with some frequency. Management is centralized and decision making is clearly defined.

Continuity of Existence—The death or withdrawal of a corporate shareholder will not cause the termination of the corporation (as opposed to a partnership, where the death or withdrawal of a partner can end the partnership).

Simple Transferability of Ownership—The corporate stock may be transferred or sold to persons practicing the same profession.

Limitation of Legal Liability—The corporation is ultimately liable for the actions of its employees, and the liability of shareholders is limited to their investment in the corporation. Thus there are limitations to liability not found in other forms of business.

Deferred Compensation Plans for Estate Planning—The professional corporation has offered the most versatile means of deferring income for estate planning purposes; profit-sharing and pension plans have been the leading methods employed to create an estate. The new tax laws have had an effect on this benefit of incorporation, however, and noncorporate plans have become quite similar.

Although the preceding list is an impressive one that causes incorporation to be regarded as very desirable, there are disadvantages that offset these favorable factors and—for many practitioners—outweigh them.[10]

Cost—The organizational costs for a corporation and for the establishment of a corporate retirement plan exceed those for individuals in a partnership. Operating costs of a corporation and the expense of getting a corporation started (especially attorneys' and accountants' fees) are also expensive.

Increased Taxes—There are several taxes that will increase for the incorporated practitioner: social security taxes, unemployment taxes, worker's compensation rates, and even the federal income tax (for the corporation must pay a higher rate than an individual). The cumulative effect will be to create a larger tax liability than for a self-employed practitioner.

Accumulated Earnings Tax—Salaries paid to corporate employees that are not reasonable will be construed, in part, as being dividends, for which the corporation will receive no tax deduction. Thus there is some motivation for the corporation to retain excess income rather than to pay it out in salaries. In order to prevent the corporation from retaining unreasonable amounts of income, however, the accumulated earnings tax is imposed; a corporation may not accumulate more than $150,000 unless such moneys are needed for reasonable present or future business plans. Amounts used to purchase most employee benefit plans are secure from the accumulated earnings tax.

Personal Holding Company Tax—This tax was created to prevent individuals from forming corporations solely for the purpose of creating an additional tax entity in order to lower income taxes. To prevent this possibility, a penalty is imposed on corporate income that is deemed to be personal holding company income. At this time the typical professional corporation will not be considered a personal holding company and subject to the penalty; however, in order to be assured that neither the personal holding penalty tax nor the accumulated earnings tax would be levied on the corporation, the major portion of the corporate income must be distributed, either as salary or as benefits. Thus tax planning is an essential aspect of incorporation.

Increased Retirement Plan Costs—When a doctor incorporates his practice and establishes a pension plan, he may be required to include all employees within the provisions of the plan, which could be more costly than like benefits offered by an unincorporated Keogh Plan.

Greater Business Complexity—A corporation is more complex than a partnership or individual proprietorship. Since it is a separate tax entity, it requires more careful documentation of how money is being used. Stockholders' and directors' meetings must be held periodically and minutes carefully maintained. A legal or tax advisor will be needed to ensure compliance with the legal requirements associated with incorporation.

Limited Investment Opportunities—The corporate retirement benefits usually substitute for the personal investments that a doctor would otherwise make. The money diverted into corporate plans reduces the opportunity for other investments, when compared to an individual proprietorship or partnership.

Enjoyment of Benefits Requires Retirement—The major advantage of incorporation, income during retirement, is lost if the practitioner does not in fact retire. This is because tax-deferred income is nothing more than enforced savings if the taxpayer is not in a lower tax bracket at the time the tax-deferred money is withdrawn. Of course, everyone should plan for retirement because it may be forced upon an unwilling practitioner due to any of a variety of reasons.

Loss of Independence—In more than one-person corporations, there is a loss of individual control over business affairs that is not found in sole proprietorships. Also, financial planning will have to reflect the needs and desires of all employees and not those of just one practitioner.

Disclosure Requirements—Professional corporations are sometimes subject to disclosure requirements (both governmental and private) that do not apply to individual proprietorships and partnerships.

As the preceding lists point out, the decision to incorporate is primarily financial in nature, although there are personal factors that must also be weighed. For the majority of practitioners, the decision to incorporate centers around the amount of money that may be set aside for retirement through the tax shelters available to self-employed individuals. Before the early 1980s there was a significant difference between the amount of money that could be placed into pension and profit-sharing plans and into Keogh Plans. Professionals earning higher incomes found incorporation to be financially inviting because more income could be sheltered. With the growing similarity between the two types of plans, however, the advantages of pension and profit-sharing plans are open to question.[11]

With the formalities that must be observed in incorporated practices, the costs that must be borne to fund incorporated retirement plans for all eligible employees, and the substantial earnings that must be achieved in order to realize the full tax benefits possible under incorporated plans, the decision to incorporate requires thoughtful deliberation and astute financial advice from a competent professional counselor.[12]

Organization

Under many of the original state professional corporation enabling statutes, three persons were needed to form the corporation, but most of these laws have been amended to permit two and, in many states, one incorporator, thus making it possible for an individual proprietor to incorporate himself. In order to establish a corporation, there are certain legal formalities that must be observed. Typically, a set of documents known as the articles of incorporation or articles of association must be filed with the office of the Secretary of State in the state capital. These articles describe the type of profession that is to be practiced, list the names and addresses of the stockholders of the corporation or association (and of the officers in some states), contain an averral that all incorporators are licensed to practice the profession in the state, and identify the regulatory board to which the incorporators are subject. A fee is charged for filing the papers. But this is only the start of the formation process. Some of the activities that must be undertaken to initiate the corporation are summarized below.[13]

1. The corporation should comply fully with all state statutory requirements necessary to form a professional corporation.
2. The corporation should secure its own federal and state employer identification number.
3. The corporate name should be used on office doors, professional listings, telephone listings, stationery, invoices, checks, business cards, announcements, and all other documents.
4. All contracts, leases, deeds, and other legal documents should be negotiated by the corporation and executed by it in its own name.
5. All business assets transferred to the corporation and all insurance policies should be held in the corporate name.
6. The corporation should open its own bank accounts.
7. All fees for services should be paid to the corporation and deposited in the corporate bank account. Avoid depositing any fees in an individual employee's account.
8. Expenses of the corporation should be paid by the corporation with its own checks out of its own bank account.
9. All patients should promptly be notified of

the incorporation and be advised to make all payments to the corporation. Any existing contracts with patients should promptly be assigned to the corporation and any new contracts should be negotiated by the corporation and executed in the name of the corporation.

10. The professional corporation should obtain a corporate seal and stock book. There should be a bona fide issuance of stock and accurate stock records should be kept. Organizational minutes should be adopted which reflect, among other things, the election of the board of directors and officers of the corporation, the adoption of bylaws, the date for annual directors' and shareholders' meetings, the adoption of a fiscal year, the authorization to the corporation to employ professionals and nonprofessionals, the authorization to pay salaries to the corporate employees, approval of the form of stock certificates, a description of the characteristics of the stock, the authorization to the corporation to adopt a qualified retirement plan, and the selection of an accountant and attorney.
11. The corporation should obtain a corporate minute book in which to keep the articles of incorporation, bylaws, and other significant documents, including employment agreements.
12. Meetings of the board of directors and shareholders should be held at least annually and probably more frequently. At these meetings, the board of directors should be elected and officers designated. Formal minutes of these meetings should be adopted and placed in the minute book.
13. At the meetings of the board of directors, the directors should adopt resolutions establishing salaries, bonuses, and contributions to qualified retirement plans, authorizing all important contracts, and authorizing all important corporate activity. The board of directors should be as active as possible in supervising and directing corporate policies.
14. The corporation should engage in a meaningful business activity. It should hold some assets and conduct its business like a corporation.
15. Written employment agreements should be adopted and executed by both professional and nonprofessional employees. These agreements should contain provisions concerning compensation levels, or formulas for determining compensation, that are as specific as possible, as well as being reasonable and realistic. These agreements should also contain provisions requiring that all fees be turned over to the corporation and that the employees devote all of their time and attention to the conduct of their services for the corporation. The agreements may contain provisions dealing with periodic review of the quality of services and compensation.
16. Written buy-sell agreements should be executed dealing with the death, retirement, withdrawal and admission of stockholders. The agreement should also contain provisions regarding the funding for these purchases.
17. All appropriate federal and state income taxes should be properly and timely paid. The corporation should pay Social Security and state and federal withholding taxes regarding its employees and, if required by law, should cover them under state and federal unemployment compensation arrangements. The corporation should also pay all state, franchise and ad valorem taxes and file annual reports.
18. The corporation should maintain complete and accurate accounting records.
19. The corporation should avoid paying the non-business expenses of shareholder-employees.

Once the corporation has been formed, the daily management of corporate affairs is left to the officers of the corporation, who are elected by the board of directors. In many states the officers and directors do not have to be licensed professionals (although the owners, i.e., the shareholders, do). If there is only one incorporator, he may become the sole director of the corporation, but nonprofessionals can serve as officers. In some states the sole incorporator may be required to be the president of the corporation and nonprofessionals can serve in other positions, such as secretary or treasurer. The officers perform the short-term decision-making and conduct the scheduled meetings and other formalities necessary to doing business as a corporation.

With so many different classes of persons involved in a corporation—the shareholder-owners, the board of directors, the corporate officers, and the other employees of the corporation—there is some question as to just who is responsible for corporate liabilities. We will address this issue in the following section.

Liability

There are two types of liability claims that are of significance to incorporated practitioners: those

Table 39.2. Liabilities of Business Organizations

	Individual Proprietorship	Partnership	Professional Association or Corporation
Contracts	The optometrist is liable for business contracts.	The partners are jointly liable for partnership contracts.	The corporation is liable for business contracts.
Negligence of the optometrist	The optometrist is liable for his own negligence.	The partners are jointly liable for the negligence of each other.	The corporation is liable for the negligence of its employee-optometrists.
Negligence of other employees	The optometrist is liable for the negligence of employees.	The partners are liable for the negligence of employees.	The corporation is liable for the negligence of other employees.
Products liability	The optometrist is liable for the products dispensed by the proprietorship (and the manufacturer may be liable as well).	The partners are jointly liable for the products dispensed by the partnership (and the manufacturer may be liable as well).	The corporation is liable for the products its employees dispense (and the manufacturer may also be liable).

that arise out of contract and those that are due to personal injury.

Because the professional corporation may contract in its own name, it is customary for officers authorized to execute contracts on behalf of the corporation to do so in their official capacity. The officer's signature binds the corporation, which is solely responsible for any breach or failure to comply with contract terms that results in damages to the other contracting party. If damages must be paid, they must come from the assets (or the insurance) held by the corporation. Neither the officers nor the shareholders will be held liable. If the corporation fails, the loss to the shareholders will be the money invested by them in the business enterprise. Their personal assets will not be vulnerable (unless they were obligors as individuals along with the corporation). Thus a corporation affords some protection from contractual liability that the individual proprietorship and the partnership do not.

If the employee of a corporation commits an act that results in injury to the person or property of another, and the employee is held to have been legally at fault, not only is the employee responsible for the resultant damages but the employer may also be held responsible if the employee was acting within the line and scope of his duties at the time of the injury[14] (see Chapter 21). In this respect the liability of a corporation is no different from that of any other business organization. As with contracts, the liability of the corporation is limited to the extent of its assets. Professional corporations, however, may purchase liability insurance for indemnification in the event of such claims, and in the usual case the damages are paid by the insurance that is purchased by the corporation for the protection of its employees. If the insurance coverage is adequate to pay the claim, corporate employees are shielded at least to this extent in the incorporated practice. In a sole proprietorship the individual owner is liable; in a partnership the partners are liable both individually and as a group. (See Table 39.2 for a summary of the liabilities of the various forms of business organizations.)

Benefits

Perhaps the leading reason for incorporating has been the anticipated tax benefit to be enjoyed from the establishment of a qualified retirement plan. Like IRAs and Keogh Plans, these plans permit income to be tax deferred and for the money so set aside to accumulate interest and to grow without taxation until it is actually withdrawn during retirement.

The basic types of retirement plans available to a professional corporation are profit sharing, defined contribution pension plans, defined benefit pension plans, and combination profit-sharing and pension plans. In addition, 401(k) plans and simplified employee pensions (SEPs) may be used by incorporated practitioners.

Profit-Sharing Plans—Profit sharing allows a corporation to make substantial contributions without a fixed annual commitment. The corporation may deduct up to 15 percent of its payroll out of current or accumulated profits for contributions to a corporate profit-sharing plan. An employee can contribute another 10 percent of the employee's income voluntarily to such a plan. Each year the corporation's board of directors determines the amount to be contributed to the profit-sharing plan; if the board so decides, no allocation need be made.

Defined Contribution Pension Plans—This plan is merely a promise to commit an agreed-to fixed sum of money each year to each eligible employee's account. There are no promises about future benefits or about how much money will be available upon retirement. The retirement benefit will be based on the amount that has been accumulated in the individual's account over the years. The corporation may contribute and take a tax deduction on contributions up to 25 percent of payroll. Up to 25 percent of an individual's salary may be contributed, not to exceed $30,000 in any one year. This plan allows for a greater potential tax deduction than the profit-sharing plan, but it lacks the flexibility of profit sharing since the board of directors is not free to change the amount that is contributed from year to year.

Defined Benefit Pension Plans—This type of plan is much more complex than a defined contribution plan, requiring the employer to provide systematically for the payment of definitely determinable benefits to eligible corporate employees at retirement. An enrolled actuary determines the contributions that will be necessary so that the promised future benefits can be determined and the proper deductions made. Expenses are normally higher than for defined contribution plans because of the extra services that are required. Contributions to a defined benefit plan consider salary, age, and other factors. The older an employee is when enrolled in the plan, the shorter the period of time over which money can accumulate in order to provide the promised benefit. Thus, the defined benefit plan can be advantageous for the older optometrist, who may put up to 100 percent of compensation annually into the retirement fund. Conversely, it can be very disadvantageous to a young optometrist who has just become a shareholder/employee in the corporation.

Combination Profit-Sharing and Pension Plans—This approach generally combines a 15 percent maximum contribution for profit-sharing with an additional 10 percent maximum defined contribution pension plan. The corporation is afforded the opportunity to claim a tax deduction of up to 25 percent of its payroll. Yet, the corporation retains the substantial flexibility inherent in a profit-sharing arrangement. Many corporations are attracted by the simplicity and flexibility of the combination plan, and employees like them because these plans allow for sizeable contributions by individuals.

Simplified Employee Pensions—An SEP is an individual retirement arrangement into which an employee may contribute up to 15 percent of compensation to a maximum of $30,000. These accounts are much easier to administer than qualified pension or profit-sharing plans and so they are popular with employers. Because the contributions to an SEP-IRA are deductible on the employee's tax return, they are popular with employees. See Chapter 37 for a further discussion.

401(k) Plans—Although these salary reduction plans were not authorized by the U.S. Congress until 1978, they have become a popular means of providing for employee retirement savings. Sometimes referred to as cash or deferred arrangements, 401(k) plans allow employees to contribute up to 25 percent of compensation (to a maximum of $7,000) to a retirement fund. The employer determines the percentage that may be contributed to the plan. The 401(k) plans permit employees who are not eligible to claim tax deductions for IRAs to receive a favorable tax benefit because the amount deposited in the fund is not taxed as income (although it is subject to social security taxes) and grows tax-free until withdrawn. The 401(k) account is usually invested by a financial institution hired by the employer to administer the plan. Beginning in 1988 the $7,000 ceiling will be increased for inflation. But for higher-paid employees there are special restrictions that can apply, depending on the amounts contributed by other employees in the plan. Withdrawals are generally permitted when the employee retires, leaves the practice, reaches the age of $59\frac{1}{2}$, becomes disabled, or suffers financial hardship. Early withdrawals are subject to a 10 percent penalty, and there are limits to withdrawals for special circumstances, such as hardship.

The provisions of these various retirement plans are summarized in Table 39.3.

Since it was first acknowledged by the IRS that professionals could receive the tax benefits of incorporation, the retirement plans available to incorporated practitioners have been distinguished by their flexibility and opportunity to realize maximum retirement savings. But tax reform acts enacted by

Table 39.3. Comparison of Retirement Benefits Available to Incorporated and Nonincorporated Practitioners

Plan	Participant	Summary of Benefits
Keogh	Self-employed practitioners	*Defined contribution plans*: up to $30,000 annually or 25% of earned income, whichever is less *Defined benefit plans*: up to 100% of income may be contributed in order to fund an annual defined benefit at retirement (which may be up to $90,000)
Corporate pension	Employees of a professional corporation or association who qualify	*Defined contribution plans*: up to $30,000 annually or 25% of earned income, whichever is less *Defined benefit plans*: up to 100% of income may be contributed in order to fund an annual defined benefit at retirement (which may be up to $90,000)
Corporate profit-sharing	Employees of a professional corporation or association who qualify	Up to 25% of income for qualified profit-sharing plans (up to 15% from the employer and up to 10% from the employee)
Simplified employee pension	Self-employed practitioners; and employees of a professional corporation or association who qualify	Up to $30,000 annually or 15% of income, whichever is less
Corporate 401(k)	Employees of a professional corporation or association who qualify	Up to $7,000 annually or 25% of income, whichever is less
Individual retirement account	All employers and employees qualify; but the tax deductibility of contributions depends on participation in other retirement plans and level of income	Up to $2,000 annually or 100% of income, whichever is less; if married to a nonworking spouse, up to $2,250

the federal congress in 1981[15] and 1982[16] have significantly reduced the advantages that these plans offer. The two laws eliminate the difference between the benefits allowed corporate employees and those allowed for self-employed individuals.

Under the Tax Equity and Fiscal Responsibility Act of 1982 (TEFRA) the contributions made by nonincorporated practitioners to defined contribution Keogh plans are increased while at the same time the contributions allowed to defined contribution pension plans are reduced to the same level. Likewise, contributions to defined benefit Keogh plans by nonincorporated individuals are allowed to be computed in the same manner as those made by corporate employees to defined benefit pension plans, with the maximum annual benefits possible under corporate plans being reduced as well.

Another key set of restrictions applies to pension plans that are "top heavy" in favor of key employees.[17] Top-heavy plans are defined as those pension plans under which more than 60 percent of the accrued benefits (or contributions) are provided for key employees. Key employees are identified as officers, 5 percent owners, and 1 percent owners with compensation in excess of $150,000, or those employees who own the ten largest interests in the corporation (i.e., the shareholders).

Those pension plans that are not considered top heavy are permitted to continue to operate subject to certain modifications.[18] The end result of these far-reaching changes has been to raise serious questions concerning the need for incorporation.[19] The law even provides special tax breaks for corporations that are liquidated.[20]

In addition to retirement plans, there are certain fringe benefits that can be established through the use of insurance. They are attractive to the incorporated practitioner because they can be purchased with pre-tax dollars, whereas an individual proprietor or a partnership would have to finance them with after-tax dollars.

One popular fringe benefit is group term life insurance. The corporation may deduct the cost of insurance premiums for employees up to $50,000 of coverage. If a policy is paid to an employee's beneficiary, the proceeds are not taxable. If coverage exceeds $50,000, the excess is taxed to the employee (discussed in Chapter 52).

Health and accident insurance is another often-purchased benefit for corporate employees. The cost of premiums is deductible by the corporation, and benefits paid by the insurer to the employee are not taxable as income (see Chapter 41).

Disability insurance can also be provided to corporate employees, and the cost of premiums may be deducted by the corporation. The use of disability insurance is a complex issue that should be investigated carefully before a program is instituted (see Chapter 53).

There are two additional benefits of incorporation that require mention: the use of trade names and the ability of incorporated practitioners to form partnerships between corporations.

Trade Names

One consideration when forming a corporation is the use of a trade name. The right to employ a trade name is regulated by state statute, and states may lawfully prohibit the use of trade names by optometrists.[21] These state laws are among those commercial practice restrictions that the Eyeglasses II rule seeks to eliminate; see Chapter 4.

When a trade name is used, it is usually necessary for the name of the practitioner (or practitioners) to be listed along with it. This requirement is intended to put the public on notice as to the identity of the practitioner performing services under the guise of a trade name. Failure to observe the legal requirements established by state law as to the appropriate use of a trade name can subject the optometrist to discipline by the state board of optometry.

Partnerships of Professional Corporations

One much-discussed use of professional corporations has been to form partnerships comprised of these entities. Incorporated practitioners have used these partnerships as a means to limit the antidiscrimination provisions applicable to pension plans and have been successful in several cases that resulted in litigation.[22] When the federal congress enacted tax reform in 1982, however, it was provided that the IRS may allocate income, deductions, or other tax items of the corporation if it could be shown that the principal purpose of the partnership was simply to avoid federal income taxes.[23] Therefore, if challenged by the IRS, the partnership must be able to demonstrate significant nontax reasons for its formation, such as: permitting different philosophies to be employed by the partners as to whether to accumulate or pay out income, allowing the various practitioners to choose different types of qualified retirement plans, and enabling the selection of different types of fringe benefits for the employees of the two (or more) corporations. As a consequence of this provision by TEFRA, there have been relatively few of these partnerships among optometrists.

Tax Considerations

The professional corporation is treated by law as a separate tax entity, which results in both advantages and disadvantages. The tax rate for a professional service corporation, effective January 1, 1988, is considerably higher than those for individual taxpayers. Although the tax rates for other types of corporations range from 15 percent to 39 percent, professional service corporations (i.e., PAs and PCs) must pay a 34 percent tax on all net income. Since both the corporation and the employee-shareholder are subject to income taxation, it may be considered disadvantageous that a double tax can be imposed on an incorporated practitioner. But the tax deductions permitted to professional corporations frequently reduce the taxable income to zero, or result in the taxation of a minimum amount of income, leaving the employee-optometrist's salary as the major item subject to taxation.

The distribution of corporate income takes the form of salary (or bonuses) or dividends. Dividends are a distribution of any profit remaining after the costs and expenses of running the corporation have been paid.[24] Since dividends are not tax deductible and the salaries paid to employees are a major deduction for any business, the preferable distribution is a salary. Salaries paid to corporate employees (and particularly to professional employees) must be reasonable; income that is in excess of what is considered reasonable may be treated as a dividend by the IRS and hence may be refused as a deduction for the corporation. Determining the reasonableness of salaries is a difficult task since it is one of the least-defined concepts in tax law, but this is the task that faces a corporation that generates a profit in excess of expected expenditures.

If the salaries paid by the corporation to the professional employees have reached the maximum level of reasonableness, the shareholders (who are, of course, also the employees in a professional corporation) may not feel that further income can be justifiably distributed. In this event the shareholders may wish to retain the profits and leave them in the corporation.

To prevent shareholders from using the corpora-

Table 39.4. Comparisons between Corporations/Associations and Partnerships

	Partnership	Corporations/Associations
Ownership	Shared on a percentage basis by the partners	Based upon ownership of shares of stock or membership interest by the optometrists
Assets	May be owned by the partners	May be owned by the corporation
Business decisions	Determined jointly by the partners	Determined by the Board of Directors and officers of the corporation
Income	Profit is divided on the basis of ownership or according to the provisions of the partnership agreement; salary is received as a draw against expected profits.	Each optometrist-employee is paid a salary by the corporation.
Ownership of records	Owned by the partners in accordance with the provisions of the partnership agreement; if not specified in the agreement, owned jointly	Usually owned by the corporation
Insurance	Life and disability premiums for the partners are not tax deductible; health insurance premiums are partially deductible; professional liability insurance is deductible.	The corporation may deduct group life insurance, health, disability, and professional liability insurance premiums paid for optometrist-employees.
Retirement benefits	Keogh plans; simplified employee pensions; IRAs	Profit-sharing and pension plans; simplified employee pensions; 401(k) plans; IRAs
Income taxes	The partnership is not a taxable entity; the partners are taxed on their shares of the profits at their individual tax rates.	The corporation is taxed on net income at the corporate tax rate; employees are taxed on salaries at their individual tax rates.
Continuity	Ended at the death or disability of the partners	Maintained by the transfer of shares of stock to new shareholders

tion to avoid income taxes by retaining corporate earnings, the IRS imposes the accumulated earnings tax and, effective in 1988, the 34 percent tax bracket. While questions may abound concerning some uses of retained earnings, income that is used to purchase employee benefit plans are, in general, safe from the accumulated earnings tax, which is an additional tax incentive for the utilization of these plans by the incorporated practitioner.[25]

The major tax-deductible benefits that may be claimed by a professional corporation have already been described. More information on business-related tax items may be secured from tax and legal counsel.

Every corporation, unless it is specifically exempt or has dissolved, must file a tax return even if it had no taxable income for the year. The federal income tax form for corporations is IRS Form 1120.

Every corporation whose estimated tax is expected to be $40 or more is required to make estimated payments of tax. A corporation's estimated tax payments must be deposited with an authorized depository of a Federal Reserve Bank. The due date of deposits and the number of installments to be deposited depends on the earnings of the corporation, but generally the payments will be in four installments, made on a quarterly basis.

Corporate employees are paid a salary by the corporation, which is responsible for withholding of taxes. The employee will receive an annual summary of salary and withholding on the W-2 form issued by the corporation. The employee reports this income on his Form 1040 and attaches the W-2 to it.

A comparison of several of the key aspects of corporations and partnerships can be found in Table 39.4.

Subchapter S Corporations

A professional corporation may elect to be taxed under Subchapter S of the tax code, an election that is most often made by smaller corporations. The decision to seek S Corporation status has traditionally not been a popular one. The decision, when made, is primarily motivated by a desire to escape the double taxation found in the corporate earnings structure. S Corporations pay no income tax, rather being taxed in a manner that is more like a partnership. However, the S Corporation is still entitled to corporate tax benefits, such as contributions to retirement plans, premiums paid for insurance coverage, and other tax-deductible items utilized by professional corporations.[26]

The S Corporation also enjoys other advantages, including elimination of the problem of the accumulated earnings tax, the controversy over whether or not compensation to employees is salary or a dividend, and the difficulty of determining if compensation is reasonable.

In order to elect Subchapter S status, a corporation must meet certain requirements.[27] The most important of them are listed below:

- The election must be unanimous among the shareholders.
- The election must be made during the first month of the tax year (or in the month preceding).
- There must be no more than 35 shareholders.
- Not more than 20 percent of the corporate income may be passive investment income (e.g., from royalties, rents, dividends, and annuities).

One major problem with these corporations has been the highly technical requirements necessary to maintain the Subchapter S status, which, if lost through some unintended act, could have consequential and undesirable tax ramifications for the shareholders.[28] But the largest failing of these business entities has been the generally restricted savings allowable under tax-deferred retirement plans. The contributions permitted to S Corporation employees have been a pale imitation of those allowed employees of professional corporations. But the tax reform act of 1982 has removed this objection.[29]

Under the Tax Equity and Fiscal Responsibility Act of 1982, S Corporations were recognized as eligible to participate in the newly established limits for defined benefit and defined contribution Keogh plans, which, as already described, were raised in order to make them comparable with the limits allowed under corporate profit-sharing and pension plans. Therefore, S Corporations have received a tax-favored boost that may increase their popularity. In some circumstances they may provide a tax break for practitioners, such as using an S Corporation as the form of business for an optical dispensary.[30] Of course, significant tax decisions should not be made without first discussing them carefully with competent tax counsel.

Notes

1. *United States v. Kintner*, 216 F.2d 418 (9th Cir. 1954).
2. *Galt v. United States*, 175 F. Supp. 360 (D.C. Tex. 1959); and *Foreman v. United States*, 232 F. Supp. 134 (D.C. Fla. 1964).
3. *Treasury Dept. Regs.* §301.7701-2.
4. *Empey v. United States*, 406 F.2d 157 (10th Cir. 1959); *O'Neill v. United States*, 410 F.2d 888 (6th Cir. 1969); *Kurzner v. United States*, 413 F.2d 97 (5th Cir. 1969).
5. Although laws permitting corporate practice by professionals have been enacted in all jurisdictions, there are differences from state to state that make it necessary for the optometrist to consult competent legal and tax counsel prior to making the determination to form a professional association or corporation.
6. *Roubik & Roubik v. Commissioner*, 53 T.C. 365 (1969).
7. The effect of recent tax changes must be taken into consideration when a practitioner is debating the switch to a professional corporation. It should be noted that federal tax reform acts have become a staple of congressional life, including the Employee Retirement Income Security Act of 1974, the Tax Reform Act of 1976, the Revenue Act of 1978, the Economic Recovery Tax Act of 1981, the Tax Equity and Fiscal Responsibility Act of 1982, and the Tax Reform Acts of 1984 and 1986. See Taxes: To Incorporate or Not?, *Review of Optometry*, vol. 121, no. 4, 1984, p. 23.
8. 1987 AOA Economic Survey, published in the *AOA News*, Mar. 1, 1988.
9. Eaton, B.C., *Business Organizations*, Matthew Bender, New York, 1980, vol. 17C, pp. B-380–381.
10. Adopted from Milkie, G., *Partnerships and Professional Corporations*, Optometric Development Enterprises, St. Louis, 1972.
11. Amaon, G.P., and F.J. Tuthill, Most Tax Advantages of Professional Service Corporations Eliminated, But Some Benefits Remain, *Taxation for Lawyers*, vol. 12, no. 4, July-Aug. 1983, pp. 10–14.
12. See Funk, T.E., and M.A. Brauer, Strategies for Use of Qualified Retirement Plans of Corporations in Light of TEFRA, *Taxation for Lawyers*, vol. 11, no. 3, Nov.–Dec. 1982, pp. 140–144.
13. Martus, C., Nineteen Formalities Necessary to Incorporate, correspondence with the author.
14. For a discussion of vicarious liability, see Gabel, W., Vicarious Liability, *Journal of the American Optometric Association*, vol. 58, no. 7, 1987, pp. 599–601.
15. Economic Recovery Tax Act of 1981.
16. Tax Equity and Fiscal Responsibility Act of 1982.
17. Id. §207.
18. See Goldberg, M.A., Disincorporate? How to Unscramble the Eggs, *Optometric Management*, vol. 19, no. 2, 1983, pp. 37–42.
19. Ibid.
20. Ibid.
21. *Kiddie v. Commissioner*, 69 T.C. 1055 (1978); *Garland v. Commissioner*, 73 T.C. 5 (1979); and *Keller v. Commissioner*, 77 T.C. 1014 (1981).
22. Tax Equity and Fiscal Responsibility Act of 1982 §269A.
23. *Friedman v. Rogers*, 440 U.S. 1, 99 S. Ct. 887 (1979).
24. For a discussion of how corporations distribute income and of the many tax ramifications that accompany these decisions, see Brosterman, R., *The Complete Estate Planning Guide*, Mentor, New York, 1987.

25. Internal Revenue Service tax guide 542, *Tax Information on Corporations.*
26. Internal Revenue Service tax guide 589, *Tax Information on Subchapter S Corporations.*
27. Ibid.
28. Ibid.
29. Weil, F.B., and R.W. Wood, Subchapter S Corporations Made Simpler by New Law, But Not All Changes Are Improvements, *Taxation for Lawyers*, vol. 11, no. 4, Jan.–Feb. 1983, pp. 196–201; and Weil F.B., and R.W. Wood, New S Corporation Rules Revised and Explained by Technical Corrections Act, Temporary Regs., *Taxation for Lawyers*, vol. 11, no. 5, Mar.–Apr. 1983, pp. 272–276.
30. See Wass, V.G., Make Your Dispensary a Tax Shelter, *Optometric Management*, vol. 20, no. 4, 1984, pp. 35–39.

PART ELEVEN

TAXES

Chapter 40

Individual Income Tax

The Congress shall have power to lay and collect taxes on income, from whatever source derived, without apportionment among the several states, and without regard to any census or enumeration.
—Sixteenth Amendment, *Constitution of the United States*

The Federal Revenue System

At the time of the birth of the United States, the English government drew the ire of those in the colonies through the use of an import tariff, the purpose of which was to create a favorable balance of trade (i.e., exports were not subject to the tariff, but imports were charged a duty that was, ultimately, paid by the American consumer). The Boston Tea Party was a result of the perception by the citizens of the colonies that the tariff was unfair. Yet, one of the first acts of the new U.S. Congress was to impose an internal tariff on imports to America. Thus began a widespread system of duties on imports, rather than a true tax, because of the provisions of the U.S. Constitution, which limited the ability of the federal government to tax the U.S. citizenry.

The general taxing power permitted Congress by the Constitution was that "The Congress shall have power to lay and collect taxes, duties, imports and excises, to pay the debts and provide for the common defense and general welfare of the United States."[1]

As far as internal revenue was concerned, there were only two sources of income provided for by the Constitution:

1. Duties, imports, and excise taxes were permitted, but could not be higher in one part of the country than in another.[2]
2. No direct tax could be levied on the income of individual citizens unless it was applied in proportion to the population of the states, so that each state would have a different tax rate, a cumbersome and impractical system that made the collection of direct taxes a slow and grossly unequal operation.[3]

Attempts during the 1800s and early 1900s to impose an income tax met with limited success, with the most important development being a 1 percent tax on income over $5,000 earned by corporations organized for profit.[4] Then, in 1913, the U.S. Congress proposed an amendment to the Constitution that would allow a tax on all incomes without apportionment. Its ratification allowed an income tax to be levied on individual citizens.[5] The tax consisted of two parts: a normal tax, which was a flat 1 percent of the net income in excess of the personal exemption; and a surtax that was a progressive tax levied on net incomes in excess of $20,000 (for which another 1 percent was collected) up to a maximum of $500,000 (for which a 6 percent maximum tax was imposed). Thus, a married man with a net income of $80,000 in 1913 paid a total tax of $1,710. Subsequent changes in the rates and system of taxation have created dramatic differences in the tax burden incurred by American citizens: by 1980, this same married man would have to pay an income tax of $26,914.[6] Of such things is tax reform born, and the result has been the most remarkable series of tax reform acts ever passed by the federal congress: the Economic Recovery Tax Act of 1981 (ERTA), the Tax Equity and Fiscal Responsibility Act of 1982 (TEFRA), the Tax Reform Act of 1984, and the most revolutionary of all, the Tax Reform Act of 1986.

In fact, tax reform has become such a favorite pastime of the federal government that tax counsel should be consulted whenever financial decisions must be made. One year's tax laws rapidly give way to another's, and the wise optometrist will always seek professional advice before making personal or business decisions that have tax ramifications.

Even so, it is necessary for every optometrist to possess a reasonable understanding of the tax process. Given the significance of taxes as an item of both personal and business expense, contemporary practitioners can ill afford to live in ignorance of the basic provisions of tax law. Once these fundamental concepts are understood, the process of revision becomes less confusing, and the significance of proposed changes more apparent.

The tax base to which the income tax rates are applied is called the *taxable income*. To determine an individual's taxable income, the *gross income* must be calculated, from which *deductions* are subtracted, resulting in an intermediary sum known as the *adjusted gross income*. From this there are certain *itemized deductions* allowed, which may be used to further reduce the adjusted gross income, and which, when subtracted, results in the individual's *taxable income*. From this the *tax table tax* can be determined. *Credits* are then deducted, resulting in the actual tax owed (see Fig. 40.1 for a schematic representation of the process).

The income tax rates for individuals are graduated, i.e., they increase as the level of taxable income increases. The fourteen rates on taxable income that were imposed before the recent series of tax reform acts ranged from a minimum of 14 percent in the lowest bracket to a maximum of 70 percent. The 1986 law provides for a dramatic reduction in both the number of brackets (two) and the rates to be applied (15 percent and 28 percent). These rates are effective for the 1988 tax year and thereafter, unless modified by Congress.[7]

The purpose of this chapter is to illustrate the process by which an individual's taxable income is determined, e.g., the stepwise determination of an individual's tax. The acutal computation is performed on Internal Revenue Service (IRS) Form 1040, the standard tax form (see Fig. 40.2).

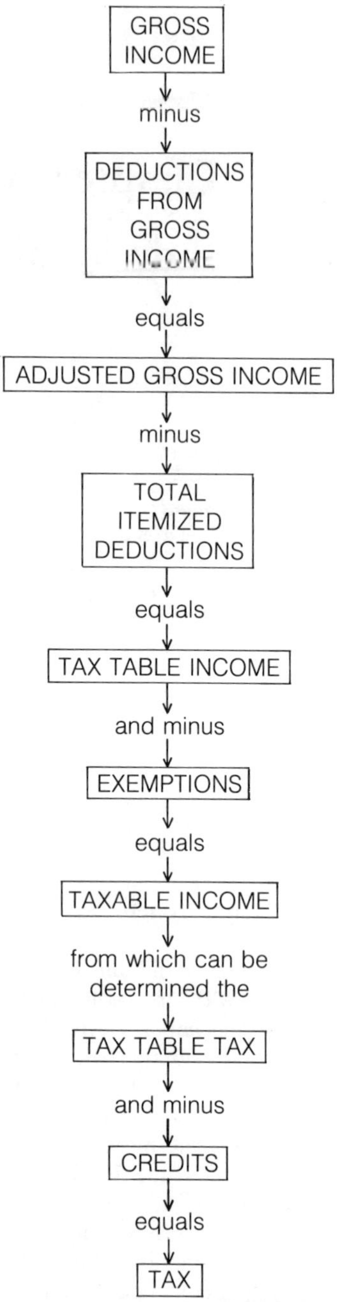

Figure 40.1. Schematic of the Tax Process

Gross Income

Every income tax return begins with gross income, which is defined as "all income from whatever source derived."[8] This rather all-inclusive phrase embraces such diverse means of income as compensation for

Form 1040 Department of the Treasury—Internal Revenue Service
U.S. Individual Income Tax Return 1987 (0)

For the year Jan.–Dec. 31, 1987, or other tax year beginning , 1987, ending , 19 . OMB No. 1545-0074

Label

Use IRS label. Otherwise, please print or type.

Your first name and initial (if joint return, also give spouse's name and initial) John G. and June	Last name O'DEE	**Your social security number** 123 45 6789
Present home address (number and street or rural route). (If you have a P.O. Box, see page 6 of Instructions.) 123 Main Street		**Spouse's social security number** 987 65 4321
City, town or post office, state, and ZIP code Anytown, State 12345		For Privacy Act and Paperwork Reduction Act Notice, see Instructions.

Presidential Election Campaign

Do you want $1 to go to this fund?	X	Yes		No
If joint return, does your spouse want $1 to go to this fund?	X	Yes		No

Note: *Checking "Yes" will not change your tax or reduce your refund.*

Filing Status

Check only one box.

1		Single
2	X	Married filing joint return (even if only one had income)
3		Married filing separate return. Enter spouse's social security no. above and full name here.
4		Head of household (with qualifying person). (See page 7 of Instructions.) If the qualifying person is your child but not your dependent, enter child's name here.
5		Qualifying widow(er) with dependent child (year spouse died ▶ 19). (See page 7 of Instructions.)

Exemptions

(See Instructions on page 7.)

Caution: If you can be claimed as a dependent on another person's tax return (such as your parents' return), do not check box 6a. But be sure to check the box on line 32b on page 2.

6a [X] Yourself   6b [X] Spouse

No. of boxes checked on 6a and 6b ▶ 2

c Dependents

(1) Name (first, initial, and last name)	(2) Check if under age 5	(3) If age 5 or over, dependent's social security number	(4) Relationship	(5) No. of months lived in your home in 1987
Junior	X		son	12

If more than 7 dependents, see Instructions on page 7.

No. of children on 6c who lived with you ▶ 1

No. of children on 6c who didn't live with you due to divorce or separation ▶

No. of parents listed on 6c ▶

No. of other dependents listed on 6c ▶

d If your child didn't live with you but is claimed as your dependent under a pre-1985 agreement, check here . ▶ ☐

e Total number of exemptions claimed (also complete line 35)

Add numbers entered in boxes above ▶ 3

Income

Please attach Copy B of your Forms W-2, W-2G, and W-2P here.

If you do not have a W-2, see page 6 of Instructions.

Please attach check or money order here.

Line	Description			Line	Amount
7	Wages, salaries, tips, etc. *(attach Form(s) W-2)*			7	1,200
8	**Taxable** interest income *(also attach Schedule B if over $400)*			8	400
9	**Tax-exempt** interest income (see page 10). DON'T include on line 8	9			
10	Dividend income *(also attach Schedule B if over $400)*			10	400
11	Taxable refunds of state and local income taxes, if any, from worksheet on page 11 of Instructions			11	
12	Alimony received			12	
13	Business income or (loss) *(attach Schedule C)*			13	39,925
14	Capital gain or (loss) *(attach Schedule D)*			14	
15	Other gains or (losses) *(attach Form 4797)*			15	
16a	Pensions, IRA distributions, annuities, and rollovers. Total received	16a			
b	Taxable amount (see page 11)			16b	
17	Rents, royalties, partnerships, estates, trusts, etc. *(attach Schedule E)*			17	
18	Farm income or (loss) *(attach Schedule F)*			18	
19	Unemployment compensation (insurance) (see page 11)			19	
20a	Social security benefits (see page 12)	20a			
b	Taxable amount, if any, from the worksheet on page 12			20b	
21	Other income (list type and amount—see page 12)			21	
22	Add the amounts shown in the far right column for lines 7, 8, and 10–21. This is your **total income** ▶			22	41,925

Adjustments to Income

(See Instructions on page 12.)

Line	Description			Line	Amount
23	Reimbursed employee business expenses from Form 2106	23			
24a	Your IRA deduction, from applicable worksheet on page 13 or 14	24a			
b	Spouse's IRA deduction, from applicable worksheet on page 13 or 14	24b			
25	Self-employed health insurance deduction, from worksheet on page 14	25			
26	Keogh retirement plan and self-employed SEP deduction	26			
27	Penalty on early withdrawal of savings	27			
28	Alimony paid (recipient's last name and social security no.)	28			
29	Add lines 23 through 28. These are your **total adjustments** ▶			29	0

Adjusted Gross Income

Line	Description	Line	Amount
30	Subtract line 29 from line 22. This is your **adjusted gross income.** *If this line is less than $15,432 and a child lived with you, see "Earned Income Credit" (line 56) on page 18 of the Instructions. If you want IRS to figure your tax, see page 15 of the Instructions* ▶	30	41,925

Figure 40.2. Sample Form 1040, page 1

Form 1040 (1987) **Page 2**

Tax Computation

			Line	Amount
31	Amount from line 30 (adjusted gross income)		31	41,925
32a	Check if: ☐ **You** were 65 or over ☐ Blind; ☐ **Spouse** was 65 or over ☐ Blind. Add the number of boxes checked and enter the total here ▶ 32a			
b	If you can be claimed as a dependent on another person's return, check here ▶ 32b ☐			
c	If you are married filing a separate return and your spouse itemizes deductions, or you are a dual-status alien, see page 15 and check here ▶ 32c ☐			
33a	**Itemized deductions.** See page 15 to see if you should itemize. If you don't itemize, enter zero. If you do itemize, attach Schedule A, enter the amount from Schedule A, line 26, **AND** skip line 33b		33a	6,673
b	**Standard deduction.** Read **Caution** to left. If it applies, see page 16 for the amount to enter. If **Caution** doesn't apply and your filing status from page 1 is: Single or Head of household, enter $2,540; Married filing jointly or Qualifying widow(er), enter $3,760; Married filing separately, enter $1,880		33b	
34	Subtract line 33a **or** 33b, whichever applies, from line 31. Enter the result here		34	35,252
35	Multiply $1,900 by the total number of exemptions claimed on line 6e or see chart on page 16		35	5,700
36	**Taxable income.** Subtract line 35 from line 34. Enter the result (but not less than zero)		36	29,552
	Caution: If under age 14 and you have more than $1,000 of investment income, check here ▶☐ and see page 16 to see if you have to use Form 8615 to figure your tax.			
37	Enter tax. Check if from ☒ Tax Table, ☐ Tax Rate Schedules, ☐ Schedule D, or ☐ Form 8615		37	4,521
38	Additional taxes (see page 16). Check if from ☐ Form 4970 or ☐ Form 4972		38	
39	Add lines 37 and 38. Enter the total ▶		39	4,521

Caution: ← If you checked any box on line 32a, b, or c and you don't itemize, see page 16 for the amount to enter on line 33b.

Credits (See Instructions on page 17.)

			Line	Amount
40	Credit for child and dependent care expenses *(attach Form 2441)*	40		
41	Credit for the elderly or for the permanently and totally disabled *(attach Schedule R)*	41		
42	Add lines 40 and 41. Enter the total		42	
43	Subtract line 42 from line 39. Enter the result (but not less than zero)		43	
44	Foreign tax credit *(attach Form 1116)*	44		
45	General business credit. Check if from ☐ Form 3800, ☐ Form 3468, ☐ Form 5884, ☐ Form 6478, ☐ Form 6765, or ☐ Form 8586	45		
46	Add lines 44 and 45. Enter the total		46	
47	Subtract line 46 from line 43. Enter the result (but not less than zero) ▶		47	4,521

Other Taxes (Including Advance EIC Payments)

		Line	Amount
48	Self-employment tax *(attach Schedule SE)*	48	4,911
49	Alternative minimum tax *(attach Form 6251)*	49	
50	Tax from recapture of investment credit *(attach Form 4255)*	50	
51	Social security tax on tip income not reported to employer *(attach Form 4137)*	51	
52	Tax on an IRA or a qualified retirement plan *(attach Form 5329)*	52	
53	Add lines 47 through 52. This is your **total tax** ▶	53	9,432

Payments Attach Forms W-2, W-2G, and W-2P to front.

				Line	Amount
54	Federal income tax withheld (including tax shown on Form(s) 1099)	54			
55	1987 estimated tax payments and amount applied from 1986 return	55	9,000		
56	Earned income credit (see page 18)	56			
57	Amount paid with Form 4868 (extension request)	57			
58	Excess social security tax and RRTA tax withheld (see page 19)	58			
59	Credit for Federal tax on gasoline and special fuels *(attach Form 4136)*	59			
60	Regulated investment company credit *(attach Form 2439)*	60			
61	Add lines 54 through 60. These are your **total payments** ▶			61	9,000

Refund or Amount You Owe

			Line	Amount
62	If line 61 is larger than line 53, enter amount **OVERPAID** ▶		62	
63	Amount of line 62 to be **REFUNDED TO YOU** ▶		63	
64	Amount of line 62 to be applied to your 1988 estimated tax ▶	64		
65	If line 53 is larger than line 61, enter **AMOUNT YOU OWE.** Attach check or money order for full amount payable to "Internal Revenue Service." Write your social security number, daytime phone number, and "1987 Form 1040" on it		65	432
	Check ▶ ☐ if Form 2210 (2210F) is attached. See page 20. **Penalty:** $			

Please Sign Here

Under penalties of perjury, I declare that I have examined this return and accompanying schedules and statements, and to the best of my knowledge and belief, they are true, correct, and complete. Declaration of preparer (other than taxpayer) is based on all information of which preparer has any knowledge.

Your signature	Date	Your occupation
Jf O'Dee	15 Apr 87	Optometrist
Spouse's signature (if joint return, BOTH must sign)	**Date**	**Spouse's occupation**
June O'Dee	15 Apr 87	Homemaker

Paid Preparer's Use Only

Preparer's signature	Date	Check if self-employed	Preparer's social security no.
Sam Accountant	Apr 15, 1987	☒	111 22 3333
Firm's name (or yours if self-employed) and address: Sam Accountant, CPA, 321 Main Street, Anytown, State		E.I. No.	12 : 34 5678
		ZIP code	12345

★U.S.GPO:1987-0-183-082

Figure 40.2. Sample Form 1040, page 2

services (such as those of a doctor), business income, gains from the sale or exchange of property, interest, rents, royalties, dividends, annuities, pensions, partnership income, income from an estate or trust, prizes, alimony, and illegally obtained windfalls such as embezzlement, gambling, theft, fraud, and related offenses.

There are certain exclusions from gross income that escape taxation. These exempt classes of income should not be confused with deductions from gross income. Some of the more important exclusions are:

Life Insurance Death Proceeds—The proceeds of life insurance policies, if paid by reason of the death of the insured, are excluded from the gross income of the beneficiary. The manner in which the policy proceeds are paid is of no consequence, i.e., whether in a lump sum or in installments. Where the proceeds of a life insurance contract are paid for reasons other than the death of the insured, however, the insured is entitled to recover tax-free only what was paid for the contract.[9]

Employees' Death Benefits—The first $5,000 received by the beneficiary of an employee, paid by or on behalf of an employer because of the death of the employee, is excluded from gross income.[10]

Gifts, Bequests, and Devises—The amount of cash or the value of property received by gift or inheritance is excluded from gross income.[11] But income derived from property received by gift is taxable as income to the recipient.

Retirement Income—Social Security benefits are currently not subject to taxation as gross income.[12]

Interest on Government Securities—State and local bonds produce interest income that is not includable as gross income. Obligations of the federal government are subject to federal taxation, and the interest on U.S. Savings Bonds (Series E) is fully taxable.[13]

Compensation for Injuries or Sickness—Compensation awarded for personal rights, such as workman's compensation, damages for personal injury, damages for defamation, and damages for other legal actions intended to "make the person whole again" are excludable from gross income. A like exclusion is permitted for accident and health benefits received under a policy purchased by the policyholder.[14]

Employee's Accident and Health Plan Benefits—Amounts received by an employee as reimbursement for medical care, payments for permanent injuries or loss of bodily function, and to a limited extent, wages or payments in lieu of wages during a period of absence from work as a result of permanent and total disability are excludable from gross income.[15]

Employer's Educational Assistance Plans—Amounts paid by an employer for an employee's education, pursuant to a plan meeting certain requirements, are excludable from gross income. Amounts received that may be excluded include tuition and fees, books, supplies, and equipment. In order for an educational assistance program to qualify, it must be in writing, limited to providing employees with educational assistance, and not discriminatory in favor of certain employees or a certain class of employees.[16]

Scholarships and Fellowship Grants—Scholarships and fellowship grants are tax exempt for degree candidates but only to the extent that amounts are paid for tuition, books, and supplies; room and board and other expenses that are paid by the scholarship or fellowship are not excluded from income.[17]

Sale of Residence by 55-Year-Olds—A person fifty-five years and older who sells a residence and realizes a profit from the sale does not have to purchase another home within twenty-four months in order to avoid the capital gains tax normally applied to such sales. $125,000 of gain realized from the sale may be excluded from gross income by the seller. This is a once-in-a-lifetime exemption.[18]

Once the gross income is determined, the next step is to consider the possible nonbusiness deductions available to the taxpayer.

Deductions

The nonbusiness expenses that are deductible in the process to arrive at the adjusted gross income are those attributable to individual retirement accounts (IRAs), forfeited interest on a time-saving deposit, and alimony.

Individual Retirement Accounts (IRAs)—Contributions to an IRA can be deducted from gross income, but this deduction is limited by the provisions of the Tax Reform Act of 1986 and may not be claimed by certain taxpayers (see Chapter 37).[19]

Forfeited Interest—Interest that was previously earned on a time savings account with a bank or savings and loan and that is forfeited in a later year under the institution's rules on premature withdrawals of funds from such account or deposit is deductible from gross income.[20]

Alimony—Alimony and separate maintenance payments are deductible from gross income by the one paying them if certain criteria are met: (1) they must be made under a written decree or agreement; (2) they must qualify as periodic payments, i.e., payments that are uncertain in amount, or for an indefinite period, or for more than ten years; (3) they must not be specifically designated for the support of minor children; and (4) they must not be in the form of a lump sum payment or settlement.[21]

These three nonbusiness deductions may be used to reduce the gross income of the taxpayer. (There are other nonbusiness deductions that can be claimed by the taxpayer in order to reduce the adjusted gross income. These deductions, which are known as the itemized deductions, are tabulated on Schedule A of Form 1040, discussed *infra.*) These three nonbusiness deductions, when subtracted from gross income, produce the *adjusted gross income* (AGI), which is a term that we will refer to later when making certain calculations such as the deduction for medical expenses on Schedule A (see Fig. 40.3). The next step in the tax determination process is to figure the itemized deductions, but in order to do so we must first understand an allied concept, the standard deduction.

The Standard Deduction

The lowest bracket in each of the tax rate schedules has a tax rate of zero; this standard deduction is available to taxpayers who do not itemize. As of 1988, this amount is $3,000 for unmarried individuals; $4,400 for heads of households; $5,000 for married individuals filing joint returns and for surviving spouses; and $2,500 for married individuals who file separate returns. An additional standard deduction of $750 is allowed for individuals age sixty-five or older ($600 if married) and for individuals who are blind. Thus, a married taxpayer who is both age sixty-five and blind could claim an additional $1,200 standard deduction.

For nonitemizers, only income in excess of the standard deduction is subject to tax. If a taxpayer does itemize, it is because the total itemized deductions exceed the standard deduction. This calculation is performed on Schedule A (see Fig. 40.3). But the extra deduction for elderly and blind taxpayers cannot be claimed by itemizers.

There are two more steps to be completed in order to determine the taxable income:

1. Subtract the total itemized deductions (listed on schedule A).
2. Subtract any personal and dependency exemptions (to be discussed subsequently).

An illustration of how the itemized deductions are calculated on Schedule A is included as Fig. 40.3. It is the total ($6,673) that is subtracted from the adjusted gross income on Form 1040.

Itemized Deductions

There are several recognized categories of expenses that are commonly incurred by taxpayers and that are recognized as itemized deductions.

Personal Interest Expense—Interest paid or accrued by a taxpayer is deductible, even though incurred for a personal purpose. Examples of such interest expense are mortgage interest payments, interest on personal loans (including insurance policy loans), and interest paid on credit purchases or credit cards. Under the Tax Reform Act of 1986, however, the deduction for personal interest expense on credit cards and consumer loans will be phased out by 1991 (see Chapter 42).[22]

Personal Taxes—Certain taxes imposed on a taxpayer during the tax year may be deducted, including state, local, and foreign real property taxes; state and local personal property taxes (i.e., an automobile tag tax); and state, local, and foreign income taxes. But state and local sales taxes are no longer deductible, as of 1987.[23]

Medical, Dental, and Optometric Expenses—The deduction allowed for these expenses is limited in several respects. A taxpayer may not claim a deduction for himself, his spouse, or his dependent, for amounts that he has been compensated for by insurance. As of 1987, this deduction is limited to the amount that is in excess of $7\frac{1}{2}$ percent of the adjusted gross income[24] (see Fig. 40.3). Amounts paid for medicine and drugs may be deducted, but, as of 1984, drugs are defined as prescription drugs and insulin only.[25] Premiums for health insurance[26] and transportation costs for health care[27] are also included as deductions in this category.

SCHEDULES A&B (Form 1040)
Department of the Treasury
Internal Revenue Service (0)

Schedule A—Itemized Deductions

(Schedule B is on back)

▶ Attach to Form 1040. ▶ See Instructions for Schedules A and B (Form 1040).

OMB No. 1545-0074
1987
Attachment Sequence No. **07**

Name(s) as shown on Form 1040: John G. and June O'DEE

Your social security number: 123 : 45 : 6789

Medical and Dental Expenses (Do not include expenses reimbursed or paid by others.) (See Instructions on page 21.)	1a	Prescription medicines and drugs, insulin, doctors, dentists, nurses, hospitals, insurance premiums you paid for medical and dental care, etc.	1a	2,400		
	b	Transportation and lodging	1b	100		
	c	Other (list—include hearing aids, dentures, eyeglasses, etc.) ▶	1c			
	2	Add lines 1a through 1c, and enter the total here	2	2,500		
	3	Multiply the amount on Form 1040, line 31, by 7.5% (.075)	3	3,135		
	4	Subtract line 3 from line 2. If zero or less, enter -0-. **Total** medical and dental ▶			4	0
Taxes You Paid (See Instructions on page 22.)		**Note:** Sales taxes are no longer deductible.				
	5	State and local income taxes	5	1,400		
	6	Real estate taxes	6	763		
	7	Other taxes (list—include personal property taxes) ▶ Automobile	7	70		
	8	Add the amounts on lines 5 through 7. Enter the total here. **Total** taxes ▶			8	2,233
Interest You Paid (See Instructions on page 22.)		**Note:** If you borrowed any new amounts against your home **after** 8/16/86 and at any time in 1987 the total of **all** your mortgage debts was more than what you paid for your home plus improvements, attach Form 8598 and check here ▶ ☐				
	9a	Deductible home mortgage interest you paid to financial institutions (report deductible points on line 10)	9a	3,000		
	b	Deductible home mortgage interest you paid to individuals (show that person's name and address) ▶	9b			
	10	Deductible points	10			
	11	Deductible investment interest	11			
	12a	Personal interest you paid (see page 22) [12a] 400				
	b	Multiply the amount on line 12a by 65% (.65). Enter the result	12b	260		
	13	Add the amounts on lines 9a through 11, and 12b. Enter the total here. **Total** interest ▶			13	3,260
Contributions You Made (See Instructions on page 23.)	14a	Cash contributions. (If you gave $3,000 or more to any one organization, report those contributions on line 14b.)	14a	880		
	b	Cash contributions totaling $3,000 or more to any one organization. (Show to whom you gave and how much you gave.) ▶	14b			
	15	Other than cash. (You must attach Form 8283 if over $500.)	15	300		
	16	Carryover from prior year	16			
	17	Add the amounts on lines 14a through 16. Enter the total here. **Total** contributions ▶			17	1,180
Casualty and Theft Losses	18	Casualty or theft loss(es) (attach Form 4684). (See page 23 of the Instructions.) ▶			18	0
Moving Expenses	19	Moving expenses (attach Form 3903 or 3903F). (See page 24 of the Instructions.) ▶			19	0
Miscellaneous Deductions Subject to 2% AGI Limit (See Instructions on page 24.)	20	Unreimbursed employee business expenses (attach Form 2106)	20	0		
	21	Other expenses (list type and amount) ▶ Acct fees 200 Safe deposit box 50 Legal fees 250	21	500		
	22	Add the amounts on lines 20 and 21. Enter the total	22	500		
	23	Multiply the amount on Form 1040, line 31, by 2% (.02). Enter the result here	23	836		
	24	Subtract line 23 from line 22. Enter the result (but not less than zero) ▶			24	0
Other Miscellaneous Deductions	25	Miscellaneous deductions not subject to 2% AGI limit (see page 24). (List type and amount.) ▶			25	0
Total Itemized Deductions	26	Add the amounts on lines 4, 8, 13, 17, 18, 19, 24, and 25. Enter the total here and on Form 1040, line 33a ▶			26	6,673

For Paperwork Reduction Act Notice, see Form 1040 Instructions. **Schedule A (Form 1040) 1987**

Figure 40.3. Sample Schedule A, Form 1040

Charitable Contributions—Contributions made to or for the use of the following types of organizations are deductible:

- A state, a possession of the United States, or any subdivision of any of these
- A corporation, trust, or other organization that is operated exclusively for religious, charitable, scientific, literary, or educational purposes
- Posts or organizations of war veterans, or an auxiliary unit or society of, or trust or foundation for, any such post or organization
- A domestic fraternal society, order, or association, operating under the lodge system (if the contribution is for charitable purposes).

Charitable contributions are allowed, generally, for money or property contributed to the above qualified organizations. The amount of a contribution in property other than money is its fair market value at the time of the contribution. The Tax Reform Act of 1986, by reducing individual tax rates, has made the charitable deduction less valuable than in the past.[28] The deduction has also been eliminated entirely for those who do not itemize, but this will not be a problem for most optometrists.

Casualty Losses—A taxpayer may deduct a limited amount for casualty losses to nonbusiness property that are due to fire, storm, shipwreck, or other casualty, and which are not covered by insurance. Such a personal casualty or theft loss may be deductible to the extent by which it exceeds 10 percent of the taxpayer's adjusted gross income.[29]

Moving Expenses—The cost of moving to another location to start a new job may qualify as a deduction if certain conditions are met (see Chapter 42). The actual costs of the move may be deducted, but pre-move expenses, temporary living expenses, and expenses for the sale, purchase, or lease of a residence are limited to $3,000, and the expenses related to house-hunting trips and temporary living expenses at the new job location cannot exceed $1,500 of the $3,000.

Miscellaneous Deductions—Beginning in 1987, deductions for miscellaneous expenses are allowable only to the extent these expenses, together with certain employee business expenses, exceed 2 percent of the taxpayer's adjusted gross income.[30] Examples of the miscellaneous deductions that may be claimed are listed in Table 40.1.

Table 40.1. Miscellaneous Expenses Deductible on Schedule A

Employee Expenses	Personal Expenses
License fees	Legal and accounting fees
Dues to professional societies	Fees paid to investment counsel
Employment-related education (i.e., continuing education expenses)	Fees paid to the custodian of an IRA
Expenses of looking for a job in the same field	Custodial fees paid for income-producing property
Malpractice insurance premiums	Cost of safe deposit box rental
Subscriptions to professional journals and magazines	Cost of tax services, periodicals, or return preparation
Work clothes or uniforms	Appraisal fees for establishing a casualty loss or charitable contribution
80% of unreimbursed business-related entertainment or meal expenses	
Business-related travel and transportation expenses in excess of reimbursement by the employer	

Source: *Prentice-Hall Guide to the Tax Reform Act of 1986*, Prentice-Hall, Paramus, N.J., 1986.

These itemized deductions require careful record-keeping. Receipts, checks, and other evidence of these expenditures should be retained and stored so that proof of claimed deductions will be readily available should the IRS audit the taxpayer's return.

Exemptions

An individual is entitled to deduct the following exemptions in calculating taxable income[31]:

- $1,950 exemption for the taxpayer in 1988, increased to $2,000 in 1989; this amount will be adjusted upwards annually (for inflation) beginning in 1990
- $1,950 exemption for the taxpayer's spouse on

a joint return ($2,000 in 1989 and adjusted annually thereafter)

- $1,950 exemption for each dependent whose gross income for the year is less than $1,000 ($2,000 in 1989 and adjusted annually thereafter); the $1,000 gross does not apply to a dependent child under 19 or to one who is a student, regardless of the student's age

These exemptions are claimed line 35 of Form 1040 (see Fig. 40.2), but the calculation as to the number of exemptions is performed in the exemptions section of the form (lines 6a–e, directly below filing status). Each exemption claimed by the taxpayer has the effect of lowering the taxable income by the amount claimed.

A taxpayer can claim a deduction for the personal exemptions of a spouse if the spouse has no gross income and is not the dependent of another taxpayer (such as the spouse's parents). It should be noted that a spouse cannot be claimed as a dependent. When the exemptions of a husband and wife are claimed on one return (a joint return), it is a return of two taxpayers, rather than of one taxpayer and one dependent, even if the spouse has no income of his or her own. The exemption for a spouse is a separate entity from the deduction claimed for a dependent.

The exemptions are used in the computation of the tax, which is the next step in the tax determination process.

Computing the Tax

The computation of individual tax is based upon the tax tables prepared by the IRS. The tables are constructed according to the tax status of the taxpayer: unmarried individuals, married couples filing a joint return, married persons filing separately, and heads of households.

Under the Tax Reform Act of 1986, effective in 1988 there are two tax rates to be applied to these categories: 15 percent and 28 percent.[32] There is, however, 5 percent surtax that will apply to high-income taxpayers, and it will have the effect of phasing out the benefit these taxpayers will receive from the 15 percent bracket (see Table 40.2).

For married couples filing jointly, the 15 percent rate begins to be phased out at about $71,900 of taxable income and is completed when income reaches $149,250, so that the entire $149,250 has been subjected to a 28 percent rate when this level of taxable income has been achieved. The same result is obtained for single taxpayers at $43,150 of taxable income, for heads of household at $61,650, and for married persons filing separately at $35,950 (see Table 40.2). After the tax has been determined, the taxpayer may be entitled to claim any of a number of credits against the tax owed.

Tax Credits

Whereas deductions and exemptions reduce the amount of income that the taxpayer must report for purposes of computing the tax owed, tax credits actually reduce the tax that must be paid, by being deducted dollar-for-dollar from the tax. Thus, a tax owed of $1,250 based upon a taxable income, after deductions, of $15,000, would be reduced to a tax of $250 by a $1,000 tax credit.

Some credits are nonrefundable, i.e., they cannot be refunded to the extent that they exceed the income tax owed by the taxpayer. The credits of most importance to optometrists are categorized below:

Credit for the Elderly or for the Permanently and the Totally Disabled—This credit can be claimed by individuals age 65 or older (under 65 if government retiree) and by individuals who are permanently and totally disabled (reported on Schedule R).

Foreign Tax Credit—This credit is allowed for income taxes paid to a foreign country or to a possession of the U.S. (reported on Form 1116).

General Business Credit—This credit is a combination of various credits (e.g., jobs credit, research credit, and employee stock ownership plan credit) and is limited by the income tax to be paid by the business; the most important credit for private practitioners, the investment tax credit, was ended by the Tax Reform Act of 1986[33] (if a general business credit is allowed, it will be reported on Form 3800).

Child and Dependent Care Credit—This credit is allowed for qualified child or dependent care expenses paid for the purpose of being gainfully employed; to be eligible for such a credit, the taxpayer must meet certain requirements[34] (reported on Form 2441).

Targeted Jobs Tax Credit—This credit may be claimed by employers who employ individuals who qualify as members of certain target groups[35] (reported on Form 5884).

Some credits are refundable, i.e., can be refunded to the extent that they exceed the tax owed by the taxpayer and so are actually treated as payments of taxes. These credits are not generally applicable to optometrists.[36] In addition to credits, there are also other taxes that the optometrist may be responsible

Table 40.2. Tax Rates under the Tax Reform Act of 1986
For 1988 and Thereafter

Single Taxpayers		Married Couples Filing Jointly	
Taxable Income	**Tax Rate (%)**	**Taxable Income**	**Tax Rate (%)**
$0–$17,850	15	$0–$29,750	15
$17,851–$43,150	28	$29,751–$71,900	28
$43,151–$100,480	33	More than $71,900	33
More than $100,480	28	After phase-outs (e.g., income more than $192,930 for a family of four)	28
Married Persons Filing Separately		**Unmarried Head of Household**	
Taxable Income	**Tax Rate (%)**	**Taxable Income**	**Tax Rate (%)**
$0–$14,875	15	$0–$23,900	15
$14,876–$35,950	28	$23,901–$61,650	28
$35,951–$113,300	33	More than $61,650	33
More than $113,300	33	After phase-outs (e.g., income more than $145,630 for a family of two)	28
After phase-outs	28		

Source: Klott, G., *The New York Times Complete Guide to the New Tax Law*, Times Books, New York, 1986, pp. 34–37.

for paying. The most important are the alternative minimum tax and the self-employment tax.

Alternative Minimum Tax

To ensure that all taxpayers pay at least a minimum amount of tax, even those who take advantage of favorable provisions and special deductions, two taxes have been enacted: the minimum tax, which applies only to corporations[37]; and the alternative minimum tax, which applies to individuals, trusts and estates. The alternative minimum tax is based upon the benefits received in the form of deductions, lower tax rates, and exclusions from tax. These items are known as tax preference items because they result from the preferential treatment accorded them. Examples are losses from tax shelters, gifts to charity of appreciated stock, incentive stock options, accelerated depreciation on real property or leased personal property, and certain itemized deductions (that can result in tax liability even though they are technically not tax preference items). To calculate the tax is a complex matter requiring professional assistance.[38] For optometrists who have claimed deductions for tax preference items, the alternative minimum tax will be reported on Form 6257.

Self-Employment Tax

This tax is a social security tax for individuals who work for themselves, similar to the social security tax withheld from the pay of employees, and represents the contributions of self-employed individuals to their coverage under the social security system.[39] The calculation of the self-employment tax, which is performed on Schedule SE, is described in Chapter 41.

Once these taxes have been calculated and have been entered on Form 1040, the last step is to subtract from this total the federal income tax withheld over the course of the tax year. If the amount withheld exceeds the total tax indebtedness calculated on the return, the taxpayer is due a refund. If the amount withheld is less than the total amount owed, the taxpayer must pay an additional sum to the IRS.

Although these calculations have concerned a taxpayer's federal tax liability, there are also state and local income taxes that will have to be paid and reported. Even though they are similar to federal tax requirements, state taxes are too varied and numerous to be discussed here. Professional counsel will be needed to ensure compliance with state income tax obligations.

Filing Requirements

Taxpayers need not file a return if their gross income is *less* than the sum of the standard deduction and the allowable personal exemption. For example, in 1988 a single taxpayer is allowed a $3,000 standard deduction and a $1,950 personal exemption, and so if

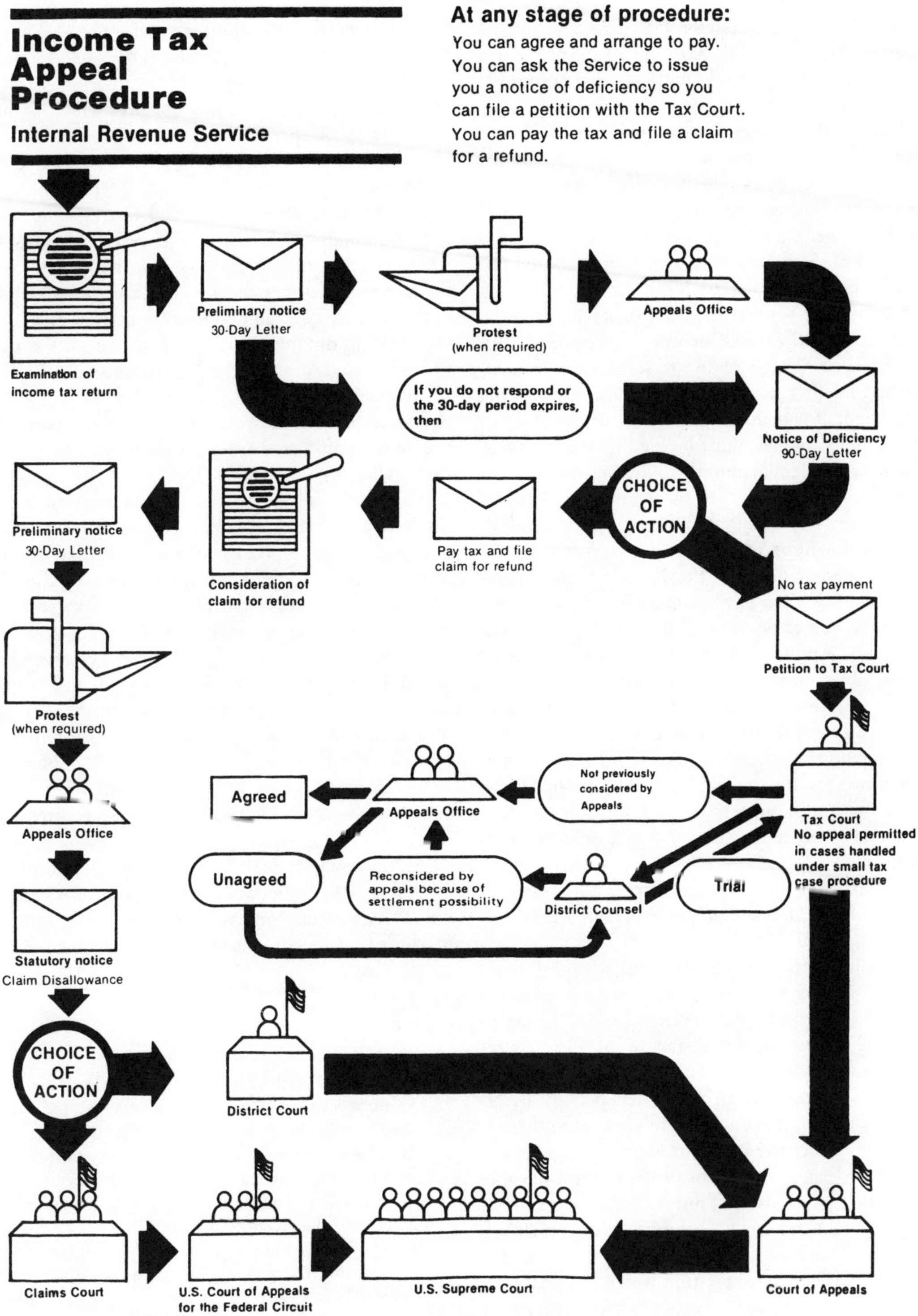

Figure 40.4. Appeals Process in Tax Disputes. (From the U.S. Government Printing Office: 1986-181-458/40031.)

this individual has less than $4,950 of taxable income then he or she does not have to file a return.[40] For a married couple filing jointly in 1988, this amount is $7,160.

A child with unearned income (such as investment income) who can be claimed as a dependent by his parents (whether or not he actually is) must file a return if his unearned income is $500 or more.[41] Earned income of a child is taxable to the child, and so he must file his own return. The parent should not report the child's earnings on his (the parent's) return. Children will be permitted to use their standard deduction to shield earned income from taxes.[42] But trusts established after 1986 are subject to stringent rules that, in effect, end such popular income-shifting arrangements for children as Clifford trusts.[43]

Individuals' returns must be filed by the 15th day of the fourth calendar month following the close of the taxable year, April 15th for a calendar year.

Taxpayers will be granted automatic two-month extensions for filing their income tax returns if they file Form 4868 on or before the due date of the return. Taxpayers must also pay a tentative estimate of the income tax due at the time of making the extension application. Applications for further extensions of time for filing must be made in writing and will be granted only in hardship cases. There are penalties for failure to file and for failure to pay by the due date.[44] In addition, there is a penalty for substantially understating the tax due, which will be applied if the unpaid amount is more than 10 percent of the final tax liability, or more than $5,000, whichever is larger.

Any taxpayer may revise a previous return to claim a refund of taxes or pay additional taxes by filing Form 1040X.[45]

In addition to the penalties already described, there is a penalty that may be imposed on frivolous returns.[46] If any part of a deficiency in tax is due to negligence or intentional disregard of IRS regulations, a penalty of 5 percent of the total amount of the deficiency, plus an additional penalty of 50 percent of the interest due, will be assessed. If there is fraud, the penalty is 75 percent of the underpayment due to fraud, and 50 percent of the interest payable on the underpayment.[47] Fraud may also be the basis for a criminal action against the taxpayer, which can result in a jail sentence of up to five years and a $10,000 fine. The period within which criminal prosecution may be started is generally three years after the commission of the offense but may be longer in many circumstances. There are other penalties that we will not discuss.[48]

Tax returns are examined by the IRS through several programs. A computer program known as the Discriminant Function System (DIF) selects most returns that are examined, by evaluating selected entries and giving the return a score, which is then reviewed by IRS personnel. Those returns deemed to have the highest probability of error are selected for audit.

Returns may also be analyzed through the Taxpayer Compliance Measurement Program (TCMP), which is a random selection system that is employed to determine correct tax liability and measure and evaluate taxpayer compliance characteristics. The information obtained through TCMP audits is used to update and improve the DIF program.

Returns may also be examined directly by IRS personnel, by assessing claims for credit or refunds of previously paid taxes or by matching tax documents, such as Forms W-2 and 1099.

The place and method of examination are determined by the IRS and may be no more than an exchange of correspondence, a more formal hearing at the taxpayer's office, or at the office of the IRS. Most taxpayers represent themselves at these meetings, and many disagreements are settled at this level. If the taxpayer does not agree with the changes proposed by the examiner, the taxpayer may appeal through the IRS or proceed to tax court. (See IRS publication 5, *Appeal Rights and Preparation of Protests for Unagreed Cases*, and IRS publication 556, *Examination of Returns, Appeal Rights, and Claims for Refund*.) The appeals alternatives are illustrated in Fig. 40.4.

An optometrist must be knowledgeable about the intricacies of business tax as well as those of individual income tax, and we will turn to the complex matter of business taxation in the next chapter.

Notes

1. Constitution of the United States, Article I, Section 8.
2. Id. provides that, "But all duties, imposts, and excises shall be uniform throughout the United States."
3. In Article I, Section 9 of the U.S. Constitution it is declared that, "No capitation, or other direct, tax shall be laid, unless in proportion to a census or enumeration hereinbefore directed to be taken."
4. In 1909 a concerted effort to provide further tax revenue for the federal government resulted in the Payne-Aldrich Tariff Act, which was expressly named a special excise tax, to be applied for the privilege of doing business as a corporation rather than as a corporate income tax. On this basis it was upheld as an excise tax by the U.S. Supreme Court. See *Flint v. Stone Tracy Co.*, 220 U.S. 107, 31 S. Ct. 342 (1911).

5. The purpose of the amendment was to eliminate the requirement of apportionment if an income tax was enacted by the federal congress, and the amendment was upheld on this basis by the U.S. Supreme Court in *Evans v. Gore*, 253 U.S. 245, 40 S. Ct. 550 (1920).
6. This example is quoted in *1980 Federal Tax Course*, Commerce Clearing House, Chicago, 1979.
7. The tax rates applied to taxpayers have fluctuated with the regularity of a yo-yo ever since the first income tax in 1913, when the top bracket was 7 percent. By 1918 it had risen to 77 percent, to sink back to 25 percent by 1925, then to spring to its highest point, 94 percent, in 1944. Therefore, one can be confident that the 28 percent top rate in 1988 represents but a temporary respite for the taxpayer, and that future tax reform will have nowhere to go but up.
8. *Internal Revenue Code of 1954*, §61.
9. Id. §§72(e)(1)(B) and 72 (e)(2)(B). Examples of payment of the proceeds of insurance other than for the death of the insured are surrender of the policy for its cash value and payments received at maturity for an endowment policy.
10. Id. §101(b).
11. Id. §102(a).
12. See Revenue Ruling 70–21.
13. The interest on federal obligations became subject to taxation under the Public Debt Act of 1941; interest on obligations of a territory, possession of the United States, the District of Columbia, or any politicial subdivision of the United States, is excluded from federal taxation under *Internal Revenue Code of 1954*, §103.
14. Id. §104.
15. Id. §105.
16. Id. §127.
17. For optometry students pursuing the O.D. degree, scholarships or fellowships are tax-free when applied to tuition, course-required fees, books, supplies, and equipment. But expenses for room, board, or incidental matters, even though paid by scholarship or fellowship funds, are subject to taxation (due to the Tax Reform Act of 1986). Nondegree candidates may no longer claim even the limited exclusion that was available prior to the tax reform act. Students who file their own tax returns and are not claimed as dependents on their parents' returns will be able to shield the first $3,000 (as of 1988) due to the standard deduction.
18. *Internal Revenue Code of 1954*, §121, as amended.
19. The full deduction for an IRA can be claimed only by individuals who are not covered by an employer-maintained retirement plan or individuals covered by an employer-maintained retirement plan who have income of less than $25,000 if single or $40,000 if married and filing jointly. These requirements, which were among the most hotly debated of the Tax Reform Act of 1986, may be changed by future tax laws.
20. *Internal Revenue Code of 1954*, §165.
21. Id. §§71 and 215.
22. Beginning in 1987, interest deductions on first and second homes will still be deductible in full, subject to certain limits. The amount that may be borrowed against is the price paid for the house plus the cost of improvements. For example, a home bought for $75,000 with $25,000 worth of improvements would be limited to mortgage interest deductions on loans up to $100,000. But if the house appreciates in value, the limit may be increased for the purpose of obtaining additional loans for college or medical bills. For example, if the home is now worth $150,000 the limit could be extended $50,000, and all interest payments on the $50,000 would be deductible, if the loan was used for the payment of qualified medical or educational expenses. See *Internal Revenue Code of 1954*, §163(h)(3). However, personal interest charges, such as those incurred on credit card or bank loans for personal items, will be phased out by 1991. Under the Tax Reform Act of 1986, deductions for personal interest will be reduced by 35 percent in 1987, 60 percent in 1988, 80 percent in 1989, and 90 percent in 1990.
23. In many states individuals will find that their state and local income tax bills have automatically gone up due to the 1986 Tax Reform Act because the state taxes are tied to the federal system of tax reporting. This increase in state taxes is one of the unhappy side effects of federal tax reform.
24. The Tax Reform Act of 1986 has made it unlikely that anyone except those with large medical expenses will be able to claim a tax deduction for these expenses. For example, if an individual has an adjusted gross of income of $40,000, that individual will be able to deduct only those medical expenses that are in excess of $3,000.
25. The Tax Reform Act of 1984 has limited the deduction for drugs to insulin or a drug "which requires a prescription by a doctor for its use by an individual." Over-the-counter drugs do not qualify for the deduction.
26. Premiums for health insurance include those paid under Part A or B of Medicare.
27. Travel to health care providers or facilities, either by public transportation or by private vehicle, may be deducted. Actual costs may be claimed or, if a private vehicle is employed, 9¢ a mile will be allowed. If a distant location is involved, lodging of up to $50 per night per person may be claimed.
28. There are a number of provisions that apply to charitable contributions of cash, appreciated property, old or used property, or services, and donors are encouraged to review IRS publication 526, *Charitable Contributions*, and IRS publication 561, *Determining the Value of Donated Property*, before claiming their donations on Form 1040.
29. The Tax Reform Act of 1986 allows the deduction only for casualty losses that are not covered by insurance, and such losses may no longer be claimed by taxpayers who choose not to claim the insurance but to write off the loss instead. Thus a tax deduction is allowed only for the amount of loss that would not have been covered by insurance, and only to the extent that this uninsured loss is greater than 10 percent of the taxpayer's adjusted

gross income.

30. The 2 percent floor for employees will doubtless affect the many optometrists in associateship or other forms of employee practice. In order to claim a tax deduction for miscellaneous business-related expenses, these optometrists will have to incur expenses in excess of $400 for a $20,000 AGI, $600 for a $30,000 AGI, $800 for a $40,000 AGI, and $1,000 for a $50,000 AGI.
31. The personal exemption is significantly increased under the Tax Reform Act of 1986, and thus large families will receive an extra tax break under the law. But elderly and blind taxpayers will no longer receive an extra personal examption, as in the past, and will receive an extra amount only if they do not itemize, as part of the standard deduction.
32. Although the effects of the tax rate changes are not fully known at the time of this writing, it has been estimated that the largest impact of the reduced brackets will be upon lower income taxpayers, who will realize a significant reduction in tax liability. This tax cut will also extend into some higher brackets so that individuals earning between $40,000 and $50,000 are expected to realize a 9.1 percent reduction in taxes, and taxpayers earning between $50,000 and $75,000 a 1.8 percent reduction. Even those earning between $75,000 and $100,000 are estimated to realize a 1.2 percent reduction in taxes by 1988. Whether or not these estimates will prove to be accurate remains to be seen.
33. The investment tax credit will be sorely missed by optometrists, who must pay reasonably large sums for equipment. None of the other business credits will usually apply to optometrists, although some optometrists may hire employees who qualify the optometrist for the targeted jobs credit. Doubtless optometrists will turn to expensing (the §179 deduction, described in Chapter 41), depreciation, and perhaps even to leasing in an effort to secure tax deductions for equipment and other capital assets needed for practice.
34. If a taxpayer pays for the care of dependents under fifteen years of age or for disabled dependents so that the taxpayer can work, a credit of up to 30 percent of these expenses may be claimed. Work-related expenses are limited to $2,400 for one qualifying person or $4,800 for two or more qualifying persons. For example, for a taxpayer with an adjusted gross income in excess of $28,000, the credit percentage is 20 percent, and if the taxpayer spends in excess of $2,400 for the care of a qualifying dependent, the maximum credit that can be claimed is $480. For more information, see IRS publication 503, *Child and Dependent Care Credit, and Employment Taxes for Household Employers.*
35. The targeted jobs credit may be claimed by optometrists who hire members of certain target groups (such as economically disadvantaged youths), and permits credits for as much as 40 percent of qualified first-year wages paid to these employees. For more information, see IRS publication 906, *Jobs and Research Credits.*
36. Credits that are refundable include the earned income credit, the credit for excess social security tax withheld, the credit from a regulated investment company, and the rebate on diesel-powered highway vehicles.
37. Although the Tax Reform Act of 1986 changed the minimum tax to be applied to corporations so that it is similar to the alternative minimum tax for individuals, in 1987 the tax for professional service corporations was changed to 34 percent, effective January 1, 1988. See IRS publications 542, *Tax Information on Corporations*, and 909, *Alternative Minimum Tax.*
38. The alternative minimum tax is computed by subtracting the taxpayer's regular tax from the gross alternative minimum tax, which is 20 percent of various items of income, less an exempt amount ($30,000 if single; $40,000 if married filing jointly). The calculation is a complicated one, to say the least, requiring professional assistance.
39. In 1988 the social security tax paid by employers for employees is 7.51 percent, whereas the self-employment tax paid by employers for themselves is 13.02 percent. In the future, the percentage of withholding for employers and employees will become equal. (The total withholding for employees, in 1988, is 15.02 percent because both employer and employee contribute 7.51 percent to Social Security. Thus the withholding for self-employed individuals will continue to rise to meet this goal, which will also continue to increase.)
40. For information on filing requirements for individuals, see IRS publication 17, *Your Federal Income Tax.*
41. The Tax Reform Act of 1986 instituted some important reforms relating to the taxation of children. For children under age fourteen, only the first $1,000 of investment income will be taxed at the child's bracket. Investment income in excess of this amount will be taxed at the tax rate of the child's parents (probably 28 percent). For children 14 or over, the tax rate will be that of the child (probably 15 percent). Regardless of age, children are allowed to use the standard deduction to shield the first $500 from taxation. Thus, for a child under fourteen years of age who has $1,500 of investment income, the first $500 would be shielded from taxation, the next $500 would be taxed at his bracket, and the last $500 would be taxed at the bracket of the child's parents.
42. Although children may no longer claim the personal exemption to shield earned income from taxation, they will benefit from the increased standard deduction authorized under the Tax Reform Act of 1986 ($3,000 in 1988). Thus, a child who earns $2,000 from a summer or after-school job will be able to exclude all his or her earnings from taxation.
43. The 1986 Tax Reform Act effectively ended Clifford trusts, spousal-remainder trusts, and other such grantor trusts by taxing the trust income at the rate of the grantor, which is typically the parent, rather than at the rate of the beneficiary, which is typically the child.
44. Interest is charged on any taxes not paid by the due

date, even if an extension of time is granted for filing. This interest rate is changed each six months. During 1986 it was 10 percent through June 30, and 9 percent from July 1 through December 31.

45. A taxpayer may file an amended return within three years from the date of the original return or within two years from the time the tax was paid, whichever is later.
46. A frivolous return is one that does not include enough information to figure the correct tax or one that shows on its face that the return is substantially incorrect. A $500 penalty is imposed, in addition to any other penalties that might have to be paid.
47. The increased penalty for fraud is effective for all returns after 1986.
48. Examples of other penalties include the penalty for failure to supply social security numbers and the penalty for failure to furnish tax shelter registration numbers.

Chapter 41

Business Taxes

Annual income twenty pounds, annual expenditure nineteen pounds and six, result happiness.
Annual income twenty pounds, annual expenditure twenty pounds ought and six, result misery.
—Charles Dickens, *David Copperfield*

Organizing for Business

A business is an activity carried on for profit, and for an activity to be considered a business, a profit motive must be present and some type of economic activity must be involved. An activity is presumed to be engaged in for profit activities if it produces a profit in any three out of five consecutive years.[1]

One of the most important decisions made when entering into business is the form of organization to use. Tax considerations are a key aspect of the decision-making process, as each business entity has different tax advantages and disadvantages. Although the individual proprietorship has been the backbone of optometry, economic and sociological factors have combined to make partnerships and group practices grow in popularity. The tax reporting requirements of the three basic types of business entities differ. For an *individual* or a *partnership*, the business itself does not pay any income taxes; the sole proprietor reports his income on his Form 1040 as business income (which is actually computed on Schedule C and attached to the Form 1040), while the partnership files its return on a Form 1065 (and each of the partners report their distributive share of the partnership income on their Form 1040); except for an S corporation, profits of a *corporation* are taxed to the corporation, which files a Form 1120, whereas the employees of the corporation—such as the doctor or doctors who are also the shareholders—report their income on their individual Form 1040; dividends, when received by a shareholder, are reported as income on Form 1040 also.

A business must have its own identification, and so each business is required to have an employer identification number which must be shown on all business tax returns. Personal tax returns, Schedule Cs included, must have the individual's social security number shown. If a sole proprietorship is incorporated, or merged with another sole proprietorship to form a partnership, then a new employer identification number is needed for the corporation or partnership. To apply for an employer identification number use Form SS-4, Application for Employer Identification Number, available from the IRS.[2]

In order to organize a business, there are three important income-related considerations that require careful planning: books and records, accounting periods, and accounting methods.

Books and Records

When starting a business, a system of recordkeeping that is suitable for the business should be established. The choice requires that the tax year and accounting method be known because the recordkeeping system should clearly show income for the accounting period that is the tax year.

The basic decision is between single-entry and double-entry bookkeeping systems. Single-entry bookkeeping is a system that is based on an income statement and not on a balance sheet. It is simple and very practical. For tax purposes the system records the flow of income and expenses through the use of a daily summary of receipts and a monthly summary of disbursements. This form of bookkeeping (often referred to as a pegboard system) is the preferred method for optometrists.[3] Double-entry bookkeeping uses journals and ledgers in which transactions are first entered in a journal and then summary totals of the transactions (usually monthly) are entered into ledger accounts for income, expenses, assets, liabilities, and net worth.

At the end of each accounting period, the business will have to prepare financial statements, which will include the income earned and the balance sheets (e.g., a statement showing the financial position of the business in terms of assets, liabilities, and net worth). These statements summarize the past business year.

All business receipts should be deposited in a separate bank account established for that purpose. All disbursements should be made by check from this account. This permits the documentation of both income and expenses. Checks payable to one's self should be written only when making withdrawals of income from the business for one's own use; checks payable to "cash" should be avoided.

A petty cash fund should be established for minor expenses, and all business expenses paid for by cash should be supported by documents showing their business purpose.

In order to document recordkeeping, observe the following rules:

Support all entries. Cancelled checks, paid bills, duplicate deposit slips, and other items that support entries in the practice books should be kept in an orderly manner.

Classify all accounts. Divide the practice accounts into five groups: income, expenses, assets, liabilities, and equity (i.e., net worth).

Keep all records. Keep all business records available for inspection by the IRS; ideally, these records should be kept in perpetuity, or, as a minimum, for a period of time that exceeds the statute of limitations.

Retain copies. Keep records supporting items on a tax return until the statute of limitations for that tax return runs out (three years after the return is due or filed or two years from the date the tax is paid, whichever occurs later). Where possible, tax records should be kept indefinitely.

Keep comprehensive employee records. Keep all records on employment taxes (income tax withholding, social security, and federal unemployment tax) for at least four years after the due date of the return or the date the tax is paid, whichever is later. Business records should always contain the employer identification number, copies of the returns filed, and the dates and amounts of deposits made.

Employment taxes will be discussed at the conclusion of this chapter.

Accounting Periods

Every taxpayer must calculate taxable income and file a tax return on the basis of an annual accounting period called a *tax year.* A tax year is usually twelve consecutive months. It may be a calendar year or a fiscal year; under certain circumstances it may be less than twelve months, a partial year.

A *calendar year* is twelve consecutive months ending on December 31. A *fiscal year* is either twelve consecutive months ending on the last day of any month other than December, or a 52- to 53-week year. To report on a fiscal year basis, the practice books must be kept on that basis. A short tax year or a *partial year* is a tax year of less than twelve months, but a short tax year return is treated as a return for a full tax year. A short tax year usually results when a taxpayer is not in business for an entire tax year. Most optometrists and small businessmen are on a calendar year accounting period. Businesses that have never filed an income tax return may adopt either a calendar or a fiscal year, but the Tax Reform Act of 1986 limits the choice to a calendar year in many cases.[4]

Accounting Methods

Taxable income is determined by using a fixed accounting period and a set of rules to decide when and how to report income and deductions.

There are two basic types of accounting methods —cash or accrual—for income and expenses of business activities.

1. *Cash method.* The cash method of accounting is used by most individuals and many small businesses with no inventories. With the cash method, all

items of income actually or constructively received during the year are included in gross income. Both property and services received must be included as income at their fair market value. Constructive receipt of income occurs when an amount is credited to the practice account or made available to the practice without restriction as to the time and manner of payment.

For example, an optometrist on the cash method of accounting renders services to a patient on December 31 but does not receive a check as payment until January 1. The payment is income reportable in the year beginning January 1.

2. *Accrual method.* Under the accrual method all items of income are included in gross income when earned, even though payment is received in another tax year. All events that fix the right to receive the income must have occurred and the amount must be able to be determined with reasonable accuracy.

For example, an optometrist on the accrual method of accounting renders services to a patient on December 31 but does not receive payment until January 1. The payment is income reportable in the year ending December 31.

There are other methods of accounting, but the cash and accrual methods are most commonly employed by optometrists; the cash method is generally preferred[5] (although it has weaknesses just as does the accrual method). An accountant should be consulted before making any decision as to the most appropriate type of bookkeeping, accounting period, or method of accounting.

Acquiring Business Assets

The optometrist in private practice who starts from scratch must purchase an expensive array of instruments; a new graduate purchasing an ongoing practice usually must allocate a significant portion of the price to instruments and equipment; an optometrist hired as an associate typically requires new equipment, purchased by the employer-optometrist; and the cost of the equipment and instrumentation needed for the practice of optometry by future graduates is not expected to decrease in the upcoming years. This property has obvious value because it contributes directly toward earning the income that supports the practice. Such property is termed a *business asset.*[6]

A business asset can be tangible real estate, such as a building or a parking lot, or tangible personal property, such as furniture, equipment, or instruments. It can also be intangible property, such as goodwill or a covenant not to compete.

The amount paid for a business asset is usually a *capital expenditure* rather than a deductible expense. Although capital expenditures cannot be deducted directly, their cost can be recovered through the use of the annual *depreciation* deduction (discussed later in this chapter). Similarly, the cost of certain assets can be recovered through *amortization* (also discussed later in this chapter). If a business asset cannot be depreciated or amortized, its cost can be recovered only when it is sold or otherwise disposed of.

A capital expenditure is actually an investment of capital, either to acquire property with a useful life of more than one year or to make permanent improvements that increase the value of property or appreciably prolong its life.[7] Any prospective purchaser should be careful to check with tax counsel so as to take full advantage of the deductions available under this category.

Business assets will have to be *classified* (this will be discussed subsequently in some detail); the accounting system will need to be able to separate these various types of assets because different methods will be used to claim deductions for these different types of property. Therefore, careful recordkeeping will be a necessity. This classification system is particularly important when purchasing a practice, especially for the seller. (The problem of the tax ramifications of the sale of an optometric practice is considered in Chapter 48.)

Basis

The *basis* of property is used when figuring the gain or loss from the sale or other disposition of property.[8] It is also used for determining the deduction for depreciation or amortization. When property is purchased, its cost is generally the original basis. If the property is received in some other manner (such as by gift or inheritance), however, then a basis other than cost must be used. And if an asset is used for business purposes and depreciation or amortization deductions are claimed by the taxpayer, then these deductions are used to calculate the *adjusted basis* of the asset. As we shall see, these deductions are useful when determining the taxable income of the taxpayer's business. They are also useful for determining gain or loss when business property is sold or exchanged. Such transactions are a common part of the decisions made by a small businessman (i.e., an optometrist).

For example, if an optometrist purchases a computer for $5,000 and uses it for a year, it will have a depreciated value of $4,000. If the optometrist sells it for $3,000, he has a $1,000 loss; if it is sold for $5,000 he has a $1,000 gain.

As the preceding example illustrates, cost serves as a beginning point for basis determination in many cases. Another important aspect of basis is the *fair market value*; it is the price at which property would change hands between a willing buyer and seller.

For example, assume that an optometrist uses an automobile exclusively for business purposes. The automobile has been depreciated by the optometrist so that it has an adjusted basis of $3,000. It has a fair market value of $4,500, however. The optometrist decides to trade it for a truck that also has a fair market value of $4,500. His basis in the truck is $3,000, the same basis as the traded automobile.

However, if the optometrist decides to trade in the truck for a new automobile that has a fair market value of $5,000 and he has to pay $1,000 in addition to the trade-in, his basis in the new car becomes $4,000 (the $3,000 basis of the old truck plus the $1,000 cash).

The effect of basis on a contemplated sale or exchange of equipment or other business assets should always be carefully considered. It is important to retain a competent accountant or tax attorney so that advice concerning the tax consequences of such a transaction can be ascertained *before* entering into the transaction.

Although the preceding examples have used tangible assets for purposes of illustration, intangible assets also have a basis that may be adjusted as required. Typical examples include:

Goodwill. The basis of goodwill is its cost when the purchase of a practice is involved; the cost of goodwill is determined by the residual method of allocating price in practice purchase arrangements, which requires an assessment of all aspects of the sales agreement (to be discussed).[9]

Covenant not to compete. Usually, the basis of a covenant not to compete is what is paid for it; if part of a sales agreement for the purchase of a practice, its cost must be listed in the contract (these covenants are discussed in Chapters 37, 38, and 39).[10]

Franchises. The basis of a franchise is its cost.

The determination of basis can become very technical and complicated, but each purchase and sale or exchange of a capital or other business asset has tax consequences that must be known in advance. In particular, the purchase of an existing practice is a transaction that hinges not only upon the price paid but also upon the way in which the various practice assets are organized for tax purposes (see Chapter 48).

Determining Gross Profit

The business of a professional such as an optometrist is to provide personal services. All compensation received for personal services, no matter what the form of payment, must be included in gross income, and must be reported as income in the year received (if on the cash basis) or in the year earned (if on the accrual basis). Such income is ordinary income, taxable at the tax table rates our government imposes.[11]

One way that personal income taxes can be reduced is through the acceptance of retirement benefits in lieu of salary increases. The retirement benefits are not taxed as income until retirement, when they are actually withdrawn by the taxpayer (and the taxpayer is usually in a lower tax bracket). These benefits are discussed in Chapters 37, 38, and 39.

To determine the gross profit of a business, the gross income (gross receipts and cost of goods sold) must be calculated. For an optometrist, there are two principal sources of income: professional services and the sale of ophthalmic materials. The gross profit from these two sources is determined before deductions from business operations can be used to reduce the taxable income.

Determining Income

All business income must be reported, whether it is in the form of cash, property, or services. Types of income other than payments for services and materials include:

Rental income. A building owned by a taxpayer-optometrist that is rented in part to others will result in business income that is reportable.

Gains from dealings in property. The sale of an asset that results in a profit is reportable as business income (assuming that it is a business asset).

Distributive shares of partnership income. A partner's share of income, gain, loss, deduction, or credit must be reported; so also must a sale or exchange of certain partnership interests (see Form 8308).

Property or services (bartering). Income received in the form of property or services must be included in income at its fair market value on the date received (including an exchange of property or services by one individual for the property or services of another individual, i.e., bartering).

An optometrist who is an individual proprietor reporting his profit on Schedule C records his income as "Gross Receipts or Sales" (see line 1a, Fig. 41.1).

Cost of Goods Sold

Personal service businesses, such as those of health-care practitioners, customarily are not required to use inventories. Their gross business income usually is the same as their gross receipts, and most optometrists use the cash method of accounting. But since optometrists also sell or charge for such items as frames, lenses, and ophthalmic supplies that are normally used in the course of the profession, optometrists must conduct inventories.

Inventories are factors in figuring the cost of goods sold and must be conducted at the beginning and end of each tax year; they must be used whenever they are necessary to clearly show income. Practitioners who dispense should always carefully maintain tax records of their inventories conducted to determine income.[12]

To arrive at a dollar amount for an inventory a method for identifying and a basis for valuing the items in the inventory are both needed. These steps will require an accountant's assistance. To show income clearly the same inventory practice must be used from year to year.

The cost of goods sold is reported on Schedule C; it is merely the beginning value of goods less the value at the end of the year, the net being the "Cost of Goods Sold" during the year (see line 2, Fig. 41.1).

Computing Gross Profit

After the gross receipts and the cost of goods sold have been calculated, the gross profit can be determined. To figure gross profit, first compute the net receipts by subtracting any returns and allowances (cash or credit refunds made to patients); then subtract the cost of goods sold from the net receipts. The result is the gross income (see line 5, Fig. 41.1).

If there is other income, it must be reported and added to the gross profit. One example of other income would be cash discounts; these are amounts that a seller allows to be deducted from the invoice price for prompt payment. For income tax purposes either of two methods may be used to account for them: they can be deducted directly from purchases or credited to a discount income account and reported at the end of the tax year as business income.[13] Once the total income for the business is determined, the deductions to which the taxpayer is entitled may be computed.

Determining Net Income

The determination between capital expenditures and ordinary business expenses now becomes important, for capital expenditures are not deductible. To be deductible, a business expense must be ordinary in the business and necessary in its operation. *Ordinary* refers to an expense that is common and an accepted practice within optometry; *necessary* expenses are those that are appropriate and helpful in developing and maintaining the optometric practice.[14]

If property is used both for business and for personal purposes (such as an automobile), then it must be determined which part of the expenses are for business and which part are for personal matters. Only the business expenses are deductible.

The following discussion of business deductions is not intended to be exhaustive; the responsibility to learn the particulars of documenting and claiming these deductions will, of necessity, be an individual responsibility that every optometrist must pursue.

The major categories of these deductions are:

- Salaries and wages and related payments
- Rent expense
- Repairs, improvements, and replacements
- Bad debts
- Travel, entertainment, and gift expenses
- Interest
- Insurance
- Taxes
- Profession-related expenses
- Miscellaneous business expenses

Salaries, Wages, and Related Expenses

Salaries, wages, and other forms of compensation paid to employees may be deductible as business expenses.

Salaries

A sole proprietor may not deduct his own salary or any other withdrawal for his personal use; partner's salaries (other than guaranteed payments) are not

SCHEDULE C (Form 1040)
Department of the Treasury
Internal Revenue Service (0)

Profit or (Loss) From Business or Profession

(Sole Proprietorship)

Partnerships, Joint Ventures, etc., Must File Form 1065.

▶ **Attach to Form 1040, Form 1041, or Form 1041S.** ▶ **See Instructions for Schedule C (Form 1040).**

OMB No. 1545-0074
1987
Attachment Sequence No. **09**

Name of proprietor: John G. O'DEE
Social security number (SSN): 123 : 45 : 6789

A Principal business or profession, including product or service (see Instructions): Optometrist

B Principal business code (from Part IV) ▶ 9 | 2 | 9 | 0

C Business name and address ▶ John G. O'Dee, O.D., 321 Main St., Anytown, State

D **Employer ID number (Not SSN)**: 8 7 | 6 5 4 3 2 1

E Method(s) used to value closing inventory:
(1) ☐ Cost (2) ☒ Lower of cost or market (3) ☐ Other (attach explanation)

		Yes	No
F	Accounting method: (1) ☒ Cash (2) ☐ Accrual (3) ☐ Other (specify) ▶		
G	Was there any change in determining quantities, costs, or valuations between opening and closing inventory? (If "Yes," attach explanation.)		X
H	Are you deducting expenses for an office in your home?		X
I	Did you file **Form 941** for this business for any quarter in 1987?	X	
J	Did you "materially participate" in the operation of this business during 1987? (If "No," see Instructions for limitations on losses.)	X	
K	Was this business in operation at the end of 1987?	X	
L	How many months was this business in operation during 1987? ▶ 12		

M If this schedule includes a loss, credit, deduction, income, or other tax benefit relating to a tax shelter required to be registered, check here. ▶ ☐
If you check this box, you **MUST** attach **Form 8271**.

Part I Income

		Line	Amount
1a	Gross receipts or sales	1a	100,000
b	Less: Returns and allowances	1b	
c	Subtract line 1b from line 1a and enter the balance here	1c	100,000
2	Cost of goods sold and/or operations (from Part III, line 8)	2	32,000
3	Subtract line 2 from line 1c and enter the **gross profit** here	3	68,000
4	Other income (including windfall profit tax credit or refund received in 1987)	4	2,000
5	Add lines 3 and 4. This is the **gross income** ▶	5	70,000

Part II Deductions

6	Advertising		23	Repairs	150
7	Bad debts from sales or services (see Instructions.)		24	Supplies (not included in Part III)	
8	Bank service charges		25	Taxes	935
9	Car and truck expenses	850	26	Travel, meals, and entertainment:	
10	Commissions		a	Travel	360
11	Depletion		b	Total meals and entertainment	200
12	Depreciation and section 179 deduction from Form 4562 (not included in Part III)	3,600	c	Enter 20% of line 26b subject to limitations (see Instructions)	40
13	Dues and publications	150	d	Subtract line 26c from 26b	160
14	Employee benefit programs	1,200	27	Utilities and telephone	1,800
15	Freight (not included in Part III)		28a	Wages	8,000
16	Insurance	1,200	b	Jobs credit	
17	Interest:		c	Subtract line 28b from 28a	8,000
a	Mortgage (paid to financial institutions)	2,000	29	Other expenses (list type and amount):	
b	Other	250		License 150	
18	Laundry and cleaning			Janitor 65	
19	Legal and professional services	2,650			
20	Office expense	555			
21	Pension and profit-sharing plans				
22	Rent on business property	6,000			215

		Line	Amount
30	Add amounts in columns for lines 6 through 29. These are the **total deductions** ▶	30	30,075
31	**Net profit or (loss).** Subtract line 30 from line 5. If a profit, enter here and on Form 1040, line 13, and on Schedule SE, line 2 (or line 5 of Form 1041 or Form 1041S). If a loss, you **MUST** go on to line 32	31	39,925

32 If you have a loss, you **MUST** answer this question: "Do you have amounts for which you are not at risk in this business?" (See Instructions.) ☐ Yes ☐ No
If "Yes," you **MUST** attach **Form 6198**. If "No," enter the loss on Form 1040, line 13, and on Schedule SE, line 2 (or line 5 of Form 1041 or Form 1041S).

For Paperwork Reduction Act Notice, see Form 1040 Instructions. **Schedule C (Form 1040) 1987**

Figure 41.1. Sample Schedule C, Form 1040

deductible; salaries paid by a professional corporation to its employees are deductible.

Payments to the Beneficiary of a Deceased Employee

These payments are deductible, and up to $5,000 is excluded as income for the beneficiary.

Bonuses

Bonuses are deductible if they are intended as additional compensation rather than as gifts.

Educational Expenses

Tuition expenses paid for employees under a qualified educational assistance program related to their employment are not considered gross income for the employees and are deductible by the business.[15]

Interview Expense Allowances

These allowances are deductible as a business expense.

Moving Expenses

Payments to employees as an allowance or reimbursement for the cost of moving to a new job site will be considered part of the employee's income (and hence deductible) if the employee is eligible for a tax deduction for the move (see Chapter 42).

Meals and Lodging

The cost of meals, lodging, and inventoriable items, furnished to employees as part of their compensation, is deductible by the employer.

Fringe Benefits

There are many forms of compensation that may be provided to employees in an indirect way, such as life or disability insurance, accident or hospitalization insurance, or reimbursements for medical care; these are referred to as fringe benefits and are deductible as business expenses if they meet certain tests.[16]

Rent Expense

If business property is leased, the rental may generally be deducted. Certain other expenses may also be deducted as rent.

Rent is the amount that is paid for the use of property that is not owned. In general, rent may be deducted as an expense only if the rent is for property that is used in the practice of optometry. If the renter has or will have equity in or title to the property, the rent is not deductible. To determine if payments may be deducted as rent, it must first be determined whether the agreement is a lease or a conditional sales contract (discussed in Chapter 49). If under the agreement the renter acquired, or will acquire, title to or equity in the property, the agreement will be treated as a conditional sales contract and hence the payments will not be deductible as rent.

If an optometrist leases business property, he may deduct as additional rent any taxes that he has to pay for or to the lessor. If a building is leased and an addition or other permanent improvements are made to it, the optometrist may be able either to depreciate or amortize the improvements.[17]

Repairs, Improvements, and Replacements

The cost of repairing, improving, or replacing property used in the practice of optometry is either a deductible expense or a capital expenditure. An expenditure necessary to keep property in a normal and efficient operating condition is a deductible expense. But if the expenditure adds to the value of the property or significantly increases its life, the cost must be capitalized rather than deducted (and, although the cost cannot be deducted right away, it can be recovered through the use of depreciation).[18]

Repairs do not add to the value or the usefulness of property, nor do they appreciably lengthen its life (e.g., repairing floors and painting). Thus, they are deductible expenses and not capital expenditures.

Improvements add to the value of property, lengthen its life, or adapt it to a different use. The cost of an improvement is a capital expenditure. Examples are a new floor, lighting renovations, and altering an office as part of a general restoration plan.

Replacements, such as the amount paid to replace parts of an instrument that only keep it in a normal operating condition, do not add to life and are deductible expenses. A replacement that stops deterioration and adds to the life of the property has to be capitalized and depreciated, however.

This is an area of practice that requires an accountant's expertise.

Bad Debts

If money is owed but the debt cannot be collected, it is known as a bad debt. Under certain circumstances, the bad debt may qualify as a business deduction. For the bad debt to qualify, there must be a true creditor-debtor relationship between the creditor and the person that owes the money. Optometrists using the accrual method normally report income that is due them as soon as it is earned. Therefore, they may take a bad debt deduction when they are unable to collect what is owed them. But if the bad debt is later recovered, all or in part, it must be reported as income in the year that it is collected. Cash method optometrists normally do not report the income that is due them until they actually receive payment. Therefore, they may not take a bad debt deduction on payments they have not received or cannot collect.

Travel, Entertainment, and Gift Expenses

Important deductions for any businessman are the travel, entertainment, and gift expenses that are related to the conduct of his business. This is an area that is carefully scrutininzed by the IRS, so record-keeping, documentation, and advisor planning are more important that ever.[19] In addition, the Tax Reform Act of 1986 has instituted some significant changes in the deduction for entertainment expenses.

Travel Expenses

Travel expenses are those ordinary and necessary expenses of foreign and domestic travel away from home for the practice of optometry. These expenses include meals and lodging,[20] transportation and baggage charges, the cost of maintaining and operating a car, cleaning and laundry expenses, telephone and telegraph expenses, and other similar expenses related to qualified travel, including tips incidental to any of these expenses.

The general rule is that if a trip was entirely for business, then the ordinary and necessary travel expenses may be deducted, but if the trip was primarily personal, no travel expenses may be deducted even if there was some business activity at the destination. If the trip was primarily for business and while at the business destination the trip was extended for vacation or other nonbusiness activities, then the expenses of travel to and from the destination may be deducted. Whether the primary purpose of the trip was business or pleasure, the expenses incurred at the destination that were related to business may be deducted.

Travel expenses that an optometrist incurs for himself (not for family members) in attending an optometric convention may be deducted. A spouse or other family member accompanying an optometrist on such a trip cannot be included within the deduction unless it can be shown that there is a business purpose and need for the other person's attendance.

Transportation expenses for business purposes may be deducted, even though the optometrist is not away from home. Transportation expenses include such items as air, train, bus, cab fares, and the expenses of driving and maintaining an automobile or other vehicle. Meals and lodging are not considered in computing transportation expenses, and commuting expenses between the home and the usual place of business are *not* deductible.[21]

If a vehicle is used entirely for business purposes, the cost of its operation may be deducted in full. The deductible items include the cost of gas, oil, repairs, insurance, depreciation, interest on a loan used to buy the vehicle, taxes, licenses, garage rent, parking fees, and tolls. If the vehicle is used for both business and personal purposes, the expenses must be divided equitably between business and personal use.

For example, assume that an automobile is used both for personal reasons and for the practice of optometry. During the year 20,000 miles are driven, 12,000 of which are for business purposes. The optometrist is entitled to deduct 60 percent (12,000/20,000) of the total cost of operating the car. Thus, if the optometrist finds that the cost of gas, oil, tires, repairs, insurance, taxes, interest on the loan needed to purchase the car, licenses, garage rent, parking fees, tolls, and depreciation total $4,000, he may claim 60 percent ($2,400) of this amount as a deduction.

If a business vehicle is leased, the lease payments may be deducted to the extent that they are related to work (just as above).

A standard mileage rate of 22½ cents a mile may be used for the first 15,000 miles of business use each year, and 11 cents a mile for each additional business mile.[22] This rate may be used instead of the actual operating and fixed expenses (and depreciation) in figuring the deductible costs of operating a vehicle. Parking fees and tolls incurred during business use are deductible in addition to the standard mileage rate. The part of interest and state and local taxes (other than gas tax) that is related to the business use of the vehicle may also be deducted, in addition to the standard mileage rate.[23]

In order to use the standard mileage rate, however, it must be chosen in the first year that the vehicle is placed in service. Failure to do so precludes the use of the standard mileage rate deduction in subsequent years.[24] If it is used in the first year, that does not prevent the use of actual expenses in the following years.[25]

For example, if the optometrist determines that parking fees, tolls, interest on the loan for the purchase of the car, and state and local taxes on the car total $500, because the car is used 60 percent of the time for business purposes he may claim a $300 deduction, which, when added to the standard mileage rate of $2,700 (12,000 × 22½) for 12,000 miles of business-related use, allows him to deduct $3,000 rather than the $2,400 based upon actual expenses.

Whether or not the standard mileage rate is used, adequate records must be kept to show when the vehicle began to be utilized for business and the cost or other basis of the vehicle.[26] The records must also show the business miles driven by the vehicle during the year, total miles driven during the year, and total miles driven by the present owner. If actual expenses are used, records documenting the other costs of operating the vehicle must be kept.

If a vehicle is leased, documentation of lease payments should be retained. For vehicles, documentation of all expenses is essential; without it, deductions will be disallowed.

Business Entertainment

Business entertainment expenses are deductible only if they are ordinary and necessary expenses of carrying on the practice of optometry and can be documented. This deduction may be taken only if the amounts spent are directly related to or associated with the active conduct of optometry, or directly precede or follow a substantial business discussion related to the practice of optometry. Furthermore, effective in 1987 only 80 percent of business-related entertainment expenses may be deducted (see Chapter 42).[27]

For example, an optometrist wishing to establish a co-op for the purpose of purchasing spectacle frames at discount takes a prospective member of the co-op to dinner, at which they discuss the details of such a business association. The cost of the meal is $100. The optometrist may deduct $80 as an entertainment expense.

Entertainment includes any activity generally considered to provide entertainment, amusement, or recreation. This covers entertaining guests at night clubs; social, athletic, and sporting clubs; theaters; and sporting events, and on yachts or hunting, fishing, or vacation trips. It may also include satisfying the personal, living, or family needs of any individuals, such as furnishing food and beverages, a hotel suite, or an automobile. Clubs are considered to be entertainment facilities. Dues and fees paid to a club are treated as being for the use of an entertainment facility, and if the club is used more than 50 percent for business purposes, that part of the dues that is directly related to the business use of the club can be deducted. If a club is used for business meals, the part of the dues or fees for this use is directly related entertainment. But an initiation fee paid only once to join is a capital expense and hence not deductible. An accountant or tax lawyer will be needed, as will documentation, when considering large expenditures for entertainment.[28]

Business Gifts

Business gifts may be deducted, but the total cost of such gifts made directly or indirectly to any person during the tax year cannot be more than $25. If a gift is not intended for the eventual personal use or benefit of a particular person or limited class of people, the gift will not be allowed.

Remember, the proof necessary to establish travel, entertainment and business gift expenses should be kept in an account book, diary, statement of expense, or similar record, supported by adequate documentary evidence, that together will support each element of an expense. For example, entries on a desk calendar, not supported by evidence, are not considered to be proper proof.

Employee Travel Expenses

Employee travel expenses that are unreimbursed by the employer may be claimed only as itemized deductions (on Schedule A) to the extent that they exceed 2 percent of the employee's adjusted gross income.[29]

For example, an associate of an optometrist in private practice attends a continuing education course, and the cost of travel, lodging, and fees for the course total $400, and the cost of meals is $100. The associate's adjusted gross income (AGI) is $20,000, and he is not reimbursed for these expenses. He may claim the $400 as travel expenses, and $80 of the cost of meals, for a total of $480. But since 2 percent of his AGI is $400, he may deduct only $80 on Schedule A (assuming he has no other miscellaneous deductions to claim).

Employee Entertainment Expenses

Employee entertainment expenses that are not reimbursed by the employer are deductible, but the employee may claim only 80 percent of these costs and only to the extent they exceed 2 percent of the employee's adjusted gross income.

For example, if the associate incurs $400 in unreimbursed entertainment expenses, he may claim $320 (80 percent) on his Schedule A which, when combined with his $80 of allowable travel expenses, brings his total deduction to $400 ($80 + $320).

Interest

Interest is the charge made for the use of money. All interest paid or accrued in the tax year on a debt that is related to business may be deducted. The interest must be on a debt under which there is a valid obligation to pay a fixed or determinable sum of money.

Generally, the amount agreed upon by the lender and the borrower as interest may be deducted when paid or accrued. Examples of deductible interest include:

- Interest on business loans used to start up or purchase a practice (or for other business purposes)
- Mortgages on real property or on personal property (chattel mortages)
- Interest on loans taken out on insurance policies
- Interest on business-related credit card charges[30]

Generally, if a taxpayer uses the cash method of accounting, he may deduct interest only in the year in which it was paid. If the taxpayer uses the accrual method of accounting, he may deduct interest in the year it accrued.

Insurance

The cost of insuring a business may be deducted as an expense, but generally the cost of life insurance cannot be deducted (there are exceptions; see Chapter 39).

Premiums paid on business insurance policies such as the following may be deducted:

- Fire, theft, flood, or other casualty insurance
- Merchandise and inventory insurance
- Employees' group hospitalization and medical plans
- Employers' liability insurance
- Malpractice insurance
- Public liability insurance covering liability for bodily injury to persons who are not employees
- Worker's compensation insurance set by state law
- State unemployment insurance fund
- Overhead insurance paid during long periods of disability to offset the costs of keeping an office open
- Employee performance bonds
- Car and other vehicle insurance
- Key person insurance

Premiums on a life insurance policy covering the employer or an employee are not deductible if the employer is directly or indirectly a beneficiary of the policy. Thus a sole proprietor cannot deduct the cost of his life insurance policy, and if a partner in a partnership purchases life insurance on his life, naming his partners as benficiaries, his premiums are not deductible.[31] But there are some exceptions. For example, group term life insurance purchased by a professional corporation for its employees is deductible. The advice of an accountant or tax lawyer will be needed in determining if such a plan is eligible for the deduction.

Taxes

Various taxes imposed by federal, state, local, and foreign governments may be deducted if they are incurred in the ordinary course of business. Federal income, estate, and gift taxes and state inheritance, legacy, and succession taxes are not deductible. Deductible taxes may be categorized as:

Real property taxes—All taxes imposed on real property that is owned and used for business purposes may be deducted.

Income taxes—State income taxes imposed on a corporation are deductible; state income taxes are not deductible for an individual as a business expense (but can be deducted on Schedule A of the individual's Form 1040).

Employment taxes—If an employer has one or more employees, generally he will be required to withhold federal income taxes from their wages; he may also be subject to social security taxes under the Federal Insurance Contributions Act (FICA) and federal unemployment tax under the Federal Unemployment Tax Act (FUTA).

Other taxes—There are other taxes that may be deducted as business expenses, including personal property taxes, sales taxes,[32] gasoline taxes, and corporate franchise taxes.

The tax accounting of employees will be discussed at the conclusion of this chapter.

Profession-Related Expenses

The ordinary and necessary expenses of conducting a private practice can be deducted, including the costs of memberships in professional organizations, subscriptions to journals, and expenses incurred for books and professional equipment that has a useful life of less than one year.[33] Legal and accounting and other professional fees incurred in the course of business are likewise deductible. Other costs that may be deducted include utility charges, such as those for heat, light, power, or water expenses for an office, the costs of telephones and telephone services, any business-related supplies and materials, licenses, and regulatory fees. The costs of attending educational seminars may also be claimed, but only 80 percent of expenses for meals is deductible.[34]

Miscellaneous Business Expenses

There are other types of expenses that may qualify for deduction. Among these are payments to charitable, religious, educational, or scientific organizations (but they must not be charitable contributions), the cost of using a home for business purposes, and amounts spent to buy a franchise, trademark, or trade name. A tax advisor should be consulted as to whether or not a particular business expense will be deductible, preferably *before* the expenditure is incurred.

After figuring business income and expenses, the net profit or net loss from the practice can be determined by subtracting business expenses from business income. If expenses are less than income, the different is a net profit, but if expenses are more than income, the result is a net loss.

For a sole proprietorship, if the Schedule C shows a net profit, it is reported as part of the individual's gross income on Form 1040 (i.e., it may boost the optometrist's taxable income even higher). If there is a net loss, it generally can be deducted from other income (and thus can reduce the income subject to taxation[35]—see Fig. 41.1).

A partnership determines its net profit or loss on Form 1065, then distributes its gain or loss to the partners. If the partnership enjoys a net profit, each partner's share is added into the partner's adjusted gross income (just as is done by the sole proprietor). If the partnership has a net loss, each partner's share is deducted when figuring the partner's adjusted gross income (i.e., the partners get a deduction in ratio to their interests in the partnership, with the result being a reduction of taxable income, just as with a sole proprietor[36]—see Fig. 41.2).

A corporation figures its net profit on Form 1120. The corporation then pays a tax on its earnings (see Fig. 41.3). Corporate employees report their wages on their individual Form 1040.[37]

Since the profit or loss statement of a business is an indicator of how well it is faring, it should always be consulted before deciding whether to enter into partnership or purchase an existing practice. The customary approach is to request copies of the Schedule C (or Form 1065 or 1120) for the five preceding years. This permits one to get a feel for the financial posture or the practice. In complicated situations the counsel of a tax expert will be needed in order to decipher the meaning (which is sometimes hidden) of the tax return.

Depreciation and Amortization

One of the most important deductions that is available to the businessman is depreciation. To a lesser extent, amortization can be used to reduce taxable income as a claimed deduction.

Depreciation

If business property that has a useful life of more than one year is purchased, its cost cannot be deducted as an expense when business income is determined for tax purposes. Instead, the cost must be spread over more than one year and deducted a portion at a time. This process is called depreciation and is a means of allowing the recovery of the cost through the use of deductions that extend over the useable lifetime of the property. Many kinds of property can be depreciated, including instruments, buildings, vehicles, patents, furniture, equipment, and professional libraries.

Depreciable property may be classified as either *tangible* or *intangible*. Tangible property is any property that can be seen or touched, whereas intangible property is just the opposite, such as a patent or a right to a franchise.

Depreciable property may also be *real* or *personal*. Personal property is anything that is not real estate, whereas real property is the land and generally anything that is erected on, growing on, or attached to it. The land itself cannot be depreciated, only the structures or other things on it.

Property is depreciable if it meets these requirements:

Form **1065** — Department of the Treasury, Internal Revenue Service

U.S. Partnership Return of Income

▶ **For Paperwork Reduction Act Notice, see Form 1065 Instructions.**

For calendar year 1987, or fiscal year beginning ______________, 1987, and ending ____________, 19 ___

OMB No. 1545-0099 — **1987**

	Use IRS label. Otherwise, please print or type.	
A Principal business activity: Optometry	Name: O'Dee and O'Dee, Optometrists	D Employer identification number: 876 54 3210
B Principal product or service: Services	Number and street (or P.O. Box number if mail is not delivered to street address): 123 Main Street	E Date business started: April 1, 1983
C Business code number: 8042	City or town, state, and ZIP code: Anytown, State 12345	F Enter total assets at end of tax year: $ 47,150

G Check accounting method: (1) ☐ Cash (2) ☒ Accrual (3) ☐ Other

H Check applicable boxes: (1) ☐ Final return (2) ☐ Change in address (3) ☐ Amended return

	Yes	No
I Number of partners in this partnership ▶ ____________		
J Is this partnership a limited partnership (see the Instructions)?		X
K Is this partnership a partner in another partnership?		X
L Are any partners in this partnership also partnerships?		X
M Does the partnership meet **all** the requirements shown in the Instructions for **Question M**?		X
N Was there a distribution of property or a transfer (for example, by sale or death) of a partnership interest during the tax year? If "Yes," see the Instructions concerning an election to adjust the basis of the partnership's assets under section 754		X

	Yes	No
O At any time during the tax year, did the partnership have an interest in or a signature or other authority over a financial account in a foreign country (such as a bank account, securities account, or other financial account)? (See the Instructions for exceptions and filing requirements for Form TD F 90-22.1.) If "Yes," write the name of the foreign country. ▶ ____________		X
P Was the partnership the grantor of, or transferor to, a foreign trust which existed during the current tax year, whether or not the partnership or any partner has any beneficial interest in it? If "Yes," you may have to file Forms 3520, 3520-A, or 926		X
Q Was this partnership in operation at the end of 1987?	X	
R Number of months in 1987 that this partnership was in operation ▶ 12		
S Check this box if the partnership has filed or is required to file Form 8264, Application for Registration of a Tax Shelter ☐		
T Check this box if this is a partnership subject to the consolidated partnership audit procedures of TEFRA. (See page 7 of the Instructions.) ☐		

Caution: *Include* **only** *trade or business income and expenses on lines 1a–21 below. See the instructions for more information.*

Income	1a	Gross receipts or sales $ ____________ 1b Minus returns and allowances $ ____________ Balance ▶	1c	312,814
	2	Cost of goods sold and/or operations (Schedule A, line 7)	2	89,781
	3	Gross profit (subtract line 2 from line 1c)	3	223,033
	4	Ordinary income (loss) from other partnerships and fiduciaries (attach schedule)	4	
	5	Net farm profit (loss) (attach Schedule F (Form 1040))	5	
	6	Net gain (loss) (Form 4797, line 18)	6	2,100
	7	Other income (loss)	7	
	8	**TOTAL** income (loss) (combine lines 3 through 7)	8	225,133
Deductions (see instructions for limitations)	9a	Salaries and wages (other than to partners) $ 29,350 9b Minus jobs credit $ ________ Balance ▶	9c	29,350
	10	Guaranteed payments to partners	10	25,000
	11	Rent	11	9,000
	12	Deductible interest expense not claimed elsewhere on return (see Instructions)	12	871
	13	Taxes	13	9,208
	14	Bad debts	14	2,250
	15	Repairs	15	2,235
	16a	Depreciation from Form 4562 (attach Form 4562) $ ____________ 16b Minus depreciation claimed on Schedule A and elsewhere on return $ ____________ Balance ▶	16c	6,083
	17	Depletion (***Do not deduct oil and gas depletion.***)	17	
	18a	Retirement plans, etc.	18a	
	b	Employee benefit programs	18b	
	19	Other deductions (attach schedule)	19	16,947
	20	**TOTAL** deductions (add amounts in column for lines 9c through 19)	20	100,944
	21	Ordinary income (loss) from trade or business activity(ies) (subtract line 20 from line 8)	21	124,189

Please Sign Here — Under penalties of perjury, I declare that I have examined this return, including accompanying schedules and statements, and to the best of my knowledge and belief, it is true, correct, and complete. Declaration of preparer (other than taxpayer) is based on all information of which preparer has any knowledge.

▶ JB O'Dee — Signature of general partner ▶ April 15, 1987 — Date

Paid Preparer's Use Only

Preparer's signature ▶	Date	Check if self-employed ▶ ☐	Preparer's social security no.
Sam Accountant	Apr 15, 1987		111 22 3345
Firm's name (or yours if self-employed) and address ▶ Sam Accountant, CPA, Debit St., Anytown, State		E.I. No. ▶	111 23 3344
		ZIP code ▶	12345

Figure 41.2. Sample Form 1065, page 1

Form 1065 (1987) **Page 2**

Schedule A Cost of Goods Sold and/or Operations

1 Inventory at beginning of year	1	8,125	
2 Purchases minus cost of items withdrawn for personal use	2	88,881	
3 Cost of labor	3		
4a Additional section 263A costs (see instructions)	4a		
b Other costs (attach schedule)	4b		
5 Total (add lines 1 through 4b)	5	97,006	
6 Inventory at end of year	6	7,225	
7 Cost of goods sold (subtract line 6 from line 5). Enter here and on page 1, line 2	7	89,781	

8a Check all methods used for valuing closing inventory:

(i) ☒ Cost

(ii) ☐ Lower of cost or market as described in regulations section 1.471-4

(iii) ☐ Writedown of "subnormal" goods as described in regulations section 1.471-2(c)

(iv) ☐ Other (specify method used and attach explanation) ▶ ....

b Check if the LIFO inventory method was adopted this tax year for any goods (if checked, attach Form 970) ☐

c Do the rules of section 263A (with respect to property produced or acquired for resale) apply to the partnership? ☐ Yes ☒ No

d Was there any change (other than for section 263A purposes) in determining quantities, cost, or valuations between opening and closing inventory? If "Yes," attach explanation ☐ Yes ☒ No

Schedule H Income (Loss) From Rental Real Estate Activity(ies)

1 In the space provided below, show the kind and location of each rental property. Attach a schedule if more space is needed.

Property A ....

Property B ....

Property C

Rental Real Estate Income		Properties A	Properties B	Properties C	Totals (Add columns A, B, C, and amounts from any attached schedule)
2 Gross Income	2				2
Rental Real Estate Expenses					
3 Advertising	3				
4 Auto and travel	4				
5 Cleaning and maintenance	5				
6 Commissions	6				
7 Insurance	7				
8 Legal and other professional fees	8				
9 Interest expense	9				
10 Repairs	10				
11 Taxes	11				
12 Utilities	12				
13 Wages and salaries	13				
14 Depreciation from Form 4562	14				
15 Other (list)					
....					
....					
16 Total expenses. Add lines 3 through 15	16				16
17 Net income (loss) from rental real estate activity(ies). Subtract line 16 from line 2. Enter total net income (loss) from all properties on Schedule K, line 2	17				17

Figure 41.2. Sample Form 1065, page 2

Form 1065 (1987) **Page 4**

Schedule L Balance Sheets

(See the Instructions for Question M Before Completing Schedules L and M.)

Assets	Beginning of tax year (a)	Beginning of tax year (b)	End of tax year (c)	End of tax year (d)
1 Cash		405		8,620
2 Trade notes and accounts receivable	7,150		10,990	
a Minus allowance for bad debts		7,150		10,990
3 Inventories		8,125		7,225
4 Federal and state government obligations		1,000		1,000
5 Other current assets (attach schedule)		10,000		10,000
6 Mortgage and real estate loans				
7 Other investments (attach schedule)		1,000		2,000
8 Buildings and other depreciable assets	16,000		8,900	
a Minus accumulated depreciation	4,000	12,000	5,583	3,317
9 Depletable assets				
a Minus accumulated depletion				
10 Land (net of any amortization)		500		1,000
11 Intangible assets (amortizable only)				
a Minus accumulated amortization				
12 Other assets (attach schedule)				
13 **TOTAL** assets		40,180		44,152
Liabilities and Capital				
14 Accounts payable		9,180		10,462
15 Mortgages, notes, bonds payable in less than 1 year		3,600		4,000
16 Other current liabilities (attach schedule)				
17 All nonrecourse loans				
18 Mortgages, notes, bonds payable in 1 year or more		14,900		14,900
19 Other liabilities (attach schedule)				
20 Partners' capital accounts		12,500		14,790
21 **TOTAL** liabilities and capital		40,180		44,152

Schedule M Reconciliation of Partners' Capital Accounts

(Show reconciliation of each partner's capital account on Schedule K-1 (Form 1065), Question I.)

(a) Capital account at beginning of year	(b) Capital contributed during year	(c) Income (loss) from lines 1,2, 3c, and 4 of Sch. K	(d) Income not included in column (c), plus nontaxable income	(e) Losses not included in column (c), plus unallowable deductions	(f) Withdrawals and distributions	(g) Capital account at end of year
12,500	1,000	124,189	1,551	650	123,800	14,790

Designation of Tax Matters Partner

The following general partner is hereby designated as the tax matters partner (TMP) for the tax year for which this partnership return is filed:

Name of designated TMP ▶ John G. O'Dee   Identifying number of TMP ▶ 123 45 6789

Address of designated TMP ▶ 123 Main Street
Anytown, State 12345

✩U.S. GOVERNMENT PRINTING OFFICE: 1987-183-165 E.I. 43-0787287

Figure 41.2. Sample Form 1065, page 4

Form **1120** Department of the Treasury Internal Revenue Service

U.S. Corporation Income Tax Return

For calendar 1987 or tax year beginning ________, 1987, ending ________, 19 ___

▶ For Paperwork Reduction Act Notice, see page 1 of the instructions.

OMB No. 1545-0123 **1987**

Check if a—
A Consolidated return ☐
B Personal Holding Co. ☐
C Business Code No. (See the list in the instructions.) 8980

Use IRS label. Otherwise please print or type.

Name: John G. O'Dee, O.D., P.A.
Number and street: 321 Main Street
City or town, state, and ZIP code: Anytown, State 12345

D Employer identification number: 987 65 4321
E Date incorporated: Oct. 1, 1982
F Total assets (See Specific Instructions.) $

G Check applicable boxes: (1) ☐ Initial return (2) ☐ Final return (3) ☐ Change in address

Section	Line	Description			Dollars	Cents
Income	1a	Gross receipts or sales 257,075 b Less returns and allowances 1,000 Balance ▶		1c	256,075	
	2	Cost of goods sold and/or operations (Schedule A)		2	84,480	
	3	Gross profit (line 1c less line 2)		3	171,595	
	4	Dividends (Schedule C)		4		
	5	Interest		5		
	6	Gross rents		6		
	7	Gross royalties		7		
	8	Capital gain net income (attach separate Schedule D)		8		
	9	Net gain or (loss) from Form 4797, line 18, Part II (attach Form 4797)		9		
	10	Other income (see instructions—attach schedule)		10		
	11	TOTAL income—Add lines 3 through 10 and enter here ▶		11	171,595	
Deductions (See instructions for limitations on deductions)	12	Compensation of officers (Schedule E)		12	80,000	
	13a	Salaries and wages 24,300 b Less jobs credit ____ Balance ▶		13c	24,300	
	14	Repairs		14		
	15	Bad debts (see instructions)		15		
	16	Rents		16	6,000	
	17	Taxes		17	7,775	
	18	Interest		18	700	
	19	Contributions (**see instructions for 10% limitation**)		19		
	20	Depreciation (attach Form 4562)	20: 8,375			
	21	Less depreciation claimed in Schedule A and elsewhere on return	21a	21b	8,375	
	22	Depletion		22		
	23	Advertising		23		
	24	Pension, profit-sharing, etc., plans		24	8,000	
	25	Employee benefit programs		25		
	26	Other deductions (attach schedule)		26	18,445	
	27	TOTAL deductions—Add lines 12 through 26 and enter here ▶		27	153,595	
	28	Taxable income before net operating loss deduction and special deductions (line 11 less line 27)		28	18,000	
	29	Less: a Net operating loss deduction (see instructions)	29a			
		b Special deductions (Schedule C)	29b	29c		
Tax and Payments	30	Taxable income (line 28 less line 29c)		30	18,000	
	31	TOTAL TAX (Schedule J)		31	2,700	
	32	Payments: a 1986 overpayment credited to 1987				
	b	1987 estimated tax payments	2,500			
	c	Less 1987 refund applied for on Form 4466	( )			
	d	Tax deposited with Form 7004				
	e	Credit from regulated investment companies (attach Form 2439)				
	f	Credit for Federal tax on gasoline and special fuels (attach Form 4136)		32	2,500	
	33	Enter any PENALTY for underpayment of estimated tax—check ▶ ☐ if Form 2220 is attached		33		
	34	TAX DUE—If the total of lines 31 and 33 is larger than line 32, enter AMOUNT OWED		34	200	
	35	OVERPAYMENT—If line 32 is larger than the total of lines 31 and 33, enter AMOUNT OVERPAID		35		
	36	Enter amount of line 35 you want: Credited to 1988 estimated tax ▶ Refunded ▶		36		

Please Sign Here

Under penalties of perjury, I declare that I have examined this return, including accompanying schedules and statements, and to the best of my knowledge and belief, it is true, correct, and complete. Declaration of preparer (other than taxpayer) is based on all information of which preparer has any knowledge.

▶ JG O'Dee — Signature of officer | Apr. 1, 87 — Date | ▶ President — Title

Paid Preparer's Use Only

Preparer's signature ▶ Sam Accountant | Date: Apr 1, 1987 | Check if self-employed ☐ | Preparer's social security number: 111 22 3344

Firm's name (or yours, if self-employed) and address ▶ Sam Accountant, CPA, Debit St., Anytown, State | E.I. No. ▶ 111 23 3445 | ZIP code ▶ 12345

Figure 41.3. Sample Form 1120, page 1

Form 1120 (1987) Page **2**

Schedule A Cost of Goods Sold and/or Operations (See instructions for line 2, page 1.)

1 Inventory at beginning of year	1	6,500	
2 Purchases	2	85,180	
3 Cost of labor	3		
4a Additional section 263A costs (see instructions)	4a		
b Other costs (attach schedule)	4b		
5 Total—Add lines 1 through 4b	5	91,680	
6 Inventory at end of year	6	7,200	
7 Cost of goods sold and/or operations—Line 5 less line 6. Enter here and on line 2, page 1	7	84,480	

8a Check all methods used for valuing closing inventory:

(i) [X] Cost (ii) [ ] Lower of cost or market as described in Regulations section 1.471-4 (see instructions)

(iii) [ ] Writedown of "subnormal" goods as described in Regulations section 1.471-2(c) (see instructions)

(iv) [ ] Other (Specify method used and attach explanation.) ▶

b Check if the LIFO inventory method was adopted this tax year for any goods (if checked, attach Form 970) [ ]

c If the LIFO inventory method was used for this tax year, enter percentage (or amounts) of closing inventory computed under LIFO 8c

d Do the rules of section 263A (with respect to property produced or acquired for resale) apply to the corporation? [ ] Yes [ ] No

e Was there any change (other than for section 263A purposes) in determining quantities, cost, or valuations between opening and closing inventory? If "Yes," attach explanation [ ] Yes [X] No

Schedule C Dividends and Special Deductions (See Schedule C instructions.)	(a) Dividends received	(b) %	(c) Special deductions: multiply (a) × (b)
1 Domestic corporations subject to section 243(a) deduction (other than debt-financed stock)		see instructions	
2 Debt-financed stock of domestic and foreign corporations (section 246A)		see instructions	
3 Certain preferred stock of public utilities		see instructions	
4 Foreign corporations and certain FSCs subject to section 245 deduction		see instructions	
5 Wholly owned foreign subsidiaries and FSCs subject to 100% deduction (sections 245(b) and (c))		100	
6 Total—Add lines 1 through 5. See instructions for limitation			
7 Affiliated groups subject to the 100% deduction (section 243(a)(3))		100	
8 Other dividends from foreign corporations not included in lines 4 and 5			
9 Income from controlled foreign corporations under subpart F (attach Forms 5471)			
10 Foreign dividend gross-up (section 78)			
11 IC–DISC or former DISC dividends not included in lines 1 and/or 2 (section 246(d))			
12 Other dividends			
13 Deduction for dividends paid on certain preferred stock of public utilities (see instructions)			
14 Total dividends—Add lines 1 through 12. Enter here and on line 4, page 1 ▶			
15 Total deductions—Add lines 6, 7, and 13. Enter here and on line 29b, page 1 ▶			

Schedule E Compensation of Officers (See instructions for line 12, page 1.)

Complete Schedule E only if total receipts (line 1a, plus lines 4 through 10, of page 1, Form 1120) are $150,000 or more.

(a) Name of officer	(b) Social security number	(c) Percent of time devoted to business	Percent of corporation stock owned (d) Common	(e) Preferred	(f) Amount of compensation
John G. O'Dee	123 45 6789	100 %	100 %	%	80,000
		%	%	%	
		%	%	%	
		%	%	%	
		%	%	%	
		%	%	%	
		%	%	%	
Total compensation of officers—Enter here and on line 12, page 1					

Figure 41.3. Sample Form 1120, page 2

Form 1120 (1987) Page **3**

Schedule J — Tax Computation (See instructions.)

1 Check if you are a member of a controlled group (see sections 1561 and 1563) . . . . ▶ ☐

2 If line 1 is checked, see instructions. If your tax year includes June 30, 1987, complete both a and b below. Otherwise, complete only b.

a (i) $ ________ (ii) $ ________ (iii) $ ________ (iv) $ ________

b (i) $ ________ (ii) $ ________

Line	Description	Ref	Amount	Line	Amount
3	Income tax (see instructions to figure the tax; enter this tax or alternative tax from Schedule D, whichever is less). Check if from Schedule D ▶ ☐			3	2,700
4a	Foreign tax credit (attach Form 1118)	4a			
b	Possessions tax credit (attach Form 5735)	b			
c	Orphan drug credit (attach Form 6765)	c			
d	Credit for fuel produced from a nonconventional source (see instructions)	d			
e	General business credit. Enter here and check which forms are attached ☐ Form 3800 ☐ Form 3468 ☐ Form 5884 ☐ Form 6478 ☐ Form 6765 ☐ Form 8586	e			
5	Total—Add lines 4a through 4e			5	
6	Line 3 less line 5			6	2,700
7	Personal holding company tax (attach Schedule PH (Form 1120))			7	
8	Tax from recomputing prior-year investment credit (attach Form 4255)			8	
9a	Alternative minimum tax (see instructions—attach Form 4626)			9a	
b	Environmental tax (see instructions—attach Form 4626)			9b	
10	Total tax—Add lines 6 through 9b. Enter here and on line 31, page 1			10	2,700

Additional Information (See instruction F.)

Item	Yes	No
H Did the corporation claim a deduction for expenses connected with:		
(1) An entertainment facility (boat, resort, ranch, etc.)?		X
(2) Living accommodations (except employees on business)?		X
(3) Employees attending conventions or meetings outside the North American area? (See section 274(h).)		X
(4) Employees' families at conventions or meetings?		X
If "Yes," were any of these conventions or meetings outside the North American area? (See section 274(h).)		
(5) Employee or family vacations not reported on Form W-2?		X
I (1) Did the corporation at the end of the tax year own, directly or indirectly, 50% or more of the voting stock of a domestic corporation? (For rules of attribution, see section 267(c).)		X
If "Yes," attach a schedule showing: (a) name, address, and identifying number; (b) percentage owned; (c) taxable income or (loss) before NOL and special deductions of such corporation for the tax year ending with or within your tax year; (d) highest amount owed by the corporation to such corporation during the year; and (e) highest amount owed to the corporation by such corporation during the year.		
(2) Did any individual, partnership, corporation, estate, or trust at the end of the tax year own, directly or indirectly, 50% or more of the corporation's voting stock? (For rules of attribution, see section 267(c).) If "Yes," complete (a) through (d)	X	
(a) Attach a schedule showing name, address, and identifying number. Enter percentage owned ▶ 100		
(b) Was the owner of such voting stock a person other than a U.S. person? (See instructions.) **Note:** *If "Yes," the corporation may have to file Form 5472.*		X
If "Yes," enter owner's country ▶ ________		
(c) Enter highest amount owed by the corporation to such owner during the year ▶ ________		
(d) Enter highest amount owed to the corporation by such owner during the year ▶ ________		
Note: *For purposes of I(1) and I(2), "highest amount owed" includes loans and accounts receivable/payable.*		
J Refer to the list in the instructions and state the principal: Business activity ▶ Optometry; Product or service ▶ Services		
K Was the corporation a U.S. shareholder of any controlled foreign corporation? (See sections 951 and 957.) If "Yes," attach Form 5471 for each such corporation.		X
L At any time during the tax year, did the corporation have an interest in or a signature or other authority over a financial account in a foreign country (such as a bank account, securities account, or other financial account)? (See instruction F and filing requirements for form TD F 90-22.1.) If "Yes," enter name of foreign country ▶ ________		X
M Was the corporation the grantor of, or transferor to, a foreign trust which existed during the current tax year, whether or not the corporation has any beneficial interest in it? If "Yes," the corporation may have to file Forms 3520, 3520-A, or 926.		X
N During this tax year, did the corporation pay dividends (other than stock dividends and distributions in exchange for stock) in excess of the corporation's current and accumulated earnings and profits? (See sections 301 and 316.) If "Yes," file Form 5452. If this is a consolidated return, answer here for parent corporation and on Form 851, Affiliations Schedule, for each subsidiary.		X
O During this tax year did the corporation maintain any part of its accounting/tax records on a computerized system?		X
P Check method of accounting: (1) ☒ Cash (2) ☐ Accrual (3) ☐ Other (specify) ▶ ________		
Q Check this box if the corporation issued publicly offered debt instruments with original issue discount ☐ If so, the corporation may have to file Form 8281.		
R Enter the amount of tax-exempt interest received or accrued during the tax year ▶ ________		
S If you are a member of a controlled group, enter the amount of taxable income for the entire group ▶ ________		

Figure 41.3. Sample Form 1120, page 3

Form 1120 (1987) Page 4

Schedule L Balance Sheets

Assets	Beginning of tax year (a)	(b)	End of tax year (c)	(d)
1 Cash		3,500		4,300
2 Trade notes and accounts receivable	2,200		2,450	
a Less allowance for bad debts				
3 Inventories		6,500		7,600
4 Federal and state government obligations				
5 Other current assets (attach schedule)				
6 Loans to stockholders				
7 Mortgage and real estate loans				
8 Other investments (attach schedule)				
9 Buildings and other depreciable assets				
a Less accumulated depreciation				
10 Depletable assets				
a Less accumulated depletion				
11 Land (net of any amortization)				
12 Intangible assets (amortizable only)				
a Less accumulated amortization				
13 Other assets (attach schedule)		11,700		12,750
14 Total assets		21,700		24,650
Liabilities and Stockholders' Equity				
15 Accounts payable		10,500		10,700
16 Mortgages, notes, bonds payable in less than 1 year				
17 Other current liabilities (attach schedule)		1,200		1,450
18 Loans from stockholders				
19 Mortgages, notes, bonds payable in 1 year or more				
20 Other liabilities (attach schedule)				
21 Capital stock: a preferred stock				
b common stock		5,000		5,000
22 Paid-in or capital surplus				
23 Retained earnings—Appropriated (attach schedule)		5,000		7,500
24 Retained earnings—Unappropriated				
25 Less cost of treasury stock		( )		( )
26 Total liabilities and stockholders' equity		21,700		24,650

Schedule M-1 Reconciliation of Income per Books With Income per Return You are not required to complete this schedule if the total assets on line 14, column (d), of Schedule L are less than $25,000.

1 Net income per books		7 Income recorded on books this year not included in this return (itemize)	
2 Federal income tax		a Tax-exempt interest $	
3 Excess of capital losses over capital gains			
4 Income subject to tax not recorded on books this year (itemize)		8 Deductions in this tax return not charged against book income this year (itemize)	
5 Expenses recorded on books this year not deducted in this return (itemize)		a Depreciation $	
a Depreciation $		b Contributions carryover $	
b Contributions carryover $			
		9 Total of lines 7 and 8	
6 Total of lines 1 through 5		10 Income (line 28, page 1)—line 6 less line 9	

Schedule M-2 Analysis of Unappropriated Retained Earnings per Books (line 24, Schedule L) You are not required to complete this schedule if the total assets on line 14, column (d), of Schedule L are less than $25,000.

1 Balance at beginning of year		5 Distributions: a Cash	
2 Net income per books		b Stock	
3 Other increases (itemize)		c Property	
		6 Other decreases (itemize)	
		7 Total of lines 5 and 6	
4 Total of lines 1, 2, and 3		8 Balance at end of year (line 4 less line 7)	

★U.S.GPO:1987-0-183-186

Figure 41.3. Sample Form 1120, page 4

- It must be used in business or held for the production of income.
- It must have a useful life that can be determined, and its useful life must be longer than one year; the useful life of a piece of property is an estimate of how long it is expected to be used in the business or for the production of income.
- It must be something that wears out, decays, gets used up, becomes obsolete, or loses value from natural causes.

In general, if property does not meet all three of these conditions, it is not depreciable.

Depreciation may only be deducted on property that is used for business purposes or held for the production of income; depreciation cannot be claimed on nonbusiness property such as a car that is used solely for commuting, vacations, or other nonbusiness activities. If property is used for both business and nonbusiness purposes, however, depreciation may be deducted for the part that is used for business. For example, a car used for both purposes is eligible for depreciation, but only that percent of its use that is related to business (discussed on page 504).

Depreciable property includes:

- Ophthalmic instruments
- Ophthalmic equipment
- Motor vehicles
- Furniture
- An office building
- Professional libraries
- Repairs or replacements to property that lengthen its life, make it more useful, or increase its value
- Patents and copyrights
- Covenants not to compete
- Franchises

Property that cannot be depreciated includes:

- Land
- Rented property
- Inventory
- Goodwill
- Trademarks or trade names that are already in existence when purchased

To calculate depreciation, there are three things that must be known about the property: its basis, the date it was placed in service, and the method of depreciation that is to be used.

Basis

For property that is purchased, the original basis is its cost. Events will often change the basis of a piece of property to a value called the *adjusted basis*. Some events (e.g., permanent repairs or improvements) improve basis; others (e.g., casualty losses) decrease basis. If basis is adjusted, the depreciation deduction may also have to be changed. The assistance of a tax advisor is needed in order to make such determinations.

Placed in Service

Property is considered to be placed in service when it is in a condition or state of readiness and availability for a specifically assigned function in a business. Depreciation begins when the property is first ready for service.

Method of Depreciation

The Economic Recovery Tax Act of 1981 instituted some significant changes in the traditional methods used to calculate depreciation. Under this law, the Accelerated Cost Recovery System (ACRS) was introduced to be used for tangible property placed in service after 1980.[38] The Tax Reform Act of 1986 modified the ACRS, repealing the investment tax credit and instituting extended recovery periods for tangible property, as well as providing for an increased first year writeoff known as expensing.[39] Beginning in 1987, tangible property must be depreciated over a three-year, five-year, seven-year, ten-year, or fifteen-year recovery period, depending on the type of property (see Table 41.1). For the purposes of optometrists in private practice, the most important are the five- and seven-year recovery periods.

Table 41.1. Selected Recovery Periods under the Modified Accelerated Cost Recovery System

5-Year Property	7-Year Property
Automobiles and other vehicles used for business	Office furniture and fixtures (e.g., desks and files)
Computers and peripheral equipment	Ophthalmic equipment and instruments
Office machinery (e.g., typewriters and calculators)	Patient records

Source: Tax Reform Act of 1986.

Table 41.2. Annual Percentages for 5- and 7-Year Property under the Accelerated Cost Recovery System

5-Year Property		7-Year Property	
Year	% Deductible	Year	% Deductible
1	20	1	14
2	32	2	25
3	19	3	17
4	12	4	13
5	12	5	9
6	6	6	9
		7	9
		8	4

Source: Klott, G., *The New York Times Complete Guide to the New Tax Law*, Times Books, New York, 1986, pp. 178–179.

The deduction under the modified ACRS is calculated by multiplying the unadjusted basis in the property by a certain percentage that varies from year to year during the recovery period. The annual percentages for the five- and seven-year recovery periods are listed in Table 41.2. The depreciation deduction is computed on Form 4562 (see Fig. 41.4).

The unadjusted basis is the same amount that would be used to compute a gain on a sale of the property without adjustment for depreciation. For example, assume that in April of 1987 an optometrist purchased a slit lamp at a total cost of $3,000. It is seven-year property, and its unadjusted basis is $3,000. The modified ACRS deduction in 1987 is 14 percent or $420; in 1988 this is increased to $750 ($3,000 × 25 percent).

There is an alternative to the modified ACRS, based on a straight line method of depreciation, which allows equal annual deductions to be made for a class of property. Under some circumstances a taxpayer may elect to use this alternate modified ACRS, but once chosen it cannot be changed.[40]

Straight Line Method

The conventional methods of depreciation, of which the straight line method is the best known,[41] differ from the ACRS in three ways:

1. Instead of taking depreciation deductions over a specified recovery period, they are taken over the useful life of the property.
2. The deduction that would be allowed for a full year must be determined and then it must be prorated for the portion of the year the property is actually in service.
3. Instead of figuring deductions using the full amount of the property's basis, salvage value must be taken into account (salvage value is the estimated value of property at the end of its useful life; it is the amount expected from the sale or other disposition of the property when the property is no longer used).[42]

The straight line method allows the same annual deduction to be claimed for the useful life of the property. To calculate a straight line deduction, first determine the property's basis, salvage value, and estimated useful life. Subtract the salvage value from the basis; the balance is the total amount of depreciation that may be claimed. Divide this amount by the number of years of useful life; this will provide the yearly depreciation deduction.

Occasionally property subject to conventional methods of depreciation will be encountered, but all tangible business property placed in service after January 1, 1987 will be subject to the modified ACRS.

Expensing

A taxpayer may choose to treat the cost of depreciable property as an expense rather than as a capital expenditure. If the taxpayer elects to deduct the property as an expense (known as a *section 179 deduction*),[43] as of 1987 up to $10,000 may be claimed in the first year the property is placed in service. This deduction may be claimed only once, in the first year of service, and the amount elected under the section 179 deduction is subtracted from the basis of the property, thereby reducing the depreciation available in later years.[44]

For example, assume an optometrist purchased $20,000 worth of ophthalmic equipment in 1987, which he put into service at a branch office. He elects to expense the maximum amount allowable, $10,000, and this deduction reduces his taxable income for 1987 by this amount. His adjusted basis in the equipment becomes $10,000 (the cost, $20,000, less the section 179 deduction of $10,000), and in 1988 he uses the ACRS to claim depreciation of $2,500 for the equipment ($10,000 × 25 percent, the allowable second year depreciation under the ACRS).

There are limitations on the amount that may be claimed for depreciation and the section 179 deduction for automobiles[45] (see Chapter 42). The expensing deduction is figured, along with other depreciation deductions, on Form 4562 (see Fig. 41.4).

Real Property

Under the modified ACRS enacted in 1986, depreciation allowances for real property are $27\frac{1}{2}$ years for

Form **4562** — **Depreciation and Amortization**

Department of the Treasury
Internal Revenue Service (O)

▶ See separate instructions.
▶ Attach this form to your return.

OMB No. 1545-0172
1987
Attachment Sequence No. 67

Name(s) as shown on return: John G. O'DEE — Identifying number: 123 45 6789

Business or activity to which this form relates: Optometry

Part I Depreciation (Do not use this part for automobiles, certain other vehicles, computers, and property used for entertainment, recreation, or amusement. Instead, use Part III.)

Section A.—Election To Expense Depreciable Assets Placed in Service During This Tax Year (Section 179)

(a) Description of property	(b) Date placed in service	(c) Cost	(d) Expense deduction
1			

2 Listed property—Enter total from Part III, Section A, column (h)	
3 Total (add lines 1 and 2, but do not enter more than $10,000)	
4 Enter the amount, if any, by which the cost of all section 179 property placed in service during this tax year is more than $200,000	
5 Subtract line 4 from line 3. If result is less than zero, enter zero. (See instructions for other limitations)	

Section B.—Depreciation

(a) Class of property	(b) Date placed in service	(c) Basis for depreciation (Business use only—see instructions)	(d) Recovery period	(e) Method of figuring depreciation	(f) Deduction
6 Accelerated Cost Recovery System (ACRS) (see instructions): *For assets placed in service* **ONLY** *during tax year beginning in 1987*					
a 3-year property					
b 5-year property Auto		4,080	5	20	816
c 7-year property Eqpt		20,000	7	14	2,800
d 10-year property					
e 15-year property					
f 20-year property					
g Residential rental property					
h Nonresidential real property					

7 Listed property—Enter total from Part III, Section A, column (g)	
8 ACRS deduction for assets placed in service prior to 1987 (see instructions)	

Section C.—Other Depreciation

9 Property subject to section 168(f)(1) election (see instructions)	
10 Other depreciation (see instructions)	

Section D.—Summary

11 Total (add deductions on lines 5 through 10). Enter here and on the Depreciation line of your return (Partnerships and S corporations—Do NOT include any amounts entered on line 5.)		3,616
12 For assets above placed in service during the current year, enter the portion of the basis attributable to additional section 263A costs. (See instructions for who must use.)		

Part II Amortization

(a) Description of property	(b) Date acquired	(c) Cost or other basis	(d) Code section	(e) Amortization period or percentage	(f) Amortization for this year
1 Amortization for property placed in service **only** during tax year beginning in 1987					
2 Amortization for property placed in service prior to 1987					
3 Total. Enter here and on Other Deductions or Other Expenses line of your return					3,616

See Paperwork Reduction Act Notice on page 1 of the separate instructions. Form **4562** (1987)

Figure 41.4. Sample Form 4562, page 1

Form 4562 (1987) Page 2

Part III **Automobiles, Certain Other Vehicles, Computers, and Property Used for Entertainment, Recreation, or Amusement (Listed Property).**

If you are using the standard mileage rate or deducting vehicle lease expense, complete columns (a) through (d) of Section A, all of Section B, and Section C if applicable.

Section A.—Depreciation (If automobiles and other listed property placed in service after June 18, 1984, are used 50% or less in a trade or business, the Section 179 deduction is not allowed and depreciation must be taken using the straight line method over 5 years. For other limitations, see instructions.)

Do you have evidence to support the business use claimed? ☒ Yes ☐ No If yes, is the evidence written? ☒ Yes ☐ No

(a) Type of property (list vehicles first)	(b) Date placed in service	(c) Business use percentage (%)	(d) Cost or other basis (see instructions for leased property)	(e) Basis for depreciation (Business use only—see instructions)	(f) Depreciation method and recovery period	(g) Depreciation deduction	(h) Section 179 expense
Chevrolet	1-1-87	51	8,000	4,080	ACRS-5yrs	816	
Total (Enter here and on line 2, page 1.)							
Total (Enter here and on line 7, page 1.)						816	

Section B.—Information Regarding Use of Vehicles

Complete this section as follows, if you deduct expenses for vehicles:

- *Always complete this section for vehicles used by a sole proprietor, partner, or other more than 5% owner or related person.*
- *If you provided vehicles to employees, first answer the questions in Section C to see if you meet an exception to completing this section for those items.*

	Vehicle 1		Vehicle 2		Vehicle 3		Vehicle 4		Vehicle 5		Vehicle 6	
1 Total miles driven during the year	14,000											
2 Total business miles driven during the year	7,140											
3 Total commuting miles driven during the year	2,400											
4 Total other personal (noncommuting) miles driven	4,460											
	Yes	No	Yes	No	Yes	No	Yes	No	Yes	No	Yes	No
5 Was the vehicle available for personal use during off-duty hours?	X											
6 Was the vehicle used primarily by a more than 5% owner or related person?	X											
7 Is another vehicle available for personal use?		X										

Section C.—Questions for Employers Who Provide Vehicles for Use by Employees.

(Answer these questions to determine if you meet an exception to completing Section B. **Note:** *Section B must always be completed for vehicles used by sole proprietors, partners, or other more than 5% owners or related persons.)*

	Yes	No
8 Do you maintain a written policy statement that prohibits all personal use of vehicles, including commuting, by your employees?		
9 Do you maintain a written policy statement that prohibits personal use of vehicles, except commuting, by your employees? (See instructions for vehicles used by corporate officers, directors, or 1% or more owners.)		
10 Do you treat all use of vehicles by employees as personal use?		
11 Do you provide more than five vehicles to your employees and retain the information received from your employees concerning the use of the vehicles?		
12 Do you meet the requirements concerning fleet vehicles or qualified automobile demonstration use (see instructions)?		

Note: *If your answer to 8, 9, 10, 11, or 12 is "Yes," you need not complete Section B for the covered vehicles.*

★U.S.GPO:1987-0-183-245

Figure 41.4. Sample Form 4562, page 2

residential rental property and $31\frac{1}{2}$ years for nonresidential rental property.[46] The law also restricts the type of depreciation to the straight line method.[47] Thus, optometrists who seek to write off office buildings will have to do so over longer periods of time than in the past.

Amortization

In addition to depreciation, an optometrist may be able to amortize certain costs of practice. Amortization allows the deduction of certain capital expenditures in a way that is similar to the straight line method of depreciation. But only certain specified expenditures may be amortized for federal income tax purposes.[48]

Probably the most important category for optometrists is that of business start-up costs. If an optometrist enters into private practice "cold" or purchases an ongoing practice, certain costs incurred in connection with setting up or purchasing the practice may be amortized over a 5 year (or longer) period.

Start-up expenses include both what was paid for investigating a prospective business and for getting the business started, including an analysis of business facilities and the potential of the business; advertising for the opening of the business; travel and other necessary expenses for securing prospective suppliers; salaries and fees for consultants or for other professional services; and the contractually agreed upon value of a covenant not to compete.

Care must be exercised when writing a contract that includes a covenant not to compete as part of the sale of a practice.[49] If appropriately drawn, the covenant may be deducted in equal amounts over the specified period of useful life. The amortization period begins with the month that operations actually start.

For example, assume a seller of an optometric practice agrees to include a covenant not to compete as a part of the sales agreement. It is valued at $55,000. The buyer may deduct $11,000 a year for the amortization of the covenant over a sixty-month period.

Employment and Self-Employment Taxes

Optometrists routinely employ individuals to assist them in private practice. These optometrists, like all employers, will be required to withhold federal income taxes from their employees' wages. They will also be subject to social security taxes under the Federal Insurance Contributions Act (FICA) and to the federal unemployment tax under the Federal Unemployment Tax Act (FUCA).

Occasionally there is a question as to whether or not an individual is in fact an "employee". It is generally held that an individual who performs services that are subject to the control of the employer, where the employer has the legal right to determine what duties are to be performed and how they are to be performed, is an employee.[50] Whether or not the employer chooses to exercise this right is not the determining factor; nor is the description given to the individual (be it agent, partner, joint venturer, or independent contractor); nor even how the individual is paid (whether employed full-time or part-time). The determinative characteristic is the right of control, two especially important aspects of which are the right to discharge the individual and the supplying of equipment and a place to work.[51] If an individual is deemed to be an employee, then income tax withholding, social security taxes, and federal unemployment taxes will be the responsibility of the employer.

Income Tax Withholding

An employer must withhold income tax from wages paid for a payroll period. Regular payroll periods can be daily, weekly, biweekly, semi-monthly, monthly, quarterly, semi-annually, or annually. The determination of how much is to be withheld is based upon the allowances claimed by the employee on Form W-4, Employee's Withholding Allowance Certificate. In general, an employee's withholding allowances will equal the number of exemptions that the employee will be entitled to in calculating the income tax on his or her Form 1040. Each new employee should be required to submit a Form W-4 before the first day of work. This certificate is effective for the first payment of wages and will last until the employee files a new one. It is kept on file by the employer and, as necessary, revised by the employee to keep his or her withholding up-to-date.

Withholding is based upon gross wages before any deductions for social security tax, pensions, insurance or other items are made. The methods for withholding, and applicable tables, may be found in IRS Publication 15, *Circular E, Employer's Tax Guide*, available from the Internal Revenue Service.

Social Security Taxes

The social security program is a federal program of old age, survivors, disability, and hospital insurance. The system is financed through social security taxes, which are levied on both the employer and the employee. The employer has the responsibility to collect and remit the employee's part of the tax. The withholding of employees' social security taxes is performed in much the same manner as the withholding of income tax, and is described in *Circular E, Employer's Tax Guide*. The employer is also liable for his or her share of these taxes, which likewise must be remitted to the federal government.

There is an annual tax rate that determines the amount to be withheld, and there is a limit to the wages subject to the tax. Unfortunately, both the tax rate and the wage base continue to escalate. For example, in 1973 the tax rate was 5.5 percent, applied to wages up to a maximum of $10,800, which meant the total amount an employee would be required to pay (assuming he or she earned at least $10,800) was $594. By 1981 these figures had risen to 6.65 percent and $29,700, or a maximum tax of $1,975, and by 1988 to 7.51 percent and $45,000, or a maximum tax of $3,379. Furture years will continue this trend.

Generally, social security taxes and withheld income taxes are reported and paid together. Employers are required to report the employee's compensation on Form W-2, Wage and Tax Statement. The W-2 must show the total wages and other compensation paid (whether or not subject to withholding), the amounts deducted for income and social security taxes, and the total amount of advance earned income credit payments. Copies must be provided to employees no later than January 31. Employers must file Form W-2, along with Form W-3 (which is a transmittal form) with the Social Security Administration by the last day of February following the calender year for which the W-2 was prepared. These forms will be processed by the Social Security Administration, which will then furnish the IRS with the income data provided on the W-2.

In addition to the W-2, the employer must file Form 941, Employer's Quarterly Tax Return, one month after the end of each calendar quarter (Table 41.3). This form reports the deposits made of withheld social security taxes, both for the employer and for employees, and of the withheld income taxes for employees (Fig. 41.5). The employer is legally obligated to pay these taxes to the federal government, even if they are not actually collected. Therefore, if the employer deducts less than the correct tax from his employees' wages, the employer is still liable for the full amount of the tax and for any interest or penalties that may be applied.[52] The deposits are made by check to an authorized financial institution or Federal Reserve Bank, along with a federal tax deposit coupon,[53] and must be made before the tax return is due. The computation of how much must be deposited for each quarter is a complex matter and should be well understood by the employer in order to avoid the imposition of penalties for late or insufficient deposits.[54] The worst offense is failure to pay the taxes actually withheld; for this offense, the penalty can be 100 percent of the tax owed.[55]

Table 41.3. Due Dates for Employer's Quarterly Federal Tax Return

First quarter	Jan.–Feb.–Mar.	April 30
Second quarter	Apr.–May–June	July 31
Third quarter	July–Aug.–Sept.	October 31
Fourth quarter	Oct.–Nov.–Dec.	January 31

Source: *Tax Guide for Small Businesses*, Internal Revenue Service, Washington, D.C., 1987, p. 122.

Unemployment Taxes

The federal unemployment tax system, together with the various state systems, provides for payments of unemployment compensation to workers who have lost their jobs. Most employers pay both a state and a federal unemployment tax, but if there is no state tax the employer is still probably responsible for the federal tax.[56]

The federal unemployment tax is determined on the first $7,000 in wages paid to each employee but is imposed upon the employer and is not collected from the wages of employees. The federal unemployment tax rate may be offset by payments made for state unemployment taxes,[57] but if the employer is exempt from state unemployment tax, the full federal rate will be applied.

The FUTA tax is reported on Form 940, Employer's Annual Federal Unemployment Tax Return, which covers one calendar year and is generally due one month after the year ends. As with social security and withheld income taxes, however, the tax must be deposited before filing the return.[58] Deposits are made at a Federal Reserve Bank or other authorized financial institution, and are accompanied by a federal tax deposit coupon.[59]

The records substantiating the employer's withholding for income taxes, social security taxes, and unemployment taxes should be carefully maintained and stored for at least four years after the due date of the return or after the date the tax is paid, whichever is later. Records should always contain the employer identification number, the dates and amounts of deposits made, and copies of the returns filed.

Form **941** (Rev. July 1987) Department of the Treasury Internal Revenue Service

Employer's Quarterly Federal Tax Return

▶ For Paperwork Reduction Act Notice, see page 2.
Please type or print.

OMB No. 1545-0029
Expires: 8-31-88

Type or print your name, address, employer identification number, and calendar quarter of return as shown on original. ▶

Name (as distinguished from trade name): John G. O'Dee, O.D.
Date quarter ended: March 31, 1987
Trade name, if any
Employer identification number: 432 10 123
Address and ZIP code: 321 Main Street, Anytown, State

YOUR COPY

If you are not liable for returns in the future, check here . . . ▶ ☐ Date final wages paid . . . . ▶

Complete for First Quarter Only

1a	Number of employees (except household) employed in the pay period that includes March 12th ▶	1a	1
b	If you are a subsidiary corporation AND your parent corporation files a consolidated Form 1120, enter parent corporation employer identification number (EIN) . . ▶ 1b –		
2	Total wages and tips subject to withholding, plus other compensation ▶	2	2,300
3	Total income tax withheld from wages, tips, pensions, annuities, sick pay, gambling, etc. ▶	3	498
4	Adjustment of withheld income tax for preceding quarters of calendar year (see instructions) ▶	4	
5	Adjusted total of income tax withheld	5	498
6	Taxable social security wages paid $ 2,300 × 14.3% (.143)	6	329
7a	Taxable tips reported $ ____ × 7.15% (.0715)	7a	
b	Tips deemed to be wages (see instructions) $ ____ × 7.15% (.0715)	7b	
c	Taxable hospital insurance wages paid $ ____ × 2.9% (.029)	7c	
8	Total social security taxes (add lines 6, 7a, 7b, and 7c)	8	329
9	Adjustment of social security taxes (see instructions for required explanation) ▶	9	
10	Adjusted total of social security taxes (see instructions)	10	
11	Backup withholding (see instructions) ▶	11	
12	Adjustment of backup withholding tax for preceding quarters of calendar year	12	
13	Adjusted total of backup withholding	13	
14	Total taxes (add lines 5, 10, and 13) ▶	14	827
15	Advance earned income credit (EIC) payments, if any	15	
16	Net taxes (subtract line 15 from line 14). **This must equal line IV below** (plus line IV of Schedule A (Form 941) if you have treated backup withholding as a separate liability).	16	827
17	Total deposits for quarter, including overpayment applied from a prior quarter, from your records ▶	17	827
18	Balance due (subtract line 17 from line 16). This should be less than $500. Pay to IRS ▶	18	0
19	If line 17 is more than line 16, enter overpayment here ▶ $ ____ and check if to be: ☐ Applied to next return **OR** ☐ Refunded.		

Record of Federal Tax Liability (Complete if line 16 is $500 or more.) See the instructions under rule 4 for details before checking these boxes.
Check only if you made eighth-monthly deposits using the 95% rule ▶ ☐ Check only if you are a first time 3-banking-day depositor ▶ ☐

Date wages paid		Tax liability (*Do not show Federal tax deposits here.*) First month of quarter		Second month of quarter		Third month of quarter
1st through 3rd	A		I		Q	
4th through 7th	B		J		R	
8th through 11th	C		K		S	
12th through 15th	D	137.83	L	137.83	T	137.83
16th through 19th	E		M		U	
20th through 22nd	F		N		V	
23rd through 25th	G		O		W	
26th through the last	H	137.83	P	137.83	X	137.83
Total liability for month	*I*	275.66	*II*	275.66	*III*	275.66

IV Total for quarter (add lines *I*, *II*, and *III*) ▶ 827

Under penalties of perjury, I declare that I have examined this return, including accompanying schedules and statements, and to the best of my knowledge and belief, it is true, correct, and complete.

Signature ▶ 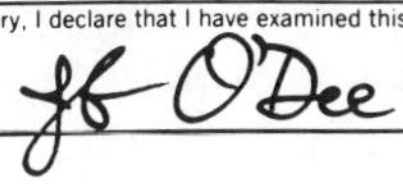 Title ▶ Employer Date ▶ Apr. 1, 1987

Figure 41.5. Sample Form 941

SCHEDULE SE (Form 1040)
Department of the Treasury
Internal Revenue Service (O)

Computation of Social Security Self-Employment Tax

▶ See Instructions for Schedule SE (Form 1040).
▶ Attach to Form 1040.

OMB No. 1545-0074
1987
Attachment Sequence No. **18**

Name of person with **self-employment** income (as shown on social security card): John G. O'DEE
Social security number of person with **self-employment** income ▶ 123 : 45 : 6789

A If your only self-employment income was from earnings as a minister, member of a religious order, or Christian Science practitioner, AND you filed Form 4361, then DO NOT file Schedule SE. Instead, write "Exempt-Form 4361" on Form 1040, line 48. However, if you filed Form 4361, but have $400 or more of other earnings subject to self-employment tax, continue with Part I and check here ▶ ☐

B If you filed Form 4029 and have received IRS approval, DO NOT file Schedule SE. Write "Exempt-Form 4029" on Form 1040, line 48.

C If your only earnings subject to self-employment tax are wages from an electing church or church-controlled organization that is exempt from employer social security taxes and you are not a minister or a member of a religious order, skip lines 1–8. Enter zero on line 9. Continue with line 11a.

Part I Regular Computation of Net Earnings From Self-Employment

		Line	Amount	
1	Net farm profit (or loss) from Schedule F (Form 1040), line 37, and farm partnerships, Schedule K-1 (Form 1065), line 14a	1		
2	Net profit (or loss) from Schedule C (Form 1040), line 31, and Schedule K-1 (Form 1065), line 14a (other than farming). (See Instructions for other income to report.) Employees of an electing church or church-controlled organization DO NOT enter your Form W-2 wages on line 2. See the Instructions	2	39,925	

Part II Optional Computation of Net Earnings From Self-Employment (See "Who Can Use Schedule SE" in the Instructions.)

See Instructions for limitations. Generally, this part may be used **only** if you meet any of the following tests:

A Your **gross** farm income[1] was not more than $2,400; **or**

B Your **gross** farm income[1] was more than $2,400 and your **net** farm profits[2] were **less** than $1,600; **or**

C Your **net** nonfarm profits[3] were less than $1,600 and your **net** nonfarm profits[3] were also **less** than two-thirds (⅔) of your **gross** nonfarm income.[4]

Note: *If line 2 above is two-thirds (⅔) or more of your gross nonfarm income[4], or, if line 2 is $1,600 or more, you may **not** use the optional method.*

[1]From Schedule F (Form 1040), line 12, and Schedule K-1 (Form 1065), line 14b. [3]From Schedule C (Form 1040), line 31, and Schedule K-1 (Form 1065), line 14a.
[2]From Schedule F (Form 1040), line 37, and Schedule K-1 (Form 1065), line 14a. [4]From Schedule C (Form 1040), line 5, and Schedule K-1 (Form 1065), line 14c.

		Line	Amount	
3	Maximum income for optional methods	3	$1,600	00
4	Farm Optional Method—If you meet test A or B above, enter the **smaller of:** two-thirds (⅔) of gross farm income from Schedule F (Form 1040), line 12, and farm partnerships, Schedule K-1 (Form 1065), line 14b; **or** $1,600	4		
5	Subtract line 4 from line 3	5		
6	Nonfarm Optional Method—If you meet test C above, enter the **smallest of:** two-thirds (⅔) of gross nonfarm income from Schedule C (Form 1040), line 5, and Schedule K-1 (Form 1065), line 14c (other than farming); **or** $1,600; **or,** if you elected the farm optional method, the amount on line 5	6		

Part III Computation of Social Security Self-Employment Tax

		Line	Amount	
7	Enter the amount from Part I, line 1, **or,** if you elected the farm optional method, Part II, line 4	7		
8	Enter the amount from Part I, line 2, **or,** if you elected the nonfarm optional method, Part II, line 6	8	39,925	
9	Add lines 7 and 8. If less than $400, do not file this schedule. (Exception: If you are an employee of an electing church or church-controlled organization and the total of lines 7 and 8 is less than $400, enter zero and complete the rest of this schedule.)	9	39,925	
10	The largest amount of combined wages and self-employment earnings subject to social security or railroad retirement tax (tier 1) for 1987 is	10	$43,800	00
11a	Total social security wages and tips from Forms W-2 and railroad retirement compensation (tier 1). **Note:** *Medicare qualified government employees whose wages are only subject to the 1.45% medicare (hospital insurance benefits) tax and employees of certain church or church-controlled organizations should **not** include those wages on this line. (See Instructions.)* — 11a			
b	Unreported tips subject to social security tax from Form 4137, line 9, or to railroad retirement tax (tier 1) — 11b			
c	Add lines 11a and 11b	11c		
12a	Subtract line 11c from line 10. (If zero or less, enter zero.)	12a		
b	Enter your medicare qualified government wages if you are required to use the worksheet in Part III of the Instructions — 12b			
c	Enter your Form W-2 wages of $100 or more from an electing church or church-controlled organization — 12c			
d	Add lines 9 and 12c	12d	39,925	
13	Enter the smaller of line 12a or line 12d	13	39,925	
	If line 13 is $43,800, enter $5,387.40 on line 14. Otherwise, multiply line 13 by .123 and enter the result on line 14		x.123	
14	Self-employment tax. Enter this amount on Form 1040, line 48	14	4,911	

For Paperwork Reduction Act Notice, see Form 1040 Instructions. **Schedule SE (Form 1040) 1987**

U.S. GOVERNMENT PRINTING OFFICE: 1987-183-120 E.I. 43-0787287

Figure 41.6. Sample Schedule SE, Form 1040

Self-Employment Tax

If an optometrist has net earnings from self-employment of $400 or more then self-employment tax must be paid on part or all of these earnings.[60] The self-employment tax is a social security tax for people who work for themselves and is similar to the social security tax withheld from the pay of employees. Social security benefits are available to people who are self-employed just as they are to wage earners, and the self-employment tax constitutes their contributions to the social security system.

To determine if a sole proprietor or partner will have to pay the tax, the following three computations must be performed[61]:

1. Net earnings from self-employment must be calculated.
2. The amount of these earnings eligible for the tax must be determined.
3. The amount eligible must be mutiplied by the tax rate.

The first step is to figure the earnings from self-employment, which is generally the net income from the practice of optometry arrived at by subtracting all allowable business expenses and deductions from gross business income.

The second step is to figure how much of these earnings is susceptible to the tax; there is both a minimum and a maximum limit. The minimum is $400; if the net income is in excess of this amount, a Schedule SE will have to be attached to Form 1040 (see Fig. 41.6). There is a limit to the amount of earnings subject to the tax, but—as with other social security taxes—this limit has steadily escalated over the years, rising to $45,000 in 1988.[62]

The third step is to multiply the amount of earnings subject to the tax by the tax rate. This rate is lower than that imposed on an employee.[63]

The preceding discussion has focused upon the difficult and complex subject of business taxes. There are some aspects of business taxes that have been omitted, however, including the state taxes that will have to be reported and paid by the optometrist. These are too numerous and varied to be discussed here. And there are also several important changes in personal and business taxes created by the Tax Reform Act of 1986, one of the most revolutionary tax acts in our nation's history. Adequate tax counsel should always be consulted to ensure that tax reporting is performed correctly.

Notes

1. Prior to the Tax Reform Act of 1986 the IRS generally presumed an activity was profit motivated if a profit was earned in two out of five consecutive years; this presumption has been made more stringent under the new law. If an activity is deemed to be a hobby, the deduction for expenses will be limited to the extent of income generated (i.e., the activity will not be able to claim a loss for tax purposes). Furthermore, hobby expenses will have to be claimed as part of miscellaneous deductions on Schedule A, which means they may not be claimed at all unless all miscellaneous expenses exceed 2 percent of the taxpayer's adjusted gross income. See IRS publication 334, *Tax Guide for Small Businesses.*
2. Ibid. Every partnership, corporation (including S corporations), and individual proprietorship that pays wages to one or more employees must have an employer identification number. New identification numbers are necessary if an existing business changes its organization or its ownership. Form SS-4 is available at IRS or Social Security offices.
3. Ibid. The pegboard system is widely used by health care practitioners and allows simultaneous entries to be made on the day sheets (which list the daily income), and the individual patient ledger cards (which list individual accounts). In addition, the pegboard system allows the practitioner to keep an ongoing total of receipts and disbursements that can be rapidly balanced at the end of the month and permits an accurate assessment of accounts receivable.
4. The Tax Reform Act of 1986 instituted some important changes in the tax year selection process. Partnerships must conform their tax years to the tax years of their partners, and S corporations must also use a calendar year unless the corporation can satisfy the IRS that there is a business purpose for selecting a different tax year. See IRS publication 921, *Explanation of the Tax Reform Act of 1986 for Business.*
5. Ibid. Although the Tax Reform Act of 1986 prohibits the use of the cash method by certain corporations, personal services corporations such as those formed by optometrists are excluded from the provisions of the law.
6. For a discussion, see IRS publication 334, supra note 1.
7. Ibid. A capital expenditure is expected to be of benefit in future periods, and possesses the elements of value and time. If the expenditure will add to the value of property or extend its useful life, it is regarded as a capital expenditure rather than as current business expense.
8. For a discussion of basis, see IRS publication 551, *Basis of Assets.*
9. The Tax Reform Act of 1986 changed the method by which goodwill may be determined in the sale of a practice. The basis for goodwill must be figured by allocating the purchase price first among the other

assets acquired. This allocation must be an amount of the purchase price proportionate to but not in excess of the fair market value for assets such as buildings, equipment, records, and other items of sale. Since the price of a practice will likely exceed the fair market value of all these tangible assets, it is probable that goodwill will be an important aspect of practice sales. See IRS publication 921, supra note 4.

10. Like goodwill, the value of a covenant not to compete must be determined by allocating the purchase price first among the tangible assets. Only then can a part of the purchase price be allocated to the covenant. Since a covenant not to compete has tax value to the purchaser, it should be given consideration in contracts to sell or buy an optometric practice. See IRS publication 921, supra note 4.
11. The Tax Reform Act of 1986 instituted a top bracket of 28 percent for individuals, but there is a 5 percent surtax on income in excess of $43,150. Although in 1987 professional corporations paid only 15 percent on income up to $50,000, effective January 1, 1988 all income for professional service corporations will be taxed at 34 percent.
12. For a discussion of accounting methods for inventories, see IRS publication 334, supra note 1.
13. Ibid. Failure to take into account cash discounts, most frequently obtained for prompt payment of bills to optical suppliers and laboratories, can result in increased tax liability and penalties if an audit is conducted.
14. Ibid. Examples of types of expenses that have been held not to be ordinary and necessary include personal or family living expenses, capital expenditures for improvements or restorations (which must be deducted through depreciation), life insurance premiums for which the taxpayer is directly or indirectly a beneficiary, and bribes or illegal kickbacks.
15. Ibid. Payment for tuition, fees, books, course supplies, and other items purchased for employees under a qualified educational program are deductible, subject to certain limits, and are not includable in the employees' taxable income, to a certain amount. Employees are entitled to an exclusion from gross income of up to $5,250 of the benefits they receive during a calendar year, and these benefits are not subject to FICA, FUTA, or income tax withholding.
16. Ibid. Examples of fringe benefits include life insurance premiums, group life insurance premiums, health insurance premiums, educational expenses, dependent care assistance programs, moving expenses, self-insured medical reimbursement programs, and compensation for injuries.
17. Ibid. If the useful life of the improvement is equal to or less than the remaining term of the lease, the improvement may be depreciated over its estimated useful life. If the useful life of the improvement is longer than the remaining term of the lease, the cost of the improvement may be amortized over the remaining term of the lease.
18. Ibid. It is important to be able to distinguish costs that are capital expenditures from those that are deductible expenses because otherwise the entire amount spent will have to be capitalized, thereby losing an immediate deduction that otherwise may be claimed.
19. Documentation requirements are strict and adequate records must be maintained. Proof may include an account book, diary, statement of expense, or similar record, supported by other documentary evidence that, together, will support each element of an expense. See IRS publication 463, *Travel, Entertainment, and Gift Expenses.*
20. The deductions for business meals have been changed by the Tax Reform Act of 1986 so that only 80 percent of the costs of these meals are now deductible. Lodging expenses for business related travel remain 100 percent deductible. See IRS publication 921, supra note 4.
21. The costs of driving or using other modes of transportation between a home and a place of business are not deductible, nor are these same expenses when traveling from work to home. Travel to a business-related function or to another place of business from an office would be deductible, however. See IRS publication 917, *Business Use of a Car.*
22. Ibid. The standard mileage rate may be used whether or not the taxpayer is reimbursed for the expenses of operating the vehicle, and whether or not the reimbursement is more or less than the amount calculated using the standard mileage rate.
23. Ibid.
24. Ibid. If the standard mileage rate is used, the car is considered to be fully depreciated after 60,000 miles of business use. For this purpose a car is considered to have been driven no more than 15,000 business miles in any one year, even if the actual business mileage is more. This depreciation reduces the basis of the car and is used to determine the adjusted basis when the car is disposed of. If a car is fully depreciated, only 11¢ a mile may be deducted for all miles attributed to business use.
25. Ibid. If the standard mileage rate is used in the first year, the taxpayer is assumed to have made an election not to use the accelerated cost recovery system and may not claim the section 179 deduction (expensing). If the taxpayer changes to the actual cost method in a later year (but before the car is fully depreciated), the straight line depreciation method must be used for what is estimated to be the remaining useful life of the car.
26. Ibid.
27. For a discussion of entertainment expenses, see IRS publication 463, supra note 19.
28. Ibid. In proving entertainment expenses, the taxpayer must have documentation to show:
    - the amount of each separate expense for entertaining, except for incidental items, such as cab fare and telephone calls, which may be totaled on a daily basis
    - the date the entertainment took place
    - the name, address or location, and type of

entertainment, such as dinner or theater, if the information is not apparent from the name or designation of the places

- the reason for the entertainment of the business benefit gained or expected to be gained from entertaining and, except for business meals, the nature of any business discussion or activity that took place
- the occupation or other information about the person or persons entertained, including name, title, or other designation sufficient to establish the business relationship with the taxpayer.

29. This change was instituted by the Tax Reform Act of 1986. See IRS publication 921, supra note 4.
30. Although deductions for personal credit card interest charges will be phased out due to the Tax Reform Act of 1986, interest paid for business-related credit card charges remains fully deductible. See IRS publication 545, *Interest Expense.*
31. Under some circumstances life insurance premiums paid on key person insurance policies may be deductible. See IRS publication 535, *Business Expenses.*
32. Even though the sales tax deduction for individuals was eliminated by the Tax Reform Act of 1986, this deduction remains available to businesses. For example, if an optometrist purchases depreciable property for use in his practice, the sales tax is added to the basis of the property and is treated as part of the cost for depreciation purposes. If a nondepreciable item is purchased as a business expense, the sales tax is still deductible as a business expense. See IRS publication 921, supra note 4.
33. Bulbs, ophthalmic drugs, parts for equipment, and similar items having a useful life of less than a year are deductible as a business expense in the year of purchase. Equipment, such as an ophthalmoscope, which has a useful life of many years and is used for the production of income, must be depreciated. See IRS publication 334, supra note 1.
34. Ibid. To obtain the deduction for containuing education, it must be shown that the education maintains or improves skills required of an optometrist or is required as a prerequisite for renewal of the optometrist's license.
35. Ibid. If deductions exceed gross income a net operating loss may result, which may be used to reduce taxable income in other years under some circumstances.
36. For a discussion of partnership tax considerations, see IRS publication 541, *Tax Information on Partnerships.*
37. For a review of the tax consequences of incorporation, see IRS publication 542, *Tax Information on Corporations.*
38. Property placed in service after 1980 as recovery property, which is tangible property of a character subject to the allowance for depreciation and which may be either new or used property that is used in a business or held for the production of income, is subject to the Accelerated Cost Recovery System. See IRS publication 334, supra note 1.
39. The Modified Accelerated Cost Recovery System applies to all property placed in service as of 1987. See IRS publication 921, supra note 4.
40. The alternate depreciation method uses a recovery percentage that is based upon a modified straight line system without considering salvage value. It allows equal deductions to be taken over the class life of the property. See IRS publication 534, *Depreciation.*
41. Ibid. The conventional depreciation methods include the double (200 percent) declining balance method, the 150 percent declining balance method, and the sum-of-the-digits method.
42. Ibid. For a discussion of useful life and salvage value when using it for purposes of straight line depreciation, see IRS publication 534, supra note 40.
43. The term section 179 deduction refers to the section of the IRS Code which describes this particular deduction. See *Internal Revenue Code of 1954, §179.*
44. Ibid. The decision as to whether or not to use the section 179 deduction requires a knowledge of the taxpayer's overall tax situation, and is a decision that should be made after detailed discussions with competent tax counsel.
45. Ibid. For automobiles placed in serivce in 1987 and thereafter, there are maximum depreciation limits, which also limit the amount that may be claimed by expensing. For example, in year one the depreciation limit is $2,560, which is thereby also the limit for the section 179 deduction that could be claimed for the automobile.
46. Prior to the enactment of the Tax Reform Act of 1986, office buildings were subject to a nineteen-year depreciation schedule, and the lengthier periods now in effect make this deduction less valuable. Real property and buildings, however, remain an important means of reducing taxable income. See IRS publication 334, supra note 1.
47. Under the Modified Accelerated Cost Recovery System, the adjusted basis of the property must be divided by the number of years in the recovery period in order to obtain the annual amount of depreciation. There is also a calculation that must be made in order to determine the correct first-year's depreciation. See IRS publication 534, supra note 40.
48. Examples of expenditures that may be subject to amortization are business start-up costs, organizational costs for a partnership, and organizational costs for a corporation. See IRS publication 535, supra note 3.
49. If a covenant not to compete accompanies the transfer of goodwill in the sale of a practice, and the purpose of the covenant is to assure the purchaser of the enjoyment of the goodwill, the IRS may argue that the covenant is an aspect of the goodwill that cannot be depreciated. But a covenant not to compete for a fixed number of years that is not, in effect, a sale of goodwill, is amortizable based upon its estimated useful life. The purchaser must be able to establish from the facts and circumstances of the particular sale that the transaction is truly an agreement not to compete rather than the

purchase of goodwill. See IRS publication 334, supra note 1.

50. For a description of the tests used by the Internal Revenue Service to determine if an individual is an employee or an independent contractor, see Regulation §31.3401(c)-1.
51. Ibid.
52. See IRS publication 334, supra note 1.
53. A federal tax deposit coupon book containing copies of IRS Form 8109, Federal Tax Deposit Coupon, is automatically sent to individuals who apply for an employer identification number. Forms are also available at local IRS offices.
54. See IRS publication 15, *Employer's Tax Guide* (*Circular E*).
55. Ibid.
56. Ibid. Optometrists are subject to federal unemployment tax on wages paid to employees if in any calendar quarter the wages totaled $1,500 or more, or if in each of twenty different calendar weeks there was at least a part of a day in which the optometrist paid wages to an employee.
57. Ibid. As of 1987, the federal unemployment tax rate is 6.2 percent, and a credit is allowed up to 5.4 percent for state unemployment tax. Therefore, an employer may pay as little as 0.8 percent to the federal government if 5.4 percent is being paid to the state.
58. Ibid. If at the end of any calendar quarter an employer owes, but has not yet deposited, more than $100 in FUTA tax, the deposit must be made by the end of the next month. If the tax is $100 or less at the end of the quarter, it does not have to be deposited but must be added to the tax for the next quarter.
59. Ibid. Each deposit must be accompanied by a federal tax deposit coupon. These coupons, IRS Form 8109, Federal Tax Deposit Coupon, are automatically provided to employers when they apply for an employer identification number.
60. See IRS publication 334, supra note 1.
61. Ibid.
62. The earnings subject to the tax are the same as for employees, and, as with other aspects of Social Security, are on an upward track. See IRS publication 15, supra note 54.
63. Ibid. In 1988 the tax rate is 13.02 percent as compared to the rate of 15.02 percent for employees.

Chapter 42

The Tax Reform Act of 1986

Caution: At the time this publication was printed, Congress was considering legislation that would change or modify the tax treatment described in some of the discussions presented here.
—Notice on the cover of IRS publication 920, *Explanation of the Tax Reform Act of 1986 for Individuals*

Individual Tax Changes

Tax reform in 1986 brought about the most significant changes in fifty years, as the tax code was revised to permit the shifting of billions in taxes from individuals to businesses. Although it will require years before the effects of the revision will be clear, it seems that these changes will increase the tax burden of certain types of businesses, including those that require the purchase of expensive equipment in order to begin or improve services. Practitioners of optometry will therefore have to devise tax strategies to deal with this increased tax burden.[1]

This chapter summarizes many of the important provisions of the 1986 law.[2] Because it seems likely that further modifications of the federal tax code will be forthcoming, optometrists should always consult with tax counsel before making business decisions that will have significant tax ramifications.

The most-discussed tax change for individuals is the elimination of multiple tax brackets in favor of two basic rates, 15 and 28 percent, effective in 1988, although a surtax of 5 percent will be applied to certain high earners (see Chapter 40). Another important change is an increased standard deduction, available both to persons who itemize and to those who do not, which in 1988 becomes \$3,000 for single taxpayers and \$5,000 for married couples filing jointly (see Chapter 40). The standard deduction is increased by \$750 for single persons over 65 or blind and by \$600 for married persons who fall into either of these categories (see Chapter 40). For blind or elderly taxpayers who itemize on Schedule A, however, these deductions are no longer available. In fact, the Tax Reform Act of 1986 effected some key changes for itemizers, which are summarized in Table 42.1.[3] The 1986 law also made significant changes in a number of personal tax items, which are summarized below[4]:

1. *Capital gains*—The 60 percent net long-term capital gain exclusion is ended, and taxpayers must treat long-term capital gains, i.e., profit derived from property held for more than six months, like ordinary income. The top bracket for capital gains in 1988 and thereafter is the same as for ordinary income, i.e., 15, 28, or 33 percent.[5]
2. *Deduction for two-earner married couple*—This deduction, which allowed married couples to deduct up to \$3,000 in 1986, is repealed for 1987 and the following years.
3. *Income averaging*—Income averaging, which aids taxpayers whose income fluctuates from year to year, is ended by the 1986 law.[6]
4. *Credit for political contributions*—The credit for contributions made to political candidates and

Table 42.1. Individual Changes under the Tax Reform Act of 1986

Deduction	Former Status	Under Tax Reform Act of 1986
Mortgage interest	Fully deductible	Only first and second homes
Interest on credit cards and consumer loans	Fully deductible	Only 65% can be deducted in 1987; 40% in 1988; 20% in 1989; 10% in 1990; no longer deductible in 1991
Real and personal property taxes	Fully deductible	Unchanged
State and local income taxes	Fully deductible	Unchanged
Medical expenses	Amount in excess of 5% of AGI	Amount in excess of $7\frac{1}{2}$% of AGI
Charitable contributions	Fully deductible	Unchanged
Dividend income	$100 per person exclusion from income	Repealed
Sales taxes	Fully deductible	Repealed
Miscellaneous deductions (dues, C-E, professional fees, insurance)	Fully deductible	Amount in excess of 2% of AGI only
Casualty losses	Amount in excess of 10% of AGI	Amount in excess of 10% of AGI for which not reimbursed or eligible for reimbursement by insurance

Source: *Prentice-Hall Guide to the Tax Reform Act of 1986*, Prentice-Hall, Paramus, N.J., 1986, pp. 1–6.

organizations (currently one half of the dollar amount contributed, up to $50 per person, $100 for joint returns) is ended.

5. *Lump-sum insurance payouts*—Formerly, a spouse who chose to take an installment payout of life insurance proceeds could receive annually up to $1,000 of interest tax-free, but this interest exclusion has been repealed by the 1986 law.

6. *Clifford trusts and other income-splitting shifts*—One way for a parent to shift income is to give a child a gift of income-producing property (ophthalmic equipment, for example). This is frequently accomplished through the use of a Clifford trust, in which the equipment is transferred to a trust that lasts for more than ten years. The trust income is distributed and taxed to the lower-bracket child (usually when the child goes off to college). The property reverts to the parent when the trust terminates. This tactic is undercut by the 1986 Tax Reform Act, which taxes the trust income at the bracket of the person who funds the Clifford trust. Furthermore, under the 1986 law, any investment income received by a child under fourteen years of age can be taxed at the parent's top rate, regardless of the source of the investment property (see Chapter 40 for a further discussion).

7. *Health insurance for self-employment taxpayers*—Under the new law, a self-employed individual is allowed to deduct 25 percent of what he pays for an insured or self-insured health plan. The remaining 75 percent of premium payments may be used as a deduction on Schedule A. This deduction is not available if the individual is eligible to participate in a health plan furnished by his spouse's employer.

8. *Child care*—Parents who work may claim a tax credit to offset daycare expenses for children under age fifteen. The amount of the credit depends upon the taxpayer's income, but may be as much as 30 percent of the amount paid, up to $2,400 for one child and $4,800 for two or more (also discussed in Chapter 40).

9. *Employee moving expenses*—The cost of moving from one location to another to start a new job may qualify as a deductible expense (within certain limits), but under the 1986 law only employees who itemize deductions on Schedule A may claim the allowable amount. However, this deduction is not considered to be a miscellaneous deduction (which must exceed 2 percent of the adjusted gross income before it is of benefit) but may be claimed separately.[7] Since this deduction has obvious applicability to employee optometrists, we will discuss it in some detail.

An employee or self-employed individual may deduct from gross income the reasonable expenses of moving from one location to another if the move is incident to the commencement of work in a new location.

A deduction is allowed from gross income under specified conditions for the following job-related moving expenses[8]:

- Costs of transporting the taxpayer and members of his household from the old to the new residence
- Costs of transporting their household goods and personal effects (insurance and charges for storage of goods are also included)

- Costs of meals and lodging en route
- Temporary living expenses (lodging and meals for up to thirty days) at a new job location
- Expenses of traveling (including meals and lodging) after obtaining employment, to and from the former residence to the general location of the new place of work, for the principal purpose of searching for a new residence
- Qualified expenses incident to a sale, purchase, or lease of a residence (including broker's commissions, attorney's fees, and points to the extent the latter does not represent interest)

Premove expenses, temporary living expenses, and expenses for the sale, purchase, or lease of a residence are limited to an overall deduction of $3,000, and the expenses related to house-hunting trips and temporary living expenses at the new job location may not exceed $1,500 of the $3,000. Where a husband and a wife both begin work at a new principal place of employment within the same general location, the $3,000 limit is applied as if there were only one commencement of work.

For a moving expense deduction to be available, the distance between the taxpayer's new principal place of work or business and his former residence must be thirty-five miles greater than the distance between the taxpayers' former principal place of work and his former residence. Also, the distance between the new place of work and his former residence must be measured by the shortest of the commonly traveled routes between these two points.

In order for these moving expenses to be deductible, an employee (as distinguished from a self-employed individual) must not only meet the distance requirement but also must be a full-time employee for at least three-fourths of the immediately following year (i.e., thirty-nine weeks).

In the case of a self-employed person, in addition to the distance requirement, there is a work requirement that obligates the taxpayer to perform services for a minimum of seventy-eight weeks during the twenty-four-month period immediately following arrival at the new place of business.

Moving expenses are calculated on IRS Form 3903, Moving Expense Adjustment, but are claimed on Schedule A as an itemized deduction (see Fig. 40.3).

Reimbursement or payments by an employer to an employee for the cost of moving to a new job site must be included in income but are not considered to be wages for the purpose of income tax withholding, FICA, or FUTA, if it is reasonable for the employer to believe, at the time the payments are made, that the employee will be allowed a deduction for these expenses in computing his or her income tax. Any reimbursement to an employee for moving expenses is deductible by the employer as long as it is reasonable, ordinary, and necessary.

10. *Search for employment*—In addition to moving expenses, the IRS will allow deductions for the expenses that are directly related to a search for employment in the same business, regardless of whether the search is successful or not. Thus the travel and transportation expenses incurred by an optometrist in the search for a new job may be deducted.[9] These expenses will be claimed in the Miscellaneous category of Schedule A, and so they will be of tax benefit only to the extent they (and other miscellaneous deductions) exceed 2 percent of the employee's adjusted gross income. This same tax benefit may be claimed by the working spouse of an optometrist who must move to a new location and who seeks new employment in the same field at the new location.

Allowances or reimbursements made by an employer to a job candidate for transportation or other expenses incurred in connection with interviews for possible employment are not wages subject to social security taxes, federal unemployment taxes, or income tax withholding. These expenses may be deducted by the employer if they are ordinary, necessary, and reasonable.

As with other tax matters, employers and employees must maintain adequate records to document the expenses incurred and the efforts made in the search for employment.

Individual Retirement Accounts

The 1986 Tax Reform Act makes some major changes in the tax rules for individual retirement accounts (IRAs). Taxpayers who belong to a company-funded retirement plan may lose some or all of their deduction for IRA contributions. This change affects members of corporate pension and profit-sharing plans and those with Keogh plans, for tax years after 1986.

There are three categories of deductions for IRAs under the new law[10]:

1. *Full deduction*—Deductible annual contributions of up to $2,000 may be claimed ($2,250 for a spousal IRA) if neither the taxpayer nor the taxpayer's spouse belong to a company-funded retirement plan or either taxpayer belongs to such a plan but the adjusted gross income is less than $25,000 if

single or $40,000 if married. For this purpose, the adjusted gross income does not take into account the IRA contributions.

2. *Partial deduction*—Deductible IRA contributions are reduced proportionately if the taxpayer or the taxpayer's spouse belong to a company retirement plan and have an adjusted gross income between $25,000 and $35,000 for single taxpayers or between $40,000 and $50,000 for married taxpayers. For example, a married plan member with an adjusted gross income of $45,000 can make a $1,000 deductible IRA contribution, since his income is half-way between the $40,000 and $50,000 phaseout levels.

3. *No deduction*—Plan members with adjusted gross incomes in excess of $35,000 if single or $50,000 if married cannot claim a tax deduction for an IRA contribution.

Amounts contributed to an IRA before 1987 continue to grow tax free until withdrawn, even though the taxpayer is no longer eligible to make deductible contributions. Starting in 1987 a taxpayer may make a nondeductible IRA contribution and have it grow tax free. The total contributions for the year—both deductible and nondeductible—cannot exceed the lesser of actual compensation or $2,000 ($2,250 for a spousal IRA). Nondeductible contributions will not be taxed when withdrawn, unlike the deductible contributions, which are taxed when taken out. The penalty for early withdrawals from an IRA remains at 10 percent and is applied to withdrawals made before age 59½, unless due to death or disability.

Simplified Employee Pensions

An employer can provide retirement benefits to employees by making contributions to an IRA set up and maintained by the employee. This Simplified Employee Pension (SEP) cannot discriminate in favor of higher-paid employees. The deduction limit under an SEP is the lesser of $30,000 or 15 percent of compensation.[11]

In tax years starting after 1986, some employers can give employees a choice: continue to take all their compensation in cash or have part of it contributed to an SEP. To the extent that an employee chooses to have income contributed to an SEP, he owes no income tax on this contribution.

There are three conditions that must be met in order to make such an election[12]: at least half of the employees must elect the SEP contribution; the employer cannot have more than twenty-five employees at any time during the year; and no more than $30,000 can be deferred annually.

An employer establishing an SEP must allow each employee to participate who has reached 21 years of age, performed services for the employer during at least three of the preceding five years, and has received at least $300 in compensation from the employer for the year.[13]

Changes in Retirement Plan Rules

The most sweeping changes in the 1986 tax reform act are probably those that pertain to retirement plan rules. Some of these changes are summarized below.[14]

More Plan Coverage

A qualified retirement plan cannot discriminate in favor of employees who are officers, shareholders, or higher paid. Under prior law, a plan did not discriminate against employees if it covered as few as 56 percent of all those employed, but the new law requires that at least 70 percent of the rank and file be covered by the plan, effective for plan years starting after 1988.

Quicker Vesting of Benefits

A qualified plan must provide for accrued benefits to vest (i.e., become nonforfeitable) within a certain period of time. The new law shortens the period for vesting so that employees are entitled to benefits sooner. For example, the shortest of the three vesting schedules in the prior law required full vesting upon ten years of service (no vesting required before the tenth year). The tax reform act cuts the vesting schedules dramatically. Full vesting must take place in five years or gradually over seven years (20 percent after three years and 20 percent a year for the next four years).

Minimum Benefits for Integrated Plan Members

In an integrated plan, the Social Security taxes paid by the employer are taken into account when determining if the plan satisfies the nondiscrimination rules. Under prior law, it was possible for an employer to avoid making any retirement plan contributions for lower-paid employees. For plans starting after 1988, the new law ensures that all employees will receive at least some employer-provided retirement plan benefits in addition to Social Security benefits.

Loans to Plan Members

Under prior law, a plan member could borrow up to $50,000 from the plan if repayment had to be made within five years or, if the loan was used to buy or improve a principal residence of a plan member or the member's family, within a reasonable period. For plan years starting after 1986, the new law prevents an employee from maintaining a constant loan balance of $50,000 a year, by reducing the $50,000 limit by the member's highest outstanding loan balance during the preceding twelve months.

Early Withdrawals

Under the old law, retirement plan withdrawals before age 59½, death, or disability were taxable, but there was no tax penalty if the ordinary employee wanted to use the retirement plan for personal purposes (e.g., to buy a car or to pay for college tuition for a child). Only early withdrawals from an IRA were subject to a 10 percent penalty, but under the new tax reform act a 10 percent penalty is imposed on early withdrawals from all retirement plans, effective 1987. Generally speaking, an early withdrawal is defined as one made prior to age 59½, due to death, or due to disability. There are some exceptions to this rule: there is no penalty for withdrawals rolled over into an IRA or another retirement plan; withdrawals taken as a life annuity upon separation from employment are excluded; and also exempted are distributions made to employees because of unforeseen hardship, which is limited to medical expenses.

Mandatory Withdrawals

In years starting after 1988, all members of a company plan, Keogh plan, or tax-sheltered annuity must start making plan withdrawals no later than April 1 in the year that they reach age 70½. Thus the same rules that apply to IRAs will now apply to other retirement plans.

Leased Employees

Under the prior law, an employer's retirement plan did not have to cover leased employees if the leasing firm contributed at least 71 percent of the workers' compensation to a money purchase pension plan. For services performed after December 31, 1986, an employer's retirement plan can exclude leased workers only if no more than 20 percent of the employer's workforce is leased and the leasing firm contributes at least 10 percent to a plan for all of its employees.

Cash or Deferred Plans (Section 401(k) Plans)

A cash or deferred plan allows an employee to defer up to 25 percent of compensation to a profit-sharing plan, in which the money grows without taxation. The 1986 Tax Reform Act reduces the annual ceiling on deferred income placed into such a plan, reducing this amount from $30,000 to $7,000, effective in years after 1986. Also starting in 1987 the new law applies rules to 401(k) plans to prohibit discrimination in favor of highly paid employees.

Changes in Business Deductions

The biggest change in business deductions is the repeal of the investment tax credit, an important tax item for an equipment-intensive business such as the practice of optometry. The loss of the investment tax credit will have a significant effect on the first year tax bill of practitioners who purchase practices or start out "cold."

Another important development is the reduction in tax rates for corporations (Table 42.2). Unfortunately, this tax break proved to be short-lived for professional service corporations, as legislation passed in 1987 instituted a 34 percent tax rate for these corporations, effective January 1, 1988.

Deductions for business-related travel and entertainment are more difficult to obtain under the new law. The deduction for business entertainment expenses (including meals) is limited to 80 percent of cost. The deduction for business meals on overnight travel is also reduced by 20 percent. For employees, there is more restriction to contend with: the deductible portion of employee unreimbursed travel and transportation expenses and entertainment expenses is lumped in with other deductions so that the total miscellaneous expenses are deductible only to the extent that they exceed 2 percent of the employee's adjusted gross income (see Chapter 41).

But an employer's reimbursement to the employee for business-related travel and entertainment is not subject to the 2 percent floor. The reimbursement is tax-free to the employee and deductible by the employer. But reimbursement deductions attributable to meals and business entertainment are reduced by 20 percent.

Table 42.2. Corporate Tax Rate Schedules, Effective July 1, 1987*

Taxable Income	Tax Rate (%)
$0–$50,000	15
$50,001–$75,000	25
$75,001–$100,000	34
$100,001–$335,000	39
More than $335,000	34

*Effective January 1, 1988, professional corporations or associations will be taxed at 34%.

Source: *Prentice Hall Guide to the Tax Reform Act of 1986*, Prentice-Hall, Paramus, N.J., 1986, pp. 18–19.

Another important business-related tax change is the modification of the Accelerated Cost Recovery System (ACRS).

Changes in the Accelerated Cost Recovery System

The 1986 law modifies the ACRS system of depreciation that was introduced in the 1981 tax reform act.[15] The new system is generally effective for property placed into service in 1987 and retains many of the original ACRS rules. The three-, five-, ten-, and fifteen-year classes are retained, and two new classes are added (seven- and twenty-year property). There is no distinction made between new and used property, and salvage value continues to be disregarded. Depreciation for property in the three-, five-, and ten-year classes is further accelerated, and although the investment tax credit is repealed, the expensing deduction is boosted from $5,000 to $10,000, effective for the 1987 tax year.

Business assets used in the practice of optometry will usually fall into the five- and seven-year asset classes:

Five-year property: computers, typewriters, copiers, duplicating equipment, automobiles, trucks, and other vehicles;

Seven-year property: office furniture, fixtures, equipment (including ophthalmic equipment), instruments, and patient records.

Under the new law, the depreciation period for residential rental property is $27\frac{1}{2}$ years and for commercial property is $31\frac{1}{2}$ years. Both types of real property must be written off using straight line depreciation.

Under the new rules, all modified ACRS property is treated as placed into service (or disposed of) in the middle of the year. Thus the taxpayer gets a half-year of depreciation when the property is placed into service and a half-year when the property is disposed of. The annual recovery percentages under the new system are listed in Chapter 41.

The effect of the changes in the ACRS system is to decrease the annual deduction for business assets. For example, under the original ACRS system, a $10,000 automobile that is used 100 percent for business purposes would have to be depreciated over three years, with annual writeoffs of $2,500, $3,800, and $3,700. Under the 1986 law, the ACRS writeoffs would be $2,000, $3,200, $1,920, $1,152, $1,152 and $576. Similarly, if an optometrist purchases $50,000 of depreciable equipment for use in his practice, under the old ACRS system the five-year writeoffs would be $7,500, $11,000, $10,500, $10,500, and $10,500. Under the new seven-year system they would be $7,140, $12,245, $8,745, $6,245, $4,465, $4,465, $4,465, and $2,230.

There are special "caps" for writeoffs for automobiles under the 1986 law, which are described in Table 42.3. The dollar caps listed in Table 42.3 must be reduced if the business use of the automobile is less than 100 percent, which is a virtual certainty for optometrists.

For example, assume that an optometrist who is self-employed buys a $20,000 automobile, which is used 70 percent for business purposes and 30 percent for personal driving. The depreciation deduction in the first year will be $1,792 (70 percent of $2,560).

If qualified use for business purposes does not exceed 50 percent, then the car's depreciable basis must be recovered over five years using a straight line method, which is further reduced by the adjustment for percentage of actual business use (computed as in the example above). If during the recovery period business use falls to 50 percent or less, part

Table 42.3. Depreciation Limits for Automobiles Placed in Service in 1987 and Thereafter

First year	Lesser of $2,560 or 20% of depreciable basis
Second year	Lesser of $4,100 or 32% of depreciable basis
Third year	Lesser of $2,450 or 19.2% of depreciable basis
Fourth year	Lesser of $1,475 or 11.5% of depreciable basis
Fifth year	Lesser of $1,475 or 11.5% of depreciable basis
Sixth year*	Lesser of $1,475 or 5.7% of depreciable basis

*Any depreciable basis remaining after six years is recovered at a rate that cannot exceed $1,475 a year.

Source: Klott, G., *The New York Times Complete Guide to the New Tax Law*, Times Books, New York, 1986, p. 117.

of the depreciation claimed in prior years is "recaptured" and the taxpayer must switch to straight line depreciation.[16]

To establish that an automobile has been used sufficiently to obtain the most favorable writeoff, the taxpayer should maintain an automobile log that records the miles travelled for business purposes.

Instead of the actual costs of operating a vehicle a taxpayer may deduct a flat amount, based upon the miles travelled for business purposes. The standard mileage rate is $22\frac{1}{2}$ cents a mile for the first 15,000 business-related miles and 11 cents a mile afterwards. Ordinarily, the mileage deduction will not be as large as the writeoff for depreciation and actual out-of-pocket expenses, but for some taxpayers it may be the best option. However, unless the standard mileage rate is chosen in the first year, it may not be claimed in subsequent years (see Chapter 41).

For taxpayers seeking a large first-year deduction, the new law increases the expensing deduction (section 179 deduction) to $10,000 as of 1987.[17] Thus, for the optometrist who has purchased a practice or has need of a large writeoff to offset a significant purchase of equipment, the expensing deduction may be a means of compensating for the loss of the investment tax credit. For automobiles, the limits applicable to depreciation deductions also apply to expensing, and, therefore, the section 179 deduction may not exceed these limits (see Chapter 41 for a more detailed discussion).

There are many other changes in the 1986 Tax Reform Act that are not described here. Always consult competent tax counsel before making important practice decisions that may have tax consequences.

Notes

1. For an example of tax strategy to deal with changing federal law, specifically the Tax Reform Act of 1986, see Goldberg, M.A., Year-End Tax Strategies Under Tax Reform, *Optometric Management*, vol. 22, no. 12, 1986, pp. 22–26.
2. There are numerous references available for the practitioner who wishes to research the revolutionary tax law enacted in 1986. An excellent review can be found in *U.S. News and World Report*, Oct. 6, 1986; a text that describes the major provisions of the law for laymen is Klott, G.L., *The New York Times Complete Guide to the New Tax Law*, Times Books, New York, 1986; and a detailed explanation of the law can be found by consulting the *Prentice-Hall Guide to the Tax Reform Act of 1986*, Prentice-Hall, Paramus, N.J., 1986. The Internal Revenue Service summarizes the major provisions of the act in publications 920, *Explanation of the Tax Reform Act of 1986 for Individuals*, and 921, *Explanation of the Tax Reform Act of 1986 for Businesses.*
3. *Prentice-Hall Guide to the Tax Reform Act of 1986*, Prentice-Hall, Paramus, N.J., 1986.
4. Ibid.
5. The loss of capital gains will have an effect upon the strategies devised by sellers of optometric practices, who no longer will have an incentive to bargain over the allocation of assets for tax purposes in the sale of a nonincorporated practice. Sellers of incorporated practices will feel the effects even more, since the sale of stock was taxed as a long-term capital gain. See IRS publication 920, *Explanation of the Tax Reform Act of 1986 for Individuals.*
6. Ibid. Income averaging was of benefit to most optometry school graduates since the low income of school years could be used to offset the tax incurred in the first few years of practice. Like the loss of the investment tax credit, it will be one more obstacle to entry into solo practice.
7. *Prentice-Hall Guide to the Tax Reform Act of 1986*, supra note 3.
8. See IRS publication 521, *Moving Expenses.*
9. See IRS publication 334, *Tax Guide for Small Businesses.*
10. See IRS publication 590, *Individual Retirement Arrangements.*
11. See IRS publication 334, supra note 9; and publication 921, *Explanation of the Tax Reform Act of 1986 for Businesses.*
12. Ibid.
13. Ibid.
14. *Prentice-Hall Guide to the Tax Reform Act of 1986*, supra note 3.
15. See IRS publication 921, supra note 11.
16. The recapture of depreciation is to be avoided when it is an accidental result of an exchange, sale, or other disposition of property. See IRS publication 534, *Depreciation.*
17. See IRS publication 921, supra note 11.

PART TWELVE

CONTRACTS

Chapter 43

Negotiations

"You mean there's a catch?"

"Sure there's a catch," Doc Daneeka replied. "Catch-22. Anybody who wants to get out of combat duty isn't really crazy."

There was only one catch and that was Catch-22, which specified that a concern for one's own safety in the face of dangers that were real and immediate was the process of a rational mind. Orr was crazy and could be grounded. All he had to do was ask; and as soon as he did, he would no longer be crazy and would have to fly more missions. Orr would be crazy to fly more missions and sane if he didn't, but if he was sane he had to fly them. If he flew them he was crazy and didn't have to; but if he didn't want to he was sane and had to. Yossarian was moved very deeply by the absolute simplicity of this clause of Catch-22 and let out a respectful whistle.

"That's some catch, that Catch-22," he observed.

"It's the best there is," Doc Daneeka agreed.

—Joseph Heller, *Catch-22*

A contract is formed when competent parties have reached what is referred to as a meeting of the minds, and the effort to reach this agreement is often the most difficult and trying aspect of forming a contract. Negotiations may be swiftly concluded in some cases, but in most instances the road to agreement is a lengthy and tortuous one, made the more trying by the necessity that the negotiators travel it together. Although an attorney may be hired to draft a contract, or may serve as a source of expertise when determining the points to be negotiated, the actual give-and-take that results in agreement must take place between the contracting parties themselves, often without the benefit of previous experience at negotiations. The end product is not always what was desired, either from a personal or a legal point of view.

The art of negotiating a contract is one that is best learned through experience, but it is this very learning process that many times leads to frustration and disappointment as the negotiators struggle to overcome the impasses that frequently block the pathway to agreement. Yet there are principles of law and practical aspects of negotiation upon which to construct an agreement, the most fundamental of which is fairness. Contracts between optometrists for employment, partnership, or the sale of a practice depend on the willingness of the contracting parties to live up to the agreed-upon terms, and if there is a perception by one of the parties that the agreement is unfair the contract will fail. Although the breach of a contract does allow for damages to be claimed by the injured party, a legal action of this nature is something to be avoided rather than invited, and the best means of preventing contractual disputes is to draft an agreement that is fair to both parties. A Catch-22 is less a sign of cleverness than an indication of unfairness, and so negotiators should endeavor to discuss and settle all key points prior to reducing their agreement to writing.

In this chapter, some of the basic principles of contract law and of the art of negotiation will be investigated in the hope that this information will prove useful to optometrists called on to reach agreements for associateship or partnership, form a professional corporation, or sell or purchase a practice.

Basic Principles of Contract Law

The first consideration when discussing the complexities of the law of contracts is to understand when an agreement between two or more parties is elevated to the legal status of a contract.

What Is a Contract?

A multipage legal document signed by all of the parties and a verbal agreement sealed by a firm handshake are both contracts. The two agreements are equally binding on the parties and are enforceable. But the terms of the former are more easily proved in the event of dispute than are those of the latter, a fact that some practitioners have spent an inordinate amount of money and time discovering.[1] Thus, the first consideration (and one of the most important) whenever a contract is being contemplated is *get it in writing*.

Although it is often said that a handshake is all that is needed between honorable people, such a view is unrealistic—even for associateship agreements, the simplest form of contract—because it invites conflict in the event there is disagreement over the terms of the contract. A handshake also encourages superficiality, in the sense that it many times discourages detailed discussions over the important (and potentially troublesome) provisions of a contract, such as pay increases, ownership of records and rights to patient information, termination of employment, and covenants not to compete. Difficulties often arise in verbal agreements because sufficient time was not taken during the negotiation period to ensure that a comprehensive understanding was reached. These practice arrangements frequently end unhappily both for employer and for employee. Therefore, a written contract is advantageous for both parties.

If, for some reason, an employee finds the employer unwilling to reduce their agreement to writing, a useful substitute for a contract is a letter, written from the employee to the employer, detailing the major points agreed on during negotiations. An example of such a letter is included as Fig. 43.1. A copy of this letter is retained by the employee, and if a dispute arises over the details of employment, the letter may be used to substantiate the employee's understanding of the agreement between the two parties. It is a preferable alternative to memory, which is the unreliable recourse left to those who have entrusted their association to a verbal agreement.

A contract is an agreement, upon sufficient consideration, to do or not do a particular thing.[2] In order to contract with someone, there are certain legal requirements and formalities that must be complied with, which necessitates a basic understanding of the concept of contract. The first aspect that must be discussed is the formation of a contract, which requires the following three elements:

1. Mutual Assent
   a. Offer
   b. Acceptance
2. Consideration
3. Capable Parties

Mutual Assent

Mutual assent is often said to be agreeing to the "same bargain at the same time," i.e., a meeting of the minds.[3] The process by which parties reach this meeting of the minds generally is negotiation, during which at some point one party makes a proposal (an offer) and the other agrees to it (an acceptance). An actual subjective meeting of the minds is not necessary. Rather, it is an *objective* measure that is employed, by which each party is bound to the apparent intention that he manifested to the other party. For example, where a statement is made in jest, anger, or by way of bragging, and the statement is reasonably understood in this context, it will have no legal effect. But where the statement is subjectively intended to be in jest but reasonably understood by the hearer to have been made seriously, a contract results because of the objective test.

The Offer

The one who makes the offer is called the *offeror*. The one to whom the offer is made is called the *offeree*. A legally sufficient offer must be definite and certain in its terms and should include parties, subject matter, price, and time for performance. An illusory promise is not a legally sufficient offer because although it is couched in terms of a promise, it in fact promises nothing, e.g., "I promise to buy your practice if I feel like it." There is no obligation inherent in this statement sufficient to create an offer.

To be legally sufficient, an offer must be communicated to the offeree, and the power of acceptance created by an offer ends when the offer is terminated.[4]

Dear Doctor,

Thank you for offering me a position as associate in your practice. I know I will enjoy working for you, and I hope, just as you do, that our association will evolve into partnership.

I felt it would be useful if I summarized the discussions we held concerning my responsibilities as a member of the practice and the terms of my employment. I am to begin on July 1, 1987, in your practice at 123 Main Street, Anytown, and my duties are to include general eye examinations, contact lens fittings and follow-up, specialized testing of ocular health, and other responsibilities that we may mutually agree upon. Office hours are to be from 9 A.M. to 6 P.M., Monday through Friday, and after six months I will be eligible for one week of vacation. My term of employment will run until June 30, 1988, but may be terminated by either of us upon 60 days' written notice.

My salary is to be $2,500 per month, and in addition I will receive 25 percent of the gross income in excess of $6,500 per month generated by my patient examinations and dispensings. Benefits provided by the practice include malpractice insurance coverage, dues for membership in the state association, and reimbursement for continuing education requirements necessary to renew my license.

All patient records, addresses, or lists remain the property of the practice, even those of patients seen exclusively by me. However, it is agreed that, should I leave the practice, copies of patient records will be provided to me upon appropriate written request of the patient.

Prior to the termination of my year of employment, we have agreed to discuss the feasibility of entering into partnership. Should we so agree, articles of partnership will be drawn up to reflect this new relationship.

This letter summarizes my understanding of the agreement we have reached. If I have incorrectly stated or omitted any of the provisions agreed to, please let me know as soon as possible. I want to be certain we have no disagreements.

Once more, I would like to express my appreciation for being given this opportunity. I am looking forward to July 1st!

Sincerely,
Dr. New O'Dee

Figure 43.1. Sample Letter Describing the Conditions of Employment

Mutual assent is not present if the termination occurs before acceptance is effective. The termination of the offer can be effected in any of the following ways:

- Termination by the offeror (he can communicate his revocation of the offer before the offeree can accept)
- Termination by the offeree (either by an express rejection or by a counter-offer, which has the same effect as a rejection)
- Termination by operation of law (e.g., by lapse of a reasonable period of time with no response by the offeree, death or insanity of either party, or destruction of the subject matter of the contract)[5]

The Acceptance

The acceptance is a manifestion of assent to the terms of an offer in the manner prescribed or authorized in the offer. Through this manifestion of assent, the offeree exercises the power given him by the offeror to create a contract. In order for a valid acceptance to be present, the following requirements must be met:

- Acceptance must be made by the one who has the power of acceptance (generally, only the person to whom an offer is addressed has the power of acceptance).
- A valid mode of acceptance must have been used (the acceptance must be made in the mode specified by the offer or, if no mode is specified, the mode used by the offeror to transmit the offer should be used).
- The acceptance must be absolute, unqualified, and unconditional in meeting the terms of the offer (and any adding of terms or changing of terms constitutes a counteroffer and terminates the original offer).

Consideration

Consideration is the second requirement for a contract and is a legal term for money or some thing of value, generally identified as having two elements: a bargained-for exchange (an offer or promise by one party that is made in exchange for an offer or promise from another party), and some benefit to the promisor or detriment to the promisee (both parties must gain or lose something). Without consideration, there can be no contract.[6]

Capable Parties

Capable parties is the third requirement for a contract. The validity of the contract is affected by the capacity of the parties. Whether the contract is void (not valid to either party) or merely voidable (can be disaffirmed by one party, thereby unbinding both parties) depends upon the particular form of incapacity involved. Insanity of either party renders the contract void,[7] whereas drunkenness or a drugged condition makes the contract voidable when sobriety is achieved. This is not customarily a problem for optometrists.

The purpose of the preceding explanation is to illustrate the fundamental considerations attendant to reaching a legal agreement. Since the types of contracts we will be discussing typically involve the expenditure of thousands of dollars, it is wise to secure professional advice before a contract has been entered into so as to ensure that these requirements are met. The cost of such advice is relatively modest when compared to the expense of litigation after-the-fact. Thus it is best to consult a lawyer, and, on many occasions, an accountant, at the beginning of the negotiation process. The attorney can be used as a source of advice for formulating the contract, negotiating with the opposite party, and drawing up the agreement. The accountant can provide information concerning the tax ramifications of the specific provisions being contemplated (of particular importance in buy-sell practice agreements). In long-term contracts such as those for services (associateship, partnership, or corporate agreements), failure to observe this advice may result in a contract that serves more to divide the parties than to provide them with a common framework within which to work.[8]

Negotiation Tactics

The quality of a contract is directly related to the quality of the negotiations that are instituted to formulate it. There are several general rules with regard to negotiation that should be observed whenever a contract is being considered.

1. *Begin negotiating early*—Usually, the earlier that negotiations are entered into, and the more comprehensive they are, the better the end result for both parties. A corollary of this rule is that the closer the personal relationship is between the contracting parties (e.g., the better their understanding is as to opposing interests and expectations), the greater the likelihood that the contract agreed to will be satisfactory to both parties. An optometrist who initiates his search for a practice opportunity with ample time to do so, manages to visit several practices, has discussions with various practitioners, and is able to create personal relationships with these doctors, will usually enjoy a far better offer (or offers) than will optometrists who begin late or achieve only superficial relationships.

2. *Establish negotiation goals*—It is important to set reasonable and clearly-defined goals when negotiating, whether looking to purchase a practice or seeking to find an associateship or partnership. First of all, it aids negotiations in that the optometrist knows what he must have as a minimum (in terms of remuneration) in order to discuss a contract seriously; a practical result of this is that the optometrist can end up framing the general shape of the agreement.[9] Secondly, goals will serve as a measuring stick for the offers and counteroffers that are a part of negotiating; the optometrist who has defined in writing reasonable goals has less difficulty in making up his mind whether to accept or reject an offer. Goals should be flexible, and a skillfull negotiator avoids the "take it or leave it" approach and utilizes negotiations that allow ample room for compromise.

3. *Be realistic*—A doctor who overprices the value of his practice or underprices the worth of an associate or partner usually ends up being disappointed or frustrated or both. There are various ways to determine the fair market price of a practice, and in today's economic climate an overpriced practice—like an overpriced home—will find few takers.[10] Determining the salary of an associate or partner is a complex matter, but the end result must be fair and satisfactory to the new optometrist if the relationship is to be long-term.[11] When two or more optometrists work together, personalities and practice philosophies are of paramount importance. A reasonable trial period is essential in order to ensure compatibility.[12]

4. *Initiate the contract proposal*—Whenever a contract is proposed, it is the initial version that is most often adopted—with minor changes—and thus it is the initial proposal that dictates the majority of the contract terms. Frequently, the optometrist seeking the practice opportunity is able to seize the

initiative by offering to write the first draft of the proposed contract, thereby establishing favorable or key provisions that otherwise might not have been considered. This is an opportunity that should not be squandered. A competent attorney should be used to draft the proposed contract, an expense that many negotiators may not feel they can afford, but when salary and benefits of several thousand dollars are being contemplated, it is best to spend the relatively few dollars necessary to have the agreement drawn up properly. It will be money well spent.[13]

5. *Know how to overcome an impasse*—The skillful negotiator is able to overcome disagreement by making counteroffers that are persuasive. The prepared optometrist is aware of the various bargaining options available to him and has already determined how they may be employed before entering into actual negotiations.[14] If a practice sale is stuck on the sales price (the usual problem), the negotiator should be able to offer a different price, interest amount, term of payment, or breakdown of the practice assets for tax purposes.[15] Likewise, an optometrist who feels that an offered salary is too low may be able to use fringe benefits, income incentives (such as a percent of the monthly income derived from examining all patients in excess of a certain number or above a certain gross amount per month), or a guaranteed annual percentage of ownership in order to get discussions moving again.[16] Negotiation is a skill that requires careful preparation, and any optometrist who is going to engage in negotiations involving many thousands of dollars should spend an adequate amount of time readying himself or preparing with the assistance of professionals.

Types of Contracts

There are many kinds of contracts that an optometrist will have to deal with during a professional lifetime, but for purposes of this discussion we will be concerned with those contracts that involve practice sales agreements and practice employment agreements. The types of contracts that fall under these two categories are:

Buy-Sell Agreements
1. Sale of 100% ownership
    a. Straight sale
    b. Installment sale
2. Sale of less than 100% ownership

Employment and Partnership Agreements
1. Associateship contracts
    a. Employment only
    b. Employment with option to become partner
2. Partnership contracts
    a. Beginning partnerships
        (1) by merger
        (2) senior-junior partnerships
    b. Replacement of a partner
    c. Addition of a partner

Buy-Sell Agreements

In general, all things being equal, it is better to purchase an ongoing practice than to start out cold. Since the practice has a track record, financial decisions can be more easily made and there is more assurance that the numbers are reliable (compared to guessing how a brand new practice will fare). There are two kinds of buy-sell agreements, those in which the seller divests himself of all interest in the practice and those in which the seller retains some interest that allows him to stay on in some capacity (either as a partner or as the employee of the purchaser). These contracts are discussed in Chapter 48.

Employment and Partnership Agreements

Although it would seem that employment contracts and partnership contracts are entirely different and that they should not be lumped together, in fact they are often related in that one often leads to the other, i.e., an associate will eventually become a partner in an ongoing practice.

For those optometrists who do not feel that they have the skills to become an employer (with all the headaches attendant to being a small businessman), an associate arrangement might be the more appropriate choice. Associateship agreements are described in Chapter 44. A special form of employment contract—found in professional corporations—is discussed separately in Chapter 46. Entering into partnership is a complex undertaking that requires careful preparation, a trial period to ensure compatibility, and the assistance of both tax and legal counsel. The most common provisions of partnership agreements are discussed in Chapter 45.

Notes

1. In many instances an oral contract will be valid, but certain agreements, by statute, must be in writing and signed by the parties in order to be enforceable. Verbal

contracts that must be in writing in order to satisfy this requirement, which is known as the Statute of Frauds, include:

- a promise to pay the debt of another person
- a contract creating an interest in land (i.e., sales and leases of land)
- an agreement that by its terms cannot be performed within a year (although in some jurisdictions employment agreements that allow either party to terminate the contract within a year are excluded from the Statute of Frauds)
- an agreement for the sale of goods valued at $500 or more (but some enforcement is permitted for goods sold under the provisions of the Uniform Commercial Code §2-201(3)(c))

The Statute of Frauds is satisfied if there is a writing that includes:

- the identity of the contracting parties
- identification of the subject matter of the contract
- terms and conditions of the agreement
- a recital of the consideration
- signatures of the parties

For these reasons, it is advisable to secure legal counsel to ensure that the contract is appropriately drafted.

2. Dawson, J.P., and W.B. Harvey, *Contracts and Contract Remedies*, Foundation Press, Mineola, N.Y., 1969.
3. Ibid.
4. Ibid.
5. Ibid.
6. Ibid.
7. Ibid.
8. The importance of having a competent attorney draw up the contract becomes more evident when the rules of contract construction are considered. When the courts are asked to interpret contracts, they are likely to observe the following general rules:
   - The contract will be construed as a whole; specific clauses are subordinated to the general intent of the contract.
   - Words will be used in the ordinary sense unless it is clearly shown that they are to be used in a technical sense.
   - If provisions are inconsistent, and some are printed (indicating a form contract) and others are written or typed, the latter provisions will prevail.
   - The courts will look to the custom or usage of the business and area where the contract has been made or is to be performed.
   - The courts will generally try to reach a determination that a contract is valid and enforceable, and thus they will construe provisions so as to make them operative.

   If legal action is necessary to interpret and enforce a contract, the courts will turn to the parol evidence rule in making the determination that the written contract is the complete embodiment of the parties' intention. Consequently, where the parties to a contract express their agreement in writing that the contract embodies the full and final expression of their agreement, then other admissions—written or oral—made prior to or contemporaneous with the contract will be inadmissible to vary the terms of the writing. Testimony will be permitted to explain the terms of the contract but not to effect changes that thwart the intent of the parties as expressed in the contract. See Dawson and Harvey, supra note 2.
9. For a discussion, see Gregg, J., *The Business of Optometric Practice*, Advisory Enterprises, White Plains, N.Y., 1981.
10. Ibid.
11. Ibid.
12. Ibid.
13. Classe, J., The 'Write' Way to Associateship, *Optometric Management*, vol. 23, no. 9, 1987, pp. 25–29.
14. Gregg, supra note 9.
15. Ibid.
16. Ibid.

Chapter 44

Associateship Agreements

Here are a few of the unpleasant'st words that ever blotted paper.
—William Shakespeare, *The Merchant of Venice*

Assessing Associateship

An associate is an employee who holds no ownership interest. Such a position would seem to offer little challenge in terms of drafting a contract. Many contracts have been based upon no more information than the length of employment and the amount of payment and have been sealed by the execution of no more than a firm handshake. Thus there is a frequently expressed attitude that written contracts are an unnecessary entanglement for salaried employees.

The usual associate—a young, just-licensed optometrist—needs the security of a written agreement. Most of these young practitioners are looking for a permanent practice opportunity and view the associateship as a means of undergoing a trial period. This agreement often becomes a precursor to a partnership contract. The associateship contract also specifies the benefits to be received by the employee and expresses the conditions of employment with regard to duties, fees, facilities, ownership of patient records, vacation, illness, and disability and provides for termination of the agreement. It anticipates these eventualities and provides guidance in the event they come about. It also establishes the responsibilities of the parties in the event there is litigation. Without these provisions, the agreement becomes something more like Shakespeare's description in *The Merchant of Venice*, a source of discord.

However, the first determination that must be made before considering the formality of a contract is whether a practice can support another practitioner. Factors deemed to be of significance are:[1]

- When the optometrist's appointment schedule is consistently booked a month or so in advance, with full days and even weekends being spent in the office
- When the practice population has begun to grow older, with a decreasing percentage of younger patients
- When the number of new patients represents less than 25 percent of the patient population
- When the doctor's schedule is so full that he finds it difficult to provide a full range of services (such as contact lenses, low vision, binocular vision therapy, or other specialty services) and there is no availability of qualified optometrists for intraprofessional referral
- When the doctor has had a period of poor health or is currently in poor health
- When the doctor is willing to reduce his hours in the office, willing to enjoy more frequent or more prolonged vacations, and committed to making changes in his schedule so that he may do this
- When the doctor is interested in a specialty area but must spend the majority of his time with general optometric patients and is willing to transfer the general patient load to another practitioner

- When the doctor desires to protect the equity accumulated in his practice by transferring part of the ownership to another optometrist, thus acquiring some retirement security

A major factor in the decision to increase the number of practitioners in a practice is the practice volume.[2] Both the size of the gross income of the practice and the growth curve of the practice are key considerations.[3] If the doctor has good records, it will not be very difficult to assess gross income and growth. Unfortunately, good records are the exception rather than the rule. Of course, each individual proprietor will have the basic information on Schedule C of his income tax return, but a thorough analysis requires more data than is found on a tax return.[4] It will also require the doctor's cooperation.

Although there is no magic number that can be relied on when looking at the gross income of a practice and trying to decide if it is sufficient to support another optometrist, it should be equal to or greater than the average gross income for such practices nationwide or have the potential to generate such earnings.[5] One does not have to be dogmatic about the gross income of the practice if the second key item, the growth curve, is on the upswing dramatically.

A growth curve (i.e., net income increasing rapidly) indicates that the practice has not reached its potential; a curve that has stabilized (or worse, tapered off) indicates it is already saturated and no longer growing. A word of caution when examining the practice growth curve: Because of the effects of inflation, both the gross and the net should be adjusted so that the true growth of the practice can be ascertained. The cost-of-living index can be used to make this calculation.[6]

The most thorough statistical analysis that can be made is one in which a line graph is plotted (either monthly, quarterly, or yearly) for the following information[7]:

- Gross income
- Overhead expenses
- Laboratory costs
- Net income
- Gross income from each kind of professional service
- Number of contact lens patients and the income derived from them
- Other specialty areas should be monitored in the same manner as contact lenses

In addition to this graph, an analysis of the practice could include statistics demonstrating the following[8]:

The age of the patients—Is it increasing, decreasing, skewed toward a particular age bracket?

The ratio between the number of new and former patients—Is it getting progressively smaller?

The source of patients—Are patients referred by other doctors due to the recommendations of other patients, due to office location, or due to personal contacts or personality of the doctor?

The demographics of the patient population—Are patients only from the neighborhood, are they for the most part of a certain socioeconomic status, are they from certain industries, or are they participants in third-party vision-care plans?

It may be difficult to accumulate this bountiful a store of information, but the better the data base available to assess the practice, the more informed the decision-making process will be. Because of the cost and complexity of partnership (often the ultimate aim of an associateship), the time spent collecting and analyzing information will be well spent.

Probably the most difficult decision for the employer-optometrist concerns the associate's salary.[9] There is often uncertainty over whether the optometrist's income will go down because of the extra expense of the associate.[10] Usually the income goes up, rather than down, when two or more optometrists work together.[11] There are several potential sources of income for an associate: the senior doctor's overflow, coverage during periods when the senior doctor is out of the office, a service not offered by the senior doctor (contact lenses, binocular vision, low vision, pediatric care, sports vision), medical services reimburseable under Medicare, or brand new patients brought to the practice by the new doctor are a few of the obvious possibilities.

Perhaps the most difficult question for the senior optometrist to answer is how many patients the junior doctor must see in order to pay his or her own way. The answer depends on how much the associate is being paid, of course. For example, if the associate's salary is $30,000, and the net income necessary to generate this salary is assumed to be 40 percent of the gross, then the associate must generate $75,000 of income in order to produce a net of $30,000. If each patient yields $75 (a conservative estimate), the associate must examine 1,000 patients a year to obtain the $75,000 gross. Over a five-day week, fifty weeks a year, this amounts to four patients a day, certainly not an overwhelming load either for the associate or for the practice. The senior doctor should plan to incorporate the associate into the practice so as to achieve the economic goal of allowing the younger doctor to pay his own way.[12] In most circumstances the effects of adding an associate to a practice can be successfully estimated by the senior practitioner.[13]

The salary is not a concern only for the employer; the associate quite naturally rates the remuneration that is offered as either the top or one of the top factors to be considered. But salary is not the sole factor to assess when analyzing the sufficiency of a proposed income.[14] The cost of living at the new location, the availability of employment for a spouse, and tax matters are just three of the numerous influences on income. If the take-home income offered to an associate seems insufficient, the associate should be able to document this fact with statistics.[15] Moreover, it can be advantageous to both parties to use fringe benefits rather than an actual cash increase. Such benefits as prepaid moving expenses, accident and health plans, vacation time, continuing education fees, and professional dues actually increase the associate's income past the cash equivalents of these benefits, since the associate would not only have to earn the cash to pay for them but also would have to pay the tax on this amount of income. The associate may find that fringe benefits are valuable enough to compensate for the salary that is being offered.[16] This is particularly true when the associate and the optometrist are assessing one another as potential partners.

The key to a successful associateship probably hinges on the negotiations that precede the actual agreement.[17] The earlier that negotiations are entered into and the closer the bonds between the two parties, the more likely a meeting of the minds will occur and the experience will be a good one for all concerned. The important provisions of an associateship agreement that should be negotiated are discussed in the next section. They are intended to serve as a starting point for the construction of a contract. As for the contract itself, it is best written by a competent attorney rather than by the parties. Each party will be best served if he has his own legal counsel, a policy that should be adhered to whenever contracts of any variety are being contemplated.

The Associateship Agreement

The brief discussion of associateship contracts that follows describes the structure of these types of contracts and discusses some of their important provisions. It is intended to assist in the negotiation and finalization of the contract of employment that will ultimately be drafted.

An associateship agreement is nothing more than an employment contract in which the associate agrees to provide specified services in return for a stated compensation. It is a series of clauses that defines the relationship and attempts to provide for certain situations so that the parties will know their responsibilities should the particular circumstances arise. It is signed by the parties so that there can be no question that each has read and understood its provisions. There is a certain sameness to these contracts, especially in form. Although a signed contract that identifies the parties, the length of employment, and the compensation to be paid will suffice, the more complete the contract is with regard to eventualities that arise during the term of the agreement, the less likelihood there is that the contract will be the subject of litigation. A well-drawn contract should discourage legal action by its succinctness and completeness; a poorly worded, vague, or incomplete contract may be worse than a handshake in that only a court of law can clarify its disputed terms. Keep this in mind when reviewing a proposed contract: if it is not clear, make it so. It will be worth the effort at revision.

The following sections discuss the various clauses to be found in an associateship agreement, with sample language following each clause.[18]

Recitals

Each contract begins with a recitation of the preliminary matters fundamental to the contractual arrangement, such as the identification of the parties, the purpose of the agreement, the date of the agreement, and the nature of the relationship being entered into.

> Agreement made on ________, 19___, between ________, hereinafter referred to as employer, and ________, hereinafter referred to as employee.
>
> Employer is organized under the laws of the State of ________ to render professional services through those of its employees who are duly licensed to practice optometry in the State of ________.
>
> Employee is an optometrist duly licensed and authorized to practice optometry in the State of ________.
>
> Employee desires to practice optometry as an employee of employer.
>
> Employer has offered employee employment for such compensation and other benefits and under the terms and conditions hereinafter set forth, and employee is willing to accept employment on such terms.
>
> In consideration of the above premises, it is mutually agreed as follows:

After the recitals come the basic provisions of the contract: the expected duties to be performed, term of the contract, compensation, and other necessary matters to be described. The following paragraphs illustrate these various clauses, which are the key portions of the agreement.

Employment and Duties

The contract should describe the duties expected of the employee, where the duties are to be performed, and the number of hours involved in the employment on a weekly basis.

(a) *Scope of duties.* Employer hereby employs employee, and employee accepts such employment, to render optometric services, to include examination of the eyes to determine the need for optical correction and the necessity for other related eye health care. Employer shall have the power to determine the specific duties to be performed by employee, and the means and the manner by which those duties shall be performed. Employer shall have the power to determine the assignment of patients to employee, and employee must perform services for such patients assigned to him. The power to supervise the duties to be performed, the manner of performing such duties, and the terms for performance thereof shall be exercised by the employer. The employee shall work four days during the week and one-half day on Saturday. The employee shall spend seven and one-half hours per day with patients, plus additional time for office staff meetings or other meetings called to maintain office procedure and policies.

(b) *Exclusive service.* Employee shall devote his full working time and attention to the practice of optometry for the employer. During the term of this agreement, employee shall not, without the written consent of employer, directly or indirectly render services of a professional nature to or for any person or firm for compensation or engage in any practice that competes with the interest of employer.

(c) *Professional standards.* Employee shall perform his duties under this agreement in accordance with the rules of ethics of the profession of optometry, as enunciated by the ________ Optometric Association.

If the employee wishes to be assured of the right to perform certain duties (such as the fitting of contact lenses, for example), it should be specifically mentioned in the contract. If a certain day is to be an off day, the day should be specifically mentioned (i.e., Wednesday). If evening hours are contemplated, this fact should also be specifically stated in the contract. These provisions protect both parties against arguments over where, when, and what the duties of the employee shall be.

Term

The usual period of employment is for a period of one year, although six-month contracts are occasionally used. If an associate has a family and a reasonable amount of personal goods, he may feel that a contract for less than a year is unacceptable and may reasonably request that the expenses of moving be at least partially defrayed by the employer.

The term of this agreement shall begin on ________, 19__, and shall continue for one year or until terminated as hereinafter provided.

Most contracts contain certain escape provisions for both parties in the event they (either separately or jointly) wish to break off their relationship prior to the scheduled end of the contract. These termination provisions are usually found in a separate section of the agreement.

Compensation

This key section of the contract will probably be the major subject of contention during negotiations. Both parties should ensure that the contract includes all agreed-on benefits.

(a) *Basic salary.* For all services rendered by employee under this agreement, employer shall pay employee a basic salary of $________ per year, payable monthly in twelve equal installments of $________, each beginning on the effective date of this agreement and payable on the first day of each month during the term of this agreement. The basic salary may be changed by mutual agreement of the parties at any time.

(b) *Bonus.* In addition to the compensation referred to above, employer shall, for the term of this agreement, pay employee on the last day of each month, or as soon thereafter as calculated, a bonus which is to be determined as follows: the employee shall be paid a bonus of __ percent of any income generated from his examination room over $________ gross per month.

(c) *Fringe benefits.* As further consideration for the performance by employee, employer shall, within a reasonable time after the execution of this agreement, provide for employee the following further benefits and any additional benefits that may from time to time be made available to optometrists employed by employer.

1. The expenses incurred by employee in moving his household goods and personal effects from ________ to ________, pursuant to this offer of employment.
2. An accident and health plan for the payment of employee's and employee's spouse's medical care expenses.

3. Employee's dues for the ______ Optometric Association.
4. Expenses to the ______ School of Optometry for ______ hours of continuing education.
5. A group term life insurance policy, payable to the employee's beneficiary, in the amount of $______ in the event of the death of the employee.

The sample language above presupposes that the employer is a professional corporation, hence the group life insurance policy (which is tax deductible); the corporation can also pay a $5,000 employee death benefit to the beneficiary. An additional benefit is disability insurance, which is discussed separately in this chapter. A fringe benefit package such as that listed above would add a few thousand dollars to the income of the employee, money upon which the employee would not have to pay taxes.

Malpractice Insurance

Since an associate is an employee, the standard professional liability insurance carried by most optometrists will include coverage for the associate, thus obviating the need for the associate to purchase his own insurance.

> Employer shall operate and maintain at its expense such comprehensive professional liability insurance coverage as it shall deem appropriate, covering the acts or omissions of the employee in the course of his employment.

The associate should be careful to acquire insurance that will prevent a gap in coverage should he leave the employer for another employment opportunity.

Office Facilities

An employee is not expected to bring equipment or supplies to the employer's facility in the usual case. This fact should be expressed in the contract.

> Employer shall operate and maintain facilities, and shall provide at its cost equipment, drugs and supplies, suitable to employee's position and adequate for the performance of his duties. Further, employer shall supply and pay for assistants, technicians, and other personnel reasonably needed by employee in connection with his employment under this agreement.

If an employee brings major items of equipment into the practice, it is probably best to list these items specifically as belonging to the employee and not to the employer.

Records and Files

The patient records are owned by the employer-optometrist, and it is customary for the employer to retain ownership of the records of all patients examined by the employee. There are several important negotiating points that concern these records. One would be the right of the employee, in the event he leaves the employer, to take these records with him (in the form of a copy). Another point is the right of the employee to have access to all patient records during the course of his employment. Still another is the right of the employee to retain a list of the patients seen by him during the course of employment, in the event he enters into practice on his own later in the same area. These are sensitive points to negotiate, and the employee is at a distinct disadvantage (especially if partnership is not eventually contemplated by the parties). One compromise is to allow the employee to retain copies of the records of those patients who request that he do so.

> All case records, charts, and personal files concerning patients of employer shall belong to and remain the property of employer. On termination of his employment, employee shall not be entitled to keep or reproduce employer's records or charts related to any patient unless the patient shall specifically request that his records be transmitted to employee.

The clause relating to patient records is also important when drafting contracts related to sharing of offices, partnership, and incorporation.

Fees

In an employer-employee relationship, fees are paid to the employer.

> All fees and compensation received or realized as a result of the rendition of professional services by employee shall belong to and be paid and delivered to employer.

Vacation

An important benefit for any employee is paid vacation time, and the agreement should specify the amount of time to which the employee is entitled and when the right to take a vacation accrues.

> Employee shall be entitled to a paid vacation of two weeks. Without employer's consent, vacation time may not be accumulated but must be taken in the year earned. Employee's vacation will be scheduled at those times most convenient to employer's business as deter-

mined by the employer. Employee's right to two weeks annual vacation will not accrue until he has been employed by the employer for six months.

The restrictiveness of the paid vacation time will vary from employer to employer, as will the amount of time to which the employee is entitled (another negotiating point). If it is anticipated that vacation time is desired at a particular time of year (Christmas, for example), it is best to bring this up before the contract is signed so that there will be no misunderstanding later.

Illness and Disability

A young optometrist is much more likely to be disabled than killed, and so disability is a potential problem that calls for thought on the part of the new graduate. Most employment contracts (in fact, the great preponderance of them) do not provide disability benefits for employees. The reason is that a nonworking employee is a drain on the practice income, and over the course of several months the payment of benefits (with no offsetting income) could jeopardize the financial stability of the practice. Disability insurance is an alternative of course, but it is expensive, which means that dollars spent for disability insurance will be spent to provide coverage for the employer rather than his employees. The expense of this insurance is one reason that new graduates do not purchase it themselves; unlike several kinds of life insurance, it provides no investment return, rather being only an annual expense for which the employee receives no tax deduction.

Therefore, in the usual case, the employee enters into a contractual agreement that states, in effect, that if he is permanently disabled he loses his job. Such an employee is also typically not insured and ends up ignoring the risk that he will be injured or become seriously ill during the early years of his career.

> Notwithstanding anything in this agreement to the contrary, employer is hereby given the option to terminate this agreement in the event that employee shall, during the term hereof, become permanently disabled as the term permanently disabled is hereinafter fixed and defined. Such option shall be exercised by employer giving notice to employee by registered mail, addressed to him in care of employer at ________, City of ______, State of ________, or at such other addresses as employee shall designate in writing, of employer's intention to terminate this agreement on the last day of the month during which such notice is mailed. On the giving of such notice, this agreement shall cease on the last day of the month in which the notice is so mailed, with the same force and effect as if such last day of the month were the date originally herein set forth as the termination date hereof.
>
> For the purposes of this agreement employee shall be deemed to have become permanently disabled if, during any year of the term hereof, because of ill health, physical or mental disability, or for other causes beyond his control he shall have been continuously unable or unwilling or shall have failed to perform his duties hereunder for ninety (90) consecutive days, or if, during any year of the term hereof, he shall have been unable or unwilling or shall have failed to perform his duties for a total period of ninety (90) days, irrespective of whether or not such days are consecutive. For the purposes hereof, the term *any year of the term hereof* is defined to mean any twelve (12) calendar months period commencing the date this agreement is signed, and terminating one year thereafter.

Disability insurance would be an excellent fringe benefit to place in an associateship agreement. Otherwise, the employee will have to accept something such as found in the sample language above, a 90-day period during which he receives a salary, with termination immediately thereafter. Although a permanently disabled employee is eligible for social security compensation (or worker's compensation if the employer qualifies), benefits are not payable until at least four months of disability have passed. Another aspect of this problem is the disability of the employer. The contract may provide for the purchase of the practice by the employee for a specified price if the employer is permanently disabled during the term of the contract. Similar provisions can be added for the death of the employer as well.

Covenant Not to Compete

A contract may include an agreement between the parties that the associate, upon conclusion of employment, will not practice within a specified period of time or within a certain circumscribed area in competition with the employer. This agreement, in jurisdictions where it is enforceable, allows the employer to institute legal action against the associate if there is a breach of the covenant. The remedies available to the employer include injunctive relief, which is an order from the court prohibiting the employee from continuing the competitive conduct, or liquidated damages, which is a contractually agreed upon sum that the associate must pay if found to be in violation of the covenent not to compete.

> For a period of ________ months after employee ceases to be employed by employer, employee shall not, directly or indirectly, engage in the practice of optometry on his

own account, or become interested therein, directly or indirectly, as a partner, shareholder, director, officer, or employee in competition with employer within ________ miles of the city limits of ________. In the event of breach hereof, it is specifically agreed that employer shall have all rights and remedies for relief as provided by law or in equity, including the right of injunction. Alternatively and in lieu of equitable relief, at the election of the employer, it is specifically agreed that the employer shall be entitled to liquidated damages of $________. Employee has carefully read and considered these provisions and, having done so, agrees that the restrictions set forth are fair and reasonable and reasonably required for the protection of the employer.

Even though a covenant not to compete may be included in an associateship agreement, it may not be enforceable. In several states the courts have refused to enforce these clauses,[19] whereas in others the courts will uphold them if the limits of time and place are reasonable or will reform them to make them so. Legal counsel should always be consulted whenever a covenant not to compete is being considered, so that all parties will understand their rights and obligations under the contract.[20]

Termination

Although contracts are for a stated period of time, there are circumstances that can intervene and terminate the agreement prematurely (e.g., death, bankruptcy, and loss of license). The parties may also mutually agree to terminate the relationship, and this is so even if it is not expressly stated in the contract. Many employment contracts will contain a vague catch-all phrase that gives the employer some subjective leeway in deciding to terminate the contract.

This contract shall be terminated immediately

(a) if employee becomes disqualified to practice optometry in the State of ________
(b) on the death of the employee
(c) if employer and employee shall mutually agree in writing to termination
(d) if the employer's business is discontinued
(e) if employee becomes or remains disabled as set forth above
(f) if employee fails or refuses to faithfully or diligently perform the duties of his employment and the provisions of this agreement

On termination for any reason, the salary due employee to the date of such termination shall be full compensation in payment for all claims under this agreement.

Another common approach to the termination of a contract before the end of its term is to allow either of the parties to end the relationship upon the giving of notice. The period of time the parties will remain together after the notice varies from contract to contract, but thirty or sixty days are the most frequently used.

Either party shall have the privilege to terminate this agreement at any time by the giving of thirty (30) days' written notice. At the time of such termination, the salary due employee shall be full compensation in payment for all claims under this agreement.

Severance pay can be a benefit for a terminated employee. One method is to compensate the employee for any unused vacation time at the date of termination. For example, if the employee had worked for six months, on a prorata basis he would have earned one week of vacation (out of two weeks annually), assuming that the employee had not taken any vacation time prior to termination. Thus the employee would be given a week's pay as severance compensation.

Upon termination as described herein, employee shall receive as severance compensation the amount of $________ per diem, such compensation to be paid to employee for each day of unused vacation time, not to exceed a maximum of fourteen (14) days. Unused vacation time is to be determined on a prorated basis, accrued at the rate of ________ day per month of employment. For purposes of this paragraph, employee shall receive credit for a full month of employment only if he has worked in excess of fifteen (15) business days during the calendar month. The severance compensation described herein shall be payable to employee on the date of termination.

The termination provisions of a contract should be given careful scrutiny. Although an employee cannot be forced to fulfill a personal service contract, the termination provisions must be adhered to by the employee or he will be liable to the employer for damages caused by the employee's breach of the agreement.

Miscellaneous Provisions

Most contracts will conclude with several miscellaneous provisions that are intended to clarify the applicable law and to list certain restrictions that will apply to the contract. These restrictions typically prohibit changes to the contract unless they are in writing, prohibit the associate from allowing another person to fulfill his duties under the contract, and declare that the written instrument is the entire contract that has been agreed to between the parties.

(a) *Governing law.* This agreement shall be interpreted, construed, and governed according to the laws of the State of ________.

(b) *Amendments.* No amendments or variation of the terms and conditions of this agreement shall be valid unless in writing and signed by all parties.

(c) *Assignability.* Employee's rights and obligations under this agreement are personal and not assignable.

(d) *Entire agreement; binding effect.* This agreement constitutes the entire agreement between the parties and shall bind and inure to the benefit of both employer and employee and their respective successors, heirs, and legal representatives.

These provisions are to be expected on personal service contracts.

Seal

The contract is concluded with the seal of the parties, which is no more than their signatures.

> In witness whereof, employer has caused this agreement to be signed by its duly authorized officers and its seal to be hereto affixed, and employee has executed this agreement at ________, on the day and year first above written.

The signatures can be notarized if desired. A copy of the contract should be stored in a secure location so that it cannot be lost or destroyed.

As the preceding paragraphs demonstrate, a contractual arrangement that is as straightforward as that between employer and employee contains great legal complexity and requires a considerable amount of thought and negotiation before it is actually signed. Even more complex is the contractual agreement that must be made between partners, which we will discuss in the next chapter.

Tax Considerations

The associate is paid an income in cash, and this serves as the basis for the deductions being taken by the employer. But there can be income other than cash that must be reported by the associate. Examples of these fringe benefits are included below.[21]

Sick pay received while the employee is ill or injured is taxable; however, benefits received under an accident or health insurance policy paid for by the employee are not taxable.

Medical insurance premiums, if paid for by an employer, are not included in income.

Vacation allowances are considered to be wages and are included in income.

Severance pay is taxable as income.

Moving expense allowances or reimbursements are included as gross income for the employee, but are not considered wages for purposes of income tax withholding or social security withholding.

Interview expenses paid by an employer or prospective employer are considered to be income but are not wages subject to income tax or social security withholding

Rewards and bonuses are considered to be income.

Christmas gifts, such as hams, turkeys, or other gifts of nominal value from an employer, are not considered to be income; cash, gift certificates, or like items are considered income, to the extent of their cash value.

Educational expenses paid by an employer must be included as income unless the educational courses are required by the employer as job-related, and he either pays the expenses directly or reimburses the employee after a full accounting; in this event, the expenses are not income.

Property for services received from an employer generally must be included in gross income at the fair market value of the property in the year it was received; an interest acquired in a partnership as part compensation for services rendered must generally be included as income; when negotiating a partnership interest as compensation, the employee should consult a competent tax attorney.

From the gross income of the associate the employer will withhold certain items, such as income taxes, social security taxes, and state or local taxes.

An employer withholds income tax from wages if the wages are more than the employee's withholding allowances. In general, an employee's withholding allowances equal the number of exemptions that the employee will be entitled to in figuring annual income tax. Every new employee has to file a Form W-4, Employee's Withholding Allowance Certificate, which is used by the employer to determine the correct withholding for the employee. The amount to be withheld for federal income taxes is based on gross wages before any other deductions are taken. Similarly, the employee must fill out a state withholding allowance certificate so that the correct state income tax deduction from gross income can be made. There may be a local income tax to be withheld as well. These deductions are reported to the employee (and the IRS) on Form W-2, Wage and Tax Statement.

The Federal Insurance Contributions Act (FICA)

provides for a federal system of old age, survivors, disability, and hospital insurance. This system is financed through social security taxes, also known as FICA taxes. These taxes are deducted from the employee's wages on a percentage basis up to a certain maximum income.[22]

There are other deductions that an associate could find subtracted from his paycheck, including contributions to an Individual Retirement Account, health insurance plan, or county or municipal government for various reasons related to the fact that he is a licensed professional doing business within the county or city. All deductions should be understood before entering into a contract so that at least a rough estimate as to take-home income can be ascertained.

The associate may also be able to claim certain business-related expenses as a tax deduction. In order to do so, the employee must itemize these deductions on Schedule A, as part of the miscellaneous category. They will be deductible only to the extent that they exceed 2 percent of the adjusted gross income, although some expenses—such as those for moving to a new job—may be claimed separately (see Chapters 41 and 42).

Tax planning is important, even when considering an employment opportunity. Associates should understand the applicable tax law in order to take full advantage of deductions and other means of tax avoidance.[23]

A sample associateship contract may be found in the Appendix.

Notes

1. Ready or Not for an Associate?, *Optometric Management*, vol. 16, no. 3, 1980, pp. 13–17.
2. Ibid.
3. Ibid.
4. Ibid.
5. See Baldwin, B., B. Christensen, and J. Melton, *Rx For Success*, Vision Publications, Midwest City, Okla., 1983.
6. Gregg, J., *The Business of Optometric Practice*, Advisory Enterprises, White Plains, N.Y., 1981.
7. Ibid.
8. Ibid.
9. Baldwin, R., Here's How To Take in an Associate... Painlessly, *Journal of the American Optometric Association*, vol. 53, no. 2, 1982, pp. 137–139.
10. The economic surveys conducted by the AOA have demonstrated that solo practice is the least lucrative in terms of take-home income. For example, the 1978 AOA survey revealed the following statistics:

	SOLO PRACTITIONER	PARTNERSHIP	GROUP PRACTICE
Number of exams	1,311	1,401	1,513
Gross income	$94,195	$110,331	$127,901
Net Income	$36,485	$41,749	$43,386

Every such survey seen by the author reflects the same result.

11. Ready or Not for an Associate?, supra note 1.
12. Ibid.
13. Ibid.
14. Milkie, G., *Partnerships and Professional Corporations*, Optometric Development Enterprises, St. Louis, 1972.
15. Ibid.
16. Ibid.
17. Ibid.
18. The language cited herein, and the sample contracts used in this text, are courtesy of the American Optometric Association.
19. Alabama, California, Florida, Michigan, Montana, North Dakota, and Oklahoma. From Stetler, C.J., and A.R. Moritz, *Doctor and Patient and the Law*, 4th ed., C.V. Mosby, St. Louis, 1962.
20. For a discussion of restrictive covenants as they apply to medical practice, see Stetler, C.J., and A.R. Moritz, supra note 19; and the annotations of the *American Law Reports* at 62 A.L.R. 3d 1014, 62 A.L.R. 3d 970, and 62 A.L.R. 3d 918.
21. The payments in lieu of cash that qualify as fringe benefits are described in IRS publication 334, *Tax Guide for Small Businesses.*
22. As of 1988, the maximum income that is subject to social security taxes is $45,000, which is high enough to ensure that most employee optometrists will pay 7.51 percent (the percentage applied in 1988) of their earnings to the Social Security Administration. See IRS publication 15, *Employer's Tax Guide (Circular E).*
23. For a discussion, see Classe, J., Don't Let Associateship be a Taxing Experience, *Optometric Management*, vol. 23, no. 9, 1987, pp. 32–35.

Chapter 45

Partnership Agreements

The rights and duties of the partners in relation to the partnership shall be determined, subject to any agreement between them, by the following rules:

(a) Each partner shall be repaid his contributions, whether by way of capital or advances to the partnership property and share equally in the profits and surplus remaining after all liabilities, including those to partners, are satisfied; and must contribute towards the losses, whether of capital or otherwise, sustained by the partnership according to his share of the profits.

(b) The partnership must indemnify every partner in respect of payments made and personal liabilities reasonably incurred by him in the ordinary and proper conduct of its business, or for the preservation of its business or property.

(c) A partner, who in aid of the partnership makes any payment or advance beyond the amount of capital which he agreed to contribute, shall be paid interest from the date of the payment or advance.

(d) A partner shall receive interest on the capital contributed by him only from the date when repayment should be made.

(e) All partners have equal rights in the management and conduct of the partnership business.

(f) No partner is entitled to remuneration for acting in the partnership business, except that a surviving partner is entitled to reasonable compensation for his services in winding up the partnership affairs.

(g) No person can become a member of a partnership without the consent of all the partners.

(h) Any difference arising as to ordinary matters connected with the partnership business may be decided by a majority of the partners; but no act in contravention of any agreement between the partners may be done rightfully without the consent of all the partners.

—Uniform Partnership Act §18

Assessing Partnership

There is an important connection between the success of a partnership and the contractual obligations that bind the partners together: if the contract is unfair to either party, the partnership will fail, and for this reason it is the cornerstone of the arrangement.

Partnership agreements are by nature long-term instruments seeking to formalize the association of persons desiring to derive financial benefit from a joint enterprise. Although negotiation is a necessary aspect of the formulation of these contracts, and compromise—which is the inevitable product of negotiation—may obtain a result that none of the partners regards as completely satisfactory, it is the effort to achieve balance and fairness between the contracting parties that distinguishes the successful agreement.

Partnership is a consensual relationship that, in the conduct of its internal affairs, relies on interactions that are substantially personal in nature. For this reason almost all of the general characteristics of the relationship among the partners may be established by agreement. As a result, the rights and duties of the partners may be defined by a written instrument known as the *articles of partnership* or the *partnership agreement*. Although the agreement may be oral as well as written, a written agreement is preferable since it can prevent potential disputes between the partners and can serve as proof that otherwise might be inadmissible in the event of litigation.

In the great majority of states the Uniform Partnership Act (UPA) and the Uniform Limited Partnership Act (ULPA) have been adopted by statute (see Chapter 38). The UPA provisions establish many important obligations between the partners and between the partnership and third parties (section 18 is included at the beginning of this chapter). A number of the UPA provisions, however, are qualified by the phrase *unless otherwise agreed*, which permits a written contract duly executed by the partners to become the controlling document as to these obligations. Because of the legal interrelationships between the UPA and a partnership agreement, an attorney's guidance will be necessary when drafting such an instrument. All partners should thoroughly discuss and understand the agreement's provisions prior to its ratification by the partnership.

Even though partners will turn to accountants, attorneys, or other advisors for guidance in determining the correct contractual relationship, they must realize that there is no standard partnership agreement that will be acceptable for everyone. New graduates should also be aware that partnership details that have worked for one set of doctors may be inappropriate for another group due to differences in personalities, professional philosophies, and personal economic needs. Whenever a partnership arrangement is being contemplated, individuality of effort will be an important factor, and prospective partners should realize that they need to formulate their partnership agreement so that it is tailor-made for them.[1]

Probably the most important prerequisite for a successful partnership is for the doctors involved to have a solid understanding and appreciation of how they are going to work together. If they do not basically agree on such matters as attitudes toward optometric care, sharing of patient responsibilities, and financial arrangements, their relationship is not likely to endure. Optometrists who are contemplating entering into partnership should take the time to discuss (at length) practice philosophies, responsibilities, economics, and similar subjects with their prospective partners. A thorough discussion may ward off a union that is preordained to failure, thus avoiding the heavy financial and emotional costs of a subsequent split-up.

This chapter will concentrate on the senior-junior partnership arrangement, which is usually the result of a trial period between an individual proprietor and an associate.[2] Chapter 44 discussed the factors that have to be considered when a doctor wishes to employ an associate. The successful termination of this arrangement is an offer on the part of the employer-optometrist to allow the associate to purchase part of the practice and thereby create a partnership between the two.

An associate who has spent a number of months working with an older optometrist will have acquired a familiarity with both the doctor and the practice that should enable him to make an informed decision as to whether he would like to remain with the practice and eventually make it his own. But even if an associate feels that the practice opportunity is one that would be satisfactory, there are a number of matters that must be discussed and clarified before a partnership arrangement is formalized. Foremost among these is the motivation of the employer-optometrist, including the factors that have led him to look to partnership, his financial requirements, and his expectations for the future.

Discussions that explore the feasibility of partnership will need to address a wide range of topics.[3] These topics will vary with the personalities and the needs of the individuals, but there are common subjects that all prospective partners will need to consider:

- Philosophy of practice
- Capital contributions
- Partnership income
- Partnership expenses
- Partnership benefits
- Transfer of partnership interests

Each of these matters presents unique problems.

Philosophy of Practice

There are two basically opposite philosophies that can be utilized by a partnership. The first approach requires all patients to be the patients of the partnership and not of any particular optometrist. Scheduling of patients is based upon which doctor is available, and all patient records are merged without regard to which doctor was responsible for an individual patient's care. Advantages to this approach are that all members of the partnership will acquire experience with each patient and the patient load can be divided as equitably as possible between each of the partners. A disadvantage is that each doctor will have less continuing personal contact with a single patient. Also, if any of the doctors offers specialized services that the others do not, this approach to patient care will be unfeasible since the patient load cannot be as easily divided.

The second approach is merely to continue with separate responsibilities for individual patients, which is complemented by the expanded opportunities for coverage and peer consultation that partnership offers. Thus, a patient's regular appointments will be scheduled with his usual doctor, whereas emergencies or other occasions can be covered by the doctor who is available at the time. Patient records are coded according to the doctor responsible for them. Advantages of this system include ongoing personal contact with individual patients and an easy means of separating the patient pool. Disadvantages include inequitable patient loads between partners and inability to provide certain services (if the only doctor who offers them is unavailable).

These philosophical matters *must* be considered before the doctors in a partnership begin seeing patients.[4]

Capital Contributions

When a partnership is formed, it is customary to create a partnership account and to contribute capital toward this account, which is used to pay the expenses of the business. In addition, the partners may contribute property, real or personal, to the partnership, and such contributions also serve as capital for the benefit of the business. These contributions are important for tax purposes, although no gain or loss will be recognized by a partner at the time of the contribution to the partnership. Rather, it is when a distribution of property or a withdrawal of property is made that the partner has to consider the tax ramifications. A careful record of the capital contributions of the partners will have to be made at the time the partnership is started, and each year the partner's basis in the property will have to be determined. Such determinations will have to be made by a competent accountant or tax attorney.

When the partnership is terminated due to the retirement, death, or withdrawal of a partner, the partner's interest in the partnership will have to be liquidated. Payments in liquidation, to the extent that they are made in exchange for the partner's interest in the partnership property, are treated as distributions to the partner by the partnership and hence subject to income taxation. Thus, any capital contributions must be discussed before the partnership is formed.

Partnership Income

One important subject that must be thoroughly explored and agreed upon is how the partnership income will be divided.[5] It is such an important topic that a separate section of this chapter is devoted to it exclusively. The decision-making about income does not concern merely the division of profits but goes much deeper, beginning with the determination of what income shall be shared with the partnership and what is to be considered personal income.

One approach is to designate all income, however earned, as partnership income; thus, income from teaching, writing, and outside consulting activities would be designated as going to the partnership and not to an individual.

Another approach is to designate that only the income generated within the partnership and recorded in the partnership's books (presumably only from patient care) would be partnership income. Efforts outside of the practice that earn a profit belong exclusively to the individual performing them, and the other partners do not share in this income.

How the partnership income will be divided is a topic that must be clearly understood by all the partners.

Partnership Expenses

Doctors in a partnership must determine which expenditures are to be borne by the partnership and which are to be personal. Although the usual and customary expenses (e.g., rent, utilities, and employee salaries) are clearly partnership expenditures—such items as automobile expenses, professional liability premiums, professional society dues, purchase of texts and other publications, and travel to and attendance at professional meetings and educational seminars—will create differences of opinion (not to mention entertainment expenses, which can also be a source of controversy).

Partnerships vary widely in their attitudes toward these items: some pay them through the partnership because they feel that these expenses are for the benefit of the partnership as a whole; others exclude some or all of them from the joint books because they believe that the partners should be free to spend as much or as little on the items as they wish without generating concern over the possible inequity of individual spending levels.

As a general rule, common items such as insurance premiums, subscriptions to texts and periodicals, and professional society dues can be paid by the partnership without inequity, while automobile ownership and expenses, professional meeting and educational program costs, and expenses related to entertainment are personal items that are best left to each partner. Some partnerships entitle each doctor to a stated dollar amount of expense for the common items, with any additional expenses above this amount being paid by the doctor who has incurred them.

As to continuing education meetings specifically, an alternative approach is to entitle each partner to a stated number of days of absence each year in order to attend professional meetings and educational programs. The partnership will then pay for all expenses incurred at the meetings, using as a rationale the belief that, over a period of years, these expenses will be more or less equal.

Partnership Benefits

Although we have already mentioned some benefits that may be paid for out of partnership funds, there are more complex matters that must also be discussed. Foremost among these is the issue of whether the partnership will establish a retirement fund (i.e., a Keogh plan). The decision to set up such a fund requires a lawyer's expertise and an accountant's assistance.

Another tough issue that must be discussed is disability. If a partner is disabled, what benefits can he expect to receive and for how long? If the partnership wishes to purchase disability insurance, this is another problem that must be ironed out.

Any benefit that the partnership contemplates, even one as seemingly straightforward as vacation time, must be understood by the partners. Only through meaningful discussions can this understanding be generated. An appropriate amount of time should be allocated to discuss these matters.

Transfer of Partnership Interests

Although dissolution of the partnership seems to be a poor choice of subject matter when first entering into the partnership arrangement, it is a problem that must be settled before the partnership begins. As we shall see in the next section, the senior-junior partnership creates unique financial difficulties for the junior partner. Among these difficulties is the problem of how to compensate a senior partner when he retires. And there are similar difficulties involved in determining the procedure and compensation for partners who withdraw or are disabled, and for the liquidation of the partnership itself. Again, a thorough understanding between the partners and a well-written partnership agreement will be required.

Although all these important factors influence the decision to enter into partnership, probably the most discussed item is the partnership income. This fact does not decrease the importance of personal factors in the creation, maintenance, and success of a partnership but rather points out how necessary it is for the partners to have a clear understanding of how the partnership ownership and income will be managed. We will discuss this rather complex matter in the following section.

Partnership Income

When a senior-junior partnership is contemplated, there will be numerous questions that the potential partners will ask one another about practice finances. Does the senior practitioner generate enough income to afford another employee? Will the junior doctor receive an income adequate to pay his living expenses and to permit him to buy 50 percent of the practice? If there is a profit, how will it be split? What is the fair value of the senior doctor's 50 percent that is being transferred to the younger partner? And what planning is necessary with regard to the senior doctor's remaining 50 percent interest at the time of retirement? What is its fair value?

These questions center around two major issues: the acquisition of a partnership interest by the junior partner at the outset of the arrangement and the disposal of the senior partner's remaining interest at the time of his retirement. There is no clear solution for either of these issues, merely a variety of ideas that have found applicability in individual situations. Therefore, the following discussion is limited to a general set of guidelines that, hopefully, will serve to indicate useful approaches to the solution of these complex problems.

Is There Enough Income for a Partnership?

We have already discussed the personal and financial factors that must be analyzed in a senior-junior arrangement to determine if the older doctor's practice can support an associate who is interested in becoming a partner (see Chapter 44).

Although economic factors probably create the most consternation, the willingness of the senior doctor to employ the associate fully is, in many practices, the key to success. This is especially true in sole proprietorships of long standing that have never before supported an associate. There is ample opportunity for the junior doctor to "pay his own way" and for the senior doctor to encourage him to do so (see Chapter 44).

If an analysis of the practice reveals that it can support two doctors, then the immediate problem that must be considered is how to pay the junior partner while at the same time allowing him to obtain a partnership interest.

How Is the Junior Partner's Income Determined?

In attempting to solve this problem, the partners must work out a careful agreement ahead of time to cover all issues that might cause misunderstanding and have periodic reviews of the agreement to resolve problems before they become unmanageable.[6]

The first issue that must be faced is whether the junior partner will actually have to pay money up front for his interest in the partnership or will be able to earn his interest without being called upon to actually transfer funds to the senior doctor. Some older practitioners feel that the younger doctor has a greater motivation if he actually has to part with some money (usually acquired through a loan) in order to "buy in" to the new arrangement. This sum constitutes a down payment on the part of the junior doctor and may be forfeited by the junior doctor if he breaches the partnership agreement and withdraws from the arrangement before the full partnership has been realized, such sum being regarded as liquidated damages. If the older doctor is ambivalent about such a payment, it is rather easy to demonstrate that the junior partner can earn his way without the necessity for up-front money.

There are numerous formulas that have been devised to break in the junior partner through a salary differential that pays him less than the senior doctor even though they are working equal hours. The first decision that must be made concerns the fair value of the junior partner's interest and the portion of the partnership whole that it represents. Most partnerships between two persons are on a fifty-fifty shared basis. Although partnership arrangements can be written so that the senior doctor retains a larger interest (such as fifty-one–forty-nine), if this translates into sole control by the senior doctor it may ultimately poison the relationship and thus should be avoided. Once the percent of partnership interest that the junior doctor is to purchase has been determined, the actual monetary value must be established. How to calculate the fair value of a practice is a problem to itself, and will be discussed in Chapter 48. Of course, if the junior doctor is purchasing a 50 percent interest, the price is halved.

When the price is set, the doctors know how much income the younger partner must divert to the senior doctor in order to obtain his partnership interest. This is accomplished by setting different salaries for the two doctors. Typically, the partnership agreement will specify a certain monthly draw to be paid to the doctors; the junior partner receives less salary than the older doctor even though they are working equal hours (and, if both are equally busy, generating equal income). The salary differential is at its maximum in the first year and each year becomes less until eventually (between three to six years later) the monthly draw is equal. In addition to the monthly draw, there is the profit that the partnership earns at the conclusion of the tax year; it too can be divided on an unequal basis. The profit is realized after all salaries, expenses, and taxes are paid and there is additional money remaining in the partnership account; this amount is then distributed to the partners. The customary way to divide the profit is on a percentage basis, again with the senior doctor receiving a larger share at the start and over a period of years being gradually reduced to a fifty-fifty split. The total differential over several years of inequality will constitute the younger doctor's payment for his partnership interest.

This is another means of allowing the younger doctor to contribute toward his share of the partnership, but it requires the senior doctor to be willing to cut back on his time in the office.[7] The senior doctor decides how many days he wants to be out of the office, then a credit is allocated to the junior doctor for each of the days he carries the burden alone. For example, if the senior doctor wishes to work 50 days less per year, the junior doctor could be allocated credit as follows: for the first and second year he would receive $150 per day; for the third and fourth year he would receive $200 per day; for the fifth year he would receive $250, and so on. Again, this differential would be a credit toward the purchase price that had been agreed upon by the two partners.

Obviously, the question of how to compensate the younger optometrist while allowing him to buy in is a complicated one. But it is not the end of the battle. Once the partners have reached parity, there is another problem: how to divide the income thereafter.

How Is the Income Split Between Partners?

The two basic alternative income division systems are simple percentage division and division on the basis of productivity.

Percentage

The simplest of all methods is for the partners to divide the income from their efforts equally. Or the income can be divided in fixed percentages that are not equal, based on a predetermined, fixed ratio. A percentage method has the advantage of offering the partners a group incentive: Each partner will prosper as long as the venture produces sufficient income, regardless of which doctor actually performs the work. This minimizes competition because no partner receives a direct financial reward for seeing a larger share of patients than the other partners. But if the partners do not make equal contributions to the partnership's financial success difficulties can arise, particularly as these differences become larger and larger. Inequality of time or patient load and equality of income can create an unhappy relationship; this is the primary disadvantage of a percentage distribution of income.

Productivity

The opposite approach is to compensate each member in direct proportion to the amount he has contributed to the partnership's income. The common measure of such contribution is the amount of fee charges recorded on the partnership's books. Besides rewarding a member for his financial contribution, the productivity division has the additional advantage of being self-adjusting. A partner's share of the partnership income will thus vary from year to year, just as his efforts may vary. And if the senior doctor wishes to take extra time away from the practice his compensation would decrease proportionately without negotiation. However, this type of arrangement can create competition between partners for the available work. It tends to reward partners for generating dollars while ignoring other, less measurable contributions toward patient flow. Productivity division also requires careful bookkeeping of patient charges.

Combination

A frequent solution to the problem of equitably distributing income is a combination of the two described methods. The simplest example of a combination method would be to divide half of the income of the practice among its partners equally (or on some predetermined percentage) and the other half of income on the basis of the partners' actual productivity. Variations on the fifty-fifty division are frequent, and small partnerships (two or three members) often use the combination method. This system rewards both group loyalty and individual ambition but demands good bookkeeping.

Arguments over income distribution are the most frequent cause of unhappiness among partners. It is best not to be dogmatic over any particular approach, since as circumstances change the partners may find a different system will be more equitable.

What Is the Fair Value of the Senior Partner's Remaining Interest at Retirement?

This is a problem that many beginning partnerships ignore altogether but, if possible, should be solved at the outset of the senior-junior relationship. The basic problem is how to determine a fair value at a future date that may not be known with any degree of exactness. Of course, if a specific date is known, the task is made much easier. The further the retirement date is in the future, the more speculative the price and hence the greater the reluctance of the senior partner to set a specific amount. For the junior partner this is a problem as well, for in several years' time his efforts on behalf of the partnership will have made it far more valuable, thus placing him in a position of having to pay for his own labors.

The solution is to set a fair value that is somewhat flexible. There are two basic ways to set the price, either through a set figure or through a formula. If the retirement date contemplated is not too far in the future, the price can be the other half of the agreed-on price for the junior partner's share adjusted for the effects of inflation and growth during the intervening years. The agreed upon price can be paid out over a period of years as a percentage of the gross income so that the junior doctor knows he can generate the necessary income from the practice's cash flow. If the retirement date is remote, it is probably best for the partners to establish the price for the senior partner's share on an annual basis. (This will need to be done anyway in case the senior partner dies or becomes permanently disabled.)

One other aspect of this problem is the actual purchase of the partnership interest. The junior doctor may not want to purchase it himself, rather preferring that another practitioner assume the older doctor's position as partner. This may, in fact, be accomplished through an associateship that blossoms into partnership or there may be a direct substitution of partners. In either event, the junior optometrist has an obvious interest in who becomes the new partner. The usual provision is to give the junior partner the right of first refusal on the purchase of the remaining partnership interest; if he does not want a new partner, he exercises the right and buys the remaining portion of the practice himself. If he does not exercise the option, then the senior partner may sell his share to a third party. In this event, the junior partner retains the right to approve or reject a potential buyer. But failure to settle on someone acceptable within a reasonable period automatically requires the junior partner to make the purchase himself.

When discussing income, the partners need to explore all potential problems at the outset and to incorporate into the contract the agreed-upon solutions while reserving enough flexibility to be able to meet unexpected circumstances. Nowhere is the spirit of compromise more evident than in a partnership; if all partners accept the idea that they must go more than halfway in their efforts to create harmony with their fellow practitioners, then the partnership experience will be a happy and rewarding one.

Insurance

A source of consternation among potential partners seeking to construct a partnership agreement is the necessity for insurance of various kinds. The most common type of insurance purchased is professional liability insurance and casualty insurance that protects the office and its assets and any vehicles used for partnership business. There are other insurance questions that are not as commonly resolved, however, and these concern disability and life insurance.

Insurance will be described in detail later in this text. We will limit the following discussion to buy-sell agreements that are funded by life insurance.[8] The purpose of these agreements is to provide ready cash in the eventuality one of the partners dies. The insurance proceeds are used to purchase the deceased partner's share of the partnership from his heirs, thus assuring that the partnership will continue without a sudden drain on its cash flow and that the partner's heirs will receive payment promptly for the agreed-upon value. Buy-sell arrangements are not without problems, and these disadvantages will be described.

There are basically two types of partnership buy-out agreements that are funded through insurance: entity-purchase plans and cross-purchase plans.

Entity-Purchase Plans

The entity-purchase contract customarily requires the partnership to buy out and the deceased partner's estate to sell the partnership interest held by the decreased at the time of death. The funding insurance, on the life of the deceased partner, is owned and paid for by the partnership and made payable to it. Thus, where there are three partners, the partnership would own a policy of insurance on each partner in order to satisfy its obligations, as created by the partnership buy-sell agreement. Such a plan is schematically illustrated by Fig. 45.1

There are advantages to the entity-purchase method:

- The funding of this method is rather simple since all that is required is for the partnership to purchase a policy on each partner and to designate itself as the owner or beneficiary thereof.
- If the partnership owns the policies, then it owns ready assets that can be used for cash or for collateral security should there be a sudden need for additional capital. The dollars that are set aside to fund the entity-purchase serve also as a reserve for emergencies.
- Another possible advantage of entity-purchase plans is found in partnerships in which the ages of the partners vary widely. For example, if there are two partners, aged thirty and sixty, under an entity-purchase buy-out plan, the partnership helps to equalize the premium payments, a factor that helps the younger partner because the premiums for the older partner will be far more costly than those for the 30-year-old. Since the costs are merged into the partnership, the older partner, in effect, assists the younger partner in purchasing the insurance. (As we shall see, under a cross-purchase plan, the younger partner would have to pay for the insurance of the older partner personally, which would be a difficult financial burden to

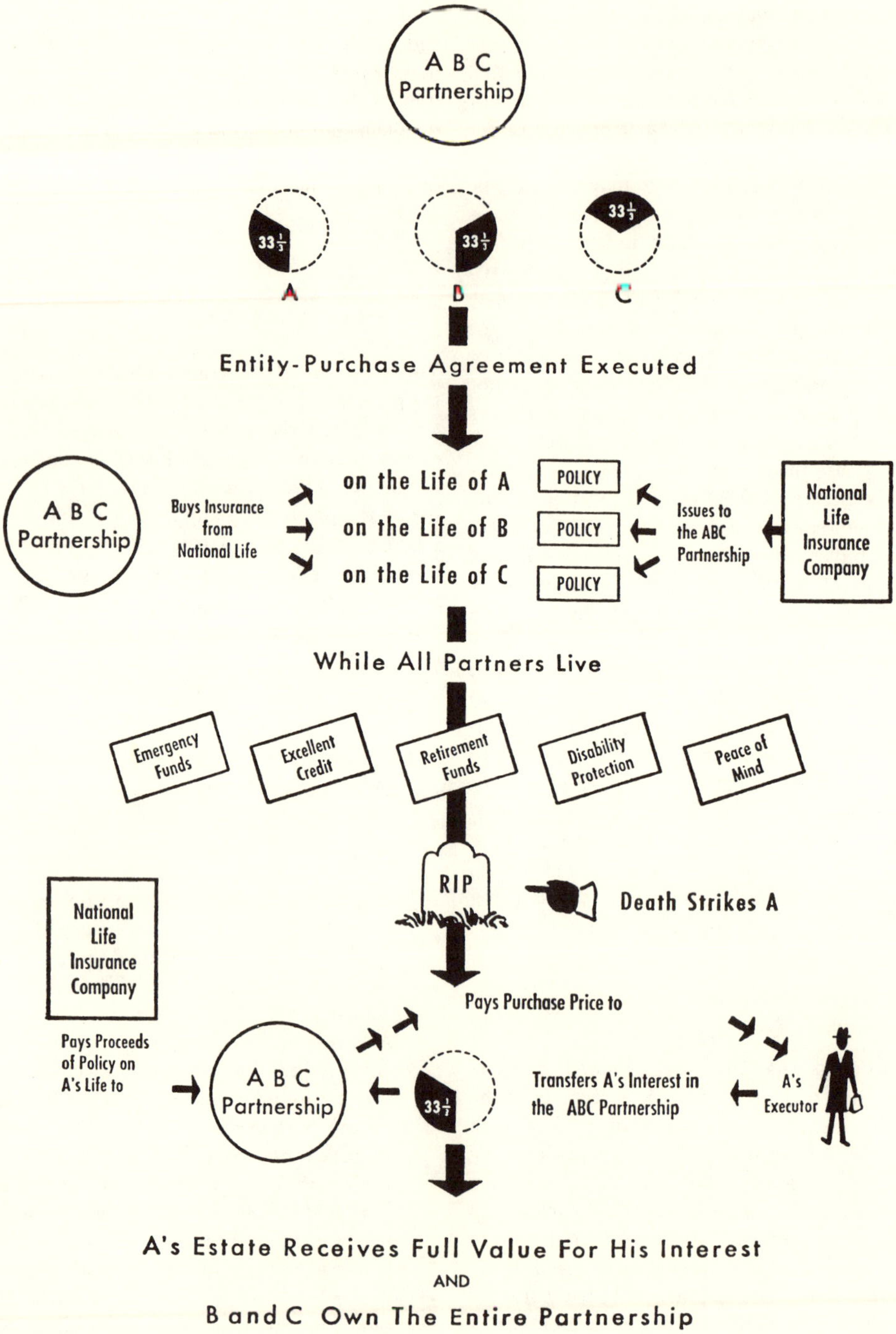

Figure 45.1. Illustration of an Entity-Purchase Plan. (Courtesy of the National Life Insurance Company)

bear.) Of course, the older partner is probably the one most in favor of the buy-sell arrangement because he is the more likely to die and can foresee the tax and planning advantages of the insurance. Thus, he can afford to defray the younger partner's costs somewhat.

There are also disadvantages to the entity-purchase method:

- When life insurance proceeds are paid to the partnership, this payment will affect the cost basis of the surviving partners in the partnership, an important tax consideration when these partners sell their interest at retirement or death. The entity-purchase method is less favorable in this regard than the cross-purchase method.
- The insurance policies owned by the partnership are assets of the partnership and therefore may be vulnerable to creditor attack.

Cross-Purchase Plans

In this type of agreement each partner agrees with the other partners that upon his death his share of the partnership will be sold to the surviving partners and the other partners agree to purchase his share, ordinarily in pro rata amounts. Of course, if there is only one survivor, he agrees to purchase the deceased partner's interest in the partnership. This arrangement requires each partner to buy insurance made payable to himself on the life of each of his colleagues. If one partner dies, his surviving partners will each have the funds required to discharge their obligations under the purchase agreement. This type of buy-sell arrangement is illustrated by Fig. 45.2, which uses a three-partner arrangement as an example. Note that when there are three partners involved, there are six separate insurance policies that must be purchased.

Advantages of the cross-purchase method include the following:

- In a small partnership (two or three persons), the cross-purchase plan has the advantage of simplicity. The individuals deal directly with the insurance company, and the partnership as an entity does not enter into consideration.
- When a surviving partner purchases his pro rata share of the interest in the partnership belonging to the deceased partner, the tax or cost basis for his interest in the partnership increases to the extent of his share of the matured insurance funding the plan. This basis will increase more than in an entity-purchase plan, thus making the cross-purchase method advantageous tax-wise for the surviving partners when they leave the partnership.
- The policies are not owned by the partnership and thus are less succeptible to creditors (although they may still be vulnerable).

Disadvantages of the cross-purchase method include the following:

- When there are a number of partners, the cross-entity method becomes extremely burdensome, both in terms of administration and in terms of cost.
- The creditors of an insolvent partner may be able to seize the policies in order to satisfy his personal debts to them, thus defeating the purpose of the buy-sell arrangement.
- In a partnership in which the ages of the partners vary significantly, there is an inequity in the premiums that the two partners pay, with the younger partner (who has insured the older partner's life) paying a much higher premium. If there are several older partners, this cost may be an impossible financial burden for a younger partner.

Most often the contingency on which the purchase agreement is based is the death of a partner. But this does not have to be only contingency; retirement at age sixty-five and permanent disability can also be used, if the agreement is so drawn. A paid-up insurance policy can fund a buy-sell plan at retirement, or disability insurance can take the place of or be added to a life insurance policy.

Disability

If disability insurance is contemplated, when drafting the buy-sell agreement the definition or test of disability should be at least as strict as the one used in a private disability insurance policy (see Chapter 53). In this event the partnership avoids the financially disastrous possibility that a partner will be disabled enough to be bought out but yet not sufficiently disabled to cause the insurance company to pay off on its policy to the partnership or the individual partner who has paid the premiums.

Another aspect of this problem is that the disability of the partner, even if it qualifies for insurance payments, may not remain until death or until he has been fully paid for his interest in the partnership. If the disabled partner—to whom installment payments

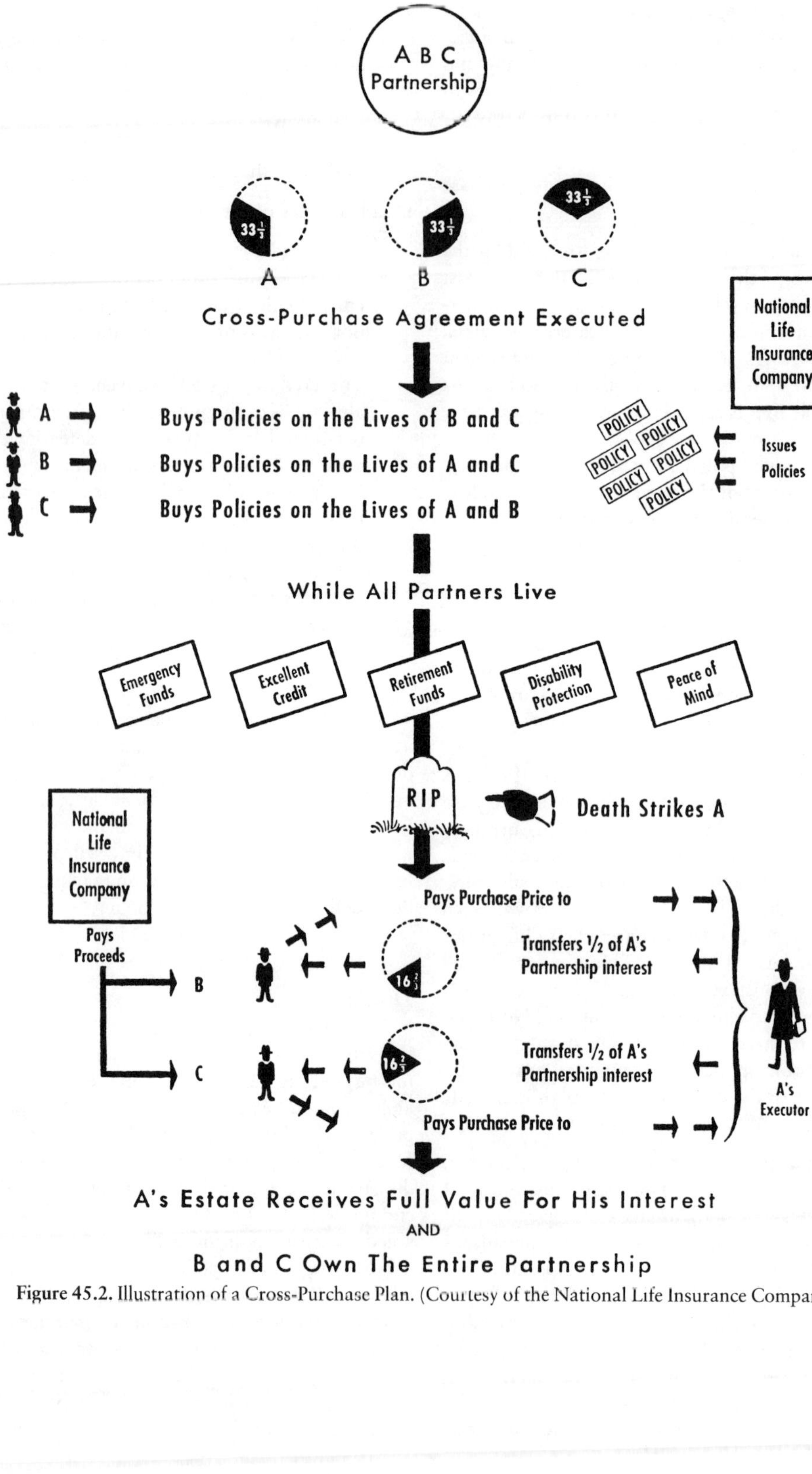

Figure 45.2. Illustration of a Cross-Purchase Plan. (Courtesy of the National Life Insurance Company)

are being made in exchange for his interest in the partnership—proceeds to recover, the agreement should specify the course to be followed. Two possible alternatives are to provide in the agreement that a partner's disability must persist for a substantial period (eighteen months to two years) before the buy-sell provisions must be instituted, or to permit the purchase price, in the event of disability, to be spread out over a prolonged period, thus reducing the size of payments and yet extending the period during which the disabled partner receives payment. In this eventuality the buy-sell agreement goes to completion even if the disabled partner recovers.

Disability insurance provisions in a partnership agreement customarily are written to protect the partnership rather than to provide a source of income for a disabled partner. The problem of disability payments and sick pay is a troublesome one that must be addressed.

Disadvantages of Insurance

Despite the widespread use of insurance as a funding vehicle for buy-sell agreements, not all authorities are in accord as to its utility. Two common points that are frequently mentioned pertain to the artificial value that life insurance places on a practice, and the actual loss the insurance premiums can represent when used to fund buy-sell agreements in a partnership.

An insurance policy purchased for the value of a practice sets the amount that the deceased partner's beneficiaries can expect to receive, but this amount may not conform to the true worth of the practice at the time of the partner's death. Furthermore, the partner to whose estate the proceeds are paid shares in the cost of the premiums. Thus the partner's estate receives an amount that was purchased with the deceased's own income, which is no more than any insured who takes out an insurance policy would expect to receive.

On the other hand, if the partner had taken out a policy personally and paid the premiums out of his partnership income (which was in effect being done when the buy-sell policy described above was purchased), he would be entitled to the proceeds of the policy and the value of the practice as well (which would be paid by the surviving partner or by a new partner assuming his partnership interest). Thus, a buy-sell agreement, although it offers some security, may not be the appropriate arrangement for those practitioners who would prefer to buy the life insurance as individuals and leave the practice purchase to some other alternative to be described in the partnership contract.

Partnership Agreements

Rather than sell their practices outright, many optometrists prefer to plan for the transition into retirement through the creation of a partnership. A younger optometrist is brought in, gradually acquires equal ownership in the practice, and at some time later the older practitioner retires and the younger doctor in turn brings in a new partner (or associate). Of course, there are reasons other than planning for retirement that cause optometrists to resort to partnership: the optometrist may wish to enjoy the increased freedom that partnership offers (compared to sole proprietorship); the optometrist may decide to merge his practice with that of another practitioner or may desire to expand services by bringing in another doctor; or the optometrist may be seeking to alter his practice in terms of location or services or be so busy that he needs another practitioner to provide efficient patient care. Each of these reasons for entering the partnership mode of practice carries with it slightly different contractual demands and requires that the written instrument describing the partnership provisions be drafted in a slightly different manner.

Optometrists may be wary of partnership because of the intensely personal nature of the arrangement, and compatibility must rightly be considered one of the key ingredients of any partnership. For this reason, there should be a period of associateship before an actual partnership is formed. The associateship does not convey any interest in the partnership to the associate, even if the associateship agreement expresses the intention of the parties to discuss partnership at the conclusion of the trial period. It is left to the partnership agreement to determine the percentage of ownership, the income to be received by each partner, how to divide partnership interests in the event of disability, dissolution, or death, and similar matters.[9]

The complexity of these issues places a large burden on the negotiations preceding the final agreement. If possible, nothing should be omitted from the written contract (probably an unreachable goal). The reason for such completeness is that legal action is often resorted to in the event the contract is itself silent or unclear and there is disagreement between the parties as to their intent at the time they entered into the contract. The common law provides for remedies if the contract is breached by either of the parties. It should be noted that the courts will not force a party who has contracted to provide personal services to continue to provide these services against his will; they may find the person liable for damages (money) but will not force him to remain at work. Thus an associate or partner who decides to leave cannot be held involuntarily.

Many disagreements between partners will be resolved by the Uniform Partnership Act (UPA), which has been adopted by statute in all states except Louisiana. The UPA is the law that will be applied in the event the partnership agreement is silent or unclear or unenforceable. Whenever partnership is contemplated, the articles of partnership should be drawn up by a competent attorney so that the intent of the parties meets the letter of the law.

The following brief discussion of partnership contracts is intended to be used as a guideline only and should be employed solely for reference purposes and not for the purpose of drafting an actual contract. That task should be left to an attorney.

Recitals

There are several preliminary matters that must be described in the agreement: The identification of the parties, the applicable state law, and the general provisions for approving additional partners being among the most significant. Another important matter is the partnership name, which should be specifically described within the agreement.

Parties. The undersigned, (name), hereinafter referred to as "Senior" and (name), hereinafter referred to as "Junior", desiring to associate themselves as partners, hereby adopt the following as their Articles of Partnership.

Law applicable. This partnership is organized subject to the laws of (state), and where there is no contrary provision in these Articles, the rights of the parties with respect to each other and with other persons shall be govered by the applicable provisions of the (state) Uniform Partnership Act, effective (date), and the (state) Surviving Partners Act, effective (date).

Name. The name of the partnership shall be and is ________.

Members and Status. The members of this partnership shall be of one class only, to wit: general.

The members and addresses of the partners are as follows: (List)

No person may be admitted as a new general partner excepting by the unanimous consent of both general partners.

In the event of any change in the membership, a suitable certificate shall be filed in the office of the (identify).

Partners may be *general* or *limited.* As the title implies, a limited partner is one who has a less-than-full obligation to the partnership. This limited obligation is usually expressed in terms of the financial liability of the partner, which cannot exceed the actual contribution to the partnership made by the limited partner. Such arrangements are signified by the title Limited or Ltd. following the partnership name.

Purposes and Powers

A key aspect of any partnership is the power to be conferred upon each partner to represent the partnership in business matters. It is typically the express intent of the partnership agreement to limit these powers so that the partnership will not be adversely affected by a profligate partner.

Section 1. *Character of the Business.* The character of the business is the practice of optometry.

Section 2. *Powers of Partners.* The partners shall participate equally in the general management of the partnership, each being constituted an agent of the partnership for the purpose of carrying on its business.

Each shall devote his entire business time to the affairs of the partnership.

Section 3. *Limitations upon Powers of Partners.*

(a) *Name and Assets.* Neither partner shall use the partnership name or assets in any way except for the transaction of the legitimate partnership business, nor shall either partner do any act in contravention of these Articles of Partnership.

(b) *Imposed by Law.* Neither partner unless authorized by the other partner shall have any power or authority to do any act prohibited by law to be done by a single partner.

The powers of partners can be a complex legal subject all in themselves, particularly when applied to the ability of partners to sign legally binding contracts based upon their apparent authority to do so. Another application of the issue of power concerns individual obligations for contractual agreements versus those incurred by the partnership entity. A partner who seeks to obligate the partnership (rather than himself personally) should always sign a contract in his official capacity ("Dr. John Jones, partner, for Jones and Smith, partnership") rather than as an individual ("John Jones"). When dealing with contracts requiring the transfer of large sums of money, a legal advisor should be consulted in order to avoid unexpected liability.

Place of Business and Responsibilities

The partnership agreement should specify the place of business (or branch offices, if it is a multisite practice) and the expected hours of business. Such provisions are especially important if one of the partners contemplates having to work at a branch office or desires to work less than full-time.

Section 1. *Place of Business.* The business to be conducted by this partnership shall be in (address), excepting as same may be moved by the unanimous agreement of both partners.

Section 2. *Responsibilities.* Each partner shall devote his full time and energies to the partnership business, and it is acknowledged by the execution of this instrument that each partner shall be a regular full-time practicing optometrist. In the event a partner desires to devote less than full time to the partnership, then his percentage entitlements as well as the other benefits as set out by this instrument shall be the subject of negotiation in an attempt to amicably provide him with compensation commensurate with the services he is performing and commensurate with his worth to the partnership.

Capital and Partner's Interests

In order to initiate the partnership, certain assets—either in cash or property—must be contributed to the business. For tax purposes, a careful record of each partner's contributions (and their value) must be maintained.

Section 1. *Total Capital.* The capital with which this partnership shall begin business is the sum of ________ Thousand Dollars ($,000). This sum is represented by a joint loan made by the partners and contributed as capital.

Section 2. *Contributions.* A financial statement reflecting the contribution of the partners is attached hereto and marked Exhibit A for identification and made a part hereof.

Section 3. *Payment before Beginning Business.* All of said items constituting capital shall be paid in, turned over, and assigned to the partnership before it commences business.

Section 4. *Books to Reflect.* A capital account reflecting the contribution made by each partner shall be maintained in the books of account of the partnership.

Section 5. *Withdrawals.* Neither partner may withdraw from the partnership any sum which will operate to diminish the contributed capital without unanimous action of all partners.

A key portion of this section will be those clauses that establish the income of each partner and the partnership interest owned by the individual partners. As discussed in this chapter, the customary arrangement between a senior and a junior doctor will provide for a gradual increase in the income to be paid the junior partner and in the percentage of ownership he enjoys. Such an arrangement requires division both of salary (paid as a draw against profits) and of any profit remaining at the conclusion of the tax year (i.e., any money remaining after all salaries, expenses, and debts of the partnership have been paid). There are several ways in which such an agreement could be constructed, with the biggest variable being the percent of the profit allocated to each partner. Since circumstances differ between partners, it is best to have the contract drawn to suit the particular circumstances of the partnership. But most contracts will require a three- to six-year period during which to divide the profits, the difference between the senior and junior partner's share being the largest during the first year and reaching equality by the last year. Likewise, the salary will reflect a difference between the two partners that favors the senior doctor initially but gradually reaches equality. This differential permits the capital contribution of the junior partner to become equal with that of the senior partner.

Section 6. *Division of Profits.* All income from the partnership shall be placed in the partnership account, and after all stipulated expenses of the partnership are paid, the net profit shall be computed as follows:

DIVISION OF PROFITS	DR. SENIOR (%)	DR. JUNIOR (%)
1st year	70	30
2nd year	65	35
3rd year	60	40
4th year	55	15
5th year	50	50

Section 7. *Drawing on Account.* The drawings on account of profits by Dr. Senior and Dr. Junior shall be as follows:

DRAWING PER MONTH	DR. SENIOR ($)	DR. JUNIOR ($)
1st year	4,000	2,000
2nd year	4,200	2,500
3rd year	4,400	3,000
4th year	4,600	3,500
5th year	4,800	4,000
Thereafter until both parties' capital contribution is equal	5,000	4,500
When the capital contribution of both parties is equal	5,000	5,000

Section 8. *Leaving Profits.* Either partner, with the consent of the other partner, may leave any portion of his share of the earnings in the business for use in con-

nection therewith; any amounts thus left shall be considered loans to the partnership and shall bear interest at the rate of ___ percent (___%) per annum.

Section 9. *Distribution of Profits.* Profits shall be distributed quarterly as soon as funds are available after the quarterly closing of the partnership books, or as the partners mutually agree.

Section 10. *Losses.* In the event the partnership sustains losses, the same shall be borne on a 50-50 basis, except that during the first four years the basis shall be the same as the profit percentage.

There are other provisions that can be included in the contract, such as those that confer extra income or a credit against the amount owed by the junior partner for his partnership interest; these clauses are frequently used when the senior partner wishes to reduce his time in the office.

Accounting

The financial records of the partnership should be provided for, both in terms of their organization and with regard to access to them by the partners.

Section 1. *Accounting Period.* Subject to change by unanimous action of the partners, the calendar year is hereby adopted as the partnership accounting period.

Section 2. *Books of Account.* Books of account accurately reflecting the partnership's business and financial status shall be kept in the partnership office located at (address). Said books shall not be removed from the office premises without the mutual consent of all partners.

Section 3. *Right of Inspection.* Each partner shall be entitled at all times to inspect the books and records of account, either personally or through attorneys or accountants.

Vacations

The right to a paid vacation is one that should be spelled out with some specificity, particularly if there is a difference in the amount of time each partner may be absent from the practice. In a senior-junior arrangement, it is not unusual to find that the vacation allowances differ between partners.

Vacations. Each partner shall be entitled to a paid vacation of the length and duration as follows:

a. Dr. Senior shall receive a vacation of four (4) weeks per year.
b. Dr. Junior shall receive a vacation of two (2) weeks during years one and two; a vacation of three (3) weeks during years three and four; and a vacation of four (4) weeks during year five and thereafter.

During said vacation each partner shall be entitled to his salary and percentage of net annual profits as hereinabove set out. If any partner takes more vacation than permitted by the terms of this section, then he shall forfeit during the extra vacation his entitlement to his weekly salary. The percentage of net annual profit entitlements for all partners shall continue during the period any partner is taking a vacation in excess of that allowed him. All vacations may be carried forward from year-to-year, and any unused vacation may be used in a subsequent year, provided however, that no more than two (2) extra weeks of vacation shall be taken in any given year.

In addition to paid vacation, there are other benefits that can be specified by the partnership agreement, such as professional dues, allowances for books and journals, and expenses for continuing education. Whether paid out of partnership funds or out of the individual funds of the partners, these are expenses that will decrease the profit to be divided by the partners at the end of the year. Thus, any inequities in the benefits allocated to the senior or the junior doctor should be carefully thought out.

Special Covenants

There are a number of problems peculiar to partnerships and the joint liability of partners that should be enumerated in the contract, such as casualty and liability insurance for the practice, limitations on the financial obligations of the partners, and restrictions on the ability of the partners to use the partnership other than for partnership business.

Each of the partners hereby covenants with the other:

Section 1. *Expenditures over $100.00.* That no single item of equipment, fixture, apparatus, or alteration or improvements to the building costing more than $100.00 shall be purchased or made without the consent of both of the partners.

Section 2. *Insurance.* That policies of insurance shall be kept in force at times as follows:

(a) Fire insurance with extended coverage upon the buildings, equipment, fixtures and inventory to the full insurable value thereof;
(b) Public liability with limits of $_______ and $_______ and property damage with limits of $_______.

Section 3. *Payment of Debts.* That neither partner will permit the capital to be impaired nor fail to pay the lawful debts for labor, merchandise, materials, and obligations for whatsoever promptly as the same falls due.

Section 4. *No Monies Lent.* That no monies or properties belonging to the partnership will be lent to any person nor used except on partnership business.

Section 5. *Suretyship.* That neither of them will become the endorser or act as surety or guarantor of the debts of any other person, firm, or corporation.

Section 6. *Personal Debts.* That neither of them will incur any indebtedness which would obligate his partner other than for normal business expenses.

Section 7. *Bonds.* That neither of them will go surety upon the bond of any person to secure his appearance in any court.

Section 8. *Margin Account.* That neither of them will buy stocks or commodities on margin or engage in any other business.

Section 9. *Banking Institution.* That the partnership shall use any banking institution that the partners mutually agree upon and at the commencement of the partnership the partners agree to use a branch bank of (bank) and that the partners agree that all checks written on the partnership checking account shall be countersigned by the partners.

Of course, partners are responsible for the negligence of one another, and this responsibility cannot be limited by the contract. But insurance can be acquired to protect the partners against this eventuality.

Covenant Not to Compete

Contracts to form a partnership frequently include covenants not to compete, which are intended to preserve the partnership patient base in the event one of the partners leaves the practice. These covenants specify that, in the event one of the partners leaves the partnership, he or she agrees not to practice within a circumscribed distance from the practice for a specific period, usually one or two years. In a few states these agreements will not be enforced by the courts, and so a departing partner cannot be legally constrained from setting up a new practice in violation of the covenant.[10] In most states, however, covenants not to compete in partnership agreements are enforceable, and the partnership may obtain an order from the court restraining the partner from violating the time and distance requirements of the covenant. In some states, the courts will enforce the covenant even if it goes beyond reasonable bounds of time and distance by reforming these restrictions to make them reasonable. Another remedy available to the partnership is to ask for the payment of liquidated damages, which may be specified in the partnership contract as an amount the departing partner agrees to pay should he or she violate the covenant not to compete. The damages must bear a reasonable relation to the injury suffered by the partnership to be enforceable.

The covenant can also prohibit the departing partner from soliciting or hiring any employees of the partnership for a period of time or from using a name, title, or phonetically similar name or title to that used by the partnership. The purpose of these restrictions is, again, to preserve the partnership.

Covenant not to compete. Dr. Junior acknowledges that his services rendered hereunder are of a special and unusual character which have a unique value to the partnership, the loss of which may not be adequately compensated by damages in an action at law. In view of the unique value to the partnership of the services of Dr. Junior for which Dr. Junior has contracted hereunder, and because of the confidential information to be obtained by or disclosed to Dr. Junior, and as a material inducement to Dr. Senior to enter into this Agreement, Dr. Junior covenants and agrees as follows:

Section 1. For a period of _____ months after he ceases to be in partnership with Dr. Senior, Dr. Junior shall not, directly or indirectly, engage in the practice of optometry on his own account, or become interested therein, directly or indirectly, as a partner, shareholder, director, officer, or employee in competition with Dr. Senior or the partnership within _____ miles of the corporate limits of the city of ________. In the event of breach hereof, it is specifically agreed that Dr. Senior shall have all rights and remedies for relief as provided by law or in equity, including the right of injunction. Alternatively and in lieu of equitable relief, at the election of Dr. Senior, it is specifically agreed that Dr. Senior shall be entitled to liquidated damages of $________.

Section 2. During Dr. Junior's association hereunder and for a period of _____ months after he ceases to be in partnership with Dr. Senior, Dr. Junior shall not, directly or indirectly, solicit for employment or employ any employee of the partnership.

Section 3. Dr. Junior further covenants and agrees that after he ceases to be in partnership with Dr. Senior, he shall not in any manner appropriate the use of, directly or indirectly, the name ________ or any facsimile or phonetically similar word, phrase or mark for use in association with, in promotion of, or in any manner connected with or related to the practice of optometry. Dr. Junior has carefully read and considered the provisions of this Article and, having done so, agrees that the restrictions set forth are fair and reasonable and are reasonably required for the protection of the partnership and Dr. Senior. In the event that, notwithstanding the foregoing, any of the provisions hereof shall be held to be invalid or unenforceable, the remaining provisions thereof shall nevertheless continue to be valid and enforceable as though the invalid or unenforceable parts had not been included therein.

Because the enforceability of covenants not to compete depends on the decisions of state courts, optometrists should always consult legal counsel whenever contemplating their usage.

Duration and Dissolution

Although a corporation can exist in perpetuity, a partnership can exist only as long as its partners. Since personal relationships frequently alter the duration of partnerships, it is necessary to include provisions for the dissolution of the business.[11] Dissolution may be mandatory (such as upon the death or insanity of a partner) or optional (such as upon the violation of the articles of partnership or by the giving of appropriate notice). In the event of dissolution, the contract must specify how the partnership property is to be divided. Of particular importance are the patient records; unless the contract is explicit as to their division, they can become a source of acrimonious debate or even of prolonged legal action.

Section 1. *Term.* The partnership hereby created shall be perpetual, subject, however, to termination as herein provided.

Section 2. *Dissolution Upon Notice.* After five (5) years, but not before, either partner by sixty (60) days' notice in writing to the other partner may require a dissolution and winding up of the partnership.

Section 3. *Dissolution Upon Death or Insanity.* The death or insanity of either partner shall cause a dissolution of the partnership.

Section 4. *Dissolution for Violation of Articles.* In the event the partners, or any of them, default in the performance of the special covenants herein provided and upon notice in writing fails to cure said default or defaults within ten (10) days, the complaining partner may cause a dissolution of the partnership as described by the (state) state statutes hereinabove mentioned.

Section 5. *Manner of Liquidation.* Upon the dissolution of the partnership by the expiration of the term for which it is organized, by unanimous agreement of the parties, or by the happening of one of the events specified in Sections 2, 3, or 4 of this Article, liquidation and winding up shall proceed in accordance with the law of (state).

Section 6. *Property Previously Held by Partners.* Upon the dissolution of the partnership by the expiration of the term for which it is organized, by unanimous agreement of the parties, or by the happening of one of the events specified in Sections 2, 3, or 4 of this Article, but not inconsistent with any "Buy and Sell Agreement" that the parties might hereinafter enter into, the parties agree as follows:

(a) All items of personal property contributed by the partners or purchased by the partnership after the execution of this agreement shall become the sole property of the partnership, except the personal refraction room equipment and the furniture and furnishings belonging to each partner before the execution of this agreement, which shall remain the exclusive property of each partner.

(b) All patient records belonging to each partner prior to the execution of this agreement shall remain the exclusive property of each of the partners, and all new records—those coming into the partnership following the execution of this agreement—shall be treated in such a way that each of said patients will be notified of the dissolution so that the patients shall have a choice of whichever doctor they elect to continue with for future treatment and service.

Special care must be given to drafting the clauses that permit a voluntary dissolution upon the giving of adequate notice. These clauses should be constructed in accordance with the individual requirements of the partners, and should provide a workable means of terminating the partnership that is fair.

Disability of Partners

One of the most important sections of the partnership deals with the possibility that one of the partners will become disabled. There are many complexities that have to be considered by the partners at the time the agreement is entered into, including the definition of temporary, permanent, and partial disability for purposes of the partnership, what income can be provided to the disabled partner, the length of time for which benefits may be paid, and the fair value of the disabled partner's share of the practice in the event it has to be purchased. Professional assistance will be required to determine the specific provisions that will be equitable given the age, earnings, and percent of ownership of each of the partners. Since disability is a more likely eventuality than death, consideration should be given to the purchase of private disability insurance.

Section 1. *Temporary Disability.* In the event that any of the partners shall become disabled so as to be unable to attend to the affairs of the partnership (that is, actively engage in the practice of optometry as normally done day-by-day), his share of the partnership profits and losses shall be reduced or treated as follows:

(a) *Less than 30 days.* A partner is entitled to a full share of partnership profits or losses.

(b) *Thirty-one (31) through sixty (60) days.* A partner shall be entitled to two-thirds (2/3) of his share of the partnership profits or losses.

(c) *Sixty-one (61) through ninety (90) days.* A

partner shall be entitled to one-third (1/3) of his share of partnership profits or losses.

(d) *Ninety-one (91) through three hundred sixty-five (365) days.* A disabled partner, in case of his disability extending beyond ninety (90) days, shall arrange for and provide for a qualified and licensed optometrist within thirty (30) days; otherwise, the able partner shall have the privilege of arranging for a qualified and licensed optometrist to substitute in the place of the disabled partner; provided, however, that in either event the salary of said replacement optometrist shall be borne by the disabled partner and deducted from the disabled partner's share of profits. The disabled partner shall be entitled to the difference between the cost and additional expenses to provide for the substitute optometrist and his share of the partnership profits.

(e) *After one (1) year of disablement.* In the event that the disability shall continue for a period of one (1) year, the remaining partner shall purchase the interest of the disabled partner. The purchase price shall be paid by the remaining partner in ______ quarterly installments, the first installment to be paid no later than three (3) months after the expiration of the one (1) year disability period, and the total amount of the stated value plus the other items, as set out in Section 3 of this Article. However, if the parties mutually agree to dissolve the partnership rather than the remaining partner purchasing the interest of the disabled partner, the mode and manner of dissolution shall be carried out as described in Article ______ of this agreement.

Section 2. *Partial Disability.* In the event of a partner's partial disability which enables his participation in the practice on a part-time basis, and if the partners mutually agree, the disabled partner's share of the partnership profits and losses shall be proportional to his productive contribution to the gross income of the partnership. Provided, however, if after one (1) year of such limited practice by a partially disabled partner the books and records of the partnership reflect that the disabled partner is unable to produce at least one third (1/3) of the total gross income of the practice, the disabled partner shall, by certified mail, notify the able partner that the partnership shall be dissolved or demand the purchase of his interest by the able partner. The able partner, within thirty (30) days after receipt of such notice, shall cooperate in the following mode and manner of dissolution as set forth in Article ______ of this agreement, or proceed with the purchase of the partnership interest as set forth in the foregoing Section 1 of this Article.

Section 3. *Stated Value of the Business.* For the purpose of this Article relating to the purchase of the disabled partner's interest by the able partner, the stated value of the business is $________, and shall remain so unless the partners mutually agree from time to time, in writing, what the stated value shall be. In addition to one half (1/2) of the stated value, the disabled partner shall also be entitled to fifty percent (50%) of all cash amounts in the bank representing partnership assets and an amount equal to forty percent (40%) of the accounts receivable reflected on the books as of the date the three hundred sixty-fifth (365th) day occurs. The disabled partner shall also be entitled to the return of his personal refraction room equipment. When this Section applies to other Articles in this agreement, the cut-off dates shall be the date of notice or the date of death, whichever is applicable.

When determining the value of the practice for purposes of a required transfer between the partners, the contract should provide for either a stated cash amount or for the use of a formula to determine the amount to be paid. If a cash value is used, the contract should require periodic evaluation (e.g., annually) so as to adjust the value in accordance with the growth (or diminution) of the practice.

Death of a Partner

As described in this chapter, the use of life insurance to provide funds in the event of the death of one of the partners has been a frequent provision of partnership agreements. Life insurance, however, may be used in any of several ways, or not at all, according to the wishes of the partners. If insurance is used, the customary policy purchased is one of term insurance, which may be for a stated amount (periodically renewed) or for a decreasing amount. If a decreasing term policy is employed, the partnership agreement must provide for a means of paying the balance between that amount covered by the insurance and the fair value of the practice as agreed upon in the partnership contract.

Section 1. *Insurance.* Each partner has insured the life of the other partner in the following mode and manner:

(a) Dr. Senior is the owner of a certain term life insurance policy on the life of Dr. Junior, issued by ________ in the amount of $________, and the monthly premiums are in the amount of $________.

(b) Dr. Junior is the owner of a certain term life insurance policy on the life of Dr. Senior, issued by ________ in the amount of $________, and the monthly premiums are in the amount of $________.

Section 2. *Purchase of Partnership Interest on Death.* Upon the death of either partner, the surviving partner shall purchase the entire interest of the deceased partner in the partnership, and the estate of the decedent shall sell such interest to the surviving partner. The entire purchase price for the interest of the deceased partner shall be paid in cash to his estate within thirty (30) days after the appointment and qualifications of the legal representative of such estate. Where the insurance proceeds are of sufficient amount to fully cover the purchase price as hereinafter set forth and the proceeds of insurance exceed the purchase price required to be paid in full, any excess shall be paid to the owner of the policy. In the event that the proceeds of insurance shall be insufficient to properly cover the purchase price, then, after applying the total proceeds from the insurance policy to the purchase price, the difference so remaining shall be paid in four (4) equal quarterly installments, beginning with thirty (30) days after the date of death of the deceased partner.

Section 3. *Purchase Price.* The purchase price of the interest of a deceased partner shall be computed in the same manner as set forth in Section ________ of Article ________ of this agreement.

Section 4. *Transfer of Partnership Interest.* Upon receipt of the purchase price the legal representative of the estate of the deceased partner shall execute and deliver to the surviving partner all documents required to evidence his purchase of the decedent's partnership interest. Simultaneously the surviving partner shall deliver to the legal representative of the estate of the deceased partner an agreement indemnifying the estate against any liabilities of the partnership.

Section 5. *Purchase of Policies Upon Death or Termination.* Upon the termination of the partnership for any reason during the lives of the partners, or upon the death of either partner, the insured partner shall have the right to purchase from the other partner or from the estate of the deceased partner all policies insuring his life taken out pursuant to this agreement. The price for such policies shall equal their cash value on the date of termination or death, plus a proportionate part of the premium last paid before such date which covers the period extending beyond such date. The price shall be paid in cash within thirty (30) days after the termination of the partnership or the death of a partner. If this right to purchase is not exercised within the thirty (30) day period, it shall lapse and all rights under the policies shall belong the owner thereof.

Section 6. *Term.* In the event of the termination of the partnership for any reason prior to the death of either partner, all rights under this Article shall terminate, except as otherwise provided in Section 5.

Section 7. *Benefit.* This Article shall bind the parties and their respective estates.

Prior to initiating any insurance agreement, the partners will have to initiate detailed discussions with insurance and financial advisors.

Obligation as Lessees

If the partnership has obligated itself to a long-term lease for office space, it is beneficial to include a clause in the partnership agreement that describes the responsibilities of the partners in the event of dissolution of the partnership or the death of a partner.

> The partners are personally liable under a certain written lease, as lessees, with ________ as lessor, and the partners agree that they shall so remain liable regardless of dissolution of the partnership. However, in the event of the death of a partner or the purchase of the entire interest of the partnership by a partner, the surviving partner agrees to assume the full responsibility of the lease covenants and agrees to save the withdrawing partner or his estate harmless from future liability for rent and other material conditions and covenants, during the present term of said lease or any extensions or renewals thereof.

The office lease is a long-term legal obligation that requires professional consultation before it is entered into (see Chapter 49).

Effective Date

The partnership agreement should specify a date on which it becomes effective.

> The effective date of this agreement is ________, 19______.

Seal

The parties to the agreement will have to sign the contract, which acts as their seal, binding them to the contract.

> In witness therefore, Dr. Senior and Dr. Junior have hereunto affixed their signatures, on this the ______ day of ________, 19______.

As the preceding paragraphs have illustrated, a partnership agreement is a lengthy and complex legal document that requires a considerable amount of thought, planning, and compromise. Since it is intended to serve as the basis for an interpersonal relationship that may exist for decades and may involve the allocation of millions of dollars, it should be drafted by a competent attorney after detailed discussions and negotiations. A well-drafted and comprehensive instrument will be well worth its cost. Optometrists who, as prospective partners, decide to draft their agreement themselves, will probably pay far more later, as they seek to extract themselves from unanticipated legal entanglements.

A sample Partnership Agreement may be found in the Appendix.

Notes

1. For other perspectives on senior-junior partnerships, see Milkie, G., *Partnerships and Professional Corporations*, Optometric Development Enterprises, St. Louis, 1972; Elmstrom, G., *Advanced Management Strategies for Optometrists*, Professional Press, Chicago, 1982; and Baldwin, B., B. Christensen, and J. Melton, *Rx For Success*, Vision Publications, Midwest City, Okla., 1983.
2. Baldwin, R., Here's How To Take in an Associate... Painlessly, *Journal of the American Optometric Association*, vol. 53, no. 2, 1982, pp. 137–139.
3. See Hubler, R., My Born-Again Practice, *Review of Optometry*, vol. 119, no. 7, 1982, pp. 41–45.
4. See Milkie, supra note 1, for a more detailed discussion.
5. See Splitting the Partnership Melon, *Optometric Management*, vol. 16, no. 3, 1980, pp. 49–53.
6. Baldwin, B., How To Make a New Partner Immediately Productive, *Journal of the American Optometric Association*, vol. 53, no. 3, 1982, pp. 231–232.
7. Ibid.
8. Guild, A., *Professional Partnership Purchase Plans*, 2d ed., National Life Insurance Co., Montpelier, Vt., 1973.
9. Hammering Out the Partnership Agreement, *Optometric Management*, vol. 16, no. 3, 1980, pp. 29–34.
10. Restrictive covenants are described by Stetler, C.J., and A.R. Moritz, *Doctor and Patient and the Law*, 4th ed., C.V. Mosby, St. Louis, 1962, and are discussed in the following annotations of the *American Law Reports*: 62 A.L.R. 3d 918, 62 A.L.R. 3d 970, and 62 A.L.R. 3d 1014.
11. What Our Group's Separation Agreement *Didn't* Cover, *Medical Economics*, vol. 57, no. 4, Feb. 18, 1980, pp. 133–138.

Chapter 46

Agreements to Form a Professional Corporation

The professional corporation may open a new avenue to accumulation of wealth beyond what would possibly be available otherwise. There is, therefore, obviously a strong incentive to incorporate. However, it is just as obvious that you should not make the move to incorporate without consideration of all of the tax as well as other non-tax advantages, disadvantages, and problems. Sound professional advice is required to thoroughly evaluate these vital considerations and to develop a stable corporate practice.
—George M. Milkie, O.D., *Partnerships and Professional Corporations*

Creating a Professional Corporation

The decision to incorporate, as Dr. Milkie points out, cannot be made strictly on the basis of anticipated financial rewards or without the benefit of sound professional advice. The problems are too technical and require tax and legal expertise that is beyond the experience of the majority of health care practitioners. Therefore, the first step in the long voyage to form a professional corporation is to resolve any doubts that incorporation is the appropriate step to take. With the changing character of tax laws, which have greatly improved retirement benefits for nonincorporated practitioners, it will be the rare optometrist who finds that incorporation is the best business organization for him. Less than 5 percent of optometrists were in incorporated practices at the start of the decade of the 1980s, and it is not likely that this figure will change substantially in the coming years.[1]

To form a professional corporation, optometrists should consult a capable attorney who has had previous experience not only with incorporation but also with the tax problems encountered by these business entities. Particularly if partnerships or well-established proprietorships containing numerous assets are to be incorporated, or where a tax-sheltered retirement plan is to be established, the attorney should be able to anticipate tax and legal problems and should provide guidance that will enable the incorporating practitioners to achieve a smooth transition.[2]

In forming the corporation and in setting it into practice, there are several documents and a number of procedural matters that must be attended to (see Chapter 39 for a summary). We will discuss the following major considerations[3]:

- The preincorporation agreement
- Preincorporation procedures
- The articles of incorporation
- Postincorporation procedures
- Corporate bylaws
- Employment contracts
- Stock-purchase agreements
- The section 1244 election
- Profit-sharing and pension plans and other benefits
- Co-ownership with a physician

The Preincorporation Agreement

Prior to incorporation the prospective shareholders should execute an agreement that sets forth their intention to form a professional corporation. In many cases it will consist of a subscription agreement that expresses the intent of the incorporators to purchase stock through a cash purchase or through the transfer of personal assets to the corporation. (Partners may transfer the partnership assets to the corporation in exchange for their individual shares of the stock.) The date of transfer should be stated.

The agreement can specify how the incorporators will be reimbursed for expenses they incur for the benefit of the corporation prior to the date of incorporation. It can also provide for the collection of accounts receivable from the prior individual proprietorship or partnership (which usually is allowed to continue for that purpose while the new corporation is functioning). Provision should also be made for the transfer of accounts payable from the private practices that are being transferred into the corporation.

There should be some means of providing for the dissolution of the corporation or of the prospective shareholders in the event the corporation is not in fact formed. Separation of assets and transfer back to the incorporators will be necessary in order to restore the practices to their prior status.

The more comprehensive the preincorporation agreement, the more certain the incorporators can be that they have in fact attained a meeting of the minds on the details of the incorporation.

Preincorporation Procedures

If real property is involved, appraisals of the property, title binders, leasehold agreements, and other legal documents should be acquired for the corporate file. If any of the incorporators are obligated under existing contracts, the effect of incorporation should be ascertained, by the corporate attorney if necessary.

Insurance policies already in effect should also be studied to determine whether transfer to the corporation is feasible. A key task during the preincorporation period is the determination of the most appropriate profit-sharing or pension plan for the various corporate employees because the attorney will need to qualify the plan with the IRS before it can be instituted.[4] Another important decision concerns the selection of corporate fringe benefits. Both tax and legal advice will be required in order to select the most affordable benefits.

The Articles of Incorporation

The articles of incorporation must be drafted by the corporate attorney and filed with the state government (Secretary of State). In those states that only permit professional associations, this document will not have to be filed.[5]

The articles of incorporation contain a statement describing the type of services that are to be rendered, the purpose of the corporation, the address of the principal office, the duration of the corporation's existence, and certain statements pertaining to the licensure of the shareholders and the recognition of governing state law. In addition, the articles should contain a statement regarding the liability of shareholders for the acts of employees and should provide procedures to be followed in the event of the death or disqualification of shareholders. All provisions should be in compliance with state law regulating professional corporations.

The articles are signed and notarized and filed with the state. In some states a copy may have to be provided to the board of optometry.

Postincorporation Procedures

Necessary items such as the corporate seal, stock certificates, and stock register must be acquired. The first board of directors meeting must be held and the minutes recorded. (The minutes will often have to be submitted to the attorney prior to filing with the state.) At the first meeting the corporate bylaws should be adopted, the officers elected, and other necessary organizational duties performed. Contracts must be prepared for corporate employees by the attorney (discussed *infra*).

Corporate Bylaws

The bylaws provide guidance for the day-to-day activities of the corporation and establish the relationships between shareholders, directors, officers, employees, and others for the conduct of business activities. The bylaws are important to the directors and officers since they state the procedure for their election, provide for their compensation, and in general provide a framework for the performance of their responsibilities. The bylaws also set forth the procedure by which they may be amended.

Employment Contracts

The corporation should offer written contracts to its employees, enumerating the salary to be paid, employee rights, and other essential aspects of employment. To avoid the prospect of having the corporation considered a personal holding company by the IRS, the contract should indicate that the corporation has the authority to control the activities of the employee (see Chapter 39 for a discussion of the personal holding tax).

As with most employment contracts, the benefits to be granted to the employee should be described, especially insurance benefits for which the corporation receives tax-favored treatment.[6] Termination of the contract should also be provided for, and the stock-purchase agreement should be in accord with the terms of the contract. A restrictive covenant may also be included.[7]

Stock-Purchase Agreements

These agreements are necessary because of state restrictions as to ownership of professional corporations. The corporation may use a separate agreement or may provide for withdrawal in the articles of incorporation or in the bylaws.

If a separate stock-purchase agreement is drafted, it will control the entry and withdrawal of shareholders. When a shareholder withdraws from the corporation, after the passage of a period of time set by law the corporation must purchase his shares of stock. The agreement should specify some method of determining the value of the shares and the basis for the amount to be paid by the corporation. Failure to exercise the option to purchase the shares may result in the dissolution of the corporation.[8]

In determining the price of the stock, the largest consideration is unrealized receivables, which may be paid directly as termination pay or included in the value of the stock (this problem is discussed separately herein).

The Section 1244 Election

Section 1244 of the Internal Revenue Code allows incorporated professionals to elect certain tax advantages if stock is sold at a loss.[9] This election may be made without penalty through a resolution of the board of directors because the resolution may be abandoned at any time.

Profit-Sharing and Pension Plans and Other Benefits

These retirement plans and fringe benefits traditionally have been the principal reason for incorporating. The plan that is adopted by the corporation should first receive a determination from the IRS that it is qualified. In order to receive federal tax advantages, the corporate contributions must be in compliance with the Employee Retirement Income Security Act (ERISA), which requires that non-shareholder employees receive no less favorable treatment than the shareholder-employees under the plan.[10] The details of profit-sharing and pension plans are described in Chapter 39.

Co-Ownership with a Physician

The original state laws recognizing the right of professionals to incorporate uniformly limited the ownership of the corporation to individuals holding the same degree, which meant that physicians were prohibited from incorporating as co-owners with other professionals, such as optometrists. These laws effectively barred optometrists from practicing with ophthalmologists on an equal basis because the ophthalmologists could point out that state law did not permit optometrists to become shareholders in a corporation owned by physicians.

As a result, optometrists were by-and-large relegated to the role of employee. During the past decade, however, several states have modified these laws to permit co-ownership by optometrists and ophthalmologists, a development of significance not only for private practitioners but also for health maintenance organizations and other health delivery systems that have relegated optometrists to nonownership roles. Consequently, an optometrist may purchase shares of stock in a professional corporation owned by an ophthalmologist in these states.[11]

If the earning power or retirement goals of the optometrist and the ophthalmologist are widely disparate, co-ownership of the corporation may not be feasible. An alternative arrangement would be to form a partnership of corporations, through which each of the practitioners obtains more flexibility in determining how to allocate income or how to provide for retirement. Such an arrangement must satisfy federal and state requirements or its tax advantages will be disallowed. Practitioners considering this alternative must consult legal and tax counsel to determine that it is reasonable in their case. This same caution is advisable in corporate partnerships between optometrists.

This impressive list of responsibilities continues throughout the life of the corporation, as shareholders change, benefits are altered, and financial transactions occur. Because of the complexity of management—all technical requirements must be complied with or the corporate structure may be questioned by the IRS—an attorney's assistance is necessary. One of the more difficult management problems the attorney will face is advising the corporation as to how to value its stock when there is a withdrawal of one of the shareholders.

Valuing Corporate Stock

State law requires the corporation to purchase the stock of a withdrawing shareholder within a specified period of time. The same event occurs if the shareholder dies or is permanently disabled. The principal problem in these transactions is the determination of a fair price, which is set by the corporation.

Many stock-purchase agreements include the book value of the corporation's equipment, furnishings, and fixtures in the price to be paid. Another approach is to base the price on the fair market value (the price for which it could be sold). Other considerations include the value of accounts receivable for the withdrawing shareholder, the use of separation pay, and life insurance.

Value of Assets

Determining the value of the withdrawing shareholder's portion of corporate assets presents a choice between two alternatives: fair market value and book value. Each has its weaknesses.

Fair market value attempts to allocate to the assets a price based upon the worth of the equipment and furnishings at the time of the withdrawal of the shareholder. In order to obtain such a determination, expert appraisal will be needed. The better-written agreement will specify some means of obtaining the appraisal, usually by requiring the use of two experts and establishing a price based upon an average of the appraisals of the two.

An alternative technique is to use book value, which is the original purchase price less the annual depreciation that has been claimed. If accelerated depreciation has been used, artificially lowering the value of the equipment, a modified book value can be achieved by using a straight line depreciation for stock valuation purposes, the straight line basis being from ten to fifteen years. The modified book value and the book value have the advantage of being easy to determine.[12]

Accounts Receivable

Since unpaid accounts can constitute a significant sum in some practices, there is often provision for payment of the withdrawing shareholder's pro rata share in the stock-purchase agreement. These uncollected receivables are frequently valued on a formula basis that is structured so that the most current accounts receive the highest value, whereas the accounts in excess of a certain period of time (six months customarily) are given a very low value, or no value. An alternative means of accomplishing this valuation is to assign an arbitrary percentage for all accounts that have had some activity within a certain period of time. For example, for all accounts of the departing shareholder for which a charge has been made or a payment received within six months of the valuation date the shareholder could receive a 90 percent reimbursement. Other percentages can be used to more accurately reflect the collections status of the corporate accounts.[13]

Separation Pay

In lieu of payment for accounts receivable, some stock purchase agreements specify the use of separation pay. These payments are made to the shareholder on a periodic basis for a stated period of time after the shareholder has left the corporation. They are tax-deductible to the corporation and are considered ordinary income for the shareholder (rather than a capital gain, which will result when the stock is sold after being owned by the partner for the required holding period).[14] Such an arrangement should be drafted by an attorney to avoid the possibility that it will be regarded as a taxable substitute for the purchase of the stock.

Life Insurance

Some stock-purchase agreements use life insurance to serve as the value of the stock in the event a shareholder dies. The insurance premiums are paid by the corporation, which holds the policies and becomes the beneficiary in the event of the death of any of the shareholders. These policies, however, tend to establish an artificial value for the stock that may be arbitrarily high or low.

If the life insurance purchased is whole life, the corporation will not receive a deduction for the premiums. Furthermore, since the deceased shareholder cannot give his stock to his family or place it in trust due to restrictions of state law, the proceeds that will be paid to his beneficiaries will be eligible for estate taxation.

There can also be economic loss to the estate of the shareholder who dies first, since had he paid for the insurance premiums himself (the corporation receives no deduction for whole life policies), his beneficiary would receive not only the insurance proceeds but also the value of the stock (see Chapter 45 for a discussion of "buy-sell" insurance arrangements). The use of insurance to artificially increase the worth of corporate stock is probably inadvisable.

Care should be taken when drafting agreements for the purchase of stock if there are also provisions in the corporate employment agreement that allow for the payment of sick pay. If serious disability is followed by death, the corporation may end up duplicating benefits, giving sick pay to the disabled shareholder for several months, then paying for the shareholder's stock after his death. A similar result can occur if a sick shareholder who has received several months of sick pay suffers a recurrence shortly after returning to work. The resulting financial strain on the corporation may be more than the shareholders intended, and so the corporate employment agreements and stock-purchase agreements should be constructed to avoid this problem.[15]

We will now turn to a description of some of the corporate contracts that are a necessary aspect of doing business as a professional corporation.

Corporate Agreements

The diversity of personal arrangements between shareholders makes it mandatory that such agreements be constructed by an able attorney who drafts the corporate documents so as to reflect the particular circumstances faced by the contracting parties. In particular, the corporate bylaws, employment contracts, and stock-purchase agreements should reflect the desires and opinions of the corporate shareholders and of their legal and financial advisors. Therefore, it would not be worthwhile to review specimen documents reflecting these agreements. Because there is a certain universality to the preincorporation agreement and to the articles of incorporation, we will briefly describe some of the necessary provisions of these contracts, illustrated by sample language, as the conclusion to this chapter.[16]

Preincorporation Agreement

The purpose of the preincorporation agreement is to commit to writing the intention of the incorporators to join together in an incorporated practice. The details are mostly organizational, describing the formation of the new business entity.

The agreement will begin with the identification of the incorporators and, if there is real property involved, with a statement as to the use of the property for the purposes of incorporation. If possible, a date by which to consummate the incorporation should be included.

AGREEMENT TO FORM A CORPORATION

Agreement made ________, 19___, between ________ and ________, doctors of optometry, all of City of ________, State of ________.

Whereas the parties have entered into an agreement for the purchase of the office building located at ________. City of ________, State of ________; and

Whereas the parties have agreed to organize a corporation to take title to and to own said property; and

Whereas the parties are members of an optometric partnership and intend to cause the corporation to lease the property to the partnership for use as optometric offices.

It is therefore agreed:

It will also be necessary to identify the applicable law, the formation of the corporation, and the name by which the corporation will be known.

1. *Formation of Corporation.* The parties shall organize a corporation under the laws of the State of ________ to be known as ________________.

Since the articles of incorporation will have to be filed with the state, mention of the requirements to be included therein—which deals with the identities of the incorporators and their stock subscriptions—is a common provision of preincorporation agreements.

Another important provision that can be included is the duration of the corporation, which, in the usual case, will be perpetual.

The purpose for which the corporation is formed should also be included.

2. *Articles of Incorporation.* The following provisions shall be included in the articles of incorporation:

(a) The initial Registered Agent shall be ________, attorney.
(b) The duration of the corporation shall be perpetual.
(c) The number of directors of the corporation shall be three.
(d) The corporation shall be authorized to issue $______ capital stock, consisting of ____ shares of common stock having a par value of $___ per share.
(e) The purposes of the corporation shall be to own an optometric office building, office furnishings, optometric equipment and such other real or personal property as the corporation may acquire from time to time; and to provide miscellaneous office and technical services to the lessees in connection with said property.

The amount of stock to be issued, the number of shares that will be purchased by each incorporator, and any restrictions dealing with its sale should also be included in the preincorporation agreement.

3. *Suscriptions.* The parties shall subscribe for the number of shares set opposite their names, and agree to pay therefor $___ per share:

Dr. ________ ___ shares
Dr. ________ ___ shares
Dr. ________ ___ shares

The subscriptions shall be payable at such time as the board of directors may determine and shall be paid by certified or bank cashier's check.

4. *Stock Restrictions.* None of the parties, nor the administrator nor executor of the estate of any party, shall transfer, pledge or sell stock in the corporation except with the written consent of all the other parties. If written consent is not obtained, a party, administrator, or executor desiring to sell stock shall notify the other parties of his offer to sell by registered mail. Each of the other parties shall have the option of purchasing said stock in proportion to his stock holdings in the corporation within 60 days. If any party shall not execute his option or any part thereof, the remaining party shall have an additional 30 days to purchase such stock as may be unsold. The purchase price shall be the book value of the stock, determined in accordance with standard accounting practice by the certified public accountant usually employed by the corporation as of the date of the registered mailing of the offer to sell. These stock restrictions shall become void in the event of the dissolution of the corporation or the death of all of the parties within a period of 90 days.

5. *Stock Certificates.* Stock certificates shall be issued only upon payment of the subscription price. Each certificate shall contain the endorsement that it is subject to the restrictions contained in paragraph 4 of an agreement executed among the parties on ________, 19___, and available for examination at the office of the Registered Agent of the corporation.

The financial obligations on which the corporation is based should be acknowledged. Any outstanding debts, such as mortgages, should be described.

6. *Ratification.* The parties shall cause the corporation to adopt and ratify the agreement for the purchase of the property at ________, the application with the ________ Bank for a purchase money mortgage in the amount of $______ upon said property, and the terms of this agreement.

The agreement may conclude with a requirement that the incorporators will provide such documents as are necessary for the implementation of the agreement.

7. *Necessary Documents.* Each of the parties shall execute and deliver in legally acceptable form any document necessary to the implementation of this agreement.

Articles of Incorporation

The articles of incorporation are composed of numerous clauses that describe the purpose of the corporation, list the individuals who are its owners and directors, and provide general guidelines for the establishment and organization of the new business enterprise. It should be remembered that this document will be filed with the Secretary of State and will be available to the public.

The articles will begin with an acknowledgment of the applicable state law.

ARTICLES OF INCORPORATION

We, the undersigned, hereby associate ourselves together for the purposes of becoming a professional corporation for profit under the provisions of Business and Professional Statutes, as amended by "The Professional Service Corporation Act" of the State of ________, pursuant to the following Articles of Incorporation:

Preliminary clauses will identify the corporation's name and state its general purpose.

ARTICLE I
NAME

The name of this corporation shall be:________.

ARTICLE II
PURPOSE

The general nature of the business to be transacted by the corporation shall be and is to engage in every aspect of the general practice of optometry. The professional services involved in the corporation's practice of optometry may be rendered only through its officers, agents and employees who are duly authorized and licensed to practice optometry in the State of ________.

This corporation shall not engage in any business other than the practice of optometry. However, this corporation may invest its funds in real estate, mortgages, stocks, bonds and other types of investments, and may own real and personal property necessary for the rendering of the professional services authorized hereby.

The stock to be issued by the corporation must be described, and the restricted nature of its sale—only to licensed optometrists in the state—should be noted as required by law.

ARTICLE III
STOCKS

The maximum number of shares of stock that the corporation is authorized to have outstanding at any time shall be ___ shares of the par value of ________ Dollars ($______) per share, all of which shall be common stock of the same class. All stock issued shall be fully paid and nonassessable. The stockholders shall have no preemptive rights with respect to the stock of the corporation, and the corporation may issue and sell its common stock from time to time without offering such shares to the stockholders then holding shares of common stock. Shares of the corporation's stock and certificates therefor shall be issued only to doctors authorized and licensed to practice optometry in the State of ________.

The capital of the corporation should be stated, as should other necessary organizational items such as the location of the corporate offices and the expected duration of the corporation.

ARTICLE IV
CAPITAL

The amount of capital with which this corporation will begin business shall be and is the sum of ________ Dollars ($______).

ARTICLE V
DURATION

The corporation shall have perpetual existence.

ARTICLE VI
OFFICES

The principal office of this corporation shall be located in the City of ________, County of ________, State of ________, and the post office address of said principal office of the corporation shall be ________, City of ________, State of ________.

The directors of the corporation are those individuals chosen by the ownership to control the long-range planning of the business. The board of directors also is responsible for the selection of the corporate officers, who direct the day-to-day activities of the corporation. The articles should identify those persons who are to be the directors, beginning with the number (which may be as low as one in some states) and then providing their names and addresses.

ARTICLE VII
DIRECTORS

The number of directors of this corporation shall be not less than three (3) nor more than five (5).

ARTICLE VIII
BOARD OF DIRECTORS

The names and post office addresses of the members of the first Board of Directors, who, subject to the provisions of the by-laws and these Articles of Incorporation, shall hold office for the first year of the corporation's existence or until their successors are elected and have qualified, are as follows:

NAMES	ADDRESSES
Dr. ________	____________________
Dr. ________	____________________
Dr. ________	____________________

The names of the persons who are initiating the corporation—the subscribers—must be included in the articles. Although the subscribers and the owners of a non-professional corporation (the stockholders) do not have to be same individuals, when a professional corporation is formed this will be the case.

ARTICLE IX
SUBSCRIBERS

The name and post office address of each subscriber of these Articles of Incorporation are as follows:

NAMES	ADDRESSES
Dr. ________	____________________
Dr. ________	____________________
Dr. ________	____________________

The subscribers certify that the proceeds of the stock subscribed for will not be less than the amount of capital with which the corporation will begin business, as set forth in Article IV hereinabove.

A large portion of the articles of incorporation will be devoted to the issue, maintenance, and transfer of the corporate stock. Due to the restricted nature of the stock of professional corporations, provisions must be included that allow for the lawful transfer of the stock to successor stockholders.

ARTICLE X
STOCKHOLDERS

The stock of this corporation may be issued, owned and registered only in the name or names of an individual or individuals who are duly authorized and licensed to practice optometry in the State of ________ and who are employees, officers or agents of this corporation. In the event a stockholder:

(a) becomes disqualified to practice optometry in this State, or

(b) is elected to a public office or accepts employment, that pursuant to law, places restrictions or limitations upon his continued rendering of professional services as a doctor of optometry, or

(c) ceases to be an employee, officer or agent of the corporation, or

(d) sells, transfers, pledges, or attempts to sell, transfer, or pledge any shares of stock in this corporation to any person ineligible by law or by virtue of these Articles to be a shareholder in this corporation, or if such sale, transfer, pledge, or attempt to sell, transfer, or pledge is made in a manner prohibited by law, or in a manner inconsistent with the provisions of these Articles, or by the By-Laws of this corporation, or

(e) suffers an execution to be levied upon his stock, or such stock is subjected to judicial sale or other process, the effect of which is to vest any legal or equitable interest in such stock in some person other than the stockholder, then the stock of such stockholder shall immediately stand forfeited and such stock shall be immediately cancelled by this corporation and the stockholder or other person in possession of such stock shall be entitled only to receive payment for the value of such stock, which said value shall be the book value thereof as of the last day of the month preceding the month in which any of the events above enumerated occurs. The stockholder whose stock so becomes forfeit and is cancelled by the corporation, shall forthwith cease to be an employee, officer, director, or agent of the corporation and except to receive payment for his stock in accordance with the foregoing, and payment of any other sums then lawfully due and owing to said stockholder by the corporation, such stockholder shall then and thereafter have no further financial interest of any kind in this corporation.

ARTICLE XI
DEATH OF STOCKHOLDER

Upon the death of a stockholder, his stock shall be subject to purchase by the corporation or by the other stockholders at such price and upon such terms and conditions and in such manner as may be provided for in the By-Laws of this corporation, in a manner consistent with law and these Articles.

ARTICLE XII
SALE OF STOCKS

No stockholder of this corporation may sell or transfer any of such stockholder's share of stock in this corporation except to another individual who is then duly authorized and licensed to practice optometry in the State of ________ and then only after the proposed sale or transfer shall have been first approved, at a stockholder's meeting specially called for such purpose, by such proportion, not less than a majority, of the outstanding stock, excluding the shares of stock proposed to be sold or transferred, as may be provided from time to time in the By-Laws. In such stockholder's meeting, the shares of stock proposed to be sold or transferred may not be voted or counted for any purpose.

The corporation's shareholders are specifically authorized from time to time to adopt By-Laws not inconsistent herewith restraining the alienation of shares of stock of this corporation and providing for the purchase or redemption by the corporation of its shares of stock.

The articles will also include provisions that describe the general organization of the corporation, the corporate officers, and the rights that they may exercise when dealing with the corporation as individuals or as officers in other companies.

ARTICLE XIII
REGULATION OF BUSINESS

In furtherance of and not in limitation of the powers conferred by statute, the following specific provisions are made for the regulation of the business and the conduct of the affairs of the corporation:

1. Subject to such restrictions, if any, as are herein expressed and such further restrictions, if any, as may be set forth in the By-Laws, the Board of Directors shall have the general management and control of the business and may exercise all the powers of the Corporation except such as may be by statute, or by the Articles of Incorporation or amendment thereto, or by the By-Laws as constituted from time to time, expressly conferred upon or reserved to the stockholders.

2. The corporation shall have such officers as may from time to time be provided in the By-Laws and such officers shall be designated in such manner and shall hold their offices for such terms and shall have such powers and duties as may be prescribed by the By-Laws or as may be determined from time to time by the Board of Directors subject to the By-Laws.

3. No contract or other transaction between the corporation and any other firm, association or corporation shall be affected or invalidated by the fact that any one or more of the directors of the corporation is or are interested in or is a member, director or officer or are members, directors or officers of such firm or corporation and any director or directors individually or jointly may be a party or parties to or may be interested in any contract or transaction of the corporation or in which the corporation is interested; and no contract, act or transaction of the corporation with any person, firm, association or corporation shall be affected or invalidated by the fact that any director or directors of the corporation is a part or are parties to or interested in such contract, act or transaction or in any way connected with such person, firm, association or corporation, and each and every person who may become a director of the corporation is hereby relieved from any liability that might otherwise exist from contracting with the corporation for the benefit of himself or any firm, association or corporation in which he may in any way be interested.

The articles usually conclude with an obligatory reference to the right of the corporation to amend the articles as it deems necessary.

ARTICLE XIV
AMENDMENTS

This corporation reserves the right to amend, alter, change, or repeal any provision contained herein in the manner now or hereafter prescribed by law, and all rights conferred on stockholders herein are granted subject to this reservation.

The corporate bylaws, stock-purchase agreements,

and employment contracts are more detailed than the preceding agreements and must be drafted by an attorney. In fact, the entire process of incorporating —formation, initiation of business, maintenance of activities, and dissolution—require the guidance and assistance of professionals knowledgeable in legal, tax, and administrative matters. Every optometrist who incorporates should secure the best advisors possible so as to obtain the maximum benefit from this complicated enterprise.

A sample corporate agreement is included within the Appendix.

Notes

1. As of 1987, this percentage was 5.3 percent. See the *AOA News* of March 1, 1988.
2. For a review of the considerations attendant to the formation of a professional association or corporation, see Milkie, G., *Partnerships and Professional Corporations*, Optometric Development Enterprises, St. Louis, Mo., 1972.
3. Webber, M.M., The Medical Corporation, in James, A.E. (ed.), *Legal Medicine*, Urban and Schwarzenberg, Baltimore, 1980, p. 173.
4. Ibid.
5. Ibid.
6. Ibid.
7. Restrictive covenants that prevent employees, partners, or corporate shareholders from entering into competition with the proprietorship, partnership, or professional corporation may or may not be enforceable in a given jurisdiction. For a review of the legal considerations, see "Validity and Construction of Contractual Restrictions on Right of Medical Practitioner to Practice, Incident to Employment Agreement," 62 A.L.R. 3d 1014, and the related annotations at 62 A.L.R. 3d 918 and 62 A.L.R. 3d 970.
8. Webber, supra note 3.
9. Ibid.
10. Ibid.
11. As of 1980, California, Iowa, Kansas, Mississippi, New York, and Pennsylvania. See Eaton, B.C., *Business Organizations—Professional Corporations and Associations*, vol. 17C, Matthew Bender, N.Y., 1987 cum. supp., pp. B-380–381.
12. See Webber, supra note 3.
13. Ibid.
14. Ibid.
15. Ibid.
16. The clauses and contracts used for purposes of illustration herein have been generously supplied to the author by the American Optometric Association.

PART THIRTEEN

ECONOMICOLEGAL CONSIDERATIONS

Chapter 47

Loans

"Take some more tea," the March Hare said to Alice, very earnestly.
"I've had nothing yet," Alice replied in an offended tone, "so I can't take more."
"You mean you can't take less,*" said the Hatter, "it's very easy to take* more *than nothing."*
—Lewis Carroll, *Alice in Wonderland*

Fundamentals of Financing
Conventional Loan Sources
Basic Provisions of Loan Agreements
Being Prepared

Fundamentals of Financing

The traditional mode of delivering optometric services (individual proprietorship) requires offices to be equipped with an array of up-to-date instrumentation, inventories of frames and contact lenses, and tasteful fixtures and furnishings, which places a heavy financial burden on practitioners seeking to practice in the time-honored way. In addition, there are operating costs that must be met (e.g., rent, taxes, utilities, and salaries), and so the average optometrist has found it necessary to obtain financing in order to afford the start-up costs of private practice.

In the usual case, financing must be acquired both for capital assets and for operating expenses. Thus the creditor may be required to loan more money than there will be collateral to serve as security, which necessitates careful planning and meticulous preparation on the part of the borrower because the creditor will have to be convinced that the risk is minimal in order to make such a partially unsecured loan. To ensure that the risk is low, the creditor will dictate the terms of the agreement and will protect his interest in the collateral as best he can. This chapter discusses the conventional devices used by creditors to secure their loans and to protect their collateral in the event of default on the part of the borrower.

The most basic aspects of financing involve the method of repayment and the type of interest. Borrowing money involves not only the act of obtaining the loan but also the repayment of principal and interest. Although there are a number of methods used for the repayment of loans and for the computation of interest, this chapter will discuss the most prevalently used techniques for both.

There are two usual methods relied upon by banks and similar lending institutions for the repayment of loans:

Renewable short-term notes—instruments that acknowledge the loaning of money for a relatively brief period (usually 90 days), with provision for renewal at the option of the lender. At the close of any 90-day period, the lender can demand payment of the balance due—in full.

Installment notes—instruments that provide for the periodic repayment of a stated sum at regular intervals, such as monthly payments, usually for a period of three, four, or five years.

Either of two interest rates may be applied to these short-term loans, simple interest or add-on interest.

Simple interest applies a fixed percentage rate to the amount borrowed for a stated period of time. An example will illustrate how it is determined (see Fig. 47.1). If the amount of interest due for a loan of

If $10,000 is borrowed at 10% simple interest on a renewable 90-day note, what would be the interest payable at the end of 90 days?

Amount borrowed	$10,000
Interest rate	× 10%
Total interest if the note was held for a year	$1,000
Interest for one quarter of a year	$250

If the note is due in 90 days without renewal, the total amount that has to be repaid is $10,250.

Figure 47.1. Sample Simple Interest Loan

a year's duration is $1,000, and the money is only borrowed for 90 days (25 percent of a year), the interest is $250.

Simple interest is one of the most advantageous ways to borrow money. Should the borrower decide to pay off the note early, he does not have to pay a prepayment penalty because the interest is *prorated* for the actual number of days that the money has been borrowed. However, renewable 90-day notes are subject to fluctuating interest rates based on the prime lending rate at the end of each 90-day period. Some notes provide for changes in the interest charged whenever the prime rate changes, without regard to the term of the note. In addition, there is the matter of renewal; the bank has no obligation to renew the note at the end of the 90-day period, (i.e., at maturity). The interest rate is guaranteed only for the life of the note, which is not automatically subject to renewal by the lender.

Add-on interest is the second method of lending money, and whereas simple interest is usually found on bank loans for equipment purchases and start-up money, add-on interest is commonly encountered on installment loans for such items as boats and automobiles. It is best illustrated by an example (see Fig. 47.2).

The reason this type of interest is called add-on is because the interest is added onto the principal to determine the total amount financed. These loans are paid in equal installments during each month of the term of the loan, which may be three, four, five, or more years.

If a borrower decides to prepay (i.e., pay before maturity) an installment loan, the interest is *shortrated* rather than prorated (as in a simple interest loan). In a simple interest note, the interest is figured on the number of days the money is borrowed and is computed on the declining balance after each payment. Shortrating means that if the borrower pays off the loan early, the lender will charge a fee for administrative expense and profit. Normally this fee is governed by the Rule of 78, which is a standard formula for figuring the interest due. A borrower should always inquire into the shortrate charge with add-on interest prior to borrowing money, if the borrower thinks there is a possibility of paying off the loan early (see Fig. 47.3 for an example.)

Early repayment of an add-on loan is usually

If $10,000 was borrowed at 10% add-on interest for a period of three years, what would be the total cost to the borrower?

Multiply $10,000	$10,000
By 10%	× .10
Yearly interest	$ 1,000
Multiply by 3 years	× 3
Finance charge	$ 3,000
Add principal	+ 10,000
Total amount financed	$13,000
Divide by 36 months	÷ 36
Monthly payments	$361.11

Figure 47.2. Sample Add-On Interest Loan

How is \$1,000 in interest computed over a 12-month period under the "Rule of 78?"

The 12-month period is summed as follows:

$$12 + 11 + 10 + 9 + 8 + 7 + 6 + 5 + 4 + 3 + 2 + 1 = 78$$

The interest is computed as follows:

First month	12/78 = 153.84
Second month	11/78 = 141.02
Third month	10/78 = 128.20
Fourth month	9/78 = 115.38
Fifth month	8/78 = 102.56
Sixth month	7/78 = 89.74
Total	\$730.74

Therefore, 73% of the interest due is paid in the first six months, leaving \$270 interest to be paid in the last six months.

Figure 47.3. Calculation of Interest under the "Rule of 78"

Table 47.1. Shortrated Interest under the "Rule of 78"

3-Year Note	4-Year Note	5-Year Note
50% of interest in 1st year	43% of interest in 1st year	36% of interest in 1st year
33% of interest in 2nd year	29% of interest in 2nd year	28% of interest in 2nd year
17% of interest in 3rd year	18% of interest in 3rd year	18% of interest in 3rd year
	9% of interest in 4th year	12% of interest in 4th year
		6% of interest in 5th year

not advantageous if the interest is shortrated. For example, in an installment note for a term of three years, 50 percent of the interest is repaid in the first year, and by the end of the second year 83 percent of the interest has been repaid. Similar results are obtained for four- and five-year installment notes (see Table 47.1).

Usual banking custom is to utilize simple interest notes for relatively small amounts and for short periods of time based upon the borrower's signature. This means that the loan is *unsecured* (not backed up by some security, such as stocks, personal property, and land). Although an unsecured simple interest loan may be obtained for the financing of equipment, in the great majority of instances the equipment will be required to serve as collateral for the loan (discussed below).

Add-on interest is used for longer term financing involving periodic payments and is normally secured by the piece of equipment or other collateral, such as an automobile, that is financed. Of course, the personal endorsement of the borrower is also obtained.

The burden is on the borrower to determine the type of financing that is being offered and whether the rate and terms of the loan are favorable and competitive for the market. Some of the loan sources available to practitioners are discussed in the section that follows.

Conventional Loan Sources

There are several types of creditors available to the optometrist seeking funds to begin a private practice. The basic decision is whether to obtain short term or long-term financing. Short-term financing is less than ten years (usually five to seven years), whereas long-term financing is for lengthy periods (usually between ten and thirty years in duration).

The most common choice is short-term financing because the total cost is less and there is a wider variety of creditors available with less restrictive loan provisions.

Short-Term Financing

The conventional sources for short-term loans are banks, credit unions and corporations, the Small Business Administration, professional development companies, and equipment dealers or manufacturers.

Banks

The leading source of funds for small businessmen is a full service bank.[1] Not only are banks able to pro-

> What is the difference in total cost for $40,000 borrowed for 5 years at 10% interest when simple interest is obtained instead of add-on?
>
> Let us assume that there will be no repayment of principal during the first year. If equal payments of principal and interest are made during the last four years of the loan, the total amount paid under a simple-interest renewable short-term note is approximately $53,000
>
> Let us assume that the add-on rate requires repayment of principal and interest in the first year and in each of the four years that follow. Over a five-year period, the repayment will be constant and will amount to approximately $60,000.
>
> Therefore, the approximate difference will be $7,000.

Figure 47.4. Comparison of Loan Interest: Simple Versus Add-On

vide substantial funds for the start-up of a practice, they are also capable of supplying funds for such necessities of life as vehicles, boats, home renovation, and many other pleasantries. Bank services include commercial checking, savings accounts, trust departments, individual retirement accounts, and the ability to assist a customer in establishing a strong credit rating. But bank loans require careful preparation on the part of the borrower and a capable presentation to the loan officer. Bank loans may be limited by law to repayment periods that are less than ten years in duration.

The primary concern of most creditors is security for the loan. Few, if any, banks will be willing to make a large loan to a beginning practitioner based merely upon the practitioner's signature. There are several customary provisions of bank loans that are intended to afford protection in the event the borrower defaults; among these are a security interest in equipment and other personal property, the assignment to the bank of a life insurance policy sufficient to cover the debt in the event the borrower dies, and, in many instances, a co-signer or additional collateral. The customary provisions of conventional loans will be discussed in the following section.

If the loan is to purchase a particular item, such as a car, the bank will not require additional collateral because no part of the loan is unsecured. But if the amount to be borrowed exceeds the value of the tangible items to be purchased with the loan proceeds —as in a loan to establish a private practice—the bank may require a co-signer or additional collateral in order to protect the unsecured portion of the loan (i.e., that part used to pay expenses and not for capitalization). This policy varies from bank to bank and from community to community.[2]

How the bank offers to finance the loan will make a substantial difference in the amount to be repaid by the borrower.

The lender may choose to place both the equipment and the working capital under one master note and charge an add-on rate for the whole amount. Or the lender may offer a simple interest renewable short-term note for both. The difference is best illustrated by an example (see Fig. 47.4). If add-on interest is required, the cost over the life of the loan will be substantially higher than if simple interest were utilized.

The interest rate itself is customarily tied to the prime lending rate nationwide; most banks will offer professionals such as optometrists 1 or 2 percent over the prime rate. This rate may float or be readjustable at periodic intervals if the loan is at simple interest; add-on interest is usually set for the period of the loan.

Some lenders may choose to lend the working capital at simple interest on a short-term renewal note and place the equipment on a three- to five-year installment note.[3] Often the simple interest is offered in terms of a draw note, which allows the borrower to draw what is needed and to pay interest only on what is drawn. This alternative is often referred to as a *line of credit*. One advantage that bank financing offers is this flexibility. Banks are often willing to allow a beginning practitioner to repay only interest in the first year and to make payments of principal and interest thereafter on a graduated basis, so that the payments increase in size as the practitioner's cash flow grows.

Although banks have been the most popular source of loans for optometrists, there are several other institutions that can provide funds at competitive rates. Among them is the federal government.

Small Business Administration

An ancillary form of bank financing (up to $500,000) is available through the Small Business Administration (SBA).[4] The SBA can guarantee loans to qualified borrowers and have the authority to make direct loans to optometrists (who can occasionally qualify).

If an optometrist has been turned down by a bank, the SBA may be an alternative source of financing.

For direct loans, the SBA gives favorable terms—seven to ten years—and offers competitive interest rates. A graduated payment scale is also allowed; this means that lower payments are made in the beginning, and over the course of time they are increased until a reasonable maximum is attained.[5]

Unfortunately, the SBA is not making direct loans at the present, and in order to obtain SBA participation the optometrist must obtain bank participation (i.e., have the bank agree to sponsor the loan), with the bank endorsing the loan proposal and forwarding it on the the SBA.[6] If approved by the SBA, the loan is guaranteed (up to 90 percent of the loan amount or a maximum of $500,000) so that the bank will not incur loss should the optometrist default; for this reason, the SBA chooses its borrowers carefully. The interest rate is a true simple interest, computed on the declining balance of the loan. But the SBA permits the bank to charge an interest rate of up to 2 percent more than prime, which means that—at today's prime interest rates—it is no bargain. However, having the SBA guarantee could mean the difference between getting a loan and not getting one. Since optometrists are not the usual applicants for SBA loans, attempting to obtain SBA backing could be both time consuming and difficult.

Credit Unions and Corporations

There are private loan institutions other than banks that can be turned to as a source of funds. Credit unions are institutions that are established to serve special groups; thus the first requirement of seeking a loan from a credit union would be to set up an account there. Credit unions, however, are limited as to types of loans and have ceilings on unsecured loans that are generally modest. They can make large secured loans, but this requires the borrower to maintain a sizable deposit within the credit union. They are most often used as a source of financing for vehicles, trailers, boats, aircraft, and the like.

Credit corporations can provide the sizable loans necessary to begin a practice. The terms and repayment provisions will be analogous to those used by a bank, although commercial finance plans offered by credit corporations may require a down payment.[7]

Professional Development Companies

During the past decade, a number of insurance companies have established offshoot businesses that offer a range of services for the professional. These services frequently include arrangements for the leasing of equipment. But leasing is just one of several services that are offered (these companies will also provide cash loans for operating expenses and insurance coverage). Under such a program, the leasing company will permit the doctor to select the equipment that is wanted, and then the company will purchase the equipment and lease it to the doctor for a period ranging from five to seven years. The leasing company, it should be noted, holds the title to the equipment. The doctor pays a straight finance charge, usually 3 to 4 percent more than the bank rate, which does not change over the period of the lease. The doctor also receives an option to purchase the equipment at the conclusion of the lease period. The purchase amount can either be a set amount (10 percent of the fair market value at the time of the purchase being typical), or it can be whatever the lessor and lessee agree on, and it can even be guaranteed in the lease, if desired. Most leases provide for a set payment, per month, for the period of the lease, but some plans escalate payments over the term of the lease.

Leasing is not particularly advantageous for a beginning practitioner who starts up cold, but the decision to buy or to lease is not always made on the basis of dollars and cents. If a beginning optometrist cannot secure bank financing, a lease arrangement may be the only alternative. If a young practitioner with a family wishes to purchase a home, he may find that the financial obligations of buying equipment will preclude him from being able to obtain mortgage financing, and so he may turn to leasing as a means of affording both while satisfying his creditors. Or, an optometrist who buys an established practice may find that leasing allows him a favorable tax write-off while at the same time freeing his personal financial statement of large obligations such as those necessary to buy major items of ophthalmic equipment. The decision to lease can be philosophical as well as financial, and under the appropriate circumstances even a beginning practitioner may find it acceptable.

Long-Term Financing

Over the past few years, various methods of achieving long-term financing for optometric practices have been attempted.[8] Each, in its own way, has met with limited success. The three most commonly used methods are:

- Direct loans offered by a federally chartered loan institution licensed under the SBA
- Direct loans made by the Federal Land Bank to qualifying landholder-applicants
- Municipal bond issues supported by small cities to finance the costs of establishing a professional office within the city

None of these methods has proved to be a panacea. They can be complicated, and individual inquiries will be necessary for those who are interested.

Direct Long-Term Loans

A national institution organized by an optometrist offers long-term financing (up to twenty years) for optometric equipment and working capital.[9] The loan program provides for five-year simple interest financing by a secured note, with—at the lender's option—renewal of the note for additional five-year periods. The interest rate is similar to that offered by banks, prime plus 1 to 2 percent. Obviously, the prevailing rate at the time the loan is entered into is of enormous importance. The applicant must have some collateral, offer the equipment as collateral, or have someone with collateral co-sign the note. There is a finance charge that must be paid at the outset of the loan.

The chief disadvantage of any long-term financing program is its cost. Although monthly payments are lower, they are spread out over a much longer period, which means that the ultimate cost is larger than with conventional financing. Also, the long term of indebtedness affects the future capability of a practitioner to seek other financing or to change modes of practice.

Federal Land Bank Loans

For landowners (realty owned free of any mortgage indebtedness), an alternative form of financing is possible. The optometrist-landowner offers the property as security for a loan from the Federal Land Bank, which in turns loans the optometrist the capital he needs to set up a private practice. The loan is limited to the fair market value of the land, but the interest rate is reasonable (below that of mortgage financing), the rate changes are limited by law to increments of 0.25 percent at a time, and financing can be spread over a thirty-year period. The chief limitation of this alternative is that only those optometrists affluent enough to own unmortgaged land may participate.

Municipal Bond Issues

A few—very few—optometrists are lucky enough to find a community that is sufficiently interested in obtaining optometric services that it will finance the cost of establishing an optometric practice through the issuance of municipal bonds.[10] The bonds are purchased by the public and return a guaranteed rate of interest to the purchasers. The money received from the sale of the bonds is used to finance the cost of setting up and starting a practice. The doctor (or doctors) who are the recipients of this largesse usually provide the land that is to be developed or purchase it from the city as part of the arrangement. Since municipal bonds are long-term instruments (typically twenty to thirty years), annual payments made by the participating doctor (for the land or other participation in the bond issue) are low.

This type of arrangement takes quite a bit of time to organize, is complicated, and can be costly for everyone if it is not properly done. Legal expertise is a must. If there is an existing plan that the city is eager to take advantage of, then the possibility of participating in such a plan should be investigated.

Basic Provisions of Loan Agreements

Since banks are the usual source of loans for optometrists, the basic provisions of bank loan agreements are deserving of some commentary. Although individual agreements may differ in their terms, there is a commonality to these contracts that permits generalizations to be made.

The basic provisions of loans agreements include:

- amount and terms
- interest rate
- collateral requirements
- limitation on additional indebtedness
- repayment structure
- acceleration clause.

Each of these provisions will be briefly discussed in the subsequent paragraphs. Sample language illustrating each of the provisions accompanies the discussion.

Amount and Terms

Any creditor will have loan limits that will not be exceeded without good cause, and will have established loan repayment terms that vary with the purpose of the loan and the amount borrowed. For example, most automobile loans are for three or four years; most practice loans are for five to seven years. There will be an upper limit on the amount loaned that can be utilized for nontangible items. The more conservative the bank, the lower the amount allowed for these expenses (i.e., working capital).

> WHEREAS, _______ (Hereinafter referred to as Borrower) hereby expressly agrees to the following terms and conditions in consideration for the extension of credit in the original principal amount of _______ ($_______) together with all renewals, extensions or increases thereof with _______ (Hereinafter referred to as Bank).

Interest Rate

If the loan is for simple interest, it is likely that the agreement will specify a short-term renewable note. In this event the interest charge will probably be a fluctuating one that is tied to the prime interest rate; the only variable will be the frequency with which the rate changes. Some banks specify a floating rate that changes whenever the prime rate rises or falls, whereas others set the rate at the renewal of the note (which is usually done quarterly or semi-annually).

> Interest on said note may change, at the Bank's option, at each maturity, but in no event shall exceed the maximum rate of interest allowed by law.

If the loan is for add-on interest, the rate is usually set at the start of the loan and does not change thereafter; add-on rates are customarily found on installment notes. If add-on interest is utilized in conjunction with a renewable short-term note, the rate can be changed at each renewal.

Collateral Requirements

There are two customary collateral requirements in practice loans: a purchase money security interest in the equipment and a life insurance policy that is assigned to the bank.

A *security interest* is a rather complicated creation of the law that requires the creditor and the borrower to follow certain procedures:

- The creditor and the borrower must agree, in writing, to the formation of the security interest, which is done through the execution of a security agreement.
- The creditor must make the loan, and the borrower must acquire the property.
- The creditor must file a financing statement, which is a document putting the public on notice that he has a financial interest in the property.

The filing requirement is necessary in order to protect the creditor from subsequent creditors; if the borrower's business fails, his creditors will then have to fight among themselves for whatever assets remain, and the creditor who has filed the earliest security interest will prevail over all others. Consequently, there is a great deal of emphasis placed on security interests by creditors.

An optometrist should always examine a security interest to determine the identity of the creditors to whom the security interest is being granted.

> Bank shall require a purchase money security interest in equipment and furnishing purchased, patient accounts receivable, assignment of life insurance (adequate to cover the loan balance), designation as loss-payee for property insurance on equipment, furnishings or other collateral given, and a Professional Practice Loan Agreement. Bank may require additional collateral, such as real estate or other assets acceptable to the bank, depending on the particular circumstances.

The bank will usually require the borrower to assign to the bank a life insurance policy sufficient to cover the loan balance in the event of the death of the borrower.

An *assignment* is the transfer of a contractual right or benefit, which operates to extinguish the right in the one making the transfer and to set the right up exclusively for the benefit of the one to whom it is transferred. Many contractual rights can be transferred in this manner.

The one making the assignment is known as the assignor; the one to whom the assignment is made is known as the assignee. Although a bank may hold a security interest in equipment, the typical loan required by a private practitioner includes items other than equipment, such as start-up costs, salaries, and professional fees. Thus there is a certain amount of the loan that the bank cannot protect through the acquisition of a security interest in equipment, furniture, and other tangible items, especially if the creditor dies. Many banks require the borrower to assign his rights under a life insurance policy to the bank, placing the bank before any other beneficiary in terms of repayment in the event the practitioner should die unexpectedly.

The practitioner will be asked to execute an assignment agreement and will have to surrender the policy to the bank, which will hold it as long as the loan is outstanding. When the loan is repaid, the assignment will be extinguished and the policy will be returned to the practitioner.

In addition to the life insurance policy, the bank may require the borrower to maintain certain other types of coverage. This typically requires the practitioner to purchase property and professional liability insurance sufficient to indemnify the bank in the event of the loss of its collateral.

> Borrowers shall maintain property and personal liability insurance (including malpractice coverage) in such amounts as may reasonably be required by Bank and deliver to Bank evidence that such policies and coverage are in force and in good order, and further designate Bank as the "loss payee" for such policies and coverage, as might be applicable.

Of course, the bank may require additional collateral, a co-signer, or other such terms as it deems necessary to protect its security adequately.

Limitation on Additional Indebtedness

In an effort to prevent borrowers from overextending themselves, some banks limit the ability of borrowers to obtain additional sums from other creditors. The limitation is usually expressed as a cash limit, not to be exceeded without the prior approval of the bank.

> Borrower, will not, during the term of this loan incur any additional indebtedness, except for obligations incurred during the normal operation of business or consumer purchases with any financing institution, nor become directly, indirectly, or contingently liable as co-maker, endorser, or guarantor for sums in the aggregate amount of $_______ per year without the prior expressed written consent of the Bank.

These limits do not usually apply to consumer purchases or to debts incurred during the course of everyday practice activities.

Repayment Structure

Repayment plans vary widely from bank to bank and with the type of note and interest charged.

Installment notes specify a stated payment per month for the period of the note. The monthly payment does not change during the repayment period, which is usually for three to five years, but may be longer.

Short-term renewable notes offer the bank more options. These loans are described as for a period of years (usually five to seven) but are actually renewable at the option of the bank, at stated intervals that are specified in the loan agreement. Renewable periods may be as brief as ninety days or may be for as long as a term of years. Notes retain a degree of flexibility that enables the bank to adjust the repayment schedule as necessary to accommodate the borrower's ability to pay. Some notes specify interest repayment only during the first year of the loan, then amortize the principal and interest over a period of several years thereafter. Other notes will allow the borrower to pay less during the first years of the repayment period.

Regardless of the type of note or repayment schedule, the bank will require the borrower to submit periodic financial statements so that the status of the borrower's practice can be assessed.

> Borrower shall furnish Bank with semi-annual financial statements to include a Balance Sheet and Statement of Profit and Loss during the first (1st) year of this Agreement and then annually thereafter, unless as otherwise may be requested by the Bank. The statements shall be prepared preferably by a certified public accountant acceptable to the Bank in such sufficient detail as may reasonably be required by the Bank. The initial maturity of the practice loan shall be six (6) months from the date of the note executed in conjunction herewith. Upon receipt and review by Bank of Borrower's financial statement as described in the paragraph above, the Bank will at its option:
>
> a. Demand payment in full of principal and all accrued and unpaid interest.
> b. Renew note and extend moratorium of principal payments for an additional period to be determined by the Bank at that time.
> c. Establish monthly installments of principal plus interest for eleven (11) months with the balance due in full in the twelfth (12th) month, then review or,
> d. Establish monthly amortization of principal plus interest over the following sixty (60) months.
>
> In any event, the entire indebtness shall be fully repaid within six (6) years of the date of said note.

Acceleration Clause

Any note will contain a so-called acceleration clause, which permits the bank to demand the full amount of the loan due and payable in the event the borrower fails to comply with the provisions of the agreement. This provision affords the bank some protection in the event the borrower cannot make the required payments because it allows the bank to claim its collateral and to proceed as necessary to collect the

!MPORTANT: Read these directions before completing this Statement.

- ☐ If you are applying for individual credit in your own name and are relying on your own income or assets and not the income or assets of another person as the basis of repayment of the credit requested, complete only Sections 1 and 3.
- ☐ If you are applying for joint credit with another person, complete all Sections providing information in Section 2 about the joint applicant.
- ☐ If you are applying for individual credit but are relying on income from alimony, child support, or separate maintenance or on the income or assets of another person as a basis for repayment of the credit requested, complete all Sections, providing information in Section 2 about the person whose alimony, support or maintenance payments or income or assets you are relying.
- ☐ If this statement relates to your guaranty of the indebtedness of other person(s), firm(s), or corporation(s), complete Sections 1 and 3.

SECTION I – INDIVIDUAL INFORMATION			SECTION II – OTHER PARTY INFORMATION		
Name			Name		
Address			Address		
City	State	Zip	City	State	Zip
Position or Occupation			Position or Occupation		
Business Name			Business Name		
Business Address			Business Address		
City	State	Zip	City	State	Zip
Res. Phone	Bus. Phone		Res. Phone	Bus. Phone	

SECTION III – STATEMENT OF FINANCIAL CONDITION AS OF ____________ 19____

ASSETS (Do not include assets of doubtful value)	In Dollars (Omit Cents)	LIABILITIES (Include All Liabilities as Co-Maker)	In Dollars (Omit Cents)
Cash on hand and in banks	$	Notes payable to banks – secured	$
U.S. Gov't. & Marketable securities –	$	Notes payable to banks – unsecured	$
See Sched. A	$	Due to brokers	$
Non-marketable securities – See Sched. B	$	Amounts payable to others – secured	$
Securities held by broker in margin accounts	$	Amounts payable to others – unsecured	$
Restricted or control stocks	$	Accounts and bills due	$
Partial interest in real estate equities	$	Unpaid Income tax	$
See Sched. C.	$	Other unpaid interest and taxes	$
Real estate owned – see Sched. D	$	Real estate mortgages payable	$
Loans receivable	$	See Sched. D.	$
Automobiles and other personal property	$	Other debts	$
Cash value - Life Insurance – see Sched. E	$		$
Other assets: (itemize)	$		$
	$		$
	$		$
	$		$
	$	TOTAL LIABILITIES	$
	$	NET WORTH	$
TOTAL ASSETS	$	TOTAL LIABILITIES AND NET WORTH	$

Source of Income for Year Ended __________ 19____.

Salary, Bonuses & Commissions	$
Dividends	$
Real Estate income	$
Other income (**Alimony, child support,**	$
or separate maintenance need not be revealed if you do not desire the Bank to consider such income in determining your credit worthiness.)	$
	$
	$
	$
	$

Personal Information

Do you have a will? If so, name of executor.
Are you a partner or officer in any other venture? If so, describe.
Are you obligated to pay alimony, child support or separate maintenance payments? If so, describe.
Are any assets pledged other than described on schedules? If so, describe.
Income tax settled through (date):
Are you a defendent in any suits or legal actions?
Personal bank accounts carried at:
Have you ever been declared bankrupt in the last 14 years? If so, describe.

Contingent Liabilities

Do you have any contingent liabilities? If so, describe.	
Liabilities as endorser or guarantor?	$
Liabilities on leases or contracts?	$
Legal claims	$
Other special debts	$
Amount of contested income tax liens	$

99/12-1702 Rev. 12/77

PLEASE COMPLETE THE REVERSE SIDE

Figure 47.5. Sample Personal Financial Statement. (Courtesy of Central Bank of Birmingham, Alabama)

Schedule A — U.S. Governments & Marketable Securities

Number of Shares or Face Value (Bonds)	Description	In Name of	Are these pledged?	Market Value

Schedule B — Non-Marketable Securities

Number of Shares	Description	In Name of	Are these pledged?	Source of Value	Value

Schedule C — Partial Interests in Real Estate Equities

Address & Type Of Property	Title in Name of	% of Ownership	Date Acquired	Cost	Market Value	Mortgage Maturity	Mortgage Amount

Schedule D — Real Estate Owned

Address & Type Of Property	Title in Name of	Date Acquired	Cost	Market Value	Mortgage Maturity	Mortgage Amount

Schedule E — Life Insurance Carried, Including Group Insurance

Name of Insurance Company	Owner of Policy	Beneficiary	Face Amount	Policy Loans	Cash Surrender Value

Schedule F — Banks or Finance Companies where credit has been obtained

Name & Address of Lender	Credit in Name of	Secured or Unsecured?	Original date	High Credit	Current Balance

The information contained in this statement is provided for the purpose of obtaining, or maintaining credit with you on behalf of the undersigned, or persons, firms or corporations in whose behalf the undersigned may either severally or jointly with others, execute a guaranty in your favor. Each undersigned understands that you are relying on the information provided herein (including the designation made as to ownership of property) in deciding to grant or continue credit.

Each undersigned represents and warrants that the information provided is true and complete and that you may consider this statement as continuing to be true and correct until a written notice of a change is given to you by the undersigned. You are authorized to make all inquiries you deem necessary to verify the accuracy of the statements made herein, and to determine my/our creditworthiness. You are authorized to answer questions about your credit experience with me/us.

Signature (Individual) ____________ Signature (Other Party) ____________

Social Security No. ____________ Date of Birth ____________ Social Security No. ____________ Date of Birth ____________

99/12-1702

Figure 47.5. *Continued.*

full amount outstanding. These clauses are a standard aspect of any financial agreement, and can only be enforced by the creditor if there is some default on the part of the borrower.

> Failure of Borrower to fully comply with any term, condition, or covenant of this Agreement of said note executed by Borrower shall constitute default under this Agreement and unless remedied within ten (10) days of such default, the Bank may, at its option, declare all indebtedness of Borrower then outstanding immediately due and payable in full.

Loan agreements are complex and comprehensive documents that typically involve the transfer of large sums of money. A potential borrower who is not knowledgeable in financial affairs would be well advised to secure professional counsel before entering into any long-term financial arrangement of which he is uncertain.

Being Prepared

The preceding pages have illustrated the many considerations involved in borrowing money. There yet remains the matter of how to obtain the necessary financing from the lender of choice. What must a borrower do in order to secure the loan for the requested amount?

The answer is straightforward: Be prepared. Unfortunately, the road to preparedness is not a simple one, and requires that the borrower spend many hours planning and documenting his loan request. For all borrowers, the beginning point is the personal financial statement (see Fig. 47.5). This is a key document in any loan proposal, but for borrowers who are seeking funds to begin an optometric practice there are other requirements:

- Three years' prior tax returns
- An estimate of the equipment costs and of the furnishings that must be purchased
- A tentative office lease
- An estimate of the cost to renovate or modify the leased office space (if necessary)
- An item-by-item statement of the disbursement breakdown (in terms of equipment, furnishings, leasehold improvements, and working capital) for the loan
- A detailed projection of income and expenses for the first year of practice
- A five-year projection of income and expenses for the practice
- A list of all insurance coverage in force or to be acquired (life, health, personal property, casualty, malpractice, and disability)

Acquiring this wealth of information will not assure acceptance of the loan proposal, but it will force the borrower to be realistic in his assessment of how much money he needs and how it is to be allocated. And it assures the borrower of being able to answer the many questions the banker will ask concerning the proposed practice.

The initiation of a practice "from scratch" is not always the best way to begin. With greater frequency young optometrists are turning to the purchase of existing practices as a means of getting started, a type of transaction that possesses its own nuances and complexities. We will discuss the legal, financial, and tax problems inherent in purchase agreements in the next chapter.

Notes

1. A description of some of the problems of short-term financing from full-service banks is described by Gregg, J., *The Business of Optometric Practice*, Advisory Enterprises, White Plains, N.Y., 1981, pp. 61–70.
2. Ibid.
3. Ibid.
4. *Business Loans From the SBA*, U.S. Small Business Administration, Washington, D.C., 1985.
5. Ibid.
6. Ibid.
7. Gregg, supra note 1.
8. Ibid.
9. See Runninger, J., Your New Wellspring of Ready Credit, *Optometric Management*, vol. 17, no. 2, 1981, pp. 27–31.
10. See Halenar, J.F., The Whole Town Financed This Medical Office Building, *Medical Economics*, vol. 56, no. 7, Apr. 2, 1979, pp. 145–149.

Chapter 48

Purchase Agreements

Buy now, pay later.
—Contemporary American philosophy

Purchasing Equipment
Buying a Practice: Some Considerations
Determining the Fair Value of a Practice
Tax Ramifications

Purchasing Equipment

The first contact that an optometrist is likely to have with a purchase agreement is when bargaining for the purchase of ophthalmic equipment. There is a tendency on the part of young optometrists to assume a rather cavalier attitude toward these agreements. This is due, in part, to the circumstances of the usual agreement: the optometrist places an order, which the seller promises to deliver at a time that is often several months in the future, the optometrist signs what is not much more than a list of the agreed-on equipment, and no money actually changes hands.

Although equipment purchase agreements would not seem to be in the same category as practice purchase agreements, which require lawyers, accountants, and a bank loan and are often accompanied by a prolonged period of hard bargaining, nothing could be further from the truth. As with agreements to purchase a practice, equipment purchase agreements are contracts that are formal, binding, and enforceable.

As long as there is mutual assent between competent parties and consideration is present, there is a legal contract that the purchaser cannot void merely because some unforeseen circumstance intervened, such as disability or the failure to obtain a license as expected. Under these circumstances, the optometrist will either have to pay damages to the seller or try and sell the equipment to another buyer himself. The damages incurred by the equipment dealer who made the contract with the optometrist may be relatively small (if another buyer can be found in a brief period of time and the buyer agrees to purchase the equipment at the same price) or they may be rather consequential (if the dealer must warehouse, advertise, transport, and eventually sell the equipment at a substantially lower price). In either event, the optometrist who breaches the original contract will be legally liable for these damages.

The only way to void a purchase contract is to place a clause within the agreement that specifies the contract will not be binding should a certain described event occur. An example of a circumstance that would satisfy this requirement would be failure to obtain an optometry license. A clause stating that the sales contract would be void if the optometrist failed to receive a license would be legal and enforceable; however, it is unlikely that the equipment seller would agree to it. Such clauses are much more commonly found in practice purchase agreements, where it would actually be against public policy to permit an unlicensed practitioner to purchase a practice that is doing business.

There are other problems related to purchase agreements for equipment. If financing is required (and it usually is), the creditor retains an interest in the equipment, which serves as collateral for the loan. This interest is a security interest, which was described in Chapter 47. In the event the borrower defaults on his loan (is not able to make his payments to the bank), the security interest allows the creditor to take back the loan collateral—the equipment—and to sell it in an effort to mitigate his loss. If there is a deficit between the amount borrowed and the amount that the collateral is sold for, the creditor may be able to claim this deficit from other assets of the borrower. This remedy will depend on a number of circumstances that cannot be discussed here.

Worst of all, if the creditor becomes insolvent, those to whom the creditor is indebted may be able to sell the equipment themselves. This can occur when the security interest signed by the optometrist is not actually between himself and the seller but between himself and the creditor of the seller.

To avoid misfortune, optometrists should deal with solvent businesses that have acquired a good reputation over a period of time, not fall prey to impulses or succumb to the allure of cut-rate prices, and always obtain competent legal advice before entering into any contract that involves the expenditure of a considerable amount of money or requires years of obligation to a person or business.

Buying a Practice: Some Considerations

All things being equal, an ongoing practice should be a better investment than starting out cold.[1] Both situations require that money be borrowed (and repaid), but a seller may be more flexible than a banker in coming to financial terms. Furthermore, the interest rate that a seller charges should be lower than that of a bank, and the term of repayment could easily be extended beyond the usual five or six years demanded by a bank. And there is already an established cash flow that can be used when determining the terms of repayment; cash flow in a practice starting from scratch is usually the reverse from that of an established practice: out rather than in. These are very good reasons to favor a practice purchase arrangement. But the decision to purchase a practice involves a number of factors.[2]

Advantages

- Immediate income is usually higher than that achieved in a practice starting out cold.
- It can entail a smaller investment than starting from scratch, if the price is reasonable.
- A trained staff and established office procedures already exist.
- An inventory of frames, tools, office equipment, instruments, and supplies is already there and ready to go.
- There is a transition period, during which the departing doctor introduces the incoming doctor to as many patients as possible.

Disadvantages

- The location of the office may not be ideal.
- The design of the office and the instrumentation may not be satisfactory.
- The fee schedule and payment policies may not be desirable.
- The office assistant(s) may be reluctant to accept a new doctor and his ideas.
- The patient flow may drop drastically with the exit of the seller.

Purchasing a practice is somewhat analogous to purchasing a used car: *caveat emptor* (let the buyer beware) applies. An optometrist should approach a potential sale methodically and conservatively, using the first meeting to get acquainted, and subsequent meetings to collect and analyze information about the practice. He should then seek out a competent advisor with whom he can discuss the situation.

The decision-making process for a practitioner who has decided to seek out a practice purchase opportunity basically centers around two questions:

- Do I want to purchase the practice?
- What is the practice worth?

The first question is philosophical; the second is financial.

The first question requires a commitment on the part of the practitioner to a particular state, city, and community. Unfortunately, purchasing a practice entails the opposite procedure from that of setting up a practice from scratch. When a doctor decides to start up a new practice, he usually decides first on the area that could support him and that he has found to be socially acceptable in terms of his personal and family needs. There is a great deal more freedom in this procedure than in the one that a potential purchaser must go through. A purchaser must first locate a practice that is for sale and then take the community that it is in as a second consideration; he goes through the opposite selection process from that of the doctor starting out cold. This can lead to some difficulties for the practitioner who has purchased a satisfactory practice but who has discovered that he does not find the community as successful a match.

The second question is strictly a business decision (once the answer to question one is yes). It is the question that has aroused the most commentary from practitioners and financial experts, but question one is still the most fundamental of the two and must be answered first. If the answer to it is no, then the time spent on question two was wasted.

The following section is a brief discussion of the answer to the second question, relying on the advice of financial experts who have attempted to analyze the rather complex matter of how to determine the fair price of a private practice.

Determining the Fair Value of a Practice

There are two legal problems that await the potential purchaser of an optometric practice: how to determine the cost of the practice and how to allocate the assets for tax purposes. Both are complex legal matters that demand the counsel of competent professionals.

Arranging the sale of an optometric practice has become a mini-industry in itself, drawing the attention of brokers, consultants, lawyers, and accountants.[3] There is good reason for this interest, however, for such sales customarily require the transfer of large sums of money and a long-term relationship between buyer and seller.

A significant hurdle for any potential sale is the price to be paid. There are numerous references in the literature as to how to establish a fair price, and so this problem will not be discussed in detail here. But the optometrist considering a practice purchase agreement should realize that he is buying two distinctly different types of assets:

- Personal property, consisting of ophthalmic equipment and instrumentation, furnishings, inventory, fixtures, and other tangible items
- The reputation, success, or good standing of the practice in the community, which is known as goodwill, an intangible asset that is perhaps best represented by the net income of the practice

The customary cost placed on tangible assets is their fair market value, although this can be altered for tax purposes. Fair market value is easily established because any tangible item has a worth in the marketplace that can be determined with reasonable certainty. Placing a cost on goodwill is not so easily accomplished because the value of a practice to a community, the patients it serves, or its owner is an individual commodity that is unique. It is this aspect of a practice sale that creates the most difficulty in determining a fair price.

A solution of sorts to this dilemma has been the introduction of formulas. A number of formulas have been devised to establish the sales price for a practice, but they are only rough guidelines. The value of a practice is what the buyer is willing to pay and what the seller is willing to accept. Formulas merely serve as a starting point for negotiation. Sample formulas include:

- The net income of the practice for the year preceding the sale or for twice this amount[4]
- A sales price determined by the performance of the practice after the sale (i.e., a contingent sales price)[5]
- One year's net income plus the fair market value of the equipment, furnishings, and other tangibles[6]
- The average net income for the three years preceding the sale, plus the value of the inventory[7]
- Various fractions of the gross income of the practice, ranging from 10 percent to 100 percent[8]

For the buyer, the average net income for the three years preceding the sale, plus the fair market value of the tangibles, is probably the most advantageous formula. For the seller, the highest price, although desirable, may not always be the best. This surprising conclusion may occur in practice sales where the seller finances the arrangement through an installment sale.

An alternative approach is to use a formula merely for the purposes of establishing price limits—a floor and a ceiling—with outside factors determining if the ultimate value lies on the high, low, or middle range of the scale. One example of this approach[9] assumes that the value of a viable optometric practice lies within the range of an average of the last three years' net income (low) to three fourths of the average of the last three years' gross income (high). The assessment of the practice's value begins with the low value (the average net income) and adds onto this base price as appropriate by considering specific factors that add to a practice's worth. A practice that receives full value for each of these factors would be worth the highest value (three fourths of the average gross income).

Factors to be considered in making this determination are as follows:

- Age of the practice (fifteen years or better brings the maximum value)
- Number of primary (full) exams per year (1,600 is the mean as of 1987); the number of days that the appointment book is filled in advance
- Practice location (e.g., parking facilities and the safety of the community)
- Scope of the practice (e.g., the fee schedule, equipment used, and quality of materials)

- Income per patient, which is determined by dividing the annual gross income by the number of full examinations; the average nationally is about $75. The higher the income per patient, the greater the loss to the purchaser if part of the practice is lost to attrition when the seller departs. Other considerations in this category include the accounts receivable (which should be no more than one and a half times the monthly gross income) and the total bad debts (which should be less than 3 percent of the monthly gross income)
- Total number of viable patient records for the past five years; repeat records are important, but new records can be used to show growth
- Salary and benefits available for practitioner and employees
- Derivation of practice income (e.g., percent from professional fees, from materials for eyeglasses, or from contact lenses)
- Practice growth, which consists of three parts: percent increase in growth over the preceding three years; percent increase in net worth over the preceding three years; and percent increase in net compared to gross over the preceding three years
- The fixed and variable expenses of the practice (can they be modified?)
- Lease and rental terms (e.g., renewable? transferable? fixed increases?)
- Office space (is it adequate? is there room for expansion? is it well designed? is it ready for the new practitioner?)
- Does the purchaser require additional capital investment in order to get the practice ready for him?
- Use of para-optometrics and other ancillary personnel; is there employment of family?
- Sources of office income (e.g., private patients, third-party eyeglass or medical reimbursement plans, Medicaid, and Medicare)
- Participation of the seller in the practice after the sale is consummated; will the seller remain for a set period of time?
- Current market value of office equipment, furnishings, and inventory (all tangible items that are being sold)
- Value of leasehold improvements (e.g., ceiling, walls, and carpeting)
- Demographics (both the city and the county ratio of eye-care practitioners per total population)
- Effects on the practice of HMOs, PPOs, union clinical care, closed panels, commercial practice, hospitals, ophthalmology, and other optometrists
- Community economics (e.g., unemployment, welfare system for the reimbursement of optometric services, diversification of industry and business, and stability and growth projections)
- Population trends (e.g., whether up or down, the effect of these trends on the need for eye care, and the increase or decrease in numbers of eye-care practitioners)
- Age of the population and their vision needs (older? younger? contact lenses? special services?)
- History of the practice and the practitioner (has there been a previous partner or associate? has the practice been up for sale before? how long has the practice been looking for a buyer?)
- The financial plan of the seller (what is the payment plan proposed by the seller?)

It should be obvious that the cost of financing a practice sale is a key consideration, and for this reason lending institutions often use a basic formula in order to safeguard against a debtor being overloaded with debt repayments: They figure that a debtor's total loan (both principal and interest) should have a debt service on a monthly basis of no more than 30 percent of his gross income. This should be considered as a guideline in determining the payments to be made by the practice purchaser.[10] Another consideration is that the attrition incurred by the buyer (due to the absence of the seller) may not be offset by his ability to attract new patients and make the practice grow during the first few years.

As difficult and complicated as setting a price is, it is not the only aspect of establishing a value for the practice that is perplexing. Of equal importance and complexity is the problem of allocating the assets of the practice for tax purposes.

Tax Ramifications

How the various assets of a practice are allocated will have a significant influence on the sale. Even if the total price agreed upon by the buyer and seller is reasonable, the fairness of the sale for the buyer may hinge upon how the assets are divided and their costs allocated.[11]

Building—An office building that is owned by the seller is an important asset that must be considered at the time of the sale; however, some sellers may wish to retain title to the building and lease it to the purchaser. Current tax laws award important tax benefits to the owner of such property.

Land—The office property must also be considered at the time of sale, and although it is transferred along with the building, it must be listed separately for tax purposes.

Equipment value—The value of the office equipment, computers, furnishings, ophthalmic instruments and equipment, accessories, and similar items constitutes an important aspect of the practice sale. Because of changes in the federal tax laws, the preferable value to ascribe to equipment is the fair market value, which is what a reasonable buyer would pay and a reasonable seller would accept for the item in a competitive market.

Inventory—Items such as frames, contact lenses, pharmaceutical agents, stationery, and the like are usually sold at their fair market value.

Accounts receivable—Fees that are due and payable but not received at the time of the transfer of the practice are valued according to how old they are. (For example, accounts sixty days or less in arrears could be valued at 100 percent, those 60 to 120 days at 50 percent, those 120 to 180 days at 25 percent, and accounts more than six months old that are not active at 0 percent.) Another approach is to set a certain percentage of value to be applied across the board to all unpaid accounts (90 percent for example).

Goodwill—This is a term that, for want of a better way of expressing its meaning, can be interpreted to mean the willingness and probability that a departing optometrist's patients will return to the newly purchased practice and the new doctor. It has most important tax ramifications for the purchaser.

Covenant Not to Compete—An agreement by the seller that he will not practice in the locality for a specified period of time after the sale is a common provision of practice sales contracts. The value for the covenant must bear a reasonable relationship to the total price being paid for the practice, which requires some careful thought on behalf of both parties. Many authorities consider a covenant not to compete as unnecessary, for they are legally unenforceable in some states (or, even if enforceable, can be reformed by a court if they are excessively restrictive). But they have utility for tax purposes because they offer a substantial tax benefit to the purchaser.

Records—The patient records may be an item of sale, but determining a reasonable value may be difficult. The preferable way to evaluate records is by age; current records are the most valuable, and the older (and more inactive) the record, the less its value to the purchaser. Patient records can be an important tax deduction for the purchaser,[12] and so an effort should be made to establish a reasonable value for them on a per record basis.

These are the major assets that must be considered in the purchase agreement. Their significance is in the value attributed to each because the Tax Reform Act of 1986 has instituted some important changes in the way practice sales are structured.

First of all, we must recognize that there is a substantial difference between the sale of an incorporated practice and the sale of one that is not (i.e., an individual proprietorship). The purchaser of an incorporated practice buys the shares of stock, and the price paid for these shares becomes the purchaser's basis in the corporation, important when the purchaser in turn sells the practice. In many instances, however, the purchaser will not wish to purchase the corporation but will be willing to purchase the corporate assets. Under these circumstances the allocation of assets is performed in the same manner as for an individual proprietorship.

Under the Tax Reform Act of 1986, purchasers of practices are required to use the residual method of allocating the purchase price. The unfortunate result of this law is to obligate the parties to use the fair market value for all tangible and intangible assets and to allocate any residual amount of the sales price to goodwill. For example, if the sales price is $100,000, and the fair market value of all tangible and intangible assets is $60,000, then $40,000 of the purchase price must be allocated to goodwill. Such an allocation would be extremely disadvantageous for the buyer, and so the parties should review the practice assets carefully and thoroughly.

Tax Ramifications for the Seller

Prior to the revolutionary 1986 tax law, a seller had a substantial interest in the way assets were allocated for tax purposes because favorable long-term capital gains could be claimed on many of the assets sold. But the new tax code does away with this tax break, which means that the seller will be taxed on the proceeds of sale at his tax bracket. As of 1988, this means that the seller will most likely face a tax rate of 28 percent and, for some, perhaps a 33 percent rate. Under the new code the allocation of assets will usually have few tax consequences for the seller, except for depreciation recapture income (discussed *infra*). Therefore, it is the manner in which the buyer will finance the purchase and the period of time over which the buyer will pay the sales price that will create the most concern. For many sellers, the best arrangement will be one in which the seller self-finances the loan through the use of an installment sale. By extending the repayment over a period of years, and by charging the buyer a reasonable rate of interest, the seller is able to maximize the financial return on the sale. Thus the sales price, the period of repayment, and the interest to be charged are most significant items for the seller.

Tax Ramifications for the Buyer

Because the buyer's allowable tax deductions depend on the manner in which the assets are allocated for sale, the buyer should emphasize this point during negotiations with the seller. Because the assets must be separated into various categories, the buyer should ensure that a careful inventory is performed and that a fair market price is allocated to all assets. It may be useful to obtain estimates of value for the various assets from knowlegeable individuals such as equipment salesmen, realtors, or laboratory representatives. It is desirable to have this supporting evidence in the event the allocations in the sales contract are challenged by the IRS. Such a challenge, if successful, would result in the allocation of part of the sales price to goodwill, for which the buyer would lose not only a future deduction but also any deduction improperly claimed in the past. Back taxes and penalties also would be the responsibility of the purchaser. The IRS requires that both buyer and seller report the allocation of the sales price on Form 8594, which is attached to their federal income tax returns for the year in which the sale occurred.[13]

There are numerous assets for which the buyer can claim a deduction (see Table 48.1). The only assets for which no tax break can be realized are goodwill and land. Buildings, equipment and instruments, records, and restrictive covenants are depreciable; accounts receivable and supplies and inventory are deductible expenses. There are two other assets that deserve mention because although they do provide a tax break for the buyer, the 1986 Tax Reform Act has greatly reduced their utility. These assets are leasehold improvements and preferential leases. Under the prior tax law they could be deducted rapidly, but the new code greatly extends the period of time over which these deductions can be claimed, which reduces them to only a fraction of their former value.

Table 48.1. Tax Considerations in the Sale of Practice Assets

Practice Asset	Tax Ramifications for Buyer
Professional building	Depreciable over $31\frac{1}{2}$ years
Equipment and instruments, computers, furnishings, and other capital assets	Depreciable over 5 years (computers) or 7 years (equipment, furnishings)
Covenant not to compete	Amortizable over 5 years or more
Patient records	Depreciable over 7 years
Supplies and inventory	Deductible
Land	Not deductible or depreciable
Goodwill	Not deductible or depreciable

There is also a problem unique to goodwill and covenants not to compete that should be avoided, the inclusion of both types of assets within the practice agreement. If a covenant not to compete accompanies the transfer of goodwill, and if the purpose of the covenant is to assure the purchaser of the enjoyment of the goodwill that he bought, the covenant becomes part of the goodwill and its cost becomes a capital asset that is treated like goodwill. It cannot be amortized by the purchaser.[14]

The tax consequences of how the assets are valued weigh heavily on the purchaser, but the seller has an obvious interest in the outcome as well. In negotiating the contract, both parties must recognize that the principle underlying the transaction must be one of fairness. Since seller-funded purchase agreements (discussed below) require long-term relationships, it is necessary for the provisions of sale to be such that both buyer and seller are able to prosper. If the contract is so burdensome for the purchaser that he is unable to meet his obligations and defaults, there is economic loss to the seller as well. Therefore, these agreements must represent a satisfactory compromise by both sides.

Method of Payment

One other aspect of the sale that requires negotiation is the method of payment. If the buyer pays the seller

Determination of practice value. There are numerous ways to determine the value of a practice. We will use the following formula: the fair market value of the tangible assets of the practice plus the average of the net income for the three years preceding the sale.

The tangible assets of the practice include equipment, instruments, furnishings, inventories of frames and lenses, and similar items. The fair market value of all the practice assets is determined to be $75,000. (This sum does not take into account the value of patient records.)

The accounts receivable of the practice amount to $5,000.

The average net income of the practice for the 3 years preceding the sale is $75,000.

Determination of the terms of sale. It is agreed that Dr. Buyer will purchase the practice for $150,000. The accounts receivable will be paid to Dr. Seller as payment is received by Dr. Buyer during the six months following the sale.

The agreement specifies that Dr. Buyer will pay $10,000 down, with the balance of $140,000 to be paid to Dr. Seller in 120 equal monthly installments (i.e., over 10 years).

If no interest was to be charged on this balance, the payments to Dr. Seller would be $14,000 a year or $1,167 per month. However, it is agreed that Dr. Buyer will also pay 10% simple interest on the unpaid balance during this period. This amounts to an extra $663 monthly, for a total of $1,830 per month, $21,960 per annum, payable by Dr. Buyer.

Therefore, over the 10 years of payments the total received by Dr. Seller will be $219,600.

The interest paid by Dr. Buyer totals $79,560, which is tax deductible. This same amount is income for Dr. Seller.

Allocation of assets for sale. The practice assets must be allocated for tax purposes. There are several ways that this could be done; the following is but one alternative that could be used to equitably distribute these assets.

Equipment, instruments, furnishings	$60,000
Supplies and inventory	$15,000
Patient records	$25,000
Covenant not to compete	$40,000

The $140,000 sales price paid to Dr. Seller will be taxed at his individual bracket (probably 28%), as will the $79,560 in interest payments.

Dr. Buyer will be able to depreciate $85,000 of the sales price (equipment, instruments, furnishings, and the patient records) by using the Accelerated Cost Recovery System. The covenant not to compete will have to be amortized ($4,000 a year) over the ten-year period of the contract. The $79,560 in interest payments will have to be deducted in accordance with customary accounting procedures (and thus the deduction will be much larger at the beginning of the loan than at the end). The $15,000 for the supplies and inventory must be deducted in the year of purchase.

Summary of income for the seller. The seller realizes a total income of $229,600, including the down payment, sales price, and interest on the loan.

Summary of tax benefits for the purchaser. In the first year, Dr. Buyer may claim a total tax deduction of $33,100 ($11,900 for depreciation; $12,200 for interest; $4,000 for the covenant; and $5,000 for the supplies and inventory). He may also be able to claim an additional interest deduction if he had to borrow the $10,000 down payment.

In the second year Dr. Buyer's deduction is $36,400 ($21,200 in depreciation; $11,200 in interest deductions; and $4,000 for the covenant).

In the fifth year the deduction has dropped to $19,800 ($7,650 for depreciation; $8,150 for interest; and $4,000 for the covenant not to compete).

By the tenth year the deduction is a mere $5,000 ($1,000 for the interest and $4,000 for the covenant). The depreciation deduction has been completely used up, at a time when Dr. Buyer's income has probably reached its highest level. Thus Dr. Buyer's biggest tax problems arise at the end of the repayment period, when his deductions are depleted.

Figure 48.1. Samples Sales Arrangement. This sample is intended to serve as an illustration of how a practice purchase agreement can be formulated that is fair to both buyer and seller. The problem presumes that the seller is a non-incorporated sole practitioner and that the buyer is a relatively new optometrist who must acquire some financing in order to effect the purchase.

the agreed-upon price in a lump sum, an unnecessary portion of the proceeds of sale may be lost to taxes. Furthermore, the buyer would probably have to borrow the money to make the lump-sum payment, which might impede his ability to acquire other loans necessary to improve the practice. These two circumstances combine to produce the most common mode of payment: the installment sale.

There are two general requirements for an installment sale[15]:

- The payments must extend over more than one tax year.
- The sale cannot be interest-free; a reasonable rate of interest must be paid at each installment on the unpaid balance of the purchase price. If the agreement does not provide for interest, it will be imputed by the IRS.

The purchaser signs a note payable to the seller for the sales price, with the length of time for repayment and the interest on the unpaid balance specified. The seller receives the security of regularly scheduled payments, which are composed of both principal and interest. He can even insure the balance against the death of the buyer by having the buyer purchase decreasing term life insurance.

For the purchaser an installment sale also has advantages. The repayment schedule can be structured so that the periodic payments to the seller are affordable, and the interest portions of the payments can be deducted as a business expense. These matters are often the subject of intense negotiations and require flexibility on the part of the negotiators. For example, if the seller wishes to receive payments over an extended period (such as ten years), the buyer may be able to negotiate a lower rate of interest. If the seller is determined to sell the practice only for a certain sum, the use of an installment sale, self-financing, and an interest charge may allow that sum to be achieved. The seller must pay income taxes on the interest received, just as with the principal amount. The buyer receives a tax deduction for the interest paid. Even so, it is desirable for the buyer to secure a clause that allows for the prepayment of the loan before the expiration of the full term, in case he wishes to pay off the loan balance early. Similarly, it is advantageous for the buyer to obtain a fixed rate loan.

The seller will most likely specify the mode of repayment. The contract may simply require a fixed monthly payment, it may specify a variable repayment schedule that requires larger payments in later years, or it may permit payment to be made as a percentage of the gross income (until the sales price is realized). The exact details will depend on the circumstances of the sale and the needs of the buyer and seller. Because practice sales arrangements can vary significantly due to personal factors, both parties should consult legal counsel to ensure that the conditions of sale will achieve the result intended.

One tax issue for the seller that requires professional expertise is depreciation recapture income. If an installment sale is used, and depreciated property (e.g., ophthalmic equipment) is sold, any depreciation recapture income must be reported in the year of sale, which can place an unexpected tax burden on the seller.[16]

A sample sales arrangement is included as Fig. 48.1.

Notes

1. For a discussion of the problems of purchasing an optometric practice, see Gregg, J., *The Business of Optometric Practice*, Advisory Enterprises, White Plains, N.Y., 1981, pp. 40–50.
2. Adopted from ibid.
3. See Hubler, R.S., How to Buy (Or Maybe Sell) An Optometric Practice, *Optometric Management*, vol. 18, no. 5, 1982, pp. 27–30.
4. Elmstrom, G., *Advanced Management for Optometrists*, Professional Press, Chicago, 1974, pp. 111–118.
5. Thal, L.S., The Practice Sale: Getting to the Bottom Line, *Optometric Management*, vol. 22, no. 6, 1986, pp. 66–67.
6. Elmstrom, supra note 4.
7. Gregg, supra note 1.
8. Elmstrom, G., *Advanced Management Strategies for Optometrists*, Professional Press, Chicago, 1982, pp. 42–49.
9. Martus, C., Private Sector for the Practice of Optometry?, *Foresight*, Apr. 1982, pp. 8–10.
10. *Guidelines for Structuring a Practice Purchase*, Pro-Med Capital Co., North Miami Beach, Fla., 1985.
11. Selling Your Solo Practice, *Review of Optometry*, vol. 121, no. 12, 1984, p. 20; and Josselson, B.H., How To Avoid the Pitfalls When Selling a Practice, *Private Practice*, Feb. 1984, p. 25.
12. The depreciation deduction for medical records is discussed in *Johnson v. United States*, 7 A.F.T.R.2d 793 (D.C. Tex. 1961).
13. IRS form 8594, Asset Acquisition Statement. For a discussion, see IRS Publication 921, *Explanation of the Tax Reform Act of 1986 for Business.*
14. The inclusion of covenants not to compete in sales contracts that also include goodwill has been a long-standing source of legal activity. See *Federal Tax Coordinator*, vol. I, for a lengthy discussion of cases. The

1986 Tax Reform Act, by requiring the residual method of allocating assets, will cause goodwill to become an aspect of many sales contracts that might also include covenants not to compete. Whether or not the IRS will be as aggressive in pursuing this issue under the new tax code remains to be seen.

15. For a discussion, see Internal Revenue Service Publication 537, *Installment Sales*.
16. Depreciation recapture income is determined as follows: Assume the ophthalmic equipment was originally purchased for $50,000 and depreciated by $19,500 under the ACRS, so that it had an adjusted basis of $30,500. If it was sold for $40,000 in an installment sale, there would be a gain of $9,500. This $9,500 gain would be depreciation recapture income, which would have to be reported as ordinary income by the seller in the year of sale, and which would require the payment of $2,660 in taxes if the seller was taxed on this income at 28 percent. None of this gain could be reported on an installment basis. Sellers should be certain that the down payment on the sale is sufficient to cover any depreciation recapture tax indebtedness. For a detailed discussion, see Internal Revenue Publication 544, *Sales and Other Dispositions of Assets*.

Chapter 49

Leases

Lease: *A contract in writing, under seal, whereby a person having a legal estate in hereditaments, corporeal or incorporeal, conveys a portion of his interest to another, in consideration of a certain annual rent or render, or other recompense.*
—Black's Law Dictionary

Basic Principles

The lease is a complex yet useful contract that has wide application within the practice of optometry. Like all contracts, it requires competent parties, consideration, and mutual assent, but there are other considerations peculiar to the lease that must be understood.

A lease is a written instrument that reflects a special relationship between the parties because it is an agreement on the part of one to convey some right that he holds in property to the other. The typical arrangement is between one who holds the right to title to property and one who seeks the right to possession of the property. Therefore, a lease does not involve a transfer of the right of ownership; rather, it is a transfer of the right of possession. The right of possession is temporary, being limited to some term specified in the agreement, but can be extended for successive terms to result in a very lengthy period. (And, as we shall see, some lease arrangements can even provide for a transfer of title.) The property that is the subject of the lease can be real or personal, and in fact optometrists commonly acquire leasehold interests in both realty and personalty. Lastly, the lease requires consideration, such that the one transferring the right of possession (called the *lessor*) receives a certain compensation from the one acquiring the right of possession (called the *lessee*).

This chapter discusses three of the most common uses of leases—for office space, ophthalmic equipment, and automobiles—and describes the provisions customarily encountered in leases for these kinds of property.

A lease is a binding document that, in the usual case, creates a long-term relationship and requires the transfer of substantial sums of money. As with all contracts, an optometrist should consult with competent legal counsel before entering into such an agreement. Leases are frequently lengthy, written in complex and stilted language, and composed of provisions that establish rights and responsibilities understandable only to those familiar with the common law. (Just like the definition at the beginning of this chapter!) Yet they should be understood before being signed.

Real Property Leases

The most common type of lease that will be encountered by optometrists is one for the possession of real estate. The contract will allow the possession of office space for a stated period of time and for a specific amount of compensation. Although the cost and duration of the lease are the two principal considerations, a lease contains numerous other provisions that relate to the relationship of lessor and lessee.[1] Since leases are customarily drafted for the benefit of the lessor, there is often little that the lessee can do in terms of modifying the contract. But the lessee can find himself in a position to bargain with the lessor under certain circumstances, such as when a long-term arrangement is contemplated or the lease property has been vacant for a long period. The lessee should always attempt to negotiate favorable lease provisions, especially those provisions that are found in this section; a lessor who is eager to lease his property may be willing to make some concessions.[2]

Although there are a multitude of clauses that could be added to a lease, this discussion is limited to several of the basic provisions that should be found in any lease.

Identification of the parties—The parties to the contract must be clearly identified; this is especially important when the lessee is a professional corporation or partnership rather than an individual.

Description of the lease property—The property must be identified by its legal description.

Term of the lease—The usual lease period is one to five years, but this is frequently open to negotiation; the lease period may be extended through the use of an option to renew, which permits both lessor and lessee to enjoy a long-term relationship.

Option to renew—Stability is obtained by including an option to renew in the lease agreement; this clause permits the lessee, at his option, to renew the lease for an additional period; the lease can contain an option to renew for several additional periods, thus assuring the lessee that, if he wishes to remain at the location, he may do so. It is customary, however, for the lessor to be permitted to adjust the rent during the option period; typically, the new rental rate is specified in the clause containing the option to renew.

Lease rental—The amount of the lease should be clearly specified but is often expressed as a base rate that can be escalated periodically; in addition, the lease should specify either the amount or the method of determining the rent during any subsequent renewal periods (discussed in more detail *infra*).

Covenant of free title—The lessor should covenant that he has title to the property and thus has the right to lease it to the lessee.

Lessor's right to enter the premises—The lessor is customarily given the right to enter the lease premises during usual working hours for the purpose of making repairs or alterations.

Right to sublet or assign—The lessee may be given the right to sublet the premises without the prior approval of the lessor, but the opposite is more commonly the rule; this can be a substantial right for the lessee, and should not be overlooked.

Responsibility for repairs—The repairs of leased premises are frequently divided between the lessor and the lessee; the more permanent repairs (e.g., rebuilding and repainting) are usually the responsibility of the lessor, while day-to-day repairs (e.g., broken windows or leaky faucets) are more likely to be the responsibility of the lessee.

Cost of utilities—The cost of utilities usually falls upon the lessee; if the lessor is responsible, the lease will typically include an escalation clause that permits the lessor to pass the cost on the lessee; (this can be a substantial expense under some circumstances, discussed *infra*).

Insurance for fire, storm, or other hazard—The lessor has the responsibility to insure the building; however, the contents of the interior (i.e., the office) will have to be insured by the lessee; casualty insurance and other types of coverage can be obtained to protect against loss (see Chapter 54).

Termination of the lease due to casualty loss—If the building is totally destroyed by fire or other casualty, the lease should automatically terminate; if only a portion of the building is lost, the lease should provide some time limit within which the building must be repaired and returned to use (or be expected to be returned to use) or the lessee may terminate the lease upon the giving of notice (see the discussion in Chapter 54).

Installation of fixtures and permanent improvements—If the lessee wishes to make structural changes in the office space prior to beginning business, he must secure the approval of the lessor; the cost of these improvements may be borne by the lessee (the usual case), the lessee and lessor jointly (a relatively common compromise), or the lessor (rare); the agreement should specify the right to make the necessary changes and who will be responsible for the costs.

Failure to pay rent within required time—The lease will provide remedies to the lessor in the event the lessee defaults in payment of the rent; several legal remedies will be available to the lessor, including acceleration of payments, monetary damages, or eviction; these will vary with the state and locality.

Notice required in writing—Any notice or demand that is required under the lease should be required to be in writing, with delivery specified for each of the parties at a particular address.

There are several potential problem areas that should be avoided if possible when an office lease is being negotiated.

Cost-of-living adjustments (COLAs)—Many leases contain provisions that allow the lessor to escalate the rental in accordance with changes in the cost of living. The lessee may find that an escalation clause based upon actual costs is a better deal. If a COLA clause is unavoidable, the lessee can obtain some protection by ensuring that the increase cannot be retroactively applied, that notice of increases must be given in advance, and that a specific dollar or percentage limit is listed.

Separate utility charges—If a building's energy bill is equally shared among lessees, a lessee who is open fewer hours or days could pay a disproportionate amount of the utility expenses. A clause providing for separate utility metering can prevent this problem.

Zoning requirements—Zoning laws and other regulations may limit the modifications that can be performed at a particular location. Historic buildings, covenants attached to realty, and inability to alter adjacent property are common difficulties.

Shopping mall offices—There are numerous provisions of shopping mall leases that can be troublesome. Some malls require both a basic rent and a charge based on retail sales; these charges should be fully understood and, if possible, avoided. Normal office hours should be specified in the mall lease; requirements for "continuous operation," or like language, should be stricken. Most malls require lessees to pay a prorated share for maintaining common areas, and partly occupied malls can result in staggering costs; if possible, these expenses should be limited in the lease. Shopping mall leases often require joint advertising or membership in a merchant's association; these provisions should also be deleted. An optometrist leasing space in a mall should insist on a clause that limits the kinds of businesses that can be located within a certain distance of his office. Mall leases can become so complicated that a lawyer's expertise will be necessary to unravel their complexities.

Leases for real property are lengthy and expensive, but an optometrist can also obligate himself for substantial amounts of money and time through a lease for ophthalmic equipment. Although optometrists have traditionally purchased ophthalmic equipment, there are occasions when leasing becomes a viable alternative to ownership.

Equipment Leases

Leases for personal property (i.e., ophthalmic equipment) differ somewhat from those for realty. There is little flexibility in the lease terms, although there are certain provisions that the lessor provides as options to be chosen by the lessee. In terms of the legal obligation, it is the same as for a lease of real property.[3]

The lease for ophthalmic equipment is often offered by a professional development company, one that specializes in offering financial plans to professionals. Leasing is but one of a series of benefits available to the practitioner, including revolving charge accounts, loans, and casualty, disability, and life insurance. These companies typically charge more than a bank for these services.

Commonly cited advantages of leasing include the following[4]:

- One hundred percent financing of the equipment
- No down payment
- One hundred percent of the lease cost may be deducted.
- After the term of the lease, the equipment does not have to be purchased; instead, a new lease for new equipment can be entered into.
- The finance charge for the lease period does not change, and so fluctuating interest rates do not affect the amount due.

Disadvantages of leasing include the following:

- Most beginning optometrists do not earn enough income to justify the full deduction that the lease bestows.
- The cost of a lease is greater than the cost of a straight purchase of the same equipment; at the end of the lease period the doctor will have to pay 10 to 15 percent of the fair market value of the equipment if he wishes to obtain title to it.
- The optometrist will not be entitled to claim the

depreciation deduction; the deduction will be taken by the lessor.

- The leased equipment must be kept for the full term of the lease, and the only exceptions are if the equipment is upgraded or equipment of a greater value is obtained; if returned to the company (for example, the doctor defaults on his payments), the equipment can be sold by the leasing company and any deficit in what is owed can then be collected from the defaulting doctor.
- The lease agreement will probably require the doctor to pay for insurance on the equipment; the doctor may also be required to pay for all repairs, although this will probaby be a matter of the warranty that the doctor receives from the equipment seller or manufacturer (and this is no different from the arrangement that a doctor receives when he purchases equipment through bank financing; usually, the only warranties for repair or servicing that the doctor receives are those made by the equipment supplier or manufacturer, and these warranties are for a limited period).

A lease agreement for ophthalmic equipment (or furniture, fixtures, or office renovation) should include the following clauses:

Identification of the parties—The lessee, if a corporation or partnership, should sign the lease as such.

Description of the lease property—The lessee will select the ophthalmic equipment that he wants to lease, and the leasing company will provide him with the economic means to obtain it from the manufacturer, and so the property will have to be described with specificity in the agreement.

Term of the lease—The usual lease term is from one to seven years, but some companies may permit even longer periods.

Option to purchase—At the end of the lease period, the lessee will have the right to purchase the equipment from the lessor; the price can be set at the outset of the agreement or may be expressed as a percentage that cannot be exceeded; if the lessee does not wish to buy the equipment, it is returned to the leasing company at the conclusion of the lease term.

Cost of the lease—The interest on the lease will be higher than that charged by a bank, but it will be stable throughout the lease period (i.e., it is set at the outset of the lease and does not fluctuate); if bank loan rates are down but subsequently go up significantly, then the interest charged by the leasing company may fall below that of the bank; also, many leasing companies offer a graduated payment schedule, whereby the lease payments are lower in the first years, gradually escalating in the later years (when the doctor has more cash flow and hence more need for the tax deduction).

Responsibility for repairs—The lease company will not provide repairs; the lessee will have to find a dealer who will perform any necessary repairs and will have to pay for these repairs himself (although the manufacturer will provide maintenance and repairs during the warranty period).

Insurance—The lessee will probably be required to purchase insurance sufficient to indemnify the lessor in the event the equipment is lost (as in a fire or other casualty).

Right of exchange—The lessee may wish to exchange certain equipment before the lease term is concluded, in order to obtain a newer model or a different piece of equipment altogether; the lease should recognize the right to do so (of course, the cost of the lease will escalate accordingly).

Failure to make payment within required time—The lease will provide certain remedies to the lessor should the lessee fail to make the lease payments as provided in the agreement. Among the remedies available to the the lessor are acceleration of payments, increased charges for late payments, and seizure and sale of the equipment. The penalties involved if payments cannot be made as the lease schedule demands should be understood (of course, the lease may be extended for an additional period, just as with a bank loan).

A lease agreement for equipment is a complicated legal document that requires consultation with an attorney, especially if the lessee is inexperienced in transactions of this nature.

Automobile Leases

One item of personal property that is leased with some frequency is the automobile. Although lease provisions for automobiles are not unlike those for equipment, there are unique provisions of automobile leasing that sets it apart. There are three basic types of leasing arrangements for automobiles.

The finance lease—This is the cheapest form of lease, but there is a charge at the end of the lease term for any wear and tear or other damage suffered by the vehicle.

The net lease—This lease is more expensive than the finance lease because there is no charge at the end of the lease term for normal wear and tear, rather this charge is factored into the cost of the lease.

The maintenance lease—This is the most expensive form of lease because it includes not only coverage for normal wear and tear but also the cost of regular vehicle service.

The advantages of leasing an automobile include the following: Bank financing is not required, which means that the lessee's personal financial statement is clear of this obligation (and, if the lessee is a professional corporation, the employee-optometrist has no personal obligation whatsoever); automobile insurance may be cheaper; transportation expenses can be more easily budgeted (of special importance for incorporated practices); the tax-deductible costs of operating a leased vehicle can be easily documented; and, at the end of the term of the lease, the automobile may be purchased by the lessee.

Optometrists who wish to retain capital for expenditures other than vehicles, or who wish to keep their personal financial statements clear for other obligations (such as buying a house), may find a vehicle lease to be an attractive alternative to purchasing.

Notes

1. Cassidy, R., New Traps To Avoid in Negotiating an Office Lease, *Medical Economics*, vol. 57, no. 17, Aug. 18, 1980, pp. 141–148.
2. Josselson, B.H., Leasing Office Space: More than Just Signing on the Dotted Line, *Private Practice*, Nov. 1984, p. 35.
3. Pinto, D., How To Succeed in Optometry Without Really Buying, *Optometric Management*, vol. 17, no. 4, 1981, pp. 29–36.
4. Adopted from Gregg, J., *The Business of Optometric Practice*, Advisory Enterprises, White Plains, N.Y., 1981, pp. 110–114.

Chapter 50

Credit

Neither a borrower, nor a lender be.
—William Shakespeare, *Hamlet*

An Overview of Consumer Credit

The famous advice offered by Polonius to his departing son, Laertes, to avoid financial transactions with others would fall upon deaf ears in the twentieth century. The majority of people in the United States own and use credit cards, and the utilization of credit by U.S. consumers has literally exploded over the past two decades, significantly affecting the national economy, the manner in which business is conducted, the expectations of consumers themselves, and leading inevitably to a mushrooming body of federal and state regulation that has already reached a pervasiveness that was unthought of as recently as the mid-1960s.

Optometrists, as providers of services, come face-to-face with credit on a daily basis and must make many decisions pertaining to consumer credit that are influenced by legal considerations. The decision to extend credit, to collect or disseminate credit information, or to pursue an overdue credit account brings the optometrist into contact with the Consumer Credit Protection Act,[1] the first major federal consumer credit legislation, and with numerous state laws directed at the regulation of some form or aspect of consumer credit. In order to serve patients fairly and to avoid conflict with legal requirements, optometrists must possess a working knowledge of applicable credit laws and must ensure that their credit policies conform to acceptable procedures.

In this chapter we will briefly review the major federal credit laws that have applicability to optometrists and how they affect the daily activities of the private practitioner. Since federal laws are uniformly applied to all states, every optometrist will feel the influence of these provisions. Although there are numerous consumer credit laws at the state level, they vary so significantly that no meaningful consensus can be drawn, and optometrists will have to obtain legal counsel to learn the local credit provisions that will have applicability to them. Several states, however, have adopted the Uniform Consumer Credit Code, and we will conclude the chapter with a description of the major provisions of this law (which establishes uniform laws in all of the states that have adopted it).

First of all, let us define credit, which can be broadly described as "any arrangement whereby a consumer purchases goods or services or borrows funds and pays what is owed at some time in the future."[2] Consumer credit is credit that is obtained for personal purposes. The Consumer Credit Protection Act, enacted by Congress in 1968, was the first and most ambitious effort to regulate consumer credit transactions. One of its most significant provisions was the Truth-in-Lending Act.

The Truth-in-Lending Act

The Truth-in-Lending Act, Title I of the Consumer Credit Protection Act, was adopted "to assure a meaningful disclosure of credit terms so that the consumer will be able to compare more readily the various credit terms available to him."[3] In order to accomplish this goal, Congress instructed the Board of Governors of the Federal Reserve Board to promulgate regulations intended to carry out the law's provisions. The result was Regulation Z,[4] which—according to the Federal Reserve Board—applied to:

> . . . doctors, dentists, and other professional people, and hospitals. In fact to any individual or organization that extends or arranges credit for which a finance charge is or may be payable or which is repayable in more than four installments.[5]

Thus Regulation Z could be applied to credit transactions involving the private practice of optometry. To comply with the requirements of Truth-in-Lending, creditors were obligated to disclose certain details related to the credit to be granted and to maintain records of the credit transaction.[6] Failure to comply with the law could result in the imposition of severe penalties upon conviction. The Truth-in-Lending Act, however, was modified by a series of laws passed by Congress during the latter half of the 1970s.

The first of these laws was the Fair Credit Billing Act, passed in 1974,[7] which dealt with a variety of problems related to the use of credit cards, particularly errors in billing. In 1976 the Consumer Leasing Act was enacted[8]; it added certain disclosure requirements to the Truth-in-Lending Act for consumer leases of personal property and imposed certain limits on a lessee's liability at the termination of a lease. And in 1980, the Truth-in-Lending Simplification and Reform Act[9] was approved by Congress, which substantially overhauled the Truth-in-Lending law, altering both its substantive provisions and its penalties for noncompliance. The simplified version of the law took full effect in October of 1982.

Under the Truth-in-Lending Simplification and Reform Act and a revised Regulation Z, optometrists can come under the provisions of the law in either of two circumstances:

- If an oral or written contract for services or materials is entered into before the services are rendered, and if a finance charge is made, the optometrist is subject to the law, provided the optometrist regularly extends consumer credit (e.g., if he extended credit more than twenty-five times in the preceding calendar year).[10]
- If a written agreement for services or materials is entered into, and if the agreement provides for no finance charge but calls for more than four installment payments (not including a downpayment), the optometrist is subject to the law.[11]

Therefore, even though an optometrist may grant credit interest free, he can still be required to comply with the extensive disclosure requirements of Truth-in-Lending and to maintain credit reports as specified by the law. Such an eventuality poses a burden of unnecessary proportions to the average practitioner of optometry.[12] In order to avoid this eventuality, the optometrist may find it advisable to bill patients for the entire amount due and to permit them to satisfy the debt as they can, rather than scheduling fixed installments for repayment. Or, if the optometrist wishes to receive payments in fixed installments, he should ensure that they number four or less.

An optometrist who applies a finance charge for unpaid balances owed by patients, and who extends credit to more than twenty-five patients in a calendar year, will fall within the scope of Truth-in-Lending.

Penalties for violation of the act are both civil and criminal.

The Fair Credit Reporting Act

Title VI of the Consumer Credit Protection Act —known as the Fair Credit Reporting Act[13]—is intended

> to require that consumer reporting agencies adopt reasonable procedures for meeting the needs of commerce for consumer credit, personnel insurance, and other information in a manner which is fair and equitable to the consumer, with regard to the confidentiality, accuracy, relevancy, and proper utilization of such information.[14]

An optometrist may employ a credit bureau to obtain information concerning the credit status of a patient and may use this information to decide whether to award the patient credit. If a patient is denied credit due to such a report, the patient is entitled under the Fair Credit Reporting Act to review his file at the issuing credit agency or consumer reporting agency. As a matter of courtesy, an optometrist who receives information that causes him to deny credit to a patient may notify the patient of the basis for his decision so that the patient may inspect his file if he so desires. If a file is in fact incorrect, and the consumer is denied credit, he may take action to have the file corrected and, in certain cases, may be eligible for damages.

Under the Fair Credit Reporting Act, any person who knowingly and willfully obtains information from a consumer reporting agency under false pretenses or provides such information to a person not authorized to receive it may be subject to a criminal penalty.

The Equal Credit Opportunity Act

The Equal Credit Opportunity Act—Title VII of the Consumer Credit Protection Act—was enacted in 1974,[15] amended in 1976,[16] and expanded by a regulation published by the Federal Reserve Board labeled "Regulation B"[17] in 1977. The purpose of this act was to prohibit discrimination in credit transactions. It prohibited discrimination on the basis of race, color, religion, national origin, sex, marital status, or age, because all or part of the applicant's income was derived from a public assistance program, or because the applicant exercised in good faith any right under the Consumer Credit Protection Act.

Regulation B implements the act's prohibitions against discrimination by setting forth the information that may be requested in connection with an application for credit, establishing guidelines for the manner in which the credit application must be evaluated, and determining the procedure that a creditor must follow when offering credit or denying an application.[18]

Optometrists may qualify as creditors under the act and must scrupulously observe its prohibitions when judging credit applications. Women, single persons, and those on public assistance are the most sensitive applicants, and the optometrist who grants credit should ensure that these individuals are considered with the same impartiality as are other applicants.

The Equal Credit Opportunity Act contains liability and enforcement provisions that are similar to those of Truth-in-Lending.

The Fair Debt Collection Practices Act

Title VIII of the Consumer Credit Protection Act, known as the Fair Debt Collection Practices Act,[19] was enacted in 1977 for the purpose of eliminating abusive debt collection practices by debt collectors. Except for a person who uses a name other than his own while attempting to collect debts owed him, the act does not apply to collection efforts instituted by an original creditor, and thus it principally affects third-party debt collectors. Any personal collection efforts are excluded. The collection practices of optometrists are regulated by state law, however, and are discussed in Chapter 51.

The Uniform Consumer Credit Code

Although state statutes regulating credit are too numerous and vary too significantly to be described here, the Uniform Consumer Credit Code (UCCC), which has been adopted by some states, will be summarized briefly.

The UCCC is a uniform state law that is broadly applied and comprehensive in scope, intending to serve as the sole authority for credit matters in the states where adopted. It modifies, repeals, or revises all statutes in the state that apply to credit, causing the state regulation of consumer credit transactions to conform to the policies of the Truth-in-Lending Act. Thus a creditor who does not apply a finance charge and permits payment in more than four installments is subject to Truth-in-Lending and must comply with disclosure and reporting requirements. In those states where the UCCC is law, optometrists will want to determine their responsibilities and obligations to those patients to whom credit is granted.

Of course, an optometrist will always want to be familiar with the provisions of state law that apply to common credit situations occurring in private practice. Legal counsel may be required in some instances, but many of these situations are amenable to the application of general rules that will be the same from state to state:

- A minor may be able to repudiate an optometrist's contract for services; for this reason, it is advisable to contract with a minor's parent or guardian.
- The children of divorced couples may live with one parent while the other parent is legally accountable for necessary medical services; responsibility for payment should be established at the time the doctor–patient relationship is established.
- A divorced spouse may wish to have the ex-spouse billed for an optometrist's services; the recommended policy in this event is to have

the person receiving the services responsible for the bill; that person can in turn obtain reimbursement from the former spouse.

- Postdated checks, although valid, should be accepted with caution if the date is remote; there is always the possibility that payment on such a check will be stopped.
- The words "paid in full" on a check pose a legal problem, especially if the check is for less than the full amount owed; even if the one executing the check crosses these words out, it is preferable not to deposit the check; the better policy is to have another check drawn without the words or to refuse to accept a partial payment.
- If a check is returned by the bank marked "insufficient funds," it is possible in some circumstances to redeposit the check and to arrange for the bank to hold the check until sufficient funds have been deposited to cover it.

Experience in credit matters will permit an optometrist to more ably fulfill his obligation to award credit fairly and to comply with federal and state disclosure and reporting requirements.

A legal matter closely allied with credit is the problem of collections. We will discuss the legal restrictions applied to collection efforts in the following chapter.

Notes

1. Consumer Credit Protection Act, P.L. No. 90–321, 82 Stat. 146 (May 29, 1968, amended in 1976).
2. Geltzer, R.L., *Federal Regulation of Consumer Credit*, Warren, Gorham and Lamont, Boston, 1981, pp. 1–3.
3. 15 U.S.C. §§1601 et seq.
4. Regulation Z, Truth-in-Lending, 12 C.F.R. §226.
5. Quoted in Rice, E.W., Regulation Z: New Paper Work Burden?, *Physicians Management*, July 1969, p. 39.
6. Truth-in-Lending Act 102(a), 15 U.S.C. §1601(a).
7. In consumer credit transactions the creditor must disclose basic terms, including the interest to be charged —the finance charge—and must use a standard measurement of the cost of credit, the annual percentage rate (APR). The act also requires that periodic billing statements be sent to the consumer when open ended or revolving credit plans are entered into. See Geltzer, supra note 2, at Sec. 3.03.
8. Consumer Leasing Act, chap. 5 of the Truth-in-Lending Act, 15 U.S.C. §1601 et seq.
9. Truth-in-Lending Simplification and Reform Act, 15 U.S.C. §1601 et seq.
10. Regulation Z, Truth-in-Lending, 12 C.F.R. §226.2.
11. Ibid.
12. See Rice, supra note 5.
13. Fair Credit Reporting Act, 15 U.S.C. §1681 et seq.
14. Fair Credit Reporting Act, §602(b), 15 U.S.C. §1681(b).
15. Equal Credit Opportunity Act, 15 U.S.C. §1691 et seq.
16. Act of March 23, 1976, P.L. No. 93–239, 90 Stat. 251.
17. 12 C.F.R. §202 (1977).
18. Regulation B contains constraints that must be applied when questions are posed pertaining to the applicant's spouse or marital status. The regulation also applies to the manner in which applications must be evaluated, the manner in which credit must be offered, the notification procedure that must be followed by creditors who deny credit to applicants, and certain matters related to how credit must be reported. See Geltzer, supra note 2, at Secs 2.01 and 2.02.
19. Fair Debt Collection Practices Act, 15 U.S.C. §1692 et seq.

Chapter 51

Collections

I'm arm'd with more than complete steel—The justice of my quarrel.
—Christopher Marlowe, *Lust's Dominion*

In-Office Collections

Although there are obvious advantages to operating on a cash basis, it may be impractical at times and is against the current financial trend, which favors the utilization of credit.[1] Indeed, many optometrists have found that operating on a cash-only basis—particularly in small communities—is not advantageous for them or for their patients. Credit, in some form or another, invariably creeps into the financial dealings of the private practitioner.[2] The increased popularity of vision service plans has also contributed to the credit-oriented philosophy of many optometrists. In third-party vision service plans, payment is guaranteed, even though it may arrive a lengthy period after services have been rendered. With patients who are not covered by third-party plans, there is no such guarantee.

There are several ways in which an optometrist can provide for the collection of fees[3]:

Advance payment—The entire amount due is paid after the examination but before the ophthalmic materials are received.

Step payment—As each service or material is received, it is paid for.

Deposit and balance—A portion of the fee is paid after the examination and the balance is paid after the delivery of the ophthalmic materials; this has been the traditional method employed by optometrists.

Billing—The amount due (beginning with the total) is billed to the patient on a monthly or other regular basis, and the patient makes payments to reduce the balance.

Installment payments—The patient agrees to pay the amount due in installments over a specified period of time.

Of these methods, the first three are more oriented toward a cash-basis philosophy because they require the payment of at least a portion of the fee by the patient concurrently with the performance of professional services. For this reason they are the preferred collections processes, especially in light of the rather substantial expenditures that optometrists must incur for the purchase of ophthalmic materials. Efficient practice management requires that optometrists obtain sufficient payment in advance so that the cost of obtaining these materials will be covered in the event of nonpayment of the total amount due by the patient.[4]

Whenever billing is used, a true credit transaction has occurred; but if payment is received prior to the second billing, there is no significant expenditure of time or effort required, nor is there any real financial loss incurred when installment payments are received as promised. It can be anticipated that approximately 70 percent of patients will pay on the first statement, and about 25 percent will require extra efforts such as additional billings and budget arrangements.[5] The remaining 5 percent represent those who cannot or will not pay. Thus, in a well-run practice, the uncollected bills should constitute no more than 5 percent of patients seen.[6] In such a practice the amount of accounts receivable would be relatively modest.

There have been many commentaries on how in-office collections should be managed.[7] Through experience most practitioners arrive at a system of collections that, depending on their personalities, location, personnel, and management abilities, reaches some level of efficiency that they find workable. But some systems are more efficient than others.[8] A few general guidelines useful to health-care practitioners are described below.[9]

A doctor should review his office philosophy with regard to billing and collections and consider—in light of economic factors—whether payment arrangements should be modified to reflect the individual needs of his patients; a collections system should be sufficiently flexible to permit a patient, who is trying to pay, a reasonable opportunity to do so.

A patient information form should be required of every patient, and it should include such basic information as where the person lives, where he works, how he can be reached by phone, name and workplace of spouse, insurance coverage, and other essential items (see Chapter 13 for an example). If someone other than the patient will be paying the bill, additional information about that individual or company will be required.

Patients should be fully informed about the practice's financial policy. Preferably, a statement of financial policy will accompany the patient information form (see Chapter 13). Otherwise, the financial policy should either be posted in a conspicuous place or some provision for discussing it with patients should be made.

Billing and collections procedures should be periodically reassessed. A timetable should be established for following up on outstanding bills. One common technique is to use reminder letters.[10] These letters are sent out at certain intervals and are intended to encourage payment. Many practices divide them into first letter (Fig. 51.1), second letter (Fig. 51.2), and third letter (Fig. 51.3) sequences that, if disregarded, result in some form of legal action.

In some instances it may be advisable to telephone the patient to find out why the bill has not been paid. If the telephone is used, however, the person making the call should have a clear understanding of the legal proscriptions that surround

Dear Mr./Ms.________,

We have not heard from you with regard to our recent statement concerning your account with this office.

If the enclosed account is in error, please contact us so that we may make the appropriate adjustment.

If it is correct, we would enjoy hearing from you soon.

Sincerely,
________ O.D.

Figure 51.1. First Collection Letter

Dear Mr./Ms.________,

We are disappointed in the fact that we have not received a response to the letter and statement mailed to you last month.

However, we are aware that unexpected developments can make it difficult to meet financial obligations from time to time.

Please consider how you wish to take care of the enclosed statement of account, and contact this office within the next few days so that may discuss this matter with you.

Sincerely,
________ O.D.

Figure 51.2. Second Collection Letter

Dear Mr./Ms.________,

In our previous efforts to contact you concerning your overdue account, we have evidently failed to make it clear that this is a matter requiring your immediate attention.

Much to our regret, unless we hear from you about the enclosed statement, we will be compelled to take an alternative course of action.

Contact this office immediately so that we may resolve this matter.

Sincerely,
________ O.D.

Figure 51.3. Third Collection Letter

the use of telephone collections efforts. It is also important that the person be capable of tactfully discussing the problem.[11]

Overdue accounts should be followed carefully. A credit analysis chart should be maintained in order to keep abreast of accounts that have gone thirty, sixty, and ninety days without payment. Accounts that are most likely to be uncollectible should be identified as early as possible.

Delinquent accounts may be turned over for collection. There are several alternatives available: small claims court, collections lawyers, and collections agencies. The determination of when an account is sufficiently delinquent to institute legal action is an individual decision, but accounts that have been inactive for six months are rarely collectible.[12]

Third-party vision service plans have become increasingly important as a source of payment for patient fees. Depending upon the provisions of the plan, the optometrist may receive a predetermined fee or a fee established on the basis of a formula. Disagreements with third-party providers can delay payment, as can failure to submit claims promptly. The policy for managing third-party forms should be clearly understood by all persons having the responsibility for processing them.

Failure to pay may indicate dissatisfaction on the part of the patient. There should be some mechanism for managing patient complaints, including—where appropriate—the cessation of collections efforts. Personal communication with the patient is usually necessary in this situation.

Under circumstances of hardship, it may be preferable to write off a patient's bill. The decision should be left to the doctor when cases of financial hardship come to the attention of the office staff.

One particular aspect of collections that deserves special mention is the return of a check for insufficient funds.

Returned Checks

If a patient's check is returned from the bank because there are insufficient funds on deposit in the patient's account, it is not necessary for the optometrist to turn to an attorney for collection if the optometrist is willing to act quickly.[13]

If the check is returned and marked "closed account" or "no account," the optometrist should call the patient immediately and ask that cash payment be made for the amount due. Upon receipt of the payment, the check will be returned to the patient. Compliance may require an aggressive effort on the part of the practitioner or staff.[14] If the check is returned and marked "returned for insufficient funds," it should be redeposited; if it is returned a second time because funds have not been deposited in the account, the optometrist should call the patient to determine the cause of the lack of funds. The optometrist may also want to call the bank to ensure that funds are in fact insufficient and that no interim deposits have been made since the time the check was initially presented to the bank. Even if the check is returned a second time, this procedure may be repeated. Or, if funds become available to cover the check, the optometrist should consider taking the check to the bank and picking up certified funds (a certified check) for deposit in his own bank.

If a check is more than six months old, it is considered stale and the bank upon which it is drawn may legally refuse to honor it. In this eventuality, the optometrist should discuss the situation with a bank officer. Once the details of the collection effort are explained, the bank may be willing to honor it.

The optometrist should always act quickly when a check is returned, and if the bank upon which the

Dear Mr./Ms.________,

The purpose of this letter is to inform you that your check number __ and dated ____ in the amount of $____ has been returned to this office marked ("insufficient funds," "no account," or other reason is described here).

It is customary for banks to notify customers when a deposited check does not clear so that this problem can be remedied immediately.

Please contact us within five days so that we can take the proper steps to rectify the situation. Failure to contact us as requested will leave us no choice but to take such action as is necessary to protect our interests.

Sincerely,
________ O.D.

Figure 51.4. Sample Letter Notifying Patient of a Bad Check

check is drawn is different from the optometrist's bank, he may take the check to his bank and ask that it be placed as a collection item with the patient's bank. Although there is a small charge for this service, the check will be applied against the first deposit the patient makes during a ten-day period.[15] The optometrist will then be able to collect the amount due. The check may also be sent for collection to the bank at which the patient makes his deposits. A small fee will again be charged to hold the check until sufficient funds have been deposited to cover it, but when funds are on hand the optometrist may go to the bank and collect the amount owed.

When discussing a bounced check with a patient, the best means of communication is face-to-face. If personal efforts are to no avail, the optometrist may wish to send the patient a letter. The purpose of the letter is to put the patient on notice that payment is expected within a specified period of time and, failing that, action will be taken to collect the amount due. A sample letter is illustrated in Fig. 51.4.

If, despite these efforts, the optometrist is left holding a bad check he should resort to legal counsel. Since all states have bad check laws, the efforts of the attorney may prompt payment, even when all he does is write a letter.

Small Claims Court

When an optometrist encounters a patient who steadfastly refuses to pay for services or materials (or both), and it is apparent that in-office collection efforts will not be successful, the optometrist can choose between three options: to pursue the collection himself in small claims court, to turn the account over to a collections attorney for resolution, or to employ a collections agency. In certain circumstances the optometrist will consider recourse to small claims court to be the best alternative.[16]

In order to use the small claims court[17]:

- the optometrist must live within a community that provides a court for small claims
- the amount owed must be sufficiently large to justify the expenditure of time and money necessary to pursue the claim
- the former patient must be within the jurisdiction of the court
- there must be a reasonable expectation of collection from the former patient if a judgment in the optometrist's favor is rendered
- the optometrist must be willing to go to court

To economize time and effort, it is advisable to file several claims at once. The suit is initiated by the filing of a complaint that specifies the injured party's claim (see Fig. 51.5). If the optometrist's contract with the patient permits the collection of court costs, attorney's fees, or interest in the event litigation must be instituted to collect a delinquent account, the optometrist may claim an amount that includes the allowable costs that are in addition to the fees owed (see Chapter 13). The suit is filed with the court, along with a check for the filing costs, which are relatively modest.

Either at the time of filing or within a short period thereafter the claim will be assigned a date on the court calendar. When the date is determined, it is best to prepare a reminder or a calendar that indicates the date and time of each hearing and other such details as are pertinent. A checklist of items that will be needed at the hearings is another worthwhile idea.

The complaint, along with a summons that announces the court of jurisdiction and time and place of the hearing, will have to be served on the patient. If it is not delivered by a specified time prior to the

State of Alabama Unified Judicial System Form SM-1-J Rev. 2/79	**STATEMENT OF CLAIM** **(Complaint)** **General**	**Case Number** SM ___ ___ ID YR Number

IN THE SMALL CLAIMS COURT OF JEFFERSON COUNTY

Plaintiff Address	John G. O'Dee 123 Main Street Anytown, State 12345	Against	Defendant Address	Joe Patient 1122 Residence Street Anytown, State 54321
Attorney Address			Additional Defendant	

Date of Filing April 1, 1987

NOTICE TO EACH DEFENDANT — READ CAREFULLY

YOU ARE BEING SUED IN THE SMALL CLAIMS COURT BY THE PLAINTIFF(S) SHOWN ABOVE. THE JUDGE HAS NOT YET MADE ANY DECISION IN THIS CASE, AND YOU HAVE THE RIGHT TO A TRIAL TO TELL YOUR SIDE.

HOWEVER, IF YOU, OR YOUR LAWYER, FAIL TO FILL OUT THE ENCLOSED ANSWER FORM AND DELIVER OR MAIL IT TO THE CLERK AT THE ADDRESS SHOWN BELOW, SO THAT IT WILL GET TO THE CLERK'S OFFICE WITHIN FOURTEEN (14) DAYS AFTER YOU RECEIVE THESE PAPERS, A JUDGMENT CAN BE TAKEN AGAINST YOU. ONCE A JUDGMENT HAS BEEN ENTERED AGAINST YOU, YOUR PAYCHECK CAN BE GARNISHED AND/OR YOUR HOME OR PROPERTY SOLD TO SATISFY THAT JUDGMENT.

COMPLAINT

1. I claim the defendant owes the plaintiff the sum of $ 500.00 because:

   Defendant contracted with plaintiff on August 9, 1986, for plaintiff to perform an eye examination and to fit defendant with spectacles, the reasonable cost of which was $200. On August 23 defendant contracted with plaintiff for plaintiff to perform an examination and fit defendant with contact lenses, the reasonable cost of which was $300. Defendant has breached these contracts with plaintiff by failing to pay the agreed upon amounts.

2. Plaintiff also claims from the defendant court costs in the sum of $ 37.00 (see note below), plus $____ for interest and $____ for lawyers fees (**only** if plaintiff is represented by a licensed, practicing attorney and if the contract or note you signed so provides.)

NOTE: The total amount of court costs may be more than this amount when the case is finally settled. The clerk will inform you of any additional costs at the close of the case.

By: ____
Clerk

J.G. O'Dee
Plaintiff or Attorney (Signature)
John G. O'Dee

CLERK ADDRESS:

PHONE NO.

PHONE NO.

SEE INSTRUCTIONS ON THE BACK

COURT RECORD (White) PLAINTIFF (Green) DEFENDANT (Yellow) ROBERTS & SON, INC., P. O. BOX 1807, BIRMINGHAM, ALABAMA 35201 TELEPHONE 822-3122

Figure 51.5. Sample Statement of Claim, page 1. (Courtesy Small Claims Court of Jefferson County, Alabama)

INSTRUCTIONS TO THE PLAINTIFF(S)

This is your case, and if you are acting as your own lawyer, you are responsible in seeing that your claim is successfully presented at each stage of the procedure until it is concluded.

The Clerk of the Court has a handbook which tells you how to handle a Small Claims case. That book is free to you on request. If you need any additional help, ask the Clerk assigned to Small Claims cases.

1. You must complete one of these forms for each defendant you wish to sue. Each defendant must be described by his correct legal name and address (not a post office box). Be as brief as possible but include every important name, date and place.

2. To start your case you must file the completed form with the Clerk assigned to Small Claims cases. The Clerk will stamp a copy for you to show that the case has been filed and will insert the number of the case on the front of this form.

3. You are responsible for seeing that each defendant receives a copy of this form. If you haven't heard from anyone about the case in about fourteen days, then check with the Clerk's office, to make sure that each defendant has been served.

4. If any of the defendants ask for a trial, you will be notified of the place, the date, and the time. You must be present or your case will be dismissed. You may take a judgment by default fourteen (14) days after the defendant has received a copy of this form, if the defendant fails to file his Answer.

5. You are responsible to see to the enforcement of any judgment that is awarded to you. The Small Claims Handbook will tell you how to go about recovering your money.

ANY TIME YOU CONTACT THE CLERK ABOUT THIS CASE YOU MUST REFER TO THE CASE NUMBER ON THE FRONT.

SUMMONS

INSTRUCTIONS TO SHERIFF OR PROCESS SERVER

To Any Sheriff or Any Person Authorized By Rule 4.1(b)(1) or 4.1(b)(2) of the Alabama Rules of Civil Procedure to Effect Service in the State of Alabama:

You are hereby commanded to serve this summons and a copy of the Statement of Claim in this action upon the defendant named on the reverse side and make proper return to this court.

Date Received ____________________ ____________________ By: ________
Clerk

Served on the defendant(s) named ____________________

____

by delivering a copy of the Summons and Statement of Claim to him in ____________________ County, Alabama.

Date Served ____________________ ____________________
Process Server Signature

This service by Certified Mail of this Summons and Statement of Claim is initiated upon the request of ____________________ pursuant to Rule 4.1(c) of the Alabama Rules of Civil Procedure.

Date Requested ____________________ Date Mailed ____________________

Return Receipt Date ____________________ ____________________ By: ________
Clerk

Figure 51.5. Sample Statement of Claim, page 2

date of the hearing (usually a stated number of days), the claim will be dismissed. In order to obtain service, a professional process server may have to be employed, or a small fee may be required to have the sheriff serve the papers. A valid address or place of work will assist the process of serving the lawsuit papers immeasurably. Once the papers are served, the optometrist should note the date of service.

After the patient has been served, the optometrist should consider sending a letter that offers to settle the case before trial upon the payment by the patient of the amount of the bill plus the costs incurred for the suit. In a number of instances the case will be settled by the patient.[18] If a check is offered as payment, the lawsuit should not be dismissed until the check has been cleared by the optometrist's bank.

If the patient does not respond to the letter, or indicates his willingness to go to court, the optometrist should prepare for the trial. If the patient contract permits the collection of attorney's fees, the optometrist will have the benefit of legal counsel. Otherwise, the optometrist may represent himself, which is not uncommon in small claims court. In the usual case, the patient will not be represented by counsel and will be forced to conduct his defense by himself. The optometrist may wish to have his bookkeeper present at the trial as well, or, in some circumstances, may feel that someone from the office other than himself can present the case adequately. Attorneys are not required in small claims court.

Documentary evidence will be needed in the presentation of the optometrist's claim, and he should be certain to bring the patient's financial records and examination chart and any correspondence or other documents having a bearing on the case.

When the case is called, if the patient does not appear the judge will enter a default judgment in the optometrist's favor. If the patient answers, he has several options: he can admit the claim and pay it; he can admit the claim but dispute the amount; he can admit the claim and amount and request that a payment schedule be arranged; or he can dispute the claim and ask for a trial.

A trial in small claims court between two nonlawyers is conducted on a less formal basis than the popular entertainments staged by television advocates. The optometrist will be asked to present his case first and will be required to show that the patient was seen on certain dates, professional services were rendered, reasonable charges were made for these services, and despite attempts to collect the amount due, the debt remains outstanding. The patient will then be given an opportunity to contest the amount claimed, in which case the office procedures and the method for determining charges will have to be explained by the optometrist. If the patient attempts to argue that the treatment was ineffective, it will be disregarded by the judge; his argument will most likely be limited to the mistakes that he believed were made in the amount billed.

Once both sides have been heard, the judge may render a decision or take the case under advisement to be decided later. If there is a dispute over evidence or testimony, he may require that further documents be turned over to the court or that another hearing be held. His decision, once rendered, will be mailed to both parties if it was not decided immediately.

If the optometrist receives a judgment in his favor for a stated amount, he should write to the patient, requesting satisfaction as per the order of the court. The patient may then pay the judgment, appeal the case to a higher court, or attempt to avoid payment by not responding. For the last alternative the optometrist will have to resort to the legal process again in an attempt to find assets of the patient that can be used to satisfy the judgment. The most-used means of obtaining satisfaction are garnisheeing wages, attaching a bank account or other personal property (such as a car), or having a payment schedule ordered by the judge. The last alternative has the advantage of the power of the court behind it; if the patient does not comply, the judge can order him jailed for contempt.

Once a judgment is paid in full, a satisfaction of judgment form must be filed with the court.

If an optometrist does not wish to use small claims court or is not able to, he may turn the unpaid bill over to a third party for collection. In so doing, he must make a choice between the use of an attorney or the employment of a collections agency.

Third-Party Collections

In those cases in which an optometrist's best efforts are unable to produce any tangible results, he may decide to employ a third party to make the collection for him. Some attorneys specialize in collections and will pursue even relatively modest claims, charging from one third to one half of the accounts that they actually collect as their fee. The alternative is a collections agency; these organizations generally charge a start-up fee plus a percentage of any collections that they make.[19] Prior to referring an account to an attorney or a collections agency, the optometrist should determine whether legitimate and reasonable methods are employed in collections efforts. The conduct of the third party will reflect on the optometrist, particularly any unfortunate side effects resulting from an ill-conceived collections effort by a third-party employee.

If a collection agency is hired, the optometrist should be aware of the legal constraints under which the agency must conduct its collections efforts on his behalf. Independent collections agencies are subject to the Fair Debt Collection Practices Act, which became effective in 1978.[20] The act only regulates the activities of these agencies, expressly exempting the conduct of in-house (creditor) collectors and collection attorneys from its provisions. This legislation establishes the practices and procedures that a collection agency may engage in while attempting to collect a past-due account. These procedures are rather stringent, and penalties for violation can be significant. If an optometrist uses a name other than his own while attempting to collect debts owed him, he may come under the provisions of the act.

Although the activities of optometrists and attorneys working on their behalf are not regulated by federal law, in every state there are common law or statutory remedies available to persons who have been the victims of improper collections efforts. Examples of such actions are those for invasion of privacy and for harassment. Some of the activities that courts have declared to be improper conduct during collections include continual and repeated calls at the home of the debtor, at unreasonable times and in substantial numbers; the contact or calling of a debtor at the debtor's place of business or employment; threats or demands that tend to frighten or upset the debtor; contacts with the debtor's friends, neighbors, or associates designed to humiliate the debtor and to coerce him to pay his delinquent account; or any systematic campaign of harassment directed at the debtor. Of course, collection agencies are subject to these state laws as well.

When deciding to pursue an unpaid account, an optometrist should consider the advantages that third-party collectors—attorneys or agencies—offer as a resource to help recapture income that would otherwise be lost. Optometrists should choose their collectors carefully; unethical conduct can cost a practitioner considerably more than is collected. Furthermore, optometrists should assess their own in-house collection practices to be sure that their personnel are using collection techniques that are appropriate, legal, and ethical.

Notes

1. The use of credit may decline due to the gradual loss of the tax deduction for personal interest charges instituted by the Tax Reform Act of 1986.
2. For contemporary views of the ongoing debate over cash versus credit, see Robert, L., Optometry's Ongoing Credit Card, *Optometric Management*, vol. 20, no. 10, 1984, pp. 39–47; Gottleib, D., Why You Need a Superbill, *Optometric Management*, vol. 20, no. 8, 1984, pp. 39–45; Meyers, J.G., Cashing in on Your Patient's Credit Cards, *Optometric Management*, vol. 13, no. 6, 1977, pp. 61–68; Veach, J.E., Take the Cash and Let the Credit Go!, *Optometric Management*, vol. 17, no. 8, 1981, pp. 45–47; and Wills, J., Credit Zero, *Optometric Management*, vol. 19, no. 3, 1983, pp. 91–95.
3. Elmstrom, G., *Advanced Management for Optometrists*, Professional Press, Chicago, 1974, pp. 211–214.
4. See Baldwin, B., B. Christensen, and J. Melton, *Rx for Success*, Vision Publications, Midwest City, Okla., 1983, pp. 81–94.
5. Elmstrom, supra note 3, at 412.
6. Ibid.
7. For representative commentaries, see Parness, W.D., Tracking Down the Deadbeats, *Optometric Management*, vol. 17, no. 6, 1981, pp. 43–47; Scroggins, C.L., The Doctor as Boss: Teaching the Subtle Art of Collections, *Medical Economics*, vol. 56, no. 13, June 25, 1979, pp. 79–90; Chapman, S., How You Can Collect More of Your Fees, *Legal Aspects of Medical Practice*, vol. 10, no. 6, 1980, p. 32; and Wilson, J., Getting Along Without a Collection Agency, *Medical Economics*, vol. 57, no. 20, Sept. 29, 1980, pp. 99–117.
8. Lerner, M., How We Collect Every Dollar We've Earned, *Medical Economics*, vol. 57, no. 22, Oct. 27, 1980, p. 75.
9. From Lane, M., *The Doctor's Lawyer*, W.B. Saunders, Philadelphia, 1979, pp. 71–73.
10. Ibid.
11. Wilson, J., Getting Along Without a Collection Agency, *Medical Economics*, vol. 57, no. 20, Sept. 29, 1980, pp. 99–117.
12. Elmstrom, supra note 3, at 411–417.
13. Feld, L.G., What Can You Do When a Patient's Check Bounces?, *Legal Aspects of Medical Practice*, vol. 6, no. 10, 1978, pp. 28–30.
14. Ibid.
15. Ibid.
16. A list of small claims courts and information as to the filing of claims can be found in Elmstrom, supra note 3, chap. 16.
17. Marco, C.H., How to Use Small Claims Court to Collect Overdue Accounts, *Legal Aspects of Medical Practice*, vol. 10, no. 6, 1980, pp. 37–39.
18. Ibid.
19. For a practitioner's view of collection efforts, see Gregg, J.R., *The Business of Optometric Practice*, Advisory Enterprises, New York, 1975, pp. 178–184.
20. 15 U.S.C. §1692 et seq.

PART FOURTEEN

INSURANCE

Chapter 52

Life Insurance

Down went the owners—greedy men whom hope of gain allured;
Oh, dry the starting tear, for they were heavily insured.
—Sir William Gilbert, *The "Babs" Ballads*

Types of Life Insurance
Uses
Riders
Settlement Options
Taxation

Life insurance is an essential part of both professional and personal planning. Creditors will insist on life insurance as a prerequisite for business loans; an optometrist may want to insure himself and his partner's lives so that, if one partner dies, there will be ready money to purchase his share of the partnership from his heirs; and an optometrist will want to provide some security for his family in the event he should prematurely die. Life insurance is indispensible in today's complex society, and most optometrists will be forced to purchase some form of life insurance (if they have not already) as a matter of personal or business necessity.

Although life insurance offers a range of costs to suit all pocketbooks, and has more options than ever to choose from (discussed *infra*), selecting the right policy with the most cost-effective coverage remains a difficult chore for many professionals. It is the purpose of this chapter to clarify the basic types of life insurance policies currently available and how they may best be used.

Life insurance may be defined as

> that kind of insurance in which the risk contemplated is the death of the particular person; upon which event (if it occurs within a prescribed term, or, according to the contract, whenever it occurs) the insurer agrees to pay a stipulated sum to the legal representatives of such person, or to a third person having an insurable interest in the life of such person.[1]

Before discussing the types of life insurance available, the types of life insurance companies that offer policies will be described.[2]

Life Insurance Companies

Life insurance—although sold to provide guaranteed protection over long periods of time—is provided without the insurer knowing at the time of granting the policy exactly how much the costs of providing the insurance will be. There are two basic approaches that are used to solve this problem. Under one approach, companies sell *participating policies*, which means that, as the actual costs of providing the insurance become known, they are shared with the policyholders. If the premiums charged for insurance coverage prove to be more than is actually needed, portions are returned annually in the form of policy dividends. Under the other approach, stock life insurance companies sell *nonparticipating policies*. If the premiums charged to policyholders prove to be more than are actually needed, the company has a profit; if the premiums instead prove to be inadequate, the company suffers a loss. In neither case does the policyholder participate. The premiums for participating policies are higher than those for corresponding nonparticipating policies. But the dividends paid by participating companies give the policyholders a choice of several extra options (to be discussed) that tend to compensate for the increased cost.[3]

There are two types of insurance companies: stock companies and mutual companies. *Stock companies* are owned by stockholders; they finance its operation and assume the risks and responsibilities of ownership and management. Most stock companies issue only nonparticipating policies; a few also issue participating policies. *Mutual companies* have no stockholders. Management is directed through a board, which is elected by the policyholders for whose benefit the company is operated. Nearly all mutual companies issue only participating policies; a few also issue policies on a nonparticipating basis, but the owners of these policies have no voice in the company management.[4]

Types of Life Insurance

There are four basic types of life insurance: term, whole life, endowment, and universal life. Each has its own particular distinctions,[5] but term insurance differs from the others by being a temporary rather than a permanent type of insurance. Premiums for term policies also differ from those of whole life, universal life, and endowment policies because they periodically jump in cost as a term expires and the policyholder has become older. But term insurance is—at least initially—much cheaper.[6]

Term

Term insurance exists for a stated period of time, usually one year or five years. The premium is fixed for the term of the policy, and at the expiration of the policy term the insurance coverage expires. The policyholder may choose to renew the policy for another term, but the premium for the new term will be more because the policyholder will be older. The premium will rise at each renewal, but the renewal option is usually not offered past age 65. For an additional premium charge, the policyholder may obtain an option to renew that cannot be cancelled by the insurance company, no matter what the policyholder's state of health. A term policy can also be converted to permanent insurance if this option is paid for by an additional premium. The policyholder then has the right to convert the policy without a physical examination whenever he desires to do so.

Since term is straight insurance, it is cheaper than any other type, at least over the short run. But over a lengthy period of years, term will actually cost more than permanent insurance, and it suffers from the inability to be renewed past 65 years of age. Because of its initial low cost, term is often the choice of young persons purchasing their first insurance, or of young married persons looking for maximum protection.[7] Term also offers other advantages: it can be purchased for mortgage protection; it can be utilized for short-term buy-sell agreements; it can be employed to protect the unpaid balance of a practice purchase agreement; and it can be used to supplement permanent insurance. Whenever there is a short-term insurance need that must be satisfied, term insurance should be given first consideration.

Whole Life

Whole life is permanent insurance that offers coverage "for a person's whole life." The premiums are paid in equal installments, but the length of time that installments must be paid can be varied.

An *ordinary life* policy requires that a set premium be paid for the whole of a person's life. The premiums are divided into two parts: protection and investment. The protection is provided by term insurance; the investment is provided by cash value, or savings, that accumulates above the cost of the term insurance. During the first few years of a policy, most of the premium is devoted to the cost of providing insurance and little is used for investment. Gradually, as the cash value increases, a proportionally greater and greater part of the premium is used for investment, further adding to the cash value of the policy. As a result, after a period of years the annual increase in cash value (including dividends) can exceed the cost of the premium. This gradual rise in cash value is usually free of income taxation. The cash value can be borrowed—at rates that are established at the time the policy is taken out and that are quite reasonable (typically less than 10 percent)—and it can be collected whenever the policy is cashed in. Tax is paid only on the amount that exceeds the total premiums paid, less dividends. Therefore, an ordinary life policy can be used as a form of investment. (*Variable life*, which is similar to ordinary life, allows the insured to invest in stocks, bonds, money market funds, and similar investment alternatives.)[8]

Limited payment life is another variety of whole life policy, and as its name implies it requires premium payments for a limited period, usually ten to twenty years or until a certain age is attained. After premiums have been paid for the requisite length of time, the policy is paid up and remains in force for the full face amount. Premiums are higher than those of ordinary life because of the shortened period for premium payment, but the cash value escalates at a much higher rate than would the cash value of a comparable ordinary life policy.[9] Otherwise, it is similar to an ordinary life policy.

There are several payment options available to a policyholder or the beneficiary of a whole life policy, and they will be discussed in a subsequent section.

Endowment

An endowment policy is permanent insurance, and like limited payment life it is purchased for a specific period (ten, twenty, thirty, or the number of years desired). At the conclusion of the period, the policy is redeemable for the face amount; if the insured dies before the period has run, the face amount is paid to the beneficiary. It provides both insurance protection and investment but differs from limited payment life because the face amount of the policy must be accumulated, which means a greater portion of the premium must be devoted to savings and less to term insurance. This necessitates a larger premium than with other types of insurance, but the cash value rises correspondingly faster because of the increased savings. At the conclusion of the period of time for which the policy has provided insurance protection, the face value is paid out to the beneficiary. Since this amount is always more than the amount of premiums paid into the policy, the beneficiary will have to pay an income tax. These policies are used to fund such expenditures as the costs of a college education, income for a retirement fund, and principal for a trust.[10] Since the cost is fairly expensive compared to other types of insurance, endowment policies are not frequently purchased.[11]

Universal Life

This relatively new type of life policy (first sold in the mid-1970s) makes permanent insurance a much better investment.[12] The policy combines renewable term insurance with a cash-value account resembling a money-market fund; either element of the policy can be adjusted, thus allowing the policyholder to change the amount of insurance coverage and the investment yield as needed.[13] The investment return on these policies is substantially higher than that of whole life policies (although variable life also offers a reasonable investment return), which permits the policyholder to earn interest at money-market rates (but there are minimum levels of insurance coverage that must be maintained in order to enjoy tax-free withdrawls). At other times the money can be withdrawn, at no cost, to meet major expenses. As in a whole life policy, all earnings of the cash-value account are tax sheltered: No income tax is paid until more money is withdrawn than has been put into the policy. (The Tax Equity and Fiscal Responsibility Act of 1982 established several important guidelines in this respect.[14])

Universal life policyholders get annual statements of how much insurance protection and cash value they have, what interest rate is being paid on the investment portion, and how much of their money has gone for insurance, investment, and company fees. (Universal life companies charge a fee for management.) These disclosures are a major innovation in life insurance. Probably the largest obstacle to a universal life policy is getting started: the minimum policy amount may be substantial and so may be the early premiums (but after a few years the premiums can be paid out of the policy's cash value). Not all companies offer this type of insurance because of its recent origin, but it does seem to be a promising alternative to the more conventional types of permanent insurance.

The preceding discussion of the types of life insurance omits the important subject of its use. Life insurance can be used to achieve three important goals: protection, funding, and investment.[15]

All three of these uses of life insurance will doubtless be considered by the astute planner. Although protection is the most common reason for obtaining life insurance, particularly among married persons, the capacity for funding that life insurance offers in an optometric partnership should not be overlooked. Oftentimes life insurance policies are offered as a fringe benefit to a practitioner or are part of the inducement to join a particular partnership or professional corporation. The use of the buy-sell agreement in an optometric partnership or for stockholder cross-purchase agreements in a professional corporation is rather common. The use of insurance for investment purposes is probably the least employed, but universal life policies seem to offer a viable means of participating in a semicompulsory investment plan.

Uses

When considering the uses to which insurance can be applied, there are three basic questions that must be answered:

1. What kinds of insurance coverage are needed?
2. When should they be purchased?
3. How much of each is necessary?

Unfortunately, there are no set answers that can be applied to everyone.[16] However, virtually every professional is linked through the common insurance problems that are part and parcel of a professional career. From the days of optometry school to the time of retirement, there is a commonality to life insurance needs that can be used to suggest some general answers to the three questions posed above.

Studenthood

Most professionally oriented individuals have their first contact with life insurance during their college years. Few have a clear understanding of life insurance, it uses, or whether or not they are getting a good deal, but many end up purchasing it anyway. Frequently, the insurance acquired is of the buy-now, pay-later type and requires a personal note for the first few years' premiums until the policy has built up enough cash value to secure the note. As a result, on a cost basis it probably is not much of a bargain, and the coverage is typically rather modest since the usual policy is a whole life policy and, therefore, relatively expensive. But—looking at the bright side—it does provide insurance protection for the purchaser.

During the student years a less expensive alternative that could provide adequate protection is term insurance, bought either as a group policy or as individual coverage. Term provides a lot more coverage for the same insurance dollar paid for whole life and can thereby satisfy two pressing needs: an instant estate in the event of death and less cost, which translates into more money for living expenses, the costs of education, and other financial obligations. Of course, the decision to obtain insurance depends on the personal circumstances of the individual: A married person would have more need than would a single person, and a married person with children would have more need than both. Term can provide adequate protection against untimely death, whatever the status of the policyholder, and can even be converted into permanent insurance at a later time if a convertible term policy is purchased. Flexibility to meet changing insurance needs is always a desirable aspect of any insurance policy. Convertible term offered by a mutual company, although more expensive than comparable insurance offered by a stock company, allows the policyholder to convert later to whole life and to participate in any dividends earned by the company (which usually more than make up for the greater expense of the mutual company policies).

What is a realistic amount of insurance in these early years? The answer lies in the individual circumstances of the purchaser; if single, he may need to insure only his debts and any expenses connected with his death; if married, he may wish to insure not only his indebtedness but also the living expenses needed by his survivors; a commonly cited figure is four to five years worth of income.[17] Economics no doubt plays a role in the amount of insurance that can be secured; whatever the amount, the best buy at this stage probably is term.[18]

Early Career

For most young practitioners, the beginning years coincide with plans to purchase a home, get married, and have a family, decisions that have significant insurance ramifications. These are the years in which financial obligations incurred during the optometrist's professional education must be repaid as well, further adding to the financial burden. Despite these expenses, the early years of practice are the optimum time to initiate a permanent insurance program because as the practitioner gets older the cost of insurance gets higher. Permanent insurance is useful to a professional for two reasons: the loan value is a source of low-interest cash, and the paid-up policy provides ready cash for estate taxes and administration costs at the time of death. But the cost of permanent insurance is rather substantial when compared to term.

Policy premiums for permanent insurance do vary from insurer to insurer, but some policy dividends and cash values may be so poor as to make the lowest-premium policy anything but a bargain. Caution must be exercised when comparison shopping for insurance: the size, assets, and reputation of an insurer deserve careful consideration along with the cost of insurance.

If convertible term has already been purchased, then an obvious alternative available to the policyholder is to go ahead and convert to permanent insurance. The policyholder should be cautious to convert into permanent insurance an amount that is affordable. Some term coverage can be retained in order to keep overall coverage at an acceptable level. And a decreasing term rider can be added to permanent insurance to protect the mortgage amount outstanding on a home.

Still another alternative is the purchase of universal

life insurance. Premiums are substantial at the start of the policy but can be paid out of the cash value in later years. It is the utility of universal life for financial needs that arise later in life that makes it worth considering here.

Whatever type of insurance best fits the needs of the young practitioner, serious consideration must be given to initiating a planned insurance program.[19]

Mid-Career

At this stage in life the practitioner has traded in the financial obligations of earlier years for new ones, the most common being the costs of educating children and initiating an investment program. Since the earnings of the optometrist have (it is hoped) escalated substantially over the intervening years, tax considerations have become very important, as have the permanent life insurance policies begun several years earlier.[20]

Over the years the cash value of these policies will have grown, and this money can be borrowed and put to use.[21] One obvious use is to defray the cost of insurance: To pay the premium on existing permanent insurance policies or purchase new coverage (called minimum deposit insurance). The interest on such an insurance loan is tax deductible (fully if for business purposes and partially if for personal use) if the premiums of the permanent insurance policy were paid for with unborrowed money at least four out of the first seven years the policy was in force. This is one reason the buy-now, pay-later policy of school days may not be such a bargain in the long run. Although the interest on insurance policy loans is relatively modest and the amount borrowed must be deducted from the policy value should death occur, the cash value of permanent insurance is a resource that can be tapped to meet the financial exigencies of mid-career. A universal life policy is especially good in this regard. But it is not advisable to plunge this borrowed cash into a speculative venture. To do so could spell disaster for an otherwise carefully constructed insurance program. Rather, it would be preferable to maximize the return from the investment and to minimize the risk to be incurred. One type of investment that could be utilized is the single premium deferred annuity.[22]

A single premium deferred annuity is purchased in a lump sum and increases in value at a reasonable rate of interest (and a guaranteed minimum) until such time as the annuity is scheduled to begin paying benefits to the contract holder (annuitant).[23] The interest accrued by the annuity is tax deferred, and the annuity can increase substantially in value by retirement, when payments to the annuitant are scheduled to begin (and the annuitant may be in a lower tax bracket). Furthermore, the loan used to purchase the annuity is not income and hence is not taxable to the purchaser. The annuity also protects the death benefits of the insurance policy from which the cash was borrowed. If $5,000 is borrowed from a whole life policy and a single premium deferred annuity is purchased, the face value of the annuity—$5,000—becomes payable as a death benefit and makes up for the deficit.

Whenever cash is borrowed from an existing insurance policy, the loan does not have to be repaid, only the annual interest. The interest can be deducted completely if the loan is used for business purposes and partially—until 1991—if the loan is used for personal purposes.

Late Career

With advancing age there is usually some relief from debt; childrens' educations, mortgages, and most major purchases have been completely or nearly paid for. Over the years insurance coverage has been increased to the necessary levels and cash values of permanent insurance have been used to supplement retirement plans. This permanent insurance coverage has probably been strenthened by continued usage of some term, bought through a group plan or as an individual policy. As a practitioner approaches age 60, however, the cost of term becomes rather expensive, and a decision as to whether or not to continue term coverage inevitably must be made.[24] After 65 years of age, term insurance will no longer be sold by the insurer. Premium money may be better put to use if added to an annuity or other investment vehicle that the practitioner has initiated.

Since the optometrist's income has risen while expenses presumably have lessened, participation in some form of investment program in which income is tax-deferred becomes a must. Keogh, 401(k), or professional corporation pension or profit-sharing plans are the most likely alternatives. No matter which program is used, the purpose is to defer taxes on income until after retirement, when a lower income tax bracket usually prevails. As these programs grow, reliance on life insurance lessens; inevitably, the point is reached at which the optometrist must decide whether to drop the whole life policies.

The decision and manner in which to end a permanent insurance policy are significant matters that call for professional consultation. As an estate grows, so does the concomitant tax liability that arises at the time of transfer. Permanent insurance may have to be retained in order to assure adequate cash to pay estate taxes at death; it may constitute an important part of an overall estate plan, such as the conversion of a paid-up insurance policy into an annuity. These are considerations that have their beginnings back in early or mid-career and that are most easily resolved when clear planning and unbroken execution lead to an expected conclusion late in the optometrist's professional life. Since retirement is an anticipated goal of most professionals, the retirement income to be enjoyed by the optometrist and his family is of paramount importance. A well-planned life insurance program can add significantly to the realization of this goal.

In establishing a well-planned life insurance program, the optometrist should be careful to consult insurance agents who are competent.[25] The selection of the appropriate agent, like the selection of the appropriate insurance, must be undertaken with deliberation and caution.[26]

Riders

There are five commonly used riders that are purchased to supplement a basic insurance policy.

1. *Mortgage protection*—A decreasing term insurance policy can be added onto the basic policy, thereby providing a homeowner with insurance protection for the mortgage balance. Actually, the benefits are paid to the policy beneficiary directly and may be used to pay the mortgage if the beneficiary desires to do so, but this is not mandatory. The money can be applied as the beneficiary sees fit.

2. *Insurability protection*—A young policyholder can acquire the right to purchase additional insurance at specific intervals, even though the health of the policyholder is poor, and without the necessity for a physical examination, thereby guaranteeing that additional insurance can be acquired at stated times to supplement the basic policy. These riders usually limit the option to add such insurance to age 40 or below, so that a 30-year-old policyholder would be able to exercise the option to purchase the additional insurance at stated intervals over a 10-year period.

3. *Family income protection*—A monthly income can be provided to the policyholder's family should the policyholder die within a stated period of time. The monthly benefits are paid for a certain period, and then the face amount of the ordinary life policy is paid out to the beneficiary in a lump sum or as an option of some kind. This rider is actually a form of decreasing term insurance, but the premium is less expensive when it is purchased as a rider to a basic insurance policy.

4. *Accidental death protection*—A policy's face amount will be doubled in the event of accidental death if this rider is purchased by the policyholder. Some policies will triple the face amount if death occurs while traveling on a common carrier (e.g., plane, train, bus).

5. *Disability protection*—A policyholder who is disabled for six months or longer can protect his life insurance policy by providing for payment of the policy premiums during the period of disability. If the policyholder is totally and permanently disabled, the insurance premiums will be paid for him rather than waived. In this event, the cash value of the life insurance policy continues to grow in amount, even though the disabled policyholder is contributing nothing. If the disability is temporary but lasts for more than six months, the waiver of premium payments is retroactive to the beginning of the disability and lasts for as long as the disability does. These disability benefits are available only for policyholders below 60 or 65 years of age (depending on the age limit allowed by the insurance company issuing the policy).

Whether to add these riders to an individual policy depends on the needs of the individual and the cost of the added coverage. Therefore, the decision to purchase a rider is a matter of personal judgment.

Settlement Options

There are several options available to a policyholder or a policy beneficiary as to how the policy proceeds are to be received[27]:

Lump sum payment—The entire face value of the policy is paid out to the policy beneficiaries, whether the policy be a term policy or a whole life, endowment, or universal life policy.

Fixed period payment—The face value of the policy is paid out in equal installments, usually monthly, over a stated number of years. Since part of the insurance policy principal is being held by the insurance company, the company agrees to pay a stated amount of interest on this principal. Therefore, payments to the beneficiary include both interest and principal. Payments are made regardless of whether the policy was a term policy or a whole life, endowment, or universal life policy.

Fixed income payment—The face value of the policy is paid out in equal installments that are fixed until the proceeds of the policy are depleted. Again, since part of the policy principal is being held by the insurance company, interest will also be paid to the beneficiary.

Interest income payment—The face value of the policy may be retained by the insurance company, with payments to the beneficiary consisting of interest only, the amount of interest to be specified by the policy. This provision, when used, is employed to prevent creditors from obtaining any rights in the insurance proceeds received by a beneficiary (often called a spendthrift clause because it prevents a beneficiary from dissipating the insurance principal and keeps it out of the hands of the beneficiary's creditors as well).

Life income payment—The beneficiary may receive periodic payments for as long as the beneficiary lives, the size of the payments depending on the face value of the insurance policy and the life expectancy of the beneficiary. Such an option is much like an annuity.

The settlement option that is most appropriate depends on the nature of the policyholder's estate plan and the needs of his survivors. Since the various options may present a rather bewildering choice to the policyholder's beneficiaries, the decision as to which settlement option is the most appropriate should be made during the lifetime of the policyholder and, as necessary, revised to reflect changing goals or situations.

Taxation

Life insurance proceeds paid as the result of the death of the insured are exempt from income taxation. Therefore, the beneficiary of life insurance proceeds pays no income tax on the amount received. There is one exception to this rule: it occurs whenever a life insurance policy is sold or exchanged for a valuable consideration. For example, a partner or a stockholder in a private practice who purchases a life insurance policy from the partnership or corporation could incur the income tax when the policy proceeds are paid out.[28] A tax advisor should be consulted prior to initiating this type of purchase.

Even though life insurance proceeds are exempt from income taxation, they are not necessarily exempt from estate taxation. If the proceeds are payable to the estate of the insured, such proceeds are taxable to the estate.[29] If the insured has retained incidents of ownership in the policy, even though the insured's spouse is the beneficiary, the face value of the policy will be includable in the taxable estate of the insured and hence subject to the estate tax.[30] Incidents of ownership include such matters as the right to borrow against the insurance policy, change the beneficiary, assign the policy, and cash in the policy. In order to avoid estate taxation of life insurance proceeds, the insured must relinquish all rights in the policy to someone else (usually the insured's spouse). Such a transfer is rarely a taxable event in itself, although a gift tax can be incurred if the policy has sufficient cash value.[31] The transfer is a permanent event, one that removes the insured's rights in the policy forever. If the policy is given to the insured's spouse, and the spouse dies before the insured, then the spouse's estate incurs the estate tax on the insurance proceeds at death.

The preceding discussion has attempted to single out several of the important considerations attendant to the purchase of life insurance. Most young professionals initiate their insurance program with the purchase of some form of life insurance, even though the risk of death is less consequential than the risk of disability. This important subject—disability coverage—is addressed in the next chapter.

Notes

1. *Black's Law Dictionary*, 4th ed., West, St. Paul, Minn., 1968. For a general reference source on life insurance, see the *Life Insurance Fact Book*, American Council of Life Insurance, Washington, D.C., published annually.
2. A detailed analysis of life insurance policies and coverage can be found in *Medical Economics*, which has published numerous articles describing insurance problems and solutions: Don't Get Stuck with the Wrong Life Insurance, vol. 55, no. 4, Feb. 20, 1978; Life Insurance: A Fresh Look at What You Really Need, vol. 56, no. 23, Nov. 5, 1979; Why You May Need Less Life Insurance These Days, vol. 57, no. 10, May 12, 1980; Insurance: The Right Coverage at the Right Cost, vol. 58, no. 22, Nov. 2, 1981; Life Insurance: Measure Your Needs and Pick Your Options, vol. 59, no. 22, Nov. 1, 1982; Best and Worst Bets in Those New Life Insurance Options, vol. 59, no. 16, Aug. 9, 1982. Other discussions can be found in Elmstrom, G., *Advanced Management for Optometrists*, ch. 16, Professional Press, Chicago, 1974; and Lane, M., *The Doctor's Law Guide*, W.B. Saunders, Philadelphia, 1979, pp. 86–95.
3. *Understanding Your Life Insurance*, American Council of Life Insurance, New York, 1980, pp. 12–13.

4. Id. at pp. 13–14.
5. For an overview of life insurance needs, see Faber, L., Don't Get Stuck with the Wrong Life Insurance, *Medical Economics*, vol. 55, no. 4, Feb. 20, 1978, pp. 124–132; 1980 Financial Planning Guide: Life Insurance: A Fresh Look at What You Really Need, *Medical Economics*, vol. 56, no. 23, Nov. 5, 1979, pp. 215–222; and 1983 Financial Planning Guide: Life Insurance: Measure Your Needs and Pick Your Options, *Medical Economics*, vol. 59, no. 22, Nov. 1, 1982, pp. 95–111.
6. Although term insurance is less expensive than permanent insurance in every age bracket when a policy is initially taken out, a term policy escalates in cost at each renewal, and as the policyholder gets older, the cost of term surpasses the premiums being paid for a permanent insurance policy initially purchased at the same time as the term coverage. See Elmstrom, G., *Optometric Practice Management*, Chilton, Philadelphia, 1963, pp. 298–302.
7. Statistics show that permanent insurance continues to be the most frequently purchased insurance coverage, but during the decade of the 1970s, the volume of term insurance rose consistently, and there is a clear trend toward increased utilization of this type of insurance. (In 1968, term amounted to 43 percent of the volume of policies sold; by 1978 it had risen to 52 percent. *1980 Life Insurance Fact Book*, supra note 1, at 15–16.)
8. For a discussion of the merits and demerits of permanent insurance, see Brosterman, R., *The Complete Estate Planning Guide*, McGraw-Hill, New York, 1987, pp. 23–44.
9. Ibid.
10. Ibid.
11. As of 1977, endowment policies purchased by individuals constituted but 4 percent of policies in force. *1980 Life Insurance Fact Book*, supra note 1, at 22.
12. Goldberg, J.H., Life Insurance Coverage that Keeps Pace with Inflation, *Medical Economics*, vol. 58, no. 6, Mar. 16, 1981, pp. 123–129; Cohn, S., A New Life to Life Insurance?, *Optometric Management*, vol. 19, no. 3, 1983, pp. 85–90.
13. For a discussion of how the universal life policy can be used to suit the life needs of a policyholder, see Runde, R., At Last—An Almost Ideal Policy, *Money*, July 1981, pp. 98–100. For another view, read Universal Life Insurance: All that Meets the Eye?, *Medical Economics*, vol. 58, no. 21, Oct. 26, 1981, p. 87.
14. For a synopsis of TEFRA, see *Concise Explanation of the Tax Equity and Fiscal Responsibility Act of 1982*, Prentice-Hall, Englewood Cliffs, New York, 1982, or the most recent edition of the Prentice-Hall or Commerce Clearing House *Federal Tax Course*. A discussion of some of the tax changes as they relate to universal life can be found in Kaufman, S., Annuities and Universal Life Lose Some Glitter, *Medical Economics*, vol. 59, no. 26, Dec. 20, 1982, p. 117. The intent of TEFRA tax law changes was to make level premium whole life insurance more competitive with universal life by requiring a certain minimum amount of insurance protection to be in force under universal life policies. Failure to maintain the required minimum results in the death proceeds of universal life policy being taxed. There are also circumstances under which cash value withdrawals from a universal life policy can be taxed. An insurance or tax adviser should be consulted in order to be certain that a policy satisfies all federal tax requirements.
15. See Brosterman, supra note 8; and Estate Planning: Make Sure Your Money Goes Where You Intend, *Medical Economics*, vol. 55, no. 23, Nov. 6, 1978, pp. 149–176.
16. There is a commonality of needs among certain classes of individuals and certain age groups that makes the task of selecting the appropriate insurance not as formidable a task as it might seem. One approach to this problem can be found in Life Insurance: Measure Your Needs and Pick Your Options, *Medical Economics*, vol. 59, no. 22, Nov. 1, 1982, pp. 95–111.
17. Janeway, E., *Prescriptions for Prosperity*, Times Books, New York, 1983.
18. An alternative that offers some promise to young and early-career professions is a relatively recent policy known as adjustable life, which allows the policyholder to purchase either term or permanent insurance and to switch back and forth between the two as circumstances dictate. This flexibility is intended to allow one policy to provide for the changing insurance needs of a policyholder. These policies must be held for a minimum term and are relatively expensive, significant drawbacks for persons who are already insured or who are seeking a first policy. But a young professional who needs adequate coverage may find this an attractive alternative to straight term. For a further discussion, see Munn, H., What's New in Life Insurance?, *Optometric Management*, vol. 14, no. 12, 1978, pp. 71–75.
19. For a testimonal to the importance of estate planning and adequate insurance, see Foster, J.H., Is Estate Planning Important? Ask a Doctor's Widow, *Medical Economics*, vol. 57, no. 25, Nov. 24, 1980, pp. 96–108.
20. Policies of life insurance should be changed or terminated only for well-reasoned purposes or clearly superior alternatives. See Untermeyer, I., Don't Drop that Life Insurance Policy!, *Optometric Management*, vol. 15, no. 7, 1979, pp. 89–97.
21. For a description of cash values and borrowing against these values, see Martinson, R., The Cheapest Cash Money Can Buy, *Optometric Management*, vol. 15, no. 12, 1979, pp. 77–81.
22. Harsham, P., Single Premium Annuities: They May Actually Make Sense Now, *Medical Economics*, vol. 56, no. 1, Jan. 8, 1979, p. 195. TEFRA has exerted an influence on annuities also. See Kaufman, S., Annuities and Universal Life Lose Some Glitter, *Medical Economics*, vol. 59, no. 26, Dec. 20, 1982, p. 117.
23. An annuity provides an income to the policyholder for

as long as the policyholder may live. This is the reverse of life insurance, which provides financial protection after—not before—death. The most common form of annuity is the single-premium immediate annuity. Under this arrangement, the policyholder makes a single payment to the insurance company, in return for which a monthly income is received from the company for as long as the policyholder may live. The older the policyholder is when the annuity is purchased, the more than resulting monthly income will be. The reason for this is because the insurance company expects to have to make fewer payments to an older person. A second popular type of annuity is known as the annual premium deferred annuity. Under this plan premium payments to purchase the annuity are spread over the years prior to retirement, instead of being paid in one lump sum. Benefits are paid as before, a fixed monthly amount that is received as long as the policyholder is alive. For a discussion of the use of annuities, see Annuities: Put Some Certainty into an Uncertain Future, *Medical Economics*, vol. 57, no. 23, Nov. 3, 1980, pp. 131–142.

24. Decisions that concern insurance are inevitably interrelated with estate planning. For commentaries on estate planning problems, see Klaff, M., Yes, You Can Take It with You, *Optometric Management*, vol. 15, no. 1, 1979, pp. 47–48; Ginsberg, L., Thinking About the Unthinkable, *Optometric Management*, vol. 16, no. 1, 1980, pp. 53–57; Ginsberg, L., Thinking About the Unthinkable: The Aftermath, *Optometric Management*, vol. 16, no. 2, 1980, pp. 109–113; Gray, J., How To Make Your Retirement Dreams Come True, *Optometric Management*, vol. 17, no. 10, 1981, pp. 17–21; Gregg, J.R., Your Practice Profile: Retirement Income, *Optometric Management*, vol. 17, no. 10, 1981, pp. 25–31; Martinson, R., Make the Most of the New Estate Tax Rules, *Optometric Management*, vol. 18, no. 4, 1982, pp. 41–47; Steinbert, H., Cashing in on Your Retirement Plan, *Optometric Management*, vol. 19, no. 1, 1983, pp. 31–37.
25. See Kaufman, S., Life Insurance: Little White Lies an Agent Might Tell You, *Medical Economics*, vol. 59, no. 2, Jan. 18, 1982, pp. 170–179.
26. Drake, K.B., How To Find an Insurance Agent Who's on Your Side, *Medical Economics*, vol. 56, no. 1, Jan. 8, 1979, pp. 195–202.
27. Settlement options have a significant influence on estate planning since insurance proceeds are often the single largest source of liquid assets available to the estate. This discussion omits the important subject of life insurance trusts, which can be a necessary means of avoiding estate and income taxes. For a discussion of this topic, see Brosterman, supra note 8, at 187–191.
28. *IRS Code of 1954*, Subtitle A, Chapter 1B, Part III, §101(a).
29. *IRS Code of 1954*, Subtitle B, Chapter 11A, Part III, §2042.
30. Ibid.
31. *IRS Code of 1954*, Subtitle B, Chapter 12A, §2502.

Chapter 53

Disability Insurance

Federal studies show that almost half of all home mortgage foreclosures result from homeowners being disabled. Statistics show the much greater likelihood of one's becoming disabled rather than dying during working years. . . . Don't find out the hard way that choosing the right disability policy might become one of the most important decisions you make in your life.
—Robert A. Seibel, *Disability Insurance: Caveat Emptor, Journal of the American Bar Association*

Types of Disability Insurance
Uses
Office Overhead Insurance
Riders
Taxation

Disability is a distinct and sobering possibility when analyzed statistically. There is a 90 percent probability that one in three persons 25 years of age will be disabled for at least three months before reaching age 65; a 92 percent probability that one in four persons 40 years of age will be disabled for at least three months before reaching age 65; and a 91 percent probability that one in five persons 50 years of age will be disabled for at least three months before reaching age 65 (see Table 53.1). Professionals are not exempt from these rather surprising odds.[1]

Studies have demonstrated that long-term disability (i.e., that in excess of ninety days within a twelve-month period) is far more likely than death, although death is the more commonly provided-for eventuality (see Table 53.2).

The chance of disability is not the sole statistic that creates concern: the likelihood that disability will be long-term is also significant. For example, of 35-year-olds who have been disabled for a year, 60 percent will still be disabled at the end of two additional years, and more than 40 percent will still be disabled at the end of five additional years. This genuine risk has to be considered when entering into practice (see Table 53.3).

Table 53.1. Mortality Versus Disability for Men

	No. of Men in Group					
Age	1 (%)	2 (%)	3 (%)	4 (%)	5 (%)	6 (%)
	Probability of at Least One Death Prior to Age 65[a]					
25	30	51	66	76	83	88
30	29	50	65	75	82	88
35	29	49	63	74	81	87
40	27	47	62	72	80	85
45	26	45	59	70	78	83
50	23	41	55	65	73	80
	Probability of at Least One Long-Term Disability* Prior to Age 65[b]					
25	53.7	78.6	90.1	95.4	97.9	99.0
30	52.2	77.1	89.1	94.8	97.5	98.8
35	50.3	75.3	87.7	93.9	97.0	98.5
40	47.7	72.7	85.7	92.5	96.1	98.0
45	44.3	69.0	82.7	90.4	94.6	97.0
50	39.4	63.2	77.7	86.5	91.8	95.0
55	32.1	53.8	68.6	78.7	85.5	90.2

*Disability lasting at least 90 days.
[a]Source: 1958 C.S.O. Mortality Table, age last birthday basis.
[b]Source: 1964 Commissioners Disability Table.

Disability insurance is a difficult problem for practitioners because the possibility of disability cannot be ignored, but the insurance coverage is expensive. In considering disability insurance, there are four basic questions that can be used to reveal the important provisions of any disability policy:

Table 53.2. Probability of Long-Term Disability

At Age	Disability of 90 days or more in year indicated is (multiple) more likely than death
22	7.46
27	6.70
32	6.59
37	5.84
42	4.26
47	3.41
52	2.73
57	2.35
62	2.10

Possibility of at Least One Disability Lasting 90 Days or More Before Age 65

At Age	Of 1,000 lives, number disabled before 65
20	789
25	756
30	723
35	685
40	635
45	573
50	489
55	377
60	221

Source: Society of Actuaries, 1980.

1. How long must the disability last before the insurance begins?
2. How long does the disability coverage continue?
3. What type of disability is covered?
4. What is the cost of the policy?

Before considering these questions, the practitioner must acquire an understanding of the types of disability insurance that are available.[2]

Types of Disability Insurance

There are three major sources of disability insurance that can be utilized by an optometrist: government plans, occupational plans, and private plans.

Government Plans

Among the major providers of disability protection are federal and state governments. Benefits can be obtained from any of five programs: Social Security,[3] worker's compensation, sickness disability, veteran's disability, and G.I. insurance. For the individual who qualifies, these will be an important source of disability income.

Occupational Plans

A common source of disability insurance for optometrists is the job-related plan, which can come from contractual disability compensation plans, self-

Table 53.3. Probability of Continuing Disability

Age When Disabled	At the End of 2 More Years: This % Will Still Be Disabled	This % Will Have Died	This % Will Have Recovered	At the End of 5 More Years: This % Will Still Be Disabled	This % Will Have Died	This % Will Have Recovered
If Disability Has Continued for One Year						
25	54.0	5.6	40.4	35.2	9.4	55.4
35	59.2	7.7	33.1	42.1	12.7	45.2
45	65.2	11.8	23.0	48.8	20.7	30.8
55	73.3	15.5	11.2	54.5	29.2	16.3
If Disability Has Continued for Two Years						
25	64.7	5.3	30.0	46.2	9.7	44.1
35	69.9	6.8	23.3	53.7	12.3	34.0
45	74.6	10.4	15.0	58.6	19.9	21.5
55	78.0	14.1	7.9	59.7	28.5	11.8

Source: Society of Actuaries, 1980.

employed retirement plans, profit-sharing plans, pension plans, or group health insurance plans. A brief discussion of each of these alternatives follows.

- Contractual disability compensation plans may be included within partnership agreements to allow a disabled partner to received disability income for a stated period of time, often at a percentage of the base salary the partner was earning prior to being disabled (see Chapter 45). Benefits usually decrease on a percentage basis during the term of disability, so that after a year the partner's disability income is reduced to zero. An employer may voluntarily pay a disabled employee disability income or may supplement disability payments made by the government, but, in the absence of some contractual obligation, payments are made at the generosity of the employer and can be terminated at any time.
- Self-employed retirement plans may be used by a disabled individual who qualifies in order to provide income during the period of disability. The retirement act for the self-employed (ERISA) permits such withdrawals to be made without penalty. Of course, doing so initiates the gradual depletion of the individual's retirement fund, a course of action that should not be undertaken without necessity.
- Profit-sharing plans are often an important fringe benefit of the professional corporation or association. Qualified plans can include provisions for disability income, with benefits payable either periodically or as a lump sum.
- Pension plans may provide for payment of retirement funds in the event of total and permanent disability, but there can be major differences in the benefits to be paid out, depending on how closely related the retirement and disability provisions are. Some plans determine the amount of disability benefits to be paid in accordance with the pension rights that have vested prior to the time of the disability; others reduce benefits if disability payments are received through Social Security or other government plans; the best plans clearly separate retirement and disability income so that both can be received.
- Group health insurance plans not only may offer the usual medical, surgical, and hospital care but also may include provisions for disability. These benefits are typically expressed as a percentage of salary, with the percentage declining over the term of the disability to some minimum. An alternative form of payment is a strict percentage of salary, payable for a term of years or until age 65. The funding of these plans has significant tax ramifications that must be understood by both employer and employee.

Although government and occupational plans are important to disability protection, most optometrists find it necessary to obtain supplemental coverage through private sources, especially young optometrists who are beginning their careers and have little or no occupational coverage.

Private Plans

Private disability insurance plans offered to professionals vary significantly from insurer to insurer, and the only truly adequate way to assess policy differences is to examine them on the basis of the four basic questions posed at the beginning of this chapter. The discussion that follows of the alternative private plans currently available to optometrists uses these four questions to analyze policy provisions.[4]

How Long Must the Disability Last before the Insurance Begins?

The period before benefits begin is called the elimination period; the longer this period is, the cheaper the policy will be. Of course, a lengthy elimination period may mean no income at a time when money is sorely needed, and so the economic advantages and disadvantages of a policy's elimination period must be given careful consideration.

How Long Does the Disability Coverage Continue?

The benefit payment period may be a year, five years, or even until age 65; the longer the period during which benefits will be received, the greater the value of the policy (and the greater its expense). Rarely do policies pay benefits for life (except for disabilities due to accident). The definition of disability under the policy plays a key role in determining whether full benefits will be received. Some policies require that the disabled individual be confined to home in order to qualify for payments; others may pay only partial benefits (or none at all) if the individual can work at any occupation. A recurrent injury is a potentially troublesome problem for both insured and insurer; whether or not a policy awards full compensation for recurrent disability should be ascertained.[5]

What Type of Disability Is Covered?

How a policy defines disability establishes the value of coverage.[6] It is best described as being "an inability to perform the duties of one's regular occupation"; an alternative definition is "an inability to work at any gainful occupation for which one might be considered reasonably fitted by education or training"; an even broader definition is "an inability to work at any occupation." The less specific the definition, the less likely that the insured will be able to draw full benefits for an extended period of time. Certain conditions may be excluded from the definition (such as mental illness) or be excluded from coverage if they did not originate after the insurance began. For this reason, the best policies cover illness that manifests itself after the policy is issued (rather than illness that originates after the policy has been taken out). Another aspect of the definition that merits investigation is the type of disability being covered: whether it is total, partial, or both has a significant influence on the value of the benefits. In addition, a policy that offers an incentive to return to work can provide for the cost of rehabilitation programs that speed recovery. And a policy that includes residual benefits will pay partial benefits in the event the policyholder is able to return to work part-time. However, years of part-time benefits are likely to be eroded severely by inflation; fortunately, some policies raise the earnings limit each year and thus defray the effects of inflation. Cost of living adjustments can also be included to adjust policy benefits upward annually, but they are an expensive addition to a basic policy.

What Is the Cost of the Policy?

The foregoing considerations are of obvious importance when discussing cost because the policies with the better benefits will cost more than their less comprehensive competitors.[7] And there are costs that are not as obvious as the premium to be paid. For example, if the cancellation clause permits, an insurer may be able to cancel the policy, refuse to renew it, or increase the premium by a substantial margin. Thus one of the most expensive types of policies is one that is "guaranteed renewable and noncancellable"; no matter what the state of the policyholder's health, the insurer cannot cancel the policy or alter the premium (although premiums may systematically increase at stated ages). A "guaranteed renewable" policy is cancellable, but the policyholder can renew the policy even though there is a risk that the insurer may raise the premium for the policyholder's risk class. The worst policies are those that are "optionally renewable"; they only require the insurer to keep the policy in force until the next premium is due to be paid. Note that the benefits to be paid in the event of disability may be substantially raised by the insurer even during the period of guaranteed renewability, thus increasing the premium cost. Also, the policy may contain a provision that does not waive the payment of premiums during the period of disability, thereby reducing the value of the benefits actually received.

Uses

The obvious use of any type of disability insurance is to supply income during an extended period of sickness or injury. Since disability income can arise from any or all of three types of insurance—governmental, occupational, or private—it is important to understand the interrelation of these three sources of disability benefits and how they can be used to maximum advantage.[8]

The first step in planning the use of disability insurance is to assess the income that would be needed should serious and debilitating illness or injury intervene. During the period of disability, certain expenses could be expected to decline: travel, entertainment, clothing, charitable contributions, and other nonnecessary budget items. Taxes would also be reduced. At the same time, medical expenses could be expected to increase. Careful planning—such as waiver of premium riders on life insurance—can reduce some expenses. But some contingencies cannot be totally anticipated. For instance, a working spouse may find it necessary to work less or to give up working altogether in order to look after a disabled mate. Although individual needs may differ, the actual amount required to maintain a family during a period of disability for the breadwinner may be less than two thirds of the family's predisability income.

Once the amount of income necessary to support the family is determined, the next step is to identify the sources of disability income that can be relied upon, particularly during the first year of disability. These sources include accounts receivable, disability insurance (occupational or private), social security, cash reserve, and personal investments.

Accounts Receivable

For optometrists who operate on other than a cash-only basis—which is the overwhelming majority—some income can be expected during the first three months of disability (or perhaps even longer) because of patient fees that are due and owing. Of course, some of this income will be needed to cover the costs of office overhead (unless office overhead insurance is purchased; discussed *infra*). The cost of operating the office during this period, including hiring a temporary stand-in, and the income that can be anticipated from collecting receivables should be analyzed.

Disability Insurance

Since Social Security benefits require a five-month waiting period (and a disability that is expected to last more than a year), and accounts receivable can probably provide only about three months (if that) of income, there is an obvious need for some form of insurance protection during these first few months. Occupational disability plans often fulfill this function: Partnership agreements and pension and profit-sharing plans are used to provide income to a disabled partner or shareholder, typically on a decreasing basis as the disability persists over an extended period of time. Since there are other practitioners available to cover for the disabled partner or shareholder, the optometrist's practice continues on despite his absence. But the individual proprietor is often faced with the twin problems of no occupational insurance and no one to cover the practice, and may be able to plan for these eventualities only through the purchase of personal insurance. Two policies could be used to alleviate this situation: one, with a ninety-day elimination period, could pick up after accounts receivable had ended and could provide needed income until Social Security benefits began; the other, with a six-month or one-year elimination period (which would make it considerably cheaper), could restore income to needed levels in the event a long-term disability is incurred. During the three- to nine-month period that only one insurance policy was paying benefits, it might be necessary for the optometrist to supplement his income with money withdrawn from a cash reserve.

Social Security

There are two major hurdles that must be passed before Social Security benefits for disability can be secured: the disabled optometrist must prove that the disability will last for more than a year (or will result in death), and the five-month waiting period must elapse before benefits begin during the sixth month of sickness or injury. If the optometrist was injured while on the job and has a worker's compensation claim pending, the Social Security benefits may be reduced and/or their payment delayed. Once begun, however, the Social Security benefits will continue as long as the disability. Unfortunately, they will be rather meager.

Cash Reserve

The purpose of a planned-for and adequately funded cash reserve[9] is to provide ready cash for eventualities such as disability. If not enough income is realized during the first few months following sickness or injury, this fund may have to be used so that other sources of revenue (such as investments, retirement accounts, and prized assets) will not have to be liquidated.

Personal Investments

If no other source of income is available, investments may have to be turned to; such a move should be a last resort because the result is an invasion of the optometrist's retirement plan. In many instances the sale of investments may not be harmful since the disabled optometrist's tax bracket will doubtless be low. Money market funds should be sold with great caution because of early withdrawal penalities for Certificates of Deposit cashed before maturity and because it might be difficult to return to a fund after recovery. For a sole proprietor who has initiated a Keogh plan or an IRA, withdrawals made prior to retirement due to disability are not subject to penalty and neither are similar withdrawals made from corporate retirement plans. Of course, reducing the amount of money set aside for retirement may have rather significant consequences as the years pass.

When income is not sufficient to meet anticipated expenses, an income gap can arise that must be filled from some source. Planning for such an eventuality requires care and is frequently a long-term proposition. Analogous to these personal considerations is the equally difficult problem of how to keep a practice open and running when the primary source of income—the optometrist—is no longer able to work. The most vulnerable practitioner is the individual proprietor.

The Disabled Practice

Since optometry is primarily composed of individual practitioners, the spectre of disability is an ominous one for most members of the profession.[10] If an optometrist in solo practice becomes disabled, the ability of the practice to generate new income is likewise disabled. Yet, in order to keep the practice running, there are overhead expenses that must be paid. No private disability insurance policy offers the payment of overhead expenses as a benefit. This form of indemnification can only be obtained through the purchase of office overhead insurance (discussed subsequently).

If the disability of the optometrist is short-term—lasting but a few months—the optometrist will want to keep the practice open to collect any accounts receivable and to render any services that can be offered. Most optometrists would consider the financial burden of doing so as much an obligation to their patients and employees as an economic necessity. Of course, if the accounts receivable are substantial (and collectable), they may not only be able to keep the office doors open but also be able to provide some income for the disabled optometrist.

Many practitioners prefer not to allow substantial accounts receivable to accumulate, which can make the cost of maintaining the practice during disability prohibitive even though office personnel are reduced to a minimum. One way to generate new income is to have a substitute practitioner, an eventuality that can be planned for. But the substitute may not be able to produce enough income to pay both the office overhead and his salary, and office overhead insurance does not provide for a substitute's salary. For the individual practitioner, the longer the disability lasts, the smaller an asset his practice becomes. A long-term disability (which the optometrist knows will last over a period of years) will most likely result in an effort to sell the practice, because the longer the practice goes unattended, the fewer the number of patients who will remain loyal, with a corresponding diminution in the value of the practice.[11]

Office Overhead Insurance

One type of private disability coverage is office overhead insurance.[12] It is a limited form of insurance that reimburses a disabled doctor for those fixed expenses that are normal and customary to his practice and office. In order to qualify for benefits, the doctor must be totally disabled—the definition of which will be found within the policy—and satisfy the elimination period (usually half a month or an entire month). The benefits are limited to the actual overhead expenses incurred by the practice, for which the doctor will be reimbursed up to 100 percent (or to the policy limits).

Office overhead expenses are rent, electricity, heat, water, laundry, employee's salaries, and other fixed expenses. Excluded are the doctor's salary (or any other remuneration payable to the disabled doctor), substitute fees, cost of frames, lenses, instruments, or equipment. The expenses that will be paid are only those that are actually incurred; if the office staff becomes reduced and overhead is thereby cut, the insurance only compensates the disabled doctor for the expenses required to maintain the reduced staff and overhead. Benefits are payable for a stated period of time and may or may not be retroactive to the first day of disability, depending on the policy (eighteen months to two years is customary). Like disability policies, there are several provisions that should be examined, including the right to cancel, waiver of policy premiums during disability, option to convert the policy into disability insurance, and extended benefits in the event of death.

Riders

Disability policies vary in cost due to the presence or absence of various riders.[13] Most of the available riders have been discussed in the preceding chapter on life insurance, but a brief summary of the most important ones is included below.

Disability period—Some plans offer extended benefits (payable for life or until age 65 or 70) for both accidental disability and disability due to sickness.

Recurrent disability—The more liberal policies will provide that a recurrent disability is a new disability (thereby extending the period of benefits) after a relatively brief period of recovery.

Residual benefits—Partial benefits may be offered to a practitioner who can return to work part-time, with guaranteed escalation in the annual earnings limit so that the total loss of insurance benefits is delayed.

Right to renew—The best policy is one that is guaranteed renewable and noncancellable.

Cost-of-living adjustment—Since inflation erodes income, some policies offer annual adjustments to the benefits being paid the disabled policyholder.

Limited exclusions—The fewer the exclusions (for illness or accident), the more comprehensive the policy.

Waiver of premium—In the event of total disability lasting for a stated period of months, the premiums for the disability insurance policy will be waived for the remainder of the period for which benefits are payable.

Although cost is a major consideration when evaluating a policy, it is the overall package of benefits for that cost that must be assessed before deciding that one particular policy is a better buy than another.[14]

Taxation

The disability income that an individual receives as the result of insurance coverage purchased with his money is not taxable as income because it is considered to be compensation for injury. The premiums paid for the insurance are not deductible.[15]

If disability benefits are received as the result of an employer-purchased plan, then the tax considerations are somewhat more complicated and an accountant's advice will be needed. Any premiums paid by an employer for an employee's disability insurance policy may be deducted as a business expense. The premiums are not considered to be income for the employee.[16]

Disability insurance will have more appeal for solo practitioners, older optometrists (who are more at risk to be disabled), and practices for which the tax considerations are favorable. But because the likelihood of long-term disability is a statistically significant one, this form of insurance will deserve consideration at one time or another by virtually all optometrists.

Notes

1. See Harsham, P., Retirement Your Way: What if a Disability Cuts You Down, *Medical Economics*, vol. 59, no. 7, Mar. 29, 1982, pp. 68–76.
2. For a general discussion of the types of disability insurance, see Brosterman, R., *The Complete Estate Planning Guide*, McGraw-Hill, New York, 1987, pp. 128–136.
3. Social Security is a major source of disability compensation, and even this program can be insured. See Lance, J.F., Now You Can Insure Your Social Security Disability Benefits, *Medical Economics*, vol. 55, no. 25, Nov. 27, 1978, pp. 137–140. Social Security requirements and guidelines can be ascertained by obtaining the *Social Security Handbook*, U.S. Government Printing Office, Washington, D.C.
4. For an assessment of private plans, see Geier, A., Your Best Buy in Disability Insurance, *Optometric Management*, vol. 19, no. 2, 1983, pp. 75–83; Kaufman, S., Why Your Disability Insurance Might Not Pay Off, *Medical Economics*, vol. 59, no. 13, June 21, 1982, pp. 251–259; and Disability Insurance, *Consumer Reports*, Mar. 1983, p. 122.
5. For example, the AOA Income Insurance Plan, which offers lifetime accident benefits and a choice of three sickness plans, provides that "successive periods of disability due to the same or a related cause and not separated by a return to full-time active practice for six consecutive months shall be considered as one disability." Thus recurrent disability compensation is accounted for under the AOA group plan. For a summary of the AOA plan provisions, see Geier, supra note 4.
6. The definition of disability is a major consideration when assessing a policy. See Goldberg, M.A., They've Taken the Disability Out of Disability Insurance, *Medical Economics*, vol. 56, no. 16, Aug. 10, 1981, pp. 133–141; Kaufman, supra note 4; and Geier, supra note 4.
7. For a discussion of the relative costs of contemporary policies, see Geier, supra note 4.
8. An analysis of disability benefits and how to integrate them into a coherent plan can be found in 1981 Financial Planning Guide: Disability Insurance: You'll Be Surprised How Little You Need, *Medical Economics*, vol. 57, no. 23, Nov. 3, 1980, pp. 169–184.
9. A cash reserve is one of the basic requirements of estate planning. Other basic requirements are generally considered to be a residence, a source of income, and adequate life insurance. For a guide to the principles of estate planning, see Brosterman, supra note 2, pp. 15–22.
10. See Miller, P., While You're Recovering, Who Will Cover the Office?, *Optometric Management*, vol. 17, no. 2, 1981, pp. 97–101.
11. There can be little doubt that a practice allowed to wither on the vine experiences a steady decline in its value. See the discussion in Elmstrom, G., *Advanced Management Strategies for Optometrists*, Professional Press, Chicago, 1974, pp. 111–122.
12. See Miller, supra note 10.
13. See Geier, supra note 4.
14. For an analysis, see *Consumer Reports*, supra note 4.
15. *IRS Code of 1954*, Subtitle A, Chapter 1B, Part III, §§104, 105, 106.
16. Ibid.

Chapter 54

Professional Liability Insurance

Hell, yes, we'll sue doctors who go bare.
—Title of article by John Carlova, describing the attitude of plaintiff's lawyers toward physicians who do not have professional liability insurance, *Medical Economics*, April 14, 1980

Besides insuring against death and disability, an optometrist will want to protect his practice from loss. The potential hazards that await a private practitioner can involve his person (malpractice, defamation), his employees (malpractice, embezzlement), his frames and lenses (product liability), his office and equipment (premises liability), or loss due to fire, burglary, theft, and other perils. With so much at stake, and the cost of professional insurance relatively low, it is little wonder that practice-related insurance has become a high priority for most optometrists. Unfortunately, both the cost of professional insurance and the number and likelihood of claims have escalated over the course of the past decade.[1] The trend toward increased exposure to liability can only be expected to increase in the years to come,[2] and so adequate professional coverage has become a necessity for all optometrists.[3]

The following chapter discusses the types of policies currently available, their usual provisions, the extent of coverage generally considered necessary, and the tax ramifications of purchasing liability insurance.

Types of Professional Insurance

Since the potential for loss touches on so many areas of optometric practice, professional liability insurance policies must protect against a wide range of risks. For the purposes of this discussion insurance coverage will be divided into three categories: personal liability insurance, fire insurance, and other property insurance.[4]

Personal Liability Insurance

The optometrist can be personally liable for injuries to patients that arise out of malpractice, defamation, product liability, premises liability, or the negligence of employees (vicarious liability). Indemnification can be obtained for each of these potential sources of liability.

Malpractice insurance pays for all costs of a legal defense and for any judgments or settlements arising out of a malpractice claim or a claim of breach of contract (up to the stated policy limits).[5] Policies no longer routinely require the approval of the doctor before any settlement can become legally binding, which means that an optometrist can no longer insist on his day in court if he considers a claim to be unwarranted.[6] Coverage also includes claims against employees who are acting within the line and scope of their duties, which means that technicians, assistants, opticians, or associates are provided with protection. Partners who are legally liable for one another's malpractice can indemnify themselves against such an eventuality through the purchase of the appropriate coverage. The employees of professional corporations can obtain coverage through a policy taken out by the corporation.

Defamation insurance provides all legal fees and

pays all judgments or settlements (up to the limits of the policy) for any injury to the reputation of another person that arises out of the optometrist's professional activities. The defendant doctor's approval is not necessary for settlement of a claim. The persons covered under a standard policy are the same as those enumerated in the preceding paragraph.

Product liability insurance indemnifies the optometrist (up to the stated policy limits) against any claim arising out of a defect in a lens or frame that results in damage to a patient's person or property; the optometrist's approval is not necessary for the settlement of a claim.

Premises liability insurance protects (to the policy limits) against any claims by a patient that result from injury while in the optometrist's office or on the office premises. These claims include injuries from equipment as well as injuries from falls, shocks, and similar mishaps.

Medical payments insurance pays for the reasonable medical expenses (up to the policy limits) incurred by persons injured while on the optometrist's office premises, no matter who is at fault.

All of the foregoing are considered part of the basic coverage required for private practice. Additional coverage can also be obtained, to insure against other eventualities:

- Employees can be insured against personal injuries that arise while the employee is acting within the line and scope of his or her duties on behalf of an optometrist.
- Automobiles used to conduct optometrist business can be insured against accident claims arising out of negligence of an employee-driver.
- Fire loss to leased or rented premises due to the negligence of an optometrist or his employees can also be covered.

There are other eventualities that can be provided for as optional coverage, and individual insurers will have to be consulted whenever special liability needs are contemplated.

Fire Insurance

Although liability insurance can protect against negligence that causes fire loss, to be fully indemnified for loss of instrumentation, equipment, records, furniture, supplies, and other items damaged by fire an optometrist must acquire fire insurance.[7] There are two fire insurance problems that an optometrist faces when leased office space is occupied: adequate insurance for all property located within the office, and adequate insurance for the building in which the office is located. Unless the optometrist owns the building, the only problem he can solve directly is the first, by adequately insuring all the personal property he uses in his practice. But there is still the worry that the structure within which his office is located may not be adequately insured. The best way to obviate this problem is to be certain that the office lease contains a clause requiring the lessor to insure the building adequately. (See Chapter 49 for typical provisions of a lease of professional office space.)

As for the insurance itself, insurance companies usually require that a building be insured to a prescribed minimum of its value, often 80 percent, in order for full benefits to be paid in the event of its loss.[8] As long as the 80 percent minimum is adhered to, a full 100 percent of any fire loss will be paid by the insurer, no matter whether the loss is partial or total. But if the insurance on the building falls below 80 percent of its value (which it can easily do if fire insurance policies are not adjusted for structure appreciation each year), the insurer is no longer obliged to pay 100 percent of the claim, reducing its liability in proportion to the percent of underinsurance. This can hinder repairs of partially damaged areas by the lessor and seriously impair an optometrist's ability to keep his office functioning.

The same considerations are involved in the optometrist's leased office space. The lessee must act as a co-insurer with the lessor and must acquire fire insurance for all property located within the office, such insurance amounting to a minimum of 80 percent of the property's value. Failure to do so results in only partial insurance coverage, just as with the building. Again, yearly review of fire insurance coverage is a must because new equipment additions can substantially boost a practice's property value.[9]

Acquiring a policy for an adequate amount is only the first step. There are three other problems that must be considered: documentation, compensation for damaged or lost property, and coverage for interrupted business losses.

Documentation of purchased items should be accomplished in two ways: all sales receipts and check stubs should be retained and stored for safekeeping, and photodocumentation of all new office contents should be performed routinely. Proof of loss is a burden that rests solely on the policyholder, and the contractual requirements to document loss under most fire insurance policies are formidable.[10]

The money paid for a claim can either be used to restore an item or to purchase a new one. Restoration costs will be paid in full by the insurer, but insurance checks for totally damaged items will not be adequate to purchase a brand-new replacement. Rather, replacement cost is considered to be the fair market value of the item at the time of the loss, which means that an instrument or piece of equipment that is several years old will be reduced in value according to its age. To obtain the cost of a new item, replacement value insurance must be obtained.[11]

Interrupted business losses—those losses incurred by virtue of the disruption of practice from the fire—can also be included in a policy, but proof of loss can again be a substantial burden for the policyholder.[12]

Other Property Insurance

Besides premises liability and medical payments insurance, which are considered basic necessities for a private practitioner, there is optional property coverage that can be purchased.[13] Among the most important risks faced by a practitioner are burglary[14] and embezzlement.[15]

Professional equipment as well as furniture and office equipment can be insured against loss on a replacement cost basis (discussed *supra*), which means that in the event of loss new items will be paid for in full, without regard for depreciation, as long as the policy limits reflect the current replacement cost value.[16] Improvements and alterations of an office (such as paneling, fixtures, and like changes) can also be insured on a replacement cost basis.

Examples of other property insurance available to optometrists include the following:

- Transit coverage can be obtained for equipment while it is away from the office at another location or while it is in transit.
- Personal effects of the optometrist, the staff, and patients can be insured against loss by perils such as fire, theft, and burglary.
- Extra expenses required to continue a practice after damage to equipment can also be provided for as an optional benefit.
- Office records can be insured for the costs of reproduction.
- Accounts receivable can be insured against loss or destruction and subsequent uncollectibility; typically, the accounts receivable that are uncollected after ninety days will be paid for by the insurer.
- Loss from burglary, theft, and robbery can be protected against through the purchase of federally sponsored crime insurance.
- Loss from embezzlement can be a shock for an unsuspecting optometrist, but the traditional method of protecting against such loss—by bonding of employees—is generally distasteful to an office staff; fortunately, insurance providing for bonding of all employees can be purchased without the stigma that actual bonding confers.[17]
- Office overhead insurance can be acquired (discussed in Chapter 53).
- Owner, landlord, and tenant liability offers protection against claims that arise from an optometrist's ownership or operation of a building.
- Multiperil insurance is a package policy that provides coverage for fire, burglary, theft, office contents, professional equipment, general liability, and other perils; comprehensive coverage under such a package can sometimes be cheaper than purchases of individual policies for various contingencies.[18]

The biggest decision facing the optometrist is how much protection he should acquire. Fortunately, professional liability insurance for optometrists is relatively cheap. A practitioner can easily afford not only basic coverage but also "umbrella" coverage, which extends the personal liability provisions of the basic policy. Umbrella coverage also extends the amount of protection well beyond that found in a standard policy, usually to one million dollars. The cost of this extended coverage is typically less than 1 percent of the average practitioner's net income.[19]

Extent of Coverage

Professional liability exposure can continue for a long period of time after the optometrist has left private practice. There is a risk that a lawsuit will be filed after the insurance coverage has ended and the optometrist has found another job (e.g., teaching) or has retired. This period of vulnerability after policy premiums are no longer being paid is known as the "risk tail," and coverage should be acquired to protect the optometrist during this period. With an *occurrence* type policy, all errors and omissions are covered, provided the incident occurred during the policy period, even if the claim is made after the policy has been terminated. Under the more common *claims-made* form of policy, the optometrist usually has the right to purchase an extended reporting endorsement or nonpracticing policy within a stated period after terminating the basic policy, and this additional coverage is intended to protect against the risk tail.

There are several points to consider when choosing the type of policy for private practice:

- Although an occurrence form of policy does not require the purchase of additional risk tail protection, it is more expensive than the claims-made policy, may have less broad coverage, and thus may be a less desirable choice.
- The right to purchase risk tail coverage should be guaranteed in the claims-made policy, irrespective of whether the policy is terminated by the insurer or by the policyholder and regardless of the reason for termination.
- The cost of the extended reporting endorsement for the risk tail should be stated in the claims-made policy, either as a specific amount or a definite percentage of the basic policy.

The wise optometrist will select the type of policy that best suits his needs and will acquaint himself fully with its provisions.

Taxation

Liability insurance coverage is a necessary aspect of the practice of optometry, and as such it is a necessary business expense for tax purposes. Thus an optometrist may claim a tax deduction for the premium, whether it is for basic or for optional coverage.[20]

Should an optometrist be unfortunate enough to have to file an insurance claim under any of the policies providing property coverage, the reimbursement to the optometrist by the insurer is not taxable. In the event the insurance payment is less than the fair market value of the property at the time of the loss, the optometrist can claim a deduction for the amount of loss in excess of the insurance proceeds. But this deduction has been limited by the Tax Equity and Fiscal Responsibility Act of 1982.

If an optometrist is a defendant in a professional liability lawsuit, the insurer will provide an attorney and will pay the attorney's fees and any costs of litigation. If the optometrist decides to hire a personal attorney, the cost of this additional counsel can be deducted. Any judgment that an optometrist is ordered to pay that is in excess of the optometrist's insurance coverage would likewise qualify as a deduction.

Notes

1. In comparison to the modest coverage and premiums necessary to insure optometrists at the start of the 1970s, the claims paid and premiums collected as the decade progressed show a steady escalation. For a review, see Elmstrom, G., Malpractice: What Can OD's Expect?, *Optical Journal and Review of Optometry*, vol. 114, no. 1, 1977, pp. 42–52. During the 1980s, more of the same is in store for the profession. For commentaries on the prospects for the future, see Guerrein, R., Editorial, *Review of Optometry*, vol. 119, no. 12, 1982, p. 18; and My Malpractice Nightmare, in the section entitled Avoiding Malpractice, *Review of Optometry*, vol. 119, no. 12, pp. 29–34. For a general analysis of malpractice claims and premiums during the 1970s, see Greenspan, N., Medical Malpractice Insurance Premiums, *Group Practice Journal*, vol. 29, no. 6, June 1980, pp. 17–20.
2. For commentaries on the increased exposure to professional liability claims, see Elmstrom, G., *Advanced Management Strategies for Optometrists*, Professional Press, Chicago, 1982, pp. 172–173; Editorial, Pathology: The Prospect of Malpractice, *Optical Journal and Review of Optometry*, vol. 114, no. 1, 1977, p. 6; Elmstrom, supra note 1; Morgan, E., The Professional Liability Problem and Optometry, *Journal of the American Optometric Association*, vol. 42, no. 2, 1971, pp. 161–164; My Malpractice Nightmare, *Review of Optometry*, vol. 119, no. 12, 1982, pp. 29–34; and Pecorino, J., Perspectives on Malpractice, *New England Journal of Optometry*, vol. 27, no. 5, 1976.
3. As has been pointed out in Chapter 2, optometric malpractice is a relatively recent phenomenon—developing after liability law had already been well established by numerous precedent-setting cases filed against physicians—and the lessons learned by physicians over the past several decades are now beginning to have applicability to optometrists. In the area of liability insurance coverage, there is ample precedent to support the proposition that adequate protection is a necessity for the contemporary practitioner. Failure to carry insurance—referred to euphemistically as "going bare"—has been demonstrated to be a practicularly poor way of doing business. See Carlova, J., Hell, Yes, We'll Sue Doctors Who Go Bare, *Medical Economics*, vol. 57, no. 7, Apr. 14, 1980, pp. 45–59; and Carlova, J., What Going Bare Means When the Patient Gets $200,000, *Medical Economics*, vol. 57, no. 18, Sept. 1, 1980, pp. 92–100.
4. The author is indebted to John Pecorino, formerly of Aetna Life & Casulty Co., and AOA counsel Tom Eichhorst for freely giving of their time and expertise in discussing optometric liability insurance.
5. An insurance company's obligation extends only to the limits of the policy, which may be less than the claim. In this event, a conflict of interest may arise that obligates the insurance company to issue a "reservation of rights" letter. In some states (such as California) the policyholder may hire an independent counsel at the insurance company's expense (a so-called "Coumis counsel"). This attorney can, in fact, direct the defense

of the case. For a discussion, see Gerber, P.C., What to Do When a Patient Plans to Sue, *Optometric Management*, vol. 23, no. 5, 1987, pp. 36–42.

6. This provision has been upheld in a case involving a physician who sued his insurance carrier for settling a case without his approval, alleging that the settlement resulted in a loss of patients and increased premiums. The court ruled that such a provision gave the insurance carrier the right to effect a settlement, despite its ramifications for the insured. See *Rogers v. Robson, Masters, Ryan, Brumund and Belom*, 392 N.E.2d 1365 (Ill. App. 1979).
7. Fire insurance has generated frequent commentary, much of it from practitioners who have learned "the hard way." See Tracht, M.E., Burned!, *Medical Economics*, vol. 55, no. 5, Mar. 6, 1978, pp. 164–175; Aldrich, C.K., We Learned About Fires—and Insurance—the Hard Way, *Medical Economics*, vol. 57, no. 8, Apr. 14, 1980, pp. 174–179; Levoy, R.P., Fire Insurance Is Not Enough!, *Optometric Management*, vol. 14, no. 1, 1978, pp. 105–109; Hauser, P., Beware of Fire and Fire Insurance!, *Optometric Management*, vol. 18, no. 2, 1982, pp. 27–29; and Krause, R., Invitation to a Lawsuit, *Optometric Management*, vol. 18, no. 2, 1982, pp. 30–33. Since fire can have such serious consequences for a practitioner, it is imperative that an adequate policy be obtained from a reputable company, and that policy provisions be reviewed annually.
8. Ibid.
9. Ibid.
10. For a review of this problem see Krause, R., Invitation to a Lawsuit, *Optometric Management*, vol. 18, no. 2, 1982, pp. 30–33.
11. The failings of "cost" insurance are reiterated by Levoy, supra note 7; and Houser, supra note 7.
12. Ibid.
13. For an overview of optional coverage available to optometrists, see Elmstrom, supra note 2, at 418–425.
14. See Huston, P., Five Lessons My Burglar Taught Me, *Medical Economics*, vol. 59, no. 2, Jan. 18, 1982, pp. 259–266; Burglars Target Doctors, *Review of Optometry*, vol. 119, no. 12, 1982, p. 3; and Adams, B., Easy Ways to Burglarproof, *Review of Optometry*, vol. 116, no. 3, 1979, p. 6.
15. See Hubler, R., That Helping Hand—Helping Itself?, *Optometric Management*, vol. 13, no. 12, 1977, pp. 47–53; Dirby, W.D., How the IRS Turned Up Our $360,000 Embezzler, *Medical Economics*, vol. 56, no. 6, Mar. 19, 1979, pp. 139–144; and Barker, D.E., Biting the Hand that Thieves You, *Optometric Management*, vol. 15, no. 10, 1979, pp. 103–111.
16. See Anonymous, Don't Lose Your Valuables to a Thief *and* Inflation, *Medical Economics*, vol. 57, no. 4, Feb. 18, 1980, pp. 170–173.
17. For a discussion, see Elmstrom, supra note 2, at 423–424.
18. For commentary on this type of policy, see Lane, M., *The Doctor's Law Guide*, W.B. Saunders, Philadelphia, 1979, pp. 86–95.
19. For a discussion, see Elmstrom, supra note 1.
20. *IRS Code of 1954*, Subtitle A, Chapter 1B, Part VI, §162.

Chapter 55

Personal Insurance

Protection is not a principle, but an expedient.
—Benjamin Disraeli, *Speech Before the House of Commons, March 17, 1845*

Types of Personal Insurance
Uses
Taxation

Types of Personal Insurance

This text's discussion of insurance needs would not be complete without some mention of the personal coverage that each individual requires in order to protect three very important aspects of life: health, home, and transportation. Thus we will divide personal insurance needs into three categories: health insurance, homeowner's insurance, and vehicle insurance.[1]

Health Insurance

Prior to 1965, when Medicare was authorized by the U.S. Congress, health insurance provided lifetime care that was guaranteed to be renewable. Today, however, most policies terminate at age 65, when Medicare benefits begin, and so the average optometrist will need a health plan for about four decades (ages 25 to 65).[2]

The usual health insurance purchased by optometrists is major medical coverage. Such a plan is intended to defray the cost of catastrophic illness, which can be financially devastating for the uninsured. There are two basic provisions to major medical coverage: there is an annual deductible, which the insured must pay out of his own pocket before the major medical coverage applies; and medical expenses that qualify under the plan and that exceed the deductible will be paid by the insurer up to a stated percentage, usually 80 percent; in addition, some plans will pay 100 percent of eligible expenses once a certain level is reached.

Hospital indemnity insurance is a supplemental insurance plan that can be used to provide protection for hospital expenses, and it can be added onto preexisting major medical or other health insurance. Benefits are typically paid directly to the recipient, beginning with the first day of hospitalization and paying for as much as a year of continuous confinement. Benefits are often increased for a limited period if intensive care is required. There are limitations to such policies (60 or 65 being the customary ages beyond which no insurance can be obtained), and there are several important exclusions that are usually present in the policy (e.g., suicide, pregnancy, nursing-home services, or preexisting conditions).

Health insurance has become an extremely important aspect of U.S. life; more than 90 percent of the population has some form of health insurance, and with the burdensome financial debt that major illness represents, there is little wonder why.[3]

Homeowner's Insurance

There are three important types of homeowner's insurance[4]: mortgage insurance, personal liability insurance, and dwelling, unscheduled personal property, and living expense insurance. Mortgage insurance is usually purchased as a decreasing term rider on a permanent insurance policy, but it can be purchased separately. Personal liability insurance and dwelling, unscheduled personal property, and living expense insurance are both includable within a standard homeowner's policy.

Mortgage insurance protects a spouse against the eventuality that, with the insured's sudden death, the spouse will no longer have the income to meet the mortgage payments. Mortgage insurance pays off the mortgage balance in the event the insured dies, thus assuring that the home will be unencumbered (also discussed in Chapter 52).

Personal liability insurance will provide an insured with protection against legal liability for any nonvehicular accidents that might occur on his property. The usual type of eventuality is a slip-and-fall injury.

Dwelling, unscheduled personal property, and living expense insurance covers a number of perils that involve an insured's home. It protects the home against fire, lightning, and other catastrophe; in addition, extended coverage against hail, windstorm, explosion, riot, falling trees, or crashing cars can be obtained. Coverage can also be provided for the theft or loss of personal items. As an adjunct to such insurance the policyholder needs to keep the receipts of all major purchases or to take photographs of these items in his house or apartment. (An inventory is also a good idea.) The owner of items of special value (e.g., jewelry, art, antiques) should check with his insurer to make certain that they are covered (discussed *infra*). If there is a homeowner's policy, the personal goods in the home may be insured for a percentage of the homeowner's insurance (usually 50 percent), but this coverage may not be sufficient for extra-valuable items. In the event that a home is damaged and made unfit for habitation, living expense insurance provides coverage for the period of time that the insured and his family are forced to live outside the home while it is being repaired, but the extent of these payments is rather limited.

To these basic homeowner's provisions there may be added a fourth type of coverage: *scheduled property*. All standard homeowner's policies will limit financial reimbursement for the loss of certain items, such as jewelry, silverware, works of art, antiques, and similar items. To insure this property, the individual items (e.g., a wedding ring, silver flatware, or original paintings) will have to be valued separately, or scheduled, on the policy. The item will be protected for its appraised value in the event of theft, loss, or destruction. Of course, the premium cost escalates when there is increased insurance coverage, and the policyholder will have to weigh this added cost and the risk of loss before deciding to schedule such items. Before purchasing a homeowner's policy, care should be taken to ensure that it is adequate for the policyholder's needs.[5]

Vehicle Insurance

An optometrist must adequately insure any vehicle that is used in his practice, especially if employees are permitted to drive it.[6] A personal vehicle also deserves adequate insurance. The types of coverage that should be acquired for a personal vehicle include liability, collision, comprehensive, medical payments, and uninsured motorist coverage.

Liability insurance protects the insured if he or other insureds cause an accident that results in personal injury, property damage, or both. The insurance company will defend the policyholder in court and pay all claims against him up to the policy limit. The policy limit is expressed as a ratio, such as $100,000/300,000; this means that coverage extends up to $100,000 per claimant, and up to an aggregate total for all claimants of $300,000.

Collision insurance reimburses the insured for damage done to his vehicle (less a deductible), even if he is at fault.

Comprehensive insurance protects an insured against virtually all hazards (e.g., fire and theft) except collision and is usually inexpensive. Deductible coverage is probably the best form in which to purchase this coverage.

Medical payments insurance covers the expenses that the insured and his passengers will incur if injured in an accident—even the ambulance bill—no matter who is responsible for the accident. These benefits are usually limited in amount.

Uninsured motorist insurance protects the insured against personal injury by a motorist who has no insurance himself. It even provides coverage in the event the insured is injured by a hit-and-run noncontact accident. The insured may not have to be in the car to be covered; if there is personal injury caused by an uninsured motorist, there may be coverage.

An optometrist should not neglect his own insurance needs in favor of those for his practice. Premium costs can be controlled by a knowledgeable purchaser.[7]

Uses

Since individual needs and circumstances vary, trying to predict the insurance coverage appropriate for all persons would be an impossible undertaking. Therefore, the following discussion concerns only the most common usages of personal insurance and describes insurance provisions only in general terms.

Vehicle Insurance

Most individuals have their first exposure to insurance when they insure an automobile, and over the course of years the ownership of automobiles (or other vehicles) will result in the contribution of many thousands of dollars for insurance protection. Nevertheless, because of the risk of loss, automobile insurance is an absolute necessity, including uninsured motorist coverage, which is optional in some states.

A long-term proposition such as vehicle insurance requires selectivity on the part of the individual seeking coverage. Insurers vary tremendously in terms of coverage offered, cost, renewability, and reputation, and policies should be selected with great care. Vehicle policies generally fall into one of two categories:

Family policies—Insurance protection exists whether or not the insured is driving his vehicle, a vehicle belonging to someone else, or a rented one. These policies also extend protection to members of the household when they drive an insured vehicle and to others who drive the vehicle with permission. Additional coverage may protect members of the household when they drive someone else's vehicle.

Special policies—Insurance protection is offered as a package at rates below those of family policies. Benefits automatically include medical payment coverage, death benefits, and uninsured motorist coverage. The addition of comprehensive or collision insurance brings with it personal property coverage and towing coverage as well. Special policies do not usually pay for injuries that are covered by other insurance.

Family policies that are not markedly more expensive than special policies should be given preference because they will provide some coverage that special policies cannot. Another consideration is the insurance: If all casualty insurance—automobile, homeowners, practice—is purchased from one insurance company, the optometrist with a valid claim has a little more leverage to exert than he would otherwise.

Health Insurance

Health insurance in general, and major medical coverage in particular, is most commonly purchased through a group plan because of the reduced cost. The best policies are those that provide virtually unlimited maximums and that are offered by large, stable companies. If coverage other than major medical is desired, care should be exercised. Certain limited policies—such as those paying benefits only for certain diseases (cancer, for example)—may be duplicative and unnecessary. Probably the biggest decision in this regard comes when the optometrist has reached age 65 and is eligible for Medicare; extra insurance may be required to "plug the gaps" in Medicare coverage.

Homeowner's Insurance

Homeowner's insurance should be reviewed annually to ensure that the policy limits are adequate, particularly in the event there is a total loss. Since the premiums are paid as part of the monthly mortgage, it is easy to forget about policy details. Property appreciation and inflation make such an omission a serious mistake.

Familiarity with the homeowner's policy is also necessary in order to understand the type of eventualities for which there is coverage, the applicable deductibles, and the maximum coverage for each type of loss. Of particular interest are the types of casualty discussed previously: mortgage protection; personal liability; dwelling, unscheduled personal property, living expense coverage; and scheduled property insurance.

The tax reform law enacted in 1982 significantly reduced the ability of a homeowner to deduct personal casualty and theft losses that are not covered by insurance and made adequate insurance protection more important than ever.[8]

Taxation

Self-employed optometrists may deduct 25 percent of premiums paid for health insurance coverage for themselves, their spouses, and their dependents.[9] The remaining 75 percent may be claimed as an itemized deduction on Schedule A. In addition, the health insurance premiums purchased by an optometrist for the benefit of employees are deductible.[10]

There is no deduction permitted for insurance premiums paid for an individual's vehicle insurance. Premiums for business premises or for business vehicles may be deducted as a necessary business expense. The extent of the deduction depends on the extent of the vehicle's use for business purposes.[11]

A homeowner cannot deduct the cost of the premiums paid for homeowner's insurance. Uninsured casualty losses may be deducted if they exceed 10 percent of the homeowner's adjusted gross income, and if they are not compensable by insurance.[12]

Notes

1. An assessment of personal insurance needs can be found in Elmstrom, G., *Advanced Management for Optometrists*, Professional Press, Chicago, 1974, pp. 425–433.
2. A philosophical review of health insurance as social policy is described by Shulman, A.N., Health Economics and Financing, in Newcomb, R., and J. Jolley, (eds.), *Public Health and Community Optometry*, Thomas, Springfield, Ill., 1980, pp. 229–252.
3. For an overview of insurance coverage, including health insurance, see Insurance: Buying All the Coverage You Need—For Less, *Medical Economics*, vol. 55, no. 23, Nov. 6, 1978, pp. 249–258. See also Elmstrom, supra note 1, at 431–432.
4. Another aspect of insurance, home security, is reviewed by Rhodes, R.C. (eds.), *Homeowner's Security Handbook*, American Society for Testing and Materials, Philadelphia, 1977.
5. Homeowner's policies can vary considerably in their terms, and have evoked numerous commentaries. See Drake, K.B., Homeowner's Coverage that Keeps Pace with Inflation, *Medical Economics*, vol. 55, no. 3, Feb. 6, 1978, pp. 137–141; Drake, K., Your Home: And Finally: Get the *Right* Home Insurance, *Medical Economics*, vol. 55, no. 20, Oct. 2, 1978, pp. 237–246; and Egerton, J., Watching the Water Rise Inside Our Dream House, *Medical Economics*, vol. 59, no. 8, Apr. 12, 1982, pp. 278–288. See also Elmstrom, supra note 1, at 432–433.
6. See Lane, M., *The Doctor's Law Guide*, W.B. Saunders, Philadelphia, 1979, pp. 86–95; and Elmstrom, supra note 1, at 432–433.
7. See Forster, J.F., Buying the Right Car Can Mean Big Insurance Savings, *Medical Economics*, vol. 57, no. 16, Aug. 4, 1980, pp. 97–102; and Enright, S.B., Auto Insurance: Five Ways to Cut Your Premium, *Medical Economics*, vol. 59, no. 2, Jan. 18, 1982, pp. 248–251.
8. The Tax Equity and Fiscal Responsibility Act of 1982 instituted a floor on noninsured casualty losses; if the loss does not exceed 10 percent of the adjusted gross income, there can be no deduction.
9. This deduction was authorized by the Tax Reform Act of 1986. The deduction cannot be claimed if the optometrist is eligible to participate in a subsidized health plan of another employer or through his spouse's employer. See IRS publication 921, *Explanation of the Tax Reform Act of 1986 for Business.*
10. *IRS Code of 1954*, Subtitle A, Chapter 1B, Part VI, §162.
11. If a vehicle is used exclusively for business purposes, the cost of operating the vehicle can be deducted (e.g., gas, oil, repairs, insurance, depreciation, interest paid on a loan to purchase the car, taxes, garage rent, parking fees, and tolls). If the vehicle is used for personal purposes, only the percentage of expenses attributable to business use can be deducted. The Tax Reform Act of 1984 imposed limitations on depreciation deductions and the Tax Reform Act of 1986 has done likewise. See IRS publication 921, supra note 9. An optometrist should seek adequate tax counsel concerning the complexities of this important deduction.
12. The deduction for the casualty loss cannot be claimed if there is insurance to reimburse the optometrist for the loss but the optometrist chooses not to file for it. This provision was instituted by the Tax Reform Act of 1986 and doubtless will end the practice (on the part of some taxpayers) of filing a claim for the tax loss rather than for the insurance coverage. See IRS publication 921, supra note 9.

Table of Reported Cases By Alphabetical Order

Abelson's, Inc. v. New Jersey State Board of Optometrists, 5 N.J. 412, 75 A.2d 867 (1950). Ch. 9, n. 32, 38; Ch. 11, n. 72; Ch. 16, n. 10.

Acupuncture Society of Kansas v. Kansas State Board of Healing Arts, 226 Kan. 639, 602 P.2d 1311 (1979). Ch. 26, n. 35.

Adam v. Connecticut Medical Examining Board, 137 Conn. 535, 70 A.2d 350 (1951). Ch. 11, n. 59.

Adkins v. Ropp, 14 N.E.2d 727 (Ind. 1938). Ch. 19, n. 24.

Aetna Casualty and Surety Co. of Illinois v. Medical Protective Co., 575 F. Supp. 901 (D.C. Ill. 1983). Ch. 28, n. 33.

Agnew v. Parks, 343 P.2d 118 (Cal. 1959). Ch. 14, n. 14.

Aiken v. Clary, 396 S.W.2d 668 (Mo. 1965). Ch. 22, Table 1.

Alabama Board of Optometry v. Eagerton, 393 So.2d 1373 (Ala. 1981). Ch. 7, n. 26; Ch. 9, n. 37; Ch. 12, n. 31.

Alabama Great Southern Railway Co. v. Hunt, 204 Ala. 504, 86 So. 100 (1920). Ch. 14, n. 16.

Alexander v. Knight, 197 Pa. Super 79, 177 A.2d 142 (1962). Ch. 20, n. 14.

Alexander v. Menefee, 64 S.W. 855 (Ky. 1901). Ch. 33, n. 22.

Allison v. State, 76 S.W.2d 527 (Tex. Crim. App. 1934). Ch. 9, n. 9.

American General Insurance Co. v. Florez, 327 S.W.2d 643 (Tex. Civ. App. 1959). Ch. 33, n. 50.

American Medical Association v. Federal Trade Commission, 638 F.2d 443 (2d Cir. 1980), *affirmed* 455 U.S. 676, 102 S.Ct. 1744 (1982). Ch. 3, n. 18, 19; Ch. 5, n. 40.

American Optical Co. v. Wiedenhamer, 404 N.E.2d 606 (Ind. App. 1980). Ch. 2, n. 14; Ch. 27, n. 35.

American Optometric Association v. Federal Trade Commission, 626 F.2d 896 (D.C. Cir. 1980). Ch. 1, n. 187, Table 4; Ch. 4, n. 48, 53, Table 3; Ch. 7, n. 15; Ch. 16, n. 20.

Anderson v. Board of Medical Examiners, 117 Cal. App. 113, 3 P.2d 344 (1931). Ch. 11, n. 59.

Archer v. Galbraith, 18 Wash. App. 369, 567 P.2d 1155 (1977). Ch. 22, n. 15.

Arshanasky v. Royal Concourse Co., 28 A.D.2d 986 283 N.Y.S.2d 646 (1967). Ch. 13, n. 22.

Attorney General v. Kenco Optics, 340 N.E.2d 868 (Mass. 1976). Ch. 9, Table 2.

Bacardi v. Holzman, 182 N.J. Super. 422, 442 A.2d 617 (1981). Ch. 28, n. 40.

Bailey v. Harmon, 74 Colo. 390, 222 P. 393 (1924). Ch. 27, n. 43.

Baker v. Texas, 240 S.W. 924 (Tex. Crim. App. 1921). Ch. 1, n. 45, 51, 60, Table 1.

Barbee v. Rogers, 425 S.W.2d 342 (Tex. 1968). Ch. 2, n. 16, Table 2; Ch. 21, n. 6; Ch. 27, n. 40, 56; Ch. 30, n. 21.

Barber v. Time, Inc., 159 S.W.2d 291 (Mo. 1942). Ch. 20, n. 36.

Barnes v. Bovenmeyer, 122 N.W.2d 312 (Iowa 1963). Ch. 19, n. 34; Ch. 26, n. 17.

Barry v. Moench, 8 Utah 2d 191, 331 P.2d 814 (1958). Ch. 20, n. 25.

Barsky v. The Board of Regents of the University of the State of New York, 347 U.S. 442, 74 S.Ct. 650 (1954). Ch. 11, n. 45, 49.

Bates v. State Bar of Arizona, 433 U.S. 350, 97 S.Ct. 2691 (1977). Ch. 1, n. 183, Table 4; Ch. 4, Table 3; Ch. 5, n. 23; Ch. 9, n. 35.

Baum v. Turel, 206 F.Supp. 490 (D.C. N.Y. 1962). Ch. 20, n. 41.

Baxter v. Ford Motor Co., 168 Wash. 456, 12 P.2d 409, *affirmed* 15 P.2d 1118 (1932). Ch. 21, n. 4.

Beaman v. Schwartz, 738 S.W.2d 632 (Tenn. App.

633 (1980). Ch. 27, n. 43.

Clark v. Geraci, 208 N.Y.S.2d 564 (1960). Ch. 20, n. 18.

Clark v. Piedmont Hospital, 162 S.E.2d 468 (Ga. 1968). Ch. 19, n. 43.

Clayman v. Bernstein, 38 Pa. D&C 543 (1940). Ch. 20, n. 33.

Clifford v. Hughes, 139 A.D. 730, 124 N.Y.S. 478, (1910). Ch. 35, n. 16.

Cobbs v. Grant, 8 Cal. 3d 229, 104 Cal. Rptr. 505, 502 P.2d 1 (1972). Ch. 22, n. 4, Table 2.

Cochran v. Sears-Roebuck and Co., 34 S.E.2d 296 (Ga. 1945). Ch. 20, n. 30.

Collins v. American Optometric Association, 693 F.2d 636 (7th Cir. 1982). Ch. 2, n. 7, 23; Ch. 23, n. 33.

Colorado State Board of Medical Examiners v. Palmer, 400 P.2d 914 (Colo. 1965). Ch. 11, n. 57, 59.

Colorado State Board of Medical Examiners v. Weiler, 402 P.2d 606 (Colo. 1965). Ch. 11, n. 53.

Commonwealth v. Houtenbrink, 235 Mass. 320, 126 N.E. 669 (1920). Ch. 1, n. 65; Ch. 9, n. 7.

Commonwealth v. S.S. Kresge Co., 267 Mass. 145, 166 N.E. 558 (1929). Ch. 9, n. 18.

Commonwealth v. Stemet, 21 Pa. D&C 2d 295 (1959). Ch. 11, n. 106.

Congrove v. Holmes, 37 Ohio Misc. 95, 308 N.E.2d 765 (1973). Ch. 22, Table 2.

Cook v. Thomas, 25 Wis. 2d 467, 131 N.W.2d 299 (1964). Ch. 14, n. 16.

Cooper v. Roberts, 220 Pa. Super. 260, 286 A.2d 647 (1971). Ch. 22, n. 4, Table 2.

Copeland v. Kansas State Board of Examiners in Optometry, 518 P.2d 377 (Kan. 1974). Ch. 11, n. 71.

Corn v. French, 71 Nev. 280, 289 P.2d 173 (1955). Ch. 22, Table 3.

Cornfeldt v. Tongen, 262 N.W.2d 684 (Minn. 1977). Ch. 22, Table 2.

County of Campbell v. Howard, 133 Va. 19, 112 S.E. 876 (1922). Ch. 35, n. 16.

Cunningham v. Yankton Clinic, 262 N.W.2d 508 (S.D. 1978). Ch. 22, Table 3.

Curry v. Corn, 52 Misc.2d 1035, 277 N.Y. S.2d 470 (1966). Ch. 20, n. 29.

Custodio v. Bauer, 251 Cal. App. 2d 303, 59 Cal. Rptr. 463 (1967). Ch. 13, n. 8; Ch. 27, n. 41.

Dahl v. Turner, 80 N.M. 564, 458 P.2d 816 (1969). Ch. 14, n. 18.

Dameron v. Harris, 281 Mo. 247, 219 S.W. 954 (1920). Ch. 33, n. 36.

Davis v. Board of Medical Examiners, 108 Cal. App. 2d 346, 239 P.2d 78 (1951). Ch. 11, n. 59.

Davis v. Calderwood, et al., Board of Registration in Medicine, 251 Mass. 283, 146 N.E. 708 (1925). Ch. 11, n. 59.

Dean v. Dyer, 64 Cal. App. 2d 646, 149 P.2d 288 (Cal. 1944). Ch. 29, n. 18.

Deaton v. Delta Democrat Publishing Co., 326 So.2d 471 (Miss. 1976). Ch. 20, n. 37.

De Gaetini v. Driskell, et al., State Board of Medical Examiners, 139 Fla. 49, 190 So. 461 (1939). Ch. 11, n. 59.

Degnan v. Ransom, 31 N.Y.S. 966 (1894). Ch. 33, n. 22.

De Groot v. Winter, 261 Mich. 660, 247 N.W. 69 (1933). Ch. 33, n. 52.

Delaware Optometric Corp. v. Sherwood, 36 Del. Ch. 223, 128 A.2d 812 (1957). Ch. 1, n. 94; Ch. 9, n. 43.

DeMay v. Roberts, 9 N.W. 166 (Mich. 1881). Ch. 20, n. 35.

Demers v. Gerety, 92 N.M. 396, 589 P.2d 180, *reversed* 92 N.M. 749, 595 P.2d 387 (1978). Ch. 22, Table 2.

Derrick v. St. Paul City Railroad Co., 252 Minn. 102, 89 N.W.2d 629 (1959). Ch. 33, n. 49.

Dickson v. Flynn, 273 N.Y. 72, 6 N.E.2d 102 (1937). Ch. 9, n. 23.

DiFebo v. Keve, 395 F. Supp. 1350 (D.C. Del. 1975). Ch. 2, n. 10.

DiFilippo v. Preston, 53 Del. 539, 173 A.2d 333 (1961). Ch. 22, Table 1.

Doane v. Doane, 238 Mass. 106, 130 N.E. 484 (1921). Ch. 33, n. 36.

Doerr v. Movius, 154 Mont. 510, 463 P.2d 477 (1970). Ch. 22, Table 1.

Donnell v. Board of Registration in Medicine, 123 Me. 523, 149 A. 153 (1930). Ch. 11, n. 84.

Dorr v. Headstream, 173 Ark. 1104, 295 S.W. 16 (1927). Ch. 35, n. 7.

Downer v. Villeux, 322 A.2d 82 (Me. 1974). Ch. 22, Table 3.

Dred Scott v. Sandford, 60 U.S. (1 How.) 393 (1857). Ch. 7, n. 12.

DuVall v. Board of Medical Examiners of Arizona, 49 Ariz. 329, 66 P.2d 1026 (1937). Ch. 11, n. 92.

Dvorine v. Castleberg Jewelry Corp., 185 A. 562 (Md. 1936). Ch. 9, n. 23.

Eder v. Beal, 609 F.2d 695 (3d Cir. 1979). Ch. 12, n. 14.

Edmunds v. Board of Examiners in Optometry, 9 Alas. 482 (1939). Ch. 11, n. 70.

Edsall v. Rockland Paper Co., 38 Del. 495, 194 A.

115 (1937). Ch. 33, n. 36.

Eisensmith v. Buhl Optical Co., 178 S.E. 695 (W. Va. 1934). Ch. 9, n 22.

Empey v. United States, 406 F.2d 157 (10th Cir. 1959). Ch. 39, n. 4.

Engel v. Clarke, 346 S.W.2d 13 (Ky. 1961). Ch. 13, n. 27.

Epstein v. Board of Regents of the University of the State of New York, 295 N.Y. 154, 65 N.E.2d 756 (1946). Ch. 11, n. 59.

Evans v. Gore, 253 U.S. 245, 40 S.Ct. 550 (1920). Ch. 40, n. 5.

Evers v. Buxbaum, 102 App. D.C. 334, 253 F.2d 356 (D.C. Cir. 1958). Ch. 2, n. 4, Table 1; Ch. 19, n. 32; Ch. 21, n. 29; Ch. 24, n. 6.

Ex parte Rust, 181 Cal. 73, 183 P. 548 (1919). Ch. 1, n. 64; Ch. 9, n.8.

Ezell v. Ritholz, 188 S.C. 39, 198 S.E. 419 (1938). Ch. 5, n. 11; Ch. 9, n. 22; Ch. 11, n. 69.

Fairchild v. Brian, 354 So. 2d 675 (La. App. 1977). Ch. 2, n. 19, 22, 24, Table 1; Ch. 18, n. 21; Ch. 21, n. 32; Ch. 24, n. 7, 8, 10, 11; Ch. 25, n. 9, 10, 11; Ch. 33, n. 16.

Falcone v. New York State Education Dept., 50 N.Y.2d 854, 407 N.E.2d 1335 (1980). Ch. 11, n. 70, 72, 90.

Favalora v. Aetna Casualty Co., 144 So.2d 544 (La. 1962). Ch. 19, n. 27.

Feeney v. Young, 191 A.D. 501, 181 N.Y.S.481 (1920). Ch. 20, n. 34.

Felis v. Greenberg, 51 Misc.2d 881, 273 N.Y.S.2d 288 (1966). Ch. 20, n. 27.

Ferrara v. Galluchio, 5 N.Y.2d 16, 152 N.E.2d 249 (1958). Ch. 18, n. 33.

Ficklin v. MacFarlane, 550 P.2d 1295 (Utah 1976). Ch. 22, Table 1.

Fields v. District of Columbia, 232 A.2d 300 (D.C. App. 1967), *adhered to* 244 A.2d 643 (D.C. App. 1968), *appeal denied* 131 App. D.C. 346, 404 F.2d 1323 (1967). Ch. 1, n. 94; Ch. 9, n. 45; Ch. 11, n. 107.

Filler v. Rayex Corp., 435 F.2d 336 (7th Cir. 1970). Ch. 2, n. 11, Table 1; Ch. 21, n. 6; Ch. 27, n. 26, 29.

Fink Jewelry Co. v. State, 50 P.2d 945 (Ariz. 1935). Ch. 9, n. 22.

Finlay Straus, Inc. v. University of the State of New York, 270 A.D. 1060, 62 N.Y.S.2d 892 (1946). Ch. 9, n. 31.

Flint v. Stone Tracy Co., 220 U.S. 107, 31 S.Ct. 342 (1911). Ch. 40, n. 4.

Florida Association of Dispensing Opticians v. Florida State Board of Optometry, 238 So.2d 839 (Fla. 1970), *conformed to* 239 So.2d 520 (Fla. App. 1970). Ch. 1, n. 94; Ch. 9, n. 45; Ch. 11, n. 106.

Florida Society of Ophthalmology v. Florida Optometric Association, 489 So.2d 1118 (Fla. 1986), *reversing* 465 So.2d 1319 (Fla. 1985). Ch. 11, n. 1, 112.

Flynn v. Stearns, 145 A.2d 33 (N.J. 1958). Ch. 19, n. 43.

Folger v. Corbett, 394 A.2d 63 (N.H. 1978). Ch. 22, Table 1.

Foreman v. State Board of Health, 157 Ky. 123, 162 S.W. 796 (1914). Ch. 11, n. 52.

Foreman v. United States, 232 F. Supp. 134 (D.C. Fla. 1964). Ch. 39, n.2.

Forthofer v. Arnold, 60 Ohio App. 436, 21 N.E.2d 869 (1938). Ch. 35, n. 7.

Frank v. Board of Regents of the University of the State of New York, 24 A.D.2d 909, 264 N.Y.S.2d 413 (1965). Ch. 11, n. 59.

Freeman v. Lockhart, 503 F.2d 1016 (8th Cir. 1974). Ch. 2, n. 9.

Freeman v. State Board, 54 Okla. 531, 154 P. 56 (1916). Ch. 11, n. 59.

Freese v. Lemon, 210 N.W.2d 576 (Iowa 1973). Ch. 32, n. 11.

Friedman v. Rogers, 438 F. Supp. 428 (D.C. Tex. 1977), *reversed* 440 U.S. 1, 99 S.Ct. 887 (1979). Ch. 1, n. 190, 191, Table 4; Ch. 5, n. 31; Ch. 7, n. 15; Ch. 11, n. 6, 59, 77; Ch. 39, n. 23.

Furnish v. Board of Medical Examiners, 149 Cal. App. 2d 326, 308 P.2d 924 (1957). Ch. 11, n. 92.

Gaines v. Schneider, 323 S.W.2d 401 (Mo. App. 1959). Ch. 33, n. 30.

Galt v. U.S., 175 F. Supp. 360 (D.C. Tex. 1959). Ch. 39, n. 2.

Garland v. Commissioner, 73 T.C. 5 (1979). Ch. 39, n. 21.

Garlock v. Cole, 199 Cal. App.2d 11, 18 Cal. Rptr. 393 (1962). Ch. 20, n. 41.

Gates v. Jensen, 92 Wash.2d 246, 595 P.2d 919 (1979), *reversing* 20 Wash. App. 81, 579 P.2d 374 (1978). Ch. 2, n. 27, 31, Table 1; Ch. 22, n. 17, Table 2; Ch. 23, n. 12.

Gates v. Preston, 41 N.Y. 113 (1869). Ch. 19, n. 61.

Gaut v. Quast, 505 S.W.2d 367 (Tex. Civ. App. 1974). Ch. 22, Table 1.

Gaynes v. Allen, 128 Mich. App. 42, 339 N.W.2d 678 (1983). Ch. 20, n. 9.

Georgia Board of Examiners v. Frieman's Jewelers, 189 S.E.238 (Ga. 1936). Ch. 9, n. 23.

Getchell v. Mansfield, 260 Or. 174, 489 P.2d 953 (1971). Ch. 22, Table 1.

Gibson v. Berryhill, 331 F. Supp. 122 (D.C. Ala. 1971), *affirmed* 441 U.S. 564, 93 S.Ct. 1689 (1973). Ch. 1, n. 180, 181, Table 4; Ch. 5, n. 21; Ch. 7, n. 15; Ch. 11, n. 5, 59.

Gilbert v. Louis Pizitz Dry Goods Co., 237 Ala. 249, 186 So. 179 (1939). Ch. 2, n. 3; Ch. 27, n. 47, 54.

Gleitman v. Cosgrove, 49 N.J. 22, 227 A.2d 689 (1966). Ch. 22, Table 1.

Glenn v. Colorado State Board of Medical Examiners, 131 Colo. 586, 284 P.2d 230 (1955). Ch. 11, n. 86.

Globe Indemnity Co. v. Reinhart, 152 Md. 439, 137 A. 43 (1927). Ch. 33, n. 36.

Golding v. Shubach Optical Co., 70 P.2d 871 (Utah 1937). Ch. 9, n. 23.

Gooden v. Tips, 651 S.W.2d 364 (Tex. Civ. App. 1983). Ch. 32, n. 10.

Govin v. Hunter, 374 P.2d 421 (Wyo. 1962). Ch. 22, Table 1.

Graddy v. New York Medical College, 19 A.D.2d 426, 243 N.Y.S.2d 940 (1963). Ch. 21, n. 36.

Graham v. Richardson, 403 U.S. 365, 91 S.Ct. 1848 (1971). Ch. 11, n. 26.

Graham v. Whitaker, 321 S.E.2d 40 (S.C. 1984). Ch. 18, n. 38; Ch. 28, n. 23; Ch. 29, n. 12.

Gravis v. Physicians and Surgeons Hospital of Alice, 415 S.W.2d 674 (Tex. Civ. App. 1967). Ch. 22, Table 1.

Green v. Hussey, 127 Ill. App. 2d 174, 262 N.E.2d 156 (1970). Ch. 22, Table 1.

Green v. Shaw, 136 S.C. 56, 134 S.E. 226 (1926). Ch. 33, n. 22.

Greenman v. Yuba Power Products, 59 Cal. 2d 57, 27 Cal. Rptr. 697, 377 P.2d 897 (1963). Ch. 21, n. 8, 10.

Griffin v. Medical Society of the State of New York, 11 N.Y.S.2d 109 (1939). Ch. 20, n. 33.

Griswold v. Connecticut, 381 U.S. 479, 85 S.Ct. 1678 (1965). Ch. 20, n. 32.

Grosjean v. Spencer, 258 Iowa 685, 140 N.W.2d 139 (1966). Ch. 22, Table 3.

Gross v. Partlow, 68 P.2d 1034 (Wash. 1937). Ch. 13, n. 5.

Gwynn v. Wilhelm, 360 P.2d 312 (Or. 1961). Ch. 19, n. 62.

Hachat v. Hachat, 71 N.E.2d 927 (Ind. 1947). Ch. 13, n. 14.

Hackler v. Ingram, 196 S.W. 279 (Tex. Civ. App. 1917). Ch. 33, n. 22.

Haffner v. Indiana State Board of Registration in Optometry, 333 N.E.2d 312 (Ind. App. 1975). Ch. 11, n. 72.

Hagler v. Major, 186 S.W.2d 564 (Mo. 1945). Ch. 20, n. 13.

Hague v. Williams, 37 N.J. 328, 181 A.2d 345 (1962). Ch. 20, n. 25, 27.

Hake v. Arkansas State Medical Board, 237 Ark. 506, 374 S.W.2d 173 (1964). Ch. 11, n. 59.

Hales v. Pittman, 118 Ariz. 305, 576 P.2d 493 (1978). Ch. 22, Table 1.

Hammer v. Polsky, 233 N.Y.S.2d 110, 36 Misc. 2d 482 (1962). Ch. 20, n. 31.

Hammond v. Aetna Casualty Co., 237 F. Supp. 96 (D.C. Ohio 1956). Ch. 20, n. 28.

Hampton v. Brackin's Jewelry and Optical Co., Inc., 237 Ala. 212, 186 So. 173 (1939). Ch. 1, n. 106; Ch. 2, n. 2, 23, Table 1; Ch. 5, n. 51; Ch. 19, n. 4.

Hanks v. Drs. Ranson, Swan and Burch, Ltd., 359 So. 2d 1089, *writ denied* 360 So. 2d. 1178 (La. 1978). Ch. 22, Table 2.

Hanley v. Spencer, 115 P.2d 399 (Colo. 1941). Ch. 19, n. 42; Ch. 26, n. 13.

Harris v. Bales, 459 S.W.2d 742 (Mo. App. 1970). Ch. 18, n. 21.

Harris v. Groth, 99 Wash.2d 438, 663 P.2d 113 (1983). Ch. 2, n. 27.

Harris v. State Board of Optometrical Examiners, 287 Pa. 531, 135 A. 237 (1926). Ch. 1, n. 85, Table 2; Ch. 9, n. 10.

Hartford Accident and Indemnity Co. v. Barfield, 89 Ga. App. 562, 80 S.E.2d 84 (1954). Ch. 26, n. 29.

Hartman v. Commonwealth, 454 A.2d 1150 (Pa. 1983). Ch. 11, n. 63.

Harwick v. Harris, 166 So. 2d 912 (Fla. 1964). Ch. 13, n. 19.

Haskins v. Howard, 16 S.W.2d 20 (Tenn. 1929). Ch. 20, n. 41.

Hawker v. People of New York, 170 U.S. 189, 18 S. Ct. 573 (1893). Ch. 11, n. 49.

Hawkins v. McGee, 84 N.H. 114, 146 A. 641 (1929). Ch. 27 n. 43.

Hawkins v. Richardson, 29 Ill. App. 3d 597, 331 N.E.2d 201 (1975). Ch. 18, n. 31.

Head v. New Mexico Board of Examiners in Optometry, 70 N.M. 90, 370 P.2d 811, *affirmed* 374 U.S. 424, 83 S. Ct. 1759 (1963). Ch. 1, n. 139, Table 3; Ch. 5, n. 18.

Head v. Russell, 307 S.W.2d 557 (Ky. 1958). Ch. 33, n. 51.

Helling v. Carey, 83 Wash.2d 514, 519 P.2d 981 (1974). Ch. 2, n. 27, Table 1; Ch. 21, n. 34; Ch. 23, n. 6, 7, 20; Ch. 30, n. 20.

Henderson v. Mason, 386 S.W.2d 879 (Tex. Civ. App. 1964). Ch. 26, n. 17.

Henningsen v. Bloomfield Motors, Inc., 32 N.J. 358, 161 A.2d 69 (1960). Ch. 21, n. 5.

Hess v. Lowery, 122 Ind. 225, 23 N.E. 156 (1890).

Ketring v. Sturges, 372 S.W.2d 104 (Mo. 1963). Ch. 1, n. 94; Ch. 11, n. 106.
Kiddie v. Commissioner, 69 T.C. 1055 (1978). Ch. 39, n. 21.
Kime v. Aetna, 66 Ohio App. 277, 33 N.E.2d 1008 (1940). Ch. 2, n. 21; Ch. 26, n. 30, 31, 32.
Kirkpatrick v. Wells, 319 Mo. 1040, 6 S.W.2d 591 (1928). Ch. 33, n. 36.
Klema v. St. Elizabeth's Hospital of Youngstown, 170 Ohio St. 519, 166 N.E.2d 765 (1960). Ch. 19, n. 55.
Kopp v. C.C. Caldwell Optical Co., 547 S.W.2d 872 (Mo. App. 1977). Ch. 2, n. 11; Ch. 27, n. 27.
Kosak v. Boyce, 201 N.W. 757 (Wis. 1925). Ch. 26, n. 9, 10.
Kramer v. John Hancock Mutual Life Insurance Co., 336 Mass. 465, 146 N.E.2d 357 (1957). Ch. 33, n. 28.
Kraus v. Spielberg, 37 Misc. 2d 519, 236 N.Y.S.2d 143 (1962). Ch. 18, n. 33.
Kresge v. Ottinger, 29 F.2d 762 (2d Cir. 1928). Ch. 1, n. 86.
Kurzner v. United States, 413 F.2d 97 (5th Cir. 1969). Ch. 39, n. 4.

Lambert v. Park, 597 F.2d 236 (10th Cir. 1979). Ch. 22, Table 2.
Landon v. Kansas City Gas Co., 10 F.2d 263 (8th Cir. 1926). Ch. 13, n. 4.
Lane v. Calvert, 138 A.2d 902 (Md. 1958). Ch. 27, n. 42.
Lawrence v. Biry et al, Board of Registration in Medicine, 238 Mass. 424, 132 N.E. 174 (1921). Ch. 11, n. 47.
Lawson v. Conaway, 16 S.E. 564 (W. Va. 1892). Ch. 19, n. 61.
Le Bow v. Optometry Examining Board, 52 Wis. 2d 569, 191 N.W.2d 47 (1971). Ch. 11, n. 94.
Lee v. Dewbre, 362 S.W.2d 900 (Tex. Civ. App. 1962). Ch. 13, n. 30.
Lee v. State, 490 P.2d 1206 (Alas. 1971). Ch. 14, n. 18.
Leyra v. Denno, 113 F. Supp. 556 (D.C. N.Y. 1950), *affirmed* 208 F.2d 605 (2d Cir. 1954), *reversed* 347 U.S. 556, 74 S.Ct. 716 (1954). Ch. 20, n. 16.
Lieberman v. State Board of Optometry, 34 A.2d 213 (Conn. 1943). Ch. 5, n. 10.
Lilly et ux v. Commissioner of Internal Revenue, 343 U.S. 90, 72 S.Ct. 497 (1951). Ch. 3, n. 32.
Lippold v. Kidd, 269 P. 210 (Or. 1928). Ch. 26, n. 16.
Lloyd v. Kull, 329 F.2d 168 (7th Cir. 1964). Ch. 22, Table 1.
Longmire v. Hoey, 512 S.W.2d 307 (Tenn. 1974). Ch. 22, Table 1.
Louisiana State Board of Optometry Examiners v. Pearle Optical, Inc., 177 So.2d 164, *annulled* 184 So.2d 10 (La. 1965). Ch. 1, n. 94.
Luka v. Lowrie, 136 N.W. 1106 (Mich. 1912). Ch. 13, n. 15.
Lundberg v. Bay View Hospital, 175 Ohio St. 133, 191 N.E.2d 821 (1963). Ch. 13, n. 6.
Lundgren v. Eustermann, 356 N.W.2d 762 (Minn. App. 1984). Ch. 35, n. 7.

Macomber v. State Board of Health, 28 R.I. 3, 65 A. 263 (1906). Ch. 11, n. 59.
Mallett v. Pirkey, 171 Colo. 271, 466 P.2d 466 (1970). Ch. 22, Table 1.
Marbury v. Madison, 5 U.S. (1 Cranch) 137 (1803). Ch. 7, n. 11.
Marchlewicz v. Stanton, 50 Mich. App. 344, 213 N.W.2d 317 (1973). Ch. 22, n. 1.
Marsh v. Arnold, 446 S.W.2d 949 (Tex. Civ. App. 1969). Ch. 22, Table 1.
Martin v. Baldy, 249 Pa. 253, 94 A. 1091 (1915). Ch. 1, n. 4, 41, 42, Table 1; Ch. 9, n. 41; Ch. 10, n. 7.
Matter of Pace, 156 N.Y.S.641, 154 Misc. 609 (1915). Ch. 9, n. 25.
Matter of Weiss, 208 Misc. 1010, 147 N.Y.S.2d 455 (1955). Ch. 16, n. 16.
Matthews v. Murphy, 23 Ky. 750, 63 S.W. 785 (1901). Ch. 11, n. 53.
Mazetti v. Armour and Co., 75 Wash. 672, 135 P. 633 (1913). Ch. 21, n. 3.
McCrory v. Wood, et al., State Board of Medicine, 171 So.2d 241 (Ala. 1965). Ch. 11, n. 72.
McGarry v. J.A. Mercier Co., 272 Mich. 501, 262 N.W. 296 (1935). Ch. 16, n. 7.
McGray v. Cobb, 152 N.W. 262 (Minn. 1915). Ch. 21, n. 33.
McKay v. State Board of Medical Examiners, 103 Colo. 305, 86 P.2d 232 (1938). Ch. 11, n. 59.
McMahon v. Glixman, 393 N.E.2d 875 (Mass. 1979). Ch. 2, n. 7, 23; Ch. 23, n. 33.
McMurdo v. Getter, 10 N.E.2d 139 (Mass. 1937). Ch. 9, n. 22.
McNaughton v. Johnson, 242 U.S. 344, 37 S.Ct. 178 (1917). Ch. 1, n. 61, 62, Table 1; Ch. 9, n. 6; Ch. 10, n. 8.
Medical Examining Board v. Stewart, 46 Wash. 79, 89 P. 475 (1907). Ch. 11, n. 59.
Meeks v. Marx, 15 Wash. App. 571, 550 P.2d 1158 (1976). Ch. 1, n. 179; Ch. 2, n. 27.
Meffert v. State Board of Medical Registration and Education, 66 Kan. 710, 72 P. 247 (1903), *affirmed* 195 U.S. 625, 25 S.Ct. 790 (1903). Ch.

133 S.E.2d 374 (1963). Ch. 9, n. 38; Ch. 12, n. 32.

Peddicord v. Lieser, 105 P.2d 5 (Wash. 1940). Ch. 18, n. 39.

Pegram v. Sisco, 406 F. Supp. 776, *affirmed* 547 F.2d 1172 (8th Cir. 1976). Ch. 22, Table 1.

Pennison v. Provident Life Insurance Co., 154 So. 2d 617 (La. 1963). Ch. 20, n. 29.

Pennsylvania Optometric Association v. DiGiovanni, 45 Pa. D&C 2d 245 (1968). Ch. 1, n. 94; Ch. 9, n. 43; Ch. 11, n. 106.

People v. Brown, 49 Cal. 2d 577, 320 P.2d 5 (1958). Ch. 33, n. 30.

People v. Fowler, 84 P.2d 326, 32 Cal. App. 2d Supp. 737 (1938). Ch. 26, n. 29.

People v. Griffith, 280 Ill. 18, 117 N.E. 195 (1917). Ch. 1, n. 66; Ch. 9, n. 17; Ch. 11, n. 105.

People v. Singh, 136 Cal. App. 233, 28 P.2d 416 (1934). Ch. 33, n. 47.

People v. Witte, 315 Ill. 282, 146 N.E. 178 (1924). Ch. 9, n. 14.

People of the State of Michigan v. Baker, 94 Mich. App. 365, 288 N.E.2d 430 (1980). Ch. 16, n. 37.

People Use of the State Board of Health v. Smith, 208 Ill. 31, 69 N.E. 810 (1904), *affirming* 108 Ill. App. 499 (1903). Ch. 1, n. 30, 31, 32, Table 1.

Percle v. St. Paul Fire and Marine Insurance Co., 349 So. 2d 1289 (La. 1977). Ch. 22, Table 2.

Peterson v. Richfield Plaza, Inc., 252 Minn. 215, 89 N.W.2d 712 (1958). Ch. 33, n. 30.

Phillips v. Delta Motor Lines, Inc., 235 Miss. 1, 108 So. 2d 409 (1959). Ch. 14, n. 16.

Physicians' Education Network v. Department of Health, Education, and Welfare, 653 F.2d 621 (D.C. Cir. 1981). Ch. 1, n. 160; Ch. 12, n. 10.

Pike v. Honsinger, 49 N.E. 760 (N.Y. 1898). Ch. 18, n. 18.

Podvin v. Eickhorst, 373 Mich. 175, 128 N.W.2d 523 (1964). Ch. 13, n. 17.

Porter v. Michigan State Board of Examiners in Optometry, 41 Mich. App. 150, 199 N.W.2d 666 (1972). Ch. 11, n. 100.

Porter v. Powell, 79 Iowa 151, 44 N.W. 295 (1890). Ch. 13, n. 14.

Poulin v. Zartman, 542 P.2d 251 (Alas. 1975). Ch. 22, Table 2.

Price v. State, 168 Wis. 603, 171 N.W. 77 (1919). Ch. 9, n. 13; Ch. 11, n. 105.

Pushkin v. Califano, 600 F.2d 486 (5th Cir. 1979). Ch. 1, n. 197; Ch. 8, n. 46; Ch. 12, n. 8.

Pushkin v. Lombard, 279 So. 2d 79 (Fla. App. 1973). Ch. 11, n. 72.

Radtke v. Taylor, 105 Or. 559, 210 P. 863 (1922). Ch. 33, n. 36.

Ramsey v. Shelton, 329 Ill. 432, 160 N.E. 769 (1928). Ch. 11, n. 59.

Ranier v. Grossman, 31 Cal. App. 3d 539, 107 Cal. Rptr. 469 (1973). Ch. 13, n. 11.

Rayburn v. Minnesota State Board of Optometry, 247 Minn. 520, 78 N.W.2d 351 (1956). Ch. 5, n. 38; Ch. 11, n. 73.

Reed v. Church, 8 S.E.2d 285 (Va. 1940). Ch. 19, n. 26; Ch. 28, n. 4, 9.

Reid v. New Mexico Board of Examiners in Optometry, 92 N.M. 414, 589 P.2d 198 (1979). Ch. 11, n. 87.

Reidinger v. Optometry Examining Board, 81 Wis.2d 292, 260 N.W.2d 270 (1977). Ch. 11, n. 84.

Reynier v. Delta Women's Clinic, Inc., 359 So. 2d 733 (La. 1978). Ch. 22, Table 2.

Rhode Island Ophthalmological Society v. Cannon, 317 A.2d 124 (R.I. 1974). Ch. 1, n. 170, Table 4; Ch. 3, n. 47; Ch. 9, n. 50; Ch. 10, n. 29, 30.

Rice v. Evatt, 144 Ohio St. 483, 59 N.E.2d 927 (1945). Ch. 12, n. 30.

Rice v. Rinaldo, 119 N.E.2d 657 (Ohio 1951). Ch. 14, n. 14.

Ricks v. Budge, 64 P.2d 208 (Utah 1937). Ch. 13, n. 34.

Riedinger v. Colburn, 361 F. Supp. 1073 (D.C. Idaho 1973). Ch. 22, Table 1.

Ritholz v. Arkansas State Board of Optometry, 177 S.W.2d 410 (Ark. 1944). Ch. 5, n. 11; Ch. 11, n. 69.

Ritholz v. Commonwealth, 184 Va. 339, 35 S.E.2d 210 (1945). Ch. 9, n. 29; Ch. 11, n. 69.

Ritholz v. Indiana State Board of Registration and Examination, 45 F. Supp 423 (D.C. Ind. 1937). Ch. 9, n. 28; Ch. 11, n. 69.

Ritholz v. Johnson, 246 Wis. 442, 17 N.W.2d 590 (1945). Ch. 9, n. 30; Ch. 11, n. 69.

Roberts v. Woods, 206 F. Supp. 579 (D.C. Ala. 1962). Ch. 22, Table 1.

Roberts v. Young, 369 Mich. 113, 119 N.W.2d 627 (1963). Ch. 22, Table 1.

Robertus v. State, 119 Tex. Crim. Rep. 370, 45 S.W.2d 595 (Tex. Crim. App. 1931). Ch. 9, n. 9, 14.

Robins v. Finestone, 308 N.Y. 543, 127 N.E. 2d 330 (1955). Ch. 27, n. 43.

Roe v. Wade, 410 U.S. 113, 93 S.Ct. 705 (1973). Ch. 7, n. 4; Ch. 32, n. 21.

Rogers v. Canfield, 262 N.W. 409 (Mich. 1935). Ch. 21, n. 37.

Rogers v. Medical Association of Georgia, 244 Ga. 151, 259 S.E.2d 85 (1979). Ch. 11, n. 7.

Rogers v. Robson, Masters, Ryan, Brumund and

Belom, 392 N.E.2d 1365 (Ill. App. 1979). Ch. 54, n. 6.

Roschen v. Ottinger, 29 F.2d 762 (2d Cir. 1928). Ch. 1, n. 86.

Roschen v. Ward, 279 U.S. 337, 49 S.Ct. 336 (1929). Ch. 1, n. 87, Table 2; Ch. 9, n. 18.

Ross v. Hodges, 234 So. 2d 905 (Miss. 1970). Ch. 22, Table 1.

Rotan v. Greenbaum, 273 F.2d 830 (D.C. Cir. 1959). Ch. 28, n. 5.

Roubik and Roubik v. Commissioner, 53 T.C. 365 (1969). Ch. 39, n. 6.

Rowe v. Standard Drug Co., 9 N.E.2d 609 (Ohio 1937). Ch. 9, n. 22.

Ruby v. Massey, 452 F. Supp. 361 (D.C. Conn. 1978). Ch. 22, Table 3.

Rusin v. Glendale Optical Co., Inc., 805 F.2d 650 (6th Cir. 1986). Ch. 27, n. 9.

Russell v. Harwick, 166 So. 2d 904 (Fla. 1964). Ch. 22, Table 1.

Ruth v. Dight, 453 P.2d 631 (Wash. 1969). Ch. 19, n. 56.

Sage-Allen Co. v. Wheeler, 119 Conn. 667, 179 A. 195 (1935). Ch. 5, n. 10; Ch. 9, n. 12, 23.

Salgo v. Stanford University Board of Trustees, 154 Cal. App. 2d 560, 317 P.2d 170 (1957). Ch. 22, Table 2; Ch. 31, n. 16.

Sandefur v. Cherry, 547 F. Supp. 418 (D.C. La. 1982), *vacated and remanded* 718 F.2d 682 (5th Cir. 1983), *certified* 721 F.2d 511 (5th Cir. 1983), *reversed* 744 F.2d 1157 (5th Cir. 1984). Ch. 1, n. 197; Ch. 8, n. 57; Ch. 12, n. 12, 24.

Sanitary District of Chicago v. Industrial Commissioner, 343 Ill. 236, 175 N.E. 372 (1931). Ch. 33, n. 53.

Saunders v. Swann, 155 Tenn. 310, 292 S.W. 458 (1927). Ch. 9, n. 10.

Scaria v. St. Paul Fire and Marine Insurance Co., 68 Wis. 2d 1, 227 N.W.2d 647 (1975). Ch. 22, Table 2.

Scarzella v. Saxon, 436 A.2d 358 (D.C. App. 1984). Ch. 27, n. 43.

Schessler v. Keck, 125 Cal. App. 2d 827, 271 P.2d 588 (1954). Ch. 20, n. 11.

Schireson v. State Board of Medical Examiners of New Jersey, 129 N.J.L. 203, 28 A.2d 879 (1942), *reversed* 130 N.J.L. 570, 33 A.2d 911 (1943). Ch. 11, n. 55, 84.

Schireson v. Walsh, 354 Ill. 40, 187 N.E. 921 (1933). Ch. 11, n. 53.

Schloendorff v. Society of New York Hospital, 211 N.Y. 125, 195 N.E. 92 (1914). Ch. 18, n. 12; Ch. 23, n. 10.

Schroeder v. Lawrence, 359 N.E.2d 1301 (Mass. 1977). Ch. 22, Table 1.

Schulz v. Commissioner, 294 F.2d 52 (9th Cir. 1961). Ch. 48, n. 7.

Schyman v. Department of Registration and Education, 9 Ill. App. 2d 504, 133 N.E.2d 551 (1956), *cert. denied* 352 U.S. 1001, 77 S.Ct. 557 (1956). Ch. 11, n. 59.

Seanor v. Browne, 154 Okla. 222, 7 P.2d 627 (1932). Ch. 27, n. 43.

Seele v. Purcell, 45 N.M. 176, 113 P.2d 320 (1941). Ch. 14, n. 16.

Seitz v. Ohio State Medical Board, 24 Ohio App. 154, 157 N.E. 304 (1926). Ch. 11, n. 84.

Semler v. Oregon State Board of Dental Examiners, 294 U.S. 608, 55 S.Ct. 570 (1935). Ch. 1, n. 100, Table 2; Ch. 4, Table 3; Ch. 5, n. 16; Ch. 9, n. 34.

Serian v. State of West Virginia, 297 S.E.2d 889 (W. Va. 1982). Ch. 11, n. 70, 89.

Shapiro v. Board of Regents of the University of the State of New York, 16 N.Y.2d 783, 262 N.Y.S.2d 503 (1965). Ch. 11, n. 59.

Shetter v. Rochelle, 2 Ariz. App. 358, 409 P.2d 74, *modified* 2 Ariz. 607, 411 P.2d 45 (1965). Ch. 22, Table 1.

Shoemaker v. Friedberg, 183 P.2d 318 (Cal. 1947). Ch. 20, n. 30.

Shulman v. Lerner, 2 Mich. App. 705, 141 N.W.2d 348 (1966). Ch. 22, Table 1.

Siefert v. Buhl Optical Co., 276 Mich. 692, 268 N.W. 784 (1936). Ch. 9, n. 29.

Silver v. Lansburgh and Brothers, 111 F.2d 518 (D.C. App. 1940). Ch. 1, n. 83; Ch. 9, n. 23.

Simonsen v. Swenson, 104 Neb. 224, 177 N.W. 831 (1920). Ch. 20, n. 30.

Simpson v. Wilson, 480 F. Supp. 97 (D.C. Vt. 1979). Ch. 12, n. 13.

Sims v. Callahan, 112 So. 2d 776 (Ala. 1959). Ch. 18, n. 21; Ch. 19, n. 28; Ch. 23, n. 32.

Sinclair v. Brunson, 212 Mich. 387, 180 N.W. 358 (1920). Ch. 13, n. 31.

Small v. Gifford Memorial Hospital, 133 Vt. 552, 349 A.2d 703 (1975). Ch. 22, Table 2.

Smart v. Kansas City, 208 Mo. 162, 105 S.W. 709 (1907). Ch. 13, n. 5.

Smith v. Department of Registration and Education of the State of Illinois, 412 Ill. 322, 106 N.E2d 722 (1952). Ch. 11, n. 59.

Smith v. Mallinckrodt Chemical Works, 212 Mo. App. 158, 251 S.W. 155 (1923). Ch. 18, n. 26.

Smith v. McComb Infirmary Association, 196 So. 2d 91 (Miss. 1967). Ch. 19, n. 55.

Smith v. People, 92 Ill. App. 22, *reversed* 199 Ill. 20, 63 N.E. 972 (1900). Ch. 1, n. 30.

Smith v. Thornhill, 25 S.W.2d 597 (Tex. 1930). Ch. 13, n. 2.
Smith v. Wharton, 154 S.E. 12 (N.C. 1930). Ch. 28, n. 46.
Speer v. State, 109 S.W.2d 1150 (Tex. Civ. App. 1937). Ch. 11, n. 92.
Stacy v. Williams, 253 Ky. 353, 69 S.W.2d 697 (1934). Ch. 13, n. 18.
Staloch v. Holm, 111 N.W. 264 (Minn. 1907). Ch. 27, n. 42.
Stammer v. Board of Regents of the University of the State of New York, 287 N.Y. 359, 39 N.E.2d 913 (1942). Ch. 11, n. 59.
State v. Broden, 181 Minn. 341, 232 N.W. 517 (1930). Ch. 9, n. 15.
State v. Etzenhouser, 223 Mo. App. 577, 16 S.W.2d 656 (1929). Ch. 11, n. 105.
State v. First Bank of Nickerson, 114 Neb. 423, 207 N.W. 674 (1926). Ch. 35, n. 16.
State v. Gus Blass Co., 105 S.W.2d 853 (Ark. 1937). Ch. 9, n. 23.
State v. Hanson, 201 Iowa 579, 207 N.W. 769 (1926). Ch. 11, n. 55, 59.
State v. Kindy Optical Co., 216 Iowa 1157, 248 N.W. 332 (1933). Ch. 1, Table 2; Ch. 5, n. 9; Ch. 9, n. 11, 22.
State v. Schaeffer, 129 Wis. 459, 109 N.W. 522 (1906). Ch. 11, n. 59.
State v. Shaw, 289 S.E.2d 325 (N.C. 1982). Ch. 16, n. 37.
State v. Viola, 82 N.E.2d 306 (1947), *appeal dismissed* 148 Ohio St. 712, 76 N.E.2d 715, *cert. denied* 334 U.S. 816, 68 S.Ct. 1070 (1948). Ch. 16, n. 37.
State Board of Medical Examiners v. Gandry, 149 S.E.2d 644 (S.C. 1966). Ch. 11, n. 59.
State Board of Medical Examiners v. Macy, 92 Wash. 614, 159 P. 801 (1916). Ch. 11, n. 52.
State Board of Optometry v. Chester, 251 Miss. 250, 169 So. 2d 468 (1964). Ch. 1, n. 94; Ch. 9, n. 45.
State by Erwin v. Goodman, 288 N.W. 157 (Minn. 1939). Ch. 9, n. 23.
State of Arizona ex rel. Board of Optometry v. Sears, Roebuck, and Co., 102 Ariz. 175, 427 P.2d 126 (1967). Ch. 11, n. 80.
State of Florida ex rel. Landis v. Simmons, 104 Fla. 487, 140 So. 187 (1932). Ch. 11, n. 59.
State of Florida ex rel. Weathers v. Davis, 143 Fla. 250, 196 So. 487 (1940). Ch. 11, n. 55.
State of Iowa ex rel. Bierring v. Ritholz, 283 N.W. 268 (Iowa 1939). Ch. 5, n. 11; Ch. 11, n. 69, 81.
State of Kansas ex rel. Beck v. Gleason, 148 Kan. 1, 79 P.2d 911 (1938). Ch. 26, n. 29.
State of Kansas ex rel. Beck v. Goldman Jewelry Co., 142 Kan. 881, 51 P.2d 995 (1935). Ch. 1, n. 83; Ch. 5, n. 8; Ch. 9, n. 21, 22; Ch. 11, n. 79.
State of Kansas ex rel. Londerholm v. Doolin, 209 Kan. 244, 497 P.2d 138 (1972). Ch. 1, n. 94; Ch. 9, n. 45.
State of Missouri ex rel. Danforth v. Dale Curteman, Inc., 480 S.W. 2d 848 (Mo. 1972). Ch. 1, n. 94; Ch. 9, n. 45; Ch. 11, n. 107.
State of Missouri ex rel. Farber v. Shot, 304 Mo. 523, 263 S.W. 804 (1924). Ch. 11, n. 59.
State of Missouri ex rel. Hurwitz v. North, et al., Board of Health of the State of Missouri, 271 U.S. 40, 46 S.Ct. 384 (1925). Ch. 11, n. 54.
State of Missouri ex rel. Johnson v. Clark, et al, State Board of Health, 288 Mo. 659, 232 S.W. 1031 (1921). Ch. 11, n. 59.
State of Missouri ex rel. McKittrick v. Gate City Optical Co., 97 S.W.2d 89 (Mo. 1936). Ch. 9, n. 23.
State of Missouri ex rel. Kerr, et al., State Board of Health v. Landwehr, 32 S.W.2d 83 (Mo. 1930). Ch. 11, n. 57.
State of Montana ex rel. Yuhas v. Board of Medical Examiners, 135 Mont. 381, 339 P.2d 981 (1959). Ch. 11, n. 59.
State of Ohio ex rel. Bricker v. Buhl Optical Co., 2 N.E.2d 601 (Ohio 1936). Ch. 9, n. 22.
State of Oklahoma ex rel. Clifton v. Reeser, 543 P.2d 1379 (Okla. 1975). Ch. 1, n. 94; Ch. 9, n. 45; Ch. 11, n. 106.
State of Oregon ex rel. Reed v. Kuzirian, 228 Or. 619, 365 P.2d 1046 (1961). Ch. 1, n. 94, 145; Ch. 9, n. 43; Ch. 11, n. 106.
State of Oregon ex rel. Sisemore v. Standard Optical Co., 188 P.2d 309 (Or. 1947). Ch. 33, n. 48.
State of Wisconsin ex rel. Harris v. Kindy Optical Co., 282 N.W. 283 (Wis. 1940). Ch. 9, n. 23.
State Medical Board v. Rogers, 109 Ark. 266, 79 S.W.2d 83 (1935). Ch. 11, n. 92.
State Medical Board of Arkansas Medical Society v. McCrary, 95 Ark. 511, 130 S.W. 544 (1910). Ch. 11, n. 51.
State Tax Commissioner v. Hopkins, 234 Ala. 556, 176 So. 210 (1937). Ch. 7, n. 25; Ch. 12, n. 28.
Steele v. St. Paul Fire and Marine Insurance Co., 371 So. 2d 843 (La. 1979). Ch. 22, Table 2.
Steele v. United States, 463 F. Supp. 321 (D.C. Alas. 1978). Ch. 2, n. 20; Ch. 24, n. 2; Ch. 31, n. 23.
Steele v. Woods, 327 S.W.2d 187 (Mo. 1959). Ch. 19, n. 43.
Stern v. Flynn, 154 Misc. 609, 278 N.Y.S. 598 (1935). Ch. 9, n. 22.
Stevens v. Hill, 74 Vt. 164, 52 A. 437 (1902). Ch. 11, n. 59.

Stohlman v. Davis, 220 N.W. 247 (Neb. 1928). Ch. 13, n. 5, 29; Ch. 21, n. 41.

Strode v. Board of Medical Examiners of California, 195 Cal. App. 2d 291, 15 Cal. Rptr. 879 (1961). Ch. 11, n. 86.

Stuhr v. Barkwill, 332 P.2d 603 (Or. 1958). Ch. 26, n. 15.

Stundon v. Stadnik, 469 P.2d 16 (Wyo. 1970). Ch. 22, Table 1.

Sugarman v. Douglas, 413 U.S. 634, 93 S.Ct. 2842 (1973). Ch. 11, n. 25.

Sullivan v. O'Connor, 363 Mass. 579, 296 N.E.2d 183 (1973). Ch. 27, n. 43.

Sunseri v. Board of Medical Examiners, 36 Cal. 553, 224 Cal. App. 2d 309 (1964). Ch. 11, n. 59.

Tadlock v. Lloyd, 65 Colo. 40, 173 P. 200 (1918). Ch. 13, n. 33.

Tapley v. Abbott, et al., State Board of Medical Examiners, 111 Cal. App. 397, 295 P. 911 (1931). Ch. 11, n. 59.

Teig v. St. John's Hospital, 387 P.2d 527 (Wash. 1963). Ch. 27, n. 42.

Tempchin v. Sampson, 262 Md. 156, 277 A.2d 67 (1971). Ch. 2, n. 5; Ch. 16, n. 41; Ch. 19, n. 29.

Terminal-Hudson Electronics, Inc. v. Department of Consumer Affairs, 407 F. Supp. 1075, *vacated and remanded* 426 U.S. 916, 96 S.Ct. 2619 (1976). Ch. 11, n. 82.

Teseshi v. Mathis, 183 A. 146 (N.J. 1936). Ch. 9, n. 22.

Texas State Board of Examiners in Optometry v. Lane, 306 S.W.2d 212 (Tex. Civ. App. 1957). Ch. 5, n. 37; Ch. 11, n. 74.

Texas State Board of Medical Examiners v. McClellan, 307 S.W.2d 317 (Tex. Civ. App. 1957). Ch. 11, n. 86.

Thaggard v. Vafes, 119 So. 647 (Ala. 1928). Ch. 28, n. 8.

Thomas v. Corso, 265 Md. 84, 288 A.2d 379 (1972). Ch. 13, n. 31.

Thornburg v. Long, 101 S.E. 99 (N.C. 1919). Ch. 20, n. 10.

Thrasher v. Board of Medical Examiners of the State of California, 44 Cal. App. 26, 185 P. 1006 (1919). Ch. 11, n. 59.

Toal v. United States, 438 F.2d 222 (2d Cir. 1971). Ch. 19, n. 58.

Tobinsky v. Board of Medical Examiners of the State of California, 49 Cal. App. 2d 591, 121 P.2d 861 (1942). Ch. 11, n. 59.

Tompkins v. Board of Regents of the University of the State of New York, 299 N.Y. 469, 87 N.E.2d 517 (1949). Ch. 11, n. 86.

Triestram v. Way, 286 Mich. 13, 281 N.W. 420 (1938). Ch. 14, n. 16.

Trogun v. Fruchtman, 58 Wis.2d 596, 207 N.W.2d 297 (1973). Ch. 22, Table 2; Ch. 28, n. 7.

Truxillo v. Gentilly Medical Building, Inc., 255 So. 2d 488 (La. 1969). Ch. 29, n. 11.

Tucker v. Tucker, 222 Ala. 595, 133 So. 714 (1931). Ch. 33, n. 36.

United States v. Kintner, 216 F.2d 418 (9th Cir. 1954). Ch. 39, n. 1.

Van Bronckhorst v. Taube, 341 N.E.2d 791 (Ind. App. 1976). Ch. 20, n. 42.

Vaughn v. Shelton, 514 S.W.2d 870 (Tenn. App. 1974). Ch. 27, n. 49.

Vigil v. Rice, 74 N.M. 693, 397 P.2d 719 (1964). Ch. 20, n. 19.

Virginia State Board of Pharmacy v. Virginia Citizens Consumer Council, 425 U.S. 748, 96 S.Ct. 1817 (1976). Ch. 1, n. 182; Ch. 5, n. 22.

Von Kesler v. Baker, 131 Cal. App. 654, 21 P.2d 1017 (1933). Ch. 35, n. 16.

Wagner v. Olmedo, 365 A.2d 643 (Del. 1976). Ch. 22, Table 1.

Walker v. North Dakota Eye Clinic, Ltd., 415 F. Supp. 891 (D.C. N.D. 1976). Ch. 22, Table 1.

Walker v. Pierce, 560 F.2d 609 (4th Cir. 1977). Ch. 22, Table 3.

Walker v. Rynd, 280 P.2d 259 (Wash. 1955). Ch. 29, n. 17.

Walker v. State Board of Optometry, 322 So. 2d 612 (Fla. 1975). Ch. 11, n. 72.

Wall v. American Optometric Association, 379 F. Supp. 175 (D.C. Ga. 1974), *affirmed* 419 U.S. 888, 95 S.Ct. 166 (1974). Ch. 11, n. 59.

Wall v. Youmans, 223 Ga. 191, 154 S.E.2d 191 (Ga. 1967). Ch. 11, n. 68.

Wallace v. Hall, 145 Ga. App. 610, 244 S.E.2d 129 (1978). Ch. 14, n. 18.

Wallace v. Yudelson, 224 Ill. App. 320 (1927). Ch. 13, n. 19.

Walstrom Optical Co. v. Miller, 59 S.W.2d 895 (Tex. Civ. App. 1933). Ch. 21, n. 11; Ch. 27, n. 13.

Welke v. Kuzilla, 144 Mich. App. 245, 375 N.W.2d 403 (1985). Ch. 2, n. 32; Ch. 32, n. 7.

Werted v. Board of Regents of the University of the State of New York, 18 A.D.2d 1032, 238 N.Y.S.2d 356 (1963). Ch. 11, n. 59.

Wharton Transport Co., Inc. v. Bridges, 606 S.W.2d 521 (Tenn. 1980). Ch. 32, n. 13.

White v. Andrews, 70 Colo. 50, 197 P. 564 (1921).

Table of Reported Cases
By Jurisdiction

Alabama

Alabama Board of Optometry v. Eagerton, 393 So. 2d 1373 (1981). Ch. 7, n. 26; Ch. 9, n. 37; Ch. 12, n. 31.

Alabama Great Southern Railway Co. v. Hunt, 204 Ala. 504, 86 So. 100 (1920). Ch. 14, n. 16.

Gilbert v. Louis Pizitz Dry Goods Co., 237 Ala. 249, 186 So. 179 (1939). Ch. 2, n. 3; Ch. 27, n. 47, 54.

Hampton v. Brackin's Jewelry and Optical Co., Inc., 237 Ala. 212, 186 So. 173 (1939). Ch. 1, n. 106; Ch. 2, n. 2, 23, Table 1; Ch. 5, n. 51; Ch. 19, n. 4.

Horne v. Patton, 291 Ala. 701, 287 So. 2d 824 (1973). Ch. 20, n. 38.

McCrory v. Wood, et al., State Board of Optometry, 171 So. 2d 241 (1965). Ch. 11, n. 72.

Sims v. Callahan, 112 So. 2d 776 (1959). Ch. 18, n. 21; Ch. 19, n. 28; Ch. 23, n. 32.

State Tax Commissioner v. Hopkins, 234 Ala. 556, 176 So. 210 (1937). Ch. 7, n. 25; Ch. 12, n. 28.

Tucker v. Tucker, 222 Ala. 595, 133 So. 714 (1931). Ch. 33, n. 36.

Thaggard v. Vafes, 119 So. 647 (Ala. 1928). Ch. 28, n. 8.

Wills v. Klingenbeck, 455 So. 2d 806 (1984). Ch. 2, n. 8, 24, Table 1; Ch. 24, n. 13, 14.

Alaska

Edmunds v. Board of Examiners in Optometry, 9 Alas. 482 (1939). Ch. 11, n. 70.

Lee v. State, 490 P.2d 1206 (1971). Ch. 14, n. 18.

Patrick v. Sedwick, 391 P.2d 453 (1964). Ch. 22, Table 2.

Poulin v. Zartman, 542 P.2d 251 (1975). Ch. 22, Table 2.

Arizona

DuVall v. Board of Medical Examiners of Arizona, 49 Ariz. 329, 66 P.2d 1026 (1937). Ch. 11, n. 92.

Fink Jewelry Co. v. State, 50 P.2d 945 (1935). Ch. 9, n. 22.

Hales v. Pittman, 118 Ariz. 305, 576 P.2d 493 (1978). Ch. 22, Table 1.

Shetter v. Rochelle, 2 Ariz. App. 358, 409 P.2d 74, *modified* 2 Ariz. 607, 411 P. 2d 45 (1965). Ch. 22, Table 1.

State of Arizona ex rel. Board of Optometry v. Sears, Roebuck and Co., 102 Ariz. 175, 427 P.2d 126 (1967). Ch. 11, n. 80.

Arkansas

Dorr v. Headstream, 173 Ark. 1104, 295 S.W. 16 (1927). Ch. 35, n. 7.

Hake v. Arkansas State Medical Board, 237 Ark. 506, 374 S.W.2d 173 (1964). Ch. 11, n. 59.

Johnson v. Order of United Commercial Travelers of America, 182 Ark. 964, 39 S.W.2d 375 (1930). Ch. 33, n. 52.

Melton v. Carter, 204 Ark. 595, 164 S.W.2d 453 (1942). Ch. 1, Table 2; Ch. 9, n. 28, 39.

Ritholz v. Arkansas State Board of Optometry, 177 S.W.2d 410 (1944). Ch. 5, n. 11; Ch. 11, n. 69.

State v. Gus Blass Co., 105 S.W.2d 853 (1937). Ch. 9, n. 23.

State Medical Board v. Rogers, 109 Ark. 266, 79 S.W.2d 83 (1935). Ch. 11, n. 92.

State Medical Board of Arkansas Medical Society v. McCrary, 95 Ark. 511, 130 S.W. 544 (1910). Ch. 11, n. 51.

California

Agnew v. Parks, 343 P.2d 118 (1959). Ch. 14, n. 14.
Anderson v. Board of Medical Examiners, 117 Cal. App. 113, 3 P.2d 344 (1931). Ch. 11, n. 59.
Bernstein v. Board of Medical Examiners, 204 Cal. App. 2d 378, 22 Cal. Rptr. 419 (1962). Ch. 11, n. 92.
Black v. Dillon, 213 Cal. App. 2d 295, 28 Cal. Rptr. 678 (1963). Ch. 19, n. 63.
Brainard v. Board of Medical Examiners of the State of California, 68 Cal. App. 2d 591, 157 P.2d 7 (1945). Ch. 11, n. 92.
California Association of Dispensing Opticians, California Board of Optometry v. Pearle Vision Center, Inc., 143 Cal. App. 3d 419, 191 Cal. Rptr. 762 (1983). Ch. 5, n. 26; Ch. 11, n. 68, 76, 83.
Cobbs v. Grant, 8 Cal. 3d 229, 104 Cal. Rptr. 505, 502 P.2d 1 (1972). Ch. 22, n. 4, Table 2.
Custodio v. Bauer, 251 Cal. App. 2d 303, 59 Cal. Rptr. 463 (1967). Ch. 13, n. 8; Ch. 27, n. 41.
Davis v. Board of Medical Examiners, 108 Cal. App. 2d 346, 239 P.2d 78 (1951). Ch. 11, n. 59.
Dean v. Dyer, 64 Cal. App. 2d 646, 149 P.2d 288 (1944). Ch. 29, n. 18.
Ex parte Rust, 181 Cal. 73, 183 P. 548 (1919). Ch. 1, n. 64; Ch. 9, n. 8.
Furnish v. Board of Medical Examiners, 149 Cal. App. 2d 326, 308 P.2d 924 (1957). Ch. 11, n. 92.
Garlock v. Cole, 199 Cal. App. 2d 11, 18 Cal. Rptr. 393 (1962). Ch. 20, n. 41.
Greenman v. Yuba Power Products, 59 Cal. 2d 57, 27 Cal. Rptr. 697, 377 P.2d 897 (1963). Ch. 21, n. 8, 10.
Hewitt v. State Medical Examiners, 148 Cal. 590, 84 P. 39 (1906). Ch. 11, n. 47.
Jacobs v. State Board of Optometry, 81 Cal. App. 3d 1022, 147 Cal Rptr. 225 (1978). Ch. 12, n. 18.
James v. Spear, 338 P.2d 22 (1959). Ch. 16, n. 46.
Kamp v. Johnson, 15 Cal. 2d 187, 99 P.2d 274 (1940). Ch. 12, n. 29.
Murphy v. Board of Medical Examiners of California, 75 Cal. App. 2d 161, 170 P.2d 510 (1946). Ch. 11, n. 59.
Myers v. Quesenberry, 144 Cal. App. 3d 888, 193 Cal. Rptr. 733 (1983). Ch. 32, n. 9.
People v. Brown, 49 Cal. 2d 577, 320 P.2d 5 (1958). Ch. 33, n. 30.
People v. Fowler, 32 Cal. App. 2d Supp. 737, 84 P.2d 326 (1938). Ch. 26, n. 29.
People v. Singh, 136 Cal. App. 233, 28 P.2d 416 (1934). Ch. 33, n. 47.
Ranier v. Grossman, 31 Cal. App. 3d 539, 107 Cal. Rptr. 469 (1973). Ch. 13, n. 11.
Salgo v. Stanford University Board of Trustees, 154 Cal. App. 2d 560, 317 P.2d 170 (1957). Ch. 22, Table 2; Ch. 31, n. 16.
Schessler v. Keck, 125 Cal. App. 2d 827, 271 P.2d 588 (1954). Ch. 20, n. 11.
Shoemaker v. Friedberg, 183 P.2d 318 (1947). Ch. 20, n. 30.
Strode v. Board of Medical Examiners of California, 195 Cal. App. 2d 291, 15 Cal. Rptr. 879 (1961). Ch. 11, n. 86.
Sunseri v. Board of Medical Examiners, 36 Cal. 553, 224 Cal. App. 2d 309 (1964). Ch. 11, n. 59.
Tapley v Abbott, et al, State Board of Medical Examiners, 111 Cal. App. 397, 295 P.2d 911 (1931). Ch. 11, n. 59.
Thrasher v. Board of Medical Examiners of the State of California, 44 Cal. App. 26, 185 P. 1006 (1919). Ch. 11, n. 59.
Tobinsky v. Board of Medical Examiners of the State of California, 49 Cal. App. 2d 591, 121 P.2d 861 (1942). Ch. 11, n. 59.
Von Kesler v. Baker, 131 Cal. App. 654, 21 P.2d 1017 (1933). Ch. 35, n. 16.
Wolfsmith v. Marsh, 337 P.2d 70 (Cal. 1959). Ch. 21, n. 33.

Colorado

Bailey v. Harmon, 74 Colo. 390, 222 P. 393 (1924). Ch. 27, n. 43.
Cardamon v. State Board of Optometric Examiners, 165 Colo. 520, 442 P.2d 25 (1968). Ch. 11, n. 70, 88.
Colorado State Board of Medical Examiners v. *Palmer*, 400 P.2d 914 (1965). Ch. 11, n. 57, 59.
Colorado State Board of Medical Examiners v. *Weiler*, 402 P.2d 606 (1965). Ch. 11, n. 53.
Glenn v. Colorado State Board of Medical Examiners, 131 Colo. 586, 284 P.2d 230 (1955). Ch. 11, n. 86.
Hanley v. Spencer, 115 P.2d 399 (1941). Ch. 19, n. 42; Ch. 26, n. 13.
Mallett v. Pirkey, 171 Colo. 271, 466 P.2d 466 (1970). Ch. 22, Table 1.
McKay v. State Board of Medical Examiners, 103 Colo. 305, 86 P.2d 232 (1938). Ch. 11, n. 59.
Mudd v. Dorr, 574 P.2d 97 (1977). Ch. 22, Table 1.
Tadlock v. Lloyd, 65 Colo. 40, 173 P. 200 (1918). Ch. 13, n. 33.
White v. Andrew, 70 Colo. 50, 197 P. 564 (1921). Ch. 11, n. 50.
Winograd v. Johnson, 561 P.2d 1274 (Colo. App. 1976). Ch. 1, n. 95, 174, 175, Table 4; Ch. 8, n. 25; Ch. 9, n. 46.

Connecticut

Adam v. Connecticut Medical Examining Board, 137 Conn. 535, 70 A.2d 350 (1951). Ch. 11, n. 59.
Camposano v. Claiborn, 2 Conn. Cir. 135, 196 A.2d 129 (1963). Ch. 27, n. 43.
Jaffe v. State Department of Health, 135 Conn. 339, 64 A.2d 330 (1949). Ch. 11, n. 59.
Lieberman v. State Board of Optometry, 34 A.2d 213 (1943). Ch. 5, n. 10.
Paley v. Connecticut, 142 Conn. 522, 115 A.2d 448 (1955). Ch. 11, n. 59.
Sage-Allen Co. v. Wheeler, 119 Conn. 667, 179 A. 195 (1935). Ch. 5, n. 10; Ch. 9, n. 12, 23.

Delaware

Delaware Optometric Corp. v. Sherwood, 36 Del. Ch. 223, 128 A.2d 812 (1957). Ch. 1, n. 94; Ch. 9, n. 43.
DiFilippo v. Preston, 53 Del. 539, 173 A.2d 333 (1961). Ch. 22, Table 1.
Edsall v. Rockland Paper Co., 38 Del. 495, 194 A. 115 (1937). Ch. 33, n. 36.
Wagner v. Olmedo, 365 A.2d 643 (1976). Ch. 22, Table 1.

District of Columbia

American Optometric Association v. Federal Trade Commission, 626 F.2d 896 (D.C. Cir. 1980). Ch. 1, n. 187, Table 4; Ch. 4, n. 48, 53, Table 3; Ch. 7, n. 15; Ch. 16, n. 20.
Canterbury v. Spence, 464 F.2d 772 (D.C. Cir. 1972). Ch. 22, n. 4, Table 2.
Carr v. Shiflette, 82 F.2d 874 (D.C. App. 1936). Ch. 20, n. 35.
Evers v. Buxbaum, 102 App. D.C. 334, 253 F.2d 356 (D.C. Cir. 1958). Ch. 2, n. 4, Table 1; Ch. 19, n. 32; Ch. 21, n. 29; Ch. 24, n. 6.
Fields v. District of Columbia, 232 A.2d 300 (D.C. App. 1967), *adhered to* 244 A.2d 643 (D.C. App. 1968), *appeal denied* 131 App. D.C. 346, 404 F.2d 1323 (1967). Ch. 1, n. 94; Ch. 9, n. 45; Ch. 11, n. 107.
Kemp v. Board of Supervisors, 45 App. D.C. 173 (D.C. App. 1917). Ch. 11, n. 92.
Physicians' Education Network, Inc. v. Department of Health, Education, and Welfare, 653 F.2d 621 (D.C. Cir. 1981). Ch. 1, n. 160; Ch. 12, n. 10.
Rotan v. Greenbaum, 273 F.2d 830 (D.C. Cir. 1959). Ch. 28, n. 5.
Scarzella v. Saxon, 436 A.2d 358 (D.C. App. 1984). Ch. 27, n. 43.
Silver v. Lansburgh and Brothers, 111 F.2d 518 (D.C. App. 1940). Ch. 1, n. 83; Ch. 9, n. 23.

Florida

Bowers v. Talmadge, 159 So. 2d 888 (1963). Ch. 22, Table 1.
DeGaetini v. Driskell, et al., State Board of Medical Examiners, 139 Fla. 49, 190 So. 461 (1939). Ch. 11, n. 59.
Florida Association of Dispensing Opticians v. Florida State Board of Optometry, 238 So. 2d 839 (1970), *conformed to* 239 So. 2d 520 (1970). Ch. 1, n. 94; Ch. 9, n. 45; Ch. 11, n. 106.
Florida Society of Ophthalmology v. Florida Optometric Association, 489 So. 2d 1118 (1986), *reversing* 465 So. 2d 1319 (1985). Ch. 11, n. 1, 112.
Harwick v. Harris, 166 So. 2d 912 (1964). Ch. 13, n. 19.
Page v. State Board of Medical Examiners of Florida, 141 Fla. 294, 193 So. 82 (1940). Ch. 11, n. 84.
Pushkin v. Lombard, 279 So. 2d 79 (1973). Ch. 11, n. 72.
Russell v. Harwick, 166 So. 2d 904 (1964). Ch. 22, Table 1.
State of Florida ex rel. Landis v. Simmons, 104 Fla. 487, 140 So. 187 (1932). Ch. 11, n. 59.
State of Florida ex rel. Weathers v. Davis, 143 Fla. 250, 196 So. 487 (1940). Ch. 11, n. 55.
Walker v. State Board of Optometry, 322 So. 2d 612 (1975). Ch. 11, n. 72.

Georgia

Brewer v. Henson, 96 Ga. App. 501, 100 S.E.2d 661 (1957). Ch. 33, n. 28.
Clark v. Piedmont Hospital, 162 S.E.2d 468 (1968). Ch. 19, n. 43.
Cochran v. Sears-Roebuck and Co., 34 S.E.2d 296 (1945). Ch. 20, n. 30.
Georgia Board of Examiners v. Frieman's Jewelers, 189 S.E. 238 (1936). Ch. 9, n. 23.
Hartford Accident and Indemnity Co. v. Barfield, 89 Ga. App. 562, 80 S.E.2d 84 (1954). Ch. 26, n. 29.
Kahn v. Shaw, 65 Ga. App. 563, 16 S.E.2d 99 (1941). Ch. 2, n. 18; Ch. 28, n. 26; Ch. 31, n. 22; Ch. 35, n. 8.
Keen v. Coleman, 20 S.E.2d 175 (1942). Ch. 20, n. 41.

Mott v. Georgia State Board of Examiners in Optometry, 148 Ga. 55, 95 S.E. 867 (1918). Ch. 11, n. 58, 66.

Pearle Optical of Monroeville, Inc. v. Georgia State Board of Examiners in Optometry, 219 Ga. 364, 133 S.E.2d 374 (1963). Ch. 9, n. 38; Ch. 12, n. 32.

Rogers v. Medical Association of Georgia, 244 Ga. 151, 259 S.E.2d 85 (1979). Ch. 11, n. 7.

Wall v. Youmans, 223 Ga. 191, 154 S.E.2d 191 (1967). Ch. 11, n. 68.

Wallace v. Hall, 145 Ga. App. 610, 244 S.E.2d 129 (1978). Ch. 14, n. 18.

Young v. Yarn, 136 Ga. App. 739, 222 S.E.2d 113 (1975). Ch. 22, Table 1.

Hawaii

Nishi v. Hartwell, 52 Hawaii 188, 473 P.2d 116 (1970). Ch. 22, Table 1.

Idaho

Holmes v. Iwasa, 104 Ida. 179, 657 P.2d 476 (1983). Ch. 2, n. 7, 23; Ch. 19, n. 52; Ch. 23, n. 33.

Illinois

Berlin v. Nathan, 21 Ill. 682, 64 Ill. App. 3d 940, 381 N.E.2d 1367 (1978). Ch. 19, n. 65.

Carroll v. Grabavoy, 77 Ill. App. 3d 895, 396 N.E.2d 836 (1979). Ch. 27, n. 47.

Cirafici v. Goffen, 85 Ill. App. 3d 1102, 407 N.E.2d 633 (1980). Ch. 27, n. 43.

Green v. Hussey, 127 Ill. App. 2d 174, 262 N.E. 2d 156 (1970). Ch. 22, Table 1.

Hawkins v. Richardson, 29 Ill. App. 3d 597, 331 N.E.2d 201 (1975). Ch. 18, n. 31.

House of Vision, Inc. v. Watson, 59 Ill. 2d 508, 322 N.E.2d 15 (1974), *cert. denied* 422 U.S. 1008, 95 S. Ct. 2631 (1974). Ch. 11, n. 65.

People v. Griffith, 280 Ill. 18, 117 N.E. 195 (1917). Ch. 1, n. 66; Ch. 9, n. 17; Ch. 11, n. 105.

People v. Witte, 315 Ill. 282, 146 N.E. 178 (1924). Ch. 9, n. 14.

People Use of the State Board of Health v. Smith, 208 Ill. 31, 69 N.E. 810 (1904), *affirming* 108 Ill. App. 499 (1903). Ch. 1, n. 30, 31, 32, Table 1.

Ramsey v. Shelton, 329 Ill. 432, 160 N.E. 769 (1928). Ch. 11, n. 59.

Rogers v. Robson, Masters, Ryan, Brumund and Belom, 392 N.E.2d 1365 (Ill. App. 1979). Ch. 54, n. 6.

Sanitary District of Chicago v. Industrial Commissioner, 343 Ill. 236, 175 N.E. 372 (1931). Ch. 33, n. 53.

Schireson v. Walsh, 354 Ill. 40, 187 N.E. 921 (1933). Ch. 11, n. 53.

Schyman v. Department of Registration and Education, 9 Ill. App. 2d 504, 133 N.E.2d 551 (1956), *cert. denied* 352 U.S. 1001, 77 S. Ct. 557 (1956). Ch. 11, n. 59.

Smith v. Department of Registration and Education of the State of Illinois, 412 Ill. 322, 106 N.E.2d 722 (1952). Ch. 11, n. 59.

Smith v. People, 92 Ill. App. 22, *reversed* 199 Ill. 20, 63 N.E. 972 (1900). Ch. 1, n. 30.

Wallace v. Yudelson, 224 Ill. App. 320 (1927). Ch. 13, n. 19.

Indiana

Adkins v. Ropp, 14 N.E.2d 727 (1938). Ch. 19, n. 24.

American Optical Co. v. Wiedenhamer, 404 N.E.2d 606 (Ind. App. 1980). Ch. 2, n. 14; Ch. 27, n. 35.

Board of Medical Registration and Education of Indiana v. Armington, 242 Ind. 436, 178 N.E.2d 741 (1961). Ch. 11, n. 86.

Cassidy v. Cain, 251 N.E.2d 852 (Ind. App. 1969). Ch. 11, n. 98.

Cassidy v. Indiana State Board of Registration and Examination in Optometry, 244 Ind. 137, 191 N.E.2d 492 (1963). Ch. 11, n. 98.

Grosjean v. Spencer, 258 Iowa 685, 140 N.W.2d 139 (1966). Ch. 22, Table 3.

Hachat v. Hachat, 71 N.E.2d 927 (1947). Ch. 13, n. 14.

Haffner v. Indiana State Board of Registration in Optometry, 333 N.E.2d 312 (Ind. App. 1975). Ch. 11, n. 72.

Hess v. Lowery, 122 Ind. 225, 23 N.E. 156 (1890). Ch. 21, n. 33.

Hurley v. Eddingfield, 59 N.E. 1058 (1901). Ch. 13, n. 13; Ch. 14, n. 14.

Indiana Academy of Ophthalmology and Otolaryngology, Inc. v. Indiana State Board of Registration and Examination in Optometry, 481 N.E.2d 179 (1985). Ch. 1, n. 91.

Joy v. Chau, 377 N.E.2d 670 (1978). Ch. 22, Table 1.

Van Brockhorst v. Taube, 341 N.E.2d 791 (Ind. App. 1976). Ch. 20, n. 42.

Iowa

Barnes v. Bovenmeyer, 122 N.W.2d 312 (1963). Ch. 19, n. 34; Ch. 26, n. 17.

Freese v. Lemon, 210 N.W.2d 576 (1973). Ch. 32, n. 11.

Hollenbeck v. Ristine, 86 N.W. 377 (1901). Ch. 20, n. 12.

Porter v. Powell, 79 Iowa 151, 44 N.W. 295 (1890). Ch. 13, n. 14.

State v. Hanson, 201 Iowa 579, 207 N.W. 769 (1926). Ch. 11, n. 55, 59.

State v. Kindy Optical Co., 216 Iowa 1157, 248 N.W. 332 (1933). Ch. 1, Table 2; Ch. 5, n. 9; Ch. 9, n. 11, 22.

State of Iowa ex rel. Bierring v. Ritholz, 283 N.W. 268 (1939). Ch. 5, n. 11; Ch. 11, n. 69, 81.

Kansas

Acupuncture Society of Kansas v. Kansas State Board of Healing Arts, 226 Kan. 639, 602 P.2d 1311 (1979). Ch. 26, n. 35.

Brown v. Hassig, 136 Kan. 384, 15 P.2d 401 (1932). Ch. 11, n. 59.

Copeland v. Kansas State Board of Examiners in Optometry, 518 P.2d 377 (1974). Ch. 11, n. 71.

Kansas State Board v. Foote, 200 Kan. 447, 436 P.2d 828 (1968). Ch. 11, n. 73.

Mickens v. Davis, 294 P. 896 (1931). Ch. 20, n. 13.

Natanson v. Kline, 186 Kan. 393, 350 P.2d 1093, *affirmed* 187 Kan. 186, 354 P.2d 670 (1960). Ch. 22, n. 2, Table 1.

Noel v. Pound, 189 Kan. 6, 367 P.2d 61 (1961). Ch. 27, n. 43.

State of Kansas ex. rel. Beck v. Gleason, 148 Kan. 1, 79 P.2d 911 (1938). Ch. 26, n. 29.

State of Kansas ex rel. Beck v. Goldman Jewelry Co., 142 Kan. 881, 51 P.2d 995 (1935). Ch. 1, n. 83; Ch. 5, n. 8; Ch. 9, n. 21, 22; Ch. 11, n. 79.

State of Kansas ex rel. Londerholm v. Doolin, 209 Kan. 244, 497 P.2d 138 (1972). Ch. 1, n. 94; Ch. 9, n. 45.

Yeates v. Harris, 193 Kan. 320, 393 P.2d 982 (1964). Ch. 22, Table 1.

Kentucky

Alexander v. Menefee, 64 S.W. 855 (1901). Ch. 33, n. 22.

Beauchamp v. Davis, 309 Ky. 397, 217 S.W.2d 822 (1948). Ch. 2, n. 42.

Bennett v. Graves, 557 S.W.2d 893 (1977). Ch. 22, Table 2.

Boyd v. Wynn, 286 Ky. 173, 150 S.W.2d 648 (1941). Ch. 20, n. 16.

Brents v. Morgan, 221 Ky. 765, 299 S.W. 867 (1927). Ch. 20, n. 39.

Engel v. Clarke, 346 S.W.2d 13 (1961). Ch. 13, n. 27.

Foreman v. State Board of Health, 157 Ky. 123, 162 S.W. 796 (1914). Ch. 11, n. 52.

Hoad v. Russell, 307 S.W.2d 557 (1958). Ch. 33, n. 51.

Holton v. Pfingst, 534 S.W.2d 786 (1975). Ch. 22, Table 2.

Matthews v. Murphy, 23 Ky. 750, 63 S.W. 785 (1901). Ch. 11, n. 53.

Our Lady of Mercy Hospital v. McIntosh, 461 S.W.2d 377 (1970). Ch. 19, n. 43.

Stacy v. Williams, 253 Ky. 353, 69 S.W2d 697 (1934). Ch. 13, n. 18.

Louisiana

Beaver v. Louisiana State Board of Optometry Examiners, 206 So. 2d 118 (1968). Ch. 11, n. 89.

Fairchild v. Brian, 354 So. 2d 675 (La. App. 1977). Ch. 2, n. 19, 22, 24, Table 1; Ch. 18, n. 21; Ch. 21, n. 32; Ch. 24, n. 7, 8, 10, 11; Ch. 25, n. 9, 10, 11; Ch. 33, n. 16.

Favalora v. Aetna Casualty Co., 144 So. 2d 544 (1962). Ch. 19, n. 27.

Hanks v. Drs. Ranson, Swan, and Burch, Ltd., 359 So. 2d 1089, *writ denied* 360 So. 2d 1178 (1978). Ch. 22, Table 2.

Louisiana State Board of Optometry Examiners v. Pearle Optical, Inc., 177 So. 2d 164, *annulled* 184 So. 2d 10 (1965). Ch. 1, n. 94.

Pennison v. Provident Life Ins. Co., 154 So. 2d 617 (1963). Ch. 20, n. 29.

Percle v. St. Paul Fire and Marine Insurance Co., 349 So. 2d 1289 (1977). Ch. 22, Table 2.

Reynier v. Delta Women's Clinic, Inc., 359 So. 2d 733 (1978). Ch. 22, Table 2.

Steele v. St. Paul Fire and Marine Insurance Co., 371 So. 2d 843 (1979). Ch. 22, Table 2.

Truxillo v. Gentilly Medical Bldg. Inc., 255 So. 2d 488 (1969). Ch. 29, n. 11.

Maine

Donnell v. Board of Registration in Medicine, 128 Me. 523, 149 A. 153 (1930). Ch. 11, n. 84.

Downer v. Villeux, 322 A.2d 82 (1974). Ch. 22, Table 3.

Maryland

Board of Examiners in Optometry v. Spitz, 479 A.2d 363 (1984). Ch. 9, Table 2.
Dvorine v. Castleberg Jewelry Corp., 185 A. 562 (1936). Ch. 9, n. 23.
Globe Indemnity Co. v. Reinhart, 152 Md. 439, 137 A. 43 (1927). Ch. 33, n. 36.
Lane v. Calvert, 138 A.2d 902 (1958). Ch. 27, n. 42.
Tempchin v. Sampson, 262 Md. 156, 277 A.2d 67 (1971). Ch. 2, n. 5; Ch. 16, n. 41; Ch. 19, n. 29.
Thomas v. Corso, 265 Md. 84, 288 A.2d 379 (1972). Ch. 13, n. 31.

Massachusetts

Attorney General v. Kenco Optics, 340 N.E.2d 868 (1976). Ch. 9, Table 2.
Commonwealth v. Houtenbrink, 235 Mass. 320, 126 N.E. 669 (1920). Ch. 1, n. 65; Ch. 9, n. 7.
Commonwealth v. S.S. Kresge Co., 267 Mass. 145, 166 N.E. 558 (1929). Ch. 9, n. 18.
David v. Calderwood, et al, Board of Registration in Medicine, 251 Mass. 283, 146 N.W. 708 (1925). Ch. 11, n. 59.
Doane v. Doane, 238 Mass. 106, 130 N.E. 484 (1921). Ch. 33, n. 36.
Kay Jewelry Co. v. Board of Registration, 27 N.E.2d 1 (1940). Ch. 9, n. 22.
Kramer v. John Hancock Mutual Life Insurance Co., 336 Mass. 465, 146 N.E.2d 357 (1957). Ch. 33, n. 28.
Lawrence v. Biry, et al., Board of Registration in Medicine, 238 Mass. 424, 132 N.E. 174 (1921). Ch. 11, n. 47.
McMahon v. Glixman, 393 N.E.2d 875 (1979). Ch. 2, n. 7, 23; Ch. 23, n. 33.
McMurdo v. Getter, 10 N.E.2d 139 (1937). Ch. 9, n. 22.
Schroeder v. Lawrence, 359 N.E.2d 1301 (1977). Ch. 22, Table 1.
Sullivan v. O'Connor, 363 Mass. 579, 296 N.E.2d 183 (1973). Ch. 27, n. 43.

Michigan

Blanchard v. Michigan State Board of Examiners in Optometry, 198 N.W.2d 804 (1972). Ch. 11, n. 95.
De Groot v. Winter, 261 Mich. 660, 247 N.W. 69 (1933). Ch. 33, n. 52.
De May v. Roberts, 9 N.W. 166 (1881). Ch. 20, n. 35.
Gaynes v. Allen, 128 Mich. App. 42, 339 N.W.2d 678 (1983). Ch. 20, n. 9.
In re Hyning, 257 Mich. 146, 241 N.W. 207 (1932). Ch. 11, n. 53.
Kelly ex rel. Michigan Board of Examiners v. Peterson, 4 Mich. App. 612, 145 N.W.2d 386 (1966). Ch. 1, n. 94; Ch. 11, n. 104.
Luka v. Lowrie, 136 N.W. 1106 (1912). Ch. 13, n. 15.
Marchlewicz v. Stanton, 50 Mich. App. 344, 213 N.W.2d 317 (1973). Ch. 22, Table 1.
McGarry v. J.A. Mercier Co., 272 Mich. 501, 262 N.W. 296 (1935). Ch. 16, n. 7.
People of the State of Michigan v. Baker, 94 Mich. App. 365, 288 N.E.2d 430 (1980). Ch. 16, n. 37.
Podvin v. Eickhorst, 373 Mich. 175, 128 N.W.2d 523 (1964). Ch. 13, n. 17.
Porter v. Michigan State Board of Examiners in Optometry, 199 N.W.2d 666 (1972). Ch. 11, n. 100.
Roberts v. Young, 369 Mich. 113, 119 N.W.2d 627 (1963). Ch. 22, Table 1.
Rogers v. Canfield, 262 N.W. 409 (1935). Ch. 21, n. 37.
Shulman v. Lerner, 2 Mich. App. 705, 141 N.W.2d 348 (1966). Ch. 22, Table 1.
Siefert v. Buhl Optical Co., 276 Mich. 692, 286 N.W. 784 (1936). Ch. 9, n. 29.
Sinclair v. Brunson, 212 Mich. 387, 180 N.W. 358 (1920). Ch. 13, n. 31.
Triestram v. Way, 286 Mich. 13, 281 N.W. 420 (1938). Ch. 14, n. 16.
Welke v. Kuzilla, 144 Mich. App. 245, 375 N.W.2d 403 (1985). Ch. 2, n. 32; Ch. 32, n. 7.
Wozniak v. State Board of Examiners in Optometry, 23 Mich. App. 646, 179 N.W.2d 208 (1970) Ch. 11, n. 72, 95.

Minnesota

Cornfeldt v. Tongen, 262 N.W.2d 684 (1977). Ch. 22, Table 2.
Derrick v. St. Paul City Railroad Co., 252 Minn. 102, 89 N.W.2d 629 (1959). Ch. 33, n. 49.
House v. Hanson, 72 N.W.2d 874 (1955). Ch. 19, n. 62.
Lundgren v. Eustermann, 356 N.W.2d 762 (Minn. App. 1984). Ch. 35, n. 7.
McGray v. Cobb, 152 N.W. 262 (1915). Ch. 21, n. 33.

Peterson v. Richfield Plaza, Inc., 252 Minn. 215, 89 N.W.2d 712 (1958). Ch. 33, n. 30.
Rayburn v. Minnesota State Board of Optometry, 247 Minn. 520, 78 N.W.2d 351 (1956). Ch. 5, n. 38; Ch. 11, n. 73.
Staloch v. Holm, 111 N.W. 264 (1907). Ch. 27, n. 42.
State v. Broden, 181 Minn. 341, 232 N.W. 517 (1930). Ch. 9, n. 15.
State by Erwin v. Goodman, 288 N.W. 157 (1939). Ch. 9 n. 23.
Williams v. Mack, 278 N.W. 585 (1938). Ch. 9, n. 23.

Mississippi

Deaton v. Delta Democrat Publishing Co., 326 So. 2d 471 (1976). Ch. 20, n. 37.
Mississippi State Board of Health v. Johnson, 197 Miss. 417, 19 So. 2d 445 (1944). Ch. 11, n. 59.
Phillips v. Delta Motor Lines, Inc., 235 Miss. 1, 108 So. 2d 409 (1959). Ch. 14, n. 16.
Ross v. Hodges, 234 S.2d 905 (1970). Ch. 22, Table 1.
Smith v. McComb Infirmary Association, 196 So. 2d 91 (1967). Ch. 19, n. 55.
State Board of Optometry v. Chester, 251 Miss. 250, 169 So. 2d 468 (1964). Ch. 1, n. 94; Ch. 9, n. 45.

Missouri

Aiken v. Clary, 396 S.W.2d 668 (1965). Ch. 22, Table 1.
Barber v. Time, Inc., 159 S.W.2d 291 (1942). Ch. 20, n. 36.
Boyd v. Andrae, 44 S.W.2d 891 (1932). Ch. 13, n. 32.
Cassell v. Schofield, 319 Mo. 1169, 85 S.W.2d 580 (1928). Ch. 35, n. 7.
Dameron v. Harris, 281 Mo. 247, 219 S.W. 954 (1920). Ch. 33, n. 36.
Gaines v. Schneider, 323 S.W.2d 401 (Mo. App. 1959). Ch. 33, n. 30.
Hagler v. Major, 186 S.W.2d 564 (1945). Ch. 20, n. 13.
Harris v. Bales, 459 S.W.2d 742 (Mo. App. 1970). Ch. 18, n. 21.
Ketring v. Sturges, 372 S.W.2d 104 (1963). Ch. 1, n. 94; Ch. 11, n. 106.
Kirkpatrick v. Wells, 319 Mo. 1040, 6 S.W.2d 591 (1928). Ch. 33, n. 36.
Kopp v. C.C. Caldwell Optical Co., 547 S.W.2d 872 (Mo. App. 1977). Ch. 2, n. 11; Ch. 27, n. 27.
Smart v. Kansas City, 208 Mo. 162, 105 S.W. 709 (1907). Ch. 13, n. 5.
Smith v. Mallinckrodt Chemical Works, 212 Mo. App. 158, 251 S.W. 155 (1923). Ch. 18, n. 26.
State v. Etzenhouser, 223 Mo. App. 577, 16 S.W.2d 656 (1929). Ch. 11, n. 105.
State of Missouri ex rel. Danforth v. Dale Curteman, Inc., 480 S.W.2d 848 (1972). Ch. 1, n. 94; Ch. 9, n. 45; Ch. 11, n. 107.
State of Missouri ex rel. Farber v. Shot, 304 Mo. 523, 263 S.W. 804 (1924). Ch. 11, n. 59.
State of Missouri ex rel. Johnson v. Clark, et al, State Board of Health, 288 Mo. 659, 232 S.W. 1031 (1921). Ch. 11, n. 59.
State of Missouri ex rel. McKittrick v. Gate City Optical Co., 97 S.W.2d 89 (1936). Ch. 9, n. 23.
State of Missouri ex rel. Kerr, et al., State Board of Health v. Landwehr, 32 S.W.2d 83 (Mo. 1930). Ch. 11, n. 57.
Steele v. Woods, 327 S.W.2d 187 (1959). Ch. 19, n. 43.

Montana

Doerr v. Movius, 154 Mont. 510, 463 P.2d 477 (1970). Ch. 22, Table 1.
Negaard v. Estate of Feda, 152 Mont. 47, 446 P.2d 436 (1968). Ch. 22, Table 1.
State of Montana ex rel. Yuhas v. Board of Medical Examiners, 135 Mont. 381, 339 P.2d 981 (1959). Ch. 11, n. 59.

Nebraska

Monk v. Frink, 75 Neb. 172, 106 N.W. 425 (1905). Ch. 11, n. 56, 59.
Simonsen v. Swenson, 104 Neb. 224, 177 N.W. 831 (1920). Ch. 20, n. 30.
State v. First Bank of Nickerson, 114 Neb. 423, 207 N.W. 674 (1926). Ch. 35, n. 16.
Stohlman v. Davis, 220 N.W. 247 (1928). Ch. 13, n. 5, 29; Ch. 21, n. 41.

Nevada

Corn v. French, 71 Nev. 280, 289 P.2d 173 (1955). Ch. 22, Table 3.
In re Reno, 57 Nev. 314, 64 P.2d 1036 (1937). Ch. 11, n. 59.

New Hampshire

Folger v. Corbett, 394 A.2d 63 (1978). Ch. 22, Table 1.
Hawkins v. McGee, 84 N.H. 114, 146 A. 641 (1929). Ch. 27, n. 43.
New Hampshire Board of Registration in Optometry v. Scott Jewelry Co., 90 N.H. 368, 9 A.2d 513 (1939). Ch. 11, n. 46.

New Jersey

Abelson's, Inc. v. New Jersey State Board of Optometrists, 5 N.J. 412, 75 A.2d 867 (1950). Ch. 9, n. 32, 38; Ch. 11, n. 72; Ch. 16, n. 10.
Bacardi v. Holzman, 182 N.J. Super. 422, 442A.2d 617 (1981). Ch. 28, n. 40.
Flynn v. Stearns, 145 A.2d 33 (1958). Ch. 19, n. 43.
Gleitman v. Cosgrove, 49 N.J. 22, 227 A.2d 689 (1966). Ch. 22, Table 1.
Hague v. Williams, 37 N.J. 328, 181 A.2d 345 (1986). Ch. 20, n. 25, 27.
Henningsen v. Bloomfield Motors, Inc., 32 N.J. 358, 161 A.2d 69 (1960). Ch. 21, n. 5.
Jaeckle v. Bamburger and Co., 181 A. 181 (1935). Ch. 9, n. 23.
Kaplan v. Haines, 96 N.J. Super. 242, 232 A.2d 840, *affirmed* 51 N.J. 404, 241 A2d. 235 (1968). Ch. 22, Table 1.
Kent v. County of Hudson, 245 A.2d 747 (1968). Ch. 19, n. 43.
New Jersey Optometric Association v. Hillman-Kohan Eyeglasses, Inc., 388 A.2d 1299 (1978). Ch. 11, n. 66.
New Jersey State Board of Optometrists v. Reiss, 83 N.J. Super. 47, 198 A.2d 816 (1964). Ch. 1, n. 94; Ch. 9, n. 44, 45; Ch. 11, n. 107.
Schireson v. State Board of Medical Examiners of New Jersey, 219 N.J.L. 203, 28 A.2d 879 (1942), *reversed* 130 N.J.L. 570, 33 A.2d 911 (1943). Ch. 11, n. 55, 84.
Teseshi v. Mathis, 183 A. 146 (1936). Ch. 9, n. 22.

New Mexico

Christman v. Voyer, 92 N.M. 772, 595 P.2d 410 (1979). Ch. 11, n. 62.
Dahl v. Turner, 80 N.M. 564, 458 P.2d 816 (1969). Ch. 14, n. 18.
Demers v. Gerety, 92 N.M. 396, 589 P.2d 180, *reversed* 92 N.M. 749, 595 P.2d 387 (1978). Ch. 22, Table 2.
Reid v. New Mexico Board of Examiners in Optometry, 92 N.M. 414, 589 P.2d 198 (1979). Ch. 11, n. 87.
Seele v. Purcell, 45 N.M. 176, 113 P.2d 320 (1941). Ch. 14, n. 16.
Vigil v. Rice, 74 N.M. 693, 397 P.2d 719 (1964). Ch. 20, n. 19.
Woods v. Brumlop, 71 N.M. 221, 377 P.2d 520 (1962). Ch. 22, n. 4.

New York

Arshanasky v. Royal Concourse Co., 28 A.D.2d 986, 283 N.Y.S.2d 646 (1967). Ch. 13, n. 22.
Bennett v. New York, 59 Misc. 2d 306, 299 N.Y.S.2d 288 (1969). Ch. 19, n. 43.
Bernanke v. Board of Regents of the University of the State of New York, 24 A.D.2d 910, 264 N.Y.S.2d 399 (1965). Chl. 11, n. 88.
Blair v. Bartlett, 75 N.Y. 150 (1878). Ch. 19, n. 61.
Boothe v. Weiss, 484 N.Y.S.2d 598 (1985). Ch. 2, n. 22.
Capuano v. Jacobs, 33 A.D.2d 743, 305 N.Y.S.2d 837 (1969). Ch. 13, n. 6.
Clark v. Geraci, 208 N.Y.S.2d 564 (1960). Ch. 20, n. 18.
Clifford v. Hughes, 139 A.D. 730, 124 N.Y.S. 478 (1910). Ch. 35, n. 16.
Curry v. Corn, 52 Misc. 2d 1035, 277 N.Y.S.2d 470 (1966). Ch. 20, n. 29.
Degnan v. Ransom, 31 N.Y.S. 966 (1894). Ch. 33, n. 22.
Dickson v. Flynn, 273 N.Y. 72, 6 N.E.2d 102 (1937). Ch. 9, n. 23.
Epstein v. Board of Regents of the University of the State of New York, 295 N.Y. 154, 65 N.E.2d 756 (1946). Ch. 11, n. 59.
Falcone v. New York State Education Department, 50 N.Y.2d 854, 407 N.E.2d 2335 (1980). Ch. 11, n. 70, 72, 90.
Feeney v. Young, 191 A.D. 501, 181 N.Y.S. 481 (1920). Ch. 20, n. 34.
Felis v. Greenberg, 51 Misc. 2d 881, 273 N.Y.S.2d 288 (1966). Ch. 20, n. 27.
Ferrara v. Galluchio, 5 N.Y.2d 16, 152 N.E.2d 249 (1958). Ch. 18, n. 33.
Finlay Straus, Inc. v. University of the State of New York, 279 A.D. 1060, 62 N.Y.S.2d 892 (1946). Ch. 9, n. 31.
Frank v. Board of Regents of the University of the State of New York, 24 A.D.2d 909, 264 N.Y.S.2d 413 (1965). Ch. 11, n. 59.
Gates v. Preston, 41 N.Y. 113, (1869). Ch. 19, n. 61.

Graddy v. New York Medical College, 19 A.D.2d 426, 243 N.Y.S.2d 940 (1963). Ch. 21, n. 36.
Griffin v. Medical Society of the State of New York, 11 N.Y.S.2d 109 (1939). Ch. 20, n. 33.
Hammer v. Polsky, 36 Misc. 2d 482, 233 N.Y.S.2d 110 (1962). Ch. 20, n. 31.
Karlsons v. Guerinot, 57 A.D.2d 73, 394 N.Y.S.2d 933 (1977). Ch. 22, Table 1.
Kraus v. Spielberg, 37 Misc. 2d 519, 236 N.Y.S.2d 143 (1962). Ch. 18, n. 33.
Matter of Pace, 156 N.Y.S. 641, 153 Misc. 609 (1915). Ch. 9, n. 25.
Matter of Weiss, 147 N.Y.S.2d 455, 208 Misc. 1010 (1955). Ch. 16, n. 16.
Newman v. Board of Regents of the State of New York, 270 A.D. 964, 61 N.Y.S.2d 841 (1946). Ch. 11, n. 59.
O'Neill v. Montefiore Hospital, 11 A.D.2d 132, 202 N.Y.S.2d 436 (1960). Ch. 13, n. 6, 10.
Palmer v. Spaulding, Commissioner of Education, 299 N.Y. 368, 87 N.E.2d 201 (1949). Ch. 11, n. 86.
Pike v. Honsinger, 49 N.E. 760 (1898). Ch. 18, n. 18.
Robins v. Finestone, 308 N.Y. 543, 127 N.E.2d 330 (1955). Ch. 27, n. 43.
Schloendorff v. Society of New York Hospital, 211 N.Y. 125, 105 N.E. 92 (1914). Ch. 18, n. 12; Ch. 23, n. 10.
Shapiro v. Board of Regents of the University of the State of New York, 16 N.Y.2d 783, 262 N.Y.S.2d 503 (1965). Ch. 11, n. 59.
Stammer v. Board of Regents of the University of the State of New York, 287 N.Y. 359, 39 N.E.2d 913 (1942). Ch. 11, n. 59.
Stern v. Flynn, 154 Misc. 609, 278 N.Y.S. 598 (1935). Ch. 9, n. 22.
Tompkins v. Board of Regents of the University of the State of New York, 299 N.Y. 469, 87 N.E.2d 517 (1949). Ch. 11, n. 86.
Werted v. Board of Regents of the University of the State of New York, 18 A.D.2d 1032, 238 N.Y.S.2d 356 (1963). Ch. 11, n. 59.
Winik v. Jewish Hospital of Brooklyn, 31 N.Y.2d 936, 293 N.E.2d 95 (1972). Ch. 18, n. 33.

North Carolina

Butler v. Berkeley, 25 N.C. App. 325, 213 S.E.2d 571 (1975). Ch. 22, Table 1.
Childers v. Frye, 201 N.C. 42, 158 S.E. 744 (1931). Ch. 13, n. 5.
High v. Ridgeway's Opticians, 258 N.C. 626, 129 S.E.2d 301 (1963). Ch. 1, n. 94; Ch. 9, n. 45; Ch. 11, n. 106.
Smith v. Wharton, 154 S.E. 12 (1930). Ch. 28, n. 46.
State v. Shaw, 289 S.E.2d 325 (1982). Ch. 16, n. 37.
Thornburg v. Long, 101 S.E. 99 (1919). Ch. 20, n. 10.
Wilson v. Martin Memorial Hospital, 232 N.C. 362, 61 S.E.2d 102 (1950). Ch. 21, n. 40.

North Dakota

In re Shortridge, 53 N.D. 614, 207 N.W. 442 (1926). Ch. 11, n. 59.
Winkjer v. Herr, 277 N.W.2d 579 (1979). Ch. 22, Table 1.

Ohio

Bruni v. Tatsumi, 46 Ohio St. 2d 127, 346 N.E.2d 673 (1976). Ch. 22, Table 2.
Champs v. Stone, 58 N.E.2d 803 (1944). Ch. 19, n. 41.
Congrove v. Holmes, 37 Ohio Misc. 95, 308 N.E.2d 765 (1973). Ch. 22, Table 2.
Forthofer v. Arnold, 60 Ohio App. 436, 21 N.E.2d 869 (1938). Ch. 35, n. 7.
In re Raab, State Medical Board of Ohio v. Raab, 156 Ohio 158, 101 N.E.2d 294 (1951). Ch. 11, n. 84.
Jeswald v. Hutt, 15 Ohio St. 2d 224, 239 N.E.2d 37 (1968). Ch. 29, n. 8.
Kime v. Aetna, 66 Ohio App. 277, 33 N.E.2d 1008 (1940). Ch. 2, n. 21; Ch. 26, n. 30, 31, 32.
Klema v. St. Elizabeth's Hospital of Youngstown, 170 Ohio St. 519, 166 N.E.2d 765 (1960). Ch. 19, n. 55.
Lundberg v. Bay View Hospital, 175 Ohio St. 133, 191 N.E.2d 821 (1963). Ch. 13, n. 6.
Morgan v. Sheppard, 188 N.E.2d 808 (1963). Ch. 19, n. 27.
Rice v. Evatt, 144 Ohio St. 483, 59 N.E.2d 927 (1945). Ch. 12, n. 30.
Rice v. Rinaldo, 119 N.E.2d 657 (1951). Ch. 14, n. 14.
Rowe v. Standard Drug. Co., 9 N.E.2d 609 (1937). Ch. 9, n. 22.
Seitz v. Ohio State Medical Board, 24 Ohio App. 154, 157 N.E. 304 (1926). Ch. 11, n. 84.
State v. Viola, 82 N.E.2d 306, *appeal dismissed* 148 Ohio St. 712, 76 N.E.2d 715, *cert. denied* 334 U.S. 816, 68 S. Ct. 1070 (1948). Ch. 16, n. 37.
State of Ohio ex rel. Bricker v. Buhl Optical Co., 2

N.E.2d 601 (1936). Ch. 9, n. 22.

Whitt v. Columbus Cooperative Enterprises, 64 Ohio St. 2d 355, 415 N.E.2d 985. (1980). Ch. 2, n. 6, 25; Ch. 19, n. 53; Ch. 23, n. 33; Ch. 25, n. 26.

Oklahoma

Freeman v. State Board, 54 Okla. 531, 154 P. 56 (1916). Ch. 11, n. 59.

Seanor v. Browne, 154 Okla. 222, 7 P.2d 627 (1932). Ch. 27, n. 43.

State of Oklahoma ex rel. Clifton v. Reeser, 543 P.2d 1379 (1975). Ch. 1, n. 94; Ch. 9, n. 45; Ch. 11, n. 106.

Oregon

Board of Medical Examiners of the State of Oregon v. Mintz, 233 Or. 441, 378 P.2d 945 (1963). Ch. 11, n. 59.

Getchell v. Mansfield, 260 Or. 174, 489 P.2d 953 (1971). Ch. 22, Table 1.

Gwynn v. Wilhelm, 360 P.2d 312 (1961). Ch. 19, n. 62.

Holland v. Sisters of St. Joseph of Peace, 270 Or. 129, 522 P.2d 208 (1974). Ch. 22, Table 1.

In re Buck's License, 200 Or. 488, 258 P.2d 124 (1953). Ch. 11, n. 59.

Lippold v. Kidd, 269 P. 210 (1928). Ch. 26, n. 16.

Moulton v. Huckleberry, 46 P.2d 589 (1935). Ch. 21, n. 25.

Radtke v. Taylor, 105 Or. 559, 210 P. 863 (1922). Ch. 33, n. 36.

State v. Standard Optical Co., 188 P.2d 309 (1947). Ch. 33, n. 48.

State of Oregon ex rel. Reed v. Kuzirian, 228 Or. 619, 365 P.2d 1046 (1961). Ch. 1, n. 94, 145; Ch. 9, n. 43; Ch. 11, n. 106.

Stuhr v. Barkwill, 332 P.2d 603 (1958). Ch. 26, n. 15.

Pennsylvania

Alexander v. Knight, 197 Pa. Super. 79, 177 A.2d 142 (1962). Ch. 20, n. 14.

Clayton v. Bernstein, 38 Pa. D&C 543 (1940). Ch. 20, n. 33.

Commonwealth v. Stemet, 21 Pa. D&C 2d 295 (1959). Ch. 11, n. 106.

Cooper v. Roberts, 220 Pa. Supper. 260, 286 A.2d 647 (1971). Ch. 22, n. 4, Table 2.

Harris v. State Optometrical Examiners, 287 Pa. 531, 135 A. 237 (1926). Ch. 1, n. 85, Table 2; Ch. 9, n. 10.

Hartman v. Commonwealth, 454 A.2d 1150 (1983). Ch. 11, n. 63.

Incollingo v. Ewing, 444 Pa. 263, 282 A.2d 206 (1971). Ch. 19, n. 27.

Jeffries v. McCague, 242 Pa. Super. 76, 363 A.2d 1167 (1976). Ch. 22, Table 2.

Martin v. Baldy, 249 Pa. 253, 94 A. 1091 (1915). Ch. 1, n. 4, 41, 42, Table 1; Ch. 9, n. 41; Ch. 10, n. 7.

Neill v. Gimbel Brothers, 330 Pa. 213, 199 A. 178 (1938). Ch. 9, n. 22.

Neill v. Wall and Ochs, Inc., 68 Pa. D&C 2d 429 (1973). Ch. 9, Table 2.

Pennsylvania Optometric Association v. Di Giovanni, 45 Pa. D&C 2d 245 (1968). Ch. 1, n. 94; Ch. 9, n. 43; Ch. 11, n. 106.

Wohlert v. Seibert, 23 Pa. Super. 213 (1903). Ch. 18, n. 25.

Yorston v. Pennell, 397 Pa. 28, 153 A.2d 255 (1959). Ch. 28, n. 6.

Rhode Island

Macomber v. State Board of Health, 28 R.I. 3, 65 A. 263 (1906). Ch. 11, n. 59.

Moss v. Clark, 146 A.2d 924 (1958). Ch. 33, n. 28.

Rhode Island Ophthalmological Society v. Cannon, 317 A.2d 124 (1974). Ch. 1, n. 170, Table 4; Ch. 3, n. 47; Ch. 9, n. 50; Ch. 10, n. 29, 30.

Wilkinson v. Vesey, 110 R.I. 606, 295 A.2d 676 (1972). Ch. 22, n. 4, Table 2.

South Carolina

Botehlo v. Bycura, 320 S.E.2d 59 (S.C. App. 1984). Ch. 18, n. 21; Ch. 35, n. 7.

Ezell v. Ritholz, 188 S.C. 39, 198 S.E. 419 (1938). Ch. 5, n. 11; Ch. 9, n. 22; Ch. 11, n. 69.

Graham v. Whitaker, 321 S.E.2d 40 (1984). Ch. 18, n. 38; Ch. 28, n. 23; Ch. 29, n. 12.

Green v. Shaw, 136 S.C. 56, 134 S.E. 226 (1926). Ch. 33, n. 22.

Melton v. Ezell, 250 S.C. 183, 156 S.E.2d 871 (1967). Ch. 1, n. 94.

State Board of Medical Examiners v. Gandy, 149 S.E.2d 644 (1966). Ch. 11, n. 59.

Whitfield v. Daniel Construction Co., 83 S.E.2d 460 (1954). Ch. 32, n. 7.

South Dakota

Brown v. State Board of Examiners in Optometry, 263 N.W.2d 490 (1978). Ch. 11, n. 97.

Cunningham v. Yankton Clinic, 262 N.W.2d 508 (1978). Ch. 22, Table 3.

Mordhorst v. Egert, 223 N.W.2d 501 (1974). Ch. 11, n. 71.

O'Connor v. Bonney, 57 S.D. 134, 231 N.W. 521 (1930). Ch. 35, n. 7.

Tennessee

Beaman v. Schwartz, 738 S.W.2d 632 (1986). Ch. 30, n. 30.

Bowser-Briggs v. Bennett, 224 Tenn. 565, 458 S.W.2d 729 (1970). Ch. 33, n. 48; Ch. 35, n. 4.

Haskins v. Howard, 16 S.W.2d 20 (1929). Ch. 20, n. 41.

Longmire v. Hoey, 512 S.W.2d 307 (1974). Ch. 22, Table 1.

Saunders v. Swann, 155 Tenn. 310, 292 S.W. 458 (1927). Ch. 9, n. 10.

Vaughn v. Shelton, 514 S.W.2d 879 (Tenn. App. 1974). Ch. 27, n. 49.

Wharton Transport Co, Inc. v. Bridges, 606 S.W.2d 521 (1980). Ch. 32, n. 3.

Texas

Allison v. State, 76 S.W.2d 527 (Tex. Crim. App. 1934). Ch. 9, n. 9.

American General Insurance Co. v. Florez, 327 S.W.2d 643 (Tex. Civ. App. 1959). Ch. 33, n. 50.

Baker v. Texas, 240 S.W. 924 (Tex. Crim. App. 1921). Ch. 1, n. 45, 51, 60, Table 1.

Barbee v. Rogers, 425 S.W.2d 342 (1968). Ch. 2, n. 16, Table 2; Ch. 21, n. 6; Ch. 27, n. 40, 56; Ch. 30, n. 21.

Callison v. Red, 149 S.W.2d 153 (Tex. Civ. App. 1941). Ch. 29, n. 9.

Gaut v. Quast, 505 S.W.2d 367 (Tex. Civ. App. 1974). Ch. 22, Table 1.

Gooden v. Tips, 651 S.W.2d 364 (Tex. Civ. App. 1983). Ch. 32, n. 10.

Gravis v. Physicians and Surgeons Hospital of Alice, 415 S.W.2d 674 (Tex. Civ. App. 1967). Ch. 22, Table 1.

Hackler v. Ingram, 196 S.W. 279 (Tex. Civ. App. 1917). Ch. 33, n. 22.

Henderson v. Mason, 386 S.W.2d 879 (Tex. Civ. App. 1964). Ch. 26, n. 17.

Hoffman v. Houston Clinic, 41 S.W.2d 134 (Tex. Civ. App. 1931). Ch. 18, n. 22; Ch. 26, n. 11.

Lee v. Dewbre, 362 S.W.2d 900 (Tex. Civ. App. 1962). Ch. 13, n. 30.

Marsh v. Arnold, 446 S.W.2d 949 (Tex. Civ. App. 1969). Ch. 22, Table 1.

Miles v. Harris, 194 S.W. 839 (Tex. Civ. App. 1917). Ch. 13, n. 26.

Miles v. Meadows, 309 S.W.2d 284 (Tex. Civ. App. 1958). Ch. 35, n. 7.

Miller v. Hooper, 94 S.W.2d 230 (Tex. Civ. App. 1936). Ch. 33, n. 52.

Morris v. Rousos, 397 S.W.2d 504 (Tex. Civ. App. 1965). Ch. 20, n. 18.

Muro v. Houston Fire and Gas Insurance Co., 329 S.W.2d 326 (Tex. Civ. App. 1959). Ch. 33, n. 32.

Robertus v. State, 119 Tex, Crim. Rep. 370, 45 S.W.2d 595 (Tex. Crim. App. 1931). Ch. 9, n. 9, 14.

Smith v. Thornhill, 25 S.W.2d 597 (1930). Ch. 13, n. 2.

Speer v. State, 109 S.W.2d 1150 (Tex. Civ. App. 1937). Ch. 11, n. 92.

Texas State Board of Examiners in Optometry v. Lane, 306 S.W.2d 212 (Tex. Civ. App. 1957). Ch. 5, n. 37; Ch. 11, n. 74.

Texas State Board of Medical Examiners v. McClellan, 307 S.W.2d 317 (Tex. Civ. App. 1957). Ch. 11, n. 86.

Walstrom Optical Co. v. Miller, 59 S.W. 2d 895 (Tex. Civ. App. 1933). Ch. 21, n. 11; Ch. 27, n. 13.

Utah

Barry v. Moench, 8 Utah 2d 191, 331 P.2d 814 (1958). Ch. 20, n. 25.

Ficklin v. MacFarlane, 550 P.2d 1295 (1976). Ch. 22, Table 1.

Golding v. Shubach Optical Co., 70 P.2d 871 (1937). Ch. 9, n. 23.

Moormeister v. Department of Registration of the State of Utah, 76 Utah 146, 288 P. 900 (1930). Ch. 11, n. 59.

Moormeister v. Golding, Director of Registration Department, 84 Utah 324, 27 P.2d 447 (1933). Ch. 11, n. 59.

Ricks v. Budge, 64 P.2d 208 (1937). Ch. 13, n. 34.

Vermont

Small v. Gifford Memorial Hospital, 133 Vt. 552, 349 A.2d 703 (1975). Ch. 22, Table 1.

Stevens v. Hill, 74 Vt. 164, 52 A. 437 (1902). Ch. 11, n. 59.

Virginia

Blue Cross of Virginia v. Commonwealth of Virginia, 269 S.E.2d 827 (1980). Ch. 1, n. 198, Table 4; Ch. 12, n. 23.
Bly v. Rhoads, 216 Va. 645, 222 S.E.2d 783 (1976). Ch. 22, Table 1.
County of Campbell v. Howard, 133 Va. 19, 112 S.E. 876 (1922). Ch. 35, n. 16.
Reed v. Church, 8 S.E.2d 285 (1940). Ch. 19, n. 26; Ch. 28, n. 4, 9.
Ritholz v. Commonwealth, 184 Va. 339, 35 S.E.2d 210 (1945). Ch. 9, n. 29; Ch. 11, n. 69.

Washington

Archer v. Galbraith, 18 Wash. App. 369 (1977). Ch. 22, n. 15.
Baxter v. Ford Motor Co., 168 Wash. 456, 12 P.2d 409, *affirmed* 15 P.2d 1118 (1932). Ch. 21, n. 4.
Gates v. Jensen, 92 Wash. 2d 246, 595 P.2d 919 (1979), *reversing* 20 Wash. App. 81, 579 P.2d 374 (1978). Ch. 2, n. 27, 31, Table 1; Ch. 22, n. 17, Table 2; Ch. 23, n. 12.
Gross v. Partlow, 68 P.2d 1034 (1937). Ch. 13, n. 5.
Harris v. Groth, 99 Wash. 2d 438, 663 P.2d 113 (1983). Ch. 2, n. 27.
Helling v. Carey, 83 Wash. 2d 514, 519 P.2d 981 (1974). Ch. 2, n. 27, Table 1; Ch. 21, n. 34; Ch. 23, n. 6, 7, 20; Ch. 30, n. 20.
Hinds v. Johnson, 347 P.2d 828 (1959). Ch. 33, n. 27.
Kaiser v. Suburban Transportation System, 65 Wash. 2d 461, 398 P.2d 14 (1965). Ch. 28, n. 24; Ch. 32, n. 12.
Keogan v. Holy Family Hospital, 22 Wash. App. 366, 589 P.2d 310, *cert. denied* 601 P.2d 1303 (1979). Ch. 22, Table 2.
Ketcham v. King County Medical Service Corp., 81 Wash. 2d 565, 502 P.2d 1197 (1972). Ch. 12, n. 7.
Mazetti v. Armour and Co., 75 Wash. 672, 135 P. 633 (1913). Ch. 21, n. 3.
Medical Examining Board v. Stewart, 46 Wash. 79, 89 P. 475 (1907). Ch. 11, n. 59.
Meeks v. Marx, 15 Wash. App. 571, 550 P.2d 1158 (1976). Ch. 2, n. 27.
Peddicord v. Lieser, 105 P.2d 5 (1940). Ch. 18, n. 39.
Ruth v. Dight, 453 P.2d 631 (1969). Ch. 19, n. 56.
State Board of Medical Examiners v. Macy, 92 Wash. 614, 159 P. 801 (1916). Ch. 11, n. 52.
Teig v. St. John's Hospital, 387 P.2d 527 (1963). Ch. 27, n. 43.
Walker v. Rynd, 280 P.2d 259 (1955). Ch. 29, n. 17.

West Virginia

Browning v. Hoffman, 111 S.E. 492 (1922). Ch. 13, n. 16; Ch. 19, n. 35.
Eisensmith v. Buhl Optical Co., 178 S.E. 695 (1934). Ch. 9, n. 22.
Hundley v. Martinez, 158 S.E.2d 159 (1967). Ch. 20, n. 40.
Lawson v. Conaway, 16 S.E. 564 (1892). Ch. 19, n. 61.
Mingo County Medical Society, Inc. v. Simon, 124 W. Va. 493, 20 S.E.2d 807 (1942). Ch. 11, n. 84.
Serian v. State of West Virginia, 297 S.E.2d 889 (1982). Ch. 11, n. 70, 89.

Wisconsin

Cook v. Thomas, 25 Wis. 2d 467, 131 N.W.2d 299 (1964). Ch. 14, n. 16.
Kosak v. Boyce, 201 N.W. 757 (1925). Ch. 26, n. 9, 10.
LeBow v. Optometry Examining Board, 52 Wis. 2d 569, 191 N.W.2d 47 (1971). Ch. 11, n. 94.
Miller v. Anderson, 183 Wis. 163, 196 N.W. 869 (1924). Ch. 35, n. 16.
Price v. State, 168 Wis. 603, 171 N.W. 77 (1919). Ch. 9, n. 13; Ch. 11, n. 105.
Reidinger v. Optometry Examining Board, 81 Wis. 2d 292, 260 N.W.2d 270 (1977). Ch. 11, n. 84.
Ritholz v. Johnson, 246 Wis. 442, 17 N.W.2d 590 (1945). Ch. 9, n. 30; Ch. 11, n. 69.
Scaria v. St. Paul Fire and Marine Insurance Co., 68 Wis. 2d 1, 227 N.W.2d 647 (1975). Ch. 22, Table 2.
State v. Schaeffer, 129 Wis. 459, 109 N.W. 522 (1906). Ch. 11, n. 59.
State of Wisconsin ex rel. Harris v. Kindy Optical Co., 282 N.W. 283 (1940). Ch. 9, n. 23.
Trogun v. Fruchtman, 58 Wis. 2d 596, 207 N.W.2d 297 (1973). Ch. 22, Table 2; Ch. 28, n. 7.

Wyoming

Govin v. Hunter, 374 P.2d 421 (1962). Ch. 22, Table 1.

Stundon v. Stadnik, 469 P.2d 16 (1970). Ch. 22, Table 1.

United States Supreme Court

American Medical Association v. Federal Trade Commission, 638 F.2d 443 (2d Cir. 1980), *affirmed* 455 U.S. 676, 102 S. Ct. 1744 (1982). Ch. 3, n. 18, 19.

Barsky v. Board of Regents of the University of the State of New York, 347 U.S. 442, 74 S. Ct. 650 (1954). Ch. 11, n. 45, 49.

Bates v. State Bar of Arizona, 433 U.S. 350, 97 S. Ct. 2691 (1977). Ch. 1, n. 183, Table 4; Ch. 4, Table 3; Ch. 5, n. 23; Ch. 9, n. 35.

Blue Shield of Virginia v. McCready, 649 F.2d 228 (4th Cir. 1981), *affirmed* 457 U.S. 465, 102 S. Ct. 2540 (1982). Ch. 12, n. 25.

Dred Scott v. Sandford, 60 U.S. (1 How.) 393 (1857). Ch. 7, n. 12.

Evans v. Gore, 253 U.S. 245, 40 S. Ct. 550 (1920). Ch. 40, n. 5.

Flint v. Stone Tracy Co., 220 U.S. 107, 31 S. Ct. 342 (1911). Ch. 40, n. 4.

Friedman v. Rogers, 438 F. Supp. 428 (D.C. Tex. 1977), *reversed* 440 U.S. 1, 99 S. Ct. 887 (1979). Ch. 1, n. 190, 191, Table 4; Ch. 5, n. 31; Ch. 7, n. 15; Ch. 11, n. 6, 59, 77; Ch. 39, n. 23.

Gibson v. Berryhill, 331 F. Supp. 122 (D.C. Ala. 1971), *affirmed* 441 U.S. 564, 93 S. Ct. 1689 (1973). Ch. 1, n. 180, 181, Table 4; Ch. 5, n. 21; Ch. 7, n. 15; Ch. 11, n. 5, 59.

Graham v. Richardson, 403 U.S. 365, 91 S. Ct. 1848 (1971). Ch. 11, n. 26.

Griswold v. Connecticut, 381 U.S. 479, 85 S. Ct. 1678 (1965). Ch. 20, n. 32.

Hawker v. People of New York, 170 U.S. 189, 18 S. Ct. 573 (1893). Ch. 11, n. 49.

Head v. New Mexico Board of Examiners in Optometry, 374 U.S. 424, 83 S. Ct. 1759 (1963). Ch. 1, n. 139, Table 3; Ch. 5, n. 18.

In re Griffiths, 413 U.S. 717, 93 S. Ct. 2851 (1973). Ch. 11, n. 24.

Leyra v. Denno, 113 F. Supp. 556 (D.C. N.Y. 1950), *affirmed* 208 F.2d 605 (2d Cir. 1954), *reversed* 347 U.S. 556, 74 S. Ct. 716 (1954). Ch. 20, n. 16.

Lilly et ux v. Commissioner of Internal Revenue, 343 U.S. 90, 72 S. Ct. 497 (1951). Ch. 3, n. 32.

Marbury v. Madison, 5 U.S. (1 Cranch.) 137 (1803). Ch. 7, n. 11.

McNaughton v. Johnson, 242 U.S. 344, 37 S. Ct. 178 (1917). Ch. 1, n. 61, 62, Table 1; Ch. 9, n. 6; Ch. 10, n. 8.

Meffert v. State Board of Medical Registration and Education, 66 Kan. 710, 72 P. 247, *affirmed* 195 U.S. 625, 25 S. Ct. 790 (1903). Ch. 11, n. 48, 59.

Metropolitan Life Insurance Co. v. Massachusetts, — U.S. —, 105 S. Ct. 2380 (1985). Ch. 12, n. 18.

New York Times v. Sullivan, 376 U.S. 254, 84 S. Ct. 710 (1964). Ch. 20, n. 9.

Roe v. Wade, 410 U.S. 113, 93 S. Ct. 705 (1973). Ch. 7, n. 4; Ch. 32, n. 21.

Roschen v. Ward, 279 U.S. 337, 49 S. Ct. 336 (1929). Ch. 1, n. 87, Table 2; Ch. 9, n. 18.

Semler v. Oregon State Board of Dental Examiners, 294 U.S. 608, 55 S. Ct. 570 (1935). Ch. 1, n. 100, Table 2; Ch. 4, Table 3; Ch. 5, n. 16; Ch. 9, n. 34.

State of Missouri ex rel. Hurwitz v. North, et al., Board of Health of the State of Missouri, 271 U.S. 40, 46 S. Ct. 384 (1925). Ch. 11, n. 54.

Sugarman v. Douglas, 413 U.S. 634, 93 S. Ct. 2842 (1973). Ch. 11, n. 25.

Terminal-Hudson Electronics, Inc. v. Department of Consumer Affairs, 407 F. Supp. 1075, *vacated and remanded* 426 U.S. 916, 96 S. Ct. 2619 (1976). Ch. 11, n. 82.

Virginia State Board of Pharmacy v. Virginia Citizens Consumer Council, 425 U.S. 748, 96 S. Ct. 1817 (1976). Ch. 1, n. 182; Ch. 5, n. 22.

Wall v. American Optometric Association, 179 F. Supp 175 (D.C. Ga. 1974), *affirmed* 419 U.S. 888, 95 S. Ct. 166 (1974). Ch. 11, n. 59.

Williamson v. Lee Optical of Oklahoma, 120 F. Supp. 128 (D.C. Okla. 1954), *reversed* 348 U.S. 483, 75 S. Ct. 461 (1955). Ch. 1, n. 134, 135, 136, 137, Table 3; Ch. 4, Table 3; Ch. 5, n. 17, 28; Ch. 7, n. 15; Ch. 9, n. 26; Ch. 11, n. 80; Ch. 17, n. 12.

Yarborough v. Yarborough, 290 U.S. 202, 54 S. Ct. 181 (1933). Ch. 13, n. 14.

United States Circuit Courts of Appeals (excluding the District of Columbia)

Napier v. Greenzweig, 256 F. 196 (2d Cir. 1919). Ch. 26, n. 29.

Kresge v. Ottinger, 29 F.2d 762 (2d Cir. 1928). Ch. 1, n. 86.

Roschen v. Ottinger, 29 F. 2d 762 (2d Cir. 1928). Ch. 1, n. 86.

Toal v. United States, 438 F.2d 222 (2d Cir. 1971). Ch. 19, n. 58.

Eder v. Beal, 609 F.2d 695 (3d Cir. 1979). Ch. 12, n. 14.

Panko v. Consolidated Mutual Insurance Co., 423 F.2d 41 (3d Cir. 1970). Ch. 20, n. 28.

Walker v. Pierce, 560 F.2d 609 (4th Cir. 1977). Ch. 22, Table 3.

Karp v. Cooley, 493 F.2d 408 (5th Cir. 1974). Ch. 22, Table 1.
Kurzner v. United States, 413 F.2d 97 (5th Cir. 1969). Ch. 39, n. 4.
Pushkin v. Califano, 600 F.2d 486 (5th Cir, 1979). Ch. 1, n. 197; Ch. 8, n. 46; Ch. 12, n. 8.
Sandefur v. Cherry, 547 F. Supp 418 (D.C. La. 1982), *vacated and remanded* 718 F.2d 1157 (5th Cir. 1983), *certified* 721 F.2d 511 (5th Cir. 1983), *reversed* 744 F.2d 1157 (5th Cir. 1984). Ch. 1, n. 197; Ch. 8, n. 57; Ch. 12, n. 12, 24.

O'Neill v. United States, 410 F.2d 888 (6th Cir. 1969). Ch. 39, n. 4.
Rusin v. Glendale Optical Co., Inc., 805 F.2d 650 (6th Cir. 1986). Ch. 27, n. 9.

Collins v. American Optometric Association, 693 F.2d 636 (7th Cir. 1982). Ch. 2, n. 7, 23; Ch. 23, n. 33.
Filler v. Rayex Corp., 435 F.2d 336 (7th Cir. 1970). Ch. 2, n. 11, Table 1; Ch. 21, n. 6; Ch. 27, n. 26, 29.
Lloyd v. Kull, 329 F.2d 168 (7th Cir. 1964). Ch. 22, Table 1.

Freeman v. Lockhart, 503 F.2d 1016 (8th Cir. 1974). Ch. 2, n. 9.
Landon v. Kansas City Gas Co., 10 F.2d 263 (8th Cir. 1926). Ch. 13, n. 1.
Pegram v. Sisco, 406 F. Supp 776 (D.C. Ark 1976), *affirmed* 547 F.2d 1172 (8th Cir. 1976). Ch. 22, Table 1.

Schulz v. Commissioner, 294 F.2d 52 (9th Cir. 1961). Ch. 48, n. 7.
United States v. Kintner, 216 F.2d 418 (9th Cir. 1954). Ch. 39, n. 1.

Empey v. United States, 406 F.2d 157 (10th Cir. 1959). Ch. 39, n. 4.
Iverson v. Frandsen, 237 F.2d 898 (10th Cir. 1956). Ch. 20, n. 18.
Lambert v. Park, 597 F.2d 236 (10th Cir. 1979). Ch. 22, Table 2.

United States District Courts

Roberts v. Woods, 206 F. Supp. 579 (D.C. Ala. 1962). Ch. 22, Table 1.
Steele v. United States, 463 F. Supp. 321 (D.C. Alas. 1978). Ch. 2, n. 20; Ch. 24, n. 2; Ch. 31, n. 23.
California Citizens Action Group v. Department of Consumer Affairs, 407 F. Supp. 1075 (D.C. Cal. 1975). Ch. 11, n. 75.
Ruby v. Massey, 452 F. Supp. 361 (D.C. Conn. 1978). Ch. 22, Table 3.
DiFebo v. Keve, 395 F. Supp. 1350 (D.C. Del. 1975). Ch. 2, n. 10.
Riedinger v. Colburn, 361 F. Supp. 1073 (D.C. Ida. 1973). Ch. 22, Table 1.
Aetna Casualty and Surety Co. of Illinois v. Medical Protective Co., 575 F. Supp. 901 (D.C. Ill. 1983). Ch. 28, n. 33.
Ritholz v. Indiana State Board of Registration and Examination, 45 F. Supp. 423 (D.C. Ind. 1937). Ch. 9, n. 28; Ch. 11, n. 69.
Morgan v. Aetna Casualty Co., 185 F. Supp. 20 (D.C. La. 1960). Ch. 18, n. 33.
Baum v. Turel, 206 F. Supp. 490 (D.C. N.Y. 1962). Ch. 20, n. 41.
Walker v. North Dakota Eye Clinic, Ltd., 415 F. Supp. 891 (D.C. N.D. 1976). Ch. 22, Table 1.
Hammond v. Aetna Casualty Co., 237 F. Supp. 96 (D.C. Ohio 1956). Ch. 20, n. 28.
Foreman v. United States, 232 F. Supp. 134 (D.C. Fla. 1964). Ch. 39, n. 2.
Galt v. United States 175 F. Supp. 360 (D.C. Tex. 1959). Ch. 39, n. 2.
Simpson v. Wilson, 480 F. Supp. 97 (D.C. Vt. 1979). Ch. 12, n. 13.

Tax Courts

Garland v. Commissioner, 73 T.C. 5 (1979). Ch. 39, n. 21.
Johnson v. United States, 7 A.F.T.R.2d 793 (D.C. Tex. 1961). Ch. 48, n. 8.
Keller v. Commissioner, 77 T.C. 1014 (1981). Ch. 39, n. 21.
Kiddie v. Commissioner, 69 T.C. 1055 (1978). Ch. 39, n. 21.
Roubik and Roubik v. Commissioner, 53 T.C. 365 (1969). Ch. 39, n. 6.

APPENDIX CONTENTS

Section III—Patient Management and the Problem-Oriented Record System*

Part A—Assess Your Recordkeeping System

	YES	NO
1. Your patient record is intended as one measure of your optometric competence.	____	____
2. Your patients problems are clearly defined.	____	____
3. The defined problems are listed and dated in a prominent place in the record.	____	____
4. Problems which might develop have been considered.	____	____
5. All reasonable diagnostic possibilities have been listed.	____	____
6. A progress note contains subjective review, objective testing, assessment or progress and continued plan.	____	____
7. Each progress note is indexed to refer to a specific problem.	____	____
8. Your routine data base (history and patient work-up) is sufficient to catch all pertinent problems.	____	____

SCORING

8 Yes Answers:
Excellent, your records not only offer proper guidance for effective patient care but protect you legally through proper documentation.

7 Yes Answers:
Good, your records need some work so concentrate on weak areas.

6 Yes Answers:
Fair, a serious review of your record keeping system is in order.

*Source: Scope of Practice: Patient Care and Management Manual. American Optometric Association, St. Louis, 1986. Reprinted with permission.

Part B—The Problem-Oriented Record System

The problem-oriented record system is solution oriented. It aids the doctor in logical patient management by helping define problems, plan for their resolution, and properly monitor their progress. The problem-oriented system aids the doctor in determining where best to spend his/her time in continuing education and study. It provides feedback on the management skills the doctor must continually update to best care for his/her patient population. It also aids co-management with other health care professions. It assists in optometricolegal protection by providing accurate documentation of patient care. Most importantly, the problem-oriented record system helps bring performance into line with the ideal in patient management and care.

The four steps in the problem-oriented system are:

1. **DATA BASE**
   Patient profile
   History
   Physical/Examination

2. **COMPLETE PROBLEM LIST**
   (#1) ....
   (#2) ....
   (#3) ....

3. **INITIAL PLANS**
   (#1) ....
   Diagnostic Tests
   Rx
   Patient Education

4. **PROGRESS NOTES**
   (#1) ....
   Subjective:
   Objective:
   Assessment:
   Plan:

EXAMPLES OF THE FOUR STEPS IN THE PROBLEM ORIENTED SYSTEM:

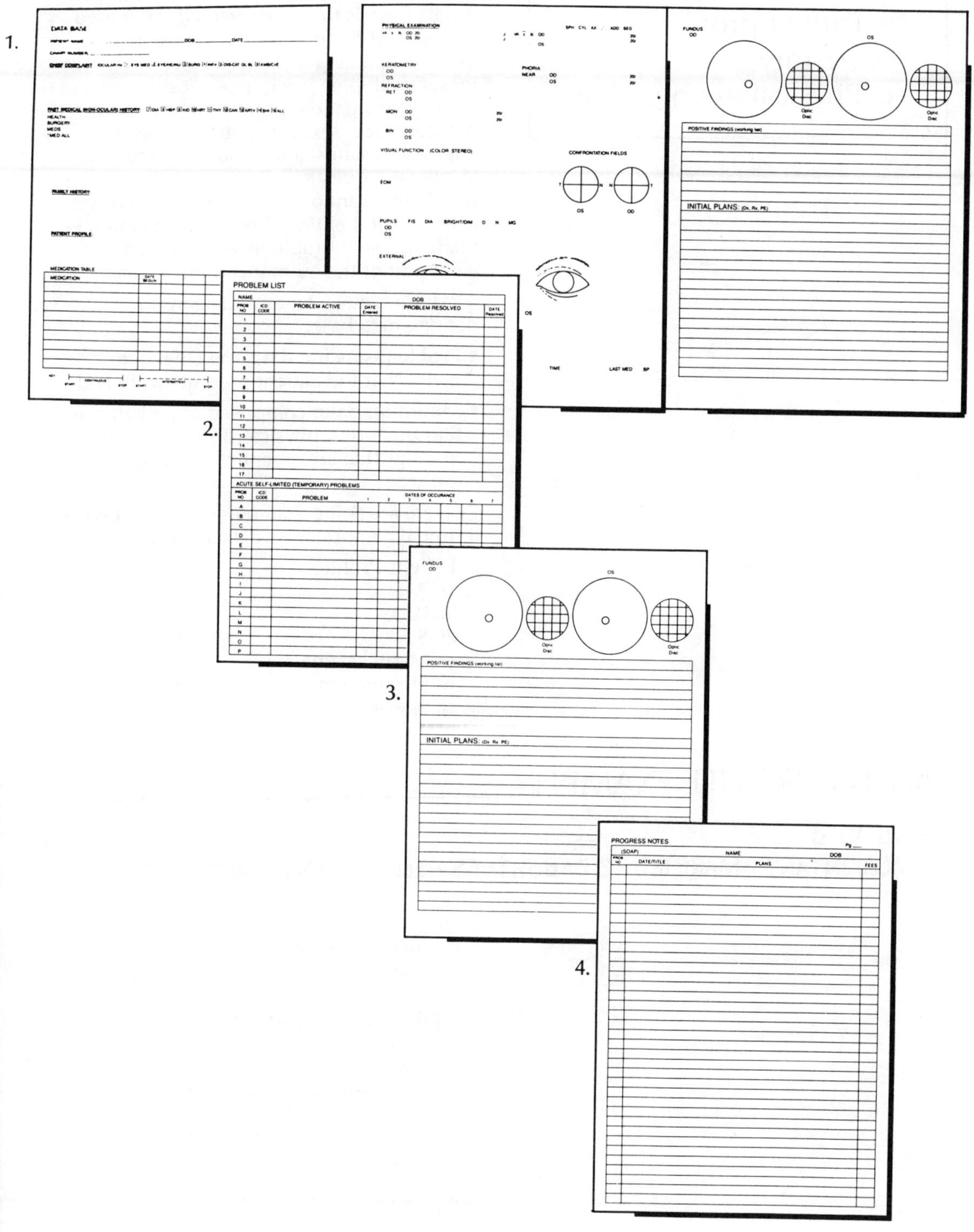

1. DATA BASE
a. Patient profile
b. History
c. Physical/examination

No comprehensive examination or data baseline is totally complete. Time, expense and patient exhaustion must be considered. A data base is therefore defined, or limited to essential findings, rather than complete, or encompassing all possible tests and findings. Developing it requires consideration of the doctor's patient population (for example, age, race, sex, occupation, geography and health status) and should affirmatively answer the question: Does this cover all the problems I cannot afford to miss? It evolves over a period of time when consideration is made for what problems were missed and what part of the exam was unnecessary.

There are two types of data in the defined data base:

- **Problem-specific data:** the chief complaint that the patient presents with; and
- **Minimum data:** comprised of patient profiles, histories, physical, and examination findings that are essential in evaluating every patient.*

Here are some examples of the data base or initial comprehensive data baseline:

a. Patient Profile:
- **i.** Age
- **ii.** Race
- **iii.** Sex
- **iv.** Marital status
- **v.** Occupation
- **vi.** Special needs

PATIENT PROFILE EXAMPLE:

54 YO W ♂
ACCOUNTANT - MARRIED - 2 DAUGHTERS - ENJOYS GOLF - WOOD SHOP

b. History
i. Chief Complaint:
What is wrong, what seems to be the trouble?
When did you first realize something was wrong?
What did you first notice?
Did the (defect) get better, worse, stay same?
Any associated signs or symptoms?

*Usually within a certain age frame: infants, school children, adults and geriatric patients will most probably require individual data bases for the initial comprehensive work-up.

CHIEF COMPLAINT EXAMPLE:

CC: BLURRED ∞ & NEAR VA NOTED 3 MO. - GETTING WORSE

ii. Past Ocular History:

Eye medication
Eye or head injury
Eye surgery
Eye infections
** Eye disease
** Amblyopia, crossed eye

OCULAR HISTORY EXAMPLE:

/ OCULAR Hx [1] EYE MED [2] EYE/HE/INS [3] SURG [4] INF// [5] DIS CAT GL,BL [6] AMB/CXE

iii. Past Health (non-ocular) History:

General health
Surgery
Medications/diet
Medication allergy
** Diabetes
** High blood pressure
** Kidney
** Heart
** Thyroid
** Cancer
** Arthritis
Shingles
Allergy

PAST MEDICAL (NON-OCULAR) HISTORY EXAMPLE:

PAST MEDICAL (NON-OCULAR) HISTORY: [7] DIA [8] HBP [9] KID [10] HRT [11] THY [12] CAN [13] ARTH [14] SHI [15] ALL

HEALTH: FAIR
SURGERY: SKIN CANCER - NOSE - 1983
MEDS: INSULIN 30 UNITS AM - 10 UNITS PM - HYDRO PRES 25 b.i.d. per DR. HANSON
*MED ALL: PENICILLIN

[7] AODM WAS ON DIET & ORALS
[8] HAS BEEN PROBLEM SINCE AGE 45
[12] FACIAL SKIN CANCERS ONLY
[14] TWO EPISODES 1964
1982 CONFINED TO CHEST

iv. Past Familial History:

** Diabetes
** High blood pressure
** Kidney
** Heart
** Thyroid
** Cancer
** Arthritis

**Indicates question applies to both patient and blood relatives.

FAMILY HISTORY EXAMPLE:

5 SISTER = CAT 7 SISTER (ADDM)

c. Physical/Examination

VA c̄ Rx, c̄ PH; VA s̄ Rx
Refraction
Color (monocular)
Confrontation fields
EOM
Pupils
External
Biomicroscopy
Tensions/BP
(Gonioscopy 4 mirror)
BIO
Hruby lens

The data base for a new patient should be able to deal with presenting complaints and screen for other common or important problems. It is a comprehensive evaluation defined by the current standard of care in the health care arena. It can be updated when new diagnostic instruments and techniques become available and if problems are being missed or if some diagnostic tests prove unproductive. Upon future patient evaluations, it can be referred to as an important baseline when compared with new findings. It is much more efficient to view one baseline than several. This is accomplished since only one initial baseline is obtained while the rest of the record becomes problem oriented through the use of a numbered problem list and corresponding numbered progress notes.

PHYSICAL/EXAMINATION EXAMPLE:

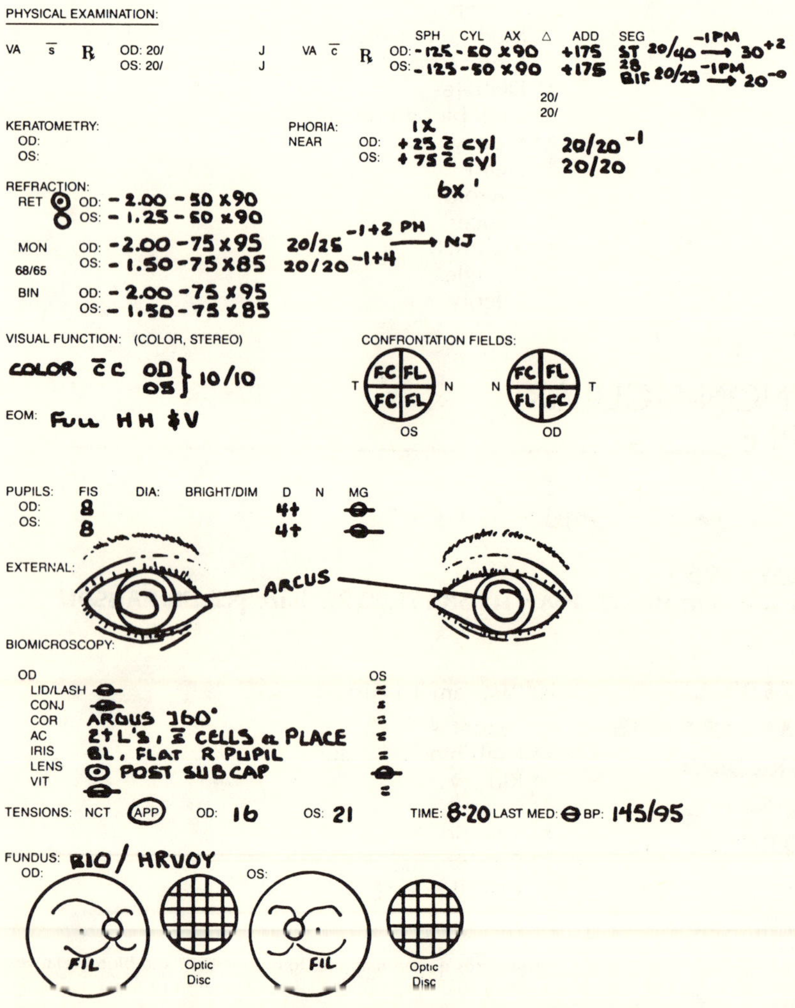

PHYSICAL EXAMINATION:

VA s̄ ℞ OD: 20/ OS: 20/ J J

VA c̄ ℞ SPH CYL AX △ ADD SEG
OD: -125 -50 x90 +175 ST 20/40 -1PM → 30+2
OS: -125 -50 x90 +175 28 BIF 20/25 -1PM → 20-0
20/ 20/

KERATOMETRY: OD: OS:

PHORIA: NEAR 1X
OD: +25 c̄ cyl 20/20-1
OS: +75 c̄ cyl 20/20
6X'

REFRACTION:
RET OD: -2.00 -50 x90
OS: -1.25 -50 x90
MON 68/65 OD: -2.00 -75 x95 20/25 -1+2 PH → NJ
OS: -1.50 -75 x85 20/20 -1+4
BIN OD: -2.00 -75 x95
OS: -1.50 -75 x85

VISUAL FUNCTION: (COLOR, STEREO)
COLOR c̄ c OD OS } 10/10

CONFRONTATION FIELDS:
T FC FL FC FL N — OS
N FC FL FL FC T — OD

EOM: FULL HH & V

PUPILS: FIS DIA: BRIGHT/DIM D N MG
OD: 8 4+ ⊖
OS: 8 4+ ⊖

EXTERNAL: ARCUS

BIOMICROSCOPY:
OD OS
LID/LASH ⊖ =
CONJ ⊖ =
COR ARCUS 360° =
AC 2+ L'S, c̄ CELLS & PLACE =
IRIS BL, FLAT R PUPIL =
LENS ⊙ POST SUBCAP ⊖
VIT ⊖ =

TENSIONS: NCT (APP) OD: 16 OS: 21 TIME: 8:20 LAST MED: ⊖ BP: 145/95

FUNDUS: BIO / HRUBY
OD: FIL Optic Disc
OS: FIL Optic Disc

2. COMPLETE PROBLEM LIST

#1 ....
#2 ....
#3 ....
#4 ....

Problem lists act as a table of contents to the patient's record. It is placed in the front of the patient's chart. A problem list assures thoroughness and reduces fragmented care. This master or complete problem list emerges from a working problem list of positive findings of the data base and their relation to one another.

Working list:

i. All positive findings in data base
ii. Relation to one another

POSITIVE FINDINGS EXAMPLE:

#1 Diabetes Hx
#2 HBP Hx
#3 Skin Cancer Hx
#4 Ref error/Presbyopia
#5 Cataract
#6 Elevated T_A

Complete problem list:

i. Kept in front of patient's chart
ii. Emerges from positive findings
iii. Numbered and titled list of every problem patient has or has had
iv. Anything that requires management or Dx work-up
v. Includes social and demographic problems
vi. List is added to as new problems develop and former problems are resolved
vii. Problem is listed as exactly what one knows—no more and no less (the clinician's highest level of understanding—he/she must not jump to conclusions without further diagnostic tests)

COMPLETE PROBLEM LIST EXAMPLE:

PROBLEM LIST

NAME: WILLIS T. WILLIAMS DOB: 6-22-30

PROB. NO.	ICD CODE	PROBLEM ACTIVE	DATE Entered	PROBLEM RESOLVED	DATE Resolved
1	250	DIABETES Hx	8-2-84		
2	401	HBP Hx	8-2-84		
3	232	SKIN CANCER Hx	8-2-84		
4	367	REFRACTIVE ERROR/PRESBYOPIA	8-2-84		
5	74331	CATARACT	8-2-84		
6	365.00	ELEVATED TA	8-2-84		
7					
8					
9					
10					
11					
12					
13					
14					
15					
16					
17					

ACUTE SELF-LIMITED (TEMPORARY) PROBLEMS

PROB. NO.	ICD CODE	PROBLEM	DATES OF OCCURANCE 1	2	3	4	5	6	7
A									
B									
C									
D									
E									
F									
G									
H									
I									
J									
K									
L									
M									
N									
O									
P									

3. INITIAL PLANS #1 .... Diagnostic Treatment Patient education

An initial plan is developed for each problem you determine to manage, co-manage with another practitioner, or direct to another practitioner for complete care independent of your services. The plan consists of additional diagnostic tests to be done, treatment that will be instituted and patient education.

Plans:

Diagnostic, treatment, patient education

Corresponding numbered plan for each problem consists of the following:

Dx: Differential, rule-outs, tests, consultations

Rx: Specifics of treatment, goals, contingency plans

PE: Instruction, advice, information, follow-up recall

INITIAL PLAN EXAMPLE:

INITIAL PLANS: (Dx, Rx, PE)
#1 DX: BIO/HRUBY & SCREEN B.S. 12MO
PE: EDUCATE ON EYE SIGNS. RTC 12MO: 8-2-85 @ 10:30
#2 DX: MONITOR B.P. & FUNDUS 12MO
PE: EDUCATE ON EYE SIGNS, RTC 12MO
#3 DX: EXTERNAL 12 MO
PE: CAUTION PT. TO WATCH SIGNS, RTC 12MO
#4 Rx: OD −2.00 −.75 x 95 @ +225 ADD 22 62/65 MENTOR-WHITE
OS −1.50 −.75 x85 ST28 TRI 54-18-135
DX: RE·CK VA's 3MO
PE: EXPLAIN Δ IN Rx c̄ Δ IN CAT, RTC 3MO: 11-2-84 @ 8:15
#5 DX: RE·CK SLEx & VA
PE: EDUCATE ON CAT, RTC 3MO
#6 DX: TA, HRUBY, (FIELDS) 1MO
PE: EDUCATE ON GLA, NEED FOR F/U, RTC 1MO: 9-15-85 @ 9:15
(FEES)

4. PROGRESS NOTES

#1 Narrative Notes

....

Subjective
Objective
Assessment
Plans

Progress notes are made on each managed problem and are numbered and titled to correspond to the complete problem list which is kept at the front of the record. The note is also dated and the SOAP format is utilized.

The SOAP format is also utilized for the work-up of the "non-appointment" new patient seeking care for a single problem (e.g. foreign body to the external eye). The first problem on the problems list should be labled: #1 Incomplete Data Base. A plan should then be developed for this problem in addition to the patient's presenting problem (foreign body).

(Problem #), (Date), (Title of problem from problem list)

S: Subjective, how patient feels, updated case history

O: Objective, measurements, test results, exam observations

A: Assessment, status of problem, progress of care, new problems

P: RX:
DX:
PE:

Progress Notes Example:

PROGRESS NOTES Pg.____

(SOAP) NAME: WILLIS T. WILLIAMS DOB: 6-22-30

PROB. NO.	DATE/TITLE PLANS	FEES
6	9-15-84 ELEVATED TA	
	S: SEEING FINE. ⊖ SX	
	O= TA @ 9:15 15/20, BP: 145/95	
	4 MIRROR: 3+6's $\bar{s}$ PIGMENT O.U.	
	FIELDS: AUTO FIELDS: ⊖ ANOMALIES O.U. (SEE CHART)	
	A= STABLE	
	P= DX RE-CK TA 2MO	
	PE: STABLE. RTC 2MO: 11-2-84 / 8:15	(FEE)
4	11-2-84 REF ERROR / PRES	
	S: ↓ VA OD @ ∞, ESP NITE DRIVE	
	O: V$\bar{c}$c OD $20/40^{-1+2}$ $\xrightarrow{PH}$ 25^{-1} OS $20/20^{-1+4}$	
	REF OD -2.75 -.75 x 90 = $20/25^{-2}$ 14B -50 w/c = $20/20^{-2}$	
	OS -1.50 -.75 x 85 = $20/20^{-1+4}$ +75 = 20/20	
	A: Δ OD ERROR	
	P: Rx: OD -2.75 -.75 x 90 ◇ +2.25 ST 25 TRI (L.O)	
	OS ⊖	
	Dx: CK VA's 3 MO	
	PE: EXPLAIN & DEMO Δ IN OD LENS. RTC 3 MO 2-10-85 @ 10:30	
5	11-2-85 CATARACT	
	O: SLEx. APPEARANCE OF OPACITY UNCHANGED	
	P: DX: RE-CK 3MO	
6	11-2-85 ELEVATED TA	
	O: TA 17/22 @ 8:25, BP 142/92	
	BIO/HRUBY: OD ⊖	
	OS 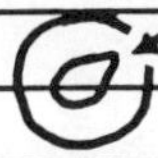 QUESTION NICKING	
	A: R/O OAG O.S.	
	P: DX: DIURNALS & FIELDS STUDY NEXT WK	
	PE: EXPLAIN POSSIBLE OAG, NEED FOR F/U. RTC 11-5-85 @ 8:00	(FEE)
6	11-5-85 ELEVATED TA	
	O: TA @ 8:00 20/26, 10:00 18/25, 1:00 16/22, 4:30 17/22	
	AUTO FIELDS: OD = ⊖ OS: INF ARCUATE SCOTOMA (SEE CHART)	
	A: ELEVATED TA $\bar{c}$ SCOTOMA	
	P: DX: CONSULT $\bar{c}$ JOHN FORD, M.D. (GLAU SPEC) + REPORT TO G.P.	
	PE: EXPLAIN NEED CONSULT (APPT 10:30/11-8-85), RTC 1WK	
	POST CONSULT: 11-15-85 @ 8:30	(FEE)

Part C—Consultation Reports

Consultation reports can easily be dictated from the information on the problem orientated record. These reports are sent to consultants and general practitioners. Following is an example of a consultation report.

OPTOMETRIC ASSOCIATES

• JOHN SMITH, O.D.
• JANE DOE, O.D.

PHONE (123) 456-7890
100 FIRST STREET
ANYWHERE, STATE

CONSULTATION REPORT

FROM:	John Smith, O.D.	DATE:	11-6-84
PATIENT:	Willis T. Williams 101 South Street Anywhere, State	EXAM: DOB:	8-2-84 6-22-30

CHIEF COMPLAINT:	Blur distance and near
PATIENT PROFILE:	54 year old white male accountant. Married, 2 daughters
OCULAR HISTORY:	Patient reports use of Visine for red eyes as needed. There is no history of eye or head injury, surgery, diseases or infection.
PAST MEDICAL (non-ocular) HISTORY:	General health is reported as fair. There is a surgical history of skin cancer of nose 1983. Medication reported for adult onset diabetic melitis, insulin 30 units AM and 10 units PM, and for HBP Hydropres 25 b.i.d. The most recent episode of shingles was in 1982. There is a history of allergy to penicillin.
FAMILIAL HISTORY:	A sister is reported to have cataracts and diabetes.
REFRACTION:	Correction for myopic astigmatism gives OD 20/25 − 1 + 2, and OS 20/20 − 1 + 4. Phorias are within normal limits.
COLOR:	Each eye identifies 10 of 10 plates correctly.
FIELDS:	Each eye is full to finger counting.
EOM:	Versions and vergences were full.

Part C—Consultation Reports (con't)

page 2

PUPILS:	Each eye reacts 4 + to light both direct and consensually. There is no Marcus Gunn pupil.
BIOMICROSCOPY:	Lids, lashes, conjunctiva were clear and corneas exhibit arcus, Anterior chambers were of normal depth with no cells or flare, angles appear 3 + open, irides are blue, flat and form round pupils O.U. OD lens shows 1 + posterior subcapsular cataract while OS is 100% clear. Vitreous is clear O.U.
TENSIONS:	Applanation tonometry was 16/21 at 8:20 AM and BP was 145/95.
OPHTHALMOSCOPY:	Posterior poles are unremarkable with foveal reflexes and .3/.3 C/D ratios.
PROBLEMS:	#1 Diabetes Hx #2 HBP Hx #3 Skin Cancer #4 Refraction error/presbyopia #5 Cataract #6 Elevated tension
FOLLOW-UP:	#6 11-5-84 Elevated tension S = Asymptomatic O = Ta 8:00 20/26 10:00 18/25 1:00 16/22 4:30 17/22 Fields (auto): OS inferior arcuate scotoma A = OS elevated Ta, scotoma P = Dx: consult with Dr. John Ford, report to Dr. Hansen. PE: Patient app. with Dr. Ford 11-8-84, 10:30 AM

Part D—Episodic Care of the Non-Appointed Patient

A comprehensive examination and the resulting patient management involves the four steps of data base, complete problem list, initial plans and progress notes as just enumerated. For some cases it is not always possible to achieve a comprehensive examination or complete data base. For example; foreign body to the external eye. In these cases episodic care for a non-appointed patient must be instituted. The work-up would involve the use of the SOAP format and "incomplete data base" would be listed in the problem list along with "exterior ocular foreign body." An initial plan would be developed for each of these problems:

For example; Episodic problems (non-appointed patient) (problem #) (date) (external f.b.)

PROGRESS NOTES

Pg. 1

(SOAP) NAME: JOHN H. JONES DOB: 7-11-64

PROB. NO.	DATE/TITLE PLANS	FEES
	8-4-84 EXT F.B.	
	S= EXTERNAL F.B. TO O.D. FOLLOWING USE OF POWER DRILL TWO	
	DAYS AGO VISINE USED, NO MED ALLERGY	
	O= VA s̄c OD 20/30 PH→ 20⁻²	
	OS 20/40 PH→ 20	
	SLEx c̄ NAFL OD: 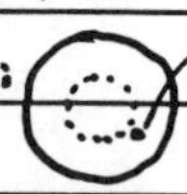 SMALL METALLIC F.B c̄ RUST RING	
	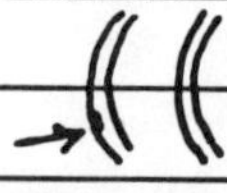 1+CELLS, EVERT LID = ⊖	
	OS: WHITE, QUIET	
	A= #1 INCOMPLETE DATA BASE	
	#2 METALLIC F.B. SUPERFICIAL EPITHELIUM O.D.	
	P= #1 Dx: SET UP COMPREHENSIVE EX FOLLOWING HEALING F.B.	
	PE: NEED FOR COMP. EX (NO PRIOR EYE CARE)	
	#2 Rx: REMOVE F.B. & RUST RING c̄ NEEDLE, INSTILL ii Gtts	
	5% HOMATROPINE SOLN, ii Gtts GARAMYCIN; DISP	
	GARAMYCIN SOLN i Gtt q.i.d WHILE AWAKE,	
	PRESSURE PATCH	
	PE: INSTRUCT ABOVE REGIMEN, INST SAFETY GOGGLES	
	RTC TOMORROW: 10:15 / 8-5-84	

Part E—Hints on Incorporating the PORS into Practice

1. Fix in your mind what you want to happen.
2. Realize that anything new that is worthwhile takes time to learn for both you and staff.
3. Don't waste time trying to create the greatest all-time data base—begin and update later.
4. Implement slowly: use with all new patients and the annual exams of former patients.
5. Remember that you won't really appreciate the system until you get the mechanics down pat. (the 4 steps)
   a. Speed comes with practice.
   b. Learn and use the accepted clinical abbreviations—it can save you valuable time.
6. Meet with staff to review records and emphasize administrative efficiency and better care of your patients through the system.
7. Review ICD codes and define your diagnostic criteria and management plans for the most common presentations.
8. Remember that an inadequate data base produces an inadequate problem list.
9. Remember that interpreting the data base findings incorrectly will produce an incorrect problem list.
10. List a problem as only what you know for sure—nothing more, nothing less.
11. Up-date your reference library and use it. Let your records (problem-oriented feedback) dictate how you spend your continuing education dollars.

SAMPLE INFORMATION FORM

PATIENT REGISTRATION (PLEASE PRINT)

WHOM MAY WE THANK FOR RECOMMENDING US?____________________

▶**PATIENT'S NAME**____________________

MARRIED ☐ SINGLE ☐ DIVORCED ☐ SEPARATED ☐ SPOUSE DECEASED ☐

ADDRESS____________________ DATE OF BIRTH____________________

STREET MONTH DAY YEAR

____________________ RESIDENCE PHONE____________________

CITY STATE ZIP

OCCUPATION____________________

\- -

RESPONSIBLE PARTY'S NAME____________________

MARRIED ☐ SINGLE ☐ DIVORCED ☐ SEPARATED ☐ SPOUSE DECEASED ☐

ADDRESS____________________

STREET CITY ZIP

RESIDENCE PHONE____________________ OCCUPATION____________________

EMPLOYER____________________ BUSINESS ADDRESS____________________

BUSINESS PHONE____________________ PREVIOUS ADDRESS____________________

YOUR SOCIAL SECURITY NUMBER ____________________

HUSBAND'S OR WIFE'S OCCUPATION____________________ EMPLOYER____________________

BUSINESS ADDRESS____________________ BUSINESS PHONE____________________

NAME AND ADDRESS OF NEAREST RELATIVE NOT LIVING WITH RESPONSIBLE PARTY____________________

NAME

____

ADDRESS

LIST THREE CREDIT REFERENCES:

1. ____________________
2. ____________________
3. ____________________

SAMPLE PROBLEM LIST

NAME:				DOB:	
PROB. NO.	ICD CODE	PROBLEM ACTIVE	DATE Entered	PROBLEM RESOLVED	DATE Resolved
1					
2					
3					
4					
5					
6					
7					
8					
9					
10					
11					
12					
13					
14					
15					
16					
17					

ACUTE SELF-LIMITED (TEMPORARY) PROBLEMS

PROB. NO.	ICD CODE	PROBLEM	DATES OF OCCURANCE 1	2	3	4	5	6	7
A									
B									
C									
D									
E									
F									
G									
H									
I									
J									
K									
L									
M									
N									
O									
P									

SAMPLE EXAMINATION FORM

PATIENT NAME________________________ DOB__________ DATE__________________

CHART NUMBER________________

CHIEF COMPLAINT /OCULAR Hx [1] EYE MED [2] EYE/HE/INJ [3] SURG [4] INF// [5] DIS-CAT, GL,BL [6] AMB/CxE

PAST MEDICAL (NON-OCULAR) HISTORY: [7] DIA [8] HBP [9] KID [10] HRT [11] THY [12] CAN [13] ART// [14] SHI [15] ALL

HEALTH:
SURGERY:
MEDS:
*MED ALL:

FAMILY HISTORY:

PATIENT PROFILE:

MEDICATION TABLE

MEDICATION	DATE BEGUN							

KEY: START |——— CONTINUOUS ———| STOP   START |– – – INTERMITTENT – – –| STOP

PHYSICAL EXAMINATION:

SPH CYL AX △ ADD SEG

VA $\bar{s}$ ℞ OD: 20/ J
OS: 20/ J

VA $\bar{c}$ ℞ OD: 20/
OS: 20/

KERATOMETRY:
OD:
OS:

PHORIA:
NEAR OD: 20/
OS: 20/

REFRACTION:
RET OD:
OS:

MON OD: 20/
OS: 20/

BIN OD:
OS:

VISUAL FUNCTION: (COLOR, STEREO)

CONFRONTATION FIELDS:

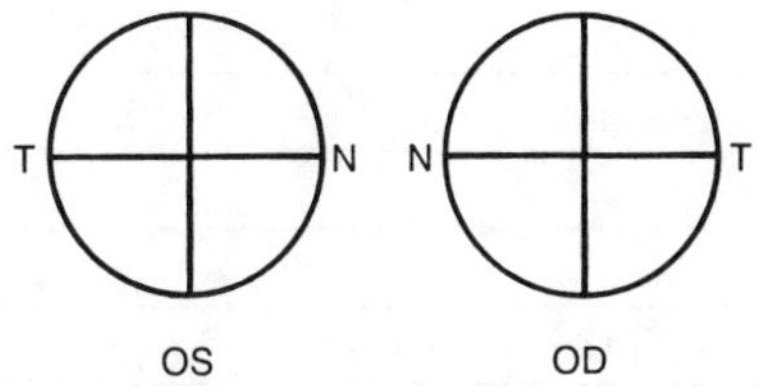

EOM:

PUPILS: FIS DIA: BRIGHT/DIM D N MG
OD:
OS:

EXTERNAL:

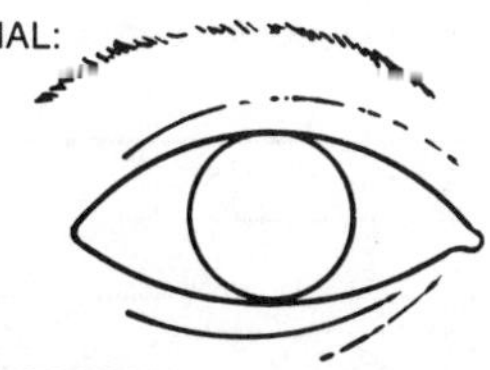

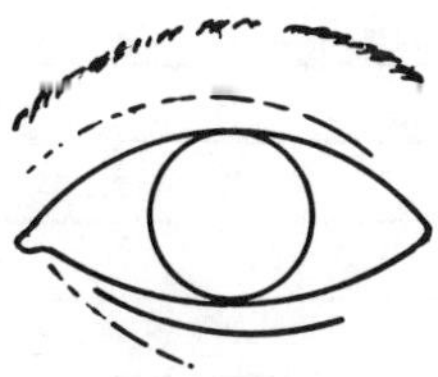

BIOMICROSCOPY:

OD
LID/LASH
CONJ
COR
AC
IRIS
LENS
VIT

OS

TENSIONS: NCT APP OD: OS: TIME: LAST MED: BP:

FUNDUS:

OD: OS:

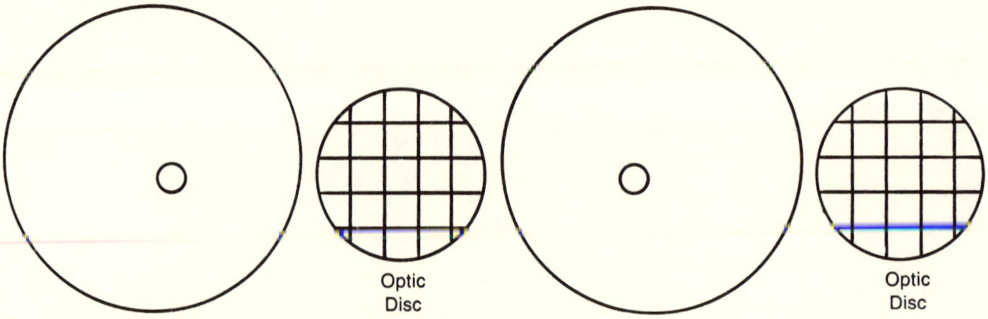

POSITIVE FINDINGS (working list):

INITIAL PLANS: (Dx, Rx, PE)

Sample Employment Agreement*

EMPLOYMENT AGREEMENT

THIS AGREEMENT, made this ___ day of ________ 19________, by and between________, a________ corporation, hereinafter called the "Company", and ________hereinafter called "Employee".

WITNESSETH:

In consideration of the covenants and agreements herein contained and the monies to be paid hereunder, the Company agrees to hire Employee and the Employee agrees to work for the Company upon the Following terms and conditions:

1. *Duties of Employee:* The Employee is employed by the Company as an Optometrist. The Employee will participate as an Optometrist in a program of clinical care requiring the Employee to observe and participate in direct patient contact involving refractions, contact lenses, eye photography, preoperative measurements, ultrasound diagnostic testing, and treatment of eye disease. The Employee will also perform such additional duties as may mutually be agreed upon by the Company and the Employee.

2. *Devotion of Full-Time to Professional Services:* The Employee shall devote substantially all of his business time to rendering services on behalf of the Company.

3. *Compensation:* The Company shall pay to the Employee as compensation for his services a salary as follows:

The sum of________Thousand Dollars ($________) as base Salary, payable in equal monthly installments of $________.

4. *Term of Agreement:* The effective date of this Agreement shall be________19________, and it shall remain and continue in force and effect for one (1) year or until terminated as hereinafter provided.

5. *Automobile:* The Employee shall purchase and own or rent the automobile used by him in the conduct of the Company's business as a condition of his employment, and shall pay for all gas, oils, repairs and maintenance, rent and insurance in connection therewith.

6. *Reimbursable Expenses:* Except as herewith otherwise provided, the Company shall reimburse the Employee for all expenses incurred by him, in and about the course of his employment by the Company. Such expenses shall include, but not be limited to:

(a) All drugs, supplies and professional equipment
(b) All premiums for malpractice insurance which the Employee might at any time carry during the course of employment by the Company
(c) License fees, membership dues in two professional associations, and subscriptions to two professional journals
(d) All ordinary necessary expenses incurred in connection with one major educational meeting

7. *Fees:* The Company shall have exclusive authority to determine the fees, or a procedure for establishing the fees, to be charged patients or customers of the Company, even though such patients or customers may be treated by the Employee in the course of his employment by the Company. All sums paid by any patient or customer of the Company in the way of fees, salary, or otherwise for medical services rendered by the Employee shall be and remain the property of the Company and shall be included in the Company's income.

8. *Patients:* The Company shall have the authority to determine who will be accepted as patients or customers of the Company. The Company shall have the authority to designate or to establish a procedure for designating which professional Employee of the Company will handle each such patient or customer.

9. *Professional Policies and Procedures:* The Company shall have the authority to establish from time to time the professional policies and procedures to be followed by the Employee in handling each individual patient or customer of the Company.

10. *Vacation:* The Employee shall be entitled to such vacation as is authorized by the Company from time to time. The Employee shall be entitled to two (2) weeks of paid vacation time during the term of this contract.

11. *Termination of Agreement:*

(a) The Employee or the Company may voluntarily elect to terminate this Agreement at any time provided that the party electing to terminate must deliver to the other party written notice of such intention to terminate not less than sixty (60) days prior to the date upon which termination is desired.

(b) The Company may terminate this Agreement at any time if the Employee becomes unfit to properly perform his services on behalf of the Company because of any good and sufficient cause or if the Employee becomes legally disqualified to render professional services with the State of________, or accepts employment that, pursuant to existing law, places restrictions or limitations upon his continued rendering of such professional services. Such termination shall be effective upon the delivery of written notice thereof to the Employee or at such later time as may be designated in said notice, and the Employee shall vacate the offices on or before such effective date.

(c) Upon termination of this Agreement as herein above provided, the Employee shall not have the right to make copies of medical records concerning any patient that he may have personally treated.

12. *Death of Employee:* In the event the Employee should die during the term hereof, the Company shall pay to the beneficiary or beneficiaries designated in writing by the Employee and delivered to the Company prior to his death, or, in the absence of such designation, to the Employee's estate, the regular unpaid salary of the Employee to the date of his death.

13. *Limitations on Authority:* Without the express written consent from the Company, the Employee shall not have apparent or implied authority to:

(a) Pledge the credit of the Company or any of its other employees;
(b) Bind the Company under any contract, agreement, note, mortgage, or otherwise;
(c) Release or discharge any debt due the Company unless the Company has received the full amount thereof;
(d) Sell, mortgage, transfer, or otherwise dispose of any assets of the Company

14. *Corporate Health, Group Life, and Retirement Plan Benefits:* The Employee shall be provided with comprehensive major medical insurance coverage for him,______Thousand Dollars ($00,000.00) of group life insurance on his life and coverage under any medical and dental reimbursement and plan which may be provided by the Company. It shall be the responsibility of the Employee to obtain the policies of insurance to which he is entitled hereby with such insurance companies as approved by the Company. He shall apply and submit to any requirement of the insurance company in order to obtain such policies. The Company will pay the premiums for such insurance. The Company is in no way responsible for the failure on the part of the Employee in the event the Employee fails to obtain the insurance. The Company is only responsible for the payment of the premiums on the policies.

15. *Non-Compete Agreement:* The Employee acknowledges that the Company would suffer irreparable harm if the Employee were to use the customer and employee relationships and contacts learned and developed while serving as an employee of the Company, sales and marketing techniques, business systems and methods, and information and knowledge, developed while serving as an employee of the Company in competition with the Company within the Area. Accordingly, the Employee makes the following covenants:

If the Employee's employment by the Company shall be terminated for any reason, the Employee agrees that he shall not practice optometry as an Employee of Physician or Optometrist as an officer, director, or shareholder of a corporation, sole proprietor, independent contractor, partner, or in any other manner after his termination of employment for a period of two years from the date of termination within a fifty (50) mile radius of the Company's office(s) at the time of termination unless an executed document is drawn whereby the Company and Employee agree upon the practice arrangement of the Employee after termination from the Company. The employee also agrees that he shall not practice optometry after his termination of employment for a period of______years from date of termination within a______(00) mile radius of the Company's offices at the time of termination. Should the Employee breach this provision, the Company shall be entitled to an injunction or such other relief as may be appropriate under the circumstances; provided, however, the Employee may practice within such ______(0) year period and within such restricted area if he shall first pay to the Company, the sum of ______Thousand Dollars ($00,000.00) as liquidated damages prior to beginning to practice Optometry within such time restricted area.

The Employee agrees that lists of contacts developed during the period of employment hereunder are the exclusive property of the Company. Employee agrees that during the period that he is employed by the Company and upon termination of his employment with Company, the Employee shall have no right to make use of any contact lists in a competing business. Employee agrees that, upon termination of his employment with the Company for any reason, he shall have no right to copy such lists and shall not solicit or contact persons named on such lists.

The Employee agrees that the covenants and agreements contained in this covenant are of the essence of this Agreement; that each of such covenants are reasonable and necessary to protect and preserve the interests and properties of the Company and the business of the Company; that irreparable loss and damage will be suffered by the Company should the Employee breach any of such covenants and agreements; that each of such covenants and agreements is separate, distinct, and severable not only from the other of such covenants or agreements but also from the other and remaining provisions of this Agreement; that the unenforceability of any such covenant or agreement shall not affect the validity or enforceability of any other such covenants or agreements or any other provision or provisions of this Agreement; and that, in addition to other remedies available to it, the Company shall be entitled to both temporary and permanent injunctions to prevent a breach or contemplated breach by the Employee of any such covenants or agreements.

In the event that the Employee shall breach any or all of the covenants set forth in this covenant, the running of the period of the restrictions set forth in such subparagraphs breached shall be tolled during the continuation(s) of any such breach(s) by the Employee, and the running of the period of such restrictions shall commence or commence again only upon compliance by the Employee with the terms of the applicable subparagraph breached.

16. *Invalid Provision:* The invalidity or unenforceability of a particular provision of this Agreement shall not affect the other provisions hereof, and the Agreement shall be construed in all respects as if such invalid or unenforceable provisions were omitted.

17. *Modification:* No change or modification of this Agreement shall be valid unless the same be in writing and signed by the parties hereto.

18. *Applicable Law and Binding Effect:* This Agreement shall be construed and regulated under and by the laws of the State of________, and shall inure to the benefit of and be binding upon the parties hereto and their heirs, personal representatives, and sucessors and assigns.

IN WITNESS WHEREOF, the undersigned have hereunto caused this Agreement to be executed the day and year first above written.

COMPANY:

BY ________________
PRESIDENT

ATTEST:

____
SECRETARY

(CORPORATE SEAL)

EMPLOYEE:

____

*Source: American Optometric Association. Adapted with permission.

Sample Articles of Partnership*

ARTICLES OF PARTNERSHIP OPTOMETRISTS

The undersigned, (name), hereinafter referred to as "Senior" and (name), hereinafter referred to as "Junior", desiring to associate themselves as partners, hereby adopt the following as their Articles of Partnership.

ARTICLE I

Law Applicable

This partnership is organized subject to the laws of (state), and where there is no contrary provision in these Articles, the rights of the parties with respect to each other and with other persons shall be governed by the applicable provisions of the (state) Uniform Partnership Act, effective (date), and the (state) Surviving Partners Act, effective (date).

ARTICLE II

Name

The name of the partnership shall be and is________.

ARTICLE III

Members and Status

Section 1. *Classes of Partners.* The members of this partnership shall be of one class only, to wit: general.

Section 2. *Present Members.* The members and addresses of the partners are as follows: (List)

Section 3. *No Additional General Partners.* No person may be admitted as a new general partner excepting by the unanimous consent of both general partners.

Section 4. *New Certificate.* In the event of any change in the membership, a suitable certificate shall be filed in the office of the (identify).

ARTICLE IV

Purposes and Powers

Section 1. *Character of the Business.* The character of the business is the practice of optometry.

Section 2. *Powers of Partners.* The partners shall participate equally in the general management of the partnership, each being constituted an agent of the partnership for the purpose of carrying on its business. Each shall devote his entire business time to the affairs of the partnership.

Section 3. *Limitations upon Powers of Partners.*

(a) *Name and Assets.* Neither partner shall use the partnership name or assets in any way except for the transaction of the legitimate partnership business, nor shall either partner do any act in contravention of these Articles of Partnership.

(b) *Imposed by Law.* Neither partner unless authorized by the other partner shall have any power or authority to do any act prohibited by law to be done by a single partner.

ARTICLE V

Place of Business

The business to be conducted by this partnership shall be in (address), excepting as same may be moved by the unanimous agreement of both partners.

ARTICLE VI

Capital and Partner's Interests

Section 1. *Total Capital.* The capital with which this partnership shall begin business is the sum of________Thousand Dollars ($,000). This sum is represented by a joint loan made by the partners and contributed as capital.

Section 2. *Contributions.* A financial statement reflecting the contribution of the partners is attached hereto and marked Exhibit A for identification and made a part hereof.

Section 3. *Payment before Beginning Business.* All of said items constituting capital shall be paid in, turned over, and assigned to the partnership before it commences business.

Section 4. *Books to Reflect.* A capital account reflecting the contribution made by each partner shall be maintained in the books of account of the partnership.

Section 5. *Withdrawals.* Neither partner may withdraw from the partnership any sum which will operate to diminish the contributed capital without unanimous action of all partners.

Section 6. *Leaving Profits.* Either partner, with the consent of the other partner, may leave any portion of his share of the earnings in the business for use in connection therewith; any amounts thus left shall be considered loans to the partnership and shall bear interest at the rate of________percent (________%) per annum.

Section 7. *Division of Capital and Profits.* Subject to priorities provided by law, both partners shall be entitled to share in the capital and profits of this partnership in the following percentages:

(a) During the first year of practice, Senior 64 per cent, and Junior 36 per cent, of the first $25,000.00 of the net profits and 50–50 per cent on the excess of $25,000.00;

(b) During the second year of practice, Senior 61.2 per cent, and Junior 38.8 per cent of the first $25,000.00 of the net profits and 50–50 per cent on the excess of $25,000.00;

(c) During the third year of practice, Senior 58.4 per cent, and Junior 41.6 per cent, of the first $25,000.00 of the net profits and 50–50 per cent on the excess of $25,000.00.

(d) During the fourth year of practice, Senior 55.6 per cent, and Junior 44.4 per cent, of the first $25,000.00 of the net profits and 50–50 per cent on the excess of $25,000.00;

(e) During the fifth year of practice, Senior 52.8 per cent, and Junior 47.2 per cent of the first $25,000.00 of the net profits and 50–50 per cent on the excess of $25,000.00; and

(f) Commencing with the sixth year of practice and thereafter, Senior 50 per cent, and Junior 50 per cent.

Profits shall be distributed quarterly as soon as funds are available after the quarterly closing of the partnership books, or as the partners mutually agree.

Section 8. *Losses.* In the event the partnership sustains losses, the same shall be borne on a 50–50 basis, except that during the first four years the basis shall be the same as the profit percentage.

Section 9. *Rights Upon Dissolution.* Upon the dissolution of this partnership by the expiration of the term for which it is organized, or by reason of any other cause provided by law, the rights of the partners shall be governed by the provisions of the laws of________.

ARTICLE VII

Accounting

Section 1. *Accounting Period.* Subject to change by unanimous action of the partners, the calendar year is hereby adopted as the partnership accounting period.

Section 2. *Books of Account.* Books of account accurately reflecting the partnership's business and financial status shall be kept in the partnership office located at (address). Said books shall not be removed from the office premises without the mutual consent of all partners.

Section 3. *Right of Inspection.* Each partner shall be entitled at all times to inspect the books and records of account, either personally or through attorneys or accountants.

ARTICLE VIII

Duration and Dissolution

Section 1. *Term.* The partnership hereby created shall be perpetual, subject, however, to termination as herein provided.

Section 2. *Dissolution Upon Notice.* After five (5) years, but not before, either partner by sixty (60) days' notice in writing to the other partner may require a dissolution and winding up of the partnership.

Section 3. *Dissolution Upon Death or Insanity.* The death or insanity of either partner shall cause a dissolution of the partnership.

Section 4. *Dissolution for Violation of Articles.* In the event the partners, or any of them, default in the performance of the special covenants herein provided and upon notice in writing fails to cure said default or defaults within ten (10) days, the complaining partner may cause a dissolution of the partnership as described by the (state) state statutes hereinabove mentioned.

Section 5. *Manner of Liquidation.* Upon the dissolution of the partnership by the expiration of the term for which it is organized, by unanimous agreement of the parties, or by the happening of one of the events specified in Sections 2, 3, or 4 of this Article, liquidation and winding up shall proceed in accordance with the law of (state).

Section 6. *Property Previously Held by Partners.* Upon the dissolution of the partnership by the expiration of the term for which it is organized, by unanimous agreement of the parties, or by the happening of one of the events specified in Sections 2, 3, or 4 of this Article, but not inconsistent with any "Buy and Sell Agreement" that the parties might hereinafter enter into, the parties agree as follows:

(a) All items of personal property contributed by the partners or purchased by the partnership after the execution of this agreement shall become the sole property of the partnership, except the personal refraction room equipment and the furniture and furnishings belonging to each partner before the execution of this agreement, which shall remain the exclusive property of each partner.

(b) All patient records belonging to each partner prior to the execution of this agreement shall remain the exclusive property of each of the partners, and all new records—those coming into the partnership following the execution of this agreement—shall be treated in such a way that each of said patients will be notified of the dissolution so that the patients shall have a choice of whichever doctor they elect to continue with for future treatment and service.

ARTICLE IX

Special Covenants

Each of the partners hereby covenants with the other:

Section 1. *Expenditures over $100.00.* That no single item of equipment, fixture, apparatus, or alteration or improvements to the building costing more than $100.00 shall be purchased or made without the consent of both of the partners.

Section 2. *Insurance.* That policies of insurance shall be kept in force at times as follows:

(a) Fire insurance with extended coverage upon the buildings, equipment, fixtures and inventory to the full insurable value thereof;

(b) Public liability with limits of $______and $______and property damage with limits of $______.

Section 3. *Payment of Debts.* That neither partner will permit the capital to be impaired nor fail to pay the lawful debts for labor, merchandise, materials, and obligations for whatsoever promptly as the same falls due.

Section 4. *No Monies Lent.* That no monies or properties belonging to the partnership will be lent to any person nor used except on partnership business.

Section 5. *Suretyship.* That neither of them will become the endorser or act as surety or guarantor of the debts of any other person, firm, or corporation.

Section 6. *Personal Debts.* That neither of them will incur any indebtedness which would obligate his partner other than for normal business expenses.

Section 7. *Bonds.* That neither of them will go surety upon the bond of any person to secure his appearance in any court.

Section 8. *Margin Account.* That neither of them will buy stocks or commodities on margin or engage in any other business.

Section 9. *Banking Institution.* That the partnership shall use any banking institution that the partners mutually agree upon and at the commencement of the partnership the partners agree to use a branch bank of (bank) and that the partners agree that all checks written on the partnership checking account shall be countersigned by the partners.

ARTICLE X

Disability of Partners

Section 1. *Temporary Disability.* In the event that any of the partners shall become disabled so as to be unable to attend to the affairs of the partnership (that is, actively engage in the practice of optometry as normally done day-by-day), his share of the partnership profits and losses shall be reduced or treated as follows:

(a) *Less than 30 days.* A partner is entitled to a full share of partnership profits or losses.

(b) *Thirty-one (31) through sixty (60) days.* A partner shall be entitled to two-thirds (2/3) of his share of the partnership profits or losses.

(c) *Sixty-one (61) through ninety (90) days.* A partner shall be entitled to one-third (1/3) of his share of partnership profits or losses.

(d) *Ninety-one (91) through three hundred sixty-five (365) days.* A disabled partner, in case of his disability extending beyond ninety (90) days, shall arrange for and provide for a qualified and licensed optometrist within thirty (30) days, otherwise, the able partner shall have the privilege of arranging for a qualified and licensed optometrist to substitute in the place of the disabled partner; provided, however, that in either event the salary of said replacement optometrist shall be borne by the disabled partner and deducted from the disabled partner's share of profits. The disabled partner shall be entitled to the difference between the cost and additional expenses to provide for the substitute optometrist and his share of the partnership profits.

(e) *After one (1) year of disablement.* In the event that the disability shall continue for a period of one (1) year, the remaining partner shall purchase the interest of the disabled partner. The purchase price shall be paid by the remaining partner in______quarterly installments, the first installment to be paid no later than three (3) months after the expiration of the one (1) year disability period, and the total amount of the stated value plus the other items, as set out in Section 3 of this Article. However, if the parties mutually agree to dissolve the partnership rather than the remaining partner purchasing the interest of the disabled partner, the mode and manner of dissolution shall be carried out as described in Article VIII of this agreement.

Section 2. *Partial Disability.* In the event of a partner's partial disability which enables his participation in the practice on a part time basis, and if the partners mutually agree, the disabled partner's share of the partnership profits and losses shall be proportional to his productive contribution to the gross income of the partnership. Provided, however, if after one (1) year of such limited practice by a partially disabled partner the books and records of the partnership reflect that the disabled partner is unable to produce at least one third (1/3) of the total gross income of the practice, the disabled partner shall, by certified mail, notify the able partner that the partnership shall be dissolved or demand the purchase of his interest by the able partner. The able partner, within thirty (30) days after receipt of such notice, shall cooperate in the following mode and manner of dissolution as set forth in Article VIII of this agreement, or proceed with the purchase of the partnership interest as set forth in the foregoing Section 1 of this Article.

Section 3. *Stated Value of the Business.* For the purpose of this Article relating to the purchase of the disabled partner's interest by the able partner, the stated value of the business is $________, and shall remain so unless the partners mutually agree from time to time, in writing, what the stated value shall be. In addition to one half (1/2) of the stated value, the disabled partner shall also be entitled to fifity percent (50%) of all cash amounts in the bank representing partnership assets and an amount equal to forty percent (40%) of the accounts receivable reflected on the books as of the date the three hundred sixty-fifth (365th) day occurs. The disabled partner shall also be entitled to the return of his personal refraction room equipment. When this Section applies to other Articles in this agreement, the cut-off dates shall be the date of notice or the date of death, whichever is applicable.

ARTICLE XI
Death of Partner

Section 1. *Insurance.* Each partner has insured the life of the other partner in the following mode and manner:

(a) Dr. Senior is the owner of a certain term life insurance policy on the life of Dr. Junior, issued by________in the amount of $________, and the monthly premiums are in the amount of $________.

(b) Dr. Junior is the owner of a certain term life insurance policy on the life of Dr. Senior, issued by________in the amount of $________, and the monthly premiums are in the amount of $________.

Section 2. *Purchase of Partnership Interest on Death.* Upon the death of either partner, the surviving partner shall purchase the entire interest of the deceased partner in the partnership, and the estate of the decedent shall sell such interest to the surviving partner. The entire purchase price for the interest of the deceased partner shall be paid in cash to his estate within thirty (30) days after the appointment and qualifications of the legal representative of such estate. Where the insurance proceeds are of sufficient amount to fully cover the purchase price as hereinafter set forth and the proceeds of insurance exceed the purchase price required to be paid in full, any excess shall be paid to the owner of the policy. In the event that the proceeds of insurance shall be insufficient to properly cover the purchase price, then, after applying the total proceeds from the insurance policy to the purchase price, the difference so remaining shall be paid in four (4) equal quarterly installments, beginning with thirty (30) days after the date of death of the deceased partner.

Section 3. *Purchase Price.* The purchase price of the interest of a deceased partner shall be computed in the same manner as set forth in Section 3 of Article X of this agreement.

Section 4. *Transfer of Partnership Interest.* Upon receipt of the purchase price the legal representative of the estate of the deceased partner shall execute and deliver to the surviving partner all documents required to evidence his purchase of the decedent's partnership interest. Simultaneously the surviving partner shall deliver to the legal representative of the estate of the deceased partner an agreement indemnifying the estate against any liabilities of the partnership.

Section 5. *Purchase of Policies Upon Death or Termination.* Upon the termination of the partnership for any reason during the lives of the partners, or upon the death of either partner, the insured partner shall have the right to purchase from the other partner or from the estate of the deceased partner all policies insuring his life taken out pursuant to this agreement. The price for such policies shall equal their cash value on the date of termination or death, plus a proportionate part of the premium last paid before such date which covers the period extending beyond such date. The price shall be paid in cash within thirty (30) days after the termination of the partnership or the death of a partner. If this right to purchase is not exercised within the thirty (30) day period, it shall lapse and all rights under the policies shall belong the owner thereof.

Section 6. *Term.* In the event of the termination of the partnership for any reason prior to the death of either partner, all rights under this Article shall terminate, except as otherwise provided in Section 5.

Section 7. *Benefit.* This Article shall bind the parties and their respective estates.

ARTICLE XII

Obligation as Lessees

The partners are personally liable under a certain written lease, as lessees, with ________ as lessor, and the partners agree that they shall so remain liable regardless of dissolution of the partnership. However, in the event of the death of a partner or the purchase of the entire interest of the partnership by a partner, the surviving partner agrees to assume the full responsibility of the lease covenants and agrees to save the withdrawing partner or his estate harmless from future liability for rent and other material conditions and covenants, during the present term of said lease or any extensions or renewals thereof.

ARTICLE XIII

Effective Date

The effective date of this agreement relates back to the ________ day of ________, 19________, and since which time the parties have substantially operated as set forth in this agreement.

In witness therefore, Dr. Senior and Dr. Junior have hereunto affixed their signatures, on this the ________ day of ________, 19________.

*Source: American Optometric Association. Adapted with permission.

Documents Required to Form a Professional Corporation*

AGREEMENT TO FORM A CORPORATION

Agreement made________, 19________, between________and________, doctors of optometry, all of City of________, State of________.

Whereas the parties have entered into an agreement for the purchase of the office building located at________, City of________, State of________; and

Whereas the parties have agreed to organize a corporation to take title to and to own said property; and

Whereas the parties are members of an optometric partnership and intend to cause the corporation to lease the property to the partnership for use as optometric offices.

It is therefore agreed:

1. *Formation of Corporation.* The parties shall organize a corporation under the laws of the State of________to be known as________.

2. *Articles of Incorporation.* The following provisions shall be included in the articles of incorporation:

(a) The initial Registered Agent shall be________, attorney.

(b) The duration of the corporation shall be perpetual.

(c) The number of directors of the corporation shall be three.

(d) The corporation shall be authorized to issue $________capital stock, consisting of________shares of common stock having a par value of $________per share.

(e) The purposes of the corporation shall be to own an optometric office building, office furnishings, optometric equipment and such other real or personal property as the corporation may acquire from time to time; and to provide miscellaneous office and technical services to the lessees in connection with said property.

3. *Subscriptions.* The parties shall subscribe for the number of shares set opposite their names, and agree to pay therefor $________per share:

Dr.________ ________shares
Dr.________ ________shares
Dr.________ ________shares

The subscriptions shall be payable at such time as the board of directors may determine and shall be paid by certified or bank cashier's check.

4. *Stock Restrictions.* None of the parties, nor the administrator nor executor of the estate of any party, shall transfer, pledge or sell stock in the corporation except with the written consent of all the other parties. If written consent is not obtained, a party, administrator, or executor desiring to sell stock shall notify the other parties of his offer to sell by registered mail. Each of the other parties shall have the option of purchasing said stock in proportion to his stock holdings in the corporation within 60 days. If any party shall not execute his option or any part thereof, the remaining party shall have an additional 30 days to purchase such stock as may be unsold. The purchase price shall be the book value of the stock, determined in accordance with standard accounting practice by the certified public accountant usually employed by the corporation as of the date of the registered mailing of the offer to sell. These stock restrictions shall become void in the event of the dissolution of the corporation or the death of all of the parties within a period of 90 days.

5. *Stock Certificates.* Stock certificates shall be issued only upon payment of the subscription price. Each certificate shall contain the endorsement that it is subject to the restrictions contained in paragraph 4

of an agreement executed among the parties on________, 19________, and available for examination at the office of the Registered Agent of the corporation.

6. *Ratification.* The parties shall cause the corporation to adopt and ratify the agreement for the purchase of the property at________, the application with the________Bank for a purchase money mortgage in the amount of $________upon said property, and the terms of this agreement.

7. *Necessary Documents.* Each of the parties shall execute and deliver in legally acceptable form any document necessary to the implementation of this agreement.

8. *Benefit.* This agreement shall be binding upon the parties and their legal representatives and successors.

ARTICLES OF INCORPORATION

We, the undersigned hereby associate ourselves together for the purpose of becoming a professional corporation for profit under the provisions of Business and Professional Statutes, as amended by "The Professional Service Corporation Act" of the State of________, pursuant to the following Articles of Incorporation:

ARTICLE I
NAME

The name of this corporation shall be:________.

ARTICLE II
PURPOSE

The general nature of the business to be transacted by the corporation shall be and is to engage in every aspect of the general practice of optometry. The professional services involved in the corporation's practice of optometry may be rendered only through its officers, agents and employees who are duly authorized and licensed to practice optometry in the State of________.

This corporation shall not engage in any business other than the practice of optometry. However, this corporation may invest its funds in real estate, mortgages, stocks, bonds and other types of investments, and may own real and personal property necessary for the rendering of the professional services authorized hereby.

ARTICLE III
STOCKS

The maximum number of shares of stock that the corporation is authorized to have outstanding at any time shall be________shares of the par value of________Dollars ($________) per share, all of which shall be common stock of the same class. All stock issued shall be fully paid and nonassessable. The stockholders shall have no preemptive rights with respect to the stock of the corporation, and the corporation may issue and sell its common stock from time to time without offering such shares to the stockholders then holding shares of common stock. Shares of the corporation's stock and certificates therefore shall be issued only to doctors authorized and licensed to practice optometry in the State of________.

ARTICLE IV
CAPITAL

The amount of capital with which this corporation will begin business shall be and is the sum of________Dollars ($________).

ARTICLE V
DURATION

The corporation shall have perpetual existence.

ARTICLE VI
OFFICES

The principal office of this corporation shall be located in the City of________, County of________, State of________, and the post office address of said principal office of the corporation shall be________, City of________, State of________.

ARTICLE VII
DIRECTORS

The number of directors of this corporation shall be not less than three (3) nor more than five (5).

ARTICLE VIII
BOARD OF DIRECTORS

The names and post office addresses of the members of the first Board of Directors, who, subject to the provisions of the By-laws and these Articles of Incorporation, shall hold office for the first year of the corporation's existence or until their successors are elected and have qualified, are as follows:

NAMES	ADDRESSES
Dr.________	________________
Dr.________	________________
Dr.________	________________

ARTICLE IX
SUBSCRIBERS

The name and post office address of each subscriber of these Articles of Incorporation are as follows:

NAMES	ADDRESSES
Dr.________	________________
Dr.________	________________
Dr.________	________________

The subscribers certify that the proceeds of the stock subscribed for will not be less than the amount of capital with which the corporation will begin business, as set forth in Article IV hereinabove.

ARTICLE X
STOCKHOLDERS

The stock of this corporation may be issued, owned and registered only in the name or names of an individual or individuals who are duly authorized and licensed to practice optometry in the State of________and who are employees, officers or agents of this corporation. In the event a stockholder:

(a) becomes disqualified to practice optometry in this State, or

(b) is elected to a public office or accepts employment, that pursuant to law, places restrictions or limitations upon his continued rendering of professional services as a doctor of optometry, or

(c) ceases to be an employee, officer or agent of the corporation, or

(d) sells, transfers, pledges, or attempts to sell, transfer, or pledge any shares of stock in this corporation to any person ineligible by law or by virtue of these Articles to be a shareholder in this corporation, or if such sale, transfer, pledge, or attempt to sell, transfer, or pledge is made in a manner prohibited by law, or in a manner inconsistent with the provisions of these Articles, or by the By-Laws of this corporation, or

(e) suffers an execution to be levied upon his stock, or such stock is subjected to judicial sale or other process, the effect of which is to vest any legal or equitable interest in such stock in some person other than the stockholder,

then the stock of such stockholder shall immediately stand forfeited and such stock shall be immediately cancelled by this corporation and the stockholder or other person in possession of such stock shall be entitled only to receive payment for the value of such stock, which said value shall be the book value thereof as of the last day of the month preceding the month in which any of the events above enumerated occurs. The stockholder whose stock so becomes forfeit and is cancelled by the corporation, shall forthwith cease to be an employee, officer, director, or agent of the corporation and except to receive payment for his stock in accordance with the foregoing, and payment of any other sums then lawfully due and owing to said stockholder by the corporation, such stockholder shall then and thereafter have no further financial interest of any kind in this corporation.

ARTICLE XI
DEATH OF STOCKHOLDER

Upon the death of a stockholder, his stock shall be subject to purchase by the corporation or by the other stockholders at such price and upon such terms and conditions and in such manner as may be provided for in the By-Laws of this corporation, in a manner consistent with law and these Articles.

ARTICLE XII
SALE OF STOCKS

No stockholder of this corporation may sell or transfer any of such stockholder's share of stock in this corporation except to another individual who is then duly authorized and licensed to practice optometry in the State of________and then only after the proposed sale or transfer shall have been first approved, at a stockholder's meeting specially called for such purpose, by such proportion, not less than a majority, of the outstanding stock, excluding the shares of stock proposed to be sold or transferred, as may be provided from time to time in the By-Laws. In such stockholder's meeting, the shares of stock proposed to be sold or transferred may not be voted or counted for any purpose.

The corporation's shareholders are specifically authorized from time to time to adopt By-Laws not inconsistent herewith restraining the alienation of shares of stock of this corporation and providing for the purchase or redemption by the corporation of its shares of stock.

ARTICLE XIII
REGULATION OF BUSINESS

In furtherance of and not in limitation of the powers conferred by statute, the following specific provisions are made for the regulation of the business and the conduct of the affairs of the corporation:

1. Subject to such restrictions, if any, as are herein expressed and such further restrictions, if any, as may be set forth in the By-Laws, the Board of Directors shall have the general management and control of the business and may exercise all the powers of the Corporation except such as may be by statute, or by the Articles of Incorporation or amendment thereto, or by the By-Laws as constituted from time to time, expressly conferred upon or reserved to the stockholders.

2. The corporation shall have such officers as may from time to time be provided in the By-Laws and such officers shall be designated in such manner and shall hold their offices for such terms and shall have such powers and duties as may be prescribed by the By-Laws or as may be determined from time to time by the Board of Directors subject to the By-Laws.

3. No contract or other transaction between the corporation and any other firm, association or corporation shall be affected or invalidated by the fact that any one or more of the directors of the

corporation is or are interested in or is a member, director or officer or are members, directors or officers of such firm or corporation and any director or directors individually or jointly may be a party or parties to or may be interested in any contract or transaction of the corporation or in which the corporation is interested; and no contract, act or transaction of the corporation with any person, firm, association or corporation shall be affected or invalidated by the fact that any director or directors of the corporation is a part or are parties to or interested in such contract, act or transaction or in any way connected with such person, firm, association or corporation, and each and every person who may become a director of the corporation is hereby relieved from any liability that might otherwise exist from contracting with the corporation for the benefit of himself or any firm, association or corporation in which he may in any way be interested.

ARTICLE XIV
AMENDMENTS

This corporation reserves the right to amend, alter, change, or repeal any provision contained herein in the manner now or hereafter prescribed by law, and all rights conferred on stockholders herein are granted subject to this reservation.

STOCK PURCHASE AGREEMENT

THIS STOCK PURCHASE AGREEMENT, is entered into as of_________, 19_______by and between________O.D. (hereinafter called "Seller") and________O.D. (hereinafter called "Buyer") with reference to the following acts:

RECITALS

WHEREAS, Seller owns all of the issued and outstanding stock of________, O.D., Inc. (hereinafter called "corporation"); and

WHEREAS, corporation is a_________corporation duly licensed to practice as an Optometric Corporation under___________Business and Professions Code Section 3161; and

WHEREAS, Buyer is currently employed by corporation; and

WHEREAS, Buyer is duly licensed to practice optometry by the State of________; and

WHEREAS, Buyer would like to purchase all Seller's stock in corporation on the terms and conditions hereinafter set forth; and

WHEREAS, Seller would like to sell all Seller's stock to Buyer on the terms and conditions hereinafter set forth.

THE PARTIES AND EACH OF THEM AGREE:

AGREEMENT

1. *Sales of Stock*—On the terms and conditions hereinafter set forth, Seller agrees to sell and Buyer agrees to purchase all Seller's stock in corporation.

2. *Effective Date*—The purchase and sale of the corporate stock shall take place as of___________, 19_____. Said date is hereinafter called "effective date".

3. *Purchase Price*—The purchase price for the corporate stock is $________, plus or minus the sum of the following items, all of which shall be determined by the parties as of the effective date.

A. *Cash*—The total amount of all corporate cash on hand and in banks on the effective date shall be added to the purchase price. Said cash shall not include any cash in the corporation's retirement plans.

B. *Accounts Receivable*—The total amount of all collectible corporate accounts receivable on the effective date shall be added to the purchase price.

C. *Deposits and Refunds*—The total amount of all corporate deposits on the effective date shall be added to the purchase price, including the prepaid rent, telephone deposits, utility deposits, prepaid federal and state income taxes, etc.

D. *Equipment*—The total depreciated value of all corporate instruments, equipment, furniture furnishings, and leasehold improvements purchased by the corporation after________, 19________shall be added to the purchase price. Said depreciated value shall be determined by the corporation's accountant by using the method of depreciation which is utilized by said accountant for federal income tax purposes.

E. *Corporate Liabilities*—The total amount of all corporate liabilities on the effective date, including payroll taxes payable, income taxes payable, accounts payable, laboratory bills, wages payable, and rent payable, etc. shall be deducted from the purchase price.

4. *Payment of Purchase Price*—Buyer shall pay the purchase price computed in conformity with Paragraph 3 hereof, as follows:

A. *Cash Payment*—On the effective date Buyer shall pay Seller $00,000.00 cash.

B. *Note Payment*—As of the effective date, Buyer shall provide Seller with a Promissory Note with principal balance equal to the total purchase price computed in conformity with

Paragraph 3 hereof, less the $00,000.00 paid Buyer to Seller pursuant to subparagraph A of this Paragraph 4. Said Promissory Note shall be executed by Buyer and Buyer's wife. Said Promissory Note shall be dated as of________, 19________. Said Promissory Note shall provide for variable interest. Said interest shall be determined with reference to the prime rate of interest charged by the Bank of America on December 31 of the year preceding the interest computation year. The interest charge for said interest computation year shall be 1% less than the prime rate of interest charged by Bank of America on the preceding December 31. For example, interest rate on the note for the period from February 1, 1980, through January 31, 1981, is 1% less than the prime rate of interest charged by Bank of America on December 31, 1979. By way of further example, interest on the note for the period from February 1, 1981, through January 31, 1982, is 1% less than the prime rate of interest charged by Bank of America on December 31, 1980. The note shall provide for 120 monthly payments due on the first day of each and every month commencing with the first day of______ 19______. The amount of each such monthly payment shall be determined by amortizing the total unpaid principal balance of the note at the beginning of the interest period over the remaining term of the entire note, in equal installments, at the interest rate applicable at the beginning of the interest period. For example, the payments for the first 12 months of the note would be determined by amortizing the total original unpaid principal balance of the note over a period of 120 months, in equal installments, at an interest rate which is 1% less than the prime rate of interest charged by Bank of America on December 31, 1979. As a further example, the monthly payments for the 13th month through the 24th month would be determined by amortizing the unpaid principal balance at the end of the 12th month over a period of 108 months, in equal installments, at an interest rate which is 1% less than the prime rate of interest charged by Bank of America on December 31, 1980. Notwithstanding the foregoing, interest on the Promissory Note for the first year (________, 19________, through ______, 19______) shall not exceed______%. The note shall also provide that the Maker of the note may not prepay principal or interest without the consent of the Holder of the Note.

In addition, the form of said Promissory Note shall be identical to the form of Promissory Note which is set forth in Exhibit "A" attached.

5. *Delivery of Stock and Security*—On the effective date Seller shall deliver fully executed stock certificates for all the corporate stock to Buyer. Buyer shall immediately cause said stock certificates to be re-registered in Buyer's name. In addition, Buyer shall cause the corporation to add Seller's name as a pledgee of said stock. Immediately following re-registration, Buyer shall return the re-registered stock and the pledge agreement which is attached hereto by Exhibit "B" to Seller. Upon Buyer's faithful performance of all of the terms and conditions of the promissory note and pledge agreement, Seller shall release the pledge and return the share certificates to Buyer.

6. *Life Insurance*—As a material part of this Agreement, Buyer agrees to insure Buyer's life in an amount equal to the full unpaid principal balance of the aforementioned promissory note and to name Seller as beneficiary on said policy. Said policy shall provide that it may not be altered, amended, or cancelled without 10 days prior written notice to Seller. Upon request, Buyer shall provide proof of said insurance to Seller. On death, the proceeds of said insurance shall be applied to the promissory note. If the proceeds of said insurance exceed the amount of said promissory note, Seller agrees to pay the excess to Buyer's wife. If Buyer's wife should be deceased at the time payment is required, then Seller agrees to pay the excess to Buyer's Personal Representative.

7. *Professional Liability and Insurance*—As a material part of this agreement, Buyer agrees to cause the corporation to insure Seller against professional liability for services rendered by Seller as an employee of corporation. The amount of said professional liability insurance shall not be less than the amount of insurance which is presently carried by corporation. Upon request, proof of said insurance shall be furnished to Seller.

8. *Resignation*—As of the effective date, Seller shall resign as a officer and director of corporation. In connection with said resignation, Seller agrees Seller will not engage in the practice of Optometry within a radius of 25 miles from corporation's present location during the period from________, 19________ through__________, 19________, without Buyer's prior written consent. Buyer's default under the Promissory note or Pledge Agreement shall automatically relieve Seller of the obligations which are imposed under this Paragraph.

9. *Governmental Agencies*—Buyer agrees to

advise the State Board of Optometry of all the corporate changes which are being made pursuant to this Agreement. Buyer further agrees to comply with all requirements of any governmental agency having jurisdiction over any term or condition of this Agreement.

10. *Seller's Warranties*—Seller hereby warrants and represents:

A. *Ownership*—Seller beneficially owns, of record, free and clear of all liens, liabilities and encumbrances, all of the outstanding stock of corporation.

B. *Breach of Agreement*—The sale and transfer of the shares of corporate stock covered by this Agreement will not constitute a breach or violation of any agreement or other instrument executed by either corporation or Seller.

C. *Corporation*—Corporation is a duly organized corporation, validly existing and in good standing under the law of the State of________.

D. *Additional Stock*—There are no outstanding stock options or stock warrants or other rights which would give any person the right to subscribe to additional corporate stock. No additional stock or stock rights or stock options will be issued by corporation prior to the effective date.

E. *Title to Assets*—As of the effective date, corporation will have marketable title to all of the assets described in paragraph 3 of this Agreement. Except as otherwise specified in paragraph 3 of this Agreement, said title will be free and clear of all liens, liabilities, and encumbrances on the effective date.

F. *Corporate Operation*—From execution of this Agreement through the effective date, corporation will not purchase any asset having a value above $1,000.00 without Buyer's consent, and corporation will not make any sale of corporate assets, except to customers in the ordinary course of business.

G. *Lease*—Buyer acknowledges that the corporation's principal place of business is leased from ________Inc. and that said lease expires on ________, 19______. Buyer further acknowledges that he has read said lease and that he approves same. Seller agrees to assist Buyer in arranging a new lease with________Inc.; but Seller does not warrant or represent that said lease is obtainable.

H. *Business Conduct*—Until the effective date, corporation will carry on its business in a diligent manner and will keep and maintain all of its records and accounts in good form. Corporation will pay all of its obligations as they become due and corporation will maintain itself in good standing under the laws of the State of________. Without in any way limiting the generality of the foregoing, corporation will not (1) amend its Article of Incorporation; (2) issue or agree to issue additional shares of capital stock or other securities or evidence of indebtedness; (3) declare any dividends or make any capital or other distributions; (4) enter into any long-term agreements of any kind whatsoever or (5) transfer any asset, except in the ordinary course of business.

I. *Best Efforts*—Corporation and Seller will each use their best efforts to consumate this transaction. In this regard corporation and Seller will promptly sign all papers and other documents which are required of Seller or Corporation.

11. *Buyer's Warranties*—Buyer hereby warrants and represents:

A. *Status*—Buyer is duly authorized by the State of________to practice optometry.

B. *Best Efforts*—Buyer will use Buyer's best efforts to consumate this transaction. In this regard Buyer will promptly prepare and file all of the papers and other documents which are required by any governmental agency in connection with the transfer of the stock contemplated by this Agreement.

12. *Effect of Representations*—The representations and warranties made by either Buyer or Seller under this Agreement (whether contained in Paragraphs 10 and 11, or otherwise) shall be deemed to have been made both as of the date of execution of this Agreement and as of the effective date. All warranties and representations shall survive consumation of the transactions contemplated by this Agreement.

13. *Miscellaneous*—Buyer and Seller further covenant, warrant, and agree:

A. *Further Documents*—Each party will execute, acknowledge, and deliver such further instruments and documents as may be necessary to complete the sale provided in this Agreement.

B. *Entire Agreement*—this Agreement contains the entire understanding of the parties with respect to the matters covered by it and as such it supercedes all prior agreements and understandings.

C. *Amendments*—This Agreement may only be amended by written document signed by all of the parties.

D. *Survival*—All of the agreements, covenants and warranties contained in this Agreement shall survive the transfer of stock covered by this Agreement.

E. *Applicable Law*—This Agreement shall be construed, interpreted, governed, and enforced according to the laws of the State of________.

F. *Attorney's Fees*—In the event of any controversy, claim, or dispute between the parties relating to any provision or term of this Agreement or any breach thereof, the prevailing party shall be entitled to receive reasonable attorney's fees, expenses, and costs from the losing party.

G. *Representation*—This Agreement was prepared by the law firm of________, a Professional Corporation. Said law firm solely represented Seller. Buyer acknowledges that Buyer was asked to seek separate independent counsel to represent Buyer in this transaction.

IN WITNESS WHEREOF, Buyer and Seller have executed this Agreement as of________, 19________.

____________________ , O.D. ____________________ , O.D.

SPOUSAL CONSENT

The wives of________, O.D. and________, O.D. do hereby consent to the foregoing Stock Purchase Agreement and said wives do hereby agree that the terms and conditions of said Stock Purchase Agreement shall be binding on any community or other interest they may have in the property covered by said agreement.

____________________ , O.D. ____________________ , O.D.

PROMISSORY NOTE

EXHIBIT A

FOR VALUE RECEIVED,________and his wife________(hereinafter called "Maker") promise to pay________or order (hereinafter called "Holder") the principal sum of $________, together with interest on the unpaid principal sum computed at the rates hereinafter set forth, in 120 monthly installments.

INTEREST AT THE FOLLOWING RATES:

A. From February 1, 1980, through January 31, 1981, interest shall be 1% less than the prime rate of interest charged by Bank of America on December 31, 1979; or______%, whichever is less;

B. Interest from February 1, 1981, through January 31, 1982, shall be 1% less than the prime rate of interest charged by Bank of America on December 31, 1980;

C. Interest from February 1, 1982, through January 31, 1983, shall be 1% less than the prime rate of interest charged by Bank of America on December 31, 1981;

D. Interest from February 1, 1983, through January 31, 1984, shall be 1% less than the prime rate of interest charged by Bank of America on December 31, 1982;

E. Interest from February 1, 1984, through January 31, 1985, shall be 1% less than the prime rate of interest charged by Bank of America on December 31, 1983;

F. Interest from February 1, 1985, through January 31, 1986, shall be 1% less than the prime rate of interest charged by Bank of America on December 31, 1984;

G. Interest from February 1, 1986, through January 31, 1987, shall be 1% less than the prime rate of interest charged by Bank of America on December 31, 1985;

H. Interest from February 1, 1987, through January 31, 1988, shall be 1% less than the prime rate of interest charged by Bank of America on December 31, 1986;

I. Interest from February 1, 1988, through January 31, 1989, shall be 1% less than the prime rate of interest charged by Bank of America on December 31, 1987; and

J. Interest from February 1, 1989, through January 31, 1990, shall be 1% less than the prime rate of interest charged by Bank of America on December 31, 1988.

Principal and interest are payable in lawful money of the United States at whatever place or places the Holder of this note, from time to time, shall designate.

Principal and interest are to be paid in monthly installments. The first such monthly installment is due________, 19________, and each successive monthly installment is due on the first day of each and every month thereafter.

MONTHLY PAYMENTS AS FOLLOWS:

1. The monthly payments for the first 12 months shall be determined by amortizing the total unpaid principal balance of the note over a period of 120 months in equal installments at the interest rate stated in Paragraph A of this note;
2. The monthly payments for the 13th month through the 24th month shall be determined by amortizing the unpaid principal balance at the end of the 12th month over a period of 108 months in equal installments at the interest rate stated in Paragraph B of this note;
3. The monthly payments for the 25th month through the 36th month shall be determined by amortizing the unpaid principal balance of the promissory note at the end of the 24th month over a period of 96 months, in equal installments at the interest rate stated in Paragraph C of this note;
4. The monthly payments for the 37th month through the 48th month shall be determined by amortizing the unpaid principal balance at the end of the 36th month over a period of 84 months, in equal installments at the interest rate stated in Paragraph D of this note;
5. The monthly payments for the 49th month through the 60th month shall be determined by amortizing the unpaid principal balance at the end of the 48th month over a period of 72 months, in equal installments at the interest rate stated in Paragraph E of this note;
6. The monthly payments for the 61st month through the 72nd month shall be determined by amortizing the unpaid principal balance at the end of the 60th month over a period of 60 months, in equal installments at the interest rate stated in Paragraph F of this note;
7. The monthly payments for the 73rd month through the 84th month shall be determined by amortizing the unpaid principal balance at the end of the 72nd month over 48 months, in equal installments at the interest rate stated in Paragraph G of this note;
8. The monthly payments for the 85th month through the 96th month shall be determined by amortizing the unpaid principal balance at the end of the 84th month over a period of 36 months, in equal installments at the interest rate stated in Paragraph H of this note; and
9. The monthly payments for the 97th month through the 108th month shall be determined by amortizing the unpaid principal balance at the end of the 96th month over a period of 24 months, in equal installments at the interest rate stated in Paragraph I of this note.
10. The monthly payments for the last 12 months of the note shall be determined by amortizing the unpaid principal balance at the end of the 108th month over 12 months, in equal installments at the interest rate stated in Paragraph J of this note.

Each payment shall first be applied to interest which is then accrued and the remainder of said payment shall be applied to the unpaid principal balance of the note. Should interest not be paid when due, it shall thereafter bear like interest as the principal, but such unpaid interest so compounded shall not exceed an amount equal to simple interest on the unpaid principal at the maximum rate permitted by law.

Should any payment be more than 15 days past due, a late fee equal to 10% of the amount of said deliquent payment shall be due and payable with the deliquent payment.

The whole sum of principal and interest may become immediately due and payable at the option of the Holder of this note on the happening of any one of the following events: (1) on the death of________; (2) on default of any term or condition of this note; or (3) on default of any term or condition of the Pledge Agreement which secures performance of this promissory note.

All payments due hereunder are free from any and all offsets and counter claims. The Maker hereby waives any and all rights to any cross-demands which might otherwise be available to the Maker under________Code of Civil Procedure section 431.

During the first three years of this note, the Maker may not prepay principal or interest without the Holder's written consent. Thereafter, the Maker may prepay principal on 90 days advance written notice to the Holder.

The Maker hereby promises to pay all costs and reasonable attorney's fees incurred by the Holder by reason of the Maker's default under this note.

The Maker's obligations under this note are secured by a Pledge Agreement.

The Maker's obligations are joint and several.

IN WITNESS WHEREOF, this note is executed as of________, 19________at________.

________________, O.D.   ________________, O.D.

PLEDGE AGREEMENT

EXHIBIT B

THIS PLEDGE AGREEMENT is entered into between________, O.D. (hereinafter called "Buyer") and________, O.D. (hereinafter called "Seller") to cover Buyer's pledge of all of the issued and outstanding stock of________, O.D. Inc. (hereinafter called "pledged stock") as security for Buyer's performance of that certain promissory note from Buyer to Seller dated ________, 19________ (hereinafter called "promissory note"). In connection with said pledge, Buyer and Seller agree:

1. *Effect*—Until the promissory note is paid in full, this Pledge Agreement shall govern the rights and liabilities of Buyer and Seller with respect to the pledged stock.

2. *Delivery and Return*—Buyer shall cause the pledged stock to be registered in Buyer's name with Seller shown as a "pledgee". Following said registration, Buyer shall immediately deliver said pledged stock to Seller. Upon faithful performance of all the terms and conditions of this Pledge Agreement and the accompanying promissory note, Seller shall return the pledged stock, free of pledge, to Buyer.

3. *Risk of Ownership*—All risk of ownership of the pledged stock shall be borne entirely by Buyer.

4. *Voting Rights and Dividends*—Until Seller elects to foreclose for Buyer's default under this Pledge Agreement and/or the accompanying promissory note, Buyer shall be entitled to vote the pledged stock and to receive all of the dividends and other rights which are connected with same. If Seller commences foreclosure proceedings pursuant to this Pledge Agreement, effective as of the commencement of said proceedings, the voting rights and other rights attributable to the stock shall automatically pass to Seller. Any dividends which are paid to Seller before completion of the foreclosure proceedings shall be applied against Buyer's obligations under the promissory note.

5. *Buyer's Covenants*—Until the promissory note is paid in full, Buyer warrants, covenants, and agrees:

A. *Full-time and Attention*—Buyer shall devote full-time and attention to the practice of Optometry as an employee of________, O.D. Inc. (hereinafter called "corporation").

B. *Transfer of Stock*—Buyer will not sell, transfer assign, hypothecate, or further encumber the pledged stock. In addition, Buyer and/or the corporation will not enter into any joint venture agreement or profit-sharing type of agreement or arrangement with any person other than Buyer, without Seller's prior written consent.

C. *License*—At all times Buyer shall maintain Buyer's license to practice Optometry in the State of________in full force and effect. In addition, at all times Buyer shall cause corporation to maintain its license to practice Optometry in full force and effect and Buyer shall cause corporation to comply with all governmental rules and regulations applicable to corporation.

D. *Life Insurance*—Buyer shall maintain life insurance on Buyer's life in an amount equal to the unpaid principal balance of the promissory note. Said life insurance policy or policies shall name Seller as the beneficiary. Upon Seller's request, proof of said insurance shall be furnished Seller or Seller's duly authorized agent. All proceeds collected on said insurance shall be applied toward the payment of the promissory note. If the proceeds collected by Seller exceed the then unpaid balance of the promissory note, Seller shall forthwith pay the excess to Buyer's wife, providing she is then living, and if she is not then living, Seller shall pay the excess to Buyer's Personal Representative.

E. *Corporate Operations*—Buyer shall cause the corporation to carry on its business in a diligent manner and to keep and maintain all of its records and accounts in good form. Buyer will cause corporation to pay all of its obligations as they become due and Buyer will cause corporation to maintain itself in good standing under the laws of the State of ________and the regulations of the State Board of Optometry. Without in any way limiting the foregoing, Buyer will make sure that corporation does not (1) amend its Articles of Incorporation; (2) issue or agree to issue any additional shares of capital stock or securities or any evidence of indebtedness other than indebtedness connected with the purchase of additional assets or equipment; (3) make any capital distributions; (4) change its present business location; (5) open another business location; (6) make any direct or indirect payment (including contributions to profit sharing plans, retirement plans, or other fringe benefits) to or for the benefit of a shareholder employee of the corporation which would, in any way, impair the corporation's financial ability; and (7) transfer any asset except in the ordinary course of business. In addition, Buyer shall cause corporation to insure Buyer and its other employees against professional malpractice in an amount which is not less than the existing malpractice insurance carried by corporation and Buyer will cause corporation to insure all of corporation's assets against liability, casualty, fire, and theft in an amount which is not less than its existing insurance. Upon request, proof of said insurance shall be furnished to Seller.

6. *Foreclosure*—If Buyer defaults under any term or condition of this Pledge Agreement or the accompanying promissory note, Seller may, at Seller's sole option, elect to commence foreclosure proceedings on the pledged stock. To commence said foreclosure proceedings, Seller must provide Buyer with written notice of the default. If the default (payment of money or otherwise) is caused by Buyer's permanent disability, Buyer shall have a period of 180 days from receipt of the written notice to cure the default. If the default is in the payment of money (not caused by Buyer's permanent disability), Buyer shall have a period of 90 days from receipt of the written notice to cure the default. If the default is for breach of any term or condition of the Pledge Agreement or Promissory Note (other than breaches caused by Buyer's permanant disability or payment of money), Buyer shall have a period of 30 days from the receipt of the written notice to cure the default. "Permanent disability" is defined as any mental or physical ailment or disability (except alcoholism or drug abuse) which renders Buyer unable to devote a minimum of 20 hours per week to the practice of optometry for a minimum period of 120 consecutive calendar days. On Seller's request, proof of said "permanent disability" shall be furnished by a duly licensed physician authorized to practice in the State of________. If Buyer elects not to cure the default, Buyer shall have the right to require Seller to conduct a private sale of the stock covered by this Pledge Agreement. Buyer's demand for said private sale shall be delivered to Seller within the time period for curing the default and said demand shall specify the time and place of the sale. The place designated for the sale must be reasonably convenient to the Seller and the designated time must be within 20 days following expiration of the period allowed for curing the default. In addition, Buyer must advance all of the estimated costs and expenses of the sale at the time the request is made. If Buyer does request a private sale pursuant to this provision, the Seller shall conduct same as requested. All bids shall be for cash. The Seller shall be entitled to bid on the stock. Any offer of the Seller to cancel all or any portion of the unpaid balance of the promissory note shall be treated as a cash bid. The proceeds from the sale shall first be applied to the satisfaction of the indebtedness secured by this Pledge Agreement; and the excess, if any, shall be paid to Buyer. If a sale is not requested by Buyer as aforesaid, at the expiration of the time allowed for curing the default, the Seller shall acquire title to the pledged stock free and clear of all liens and encumbrances. Notwithstanding foreclosure, Seller may bring an independent action against the Buyer for the difference between the fair market value of stock acquired by the Seller through foreclosure; or, if the stock is sold, the net amount realized from the sale and the total unpaid balance of the promissory note at the date of the sale, including attorney's fees and collection costs. If the Buyer does not request a private sale, it shall be conclusively presumed that the fair market value of the stock acquired by the Seller on Buyer's default did not exceed the total unpaid balance of the promissory note upon said date.

7. *Binding Effect*—This Pledge Agreement shall be binding on the parties and their heirs and assigns. It may only be altered, amended, or revoked by written instrument signed by all of the parties.

8. *Attorney's Fees*—In the event of any controversy, claim, or dispute, between the parties relating to any provision or term of this Pledge Agreement, or any breach thereof, the prevailing party shall be entitled to receive reasonable expenses, attorney's fees, and costs from the losing party.

9. *Notices*—All notices required by this Pledge Agreement shall be given in writing, either personally or by mail. If mailed, said notices shall be deemed to have been received three days following deposit in the United States mail, postage prepaid, addressed as follows:

Buyer: ____________

Seller: ____________

10. *Notice Changes*—Either party may change the place of giving notices by written notice delivered in accordance with the immediately preceding section.

11. *Cooperation*—Seller acknowledges that the income tax laws or other laws may change and that, as a consequence, it may not always be advantageous for Buyer to conduct business in the corporate form. Notwithstanding anything in this Agreement appar-

ently to the contrary, Seller agrees to cooperate with Buyer's change of corporate form on the condition that said change will not impair Seller's security and on the further condition that Buyer will pay all of the attorney's fees and other costs incurred by Seller by reason of Buyer's requested change.

12. *Business Operations*—Seller acknowledges that Buyer has entered into an Agreement with____ ____, O.D. Pursuant to said Agreement, Buyer could spend up to 12 hours per week practicing optometry in________. Seller hereby consents to said arrangement and Seller hereby agrees that said arrangement will not constitute a violation of the warranties which are set forth in subparagraphs 5A and 5B of this Pledge Agreement, if: (1) the offices of________, O.D., Inc., are continually staffed, on a full-time basis, by a licensed Optometrist; (2) Buyer's absence from the offices of________, Inc., does not exceed 12 hours per week; and (3) the salaries charged to the corporation for licensed optrometric services do not, in any way, impair the corporation's financial condition. In addition, Seller acknowledges that Buyer may wish, for sound business reasons, to alter some of the warranties, covenants, and agreements Buyer has made under Paragraph 5 of this Pledge Agreement. Seller agrees that Seller will not unreasonably withhold Seller's consent to any such requested alteration. Notwithstanding the foregoing, said consent may only be affected by a written instrument signed by both Buyer and Seller.

IN WITNESS WHEREOF, Buyer and Seller have executed this Pledge Agreement effective as of ________, 19________.

____________________, O.D.	____________________, O.D.
"Seller"	"Buyer"
____________________	____________________
Wife of	Wife of

*Source: American Optometric Association. Adapted with permission.

How to Determine Impairment of the Whole Person Contributed by the Visual System*

Step 1. Calculate and record:

(a) percentage loss of central vision for each eye (Tables 15.1 and 15.2)
(b) percentage loss of visual field for each eye (Tables 15.3 and 15.4)
(c) percentage loss of ocular motility (Figure 15.2)

Step 2. Use the Combined Values Chart (pages 728–730) to:

(a) combine the percentage loss of central vision with the percentage loss of visual field in each eye
Example:

<u>Right Eye</u>

loss of central vision	56%
loss of visual field	32%
Combined Values Chart result	70%

<u>Left Eye</u>

loss of central vision	46%
loss of visual field	32%
Combined Values Chart result	63%

(b) combine the percentage loss of ocular motility with the combined value for central vision and visual field in the eye manifesting the greater impairment. Disregard loss of motility in the other eye.
Example:

<u>Right Eye</u>

combined value for acuity and field	70%
loss of ocular motility	25%
Combined Values Chart result	78%

Step 3. Determine the impairment of the visual system (see table on pages 731–733)
Example:

impairment of right (worse) eye	78%
impairment of the left (better) eye	63%
impairment of the visual system	67%

Step 4. Determine the impairment of the whole person that is contributed by impairment of the visual system (Table 15.5)
Example:

67% impairment of the visual system is equivalent to a 63% impairment of the whole person

*Source: *Guides to the Evaluation of Permanent Impairment*, 2nd ed., American Medical Assn., 1984, p. 147.

COMBINED VALUES CHART

The values are derived from the formula: A + B (1 − A) = combined value of A and B, where A and B are the decimal equivalents of the impairment ratings. In the chart all values are expressed as percents. To combine any two impairment values, locate the larger of the values on the side of the chart and read along that row until you come to the column indicated by the smaller value at the bottom of the chart. At the intersection of the row and the column is the combined value.

For example, to combine 35% and 20% read down the side of the chart until you come to the larger value, 35%. Then read across the 35% row until you come to the column indicated by 20% at the bottom of the chart. At the intersection of the row and column is the number 48. Therefore, 35% combined with 20% is 48%. Due to the construction of this chart, the larger impairment value must be identified at the side of the chart.

If three or more impairment values are to be combined, select any two and find their combined value as above. Then use that value and the third value to locate the combined value of all. This process can be repeated indefinitely, the final value in each instance being the combination of all the previous values. In each step of this process the larger impairment value must be identified at the side of the chart.

	1	2	3	4	5	6	7	8	9	10	11	12	13	14	15	16	17	18	19	20	21	22	23	24	25	26	27	28	29	30	31	32	33	34	35	36	37	38	39	40	41	42	43	44	45	46	47	48	49	50
1	2																																																	
2	3	4																																																
3	4	5	6																																															
4	5	6	7	8																																														
5	6	7	8	9	10																																													
6	7	8	9	10	11	12																																												
7	8	9	10	11	12	13	14																																											
8	9	10	11	12	13	14	14	15																																										
9	10	11	12	13	14	14	15	16	17																																									
10	11	12	13	14	14	15	16	17	18	19																																								
11	12	13	14	15	15	16	17	18	19	20	21																																							
12	13	14	15	16	16	17	18	19	20	21	22	23																																						
13	14	15	16	16	17	18	19	20	21	22	23	23	24																																					
14	15	16	17	17	18	19	20	21	22	23	23	24	25	26																																				
15	16	17	18	18	19	20	21	22	23	24	24	25	26	27	28																																			
16	17	18	19	19	20	21	22	23	24	24	25	26	27	28	29	29																																		
17	18	19	19	20	21	22	23	24	24	25	26	27	28	29	29	30	31																																	
18	19	20	20	21	22	23	24	25	25	26	27	28	29	29	30	31	32	33																																
19	20	21	21	22	23	24	25	25	26	27	28	29	30	30	31	32	33	34	34																															
20	21	22	22	23	24	25	26	26	27	28	29	30	30	31	32	33	34	34	35	36																														
21	22	23	23	24	25	26	27	27	28	29	30	30	31	32	33	34	34	35	36	37	38																													
22	23	24	24	25	26	27	27	28	29	30	31	31	32	33	34	34	35	36	37	38	38	39																												
23	24	25	25	26	27	28	28	29	30	31	31	32	33	34	35	35	36	37	38	38	39	40	40																											
24	25	26	26	27	28	29	29	30	31	32	32	33	34	35	35	36	37	38	38	39	40	41	41	42																										
25	26	27	27	28	29	30	30	31	32	33	33	34	35	36	36	37	38	39	39	40	41	42	42	43	44																									
26	27	27	28	29	30	30	31	32	33	33	34	35	36	36	37	38	39	39	40	41	42	42	43	44	45	45																								
27	28	28	29	30	31	31	32	33	34	34	35	36	36	37	38	39	39	40	41	42	42	43	44	45	45	46	47																							
28	29	29	30	31	32	32	33	34	34	35	36	37	37	38	39	40	40	41	42	42	43	44	45	45	46	47	47	48																						
29	30	30	31	32	33	33	34	35	35	36	37	38	38	39	40	40	41	42	42	43	44	45	45	46	47	47	48	49	50																					
30	31	31	32	33	34	34	35	36	36	37	38	38	39	40	41	41	42	43	43	44	45	45	46	47	48	48	49	50	50	51																				
31	32	32	33	34	34	35	36	37	37	38	39	39	40	41	41	42	43	43	44	45	45	46	47	48	48	49	50	50	51	52	52																			
32	33	33	34	35	35	36	37	37	38	39	39	40	41	42	42	43	44	44	45	46	46	47	48	48	49	50	50	51	52	52	53	54																		
33	34	34	35	36	36	37	38	38	39	40	40	41	42	42	43	44	44	45	46	46	47	48	48	49	50	50	51	52	52	53	54	54	55																	
34	35	35	36	37	37	38	39	39	40	41	41	42	43	43	44	45	45	46	47	47	48	49	49	50	51	51	52	52	53	54	54	55	56	56																
35	36	36	37	38	38	39	40	40	41	42	42	43	43	44	45	45	46	47	47	48	49	49	50	51	51	52	53	53	54	55	55	56	56	57	58															
36	37	37	38	39	39	40	40	41	42	42	43	44	44	45	46	46	47	48	48	49	49	50	51	51	52	53	53	54	55	55	56	56	57	58	58	59														
37	38	38	39	40	40	41	41	42	43	43	44	45	45	46	46	47	48	48	49	50	50	51	51	52	53	53	54	55	55	56	57	57	58	58	59	60	60													
38	39	39	40	40	41	42	42	43	44	44	45	45	46	47	47	48	49	49	50	50	51	52	52	53	54	54	55	55	56	57	57	58	58	59	60	60	61	62												
39	40	40	41	41	42	43	43	44	44	45	46	46	47	48	48	49	50	50	51	51	52	52	53	54	54	55	55	56	57	57	58	59	59	60	60	61	62	62	63											
40	41	41	42	42	43	44	44	45	45	46	47	47	48	48	49	50	50	51	51	52	53	53	54	54	55	56	56	57	57	58	59	59	60	60	61	62	62	63	63	64										
41	42	42	43	43	44	45	45	46	46	47	47	48	49	49	50	50	51	52	52	53	53	54	55	55	56	56	57	58	58	59	59	60	60	61	62	62	63	63	64	65	65									
42	43	43	44	44	45	45	46	47	47	48	48	49	50	50	51	51	52	52	53	54	54	55	55	56	57	57	58	58	59	59	60	61	61	62	62	63	63	64	65	65	66	66								
43	44	44	45	45	46	46	47	48	48	49	49	50	50	51	52	52	53	53	54	54	55	56	56	57	57	58	58	59	60	60	61	61	62	62	63	64	64	65	65	66	66	67	68							
44	45	45	46	46	47	47	48	48	49	50	50	51	51	52	52	53	54	54	55	55	56	56	57	57	58	59	59	60	60	61	61	62	62	63	64	64	65	65	66	66	67	68	68	69						
45	46	46	47	47	48	48	49	49	50	51	51	52	52	53	53	54	54	55	55	56	57	57	58	58	59	59	60	60	61	62	62	63	63	64	64	65	65	66	66	67	68	68	69	69	70					
46	47	47	48	48	49	49	50	50	51	51	52	52	53	54	54	55	55	56	56	57	57	58	58	59	60	60	61	61	62	62	63	63	64	64	65	65	66	67	67	68	68	69	69	70	70	71				
47	48	48	49	49	50	50	51	51	52	52	53	53	54	54	55	55	56	57	57	58	58	59	59	60	60	61	61	62	62	63	63	64	64	65	66	66	67	67	68	68	69	69	70	70	71	71	72			
48	49	49	50	50	51	51	52	52	53	53	54	54	55	55	56	56	57	57	58	58	59	59	60	60	61	62	62	63	63	64	64	65	65	66	66	67	67	68	68	69	69	70	70	71	71	72	72	73		
49	50	50	51	51	52	52	53	53	54	54	55	55	56	56	57	57	58	58	59	59	60	60	61	61	62	62	63	63	64	64	65	65	66	66	67	67	68	68	69	69	70	70	71	71	72	72	73	73	74	
50	51	51	52	52	53	53	54	54	55	55	56	56	57	57	58	58	59	59	60	60	61	61	62	62	63	63	64	64	65	65	66	66	67	67	68	68	69	69	70	70	71	71	72	72	73	73	74	74	75	75

	1	2	3	4	5	6	7	8	9	10	11	12	13	14	15	16	17	18	19	20	21	22	23	24	25	26	27	28	29	30	31	32	33	34	35	36	37	38	39	40	41	42	43	44	45	46	47	48	49	50
51	51	52	52	53	53	54	54	55	55	56	56	57	57	58	58	59	59	60	60	61	61	62	62	63	63	64	64	65	65	66	66	67	67	68	68	69	69	70	70	71	71	72	72	73	73	74	74	75	75	76
52	52	53	53	54	54	55	55	56	56	57	57	58	58	59	59	60	60	61	61	62	62	63	63	64	64	64	65	65	66	66	67	67	68	68	69	69	70	70	71	71	72	72	73	73	74	75	75	75	76	76
53	53	54	54	55	55	56	56	57	57	58	58	59	59	60	60	61	61	61	62	62	63	63	64	64	65	65	66	66	67	67	68	68	69	69	69	70	70	71	71	72	72	73	73	74	74	74	75	76	76	77
54	54	55	55	56	56	57	57	58	58	59	59	59	60	60	61	61	62	62	63	63	64	64	65	65	66	66	66	67	67	68	68	69	69	70	70	71	71	71	72	72	73	73	74	74	75	75	76	76	77	77
55	55	56	56	57	57	58	58	59	59	60	60	60	61	61	62	62	63	63	64	64	64	65	65	66	66	67	67	68	68	69	69	69	70	70	71	71	72	72	73	73	73	74	74	75	75	76	76	77	77	78
56	56	57	57	58	58	59	59	60	60	60	61	61	62	62	63	63	63	64	64	65	65	66	66	67	67	67	68	68	69	69	70	70	71	71	71	72	72	73	73	74	74	74	75	75	76	76	77	77	78	78
57	57	58	58	59	59	60	60	60	61	61	62	62	63	63	63	64	64	65	65	66	66	66	67	67	68	68	69	69	69	70	70	71	71	72	72	72	73	73	74	74	75	75	75	76	76	77	77	78	78	79
58	58	59	59	60	60	61	61	61	62	62	63	63	63	64	64	65	65	66	66	66	67	67	68	68	68	69	69	70	70	71	71	71	72	72	73	73	74	74	74	75	75	76	76	76	77	77	78	78	79	79
59	59	60	60	61	61	61	62	62	63	63	64	64	64	65	65	66	66	66	67	67	68	68	68	69	69	70	70	70	71	71	72	72	73	73	73	74	74	75	75	75	76	76	77	77	77	78	78	79	79	80
60	60	61	61	62	62	62	63	63	64	64	64	65	65	65	66	66	67	67	68	68	68	69	69	70	70	70	71	71	72	72	72	73	73	74	74	74	75	75	76	76	76	77	77	78	78	78	79	79	80	80
61	61	62	62	63	63	63	64	64	65	65	65	66	66	66	67	67	68	68	68	69	69	70	70	70	71	71	72	72	72	73	73	73	74	74	75	75	75	76	76	77	77	77	78	78	79	79	79	80	80	81
62	62	63	63	64	64	64	65	65	65	66	66	67	67	67	68	68	68	69	69	70	70	70	71	71	72	72	72	73	73	73	74	74	75	75	75	76	76	76	77	77	78	78	78	79	79	79	80	80	81	81
63	63	64	64	64	65	65	66	66	66	67	67	67	68	68	69	69	69	70	70	70	71	71	72	72	72	73	73	73	74	74	74	75	75	76	76	76	77	77	77	78	78	79	79	79	80	80	80	81	81	82
64	64	65	65	65	66	66	67	67	67	68	68	68	69	69	69	70	70	70	71	71	72	72	72	73	73	73	74	74	74	75	75	76	76	76	77	77	77	78	78	78	79	79	79	80	80	81	81	81	82	82
65	65	66	66	66	67	67	67	68	68	69	69	69	70	70	70	71	71	71	72	72	72	73	73	73	74	74	74	75	75	76	76	76	77	77	77	78	78	78	79	79	79	80	80	80	81	81	81	82	82	83
66	66	67	67	67	68	68	68	69	69	69	70	70	70	71	71	71	72	72	72	73	73	73	74	74	75	75	75	76	76	76	77	77	77	78	78	78	79	79	79	80	80	80	81	81	81	82	82	82	83	83
67	67	68	68	68	69	69	69	70	70	70	71	71	71	72	72	72	73	73	73	74	74	74	75	75	75	76	76	76	77	77	77	78	78	78	79	79	79	80	80	80	81	81	81	82	82	82	83	83	83	84
68	68	69	69	69	70	70	70	71	71	71	72	72	72	72	73	73	73	74	74	74	75	75	75	76	76	76	77	77	77	78	78	78	79	79	79	80	80	80	80	81	81	81	82	82	82	83	83	83	84	84
69	69	70	70	70	71	71	71	71	72	72	72	73	73	73	74	74	74	75	75	75	76	76	76	76	77	77	77	78	78	78	79	79	79	80	80	80	80	81	81	81	82	82	82	83	83	83	84	84	84	85
70	70	71	71	71	72	72	72	72	73	73	73	74	74	74	75	75	75	75	76	76	76	77	77	77	78	78	78	78	79	79	79	80	80	80	81	81	81	81	82	82	82	83	83	83	84	84	84	84	85	85
71	71	72	72	72	72	73	73	73	74	74	74	74	75	75	75	76	76	76	77	77	77	77	78	78	78	79	79	79	79	80	80	80	81	81	81	81	82	82	82	83	83	83	83	84	84	84	85	85	85	86
72	72	73	73	73	73	74	74	74	75	75	75	75	76	76	76	76	77	77	77	78	78	78	78	79	79	79	80	80	80	80	81	81	81	82	82	82	82	83	83	83	83	84	84	84	85	85	85	85	86	86
73	73	74	74	74	74	75	75	75	75	76	76	76	77	77	77	77	78	78	78	78	79	79	79	79	80	80	80	81	81	81	81	82	82	82	82	83	83	83	84	84	84	84	85	85	85	85	86	86	86	87
74	74	75	75	75	75	76	76	76	76	77	77	77	77	78	78	78	78	79	79	79	79	80	80	80	81	81	81	81	82	82	82	82	83	83	83	83	84	84	84	84	85	85	85	85	86	86	86	86	87	87
75	75	76	76	76	76	77	77	77	77	78	78	78	78	79	79	79	79	80	80	80	80	81	81	81	81	82	82	82	82	83	83	83	83	84	84	84	84	85	85	85	85	86	86	86	86	87	87	87	87	88
76	76	76	77	77	77	77	78	78	78	78	79	79	79	79	80	80	80	80	81	81	81	81	82	82	82	82	82	83	83	83	83	84	84	84	84	85	85	85	85	86	86	86	86	87	87	87	87	88	88	88
77	77	77	78	78	78	78	79	79	79	79	80	80	80	80	80	81	81	81	81	82	82	82	82	83	83	83	83	83	84	84	84	84	85	85	85	85	86	86	86	86	86	87	87	87	87	88	88	88	88	89
78	78	78	79	79	79	79	80	80	80	80	80	81	81	81	81	82	82	82	82	82	83	83	83	83	84	84	84	84	84	85	85	85	85	85	86	86	86	86	87	87	87	87	87	88	88	88	88	89	89	89
79	79	79	80	80	80	80	80	81	81	81	81	82	82	82	82	82	83	83	83	83	83	84	84	84	84	84	85	85	85	85	86	86	86	86	86	87	87	87	87	87	88	88	88	88	88	89	89	89	89	90
80	80	80	81	81	81	81	81	82	82	82	82	82	83	83	83	83	83	84	84	84	84	84	85	85	85	85	85	86	86	86	86	86	87	87	87	87	87	88	88	88	88	88	89	89	89	89	89	90	90	90
81	81	81	82	82	82	82	82	83	83	83	83	83	83	84	84	84	84	84	85	85	85	85	85	86	86	86	86	86	87	87	87	87	87	87	88	88	88	88	88	89	89	89	89	89	90	90	90	90	90	91
82	82	82	83	83	83	83	83	83	84	84	84	84	84	85	85	85	85	85	86	86	86	86	86	86	87	87	87	87	87	87	88	88	88	88	88	88	89	89	89	89	89	90	90	90	90	90	90	91	91	91
83	83	83	84	84	84	84	84	84	85	85	85	85	85	85	86	86	86	86	86	86	87	87	87	87	87	87	88	88	88	88	88	88	89	89	89	89	89	89	90	90	90	90	90	90	91	91	91	91	91	92
84	84	84	84	85	85	85	85	85	85	86	86	86	86	86	86	87	87	87	87	87	87	88	88	88	88	88	88	88	89	89	89	89	89	89	90	90	90	90	90	90	91	91	91	91	91	91	92	92	92	92
85	85	85	85	86	86	86	86	86	86	87	87	87	87	87	87	87	88	88	88	88	88	88	88	89	89	89	89	89	89	90	90	90	90	90	90	90	91	91	91	91	91	91	91	92	92	92	92	92	92	93
86	86	86	86	87	87	87	87	87	87	87	88	88	88	88	88	88	88	89	89	89	89	89	89	89	90	90	90	90	90	90	90	90	91	91	91	91	91	91	91	92	92	92	92	92	92	92	93	93	93	93
87	87	87	87	88	88	88	88	88	88	88	88	89	89	89	89	89	89	89	89	90	90	90	90	90	90	90	91	91	91	91	91	91	91	91	92	92	92	92	92	92	92	92	93	93	93	93	93	93	93	94
88	88	88	88	88	89	89	89	89	89	89	89	89	90	90	90	90	90	90	90	90	91	91	91	91	91	91	91	91	91	92	92	92	92	92	92	92	92	93	93	93	93	93	93	93	93	94	94	94	94	94
89	89	89	89	89	90	90	90	90	90	90	90	90	90	91	91	91	91	91	91	91	91	91	92	92	92	92	92	92	92	92	92	93	93	93	93	93	93	93	93	93	94	94	94	94	94	94	94	94	94	95
90	90	90	90	90	91	91	91	91	91	91	91	91	91	91	92	92	92	92	92	92	92	92	92	92	93	93	93	93	93	93	93	93	93	93	94	94	94	94	94	94	94	94	94	94	95	95	95	95	95	95
91	91	91	91	91	91	92	92	92	92	92	92	92	92	92	92	92	93	93	93	93	93	93	93	93	93	93	93	94	94	94	94	94	94	94	94	94	94	94	95	95	95	95	95	95	95	95	95	95	95	96
92	92	92	92	92	92	92	93	93	93	93	93	93	93	93	93	93	93	93	94	94	94	94	94	94	94	94	94	94	94	94	94	95	95	95	95	95	95	95	95	95	95	95	95	96	96	96	96	96	96	96
93	93	93	93	93	93	93	93	94	94	94	94	94	94	94	94	94	94	94	94	94	94	95	95	95	95	95	95	95	95	95	95	95	95	95	95	96	96	96	96	96	96	96	96	96	96	96	96	96	96	97
94	94	94	94	94	94	94	94	94	95	95	95	95	95	95	95	95	95	95	95	95	95	95	95	95	96	96	96	96	96	96	96	96	96	96	96	96	96	96	96	96	96	97	97	97	97	97	97	97	97	97
95	95	95	95	95	95	95	95	95	95	96	96	96	96	96	96	96	96	96	96	96	96	96	96	96	96	96	96	96	96	96	97	97	97	97	97	97	97	97	97	97	97	97	97	97	97	97	97	97	97	98
96	96	96	96	96	96	96	96	96	96	96	96	96	97	97	97	97	97	97	97	97	97	97	97	97	97	97	97	97	97	97	97	97	97	97	97	97	97	98	98	98	98	98	98	98	98	98	98	98	98	98
97	97	97	97	97	97	97	97	97	97	97	97	97	97	97	97	97	98	98	98	98	98	98	98	98	98	98	98	98	98	98	98	98	98	98	98	98	98	98	98	98	98	98	98	98	98	98	98	98	98	99
98	98	98	98	98	98	98	98	98	98	98	98	98	98	98	98	98	98	98	98	98	98	98	98	98	99	99	99	99	99	99	99	99	99	99	99	99	99	99	99	99	99	99	99	99	99	99	99	99	99	99
99	99	99	99	99	99	99	99	99	99	99	99	99	99	99	99	99	99	99	99	99	99	99	99	99	99	99	99	99	99	99	99	99	99	99	99	99	99	99	99	99	99	99	99	99	99	99	99	99	99	100
	1	2	3	4	5	6	7	8	9	10	11	12	13	14	15	16	17	18	19	20	21	22	23	24	25	26	27	28	29	30	31	32	33	34	35	36	37	38	39	40	41	42	43	44	45	46	47	48	49	50

	51	52	53	54	55	56	57	58	59	60	61	62	63	64	65	66	67	68	69	70	71	72	73	74	75	76	77	78	79	80	81	82	83	84	85	86	87	88	89	90	91	92	93	94	95	96	97	98	99
51	76																																																
52	76	77																																															
53	77	77	78																																														
54	77	78	78	79																																													
55	78	78	79	79	80																																												
56	78	79	79	80	80	81																																											
57	79	79	80	80	81	81	82																																										
58	79	80	80	81	81	82	82	82																																									
59	80	80	81	81	82	82	82	83	83																																								
60	80	81	81	82	82	82	83	83	84	84																																							
61	81	81	82	82	82	83	83	84	84	84	85																																						
62	81	82	82	83	83	83	84	84	84	85	85	86																																					
63	82	82	83	83	83	84	84	84	85	85	86	86	86																																				
64	82	83	83	83	84	84	85	85	85	86	86	86	87	87																																			
65	83	83	84	84	84	85	85	85	86	86	86	87	87	87	88																																		
66	83	84	84	84	85	85	85	86	86	86	87	87	87	88	88	88																																	
67	84	84	84	85	85	85	86	86	86	87	87	87	88	88	88	89	89																																
68	84	85	85	85	86	86	86	87	87	87	88	88	88	88	89	89	89	90																															
69	85	85	85	86	86	86	87	87	87	88	88	88	89	89	89	89	90	90	90																														
70	85	86	86	86	87	87	87	87	88	88	88	89	89	89	90	90	90	90	91	91																													
71	86	86	86	87	87	87	88	88	88	88	89	89	89	90	90	90	90	91	91	91	92																												
72	86	87	87	87	87	88	88	88	89	89	89	89	90	90	90	90	91	91	91	92	92	92																											
73	87	87	87	88	88	88	88	89	89	89	89	90	90	90	91	91	91	91	92	92	92	92	93																										
74	87	88	88	88	88	89	89	89	89	90	90	90	90	91	91	91	91	92	92	92	92	93	93	93																									
75	88	88	88	89	89	89	89	90	90	90	90	91	91	91	91	92	92	92	92	93	93	93	93	94	94																								
76	88	88	89	89	89	89	90	90	90	90	91	91	91	91	92	92	92	92	93	93	93	93	94	94	94	94																							
77	89	89	89	89	90	90	90	90	91	91	91	91	91	92	92	92	92	93	93	93	93	94	94	94	94	94	95																						
78	89	89	90	90	90	90	91	91	91	91	91	92	92	92	92	93	93	93	93	93	94	94	94	94	95	95	95	95																					
79	90	90	90	90	91	91	91	91	91	92	92	92	92	92	93	93	93	93	93	94	94	94	94	95	95	95	95	95	96																				
80	90	90	91	91	91	91	91	92	92	92	92	92	93	93	93	93	93	94	94	94	94	94	95	95	95	95	95	96	96	96																			
81	91	91	91	91	91	92	92	92	92	92	93	93	93	93	93	94	94	94	94	94	94	95	95	95	95	95	96	96	96	96	96																		
82	91	91	92	92	92	92	92	92	93	93	93	93	93	94	94	94	94	94	94	95	95	95	95	95	96	96	96	96	96	96	97	97																	
83	92	92	92	92	92	93	93	93	93	93	93	94	94	94	94	94	94	95	95	95	95	95	95	96	96	96	96	96	96	97	97	97	97																
84	92	92	92	93	93	93	93	93	93	94	94	94	94	94	94	95	95	95	95	95	95	96	96	96	96	96	96	96	97	97	97	97	97	97															
85	93	93	93	93	93	93	94	94	94	94	94	94	94	95	95	95	95	95	95	96	96	96	96	96	96	96	97	97	97	97	97	97	97	98	98														
86	93	93	93	94	94	94	94	94	94	94	95	95	95	95	95	95	95	96	96	96	96	96	96	96	97	97	97	97	97	97	97	97	98	98	98	98													
87	94	94	94	94	94	94	94	95	95	95	95	95	95	95	95	96	96	96	96	96	96	96	96	97	97	97	97	97	97	97	98	98	98	98	98	98	98												
88	94	94	94	94	95	95	95	95	95	95	95	95	96	96	96	96	96	96	96	96	97	97	97	97	97	97	97	97	97	98	98	98	98	98	98	98	98	99											
89	95	95	95	95	95	95	95	95	95	96	96	96	96	96	96	96	96	96	97	97	97	97	97	97	97	97	97	98	98	98	98	98	98	98	98	98	99	99	99										
90	95	95	95	95	96	96	96	96	96	96	96	96	96	96	97	97	97	97	97	97	97	97	97	97	98	98	98	98	98	98	98	98	98	98	99	99	99	99	99	99									
91	96	96	96	96	96	96	96	96	96	96	96	97	97	97	97	97	97	97	97	97	97	97	98	98	98	98	98	98	98	98	98	98	98	99	99	99	99	99	99	99	99								
92	96	96	96	96	96	96	97	97	97	97	97	97	97	97	97	97	97	97	98	98	98	98	98	98	98	98	98	98	98	98	98	99	99	99	99	99	99	99	99	99	99	99							
93	97	97	97	97	97	97	97	97	97	97	97	97	97	98	98	98	98	98	98	98	98	98	98	98	98	98	98	98	98	99	99	99	99	99	99	99	99	99	99	99	99	99	00						
94	97	97	97	97	97	97	97	97	98	98	98	98	98	98	98	98	98	98	98	98	98	98	98	98	99	99	99	99	99	99	99	99	99	99	99	99	99	99	99	99	99	100	100	100					
95	98	98	98	98	98	98	98	98	98	98	98	98	98	98	98	98	98	98	98	99	99	99	99	99	99	99	99	99	99	99	99	99	99	99	99	99	99	99	99	100	100	100	100	100	100				
96	98	98	98	98	98	98	98	98	98	98	98	98	99	99	99	99	99	99	99	99	99	99	99	99	99	99	99	99	99	99	99	99	99	99	99	99	99	100	100	100	100	100	100	100	100	100			
97	99	99	99	99	99	99	99	99	99	99	99	99	99	99	99	99	99	99	99	99	99	99	99	99	99	99	99	99	99	99	99	99	99	100	100	100	100	100	100	100	100	100	100	100	100	100	100		
98	99	99	99	99	99	99	99	99	99	99	99	99	99	99	99	99	99	99	99	99	99	99	99	99	100	100	100	100	100	100	100	100	100	100	100	100	100	100	100	100	100	100	100	100	100	100	100	100	
99	100	100	100	100	100	100	100	100	100	100	100	100	100	100	100	100	100	100	100	100	100	100	100	100	100	100	100	100	100	100	100	100	100	100	100	100	100	100	100	100	100	100	100	100	100	100	100	100	100

% IMPAIRMENT WORSE EYE

Worse eye \ Better eye	0	1	2	3	4	5	6	7	8	9	10	11	12	13	14	15	16	17	18	19	20	21	22	23	24	25	26	27	28	29	30	31	32	33	34	35	36	37	38	39	40	41	42	43	44	45	46	47	48	49
0	0																																																	
1	0	1																																															
2	1	1	2																																													
3	1	2	2	3																																											
4	1	2	3	3	4																																									
5	1	2	3	4	4	5																																							
6	2	2	3	4	5	5	6																																					
7	2	3	3	4	5	6	6	7																																				
8	2	3	4	4	5	6	7	7	8																																			
9	2	3	4	5	5	6	7	8	8	9																																		
10	3	3	4	5	6	6	7	8	9	9	10																																							
11	3	4	4	5	6	7	7	8	9	10	10	11																																					
12	3	4	5	5	6	7	8	8	9	10	11	11	12																																				
13	3	4	5	6	6	7	8	9	9	10	11	12	12	13																																			
14	4	4	5	6	7	7	8	9	10	10	11	12	13	13	14																																		
15	4	5	5	6	7	8	8	9	10	11	11	12	13	14	14	15																																	
16	4	5	6	6	7	8	9	9	10	11	12	12	13	14	15	15	16																																
17	4	5	6	7	7	8	9	10	10	11	12	13	13	14	15	16	16	17																															
18	5	5	6	7	8	8	9	10	11	11	12	13	14	14	15	16	17	17	18																														
19	5	6	6	7	8	9	9	10	11	12	12	13	14	15	15	16	17	18	18	19																													
20	5	6	7	7	8	9	10	10	11	12	13	13	14	15	16	16	17	18	19	19	20																												
21	5	6	7	8	8	9	10	11	11	12	13	14	14	15	16	17	17	18	19	20	20	21																											
22	6	6	7	8	9	9	10	11	12	12	13	14	15	15	16	17	18	18	19	20	21	21	22																										
23	6	7	7	8	9	10	10	11	12	13	13	14	15	16	16	17	18	19	19	20	21	22	22	23																									
24	6	7	8	8	9	10	11	11	12	13	14	14	15	16	17	17	18	19	20	20	21	22	23	23	24																								
25	6	7	8	9	9	10	11	12	12	13	14	15	15	16	17	18	18	19	20	21	21	22	23	24	24	25																							
26	7	7	8	9	10	10	11	12	13	13	14	15	16	16	17	18	19	19	20	21	22	22	23	24	25	25	26																						
27	7	8	8	9	10	11	11	12	13	14	14	15	16	17	17	18	19	20	20	21	22	23	23	24	25	26	26	27																					
28	7	8	9	9	10	11	12	12	13	14	15	15	16	17	18	18	19	20	21	21	22	23	24	24	25	26	27	27	28																				
29	7	8	9	10	10	11	12	13	13	14	15	16	16	17	18	19	19	20	21	22	22	23	24	25	25	26	27	28	28	29																			
30	8	8	9	10	11	11	12	13	14	14	15	16	17	17	18	19	20	20	21	22	23	23	24	25	26	26	27	28	29	29	30																		
31	8	9	9	10	11	12	12	13	14	15	15	16	17	18	18	19	20	21	21	22	23	24	24	25	26	27	27	28	29	30	30	31																	
32	8	9	10	10	11	12	13	13	14	15	16	16	17	18	19	19	20	21	22	22	23	24	25	25	26	27	28	28	29	30	31	31	32																
33	8	9	10	11	11	12	13	14	14	15	16	17	17	18	19	20	20	21	22	23	23	24	25	26	26	27	28	29	29	30	31	32	32	33															
34	9	9	10	11	12	12	13	14	15	15	16	17	18	18	19	20	21	21	22	23	24	24	25	26	27	27	28	29	30	30	31	32	33	33	34														
35	9	10	10	11	12	13	13	14	15	16	16	17	18	19	19	20	21	22	22	23	24	25	25	26	27	28	28	29	30	31	31	32	33	34	34	35													
36	9	10	11	11	12	13	14	14	15	16	17	17	18	19	20	20	21	22	23	23	24	25	26	26	27	28	29	29	30	31	32	32	33	34	35	35	36												
37	9	10	11	12	12	13	14	15	15	16	17	18	18	19	20	21	21	22	23	24	24	25	26	27	27	28	29	30	30	31	32	33	33	34	35	36	36	37											
38	10	10	11	12	13	13	14	15	16	16	17	18	19	19	20	21	22	22	23	24	25	25	26	27	28	28	29	30	31	31	32	33	34	34	35	36	37	37	38										
39	10	11	11	12	13	14	14	15	16	17	17	18	19	20	20	21	22	23	23	24	25	26	26	27	28	29	29	30	31	32	32	33	34	35	35	36	37	38	38	39									
40	10	11	12	12	13	14	15	15	16	17	18	18	19	20	21	21	22	23	24	24	25	26	27	27	28	29	30	30	31	32	33	33	34	35	36	36	37	38	39	39	40								
41	10	11	12	13	13	14	15	16	16	17	18	19	19	20	21	22	22	23	24	25	25	26	27	28	28	29	30	31	31	32	33	34	34	35	36	37	37	38	39	40	40	41							
42	11	11	12	13	14	14	15	16	17	17	18	19	20	20	21	22	23	23	24	25	26	26	27	28	29	29	30	31	32	32	33	34	35	35	36	37	38	38	39	40	41	41	42						
43	11	12	12	13	14	15	15	16	17	18	18	19	20	21	21	22	23	24	24	25	26	27	27	28	29	30	30	31	32	33	33	34	35	36	36	37	38	39	39	40	41	42	42	43					
44	11	12	13	13	14	15	16	16	17	18	19	19	20	21	22	22	23	24	25	25	26	27	28	28	29	30	31	31	32	33	34	34	35	36	37	37	38	39	40	40	41	42	43	43	44				
45	11	12	13	14	14	15	16	17	17	18	19	20	20	21	22	23	23	24	25	26	26	27	28	29	29	30	31	32	32	33	34	35	35	36	37	38	38	39	40	41	41	42	43	44	44	45				
46	12	12	13	14	15	15	16	17	18	18	19	20	21	21	22	23	24	24	25	26	27	27	28	29	30	30	31	32	33	33	34	35	36	36	37	38	39	39	40	41	42	42	43	44	45	45	46			
47	12	13	13	14	15	16	16	17	18	19	19	20	21	22	22	23	24	25	25	26	27	28	28	29	30	31	31	32	33	34	34	35	36	37	37	38	39	40	40	41	42	43	43	44	45	46	46	47		
48	12	13	14	14	15	16	17	17	18	19	20	20	21	22	23	23	24	25	26	26	27	28	29	29	30	31	32	32	33	34	35	35	36	37	38	38	39	40	41	41	42	43	44	44	45	46	47	47	48	
49	12	13	14	15	15	16	17	18	18	19	20	21	21	22	23	24	24	25	26	27	27	28	29	30	30	31	32	33	33	34	35	36	36	37	38	39	39	40	41	42	42	43	44	45	45	46	47	48	48	49

The values in this table are based on the following formula:

$$\frac{3 \times \text{better eye value} + \text{worse eye value}}{4} = \text{impairment of visual system.}$$

The guides to the table are percentage impairment values for each eye. The percentage for the worse eye is read at the side of the table. The percentage for the better eye is read at the bottom of the table. At the intersection of the column for the worse eye and the column for the better eye is the impairment of visual system value.

For example, when there is 60% impairment of one eye and 30% impairment of the other eye, read down the side of the table until you come to the larger value (60%). Then follow across the row until it is intersected by the column headed by 30% at the bottom of the page. At the intersection of these two columns is printed the number 38. The number (38) represents the percentage impairment of the visual system when there is 60% impairment of one eye and 30% impairment of the other eye.

If bilateral aphakia is present and corrected central vision has been used in evaluation, impairment of visual system is increased 25%. For example, a 38% impairment would be increased to 38% + (25%) (38%) = 48%

% IMPAIRMENT WORSE EYE

	0	1	2	3	4	5	6	7	8	9	10	11	12	13	14	15	16	17	18	19	20	21	22	23	24	25	26	27	28	29	30	31	32	33	34	35	36	37	38	39	40	41	42	43	44	45	46	47	48	49	
50	13	13	14	15	16	16	17	18	19	19	20	21	22	22	23	24	25	25	26	27	28	28	29	30	31	31	32	33	34	34	35	36	37	37	38	39	40	40	41	42	43	43	44	45	46	46	47	48	49	49	**50**
51	13	14	14	15	16	17	17	18	19	20	20	21	22	23	23	24	25	26	26	27	28	29	29	30	31	32	32	33	34	35	35	36	37	38	38	39	40	41	41	42	43	44	44	45	46	47	47	48	49	50	51
52	13	14	15	15	16	17	18	18	19	20	21	21	22	23	24	24	25	26	27	27	28	29	30	30	31	32	33	33	34	35	36	36	37	38	39	39	40	41	42	42	43	44	45	45	46	47	48	48	49	50	52
53	13	14	15	16	16	17	18	19	19	20	21	22	22	23	24	25	25	26	27	28	28	29	30	31	31	32	33	34	34	35	36	37	37	38	39	40	40	41	42	43	43	44	45	46	46	47	48	49	49	50	53
54	14	14	15	16	17	17	18	19	20	20	21	22	23	23	24	25	26	26	27	28	29	29	30	31	32	32	33	34	35	35	36	37	38	38	39	40	41	41	42	43	44	44	45	46	47	47	48	49	50	50	54
55	14	15	15	16	17	18	18	19	20	21	21	22	23	24	24	25	26	27	27	28	29	30	30	31	32	33	33	34	35	36	36	37	38	39	39	40	41	42	42	43	44	45	45	46	47	48	48	49	50	51	**55**
56	14	15	16	16	17	18	19	19	20	21	22	22	23	24	25	25	26	27	28	28	29	30	31	31	32	33	34	34	35	36	37	37	38	39	40	40	41	42	43	43	44	45	46	46	47	48	49	49	50	51	56
57	14	15	16	17	17	18	19	20	20	21	22	23	23	24	25	26	26	27	28	29	29	30	31	32	32	33	34	35	35	36	37	38	38	39	40	41	41	42	43	44	44	45	46	47	47	48	49	50	50	51	57
58	15	15	16	17	18	18	19	20	21	21	22	23	24	24	25	26	27	27	28	29	30	30	31	32	33	33	34	35	36	36	37	38	39	39	40	41	42	42	43	44	45	45	46	47	48	48	49	50	51	51	58
59	15	16	16	17	18	19	19	20	21	22	22	23	24	25	25	26	27	28	28	29	30	31	31	32	33	34	34	35	36	37	37	38	39	40	40	41	42	43	43	44	45	46	46	47	48	49	49	50	51	52	59
60	15	16	17	17	18	19	20	20	21	22	23	23	24	25	26	26	27	28	29	29	30	31	32	32	33	34	35	35	36	37	38	38	39	40	41	41	42	43	44	44	45	46	47	47	48	49	50	50	51	52	**60**
61	15	16	17	18	18	19	20	21	21	22	23	24	24	25	26	27	27	28	29	30	30	31	32	33	33	34	35	36	36	37	38	39	39	40	41	42	42	43	44	45	45	46	47	48	48	49	50	51	51	52	61
62	16	16	17	18	19	19	20	21	22	22	23	24	25	25	26	27	28	28	29	30	31	31	32	33	34	34	35	36	37	37	38	39	40	40	41	42	43	43	44	45	46	46	47	48	49	49	50	51	52	52	62
63	16	17	17	18	19	20	20	21	22	23	23	24	25	26	26	27	28	29	29	30	31	32	32	33	34	35	35	36	37	38	38	39	40	41	41	42	43	44	44	45	46	47	47	48	49	50	50	51	52	53	63
64	16	17	18	18	19	20	21	21	22	23	24	24	25	26	27	27	28	29	30	30	31	32	33	33	34	35	36	36	37	38	39	39	40	41	42	42	43	44	45	45	46	47	48	48	49	50	51	51	52	53	64
65	16	17	18	19	19	20	21	22	22	23	24	25	25	26	27	28	28	29	30	31	31	32	33	34	34	35	36	37	37	38	39	40	40	41	42	43	43	44	45	46	46	47	48	49	49	50	51	52	52	53	**65**
66	17	17	18	19	20	20	21	22	23	23	24	25	26	26	27	28	29	29	30	31	32	32	33	34	35	35	36	37	38	38	39	40	41	41	42	43	44	44	45	46	47	47	48	49	50	50	51	52	53	53	66
67	17	18	18	19	20	21	21	22	23	24	24	25	26	27	27	28	29	30	30	31	32	33	33	34	35	36	36	37	38	39	39	40	41	42	42	43	44	45	45	46	47	48	48	49	50	51	51	52	53	54	67
68	17	18	19	19	20	21	22	22	23	24	25	25	26	27	28	28	29	30	31	31	32	33	34	34	35	36	37	37	38	39	40	40	41	42	43	43	44	45	46	46	47	48	49	49	50	51	52	52	53	54	68
69	17	18	19	20	20	21	22	23	23	24	25	26	26	27	28	29	29	30	31	32	32	33	34	35	35	36	37	38	38	39	40	41	41	42	43	44	44	45	46	47	47	48	49	50	50	51	52	53	53	54	69
70	18	18	19	20	21	21	22	23	24	24	25	26	27	27	28	29	30	30	31	32	33	33	34	35	36	36	37	38	39	39	40	41	42	42	43	44	45	45	46	47	48	48	49	50	51	51	52	53	54	54	**70**
71	18	19	19	20	21	22	22	23	24	25	25	26	27	28	28	29	30	31	31	32	33	34	34	35	36	37	37	38	39	40	40	41	42	43	43	44	45	46	46	47	48	49	49	50	51	52	52	53	54	55	71
72	18	19	20	20	21	22	23	23	24	25	26	26	27	28	29	29	30	31	32	32	33	34	35	35	36	37	38	38	39	40	41	41	42	43	44	44	45	46	47	47	48	49	50	50	51	52	53	53	54	55	72
73	18	19	20	21	21	22	23	24	24	25	26	27	27	28	29	30	30	31	32	33	33	34	35	36	36	37	38	39	39	40	41	42	42	43	44	45	45	46	47	48	48	49	50	51	51	52	53	54	54	55	73
74	19	19	20	21	22	22	23	24	25	25	26	27	28	28	29	30	31	31	32	33	34	34	35	36	37	37	38	39	40	40	41	42	43	43	44	45	46	46	47	48	49	49	50	51	52	52	53	54	55	55	74
75	19	20	20	21	22	23	23	24	25	26	26	27	28	29	29	30	31	32	32	33	34	35	35	36	37	38	38	39	40	41	41	42	43	44	44	45	46	47	47	48	49	50	50	51	52	53	53	54	55	56	**75**
76	19	20	21	21	22	23	24	24	25	26	27	27	28	29	30	30	31	32	33	33	34	35	36	36	37	38	39	39	40	41	42	42	43	44	45	45	46	47	48	48	49	50	51	51	52	53	54	54	55	56	76
77	19	20	21	22	22	23	24	25	25	26	27	28	28	29	30	31	31	32	33	34	34	35	36	37	37	38	39	40	40	41	42	43	43	44	45	46	46	47	48	49	49	50	51	52	52	53	54	55	55	56	77
78	20	20	21	22	23	23	24	25	26	26	27	28	29	29	30	31	32	32	33	34	35	35	36	37	38	38	39	40	41	41	42	43	44	44	45	46	47	47	48	49	50	50	51	52	53	53	54	55	56	56	78
79	20	21	21	22	23	24	24	25	26	27	27	28	29	30	30	31	32	33	33	34	35	36	36	37	38	39	39	40	41	42	42	43	44	45	45	46	47	48	48	49	50	51	51	52	53	54	54	55	56	57	79
80	20	21	22	22	23	24	25	25	26	27	28	28	29	30	31	31	32	33	34	34	35	36	37	37	38	39	40	40	41	42	43	43	44	45	46	46	47	48	49	49	50	51	52	52	53	54	55	55	56	57	**80**
81	20	21	22	23	23	24	25	26	26	27	28	29	29	30	31	32	32	33	34	35	35	36	37	38	38	39	40	41	41	42	43	44	44	45	46	47	47	48	49	50	50	51	52	53	53	54	55	56	56	57	81
82	21	21	22	23	24	24	25	26	27	27	28	29	30	30	31	32	33	33	34	35	36	36	37	38	39	39	40	41	42	42	43	44	45	45	46	47	48	48	49	50	51	51	52	53	54	54	55	56	57	57	82
83	21	22	22	23	24	25	25	26	27	28	28	29	30	31	31	32	33	34	34	35	36	37	37	38	39	40	40	41	42	43	43	44	45	46	46	47	48	49	49	50	51	52	52	53	54	55	55	56	57	58	83
84	21	22	23	23	24	25	26	26	27	28	29	29	30	31	32	32	33	34	35	35	36	37	38	38	39	40	41	41	42	43	44	44	45	46	47	47	48	49	50	50	51	52	53	53	54	55	56	56	57	58	84
85	21	22	23	24	24	25	26	27	27	28	29	30	30	31	32	33	33	34	35	36	36	37	38	39	39	40	41	42	42	43	44	45	45	46	47	48	48	49	50	51	51	52	53	54	54	55	56	57	57	58	**85**
86	22	22	23	24	25	25	26	27	28	28	29	30	31	31	32	33	34	34	35	36	37	37	38	39	40	40	41	42	43	43	44	45	46	46	47	48	49	49	50	51	52	52	53	54	55	55	56	57	58	58	86
87	22	23	23	24	25	26	26	27	28	29	29	30	31	32	32	33	34	35	35	36	37	38	38	39	40	41	41	42	43	44	44	45	46	47	47	48	49	50	50	51	52	53	53	54	55	56	56	57	58	59	87
88	22	23	24	24	25	26	27	27	28	29	30	30	31	32	33	33	34	35	36	36	37	38	39	39	40	41	42	42	43	44	45	45	46	47	48	48	49	50	51	51	52	53	54	54	55	56	57	57	58	59	88
89	22	23	24	25	25	26	27	28	28	29	30	31	31	32	33	34	34	35	36	37	37	38	39	40	40	41	42	43	43	44	45	46	46	47	48	49	49	50	51	52	52	53	54	55	55	56	57	58	58	59	89
90	23	23	24	25	26	26	27	28	29	29	30	31	32	32	33	34	35	35	36	37	38	38	39	40	41	41	42	43	44	44	45	46	47	47	48	49	50	50	51	52	53	53	54	55	56	56	57	58	59	59	**90**
91	23	24	24	25	26	27	27	28	29	30	30	31	32	33	33	34	35	36	36	37	38	39	39	40	41	42	42	43	44	45	45	46	47	48	48	49	50	51	51	52	53	54	54	55	56	57	57	58	59	60	91
92	23	24	25	25	26	27	28	28	29	30	31	31	32	33	34	34	35	36	37	37	38	39	40	40	41	42	43	43	44	45	46	46	47	48	49	49	50	51	52	52	53	54	55	55	56	57	58	58	59	60	92
93	23	24	25	26	26	27	28	29	29	30	31	32	32	33	34	35	35	36	37	38	38	39	40	41	41	42	43	44	44	45	46	47	47	48	49	50	50	51	52	53	53	54	55	56	56	57	58	59	59	60	93
94	24	24	25	26	27	27	28	29	30	30	31	32	33	33	34	35	36	36	37	38	39	39	40	41	42	42	43	44	45	45	46	47	48	48	49	50	51	51	52	53	54	54	55	56	57	57	58	59	60	60	94
95	24	25	25	26	27	28	28	29	30	31	31	32	33	34	34	35	36	37	37	38	39	40	40	41	42	43	43	44	45	46	46	47	48	49	49	50	51	52	52	53	54	55	55	56	57	58	58	59	60	61	**95**
96	24	25	26	26	27	28	29	29	30	31	32	32	33	34	35	35	36	37	38	38	39	40	41	41	42	43	44	44	45	46	47	47	48	49	50	50	51	52	53	53	54	55	56	56	57	58	59	59	60	61	96
97	24	25	26	27	27	28	29	30	30	31	32	33	33	34	35	36	36	37	38	39	39	40	41	42	42	43	44	45	45	46	47	48	48	49	50	51	51	52	53	54	54	55	56	57	57	58	59	60	60	61	97
98	25	25	26	27	28	28	29	30	31	31	32	33	34	34	35	36	37	37	38	39	40	40	41	42	43	43	44	45	46	46	47	48	49	49	50	51	52	52	53	54	55	55	56	57	58	58	59	60	61	61	98
99	25	26	26	27	28	29	29	30	31	32	32	33	34	35	35	36	37	38	38	39	40	41	41	42	43	44	44	45	46	47	47	48	49	50	50	51	52	53	53	54	55	56	56	57	58	59	59	60	61	62	99
100	25	26	27	27	28	29	30	30	31	32	33	33	34	35	36	36	37	38	39	39	40	41	42	42	43	44	45	45	46	47	48	48	49	50	51	51	52	53	54	54	55	56	57	57	58	59	60	60	61	62	**100**
	0	1	2	3	4	**5**	6	7	8	9	**10**	11	12	13	14	**15**	16	17	18	19	**20**	21	22	23	24	**25**	26	27	28	29	**30**	31	32	33	34	**35**	36	37	38	39	**40**	41	42	43	44	**45**	46	47	48	49	

% IMPAIRMENT BETTER EYE

% IMPAIRMENT WORSE EYE / % IMPAIRMENT BETTER EYE

% Impairment worse eye	**50**	51	52	53	54	**55**	56	57	58	59	**60**	61	62	63	64	**65**	66	67	68	69	**70**	71	72	73	74	**75**	76	77	78	79	**80**	81	82	83	84	**85**	86	87	88	89	**90**	91	92	93	94	**95**	96	97	98	99	**100**
50	50																																																		
51	50	51																																																	
52	51	51	52																																																
53	51	52	52	53																																															
54	51	52	53	53	54																																														
55	51	52	53	54	54	55																																													
56	52	52	53	54	55	55	56																																												
57	52	53	53	54	55	56	56	57																																											
58	52	53	54	54	55	56	57	57	58																																										
59	52	53	54	55	55	56	57	58	58	59																																									
60	53	53	54	55	56	56	57	58	59	59	60																																								
61	53	54	54	55	56	57	57	58	59	60	60	61																																							
62	53	54	55	55	56	57	58	58	59	60	61	61	62																																						
63	53	54	55	56	56	57	58	59	59	60	61	62	62	63																																					
64	54	54	55	56	57	57	58	59	60	60	61	62	63	63	64																																				
65	54	55	55	56	57	58	58	59	60	61	61	62	63	64	64	65																																			
66	54	55	56	56	57	58	59	59	60	61	62	62	63	64	65	65	66																																		
67	54	55	56	57	57	58	59	60	60	61	62	63	63	64	65	66	66	67																																	
68	55	55	56	57	58	58	59	60	61	61	62	63	64	64	65	66	67	67	68																																
69	55	56	56	57	58	59	59	60	61	62	62	63	64	65	65	66	67	68	68	69																															
70	55	56	57	57	58	59	60	60	61	62	63	63	64	65	66	66	67	68	69	69	70																														
71	55	56	57	58	58	59	60	61	61	62	63	64	64	65	66	67	67	68	69	70	70	71																													
72	56	56	57	58	59	59	60	61	62	62	63	64	65	65	66	67	68	68	69	70	71	71	72																												
73	56	57	57	58	59	60	60	61	62	63	63	64	65	66	66	67	68	69	69	70	71	72	72	73																											
74	56	57	58	58	59	60	61	61	62	63	64	64	65	66	67	67	68	69	70	70	71	72	73	73	74																										
75	56	57	58	59	59	60	61	62	62	63	64	65	65	66	67	68	68	69	70	71	71	72	73	74	74	75																									
76	57	57	58	59	60	60	61	62	63	63	64	65	66	66	67	68	69	69	70	71	72	72	73	74	75	75	76																								
77	57	58	58	59	60	61	61	62	63	64	64	65	66	67	67	68	69	70	70	71	72	73	73	74	75	76	76	77																							
78	57	58	59	59	60	61	62	62	63	64	65	65	66	67	68	68	69	70	71	71	72	73	74	74	75	76	77	77	78																						
79	57	58	59	60	60	61	62	63	63	64	65	66	66	67	68	69	69	70	71	72	72	73	74	75	75	76	77	78	78	79																					
80	58	58	59	60	61	61	62	63	64	64	65	66	67	67	68	69	70	70	71	72	73	73	74	75	76	76	77	78	79	79	80																				
81	58	59	59	60	61	62	62	63	64	65	65	66	67	68	68	69	70	71	71	72	73	74	74	75	76	77	77	78	79	80	80	81																			
82	58	59	60	60	61	62	63	63	64	65	66	66	67	68	69	69	70	71	72	72	73	74	75	75	76	77	78	78	79	80	81	81	82																		
83	58	59	60	61	61	62	63	64	64	65	66	67	67	68	69	70	70	71	72	73	73	74	75	76	76	77	78	79	79	80	81	82	82	83																	
84	59	59	60	61	62	62	63	64	65	65	66	67	68	68	69	70	71	71	72	73	74	74	75	76	77	77	78	79	80	80	81	82	83	83	84																
85	59	60	60	61	62	63	63	64	65	66	66	67	68	69	69	70	71	72	72	73	74	75	75	76	77	78	78	79	80	81	81	82	83	84	84	85															
86	59	60	61	61	62	63	64	64	65	66	67	67	68	69	70	70	71	72	73	73	74	75	76	76	77	78	79	79	80	81	82	82	83	84	85	85	86														
87	59	60	61	62	62	63	64	65	65	66	67	68	68	69	70	71	71	72	73	74	74	75	76	77	77	78	79	80	80	81	82	83	83	84	85	86	86	87													
88	60	60	61	62	63	63	64	65	66	66	67	68	69	69	70	71	72	72	73	74	75	75	76	77	78	78	79	80	81	81	82	83	84	84	85	86	87	87	88												
89	60	61	61	62	63	64	64	65	66	67	67	68	69	70	70	71	72	73	73	74	75	76	76	77	78	79	79	80	81	82	82	83	84	85	85	86	87	88	88	89											
90	60	61	62	62	63	64	65	65	66	67	68	68	69	70	71	71	72	73	74	74	75	76	77	77	78	79	80	80	81	82	83	83	84	85	86	86	87	88	89	89	90										
91	60	61	62	63	63	64	65	66	66	67	68	69	69	70	71	72	72	73	74	75	75	76	77	78	78	79	80	81	81	82	83	84	84	85	86	87	87	88	89	90	90	91									
92	61	61	62	63	64	64	65	66	67	67	68	69	70	70	71	72	73	73	74	75	76	76	77	78	79	79	80	81	82	82	83	84	85	85	86	87	88	88	89	90	91	91	92								
93	61	62	62	63	64	65	65	66	67	68	68	69	70	71	71	72	73	74	74	75	76	77	77	78	79	80	80	81	82	83	83	84	85	86	86	87	88	89	89	90	91	92	92	93							
94	61	62	63	63	64	65	66	66	67	68	69	69	70	71	72	72	73	74	75	75	76	77	78	78	79	80	81	81	82	83	84	84	85	86	87	87	88	89	90	90	91	92	93	93	94						
95	61	62	63	64	64	65	66	67	67	68	69	70	70	71	72	73	73	74	75	76	76	77	78	79	79	80	81	82	82	83	84	85	85	86	87	88	88	89	90	91	91	92	93	94	94	95					
96	62	62	63	64	65	65	66	67	68	68	69	70	71	71	72	73	74	74	75	76	77	77	78	79	80	80	81	82	83	83	84	85	86	86	87	88	89	89	90	91	92	92	93	94	95	95	96				
97	62	63	63	64	65	66	66	67	68	69	69	70	71	72	72	73	74	75	75	76	77	78	78	79	80	81	81	82	83	84	84	85	86	87	87	88	89	90	90	91	92	93	93	94	95	96	96	97			
98	62	63	64	64	65	66	67	67	68	69	70	70	71	72	73	73	74	75	76	76	77	78	79	79	80	81	82	82	83	84	85	85	86	87	88	88	89	90	91	91	92	93	94	94	95	96	97	97	98		
99	62	63	64	65	65	66	67	68	68	69	70	71	71	72	73	74	74	75	76	77	77	78	79	80	80	81	82	83	83	84	85	86	86	87	88	89	89	90	91	92	92	93	94	95	95	96	97	98	98	99	
100	63	63	64	65	66	66	67	68	69	69	70	71	72	72	73	74	75	75	76	77	78	78	79	80	81	81	82	83	84	84	85	86	87	87	88	89	90	90	91	92	93	93	94	95	96	96	97	98	99	99	100

Selected References

Textbooks

Baldwin, B., Christensen, B., and J. Melton, *Rx for Success*, Vision Publications, Midwest City, Okla., 1983.

Coblens, S., *Optometry and the Law*, American Optometric Association, St. Louis, 1976.

Elmstrom, G., *Advanced Management for Optometrists*, Professional Press, Chicago, 1974.

Elmstrom, G., *Advanced Management Strategies for Optometrists*, Professional Press, Chicago, 1982.

Milkie, G., *Partnerships and Professional Corporations*, Optometric Development Enterprises, St. Louis, 1972.

Annotations of the American Law Reports

Bias of Members of License Revocation Board, 97 ALR 2d 1210.

Competency of Physician or Surgeon of School of Practice Other Than That to Which Defendant Belongs to Testify in Malpractice Case, 78 ALR 697 and 85 ALR 2d 1022.

Constitutionality of Statutes and Validity of Regulations Relating to Optometry, 98 ALR 905.

Eyeglasses and Other Optical Accessories as Subject to Sales or Use Tax, 14 ALR 4th 1370.

Failure to Administer Glaucoma Test as Malpractice, 67 ALR 3d 183.

Fitting of Contact Lenses as Practice of Optometry, 77 ALR 3d 817.

Furnishing Glasses or Optical Accessories as Sale Within Sales Tax Law, 157 ALR 578.

Liability of Optometrist or Optician for Malpractice, 68 ALR 2d 426 and 51 ALR 3d 1273.

Medical Books or Treatises as Independent Evidence, 65 ALR 2d 1102.

One Who Fills Prescriptions under Reciprocal Arrangement with Physician or Optometrist as Subject to Charge of Practice of Medicine or Optometry without License, 121 ALR 1455.

Optometry as within Statute Relating to Practice of Medicine, 22 ALR 1173.

Practicing Medicine, Surgery, Dentistry, Optometry or Podiatry without a License as a Separate or Continuing Offense, 99 ALR 2d 654.

Personal Liability of Servant or Agent to Third Person for Injuries Caused by the Performance or Nonperformance of His Duties to His Employer, 99 ALR 408.

Right of Corporation, or Individual Not Himself Licensed, to Practice Optometry through Licensed Employees, 102 ALR 343 and 128 ALR 585.

Use of Medical or Other Scientific Treatises in Cross-Examination of Expert Witnesses, 60 ALR 2d 77.

Validity and Construction of Contractual Restriction on Right of Medical Practitioner to Practice, Incident to Employment Agreement, 62 ALR 3d 970.

Validity and Construction of Contractual Restriction on Right of Medical Practitioner to Practice, Incident to Sale of Practice, 62 ALR 3d 918.

Validity of Governmental Regulation of Optometry, 22 ALR 2d 939.

What Constitutes Practice of Optometry, 121 ALR 1455, 141 ALR 883, and 88 ALR 2d 1290.

"Clinicolegal Aspects of Practice" Series: *Southern Journal of Optometry*

Classe, J., Optometrist's Duty to Test for Glaucoma, vol. 2, no. 3, 1984, pp. 6–10.

Classe, J., Liability for Use of Ophthalmic Pharmaceutical Agents, vol. 2, no. 4, 1984, pp. 43–49

Classe, J., Optometrist's Duty to Detect Ocular Tumors, vol. 3, no. 1, 1985, pp. 26–39.

Classe, J., Optometrist's Duty to Detect Retinal Detachment, vol. 3 no. 2, 1985, pp. 7–13.

Classe, J., Removal of Ocular Foreign Bodies: Optometry? Or "Surgery"?, vol. 3, no. 4, 1985, pp. 27–32.

Classe, J., Optometrist's Duty to Warn of Vision Impairment, vol. 4, no. 1, 1986, pp. 66–69.

Classe, J., Optometrist's Liability for Ophthalmic Lenses: The Law after Polycarbonate, vol. 4, no. 2, 1986, pp. 36–43.

Classe, J., Optometrist's Liability for Contact Lenses, vol. 4, no. 3, 1986, pp. 52–57.

Classe, J., Liability for Ocular Urgencies and Emergencies, vol. 4, no. 4, 1986, pp. 51–58.

Classe, J., Optometrist's Duty to Release Patient Information, vol. 5, no. 1, 1987, pp. 9–15.

Classe, J., Record-Keeping and Documentation in Clinical Practice, vol. 5, no. 2, 1987, pp. 11–25.

Classe, J., Malpractice and Optometry: A Personal Commentary, vol. 5, no. 3, 1987, pp. 26–31.

"Optometry and the Law" Series: *Journal of the American Optometric Association*

Alexander, L.J., and J.R Scholles, Clinical and Legal Aspects of Pupillary Dilation, vol. 58, no. 5, 1987, pp. 432–437.

Berglund, B., The Easy Way to Tax-Deferred Savings for Retirement, vol. 58, no. 11, 1987, pp. 931–934.

Bowers, S.A., Precedent-Setting Professional Liability Claims Involving Optometrists, vol. 57, no. 5, 1986, pp. 397–401.

Classe, J., A Review of Professional Liability Cases Affecting the Practice of Optometry, vol. 57, no. 1, 1986, pp. 66–71.

Classe, J.G., Contractual Considerations in Contact Lens Practice, vol. 57, no. 3, 1986, pp. 220–226.

Classe, J., The Right to Practice Primary Care, vol. 57, no. 7, 1986, pp. 549–553.

Classe, J., Liability and the Primary Care Optometrist, vol. 57, no. 12, 1986, pp. 926–929.

Classe, J., *Helling* Revisited: How the "Tale" Wagged the Dog, vol. 58, no. 4, 1987, pp. 343–345.

Classe, J., Legal Aspects of Prescribing for Athletes and Sportsmen, vol. 58, no. 8, 1987, pp. 674–679.

Classe, J., and M.G. Harris, Liability and Extended Wear Contact Lenses, vol. 58, no. 10, 1987, pp. 848–854.

Classe, J., and J.R. Scholles, Liability for Ophthalmic Materials, vol. 57, no. 6, 1986, pp. 470–477.

Gabel, W., Vicarious Liability, vol. 58, no. 7, 1987, pp. 599–601.

Garland, N., Optometry Parity Legislation under Medicare, vol. 58, no. 6, 1987, pp. 518–519.

Gold, A.R., Failure to Warn, vol. 57, no. 4, 1986, pp. 317–319.

Gold, A.R., Malpractice Reform, vol. 58, no. 12, 1987, pp. 1000–1003.

Harris, M.G., and R.E. Dister, Informed Consent in Contact Lens Practice, vol. 58, no. 3, 1987, pp. 230–237.

Horowitz, J.E., and R.L. Abramowitz, Adding a Partner or Associate to Your Professional Practice, vol. 57, no. 11, 1986, pp. 850–855.

Miller, P.J., Documentation as a Defense to Legal Claims, vol. 57, no. 2, 1986, pp. 144–145.

Scholles, J.R., Documentation and Record-Keeping in Clinical Practice, vol. 57, no. 2, 1986, pp. 141–143.

Scholles, J.R., Legal and Malpractice Implications of Radial Keratotomy, vol. 57, no. 8, 1986, pp. 624–627.

Scholles, J.R., A Review of Professional Liability

Claims in Optometry, vol. 57, no. 10, 1986, pp. 764–766.

Semes, L.P. and A.R. Gold, Clinical and Legal Considerations in the Diagnosis and Management of Ocular Tumors, vol. 58, no. 2, 1987, pp. 134–139.

Tiffany, D.V., Optometric Expert Testimony: Foundation for the Horizontal Gaze Nystagmus Test, vol. 57, no. 9, 1986, pp. 705–708.

Other References

Baldwin, R., Here's How to Take in an Associate . . . Painlessly, *Journal of the American Optometric Association*, vol. 53, no. 2, 1982, pp. 137–139.

Baldwin, R., How to Make a New Partner Immediately Productive, *Journal of the American Optometric Association*, vol. 53, no. 3, 1982, pp. 231–232.

Bartlett, J.D., and J.W. Wood, Optometry and the Drug Enforcement Administration, *Journal of the American Optometric Association*, vol. 52, no. 6, 1981, pp. 495–498.

Classe, J., How to be Sued for Malpractice, *Southern Journal of Optometry*, vol. 22, no. 1, 1980, pp. 16–22.

Classe, J., How Your Helper Can Help You Get Sued, *Optometric Management*, vol. 16, no. 11, 1980, pp. 61–65.

Classe, J., Legal Problems in Contract Lens Practice, *Southern Journal of Optometry*, vol. 22, no. 8, 1980, pp. 28–35.

Classe, J., The Effects of FTC Rulings on the Practice of Optometry, *Southern Journal of Optometry*, vol. 21, no. 5, 1979, pp. 347–350.

Classe, J., The "Write" Way to Associateship, *Optometric Management*, vol. 23, no. 9, 1987, pp. 25–29.

Coblens, S.L., Privileged and Confidential Communications between Optometrists and Patients, *American Journal of Optometry and Archives of American Academy of Optometry*, vol. 48, no. 12, 1971, pp. 1048–1052.

Coblens, S.L., The *Berryhill* Case: A Critique and a Prediction, *American Journal of Optometry and Archives of American Academy of Optometry*, vol. 51, no. 5, 1974, pp. 347–350.

Cohn, S., A New Life to Life Insurance?, *Optometric Management*, vol. 19, no. 3, 1983, pp. 85–90.

Colton, D.J., The O.D.-M.D. Conflict: Economic Warfare, *Optometric Management*, vol. 18, no. 7, 1982, pp. 23–27.

Drucker, S., Medical Referral—Is Our Obligation Legal or Ethical?, *Review of Optometry*, vol. 110, no. 18, 1973, pp. 35–36.

Elmstrom, G., Malpractice: What Can O.D.'s Expect?, *Review of Optometry*, vol. 114, no. 1, 1977, pp. 42–52.

Geier, A., Your Best Buy in Disability Insurance, *Optometric Management*, vol. 19, no. 2, 1983, pp. 75–83.

Gerber, P., Eyeglasses II: FTC's Latest Probe, *Optometric Management*, vol. 15, no. 10, 1979, pp. 31–37.

Gerber, P., How to Blow Your Own Malpractice Defense, *Optometric Management*, vol. 17, no. 7, 1981, pp. 19–25.

Gerber, P., New ANSI Rule and What It Means, *Optometric Management*, vol. 15, no. 2, 1979, pp. 103–107.

Gerber, P., Saving Patient Records, *Review of Optometry*, vol. 116, no. 8, 1979, pp. 3–4.

Gerber, P., When a Lawyer Calls, Don't Hang Up, *Optometric Management*, vol. 18, no. 5, 1982, pp. 71–77.

Godio, L., Ruskiewicz, J., and W. Chao, The Impact of a Court Decision on the Actual Practice of Eye Care, *American Journal of Optometry and Physiological Optics*, vol. 59, no. 3, 1982, pp. 207–210.

Gregg, J.R. How to Buy or Sell a Practice, *Optometric Management*, vol. 13, no. 4, 1977, pp. 45–52.

Hauser, P., Beware of Fire—and Fire Insurance!, *Optometric Management*, vol. 18, no. 2, 1982, pp. 27–29.

Herrin, S., and C.E. Harrold, Optometry's New Watchdogs, *Review of Optometry*, vol. 121, no. 5, 1984, pp. 35–49.

Hubler, R.S., How to Buy (or Maybe Sell) an Optometric Practice, *Optometric Management*, vol. 18, no. 5, 1982, pp. 27–32.

Irving, R., How a Broker Values a Practice, *Optometric Management*, vol. 18, no. 5, 1982, pp. 33–39.

Keller, J.T., The Risk of Angle Closure from the Use of Mydriatics, *Journal of the American Optometric Association*, vol. 46, no. 1, 1975, pp. 19–21.

Kirschen, M., Verifying Impact Resistance, *Optometric Management*, vol. 13, no. 9, 1977, pp. 55–59.

Krause, R., Invitation to a Lawsuit, *Optometric Management*, vol. 18, no. 2, 1982, pp. 30–33.

Kropiewnicki, M.E., Selling Your Solo Practice, *Review of Optometry*, vol. 121, no. 12, 1984, p. 20.

Lane, M.J., The Legal Risks You Run Prescribing Contacts, *Optometric Management*, vol. 13, no. 3, 1977, pp. 53–61.

Lane, M.J., The Malpractice Menace: What You Should Know about It, *Optometric Management*, vol. 11, no. 5, 1975, pp. 67–77.

Levoy, R.P., Fire Insurance Is Not Enough!, *Optometric Management*, vol. 14, no. 1, 1978, pp. 105–109.

Lynch, B.E., Are You Safe on Safety Glasses?, *Optometric Management*, vol. 20, no. 2, 1984, pp. 58–61.

Marks, R., Product Liability: The New Malpractice Menace, *Optometric Management*, vol. 13, no. 1, 1977, pp. 26–27.

Marks, R., Z-80.1 Standards—Can They Be Met?, *Optometric Weekly*, vol. 67, no. 46, 1976, pp. 1238–1239.

Martinson, R., The Cheapest Cash Money Can Buy, *Optometric Management*, vol. 15, no. 12, 1979, pp. 77–81.

Morgan, E., The Professional Liability Problem and Optometry, *Journal of the American Optometric Association*, vol. 42, no. 2, 1971, pp. 160–164.

Moss, H.L., "Unbreakable, Shatterproof and Safe"—The Need for a New Terminology, *Optical Journal and Review of Optometry*, vol. 108, no. 19, 1971, pp. 25–26.

Munn, H., What's New in Life Insurance, *Optometric Management*, vol. 14, no. 12, 1978, pp. 71–75.

Pavlichko, J.L., Contact Lenses by Mail—What Does the Law Say?, *Review of Optometry*, vol. 116, no. 12, 1979, pp. 16–17.

Pecorino, J., Perspectives of Malpractice, *New England Journal of Optometry*, vol. 27, no. 5, 1976, pp. 3–5.

Powell, M.X., The Legal Impact of Impact Resistant Lenses, *Optometric Management*, vol. 7, no. 12, 1971, pp. 14–21.

Robert, L., The Great Rx Giveaway: Coping with the FTC Rules, *Optometric Management*, vol. 16, no. 1, 1980, pp. 25–33.

Scholles, J., Malpractice: Watch Your Step, *Review of Optometry*, vol. 123, no. 4, 1986, p. 26.

Sherr, A.E., Industrial Safety Glasses—An Update, *Journal of the American Optometric Association*, vol. 51, no. 2, 1980, pp. 129–137.

Sloan, P.G., A "Problem-Oriented" Optometric Record?, *American Journal of Optometry and Physiological Optics*, vol. 55, no. 5, 1978, pp. 352–357.

Sposato, P., How to Buy a Practice, *Optometric Management*, vol. 13, no. 2, 1977, pp. 77–81.

Sutherland, B., and R.L. Guerrin, Partners: What Makes Buy-Ins Work, *Review of Optometry*, vol. 118, no. 2, 1981, pp. 14–20.

Swartwout, J.B., Optometry's Latest Malpractice Time Bomb!, *Optometric Management*, vol. 14, no. 6, 1978, pp. 69–73.

Tabak, S., Strengthen Your Contact Lens Practice, *Optometric Management*, vol. 20, no. 1, 1984, pp. 37–47.

Thal, L.S., *Gates v. Jensen*: Another Precedent for Glaucoma Testing, *Journal of the American Optometric Association*, vol. 52, no. 4, 1981, pp. 349–353.

Trunbull, N.R., Your Records, Your Rights, Your Responsibilities, *Optometric Management*, vol. 19, no. 7, 1973, pp. 16–19.

Wechsler, S., and J. Classe, *Helling v. Carey*: Caveat Medicus (Let the Doctor Beware), *Journal of the American Optometric Association*, vol. 48, no. 12, 1977, pp. 1526–1529.

———, FDA Regulation on Impact-Resistant

Lenses, *Optical Journal and Review of Optometry*, vol. 109, no. 7, 1972, pp. 28–31.

———, My Malpractice Nightmare, *Review of Optometry*, vol. 119, no. 12, 1982, pp. 28–34.

———, Hammering out the Partnership Agreement, *Optometric Management*, vol. 16, no. 3, 1980, pp. 29–47.

———, Ready or Not for an Associate?, *Optometric Management*, vol. 16, no. 3, 1980, pp. 13–19.

———, Splitting the Partnership Melon, *Optometric Management*, vol. 16, no. 3, 1980, pp. 49–61.

———, Swallowing the FTC's Bitter Pill, *Review of Optometry*, vol. 115, no. 12, 1978, pp. 41–45.

Index